GNRS

Geriatric Nursing Review Syllabus

2003-2005

A Core Curriculum in Advanced Practice
Geriatric Nursing

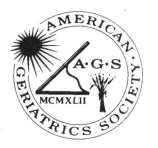

A Collaboration with
The John A. Hartford Foundation Institute for Geriatric Nursing
• New York University • Steinhardt School of Education • Division of Nursing

As new research and clinical experience broaden our knowledge of medicine, changes in treatment and drug therapy are required. This publication is intended only to facilitate the free flow of information of interest to the health care community involved in the care of older persons.

No responsibility is assumed by the editors or the American Geriatrics Society, as the Publisher, for any injury and/or damage to persons or property, as a matter of product liability, negligence, warranty, or otherwise, arising out of the use or application of any methods, products, instructions, or ideas contained herein. No guarantee, endorsement, or warranty of any kind, express or implied (including specifically no warrant of merchantability or of fitness for a particular purpose) is given by the Society in connection with any information contained herein. Independent verification of any diagnosis, treatment, or drug use or dosage should be obtained. No test or procedure should be performed unless, in the judgment of an independent qualified clinician (who is licensed to order such test or procedure), it is justified in light of the risk involved.

Inclusion in this publication of product information does not constitute a guarantee, warranty, or endorsement by the American Geriatrics Society (the Publisher) of the quality, value, safety, effectiveness, or usefulness of any such product or of any claim made about such product by its manufacturer or an author.

The editors were Ellen Flaherty, PhD(C), RN, Terry Fulmer, PhD, RN, and Mathy Mezey, EdD, RN; medical editor was Barbara B. Reitt, PhD, ELS(D); indexer was L. Pilar Wyman; managing editor was Andrea N. Sherman, MS.

Many thanks to Fry Communications for assistance in organizing the *GNRS* material onto an editorial content management website and for all production work, including typesetting, graphic design, and printing. With more than 60 years in the information industry, Fry offers printing and ancillary services to publishers and other content providers.

Citation: Flaherty E, Fulmer T, Mezey M, eds. *Geriatric Nursing Review Syllabus: A Core Curriculum in Advanced Practice Geriatric Nursing*. New York: American Geriatrics Society; 2003.

Geriatric Nursing Review Syllabus: A Core Curriculum in Advanced Practice Geriatric Nursing. Cataloging in publication data are available from the Library of Congress. Copyright © 2003 by the American Geriatrics Society

ISBN 1-886775-09-5

Printed in the United States of America

10 9 8 7 6 5 4 3 2 1

TABLE OF CONTENTS

GNRS Nursing Faculty ix
GNRS Editorial Staff. xi
Preface. xiii
Original *GRS5* Program Editorial Board and
    Chapter Authors xv
Program Guidelines xvii
Introduction. xix

GENERAL PRINCIPLES OF AGING

Chapter 1—BIOLOGY 1
Characteristics of Aging. 1
Theories of Aging. 1
Cellular Changes With Age. 3
DNA and Gene Expression During Senescence. . 3
Cellular Defense Mechanisms 5
Cell Death 6
References 7

Chapter 2—DEMOGRAPHY 7
Demographic Trends 7
Life Expectancy. 7
Socioeconomic Status. 8
Living Arrangements and Marital Status. 8
The Emergence of Assisted-Living Facilities. 9
Trends in Nursing-Home Use 9
Trends in Health and Functioning. 10
Trends in Disability 11
Trends in Health Care. 11
Other Issues. 12
References 12

Chapter 3—PSYCHOSOCIAL ISSUES 13
Stressors 13
Mediators. 14
Moderators. 16
References 17

**Chapter 4—LEGAL AND ETHICAL
    ISSUES** 18
Decisions Near the End of Life 18
Lack of Decision-Making Capacity. 19
Special Ethical Issues in Dementia. 22
Ethics in the Nursing-Home Setting. 23
Miscellaneous Issues. 24
References 25

**Chapter 5—FINANCING, COVERAGE,
    AND COSTS OF HEALTH CARE**. 26
Outpatient Care 26
Inpatient Care 30
Postacute Rehabilitation. 31
Home-Health Care. 32
Nursing-Home Care. 32
Hospice Care. 33
Changes in the Federal Financing of Health
    Care 33
References 34

Chapter 6—PHARMACOTHERAPY. 35
Age-Associated Changes in Pharmacokinetics . . . 35
Age-Associated Changes in Pharmacodynamics . . 37
Optimizing Prescribing 38
Adverse Drug Events 38
Drug Interactions 39
Drug-Disease Interactions 40
Principles of Prescribing. 40
Nonadherence 41
References 42

**Chapter 7—COMPLEMENTARY AND
    ALTERNATIVE THERAPIES** 42
Patterns of Use in the United States. 42
Reasons for Use of CAM 43
Clinical Approaches to Patients' CAM Use 43
Herbal Preparations: Regulation and Research . . 43
Specific Herbal Preparations 44
References 45

APPROACH TO THE OLDER PATIENT

Chapter 8—ASSESSMENT 47
Physical Assessment 47
Cognitive Assessment. 48
Psychologic Assessment 49
Social Assessment 49
Quality of Life. 49
Comprehensive Geriatric Assessment. 50
The Older Driver 50
Clinician-Patient Communication. 50
References 51

Chapter 9—ELDER MISTREATMENT 52
Risk Factors and Prevention 52
History. 52

Physical Assessment 53
Psychologic Assessment 54
Financial Assessment..................... 54
Self-Neglect 54
The Role of the Older Person 54
Institutional Mistreatment.................. 55
Intervention............................ 55
The Medical-Legal Interface 55
References 58

Chapter 10—PREVENTION 59
Introduction 59
Recommended Preventive Services............ 59
Other Preventive Services to Consider 62
Preventive Services Not Indicated in Older
    Adults............................. 64
Delivery of Preventive Services.............. 64
References 64

Chapter 11—PHYSICAL ACTIVITY........ 65
Preventive Health Effects.................. 65
Amount of Physical Activity 66
Sarcopenia and Resistance Training 67
Osteoporosis, Falls, Fractures, and Balance
    Training 68
Balance Training 68
Walking and Aerobic Activities 68
Reducing Sedentary Behavior 68
Physical Activity for Patients with Low Fitness .. 69
Stretching Exercises 70
Therapeutic Effects...................... 70
Promoting Physical Activity................. 70
References 71

Chapter 12—HOSPITAL CARE 72
General Principles........................ 72
Systematic Assessment of the Hospitalized
    Patient............................. 75
Strategies for Managing the Hospitalized
    Patient............................. 79
References 81

Chapter 13—REHABILITATION.......... 82
Conceptual Models for Geriatric Rehabilitation.. 82
Sites of Rehabilitation Care................. 83
Multidisciplinary Teams 84
Impacts of Comorbidities 85
Rehabilitation Strategies: An Overview 85
Assessment and Rehabilitation Planning 86
Stroke 86

Hip Fracture 88
Amputation 88
Assistive Devices, Adaptive Techniques, and
    Environmental Modifications 89
References 90

Chapter 14—COMMUNITY-BASED CARE . 91
Community-Based Services Not Requiring a
    Change in Residence 94
Community-Based Services Requiring a Change
    of Residence.......................... 95
References 96

Chapter 15—NURSING-HOME CARE 97
The Nursing-Home Population 97
Nursing-Home Availability and Financing 97
Staffing Patterns 98
Factors Associated with Nursing-Home
    Placement........................... 98
The Interface of Acute and Long-Term Care ... 98
Quality Issues 99
Medical Care Issues 99
Physician Practice in the Nursing Home........ 99
The Role of the Nurse Practitioner 101
The Role of the Medical Director 102
References 102

Chapter 16—PALLIATIVE CARE........... 103
Palliative Care and Hospice................. 103
Communicating Bad News 103
Pain.................................. 104
Pain Management........................ 106
Palliation of Nonpain Symptoms 109
Latest Developments 112
References 112

GERIATRIC SYNDROMES

Chapter 17—DEMENTIA.................. 113
Epidemiology and Societal Impact............. 113
Genetic and Other Risk Factors 114
Differential Diagnosis of Dementia 114
Assessment Methods...................... 116
Agitation.............................. 117
Treatment and Management 117
References 120

**Chapter 18—NEUROPSYCHIATRIC AND
    BEHAVIORAL DISTURBANCES IN
    DEMENTIA**........................... 121
Presentations 121

Assessment and Differential Diagnosis.......... 121
Treatments for Specific Disturbances........... 123
References 126

Chapter 19—DELIRIUM.................. 127
Incidence and Prognosis 127
Diagnosis and Differential Diagnosis........... 127
The Spectrum of Delirium 128
The Neuropathophysiology of Delirium 128
Risk Factors 129
Postoperative Delirium...................... 130
Evaluation 130
Management 130
Prevention 133
References 133

Chapter 20—URINARY INCONTINENCE . 134
Prevalence and Impact....................... 134
The Pathophysiology of Incontinence.......... 134
Clinical Types of Incontinence 135
Assessment of Urinary Incontinence 137
Management 137
References 142

Chapter 21—FALLS...................... 143
Prevalence and Morbidity 143
Causes.................................... 143
Diagnostic Approach 144
Treatment and Prevention.................... 146
Clinical Guidelines 147
References 147

Chapter 22—GAIT DISTURBANCES....... 148
Gait Assessment............................ 148
Conditions Contributing to Gait Disorders 149
Classification of Gait Disorders................ 149
Evaluation and Treatment.................... 151
References 152

Chapter 23—DIZZINESS 153
Classification 153
Prognosis 155
Evaluation 156
Management 157
References 158

Chapter 24—SYNCOPE................... 159
Natural History............................ 159
Evaluation of the Patient with Syncope 160
Treatment................................. 162
References 163

Chapter 25—HEARING IMPAIRMENT 163
Normal Hearing and Age-Related Changes in
    the Auditory System...................... 163
Epidemiology of Hearing Loss................ 164
Presbycusis................................ 164
Diagnosis of Hearing Loss 164
Treatment of Hearing Loss................... 165
References 168

Chapter 26—VISUAL IMPAIRMENT....... 169
Refractive Error and Cataract 169
Age-Related Macular Degeneration 169
Diabetic Retinopathy 170
Glaucoma................................. 171
Anterior Ischemic Optic Neuropathy.......... 172
Miscellaneous.............................. 172
Low-Vision Rehabilitation.................... 173
References 173

**Chapter 27—OSTEOPOROSIS AND
    OSTEOMALACIA**...................... 174
Definition of Osteoporosis 174
The Epidemiology and Consequences of
    Osteoporosis 174
Review of Bone Remodeling.................. 174
Bone Loss 174
Pathogenesis of Osteoporosis 175
Diagnosis of Osteoporosis and Prediction of
    Fracture 176
Prevention and Treatment of Osteoporosis 177
Working with the Patient..................... 181
Management of Vertebral Fractures........... 181
Osteomalacia 181
References 181

Chapter 28—MALNUTRITION 182
Age-Related Changes 182
Nutrition Screening and Assessment 183
Nutrition Syndromes 186
Nutritional Interventions.................... 188
Ethical and Legal Issues..................... 189
References 190

**Chapter 29—EATING AND FEEDING
    PROBLEMS**........................... 191
Swallowing in Health and Disease 191
Feeding................................... 192
References 193

Chapter 30—PRESSURE ULCERS 194
Epidemiology.............................. 194

Complications From Pressure Ulcers 194
Risk Factors and Risk-Assessment Scales 194
Prevention 195
Management 196
References 200

Chapter 31—SLEEP PROBLEMS 201
Epidemiology 201
Changes in Sleep with Increased Age 201
Evaluation of Sleep 201
Common Sleep Disorders 202
Changes in Sleep with Dementia 204
Sleep in the Nursing Home 204
Management of Sleep Problems 204
References 209

GERIATRIC PSYCHIATRY

**Chapter 32—DEPRESSION AND OTHER
   MOOD DISORDERS** 211
Epidemiology 211
Clinical Presentation and Diagnosis 211
Differential Diagnosis 212
Course 213
Treatment 314
Pharmacotherapy of Mania: Mood Stabilizers . . . 218
References 219

Chapter 33—ANXIETY DISORDERS 220
Classes of Anxiety Disorders 220
Comorbidity 222
Pharmacologic Management 222
Psychologic Management 223
References 223

Chapter 34—PSYCHOTIC DISORDERS 224
Schizophrenia and Schizophrenia-Like
   Syndromes 224
Psychotic Symptoms in Delirium 226
Psychotic Symptoms in Mood Disorder 226
Psychotic Symptoms in Dementia 226
Isolated Suspiciousness 226
Syndromes of Isolated Hallucinations 227
References 227

**Chapter 35—PERSONALITY AND
   SOMATOFORM DISORDERS** 228
Personality Disorders 228
Somatoform Disorders 232
References 234

Chapter 36—SUBSTANCE ABUSE 234
Definitions of Substance Abuse 234
Magnitude of the Problem 235
Risks and Benefits of Substance Use 236
Identifying Substance Use Disorders 237
Treatment 237
References 239

Chapter 37—MENTAL RETARDATION 240
Prevalence 240
Psychiatric and Mental Disorders in Aging Adults
   with Mental Retardation 240
Diagnosis and Treatment 241
Medical Disorders 242
Social Conditions 242
References 242

**COMMON GERIATRIC DISEASES, DISORDERS,
AND HEALTH CONCERNS**

**Chapter 38—CARDIOVASCULAR
   DISEASES AND DISORDERS** 243
Age-Related Cardiovascular Changes 243
Ischemic Heart Disease 243
Heart Failure 246
Valvular Heart Disease 250
Arrhythmias 252
Peripheral Arterial Disease 253
Venous Disorders 254
References 255

Chapter 39—HYPERTENSION 256
Epidemiology and Physiology 256
Clinical Evaluation 256
Treatment 257
Special Considerations 260
References 261

**Chapter 40—MUSCULOSKELETAL
   DISEASES AND DISORDERS** 261
Classification and Overview of Rheumatologic
   Disorders 261
Osteoarthritis 262
Back Pain and Spinal Stenosis 263
Gout 263
Chondrocalcinosis 264
Polymyalgia Rheumatica 264
Giant Cell Arteritis 265
Rheumatoid Arthritis 266
Systemic Lupus Erythematosus 267

Sjögren's Syndrome and Sjögren's Disease...... 268
Polymyositis and Dermatomyositis............ 268
References 269

Chapter 41—BACK PAIN 270
Causes of Back Pain 270
Assessment..................................... 272
Management 273
References 274

Chapter 42—DISEASES AND DISORDERS OF THE FOOT 275
Age-Related Changes and the Impact of Chronic Stress.. 275
Assessment and Treatment of Specific Disorders. 275
Systemic Diseases and the Foot 279
Special Shoes and Orthotics 280
References 281

Chapter 43—NEUROLOGIC DISEASES AND DISORDERS 281
Cerebrovascular Diseases 281
Epilepsy 283
Headaches 284
Movement Disorders 285
Myelopathy 290
Motor Neuron Disease 290
Radiculopathy 291
Peripheral Neuropathy 291
Myopathy...................................... 291
Subdural Hematoma........................... 292
Restless Legs Syndrome....................... 292
References 292

Chapter 44—INFECTIOUS DISEASES 293
Predisposition to Infection 293
Diagnosis and Management of Infections....... 294
Infectious Syndromes.......................... 295
Fever of Unknown Origin..................... 301
References 301

Chapter 45—RESPIRATORY DISEASES AND DISORDERS 302
Age-Related Alterations in Pulmonary Physiology 302
Common Respiratory Symptoms and Complaints.................................. 302
Major Pulmonary Diseases in Older Persons 302
Mechanical Ventilation in Critical Illness 305
Preoperative Pulmonary Evaluation 305
References 306

Chapter 46—ORAL DISEASES AND DISORDERS 307
The Aging of the Teeth....................... 307
Dental Decay.................................. 307
Diseases of the Periodontium 308
Toothlessness.................................. 308
Salivary Function in Aging 309
Oral Mucosal Problems 310
Chemosensory Perception..................... 311
References 311

Chapter 47—GASTROINTESTINAL DISEASES AND DISORDERS 312
Esophagus 312
Stomach 314
Biliary Disease 315
Colon 315
References 319

Chapter 48—ENDOCRINE AND METABOLIC DISORDERS 319
Thyroid Disorders............................. 320
Disorders of Parathyroid and Calcium Metabolism 322
Hormonal Regulation of Water and Electrolyte Balance 323
Disorders of the Adrenal Cortex 324
Testosterone................................... 324
Growth Hormone.............................. 325
Melatonin...................................... 326
Diabetes Mellitus 326
References 328

Chapter 49—HORMONE REPLACEMENT THERAPY 329
Treatment of Menopausal Symptoms 329
Treatment of Urogenital Symptoms 329
Prevention and Treatment of Osteoporosis 329
Prevention of Cardiovascular Disease.......... 330
Treatment and Prevention of Cognitive Disorders 331
Breast Cancer and Estrogen Replacement Therapy.................................... 331
Endometrial Cancer and Estrogen Replacement Therapy.................................... 331
Estrogen Regimens............................ 332
Androgen Deficiency 333
References 333

Chapter 50—GYNECOLOGIC DISEASES AND DISORDERS 334
History and Physical Examination 334
Urogenital Atrophy 335
Vulvovaginal Infection and Inflammation 335
Disorders of the Vulva 335
Disorders of Pelvic Floor Support 336
Postmenopausal Vaginal Bleeding............ 338
Climacteric Syndromes..................... 339
References 339

Chapter 51—DISORDERS OF SEXUAL FUNCTION.......................... 339
Male Sexuality 339
Female Sexuality 342
References 345

Chapter 52—HEMATOLOGIC DISEASES AND DISORDERS 345
Anemia 345
Coagulation 347
Vitamin B_{12}, Folate, and Homocysteine 348
References 349

Chapter 53—ONCOLOGY 349
Cancer Biology and Aging 349
Principles of Cancer Management 350
Specific Cancers.......................... 354
Principles of Management 356
References 356

Chapter 54—RENAL DISEASES AND DISORDERS........................... 357
Normal Aging Changes in Renal Function...... 357
Clinical Presentations of Renal Disease 357
Imaging Techniques and Renal Biopsy 359
Diseases of the Kidney and Vascular System..... 359
Fluid and Electrolyte Disturbances 364
References 365

Chapter 55—PROSTATE DISEASE 366
Benign Prostatic Hyperplasia................. 366
Prostate Cancer........................... 367
Prostatitis 371
References 371

Chapter 56—DERMATOLOGIC DISEASES AND DISORDERS 372
Aging and Photoaging...................... 372
Seborrheic Dermatitis...................... 372
Rosacea.................................. 373

Xerosis 373
Neurodermatitis 373
Intertrigo 374
Bullous Pemphigoid 374
Pruritus.................................. 375
Psoriasis 375
Onychomycosis 376
Herpes Zoster 377
Candidiasis 378
Scabies 378
Louse Infestations......................... 379
Actinic Keratoses.......................... 379
Squamous Cell Carcinoma.................. 379
Basal Cell Carcinoma 379
Melanoma 380
References 381

APPENDIXES

Activities of Daily Living
    Physical Self-Maintenance Scale (ADLs) 384
    Instrumental Activities of Daily Living Scale (IADLs) 385
Alcoholism: Michigan Alcoholism Screening Test—Geriatric Version (MAST-G) 386
Anticoagulation
    Oral Anticoagulation for Older Adults 387
    Reversal of Anticoagulants................. 388
    Initiation and Monitoring of Anticoagulants .. 388
    Anticoagulation When Surgical Procedure Is Planned.............................. 388
Benign Prostatic Hyperplasia (BPH): The International Prostate Symptom Score 389
Depression: The Geriatric Depression Scale (short form, GDS) 390
Falls: Recommendations from the American Geriatrics Society Guidelines for the Prevention of Falls 391
Health Survey: The SF-36 Health Survey 393
Hearing: Hearing Handicap Inventory for the Elderly—Screening Version (HHIE-S) 399
Home Safety: Checklist 400
Functional Abilities: Functional Activities Questionnaire (FAQ) 401
Geriatric Screening: Screening in Primary Care.. 402
Incontinence: Prevention and Management—Behavioral Treatment........ 403

Mobility and Movement 405
   Abnormal Involuntary Movement Scale
     (AIMS) 405
   Performance-Oriented Mobility Assessment
     (POMA) 407
NICHE Ready Sheet 409
Nutrition Screening: DETERMINE Your
   Nutritional Health Checklist 410
Pain Management
   Systematic Pharmacotherapy for Persistent Pain
     Management 411
Pressure Ulcers
   Braden Scale for Predicting Pressure Sore
     Risk 413
   The Pressure Ulcer Scale for Healing
     (PUSH) 415
Resources

What Can You Find on the AGS Web Site? . . . 417
Directory of Agencies and Organizations for
   Geriatric Clinicians 418

QUESTIONS 429

**QUESTIONS, ANSWERS AND
   CRITIQUES** 455

SUBJECT INDEX 525

**INDEX OF GRS EDITORS AND
   AUTHORS** 547

GNRS NURSING FACULTY

The *Geriatric Nursing Review Syllabus: A Core Curriculum in Advanced Practice Geriatric Nursing (GNRS)* is a collaborative effort between the American Geriatrics Society (AGS) and The John A. Hartford Foundation Institute for Geriatric Nursing.

Nursing faculty from New York University's Steinhardt School of Education, Division of Nursing and The John A. Hartford Foundation Institute for Geriatric Nursing modified the AGS's *Geriatrics Review Syllabus: A Core Curriculum in Geriatric Medicine (GRS)*, 5th edition to be used primarily by advanced practice geriatric nurses.

EDITORS

Ellen Flaherty, APRN, PhD(C), BC
Coordinator GNP/ANP Program
Co-Principal Investigator GITT
    Resource Center
New York University
Steinhardt School of Education,
    Division of Nursing

Terry T. Fulmer, PhD, RN, FAAN
New York University
Steinhardt School of Education,
    Division of Nursing
The Erline Perkins McGriff Professor
Head, Division of Nursing

Mathy Mezey, EdD, RN, FAAN
Independence Foundation
    Professor of Nursing Education
Director, The John A. Hartford
    Foundation Institute
    for Geriatric Nursing
New York University
Steinhardt School of Education,
    Division of Nursing

ADVISORY BOARD

Christine Bradway, MSN, APRN, BC
Assistant Director, Adult Health and Gerontology
    NP Programs
University of Pennsylvania School of Nursing

Elizabeth Capezuti, PhD, APRN, BC, FAAN
Associate Professor
Emory University School of Nursing

Vaunette Fay, PhD, ANP, BC
Associate Professor
University of Texas at Houston
School of Nursing

Marquis D. Foreman, PhD, RN, FAAN
Associate Professor
University of Illinois at Chicago College of Nursing

Courtney H. Lyder, ND, GNP, FAAN
University of Virginia Medical Center
    Professor of Nursing
University of Virginia School of Nursing

Lorraine Mion, PhD, RN
Director, Geriatric Nursing Program
Cleveland Clinic Foundation

Deirdre A. Mole, MSN, APRN, BC
Geriatric Nurse Practitioner
The Irving S. Wright Center on Aging
Weill Medical College of Cornell University

Barbara Resnick, PhD, CRNP, FAAN, FAANP
Associate Professor
University of Maryland School of Nursing

CONSULTANTS

Annemarie Dowling-Castronovo, APRN-BC
Clinical Assistant Professor
New York University Steinhardt School of Education
    Division of Nursing

Beth Latimer, MA, APRN, BC
Geriatric Nurse Practitioner
New York University

Elizabeth Weingast, RN, MSN
Geriatric Nurse Practitioner
Sarah Newman Center for Healthcare and
    Rehabilitation

SPECIAL ADVISOR

Perry G. Fine, MD
Professor of Anesthesiology
School of Medicine, University of Utah
National Medical Director, Vista Care

GNRS EDITORIAL STAFF

Managing Editor
Andrea N. Sherman, MS

American Geriatric Society Staff
Linda Hiddemen Barondess,
    Executive Vice President
Nancy Lundebjerg, MPA,
    Associate Vice President of
      Professional Education and Special Projects
Elvy Ickowicz, MPH,
    Associate Director, Professional Education and
      Special Projects
Linda Saunders, MSW,
    Associate Director, Professional Education and
      Special Projects
Stacia Maher, MPH
    Senior Coordinator for Professional Education
      and Special Projects

*New York University Steinhardt School of
Education, Division of Nursing*
Beverly Murphy, Administrative Assistant

Medical Editor
Barbara B. Reitt, PhD, ELS(D)

Indexer
L. Pilar Wyman, Wyman Indexing

Fry Communications, Inc.
Melissa Durborow,
    Information Services Manager
Terry Plyler,
    Content Management Architect
Jason Hughes,
    Technical Services Manager
Robyn Diven,
    Compositor

Question Scoring and Evaluation Service
Program Management Services, Inc.

PREFACE

The *Geriatric Nursing Review Syllabus: A Core Curriculum in Advanced Practice Nursing (GNRS)*, is a concise, up-to-date, and comprehensive text developed by the American Geriatrics Society in collaboration with The John A. Hartford Foundation Institute of Geriatric Nursing at New York University. The *GNRS* is based on the *Geriatric Review Syllabus, 5th edition* and adapted for advanced practice geriatric nurses.

The *GNRS*, authored by more than 100 experts in the care of older adults, contains 56 chapters covering the prevailing management strategies and recent research findings in a wide array of specialty fields. The text is divided into 5 broad areas of geriatric care: General Principles of Aging; Approach to the Older Adult; Geriatric Syndromes; Geriatric Psychiatry; and Common Geriatric Diseases, Disorders, and Health Concerns. Also included are an extensive appendix with assessment instruments and practical resources. In addition, each chapter includes references specific to nursing that allow the interested reader to pursue topics in greater depth.

The *GNRS* also includes a self-assessment program with over 100 questions. To receive Nursing Contact Hours, the participant must submit answer sheets for computer scoring and answer at least 70% of the questions correctly.

ORIGINAL *GRS5* PROGRAM EDITORIAL BOARD AND AUTHORS

This *Geriatric Nursing Review Syllabus* is based upon the *Geriatrics Review Syllabus*, 5th edition, which was developed by the following Editorial Board and chapter authors. For a complete listing of the *GRS5* Editors, Chapter Authors, and Question Writers and their professional affiliations, please see p. 000.

EDITORS

Elizabeth L. Cobbs, MD
Edmund H. Duthie, Jr, MD
John B. Murphy, MD

ASSOCIATE EDITORS

Thomas E. Finucane, MD
Howard Fillit, MD
James T. Pacala, MD, MS
Peter Pompei, MD
Peter Rabins, MD, MPH
Margaret A. Winker, MD

QUESTION REVIEW COMMITTEE

William J. Burke, MD
William J. Hall, MD
Gail M. Sullivan, MD, MPH

CONSULTING EDITORS

Pamela W. Duncan, PhD
Terry Fulmer, PhD, RN
Lisa Gwyther, MSW
Todd P. Semla, PharmD, MS
Mary E. Tinetti, MD

AUTHORS OF ORIGINAL *GRS5* CHAPTERS

GENERAL PRINCIPLES OF AGING

Biology	Donald A. Jurivich, DO, Bruce R. Troen, MD
Demography	Judith D. Kasper, PhD, Lynda Burton, ScD
Psychosocial Issues	Kenneth Hepburn, PhD
Legal and Ethical Issues	Margaret A. Drickamer, MD
Financing, Coverage, and Costs of Health Care	Chad Bout, MD, MPH, MBA
Pharmacotherapy	Todd P. Semla, MS, PharmD, Paula A. Rochon, MD, MPH
Complementary and Alternative Medicine	Melissa J. Webb, PharmD, CGP

APPROACH TO THE ELDERLY PATIENT

Assessment	Thomas M. Gill, MD
Elder Mistreatment	Terry Fulmer, PhD, RN
Prevention	Harrison Bloom, MD, Helen K. Edelberg, MD
Physical Activity	David M. Buchner, MD, MPH
Hospital Care	C. Seth Landefeld, MD
Rehabilitation	Pamela W. Duncan, PhD, Stephanie Studenski, MD, MPH, Barbara deLateur, MD,
Community-Based Care	G. Paul Eleazer, MD
Nursing-Home Care	Paul R. Katz, MD, Jurgis Karuza, PhD
Palliative Care	Stacie T. Pinderhughes, MD, R. Sean Morrison, MD

GERIATRIC SYNDROMES

Dementia	Gary W. Small, MD
Neuropsychiatric and Behavioral Disturbances in Dementia	Constantine G. Lyketsos, MD, MHS
Delirium	Edward R. Marcantonio, MD, SM
Uurinary Incontinence	Catherine E. DuBeau, MD
Falls	Douglas P. Kiel, MD, MPH
Gait Disturbances	Neil B. Alexander, MD
Dizziness	Kurt Kroenke, MD

Syncope	David Bush, MD
Hearing Impairment	Priscilla Faith Bade, MD, MS
Visual Impairment	David Sarraf, MD, Anne L. Coleman, MD, PhD
Osteoporosis and Osteomalacia	Karen M. Prestwood, MD
Malnutrition	Gordon L. Jenson, MD, PhD, James S. Powers, MD
Eating and Feeding Problems	Colleen Christmas, MD
Pressure Ulcers	Courtney H. Lyder, ND
Sleep Problems	Cathy A. Alessi, MD

GERIATRIC PSYCHIATRY

Depression and Other Mood Disorders	Barnett S. Meyers, MD
Anxiety Disorders	Javaid I. Sheikh, MD, Erin L. Cassidy, PhD
Psychotic Disorders	Peter V. Rabins, MD, MPH
Personality and Somatoform Disorders	Marc Edward Agronin, MD
Substance Abuse	David W. Oslin, MD
Mental Retardation	Andrew C. Warren, MB, BS, DPhil

COMMON GERIATRIC DISEASES, DISORDERS, AND HEALTH CONCERNS

Cardiovascular Diseases and Disorders	Wilbert S. Aronow, MD
Hypertension	Mark Andrew Supiano, MD
Musculoskeletal Diseases and Disorders	John W. Rachow, PhD, MD
Back Pain	Leo M. Cooney, Jr, MD, Michael J. Murphy, MD
Diseases and Disorders of the Foot	Arthur E. Helfand, DPM, DABPPH
Neurologic Diseases and Disorders	Elan D. Louis, MD, MS
Infectious Diseases	Kevin Paul High, MD, MSc
Respiratory Diseases and Disorders	E. Wesley Ely, MD, MPH
Oral Diseases and Disorders	Kenneth Shay, DDS, MS
Gastrointestinal Diseases and Disorders	George Triadafilopoulos, MD
Endocrine and Metabolic Disorders	David A. Gruenwald, MD, Alvin M. Matsumoto, MD, Peter Pompei, MD
Hormone Replacement Therapy	Anne M. Kenny, MD
Gynecologic Diseases and Disorders	G. Willy Davila, MD
Disorders of Sexual Function	Angela Gentili, MD , Helen Kuno, MD (with Tom Mulligan, MD)
Hematologic Diseases and Disorders	David A. Lipschitz, MD, PhD
Oncology	William B. Ershler, MD, Dan L. Longo, MD
Renal Diseases and Disorders	Catherine Lee Kelleher, MD, Robert Dean Lindeman, MD
Prostate Disease	Lisa J. Granville, MD
Dermatologic Diseases and Disorders	Sumaira Aasi, MD, Brian Cook, MD, MBA

PROGRAM GUIDELINES

NURSING CONTACT HOURS

The *GNRS* has been reviewed and approved for 50 nursing contact hours by the **New York State Nurses Association** (Activity No. 5KBNMZ-03) provided that the answers are submitted for computer scoring and at least 70% of the questions are answered correctly.

Contact hours are awarded to participants on a one-time basis after they submit an answer sheet for computer scoring and if the program is successfully completed.

Continuing education certificates will be mailed to participants who successfully complete the program.

The *GNRS* program is applicable for nursing contact hours until May 31, 2005. An extension of nursing contact hours through December 2005 is pending. These dates will be indicated on the continuing education certificates.

SELF-SCORING GUIDELINES

Performance interpretation guidelines containing self-scoring instructions and information about using and interpreting test scores are mailed to participants with the program. After the first batch of answer sheets is evaluated, question analysis will be posted on the AGS Web site: http://www.americangeriatrics.org.

INSTRUCTIONS FOR SUBMITTING ANSWER SHEETS FOR CONTINUING EDUCATION CREDIT

Your answers must be recorded on the answer sheet that accompanies the program. Directions for recording your answers are included on the answer sheet. The completed answer sheet should be submitted in the envelope addressed to Program Management Services, Inc. (PMSI). PMSI will score your answer sheet, and then an individualized performance report together with the continuing education certificate (if program is successfully completed) will be mailed to you within 6 weeks. All score results are considered confidential.

If you misplace or lose your answer sheet, a replacement may be obtained by contacting PMSI at **1-800-232-4422**. Answer sheets received *after December 31, 2005*, will not be scored, and the persons submitting them will not be eligible to receive continuing education credits.

USER EVALUATION

The AGS would appreciate participants' comments about the *GNRS* program through the enclosed user evaluation form. Comments and suggestions will be taken into consideration by those planning the next edition.

CONGRUITY OF CONTENT BETWEEN SYLLABUS AND QUESTIONS

Since the *Syllabus* chapters and the questions with critiques were written by different authors, questions may not always correlate directly with the *Syllabus*. In the event that a question's content is not addressed in the correlating chapter, its answer is fully supported in the critique.

In an effort to provide greater consistency of content between chapters and questions, editors asked the chapter authors and question writers to address topics from similar outlines of their area. However, regardless of whether the question material is covered adequately in the corresponding chapter text, the questions rely on the accompanying critiques to provide supportive information for the question content.

ERRATA

Please report any errata to:
info.amger@americangeriatrics.org,
Attention: *GNRS* Managing Editor.

Identified errata will be posted on the AGS Web site: http://www.americangeriatrics.org.

AGS GERIATRICS RECOGNITION AWARD

The GRA recognizes nurses who are committed to advancing their continuing education in geriatrics/gerontological nursing. The GRA was developed by the American Geriatrics Society to encourage nurses to acquire special knowledge and keep abreast of the latest advances in geriatrics/gerontological nursing through continuing education programs.

Credits earned from successfully completing the *GRS5* may be applied toward the GRA. To receive more information and an application, please provide your mailing address to the American Geriatrics Society CME Department, Empire State Building, Suite 801, 350 Fifth Avenue, New York, NY 10118, telephone (212) 308-1414, fax (212) 832-8646.

INTRODUCTION

The core mission of the American Geriatrics Society (AGS) is to promote the optimal health, function, and well-being of older persons. In order to accomplish this goal, AGS members must possess a current fund of knowledge that is evidence based and incorporates the most recent advances in health care. In 1989 the AGS published its first *Geriatrics Review Syllabus (GRS)*. This publication was enormously successful and has become the standard resource in the field of geriatric medicine to assist clinicians in staying current and providing the best possible care to their patients. Recognizing the need for a text specifically tailored for the advanced practice nurse, the AGS, in collaboration with The John A. Hartford Foundation Institute of Geriatric Nursing at New York University, has created the *Geriatric Nursing Review Syllabus (GNRS)*, which is based on the *Geriatrics Review Syllabus, 5th edition* and adapted for advanced practice geriatric nurses. It is with a great sense of accomplishment that the AGS publishes this first edition of the *GNRS*, authored largely by AGS members and leaders in the field of geriatrics.

The *Syllabus* text is divided into five sections: General Principles of Aging; Approach to the Older Patient; Geriatric Syndromes; Geriatric Psychiatry; and Common Geriatric Diseases, Disorders, and Health Concerns.

The *GNRS* consists of 56 chapters, each of which provides a synopsis of the current thinking about a particular topic or field. It must be recognized, however, that the *GNRS* is not intended to be a comprehensive textbook of geriatrics. Accordingly, discussion of certain subjects must be brief, and the reader is referred to more in-depth discussions in a bibliography. In addition, references specific to advanced practice nursing can be found at the end of the chapters. In compiling the bibliography, the interdisciplinary Editorial Board has made every attempt to restrict the references to journals listed in *Index Medicus*. Finally, the *GNRS* devotes little attention to topics that are core components of medicine and nursing and not unique to the care of older persons; this information can be found in standard medical texts.

The Question Review Committee, using questions drafted by a team of question writers, has developed over 100 case-oriented, multiple-choice self-study questions. These questions are designed to complement material in the chapters, and they draw on the entire knowledge base of geriatrics, rather than limiting themselves to the *GNRS* text. We recommend that participants prepare for answering these questions by first carefully reading through the *Syllabus* chapters. Any material addressed in the questions that is not discussed in the chapters is amply discussed in the critiques. It should be recognized, however, that although these questions may resemble, in format and in content, questions that appear on certifying and re-certifying examinations, they have been developed independently of any specialty board. They are not, and will not be, part of any certifying examination.

GNRS is the result of a major collaborative effort by AGS members and staff. The Advanced Practice Nursing Advisory Board has comprehensively reviewed each chapter for its relevance to advanced practice nursing.

The authors were encouraged to include information on health disparities among racial and ethnic minorities in those areas where accurate data exist. Although there has been an increase in the understanding of the health outcomes and diseases among older minorities, these populations remain insufficiently studied. Readers of the *GNRS* must recognize the differences between various ethnic groups and are encouraged to be sensitive to cultural issues in the care of older persons.

Topics for inclusion have been carefully selected by the editorial team. Authors were selected on the basis of their in-depth knowledge of a particular area and their ability to condense large amounts of information into clinically applicable, succinct essays. Editors and authors are experienced in caring for geriatric patients and emphasize the geriatric perspective in the preparation of *GNRS* content.

We hope the *GNRS* will meet our goal of improving participants' knowledge base in geriatrics and thus enhancing the practice patterns of clinicians who care for older persons by providing a self-study tool that is current, concise, scholarly, and clinically relevant. We encourage your comments and suggestions, as the AGS continually strives to better serve its members, other health professionals, and the older persons they treat.

LEARNING OBJECTIVES

At the conclusion of this program, participants will be better able to:

- Describe the general principles of aging and the biomedical and psychosocial issues of aging;

- Discuss legal and ethical issues related to geriatric medicine

- Describe the financing of health care for older persons;

- Identify the basic principles of geriatric care, including information on assessment, pharmacology, prevention, exercise, palliative care, rehabilitation, and sensory deficits, and apply them to their patient care practices;

- Describe the diagnosis and management of geriatric syndromes, including dementia, delirium, urinary incontinence, malnutrition, osteoporosis, falls, pressure ulcers, sleep disorders, pain, dysphagia, and dizziness;

- Use state-of-the-art approaches to geriatric care while providing care in hospital, office-practice, nursing-home, and home-care settings;

- Adjust patient care in the light of evidence-based data regarding the particular risks and needs of ethnic, racial, and sexual patient groups; and

- Utilize evidence-based data to increase the effectiveness of teaching geriatrics to all health professionals.

GENERAL PRINCIPLES OF AGING

CHAPTER 1—BIOLOGY

Knowledge about age-dependent changes in cellular and organ function is important in the care of older persons. The rate of physiologic aging varies from person to person, with large interindividual variations. At the cellular and molecular levels, provocative scientific findings have begun to unravel the question of why we age. Some determinants of longevity now can be understood in terms of gene expression. Importantly, temporal expression of aging resembles a rheostatic switch with small incremental changes. Attempts to answer questions about what controls the rheostatic switch and the rate of senescence have resulted in several theories on aging (Table 1.1).

CHARACTERISTICS OF AGING

Common traits of aging processes include the following:

- Mortality increases with age after maturation, and the increases become exponential with increasing age.
- The biochemical composition of tissue changes with age; examples are lipofuscin and extracellular matrix cross-linking, protein oxidation, and altered rates of gene transcription.
- Physiologic capacity decreases.
- The ability to maintain homeostasis diminishes, especially with regard to adaptive processes under physiologic stress.
- The susceptibility and vulnerability to disease increases.

One axiom of aging had been the irreversibility of changes occurring over time, and although this is generally true, the rate of aging can be influenced by environmental and genetic factors. Thus, the prevention of deleterious changes with age and the reversal of certain aspects of senescence are promising possibilities.

THEORIES OF AGING

The oxidative stress theory is one widely accepted explanation of the aging process. This theory posits that oxygen converted during metabolism into superoxide anions, hydrogen peroxide, and hydroxyl radicals causes damage over time. Untoward events are

Table 1.1—Representative Theories on Aging

Theory	Synopsis
Oxidant injury	The result of homothermia and metabolism is the accumulation of protein, lipid, and DNA damage mediated through highly reactive, oxygen-derived substances (free radicals).
Chromosomal alterations	Deletions, mutations, translocations, and polyploidy have been suggested as age-acquired chromosomal instabilities that contribute to gene silencing or expression of disease-related genes, such as those seen in cancer.
Immunologic	Time-acquired deficits, primarily in T-cell function, predispose elderly persons to infections and cancer.
Neuroendocrinologic	The cortisol surge leading to death in spawning salmon has served as a model for explaining the decline of humans after their maximal reproductive years.
Developmental-genetic	Because the maximum life span appears fixed, a genetically programmed induction of senescence is thought to occur, resulting in the activation or suppression of specific "aging" genes.

indiscriminate and cumulative. Key observations include the following:

- Free-radical damage to lipids, protein, and DNA have been found in aging heart, liver, and kidney tissue.
- Short-lived species accumulate this damage quickly.
- Transgenic animal models that concurrently overexpress copper and zinc superoxide dismutase and catalase have extended life spans.
- Antioxidant compounds such as vitamin E can enhance the average life span in animal models. Interestingly, the expression of human SOD (Table 1.2) in Drosophila neurons has been found to increase life span by 40%, which suggests that the central nervous system plays a key role in longevity.

Skeptics of the oxidative stress theory point out that knockout of the SOD gene does not accelerate

Table 1.2—Glossary of Genetic Terminology

alpha-B-crystallin	Alpha-crystallins possess genuine chaperone activity similar to that of heat-shock proteins.
alpha-2U-globulin	A protein encoded by a highly homologous multigene family and constitutively expressed.
B-Myb	A ubiquitously expressed transcription factor involved in the regulation of cell survival, proliferation, and differentiation. It is maximally expressed at G1/S boundary of cell cycle, a commitment point for senescence, apoptosis, and proliferation.
BARD1	Breast cancer 1 (*brca1*) is a tumor-suppressor gene, BARD1 is a BRCA1-associated RING domain 1 (BARD1)
bcl-2	A product of proto-oncogene *bcl-2*, named from B-cell lymphoma, which inhibits apoptosis.
CDC25B	A family of cell-division-cycle genes, including CDC25A, CDC25B, CDC25C; a protein phosphatase.
CD28	A co-receptor protein on the surface of the helper T cells.
CD152	Also known as CTLA-4, it is involved in T-lymphocyte co-stimulatory pathways modulating both humoral and cellular immune response.
CD154	CD40 ligand (CD40L), expressed by activated CD4+ T cells.
CPP32	Also known as caspase-3, a member of the interleukin-1 converting enzyme (ICE) family, considered an executioner protease in mammalian cells during apoptosis.
Cyclins	Mitotic cyclins constitute a regulatory subunit of the histone H1 kinase complex and are divided into two classes, A and B, both necessary for the mitosis.
daf-2	A homologue gene of mammalian insulin or insulin-like growth factor I (IGF-I) receptors.
Fas	Also known as CD95 or APO-1, a cell surface protein belonging to the tumor necrosis factor receptor superfamily that induces apoptosis upon interaction with Fas ligand (FasL) or agonistic antibodies.
G-regulatory protein	GTP-binding protein. When its bound GTP hydrolyzes to GDP, the GTP-binding globular domain undergoes a conformational change that inactivates the protein.
HIAP	Human inhibitor of apoptosis protein, "anti-death" factor.
HSP70	Heat-shock protein 70, a chaperone that protects newly synthesized peptides, shuttles proteins around the cells, and regulates some kinases and transcription factors.
ICE	Interleukin-1 converting enzyme (ICE), also known as caspase-1.
ICH-1	Also known as caspase-2, a member of the interleukin-1 beta-converting enzyme (ICE) protease family (caspases) in apoptosis.
NF-kB	Nuclear transcription factor kB; mediates inflammatory responses.
p16	Tumor suppressor p16 is a member of the INK4 family of inhibitors of the cyclin D-dependent kinases.
p27	A cyclin-dependent kinase inhibitor, also known as Kip1.
SOD	Superoxide dismutase, an enzyme central to converting free-radical oxygen species to less reactive forms.
ras1	A gene first identified in viruses that cause rat sarcomas.
TCR	T-cell receptor.

aging. This observation attests to redundant systems that counter damage. On a pragmatic level, no evidence exists that antioxidants delay human senescence or disease. In fact, sufficient levels of these compounds may not reach critical areas such as the brain to prevent age-associated oxidant injury.

Mitochondria play a key role in biologic aging. Damage induced by free radicals results in mitochondrial-DNA (mtDNA) mutations in muscle and brain. These lead to defective mitochondrial respiration and further oxidant injury, which creates a cycle of damage and continued loss of mitochondrial function. Mitochondrial mutations and defective respiration have been linked to neurodegeneration in conditions such as Alzheimer's and Parkinson's disease. Given maternal inheritance of mtDNA, human longevity potentially is linked to the maternal genome.

A popular perception is that longevity prevails in family members of extremely old humans. If this is true, the question is, Which genes are responsible for longevity? It has been proposed that genes regulate the rate of aging (longevity assurance) and disease acquisition (disease-resistance genes). Genes also exist for damage repair. Thus, the human life span may depend upon multiple components that counter deleterious changes. The question remains whether a "master switch" is turned on over time so as to down-regulate repair mechanisms or perhaps exude a systemic factor for aging.

Differences in life spans observed among various mammalian species suggest a developmental-genetic theory of aging. Some aspects of aging resemble developmentally regulated programs; however, it is difficult to understand why evolutionary pressures would preferentially select senescence, unless a genetically controlled program for aging might be a mechanism to assure gene-pool turnover. On the other hand, genetically regulated programs that delay the onset of aging might be selected in human evolution if this enhanced the reproductive years.

Comparable longevity between monozygotic and not dizygotic twins hints that a genetic program exists for aging. Genetic disorders leading to accelerated aging, such as that seen in Hutchinson-Gilford and Werner's syndromes, provide insight into the genetic components of processes associated with aging, such as alopecia, arteriosclerosis, osteoporosis, and skin atrophy. One of the progeria conditions, Werner's syndrome, is due to a perturbation on chromosome 8 and is linked to a gene that codes for a helicase. This enzyme is responsible for unwinding DNA during replication and repair. Chromosomal instability appears to mediate cumulative cellular pathology that contributes to death in the middle-aged adult. Clearly, progeria syndromes as well as accelerated aging observed in trisomy 21 syndrome (Down syndrome) indicate that the phenotype of human senescence has several genetic loci that can mediate the pace of aging.

Although indirect evidence supports a genetic link to the rate of aging, little direct evidence exists for a genetic program that actively triggers the aging processes. Indeed, animal models show that environmental manipulations, such as caloric restriction, can significantly extend life span. Thus, the relationship between environmental factors and gene expression appears to drive the aging process.

CELLULAR CHANGES WITH AGE

Senescence induces functional changes in cells. Perturbations are observed in cells with full replicative potential, as well as in those in a postmitotic state. Cells with proliferative capacity, such as lymphocytes and fibroblasts, typically demonstrate diminished proliferative potential over time. For instance, cultured lymphocytes from human blood start to divide after being provided a growth stimulus (plant lectin, phytohemagglutinin, and interleukin-2). The onset of proliferation is slower in old than in young donor lymphocytes, and the peak number of dividing cells is lower in elderly donor lymphocytes. The main reason for loss of lymphocyte proliferation with age is decreased secretion of interleukin-2 and expression of T-cell populations that have an altered affinity for this cytokine. Mixed populations of T cells from old donors express a high percentage of memory cells that exhibit different proliferative characteristics than naive T cells, which are more plentiful in young donor samples.

To circumvent concerns about mixed subpopulation dynamics characteristic of polyclonal T-cell cultures, researchers have stimulated single T-cell clones from young and elderly donor cells. In these instances, the cloning efficiency of T cells from old donors is reduced, with many fewer of them reaching benchmarks of 20, 30, and 40 population doublings than young donor cells that have identical cell surface markers. Thus, it appears that age alters both the population dynamics of T-cell growth and individual cellular capacity to sustain clonal expansion. The net result is diminished T-cell responses with age, which could account for the increasing infection and cancer rates observed over the human life span.

The loss of proliferation in cultured cells is broadly known as *clonal senescence*. Other cell types, such as endothelial and fibroblast cells, also exhibit loss of proliferative potential in old donors. A well-established model for replicative senescence entails serial passage of fetal or primary fibroblasts in well-defined cell culture media. At a certain point, these cells enlarge and no longer divide. Generally, old donor fibroblasts undergo fewer population doublings than do young donor cells. However, an important consideration is that the loss of replicative potential varies among aged individuals. Thus, a wide range exists whereby some young donor cells divide only a few times and old donor cells replicate comparably to many young donor cells. Skin biopsy experiments suggest an age-dependent accumulation of end-stage fibroblasts; however, the percentage of these cells in old donor skin is surprisingly small. Thus, changes in cell function other than loss of proliferation are at the root of cellular aging.

DNA AND GENE EXPRESSION DURING SENESCENCE

DNA Mutations or Deletions

The concept that age alters the integrity of DNA, primarily through mutations, originally led to the somatic mutation theory of aging. That aging results in DNA template errors, thus leading to errors in or loss of gene expression, has not held up experimentally. However, certain "hot spots" of DNA change have been observed in human and animal aging. These hypermutable DNA foci are thought to accumulate changes that produce functional cellular problems over time. Structural changes in DNA range from deletions to aberrant expansions. These changes occur in both somatic and germ cells. In the former case, rat neurons were found to have accumulated deletion mutations in the vasopressin locus, and the rate of deletion increased over time as the vasopressin activity increased. In cells that retain their mitotic potential over time, several types of deletion are observed. For example, ribosomal ribonucleic acid (rRNA) gene copies decline with age.

However, substantial rRNA redundancy appears to mask the effect of these deletions. Likewise, microsatellite loci undergo a fairly high rate of spontaneous mutations and genomic shortening in nonessential DNA segments. Importantly, several hypermutable areas are juxtaposed with key regulatory elements, such as the insulin gene and oncogene *ras1* (Table 1.2) locus. Changes over vast distances of DNA sequences can affect downstream gene activity, which suggests that age-related changes observed in nonfunctioning DNA areas can potentially exert untoward effects on critical regulatory genes.

A similar concern exits with age-dependent changes in mtDNA. The circular mtDNA is reported to undergo a mutation rate that is 10,000-fold greater in elderly than in younger adult tissue. A nearly exponential increase in mtDNA mutations occurs over time, with up to 10% of extremely old donor tissue exhibiting deletions. Because mitochondria and mtDNA are amply redundant, subtle, if any, age-dependent changes in respiratory chain activities are noticed, and it is most likely that age results in a reduced functional reserve of energy production.

Telomeres

Perhaps the most provocative data concerning DNA changes with age relates to chromosomal end points. These chromosomal tips contain redundant DNA sequences or tandem repeats that cannot be replicated by DNA polymerase. To solve this problem, a ribonucleoprotein called *telomerase* deals with end chromosomal replication.

A fundamental problem observed in aged donor cells with replicative potential is that their telomeres shorten. Telomere shortening and loss of telomerase activity has been observed during clonal senescence of fibroblasts and T cells. Telomeric DNA loss is also a function of donor age. The consequence of this diminished activity is thought to be alterations in the immune system and deficient wound healing.

Conversely, telomerase hyperactivity is linked to cellular transformation and cancer. Given the relationship of telomeres to aging and cancer, some have proposed measurement of telomere length and telomerase activity as potential clinical markers of human aging and oncogenesis. Thus, targeted disruption of telomerase activity would be important as cancer therapy, whereas reactivation of this enzyme might reverse age-dependent changes in replicative potential.

Gene Expression

Age affects gene expression at several levels. Age-related changes depend upon the cellular state, such as quiescence, proliferation, or physiologic stress. When side-by-side comparisons of gene expression from mature adult and aged donors are conducted, the rates of gene expression either decrease, stay the same, or increase in elderly donors. An important and, as yet, unresolved consideration is whether differences in gene expression with age are functionally significant. The inability of cells to withstand physiologic stress with age is the strongest evidence that changes in stress-related gene expression contribute to poor functional outcomes.

A variety of mechanisms can influence gene expression with aging. For instance, mutations in DNA sequences in or around certain genes can influence their expression. Similar effects can be expected from latent viral infections (eg, herpes viruses), as well as from accumulation of environmentally induced cell damage. Targets for altered gene expression and aging would be reduced activity of transactivators, enhanced activity of DNA silencers or repressors, and intrinsic changes in RNA polymerase activity.

Because the overall total messenger ribonucleic acid (mRNA) content does not appear to change with age, aging has been characterized as a state with a decline in mRNA turnover and transcriptional rate. RNA polymerase per se does not appear to change with age, so most of the change in mRNA expression appears to be due to changes in the gene-promoter regions. Gene promoters are areas of DNA upstream of the target gene that have constitutively and inducibly bound DNA-binding proteins. Through proper assemblage of these DNA-binding proteins, DNA conformational changes that enhance RNA polymerase recruitment and efficiency are effected. Expected age-dependent changes would include alterations in DNA-protein interactions (transcription factors), accumulation of proteins interfering with DNA-binding proteins, and unfavorable conformations of DNA during transcriptional activation. Importantly, there is no evidence that age leads to an increased error rate during transcription and translation.

In sum, the primary changes in gene expression with age are as follows:

- decreased transcription rates for key genes;
- decreased mRNA turnover;
- decreased inducibility of genes, such as immediate early genes, acute phase reactants, and stress genes.

Constitutive levels of gene expression remain intact.

Of 6000 known human genes analyzed, only 61 or 1% showed changes in expression between young and middle-aged donors. Most of these changes were reduced gene expression involving cell cycle progression and maintenance or repair of the extracellular matrix. Specific declines occurred in cyclins A, B and F

(Table 1.2), as well as certain transcription factors such as B-Myb and hepatocyte nuclear factor. Myb has a role in cell proliferation, and hepatocyte nuclear factor is a homologue of a regulatory factor in nematodes that is linked to life span. Some genes, such as the macrophage metalloproteinase, are up-regulated in middle age, as are other extracellular matrix proteins. Comparison of old and young donor cells shows that the cell cycle genes are even further down-regulated. Old donors exhibit significant drops in gene expression that are related to entry into mitosis (eg, CDC25B [Table 1.2], thymidylate synthase, RNA helicase). The functional consequence of declining gene expression related to cell cycle may predispose older individuals to increased DNA strand breaks and other chromosomal instabilities.

When gene expression in fibroblasts from progeria donors is compared with that of fibroblasts from aged donors, some interesting linkages between normal and premature aging are manifest. For example, down-regulation of bone- and joint-associated genes is found in normal aged and progeric individuals. Cathepsin C, a lysosomal protease, is similarly down-regulated sixfold in aged donors and likely contributes to dermal changes with senescence. A tumor-suppressor gene, BARD1 (Table 1.2), is down-regulated 4.5-fold with age and may account for age-related increases in breast cancer. Down-regulation with age of cyclooxygenase-2 (COX-2) expression is accompanied by changes in genes that encode for fatty-acid synthesis, which raises the possibility that age results in perturbations in lipid metabolism and possibly lipid-mediated signal transduction. Because the most extensive gene expression data are derived from human fibroblasts, additional information about tissue-specific changes in gene expression with age will reveal underlying mechanisms of senescence and increased susceptibility to disease.

Not all genes examined during senescence are found to be attenuated in their expression. Curiously, basal expression of genes related to the stress response is up-regulated in aged donor cells. One of these genes, alpha-B-crystallin (Table 1.2), is associated with the maintenance of the cellular cytoskeleton. Likewise, a heat-inducible serine protease has its basal expression increased with age, and it is found in osteoarthritic cartilage. Metalloproteinase, prostaglandin synthase, cystatin, and a matrix protein gene are all up-regulated with age by 5- to 21-fold. Cystatin is an inhibitor of cysteine proteinases, and its elevation potentially decreases an array of enzymatic activity. The consequence of up-regulation of gene expression in human aging remains to be determined. Possibly these changes are simply adaptations to accumulated ravages of environmental or metabolic (oxidative) stress.

Some of the most definitive age-dependent changes in gene expression are observed when aged donor cells are analyzed during different forms of physiologic stress. This observation is perhaps not surprising, given clinical observations that older persons often respond less well than young adults to physiologic stress, such as infections, environmental extremes, and hypoxic events.

CELLULAR DEFENSE MECHANISMS

Age results in lowered responses to physiologic stress. Cells have specific reactions to thwart injury and death. Damage may result from ultraviolet light, heat, lack of oxygen, absent nutrients, and metabolic oxidants. Cells have multiple strategies to cope with various forms of stress by means of stress-inducible transcription factors. For instance, ultraviolet radiation affects the transcription factor NF-kB (Table 1.2), whereas thermal stress causes the transcription factor heat-shock factor (HSF1) to be activated. The thermal stress response can also be evoked by hypoxia, heavy metals, and other types of injury. Damaged intracellular proteins trigger the cytoplasm-located transcription factor to translocate the nucleus and bind to a gene promoter region containing consensus nucleotide sequences GAA. HSF1 binding to the heat-shock element increases RNA polymerase activity, leading to elevated expression of mRNAs for various heat-shock proteins.

Heat-shock proteins have multiple functions. They primarily function as chaperones to allow protein trafficking and organelle transmembrane transport. Other functions include refolding damaged proteins and newly synthesized polypeptides. Heat-shock proteins interact with transcription factors, such as the steroid receptor, and serve as a type of molecular brake or attenuator of the transcription factor when conditions do not require its activation.

During stress, increased need of heat-shock proteins causes the protein synthetic machinery to exclusively translate mRNA for heat-shock proteins. Stress-induced mRNA is longer lived than other mRNA because of extended poly A tails. By inference, aging is associated with decreased turnover of mRNA and appears similar to enhanced half-lives of heat-shock protein mRNA. The accumulation of heat-shock proteins assists the tagging and transport of damaged protein to degradation pathways. Heat-shock proteins protect enzymatic function under stress. In short, heat-shock proteins assure proper protein levels and function so that cells may survive. Once overexpressed, their efficacy is sustainable, as witnessed by the increased ability of cells to withstand subsequent lethal stress.

The study of the human heat-shock response is an excellent paradigm for understanding how aging affects basic responses to cellular injury. One reason is that all species studied thus far have consistently revealed age-related decrements in various components of the heat-shock response. This fact illustrates how inducible responses, rather than constitutive responses, go awry with age.

The primary age-dependent defect of the heat-shock response occurs in the transcriptional trigger. When human fibroblast-like cells are serially passaged in tissue culture or when peripheral blood lymphocytes from old donors are analyzed, a brief thermal stress (5°C above baseline) results in only partial activation of HSF1 into its DNA-bound state. Age causes approximately a 50% reduction in observable DNA binding after stress of old donor cells. This age-dependent change in stress-inducible HSF1 binding results in marked reduction in the rate of mRNA production for all the heat-shock proteins. No one knows exactly what levels are necessary for full protection from cell death; however, levels are likely proportional to the degree and duration of cell stress. In other words, higher levels of heat-shock proteins are needed if the cellular stress is severe, whereas lower levels are capable of handling mild to moderate stress.

Loss of HSF1–DNA binding with age appears to be multifactorial. Although HSF1 is a rare, long-lived protein, levels of HSF1 protein appear to decrease in older human donor peripheral blood mononuclear cells. Another age-acquired problem in activation of HSF1 appears to be acquisition of an inhibitor to DNA binding. A well-characterized aspect of the human heat-shock response is that, despite continuous stress, HSF1–DNA binding gradually declines in normal, young cells over time. Identification of the factor responsible for HSF1 attenuation has eluded investigators, but HSF1-associated proteins, such as HSP70 (Table 1.2) and other HSF1 binding proteins, offer a clear possibility that putative attenuators of HSF1–DNA binding may be overactive or preferentially expressed with age. In support of this model, extracts from old donor lymphocytes are capable of blocking HSF1 activation. An additional consideration is that stress-mediated protein kinase and phosphatase activity affecting HSF1 is altered with age.

Most importantly, increased susceptibility to cell death results from altered heat-shock gene expression. For example, heat-shocked human lymphocytes from donors aged 75 years and older results in cell death earlier and involving more cells than in young donor lymphocytes. Despite this observation, controversy exists whether age represents a defect in apoptosis or programmed cell death. When fibroblasts are serially passaged, the cells passaged very late minimally produce heat-shock genes when thermally stressed, yet these cells are resistant to another form of death, namely, serum deprivation. These seemingly paradoxical observations are reconcilable when one considers that apoptosis can occur through several pathways, not all which are equally affected by age.

Observations regarding senescence and cell stress demonstrate an emerging principle, that inducible responses requiring enhanced gene expression are attenuated by aging. The attenuation of inducible stress responses may be due to the accumulation or overexpression of heat-shock proteins in the nonstress state, which raises a provocative question, whether senescent cells are in a state of low-grade stress.

One concern is whether age results from elevated expression of certain genes, perhaps triggered by some internal chronometer. So far, no clear evidence exists for genes that evoke the senescence phenotype. However, experiments with nematode aging show that manipulation of daf-2 (Table 1.2), a mutation that confers longevity, may result in secretion of a factor that regulates the pace of aging. Similarly, in Drosophila studies, manipulation of the methuselah gene, which is homologous with G-regulatory proteins (Table 1.2), can extend life span. By comparison, the decline in estrogen levels in aging women have been cited as a waning systemic factor that prevents bone, brain, and vascular deterioration. However, there is no hormonal factor known to extend human life span, and it is not clear whether changes in the hormonal axis with aging influence the rate of aging or merely represent an adaptive response to intrinsic tissue changes.

CELL DEATH

Experimental investigations have assessed the impact of aging on cell death. Cell death may occur by necrosis or apoptosis. In the former case, massive cell injury results in chromatin clumping and disorderly breakdown of cellular components. On the other hand, apoptosis is an active suicidal mechanism in response to external or internal stimuli. Apoptosis is essential to tissue maintenance, and it is especially important in down-regulating immune responses, such as clonally expanded lymphocytes, when infections resolve. Age-dependent problems with apoptosis could result in leukemias, lymphomas, and abnormal tissue repair.

Apoptosis is recognized by compaction and segregation of chromatin adjacent to the nuclear membrane, condensation of the cytoplasm, and nuclear fragmentation. DNA "ladders," detected in acrylamide gels, represent the orderly enzymatic degradation of DNA. Membrane-bound apoptotic bodies are phagocytized. Gene products activate and block apoptosis. For instance, cysteine proteases (ICE, CPP32, and ICH-1; see Table 1.2) initiate apoptosis, whereas bcl-2 and HIAP (Table 1.2) block or prevent apoptosis.

The exact effect of senescence on apoptosis varies according to the cell type examined. For instance, serially passaged fibroblasts are resistant to apoptosis when deprived of serum growth factors in the culture medium. In rodents, caloric restriction enhances hepatic apoptosis in aged animals, thus leading to greater cell replacement repair than in calorie-unrestricted animals. In mice, expression of Fas (Table 1.2), a cell membrane receptor responsible for initiating apoptosis, appears to decrease with age. Gene knockout experiments with Fas show that autoimmune disease prevails and the animal's life span is shortened. However, comparison of young and old donor cells indicates that human lymphocytes exposed to apoptosis-inducing thermal stress have an increased sensitivity to death. Thus, age-dependent changes in apoptosis may be evident in the initiation or signaling of cell death.

It has been suggested that apoptosis plays a role in neurodegenerative diseases associated with aging. The neuronal loss observed in Alzheimer's disease is possibly due to cytotoxicity of aggregated β-amyloid, which can induce apoptosis in cultured cells. Putative toxins such as free radicals created during neuronal transmission have also been implicated in neuronal cell death

seen in Parkinson's disease; however, the exact role of apoptosis in aging and diseases of aging remains an area of ongoing research.

REFERENCES

■ Bengtson VL, Schaie KW, eds. *Handbook of Theories of Aging*. New York: Springer Publishing Company; 1999.

■ Johnson FB, Sinclari DA, Guarente L. Molecular biology of aging. *Cell*. 1999;96(2):291–302.

■ Ly DH, Lockhart DJ, Lerner RA, et al. Mitotic misregulation and human aging. *Science*. 2000;287(5462):2486–2492.

■ Pawelec G, Adibzadeh M, Rehbein A, et al. In vitro senescence model for human T lymphocytes. *Vaccine*. 2000;18(16):1666–1674.

■ Vijg J. DNA and gene expression. In: *Encyclopedia of Geronotology*, vol 1;1996:441–453.

■ Yates FE. Theories of aging: biological. In: *Encyclopedia of Gerontology*, vol. 2;1996:545–555.

CHAPTER 2—DEMOGRAPHY

In 2000 about one in eight Americans living in the United States was aged 65 or older, but by 2030 that rate is expected to be one out of every five. This major demographic shift has prompted numerous concerns regarding U.S. social and health policy in recent years. Not only will the sheer number of older adults increase dramatically, but the composition and characteristics of the elderly population will also change. Although clinicians are primarily concerned with the needs of individual patients, some of the attributes of the older patient are a function of the cohort from which he or she is drawn. Aging baby boomers (the generation born between 1940 and 1960) are expected to have a major impact on the health and social service systems of the United States, although the exact nature of this impact remains unclear.

DEMOGRAPHIC TRENDS

In the 20th century the U.S. population under age 65 tripled, while the age group 65 years and older increased by a factor of 12, growing from 3.1 million in 1900 to 35 million in 2000. This group will more than double by the middle of the next century, to 80 million people, with most of this growth occurring

between 2010 and 2030. The United States is not unique in its growing share of older adults. At present it is surpassed by many other developed countries, including Italy, Japan, Germany, Sweden, and the United Kingdom, where the proportion of people aged 60 and older is already at 20% or above.

The older population of the United States is not evenly distributed geographically. Half of persons aged 65 or older live in nine states, led by California, Florida, and New York. The midwestern states, however, have the highest percentages of older persons living alone (30% or greater). The older U.S. population is predominantly white, but persons of other races are expected to grow from about one in ten currently, to two in ten in the next 50 years. The number of older black Americans is expected to triple in this period, whereas the size of the older Hispanic American population, which is growing much faster, may exceed that of the older black population within 30 years.

LIFE EXPECTANCY

In the United States the average life expectancy is currently highest for white women, followed by that for black women, white men, and black men (Table 2.1). Women who survive to age 65 can, on average, expect to live to age 84, and those surviving to age 85 can expect to live to age 92. Up to age 85, the life expectancy of white American men and women exceeds their black counterparts. At age 85, these race differences in life expectancy largely disappear. There is disagreement about whether these findings reflect errors in documenting age (for older black Americans) or a true cross-over in mortality rates.

The exact number of centenarians in the United States is difficult to gauge, but their numbers are growing. For persons born in 1899, the odds against living to 100 were 400 to 1; for persons born in 1980, the odds are estimated at 87 to 1.

SOCIOECONOMIC STATUS

Improvements in the Social Security system and the adoption of Medicare have had an important impact on the economic well-being of older persons in the United States. In the early 1960s, 35% of people aged 65 or older had incomes below the federal poverty level, and only 60% received Social Security pensions. By the early 1990s, 93% of older people received Social Security retirement benefits (accounting for at least 50% of income for 63% of beneficiaries, and 90% or more of income for 26%) and 97% were covered by Medicare. The percentage of older people with incomes below the poverty line today is about 10%.

Although the overall economic position of older people in the United States has improved significantly over the past three decades, these gains have not been shared by all. Poverty rates among older people are higher among black Americans (26%), Hispanic Americans (21%), persons aged 85 and older (20%), those who never finished high school (21%), those living in rural areas (13%) and central cities (14%), and those living alone (21%). Rates in some groups of older persons are much higher—half of older black American women living alone are poor, for example.

Older workers continue to decline as a share of the U.S. work force, and this trend is expected to continue. Overall, in the early 1990s, 16% of older men and 8% of older women were working. In 1990, 28% of men aged 65 to 69 were working, whereas in 1950, 60% of the same age group were still in the work force. Today, more than half of those who continue to work do so part time, and largely by choice rather than because of restricted opportunities for full-time work.

There is disagreement over whether the baby-boom retirees will be better or less well-off than today's retirees. Personal savings and retirement benefits may be lower in the future; however, a 1993 Congressional Budget Office study of baby boomers in retirement found most will have higher real incomes in retirement than their parents now have.

One of the most dramatic changes in the older U.S. population of the future will be in levels of educational attainment. Between 1970 and 1998, the percentage of those aged 65 or older who completed high school increased from 28% to 67%. By 2030, 83% will have completed high school. The percentage with a bachelor's degree or more will have increased to 24% from the current level of 15%. Education is closely related to lifetime economic status, and, as many studies have shown, those with more education generally are in better health and at lower risk of disability than those with low levels of educational attainment. There is also speculation that the better-educated older baby boomers will be both more activist health care consumers and more demanding of the health care system. Today, approximately 50% of U.S. households have personal computers, but Internet use is much more common among persons under the age of 55. Despite concerns about the accuracy of much of the health and medical information available on various Internet Web sites, use of these alternative information sources is likely to grow. In addition, pharmaceutical companies are increasingly marketing directly to consumers as a means of developing demand.

LIVING ARRANGEMENTS AND MARITAL STATUS

Among Americans living in the United States who are aged 65 to 74 years, two thirds are married and

Table 2.1—Years of Life Expectancy at Birth and Ages 65, 75, 85, by Gender and Race, 1996

	All Races			White			Black		
	Both sexes	Male	Female	Both sexes	Male	Female	Both sexes	Male	Female
At birth	76.1	73.1	79.1	76.8	73.9	79.7	70.2	66.1	74.2
Age 65	17.5	15.7	19.0	17.6	15.8	19.1	15.8	13.9	17.2
Age 75	11.1	9.8	12.0	11.1	9.8	12.0	10.3	9.0	11.2
Age 85	6.1	5.4	6.4	6.0	5.3	6.3	6.0	5.3	6.2

SOURCE: Data from *National Vital Statistics Report.* 1998; 47(13):10.

living with their spouse; in contrast, only about one fifth of those aged 85 and older are living with their spouse (Table 2.2). Not surprisingly, given women's greater life expectancy, older men are twice as likely to be married as are older women. Conversely, widowhood is much more common among older women; three in five women aged 75 to 84 and four in five women aged 85 and older are widows.

Older men and women who live alone, often having lost a spouse, usually prefer to remain independent and continue living alone as long as their health and economic means allow them to do so. Many of those who live alone have families or friends nearby, and about three in five have lived in the same place for 10 years or more. These persons may also be vulnerable, however. They are more likely than older people who live with others to use community services and to report greater levels of loneliness and social isolation.

THE EMERGENCE OF ASSISTED-LIVING FACILITIES

Assisted living represents one of the fastest-growing trends in residential settings for older people in the United States. This type of facility seeks to fill the need for greater supervision and assistance than may be possible in a private home while avoiding the detrimental aspects of institutional care. Assisted-living residences are characterized by some level of coordination or provision of personal care services, social activities, health-related services, and supervision, services provided in a homelike atmosphere that maximizes autonomy and privacy. There is considerable variation among such facilities, however. A national survey of assisted-living facilities found a range of privacy options, from private rooms to apartment units; about half would not admit residents with moderate to

severe cognitive impairment; about two thirds did not have a registered nurse on staff but did provide 24-hour staff oversight, housekeeping, two meals, and personal assistance with activities of daily living (ADLs). The transitional nature of assisted living is suggested by the average length of residency, 26 months in 1997. The most common reason for discharge was the need for nursing-home care.

Approximately 600,000 people were estimated to be living in 25,000 to 30,000 assisted-living facilities in the United States in 2000. These types of residences have not been within financial reach for older people with low or moderate incomes, however. In 1997 the average annual income of residents was approximately $31,000. Because in most states assisted-living expenses cannot be covered by Medicaid, as nursing-home costs can, some states are developing other financing mechanisms to encourage the development of affordable assisted-living residences for low-income older people. One example is Massachusetts, which, through several public and quasi-public agencies, has produced more than 1000 living units intended for older people with lower incomes.

TRENDS IN NURSING-HOME USE

The supply of nursing-home beds per 1000 people aged 75 and over has declined, from 141 per 1000 in 1987 to 117 per 1000 in 1996, creating concern that demand will outstrip supply in future years. Nationally, the percentage of older people residing in nursing homes has remained fairly constant, at about 5% overall, rising to 20% of persons aged 85 and older. The lifetime chance of ever being in a nursing home is much higher, however, at nearly 1 in 2. In part, this is due to increased use of nursing homes for short stays for recovery and rehabilitation following hospital discharge, stays that are paid for by Medicare if preceded

Table 2.2—Marital Status and Living Arrangements of Medicare Beneficiaries, by Age and Gender, 1998

	All (%)			Male (%)			Female (%)		
	65–74	75–84	85+	65–74	75–84	85+	65–74	75–84	85+
Marital Status									
Married	65.53	49.36	23.05	79.49	72.49	54.43	53.48	34.17	10.25
Widowed	20.25	41.56	68.80	7.18	19.13	37.90	31.52	56.30	81.41
Divorced or separated	9.73	5.53	3.38	8.55	4.87	3.66	10.76	5.97	3.26
Never married	4.49	3.55	4.77	4.78	3.51	4.01	4.24	3.57	5.08
Living Arrangement									
Lives alone	23.62	35.65	39.02	14.51	21.26	27.81	31.50	45.13	43.62
With spouse	62.98	45.34	18.01	76.85	67.74	43.68	51.01	30.62	7.53
With children	7.05	9.13	14.40	2.79	3.85	8.74	10.74	12.60	16.73
With others	5.01	4.80	5.43	4.58	3.57	4.17	5.38	5.61	5.95
Long-term care facility	1.34	5.08	23.14	1.27	3.57	15.60	1.37	6.03	26.17

SOURCE: Data from *Medicare Current Beneficiary Survey*, 1998; Table 1.2. Http://www.hcfa.gov/surveysmcbs/ (accessed September 2002).

by a 3-day hospital stay. The resident population is older and more disabled today. From 1987 to 1996, the proportion of residents aged 85 and older rose from 49% to 56% for women, and 29% to 33% for men; the proportion needing help with three or more ADLs rose from 72% to 83%.

In the past 10 years, nursing homes have put more resources into developing special care units, and almost one fifth of all nursing homes now have one. Two thirds of these units are for Alzheimer's disease and related dementias.

Studies comparing the performance of these units with that of traditional units have not shown that residents of special units receive more direct care or experience better outcomes.

TRENDS IN HEALTH AND FUNCTIONING

The burden of disease and disability is greater for older people than for those under age 65. In the United States in 1995, 79% of persons aged 70 or older had one or more of the seven chronic conditions most common among older people (arthritis, hypertension, heart disease, diabetes mellitus, respiratory disease, stroke, and cancer). At the same time, there is greater heterogeneity in health status among older people than is found among younger age groups. Data on self-assessed health, which has been shown in several studies to correlate highly with mortality and risk of functional decline, illustrate this (Table 2.3). Among white non-Hispanic Americans aged 65 to 74, nearly 20% regarded their health as excellent and another 32%

as very good, while 13% indicated only fair health, and 6% poor health. As might be expected, the percentages who viewed their health as only fair or poor increased with age and, within age groups, were higher for black and Hispanic Americans than for older white Americans.

Functional disability also increases with age and is closely associated with chronic disease. In the United States, a high proportion of people under the age of 85 report no difficulty in ADLs or instrumental activities of daily living (IADLs) (69% of those aged 65 to 74; 48% of those aged 75 to 84 years), but only 21% of those aged 85 and older report no difficulty (Table 2.4). Older women exhibit a higher percentage of limitations at all ages than older men do. Differences between racial and ethnic groups exist as well. Among those aged 70 and older, black Americans were 1.5 times as likely as white Americans to be unable to perform one or more ADLs.

In the United States older persons who need assistance with functioning in routine activities of daily life rely first and foremost on family. In 1995, of those providing assistance to community-dwelling persons aged 70 or older, 73% were unpaid or informal helpers. Nine out of 10 informal or unpaid caregivers were family members, one fourth were spouses, and about half were children. Half of these informal caregivers resided with the person receiving help. Estimates of the use of paid helpers vary across studies, but use is consistently found to be higher among persons living alone and to rise with increasing age.

Deaths of older persons make up nearly 75% of all deaths in the United States. About one fifth of all

Table 2.3—Perceived Health of Medicare Beneficiaries, by Age and Race or Ethnicity, 1998

	White, non-Hispanic (%)			Black, non-Hispanic (%)			Hispanic (%)		
	65–74	75–84	85+	65–74	75–84	85+	65–74	75–84	85+
Health Status									
Excellent	18.72	14.02	11.98	11.59	9.34	5.82	15.14	9.70	10.21
Very good	31.67	26.39	21.77	21.65	18.18	16.68	21.25	18.58	19.14
Good	31.01	32.68	31.53	30.59	33.58	27.40	32.40	32.04	33.09
Fair	12.89	19.15	24.26	26.35	27.48	35.20	22.50	24.18	26.76
Poor	5.70	7.77	10.47	9.82	11.42	14.90	8.71	15.50	10.80

SOURCE: Data from *Medicare Current Beneficiary Survey*, 1998; Table 2.3. Http://www.hcfa.gov/surveymcbs (accessed September 2002).

Table 2.4—Difficulty in ADLs and IADLs of Medicare Beneficiaries, by Age and Gender, 1998

	All %			Male %			Female %		
	65–74	75–84	85+	65–74	75–84	85+	65–74	75–84	85+
None	68.52	48.43	20.58	73.17	56.06	27.62	64.69	43.52	17.84
IADLs only	9.66	13.41	12.16	7.21	11.54	12.38	11.68	14.61	12.07
1–2 ADLs	15.02	23.41	28.44	13.42	21.20	27.24	16.34	24.83	28.91
3–6 ADLs	6.80	14.76	38.82	6.20	11.20	32.76	7.29	17.04	41.18

NOTE: ADLs = activities of daily living; IADLs = instrumental activities of daily living.

SOURCE: Data from *Medicare Current Beneficiary Survey*, 1998; Table 2.1. Http://www.hcfa.gov/surveymcbs (accessed September 2002).

deaths occur at age 85 or older, but this proportion is expected to grow. For many decades heart disease, cancer, and stroke have been the leading causes of death among people 65 or older, accounting for 7 out of 10 deaths (Table 2.5). Causes of death vary by race, ethnicity, and gender, however. Diabetes mellitus was the fourth leading cause of death among older Hispanic and black Americans, while ranking sixth for older white Americans. Alzheimer's disease ranked sixth among all causes of death for white American women aged 85 and older but was less common among black American women or all American men of similar age.

Some causes of death usually associated with younger people also are of concern in the older population. In the United States, older men have motor vehicle accident death rates two to three times those of older women, overall and within race and ethnic groups. The highest suicide rates among older people are for white men (43.7 per 100,000, compared with 6.5 per 100,000 for older white women), who are more likely to commit suicide than die in a motor vehicle crash.

TRENDS IN DISABILITY

There are conflicting opinions about whether rates of disability in the United States are declining among people aged 65 and over. Some studies suggest a decline in the past decade in the proportion unable to do some activities (one or more ADLs or IADLs), but there is also evidence for an increase in the proportion unable to perform one or more ADLs. Differences in study populations and measures contribute to conflicting findings. Measurement of disabilities varies across studies, and assessments of the presence and severity of

disability can differ when histories are taken from an older person, the family caregiver, or the clinician.

Trends in disability are of special interest because increases in life expectancy overall and for people aged 65 and older have led to debate over whether these additional years will be disability free. Studies of active life expectancy, which use mortality and disability estimates to project disability-free years, suggest an advantage for persons with more education. Because of their greater total life expectancy, older women also experience both greater active life expectancy and more years of disability than older men. It has also been suggested that if there is a limit to increases in life expectancy, increases in disability-free years could produce a *compression of morbidity*, with the period of disability prior to death gradually compressed as active life expectancy (or disability-free years) increases. Increases in active life expectancy must occur if compression of morbidity is to be achieved, but debate continues regarding whether there is a maximum human life span, and whether compression of morbidity is possible if total life expectancy continues to increase.

As more longitudinal studies are conducted and other evidence is brought to bear, the trend in active life expectancy among older people may become clearer. Regardless of its true direction, however, preventing and reducing disability among older people remains a major objective of much gerontologic research.

The assumption has been that disability is irreversible, but studies show that up to one third of persons who experience disability in a basic ADL recover. Age less than 85 years, good nutritional status, and greater mobility are all associated with increased likelihood of recovery from basic ADL disability.

Table 2.5—Leading Causes of Death and Numbers of Deaths, for Persons Aged 65 and Over, 1997

Rank	Cause of Death	Number of Deaths	% of Deaths
	All causes	1,728,872	100.0
1	Diseases of heart	606,913	35.1
2	Malignant neoplasms	382,913	22.1
3	Cerebrovascular diseases	140,366	8.1
4	Chronic obstructive pulmonary disease	94,411	5.5
5	Pneumonia and influenza	77,561	4.5
6	Diabetes mellitus	47,289	2.7
7	Unintentional injuries	31,386	1.8
8	Alzheimer's disease	22,154	1.3
9	Nephritis, nephrotic syndrome, and nephrosis	21,787	1.3
10	Septicemia	18,079	1.0

SOURCE: *Health, United States, 1999 With Health and Aging Chartbook.* Hyattsville, MD: US Department of Health and Human Services, National Center for Health Statistics; 1999:156 (Table 33).

TRENDS IN HEALTH CARE

On average, older adults in the United States have more contacts with health care professionals than do younger adults, from a mean of 10 per year among those aged 65 to 74, to nearly 15 per year among those aged 85 and older. Those who assess their health as fair or poor have twice as many contacts per year as do persons in excellent or good health. Although representing only 13% of the population in 1996, older people accounted for 38% of hospital discharges. The average length of stay for older patients has been declining for some time, however, from 12.1 days per stay in 1964 to 6.8 in 1996. Variations in length of stay can be considerable, however.

Diseases of the heart were the leading discharge diagnosis in the United States for older people, with heart disease and stroke together accounting for more than one fourth of all hospital discharges among men and women aged 85 and older. Malignant neoplasms were the next most frequent discharge diagnosis, followed by pneumonia and bronchitis. Fracture-related hospitalizations were more common among women than men and accounted for nearly 10% of discharges for those aged 85 and older.

Home-health care, including medical treatment, physical therapy, and homemaker services, is an alternative to institutional care for older people. Nursing care is the most commonly used service (85% of older home-health patients received nursing care in 1996), and 29% of patients use homemaker services. Medicare has been a major payer for home-health care (nearly half of expenses in 1996), and changes in payment methods have resulted in a dramatic drop in use of these services (both in the numbers of persons served and visits per user). See "Financing, Coverage, and Costs of Health Care" (p 26).

Prescription drugs have become a major component of medical treatment. Eighty percent of people in the United States aged 65 or over are using one or more prescribed medicines; among those with three to five ADL limitations, 93% use at least one.

OTHER ISSUES

The older U.S. population is among the most heterogeneous subgroups, encompassing the entire spectrum of health and functioning, from the bedridden Alzheimer's patient to the marathon runner. One of the important, unresolved questions is whether gains in longevity after age 65 are accompanied by gains or declines in years of disability-free life. It is unlikely that one answer will fit this large and diverse group. There are many questions in other areas as well. While levels of education continue to rise, so do rates of early retirement. Will the increasing numbers of better-educated, longer-lived persons contribute to the larger society, and in what ways? Will the sheer numbers of older people strain to the breaking point the medical care system and public programs that finance health care and retirement, as some analysts fear? Or will improvements in health behavior, medical breakthroughs, and financial prosperity diminish these threats?

Under any scenario, chronic illness will remain a constant in the lives of many older people. Clinicians treating this population face the challenge not only of treating chronically ill persons but of assisting all older people in preventing or at least delaying the onset of chronic disease.

REFERENCES

■ Administration on Aging. *A Profile of Older Americans*; 2002. http://www.aoa.gov/aoa/stats/profile/default.htm

■ Administration on Aging (AOA), US Department of Health and Human Services. *Profile of Older Americans*. 2001.

■ Cartwright JC. Nursing homes and assisted living facilities as places for dying. *Annu Rev Nurs Res*. 2002;20:231–264.

■ Citro J, Hermanson S, Consumer Team, Public Policy Institute Research Group. *Assisted Living in the United States*. Washington, DC: American Association of Retired People (AARP); 1999.

■ Gill RM, Robinson JT, Tinetti ME. Predictors of recovery in activities of daily living among disabled older persons living in the community. *J Gen Intern Med*. 1997;12:757–762.

■ Hawes C, Rose M, Phillips CD, et al. *A National Study of Assisted Living for the Frail Elderly: Results of a National Telephone Survey of Facilities*. Beachwood, OH: Menorah Park Center for the Aging; 1999.

■ Hobbs, FB, Damon BL. *Sixty-Five Plus in America*. Current Population Reports, Special Studies, P23–P190. Washington, DC: US Department of Commerce, Economics, and Statistics Administration, Bureau of the Census; 1996.

■ Manton KG, Stallard E, Corder LS. The dynamics of dimensions of age-related disability 1982 to 1994 in the US elderly population. *J Gerontol A Biol Sci Med Sci*. 1998;53(1):B59–B70.

■ National Center for Health Statistics. *Health, United States, 1999 With Health and Aging Chartbook*. Hyattsville, MD: US Department of Health and Human Services, National Center for Health Statistics; 1999. DHHS Pub. No. (PHS) 99–1232.

■ Stone LO. Demography of aging. In: Mezey MD, ed. *The Encyclopedia of Elder Care*. New York: Springer Publishing Company; 2001:203–206.

■ Stone R. Long-term care for the disabled elderly: current policy, emerging trends and implications for the 21st century. A special electronic report of *The Milbank Quarterly*. January, 2000.

CHAPTER 3—PSYCHOSOCIAL ISSUES

Appreciating the role and scope of psychosocial aspects of aging improves clinicians' ability to address and treat factors that have important bearing on the overall well-being of older persons. Health events have broad ramifications. When they are viewed within a framework that includes both the stressors and means to ameliorate the impact of stress, other factors besides the treatment of the disease itself can be seen to need clinical attention.

Stressors are any demands that call forth a behavioral or emotional response; often, such demands are perceived as threats. Unchecked stressors can lead to negative outcomes across the whole spectrum of physical and mental health and may also affect other domains, such as economic welfare and family life. Given the range of demands posed by the stressors, it is evident that they can greatly affect a person's physical and mental health, including every aspect of his or her well-being. The person's ability to function in the world may be reduced; the enthusiasm the person brings to and the pleasure he or she takes from interaction may also be reduced. The use the person makes of financial, health, and social service resources may also be strongly affected.

The older person's coping responses can partially filter the impact of stress. Coping may be described as having two main parts, mediators and moderators. Mediators, such as the patient's self-efficacy and the presence and strength of a social network, can offer clinicians important tools for treatment as well as targets for therapeutic intervention. Moderating behaviors, especially those in the psychosocial realm like social involvement and spirituality, can also prove effective in a broad treatment plan. Assisting older persons to see and work toward health outcomes that impact the quality of their life is an appropriate and effective clinical strategy for helping them to confront declines in physical health and the issues of mortality.

STRESSORS

The older person faces a great number and variety of stressors produced by a broad range of events and conditions. The stressors may be chronic, or they may have sudden, dramatic onset. They may be based in diseases or they may be of a more social nature. A chronic stressor may be health related (eg, the pain and mobility limitation of arthritis) or it may be psychologic (eg, the prolonged worry over a chronically ill spouse). An acute stressor might also be physical or psychologic (eg, learning of a newly diagnosed medical condition or experiencing the unexpected death of a close friend). Other stress demands include changes in social identity due to role loss in retirement or the function-driven need to move to a more supportive living arrangement. Losses in physical capacity and reserve may place demands on the person, not only because he or she perceives them as threats or increased physical demands, but also because of their accompanying psychologic component, the perception that he or she may have diminished capacity to respond to other demands. Always in the background for older persons are the various risk factors for incident or recurrent morbidity and mortality.

Some risk factors—particularly those involving behaviors over which the person (with some encouragement, teaching, and counseling) might exert control—may be modifiable. Other risk factors, such as gender and race, are not modifiable and produce accumulated assaults that may amplify other stressors. The increasing incidence of diseases with age means that the number and frequency of stressors are likely to increase as a person ages.

Caregiving

Many older persons are caregivers for a family member. Chronic diseases affect a large proportion of older persons, and much of the care they receive is provided by family members, especially spouses. The burden of caregiving for dementing disorders like Alzheimer's disease is typical. Dementia caregivers spend many hours each day in caregiving activities, and they do so for many years (20% are caregivers for more than 5 years). Such caregiving exacts a heavy toll. Caregivers are at twice the risk as their noncaregiving peers for adverse physical and mental health outcomes and more than twice as likely to be taking psychotropic medications. Social isolation, family disharmony, and economic hardships are frequent sequelae of caregiving.

Caregivers need training, information, and support, and they should be regularly observed for signs of the known effects of caregiving. Attention to family dynamics may also be useful in identifying issues contributing to stressors that are modifiable. A number of intervention programs (eg, those providing education, counseling, and cognitive behavioral therapy) have proven effective in ameliorating the stress associated with caregiving. Disease-specific support activities offer only modest relief but may be the conduit for more focused help.

Loss and Grief

Being widowed, especially for women, is a common occurrence in old age; so, too, are deaths in one's extended family and larger social network. Other losses, such as sensory and functional losses imposed by the onset of chronic or acute illnesses, also produce grief. Such losses are generally understood to be among the major negative life events, and they place a substantial demand on a person. For most, the intense experience of grief lasts 6 to 12 months, generally a time of withdrawal and depression. After about a year, a more accepting period ensues, during which a re-emergence into a social milieu occurs or a less affecting form of more permanent memorialization of the lost person is established. Acknowledgment and monitoring of the grieving process and active treatment for the depression associated with loss can help in avoiding prolongation of this process.

Role Loss and Acquisition

People typically encounter a large number of role shifts in aging. They leave work and social roles that may have provided economic rewards as well as status. Within relationships, roles may change, and wage-earning spouses, after retirement, may find themselves in significantly greater contact with each other. Grandparenthood and great-grandparenthood provide both new demands and opportunities. Functional losses may place older persons in help-seeking rather than help-providing roles, or, as noted above, another's losses may place one in a caregiving role. These role changes can be stressful and can negatively affect mental or physical health. Retirement planning can help make these positive experiences. The clinician's assessment of an older person's role loss and acquisition may suggest the need for interventions.

Social Status

Three factors are consistently associated in the United States with a broad range of negative psychosocial and physical outcomes: being nonwhite, being a woman, and being poor or poorly educated (usually a surrogate for being poor). They should serve as warnings for clinicians, as the presence of one or more of these factors may add to the person's stress load. They may also affect the kinds of coping mechanisms the person has available. Lack of disposable income, for example, may rule out the use of some formal services or involvement in community activities that come with a fee. Cultural status may present other challenges; women from some cultures, for example, may face special barriers to exercising in public.

A person's ethnic or cultural background and community context may substantially affect the outlook she or he brings to bear on a situation, the kinds of moderating activities she or he deems acceptable, and the importance she or he places on various outcomes. Older persons may understand disease through frameworks specific to other cultures, and treatment may need to include or rely principally on culturally centered options. A concept like autonomy that has become so central in issues of patient choice and advance directives has a different weight and value in cultures where choice belongs more to the community as a whole (as with some American Indian groups) or to a community or family leader (eg, in Hmong societies). Choices like hospice care may be viewed in some cultures as tantamount to wishing for and bringing about the death of the person. A procedure like autopsy may strongly violate cultural or religious beliefs. The clinician is advised to proceed attentively in cross-cultural situations.

MEDIATORS

Mediators are the internal and external resources the person can bring to bear to assess and interpret the stress and to assess his or her own capacities for addressing it; the mediators shape the person's responses to stress. Broadly, mediators can be categorized as personal qualities (eg, self-efficacy, coping skills) and external resources (eg, social network, formal services). Many key mediators are modifiable through psychosocial intervention. Instruction and information can affect the person's understanding of a situation. Various forms of psychoeducation have been shown to be effective in enhancing an older person's sense of mastery within a stress situation and in increasing his or her awareness and use of formal services. Family counseling and therapy can strengthen older person's social network.

Self-Efficacy Beliefs

A number of constructs have been studied that relate to a person's sense of his or her own ability to manage situations. The concept of self-efficacy is comparable to concepts such as mastery, internal locus of control, resilience, and competence, and although it is singled out here, it resembles these in representing a key personal quality to be considered when dealing with an older person facing any stress situation. Self-efficacy is an important consideration for the mental and physical health of older persons for two reasons.

First, there is a relationship between strong or positive self-efficacy and a number of important health and mental health outcomes (Table 3.1). A large number of longitudinal studies—most recently the MacArthur study of "successful " or healthy aging—have produced a coherent set of conclusions about self-efficacy. The way a person approaches a situation—

whether it be a specific threat, like the onset of an acute condition, or a more pervasive one, like change of life roles or decline in physical performance—affects the eventual outcome. Of particular note in Table 3.1 is the broad range of effects of strong self-efficacy beliefs, which influence physical and mental health as well as overall function. In addition, self-efficacy seems to contribute to a person's ability to be actively engaged in life, an important moderating factor.

The second reason self-efficacy is important is that it is modifiable. It can be weakened by repeated assaults and poor outcome, but it can also be strengthened. Among the strategies effective for strengthening self-efficacy are the following:

- performance accomplishment (seeing oneself succeed in a series of increasingly difficult tasks);
- vicarious learning and social modeling (seeing others like oneself succeed in a targeted area);
- encouragement (being persuaded to undertake a targeted activity); and
- reinforcement (experiencing pleasure from success).

A number of training programs aimed at improving specific performance (eg, reducing the fear of falling or increasing adherence to an exercise regimen following a heart attack) have succeeded by working to strengthen participants' self-efficacy beliefs in the targeted area. Strong self-efficacy beliefs appear to be better predictors of performance than are measures of physical ability. In falls prevention studies, for example, those with strong self-efficacy beliefs related to falling were found to show reduced fear of falling, despite low objective measures for risk of falling. Self-efficacy appears to play an important role in coping and overall

Table 3.1—Physical and Mental Health Impacts of Self-Efficacy Beliefs

Strong self-efficacy beliefs

  Buffer the effects of stress exposure on physical and mental health

  Contribute to overall physical performance, independently of ability

  Help maintain good function

  Slow functional decline among those with poor physical performance

  Contribute to good choice making, good performance, and persistence of effort (especially in women)

  Contribute to increased productivity

Weak self-efficacy beliefs

  Are associated with declines in functional status, especially in those with decreased physical performance

well-being in older persons. Clinicians should assess the older person's sense of his or her own competence and intervene, where possible, to strengthen it.

Coping Strategies

A number of theorists have studied the manner in which older persons meet and address the accumulated challenges of aging. One strategy older people may use consists of selection, optimization, and compensation. In this strategy, as people age, they begin to hone down the number and kinds of things in which they engage on the basis of what they believe they do well, selecting activities in which they are more likely to succeed. They also reframe the way they judge their own performance, looking, for example, at people their own age or older for a source of comparison. They do the selected things more, and they derive optimal credit for doing them. As losses continue and performance diminishes, people employ compensatory strategies that allow them to put their remaining performance capacities in the best light possible. A person known for preparing elaborate dinners might, for example, choose a simpler main course (selection) that she does well and has prepared many times (optimization) and surround it with numerous but very simple courses and side dishes as a way of favorably setting it off (compensation). Other coping strategies (eg, assimilation, accommodation, immunization, or resilience) also build essentially on the notion of reframing the self or one's performance in order to provide positive reinforcement and to reinforce self-esteem. Clinicians should attempt to learn how their patients typically form successful responses to challenges and help them to address new challenges in these same terms.

Social Networks

The older person's social network is a critical resource for overall well-being, and social isolation is a powerful risk factor for broad declines and mortality. The effect of their social networks on older persons' overall well-being has been extensively studied, and the results of these studies are conclusive (Table 3.2). The literature points to the importance of quality over quantity but does not discount the latter. The closeness of social relationships is most important; thus, a well-functioning marital or familial relationship—a relationship that provides a person with a confidante—will offer the kinds of support and protection suggested in Table 3.2. Dysfunctional close relationships—those characterized by negative and conflict-filled interactions—appear to work in the contrary direction. The size of an older person's social network appears to work in both

Table 3.2—Physical and Mental Health Impacts of Robust Social Networks

Reduced mortality risks

Better physical health outcomes

Better mental health outcomes

Reduced risk of ADL disability or decline

Increased likelihood of ADL recovery

Buffered impact of major negative life events

Promotion of strong self-efficacy beliefs

Assistance that does not preclude self-care but that may increase risk of new or recurrent ADL disability (especially in men)

Note: ADL = activities of daily living.

directions. On the one hand, having a larger social network offers the opportunity for greater involvement and contribution; on the other hand, it presents the likelihood of experiencing a greater number of losses within the network (because of death or increased disability).

A robust social network both mediates and moderates age-related stresses. Social networks provide emotional and instrumental help in times of crisis. Families help older persons, for example, weather the death of a spouse or close friend, but they also provide direct and indirect help when more functional losses occur. The social network can provide a person under stress with a context within which to envision and frame responses to various demands. Social networks seem to exert a positive effect on older persons by strengthening their self-efficacy beliefs (the person feels valued within the social network, and this contributes to a sense of self-value). It also provides opportunities for taking action to address demands (eg, calling on family for specific functional assistance, spending more time with children following the death of a spouse, increasing time spent with friends following retirement).

The literature is clear that the provision of such help is positive and contributes to recovery, unless it sends the wrong message. Too much instrumental assistance provided to older people (particularly men) by the social network may contribute to continued disability. Rather than being encouraged to work toward restored function, a person may receive too much help or not be encouraged to self-care and may, therefore, accept a modifiable condition as permanent. Thus, although assistance from the social network should be encouraged, it should be done with attention to promoting maximum function by the person receiving the help.

MODERATORS

Moderators—which are shaped in part by the mediators—are the behavioral and emotional responses a person employs to address demands. Moderators may be either problem focused or emotion focused. Deciding to begin an exercise program, to control diet or alcohol consumption, or to cease smoking are possible—and healthy—responses to stressors ranging from the onset of illness to a realization that one has slowed down. These healthy behaviors moderate the effect of the perceived threat or demand and contribute to better physical and mental health outcomes. Calling on one's family in a time of crisis (rather than withdrawing) may help moderate age-related demands. Becoming more involved, actively seeking out ways to contribute to and participate in the broader world, even engaging in paid work are all moderators that can lead to better outcomes. Cultivating an emotional response to a stressor can moderate its effect and produce a better outcome. Thus, invoking confidence and optimism in the face of bad news helps a person to meet the challenge and strengthens the likelihood of a positive outcome.

The literature points to three major activities that moderate stress or demand and that appear to contribute to healthy aging: social involvement, spiritual or religious activity, and engaging in healthy behaviors. Older persons' activities in these areas should be assessed regularly and encouraged, as appropriate.

Social Involvement

Like people at all ages, older persons are faced with developmental tasks and challenges. In Erikson's theory of staged development, the task of old age is integration—putting the pieces together in a way that both celebrates and continues to act on the learning and accomplishments of life. In this conception, and consistent with many other findings, involvement (sometimes termed *productivity*) plays an important role. Taking part, making a contribution—through volunteering, productive (sometimes paid) labor, active family roles (especially child care), and participation in group activities—are all associated with older persons' continued well-being.

Spiritual or Religious Involvement

Studies have consistently demonstrated two important facts about religion and older people. First, religion plays a more important part in the lives of older persons than in those of younger persons; older persons are more actively involved in attending religious services and in carrying out regular private religious practices. Second, there are consistent positive relationships between religious involvement and indicators of good health. Whether religious activity contributes to social integration, promotes involvement, or assists in the developmental tasks of aging, it seems clear that it is a positive force—at least for those already inclined to it.

Healthy Behaviors

Implementing positive behaviors (eg, exercise, controlling intake of food, tobacco, alcohol, and active relaxation or stress-reduction techniques) have all been shown to have positive effect on overall well-being, no matter at what age they are begun. Although these are physical behaviors, they often rely on and benefit from strong psychosocial mediators, particularly self-efficacy and social networks. Clinicians should use these mediators when proposing older persons begin or strengthen healthy behaviors. It can help to invoke a person's understanding of benefits and appreciation of his or her own proven ability to make change while at the same time offering suggestions about how the targeted behavior might contribute to a strong social network (eg, "you could walk everyday with your daughter," "you and your husband could take the healthy cooking class together").

REFERENCES

■ Acton, GJ, Kang J. Interventions to reduce the burden of caregiving for an adult with dementia: a meta-analysis. *Res Nurs Health.* 2001;24(5):349–360.

■ Aneshensel CS, Pearlin LI, Mullan JT, et al. *Profiles in Caregiving: The Unexpected Career.* San Diego, CA: Academic Press, Inc; 1995.

■ Bandura A. Self-efficacy mechanism in human agency. *American Psychologist.* 1982;37(2):122–147.

■ Bourgeois MS, Schulz R, Burgio L. Interventions for caregivers of patients with Alzheimer's disease: a review and analysis of content, process, and outcomes. *Int J Aging Hum Dev.* 1996;43(1):35–92.

■ Dellasega C, Zerbe TM. Caregivers of frail, rural older adults. Effects of an advanced practice nursing intervention. *J Gerontol Nurs.* 2002;28(10):40–49.

■ Schulz R, O'Brien AT, Bookwala J, et al. Psychiatric and physical morbidity effects of dementia caregiving: prevalence, correlates, and causes. *Gerontologist.* 1995;35(6):771–791.

■ Koenig HG. The healing power of faith. *Ann Long-Term Care.* 1999;7(10):381–384.

■ Koenig HG, Hays JC, Larson DB, et al. Does religious attendance prolong survival? A six-year follow-up study of 3,968 older adults. *J Gerontol A Biol Sci Med Sci.* 1999;54(7):M370–M376.

■ Lazarus RS, Folkman S. Coping and adaptation. In: Gentry WD, ed. *The Handbook of Behavioral Medicine.* New York: Guilford; 1984.

■ Rowe JW, Kahn RL. *Successful Aging.* New York: Pantheon Press; 1998.

■ Yin T, Zhou Q, Bashford C. Burden on family members: caring for frail elderly: a meta-analysis of interventions. *Nurs Res.* 2002;51(3):199–208.

CHAPTER 4—LEGAL AND ETHICAL ISSUES

DECISIONS NEAR THE END OF LIFE

Although the issues discussed in this section focus on the period near the end of life, the decision-making process and ethical principles described are the same for all medical decisions. When a person is faced with a terminal illness or a chronic, disabling, or progressive disease, decision making becomes more acute and focused. Decisions are made, consciously or subconsciously, concerning treatment of minor conditions, adherence with medical regimens, and related issues by analyzing competing values and needs. Patients, families, and clinicians must attempt to balance benefits and burdens when making many health care decisions. This difficult task is further complicated by the fact that only probabilities of the benefits and burdens can be known, not certainties.

Forgoing and Discontinuing Interventions

A patient's right to refuse unwanted treatment was confirmed by the Supreme Court of the United States in the 1991 case of *Cruzan v. Director, Department of Health of Missouri*. This refusal can occur before the intervention has been instituted or after it is in place. There is no ethical or legal distinction made between these two situations, often referred to in the more dramatic terms of withholding or withdrawing therapies. For example, in the case of uremia, a patient with renal failure may refuse to begin dialysis, thus increasing the risk of death from uremia. Alternatively, a patient may try dialysis for a period of time, even years, and then choose to stop this treatment and die from uremia. The same principle holds for discontinuing ventilatory support for a patient. The patient will die from the underlying respiratory disease whether ventilatory support is never started or it is discontinued. The act of extubating a patient with the expectation that he or she will die is difficult for many clinicians because of the proximity of the act performed by the clinician and the death of the patient, but the decision is informed by the same ethical principles as the discontinuation of dialysis or the refusal of other medical interventions.

The refusal of tube feeding and intravenous fluids is another area of some discomfort for clinicians and families. Case law, as well as the *Cruzan* case, characterizes these methods of delivering food and fluid as medical interventions; therefore, they are subject to the same ethical right of refusal that applies to any other medical interventions. Many people worry that the terminally ill patient will suffer without these interventions, but accumulated experience in hospice care has shown that it is usually easier to make someone comfortable without them. Intravenous and gastric administration of food and fluid can cause discomfort through decreased gastric emptying and gastric distention, the need to replace intravenous lines or nasogastric tubes, and fluid overload as membranes become more permeable. These interventions may dampen or eliminate some of the natural comfort measures that occur, such as the release of endorphins.

Interventions That May Hasten Death

Palliative care, defined here as interventions that are given in order to relieve discomfort or suffering, may at times have the unintended effect of hastening death. We have come to accept that there may be two effects to a treatment; one (unintended) effect is that death may come sooner than it would have had no intervention been made, and the other (intended) effect is palliation. This is sometimes referred to as *the rule of double effect*. The intention of the application of the medical intervention is not to hasten death, but to palliate symptoms. Aggressive pain management, when respiratory depression is foreseeable but not intended, is generally seen as an ethical practice. Further, most evidence shows that gradually increasing narcotic dosage does not hasten death. The rule of double effect has been extended by some to cover the use of terminal sedation (without hydration) in cases where any level of consciousness will constitute continued suffering, as is frequently the case in death from head and neck cancer, for example.

Physician-assisted suicide and euthanasia occur when an intervention is made with the clear intention of ending the patient's life. The underlying motivation of a patient who wishes to hasten death varies. In population-based surveys, fear of pain and of other suffering (such as shortness of breath, anorexia, nausea, constipation, insomnia, and anxiety) is frequently mentioned as the reason for considering physician-assisted suicide. Fear of being dependent or a burden to others is mentioned at least as often. Other circumstances that have been mentioned by physicians as motivating factors for requests for assistance in suicide are depression, problems with personal relationships, spiritual issues, grief, and sleep disorders.

In the United States, unlike in some other countries that have addressed this issue, only physician-assisted suicide (and not euthanasia) is being considered for legalization. Because suicide is an act committed by the person who will suffer the consequences, it is felt that such a death is more clearly voluntary than a death that is the consequence of another person's administration of the lethal intervention. The Supreme Court has ruled that there is not a constitutional right to physician-assisted suicide; it is not unconstitutional, either. Each state has been left to make up its own laws in this regard. Some states have yet to act; many have made physician-assisted suicide explicitly illegal. Oregon has had legalized physician-assisted suicide since 1997. Experience there has shown that relatively few terminally ill patients request physician assistance with suicide (16 persons in the first year, 27 in the second, yielding a rate of 9 per 10,000 deaths). Prominent motivating factors were loss of autonomy and determination to control the way in which one dies.

Ability to Predict Time of Death

Despite increasingly sophisticated prediction models, especially for patients who are critically ill, the clinician's judgment is still relied upon for most assessments of prognosis. Instruments such as the APACHE III (the third version of the acute physiology and chronic health evaluation scoring system), which uses a combination of age, diagnosis, cause of acute illness, and a scale of physiologic parameters to predict mortality risk in acute illness, are unable to address issues of the burden of treatment or the patient's quality of life. Long-range predictions for patients with slowly deteriorating conditions are even more difficult. Physicians must certify that a patient has 6 months or less to live in order for that patient to qualify for the Medicare hospice benefit. Similarly, the Oregon Death with Dignity Act asks physicians to predict, using reasonable judgment, whether a terminal illness will produce death within 6 months. Patients often seek a precise prognosis from their clinicians as they weigh the benefits and burdens of interventions and consider quality-of-life issues as well as survival. Unfortunately, neither clinician judgment nor prediction rules have proven accurate in predicting prognosis.

The Continuum of End-of-life Decisions Based on Goals

Decisions near the end of life are not all-or-nothing choices. The absence or presence of do-not-resuscitate orders (more accurately referred to as do-not-attempt-resuscitation orders) is often misinterpreted as instruction to the clinician either to do everything or do nothing. This is a false dichotomy.

Other medical interventions for equally seriously ill patients may have a very different outcomes. For example, a patient with New York Heart Association Class 4 congestive heart failure from a cardiomyopathy may ask not to receive cardiopulmonary resuscitation but might choose to accept placement of an automatic implantable cardiovascular defibrillator or be given a "dobutamine holiday." A patient who is dying from lung cancer may or may not feel that the relative burdens and benefits of antibiotic treatment for pneumonia will meet his or her goals and needs.

The benefits and burdens of enteral feeding are highly influenced by the condition being treated. Most studies that have been done on the utility of enteral feeding for patients who aspirate have grouped all patients with feeding tubes together, which may not be appropriate. For example:

- Patient 1 has had surgery for a localized pharyngeal cancer followed by radiation. The procedure has left the patient freely aspirating, making it difficult for him to take in eat sufficient calories by mouth. The patient's overall prognosis is still uncertain.

- Patient 2 has Parkinson's disease but is still at a very functional level. His pharyngeal muscle coordination is slow, and he recurrently chokes on his food, especially thin liquids.

- Patient 3 has end-stage Alzheimer's disease. Although she has evidence of aspiration on a swallowing examination and has had two documented pneumonias that are probably related to aspiration, she is not uncomfortable when she eats. One of her few remaining discernable pleasures is eating.

The balance between benefits and burdens is very different for each of these cases. Enteral feeding may or may not prolong their lives, and restriction of oral intake could have a different meaning for each. The recommendations by clinicians to each patient or patient's surrogate might include everything from feeding tube placement and avoidance of taking food or drink by mouth to oral intake as tolerated for pleasure and use of antipyretic medications for fevers. Before a choice is made, the patient or family must first clarify their priorities, and then the clinician can decide how different approaches can best meet these goals.

LACK OF DECISION-MAKING CAPACITY

Because of the nature of the diseases affecting older persons, clinicians are often called on to assess a person's decision-making capacity and to use other, appropriate avenues of decisional authority when that capacity is impaired. Although the focus of much of the literature has been on clinicians' assessments of patients' capacity to make medical decisions, clinicians are also called upon to render opinions on patients' ability to make decisions about other matters, such as managing money, making a will, continuing to drive, or possessing firearms. It is important to use the correct terminology in discussing the physician's or nurse practitioner's responsibility. A physician or nurse practitioner may render an opinion as to a patient's capacity to make decisions, but *competence* and *incompetence* are legal terms, and they imply that a court has taken a specific action.

Assessment of Patients' Decisional Capacity

Assessing the patient's ability to understand the consequences of a decision is the overarching principle used in making a judgment of decisional capacity. To make a medical decision, the patient must be able to understand the basic information about his or her condition and the probable outcomes of the disease process and the various interventions. This includes the ability to understand the disease process, the proposed therapy and alternative therapies, the advantages, side effects, and complications of each therapy, and the disease course without intervention. The patient needs to be able to understand the broader consequences of accepting, deferring, or rejecting a proposed intervention. Few patients can understand the full scope of complex medical decisions, since we can rarely know all the consequences of an intervention or the precise natural history of an illness. The patient should be able to make decisions that are based on his or her beliefs and values. Therefore, it is often most helpful for the clinician to explore a patient's hopes and fears and to help the patient clarify his or her goals so that sensible treatment options that are based on these goals can be offered. Such an approach helps to extract the clinician's own values from the decision-making process.

The capacity to make a living will is similar to that of being able to make treatment decisions, although it is somewhat more complicated, since the patient is being asked to think in the abstract, in a "what if?" frame of reference. The ability to choose a health care proxy (see below) is much less complex, and even fairly impaired patients can often indicate whom they want to make decisions for them.

When the issue of *testamentary competence* (the ability to make a last will and testament) arises, a clinician may be asked to render an opinion as to the person's capabilities. In general, a person's ability to decide how he or she wishes to dispose of belongings after death is felt to be preserved even when the person is very incapacitated in other ways. As long as the person can identify the individuals involved, is not delusional or in other ways psychiatrically ill in a way

that would impair judgment (including paranoia), and is capable of understanding the consequence of signing the will, he or she is considered to have testamentary competence.

Standardized Tests of Decisional Capacity

Although some attempts have been made to use standard cognitive testing to assess decisional capacity, tests have not been shown to be useful. Some deficits found on the Mini–Mental State Examination may be relevant (eg, memory, attention, language), others are not (eg, calculation, visuospatial relationships). As we come to appreciate the influence that frontal lobe dysfunction has on a patient's capacity to function, especially to perform complex activities of independent living, we are also coming to appreciate the influence that the cognitive domains tested with executive function would have on decisional capacity. Executive functions include problem solving, planning (including appreciating consequences of an action), capacity to monitor one's own behavior, initiation and inhibition of inappropriate behaviors. Published guidelines and checklists of questions are available to formally assess a patient's capacity, but the common element in all of these is how the patient operates in making the decision (reasoning, ability to understand consequences). Assessment of decisional capacity is a functional assessment, and there is no substitute for critical observation of the process itself.

Principles Governing Decision Making for Patients Who Lack Decisional Capacity

The hierarchy of decision-making strategies for incapacitated patients is as follows: 1) their last competent indication of their wishes, 2) substituted judgment, and 3) their best interest (ie, an analysis of benefits versus burden).

The last competent indication of wishes is most relevant in cases when patients are able to foresee that they will become incapacitated and also know what decisions will need to be made. Patients entering the terminal phase of an illness who know that at some point they will become confused or unconscious can give very clear advance directives (also called *advance care plans* in some contexts) as to their preferences for care. As long as the circumstances remain clear, other individuals should not reverse these decisions.

Substituted judgment is the process of constructing what the person would have wanted if he or she had been able to foresee the circumstances and give directions for care. In theory, those who knew the person best and understood what his or her fears, pleasures, and goals were (ie, what the patient's rationale for a decision would have been) could provide substituted judgment. This is usually, but not always, the next of kin. A patient can appoint someone to hold durable power of attorney for health affairs for them (this person is also referred to as a *health care agent* or *proxy*), choosing the person who could best represent the patient when and if he or she becomes incapacitated. Any such surrogate makes decisions only if the patient has become incapable of making decisions. The surrogate who holds durable power of attorney takes precedence over the next of kin.

The *best interest standard* or the *principle of beneficence* guides physicians and other team members in the process of making a medical decision for an incapacitated patient on the basis of the benefits and burdens an intervention poses to that person. When there is no expressed wish by the patient and no one to offer substituted judgment, then the surrogate decision maker will need to weigh the benefits and the burdens of treatment for that person in order to make a decision. Such analysis is best done by someone who is very aware of what gives that patient pleasure, what causes agitation, fear, pain, or discomfort, and how he or she reacts to a change in setting, use of restraints, and similar matters.

Conservatorships and Living Wills

In the absence of next of kin or durable power of attorney for a patient lacking decisional capacity, a conservator may be appointed by the court. There are usually two types of conservatorship: conservator of finance (*guardian* in some states) and conservator of person. Incompetence in matters of finance is usually determined either by the demonstrated incapacity of the patient to manage financial matters (eg, unpaid bills, uncashed checks) or through specific testing. A conservator of person is required when the patient has demonstrated an inability to make personal decisions (such as medical decisions) or an inability to care for himself or herself to the point of personal endangerment without the ability to understand and accept the need for help (self-neglect, safety).

Living wills are advance directives that attempt to demonstrate what decisions a person would make under certain circumstances. Most living wills address a couple of hypothetical clinical situations (eg, vegetative state, terminal illness) and four possible treatment options (cardiopulmonary resuscitation, respirator therapy, artificial food and hydration, and dialysis). Living wills have limited utility because of their vagueness and lack of generalizability to the types of decisions that most commonly need to be made. Nonetheless, living wills address hypothetical situations that might occur in the future and are not the same as decisions that are to be used to guide treatment at the present time. Some living wills offer a detailed set of hypothetical case scenarios and treatment decisions, but these can be difficult for patients to understand and may not expand on the rationale for decisions. A living will can be used as evidence of preferences as one is trying to construct how a patient who lacks decisional capacity might have felt about an intervention.

The Role of the Incapacitated Patient in Decision Making

Even when patients may not be fully capable of making decisions, often they can still participate in the decision making at many levels. A task assessment of decision-making ability around a specific issue is always appropriate. A patient with even a very low level of cognitive ability can give some indication when something causes discomfort or displeasure and when something brings pleasure. These indications of preferences need to be considered along with the analysis by the surrogate decision maker of the benefits and burdens of the intervention. Case law supports the idea that the patient's indications of preference should be given consideration.

The perceived relative burden of an intervention may vary from one person to the next because of differences in mental status and ability to cope with change or disability. A demented patient who is used to one environment will have a much harder time adjusting to hospitalization and may need restraints in order to undergo even something as simple as intravenous antibiotic therapy. The relative benefit of this therapy should be weighed against the increased burden of hospitalization for such a patient.

It is nearly impossible to perform some interventions without the cooperation of the patient. If the conservator recommends a cataract operation but the patient refuses, it is doubtful that the procedure could be performed. In other situations it may be hard to justify doing major invasive procedures against the will of an alert and mildly to moderately impaired person, even though it could be done. An example is a patient with frontal lobe dementia who is adamantly refusing cardiac surgery. A surrogate decision maker must take the present status of the patient and his or her wishes, concerns, pleasures, and pains into consideration when making any decision. Even though a person may not be capable of consenting to (or refusing) a treatment, his or her assent may be needed in order to carry out that treatment.

Legal and Ethical Issues **21**

Temporary Loss of Decisional Capacity

In acute confusional states, acute psychotic episodes, periods of unconsciousness from anesthesia or illness, or during an acute central nervous system event, patients may temporarily lose the ability to make decisions, but there is an expectation that they will regain this ability over time. When this is the case, the rules described above still apply. Decisions that the patient has made before becoming temporarily incapacitated should be upheld. A patient may reverse his or her do-not-resuscitate status while undergoing anesthesia with the understanding that it can be reinstated postoperatively. A patient who has stated that he would never agree to resuscitation should not have this reversed by a family member during a temporary confusional state due to an intercurrent illness.

When using either substituted judgment or best interest standards in surrogate decision making for a patient with a transient loss of decisional capacity, the decision maker should err on the side of more aggressive intervention if there are situations where the patient's wishes are not known or the circumstances are substantively different from what had been anticipated.

Informed Consent for Research

With the new emphasis being given to the quality of consent obtained for participants in research, it is imperative that the issues for the vulnerable populations of older adults be clarified and addressed. It is also imperative that research is done on dementia and related problems so that the care of these patients may improve. The two most vulnerable populations are those with cognitive impairment, by virtue of their inability to understand the study or their role in the study, and institutionalized patients who may feel a sense of coercion in the informed consent process. Research involving vulnerable populations needs to be particularly well designed and focused on issues of importance to that population.

Guidelines developed by the American Geriatrics Society for informed consent for research on cognitively impaired persons are shown in Table 4.1.

SPECIAL ETHICAL ISSUES IN DEMENTIA

Although most of the topics discussed above intimately involve the ethics of caring for cognitively impaired persons, some areas of particular concern for this population merit further discussion.

Table 4.1—AGS Guidelines for Research Using Cognitively Impaired Persons as Subjects

- The research must be justified on scientific, clinical, and ethical grounds but can be focused on conditions other than dementia itself.

- The capacity to give consent should be assessed for each individual for each research protocol since decision-making capacity is task specific and some cognitively impaired individuals will be able to give consent.

- Advance consent to participate in research given prior to the loss of decisional capacity should, in general, be respected.

- The traditional surrogates for decision making can be used to obtain consent.

- Research protocols that involve more than minimal risk or do not have a likelihood of direct benefit for the subjects should be offered only to persons who are able to consent or who have an advance directive consenting to participate in research. Exceptions might be made for exceptionally promising treatments, but this should be reviewed at a national level.

- Surrogates can refuse participation or withdraw the person from participation if the surrogate determines that the research protocol is not what the person intended to consent to or is not in the person's best interest, even if there is advance consent.

- Only in very unusual circumstances would the refusal to participate of even an incapacitated patient be overridden.

NOTE: AGS = American Geriatrics Society.
SOURCE: Data from AGS Ethics Committee. Informed consent for research on human subjects with dementia. *J Am Geriatr Soc.* 1998;46(10):1308–1310.

Truth-Telling

The ethics of truth-telling has evolved considerably through the last half of the 20th century, breaking tradition with thousands of years of paternalism in medicine that advocated withholding bad news from patients in order to do no harm. Telling a patient that he or she has a dementing illness may be the last area of controversy about truth-telling. Increasingly, today, in the United States, both professional and lay people agree that patients with dementia should be given a chance to understand what is happening to them. The opportunity for the older person with dementia to prepare legal documents (powers of attorney, a will, advance directives), to address personal issues, and to make plans is important. As therapies become available and research advances, it is imperative that persons with dementia be informed of their options and given the opportunity to voice, if not fully informed consent, at least their preferences.

Autonomy Versus Protectionism

Personal safety and avoiding harm to others are important concerns in caring for patients with dementia. They may not perceive the changes that have occurred to them and therefore would be unable to recognize their problem. Some patients with dementia may not understand the consequences of their actions and may have difficulty planning. This puts them at risk for behaviors that may endanger themselves or others, including unsafe driving, the continued possession of firearms, wandering, and inappropriate behaviors. Their care needs may exceed what their caregivers can provide, and they may be unable to understand the need for help at home, for a sitter, day care, or nursing-home care. The clinician plays a crucial role in being able to objectively recognize when this has happened and to help the family or other officials take the necessary steps to protect the patient and others.

Definition of Personhood and Advance Directives

Adults with intact decisional capacity not only have the right to make their own decisions but always have the right to change their minds. Even when they become unconscious, their last competent statement was usually made close to the event, often with full knowledge of the event; the likelihood that their rationale for the decision or that their goals, fears, and pleasures had changed significantly is low. If life experiences do mold their thinking or new interventions or approaches to problems occur, they can alter their directive to fit with these changes. A person with a slowly progressive cognitive disorder can change substantially over time. What brings pleasure and what causes fear or pain can be substantially different from year to year; almost certainly perceptions become greatly altered as the disease progresses. The demented person is unable to comprehend the future and slowly becomes more and more disconnected from the past. In some ways, the person with advancing dementia becomes suspended in time, and the connectedness to previous and future selves, the essence of what many define as personhood, fades. The demented person is tied to the decisions and perceptions of previous selves whom he or she may not even remember as the "self." The decisions made by this prior "self" may inform current decision making, even though that person did not know what he or she would need or want at this time. Therefore, there can arise a conflict between what is in the best interest of the demented patient in the here-and-now and the previous directives made by that person.

Genetic Testing and Alzheimer's Disease

Relatives of persons with Alzheimer's disease are increasingly interested in knowing their risk of having the disease. For relatives of those who have a clear autosomal dominant, known single-gene mutation, as is the case with Huntington's chorea, genetic testing has been shown to be useful when it is handled with the appropriate safeguards of counseling and follow-up. In familial early-onset Alzheimer's disease, several gene mutations have been found that cause clusters of Alzheimer's disease in families. For those clusters where the mutation is known, mapping and phenotyping may be helpful in conjunction with counseling. For most familial clusters, the gene has not been identified, and testing is not useful.

In the case of apolipoprotein E alleles that may influence a person's susceptibility or probability of having Alzheimer's disease sometime in the future, the role of testing and counseling is less certain. Many persons with the high-risk alleles do not get the disease, and many without it do get the disease. As long as there is no intervention that has been shown to significantly alter the course of the dementing process, it does not seem advisable to create anxiety when the predictive value of the test is so low. (See also "Dementia," p 113.)

ETHICS IN THE NURSING-HOME SETTING

Although the ethics that apply to the treatment of patients in other settings apply to patients in the nursing home, there are some issues that are brought more acutely into focus because of the setting and the concentration of patients with chronic and end-stage disease.

Treatment Decisions

Prior to the present attention focused on the resuscitation status of patients in nursing homes, residents were assumed not to be candidates for attempted resuscitation, and it was rarely, if ever, attempted. Studies that have looked at the outcomes of attempted resuscitation of patients in institutional long-term-care settings show it to be used infrequently and associated with low long-term survival. On the other hand, the number of patients in long-term-care settings for short-term recuperation and rehabilitation has grown, which may change the statistics concerning the utility of resuscitation in the nursing-home population.

Staff perceptions of the utility of resuscitation efforts differ by profession. Nursing staff have a strong preference for limiting interventions in this setting, especially for older patients and those with cognitive impairments. On the other hand, physicians tend to overestimate the benefit of interventions in this population and are sometimes hesitant to honor a do-not-resuscitate request for patients who are not clearly terminally ill. Patient participation in the process is variable. Federal legislation requires the systematic inquiry into advance directives for all patients in institutions receiving federal funds. With this more systematic approach to discussions about treatment status, there has been a decrease in the number of transfers to an acute-care setting and in the overall utilization of resources without a negative change in patient or family satisfaction.

The use of enteral feeding for patients in the nursing home has been encouraged by regulatory agencies to prevent nutritional deficits in patients who may be failing to take in adequate food by mouth. Although the motives for enacting these regulations were compassionate, enteral feeding, especially for patients with advanced dementia, is of questionable utility. Also, it is not ethical to use enteral feedings for patients capable of taking oral sustenance but who may not be getting enough nutrition because of their need for assistance in feeding. (See "Malnutrition," p 182.)

Restraints

The use of restraints in the long-term-care setting has become closely regulated and monitored. The use of physical restraints has been shown to be of limited, if any, value in preventing injuries from falls. Less restrictive alternatives are usually available. In decisions about the use of restraints, several factors must be examined. The risks and benefits of their use needs to be weighed by the patient's surrogate. If the patient is engaging in activities that are unsafe for other residents or staff, then the institution has a responsibility to protect others and may need to consider transferring the patient to another environment if intervention is not effective or is refused by the patient's surrogate.

Conflicts of Interest

The allocation of resources in nursing homes is closely linked to the ability of nursing-home care to prevent complications of chronic illness. Pressure sores, functional decline, depression, agitation, and the need for restraints may all be increased when staffing is decreased below a critical level. Appropriate activities to meet the patient's physical, cognitive, and emotional needs, is also part of the care of these patients.

MISCELLANEOUS ISSUES

Ethics and Health Care Financing

The ethical issues regarding the financing of health care have become much more salient in an era of rapidly rising costs and managed care. Health care professionals need to be aware of the forces, both positive and negative, exerted by payment structures on the nature of the care delivered. Ideally, providers, aware of these forces, would take maximum advantage of the positive forces and work to guard against the negative forces when caring for patients. The two major care payment structures to health care providers, fee-for-service and capitation, exert varying influences on care.

Fee-For-Service Structures

Fee-for-service (FFS) care means that the provider receives payment for each service rendered. The built-in advantage of an FFS method is that providers have an incentive of thoroughness in the diagnosis and treatment of patients; the more services a clinician provides (and documents), the more he or she is compensated financially. Patients receiving FFS care may be more reassured that everything possible is being done to care for them. The potential disadvantage of FFS care is overtreatment of patients, resulting in unnecessary iatrogenic morbidity and mortality as well as increased costs. Clinicians receiving FFS have an ethical obligation not to overtreat their patients.

About 85% of older adults receive care from "traditional" Medicare, a system that compensates nurse practitioners and physicians under an FFS arrangement (see "Financing, Coverage, and Costs of Health Care," p 26). Medicare FFS providers have relative incentives to provide covered benefits and disincentives to perform noncovered services. The primary method of controlling overall costs in an FFS system is to carefully delineate which services are covered and to discount payments for those services. Medicare discounts payments for covered services documented under the Current Procedural Terminology coding system.

Capitation Structures

Capitation means prepayment for the care of a patient population, on the basis of the number of patients in the population, regardless of the amount of care delivered. Capitation arrangements provide incentives for the prevention of serious (and costly) conditions, commonly through the use of disease management programs, health promotion efforts, and care management. Capitated care has been said to be proactive, whereas FFS has been characterized as reactive. The chief concern regarding capitation is an inherent underservice bias; the less that is spent on the patient, the more the provider or plan may profit. Providers receiving capitation, or any other incentive to restrict costs, have an ethical obligation not to undertreat their patients.

Under the Medicare Plus Choice option, which is selected by about 15% of Medicare beneficiaries, health plans (not individual providers) receive capitation from the Health Care Financing Administration (in June 2001 renamed the Centers for Medicare & Medicaid Services) on the basis of the number of enrollees (see "Financing, Coverage, and Costs of Health Care," p 26). Medicare Plus Choice plans then either provide capitation payments to providers (thereby passing on the financial risk) or pay their providers on a discounted FFS basis.

Driving

Older persons with physical and cognitive impairments have as high a risk of motor vehicle collisions per mile driven as do teen-age drivers. Clinicians face complex ethical problems when caring for older patients who endanger themselves and others by driving. The conflicting values are powerful: respect for the patient's autonomy, duty to protect the patient from harm, duty to protect others from predictable danger, and respect for patient confidentiality. Educating the patient and family members is often the key to developing a practical solution. Legal requirements vary from state to state regarding clinician reporting of unsafe older drivers. In some states, clinicians are required to report patients who may be unsafe; in other states they are permitted to do so; and in a few states, reporting may be considered a violation of patient confidentiality. (See also the section on the older driver in "Assessment," p 47.)

REFERENCES

■ AGS Ethics Committee. Informed consent for research on human subjects with dementia. *J Am Geriatr Soc.* 1998; 46(10):1308–1310.

■ Ethics and Alzheimer's Disease. *J Clin Ethics.* 1998(spring);9:1–96.

■ Mezey M, Teresi J, Ramsey G, et al. Decision-making capacity to execute a health care proxy: development and testing of guidelines. *J Am Geriatr Soc.* 2000;48(2):179–187.

■ Post SG, Whitehouse PJ. Fairhill guidelines on ethics of the care of people with Alzheimer's disease: a clinical summary: Center of Biomedical Ethics, Case Western Reserve University, and the Alzheimer's Association. *J Am Geriatr Soc.* 1995; 43 (12):1423–1429.

■ Post SG, Whitehouse PJ, Binstock, RH, et al. The clinical introduction of genetic testing for Alzheimer disease: an ethical perspective. *JAMA.* 1997;277(10):832–836.

■ Quill TE, Lee BC, Nunn S. Palliative treatments of the last resort: choosing the least harmful alternative. *Ann Int Med.* 2000;132(6):488–493.

■ Resnick B, Andrews C. End-of-life treatment preferences among older adults: a nurse practitioner initiated intervention. *J Am Acad Nurse Pract.* 2002;14(11)517–522.

■ The Hastings Center. *Guidelines for the Termination of Life-Sustaining Treatment and the Care of the Dying.* Bloomington: Indiana University Press; 1987.

CHAPTER 5—FINANCING, COVERAGE, AND COSTS OF HEALTH CARE

In 1965 the U.S. government passed legislation designed to improve access to acute health care for people who are old, disabled, or poor. During the decades that followed, the resulting Medicare and Medicaid programs expanded, evolved, and spawned thousands of supplemental commercial insurance plans. Today a complex and often confusing array of personal payments, public programs, and private insurance plans (see Figure 5.1) pays for and thereby determines much of the health care that older Americans receive.

This chapter describes, through the eyes of patients and providers, how these programs influence the day-to-day care of older people. It illustrates their effects during a year in the life of Mrs. Rose Murat, an imaginary 79-year-old retired schoolteacher who lives with her 83-year-old husband in a small older home. Mrs. Murat has hypertension, coronary artery disease, and mild congestive heart failure, for which she takes hydrochlorothiazide, diltiazem, lisinopril, and nitroglycerine. Her total out-of-pocket payments for prescription medications are $95.27 per month.

OUTPATIENT CARE

At the end of her quarterly office visit, Mrs. Murat asks for advice on joining a health maintenance organization (HMO) that has been marketing a Medicare health plan in her county. She is impressed by the HMO's offer of free eyeglasses, hearing aids, and preventive check-ups, all of which she has purchased out of pocket in the past. Her options, summarized in Table 5.1, include: staying with traditional fee-for-service (FFS) Medicare as her only coverage; keeping FFS Medicare and applying for either Medicaid or supplemental ("medigap") coverage; or exchanging her FFS Medicare coverage for membership in the Medicare HMO. Depending on the Murats' income, savings, and state of residence, they may also qualify for a Medicare assistance program that pays for some combination of their Medicare premiums, deductibles, and co-insurance costs. Some older Americans may have additional health insurance options through Veterans Affairs or through their (or their spouses') present or previous employer or union.

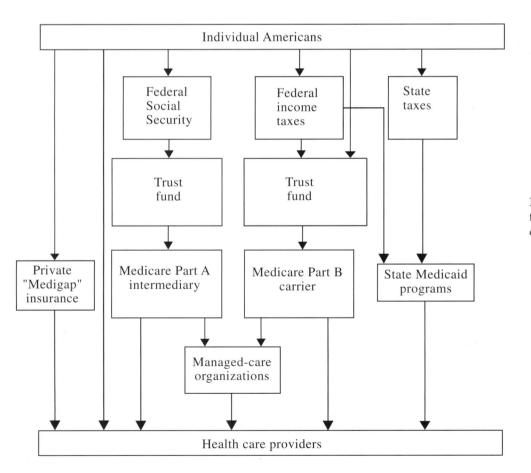

Figure 5.1—The flow of funds for the health care for older Americans.

Table 5.1—Health Insurance Coverage for Older Americans

| | FFS Medicare | | Supplemental Coverage | | Medicare HMO Plan [a] |
	Part A	Part B	Medicaid	Medigap Policy	
Covers the cost of:					
Hospitals	100% [b]	-	$776	$776	100%
Postacute care in SNF	100% [c]	-	-	-	100%
Hospice	100% [d]	-	-	-	-
Home	100%	-	-	-	100%
Durable medical equipment	80%	80% [e]	20%	20%	100%
Diagnostic tests	-	100%	-	-	100%
Physicians, nurse practitioners	-	80%	20%	20%	100%
Outpatient PT, OT, ST	-	80%	20%	20%	100%
Outpatient services, supplies	-	80%	20%	20%	100%
Emergency care	-	80%	20%	20%	100%
Ambulance services	-	80%	20%	20%	100%
Preventive services	-	[f]	20%	20%	[f, g]
Outpatient mental health care	-	50%	50%	50%	100%
Custodial care in nursing home	-	-	100%	-	-
Hearing, vision services	-	-	[h]	[h]	[h]
Outpatient medications	-	-	[h]	[h]	[h]
Additional costs to patient:					
Deductibles	$792.00 [i]	$100.00 [j]	-	[h]	[h]
Monthly premiums	-	$50.00	-	[h]	[h]

NOTE: FFS = fee for service; HMO = health maintenance organization; OT = occupational therapy; PT = physical therapy; SNF = skilled nursing facility; ST = speech therapy.

a Some Medicare Plus Choice plans require members to pay deductibles and copayments.

b After the beneficiary or secondary insurer pays the deductible amount ($792.00)

c For the first 20 days of SNF care following a hospital stay of at least 3 days.

d Patient makes copayments of $5.00 per outpatient prescription and 5% of cost of respite care.

e When patient is receiving Medicare-covered home care.

f 100% of allowed cost of fecal occult blood test, Pap smear interpretation, prostate-specific antigen test, influenza and pneumococcal vaccinations; 80% of allowed cost of mammograms and clinical examination of breast and pelvis (no deductible applies); after the annual Part B deductible has been paid, 80% of allowed cost of sigmoidoscopy or colonoscopy or barium enema, digital examination of rectum (men), measurement of bone mass, hepatitis B vaccination, and diabetic education and equipment.

g Some Medicare Plus Choice plans cover additional preventive services.

h Benefits and costs vary widely among medigap insurance plans and state Medicaid plans.

i Per benefit period (90 days following hospital admission).

j Annual.

Medicare is a federal insurance program run by the Centers for Medicare & Medicaid Services (CMS; formerly, the Health Care Financing Administration, or HCFA) that pays health professionals and organizations to provide acute health care for Americans who are 65 and older, disabled, or suffering from end-stage renal disease. As originally enacted, Medicare comprises two separate FFS plans (Part A and Part B), each of which pays predetermined amounts for specified health-related goods and services that are needed by its beneficiaries. More than 80% of older Americans are covered by these plans.

Medicare Part A uses regional insurance companies ("intermediaries") to pay hospitals, nursing homes, home-care agencies, and hospice programs for the Medicare-covered services they provide. Older Americans (and their spouses) who have had Medicare taxes deducted from their paychecks for at least 10 years are entitled to coverage through Part A without paying premiums. Others may be able to purchase Part A coverage.

Medicare Part B uses other regional insurance companies ("carriers") to pay physicians, nurse practitioners, social workers, psychologists, rehabilitation therapists, home-care agencies, ambulances, outpatient facilities, and suppliers of durable medical equipment for the Medicare-covered goods and services they provide. At age 65, people become eligible for Part B coverage if they are entitled to Part A coverage or if they are citizens or permanent residents of the United States. To obtain this coverage, eligible persons must enroll in Part B and pay premiums ($50.00 per month), usually by agreeing to have them deducted from their monthly Social Security checks.

Providers must choose whether to participate in the FFS Medicare program. For each Medicare-covered service performed, a participating provider will submit a claim to the Part B carrier, accept Medicare's fee for the service (80% of its preestablished "allowed" amount), and bill the patient or her secondary insurer for no more than a 20% co-insurance payment. For services not covered by Medicare, the provider may bill the patient, if the patient agrees in advance in writing. Providers who do not participate in Medicare can bill patients directly for up to 15% more than Medicare's allowed fees. The patients pay the providers and then submit their requests to Medicare for partial reimbursement.

Neither Part A nor Part B of the Medicare program covers outpatient medications, dental care, hearing aids, eyeglasses, foot care, orthopedic shoes, cosmetic surgery, care in foreign countries, or long-term custodial care in nursing homes. Few preventive services other than mammography, Pap smear, immunization, and bone mineral density testing are covered by FFS Medicare. Beneficiaries pay out of pocket for:

- monthly premiums for Part B ($50.00)
- annual deductible for Part B ($100.00)
- the deductible for Part A ($792.00 per benefit period, ie, the 90 days following an admission)
- co-insurance payments (usually 20%) for goods and services for which Medicare or other insurance pays only a portion, and
- the full cost of those goods and services that are not covered by Medicare or other insurance.

Medicaid is a joint federal and state program that provides supplemental health insurance to people of all ages who have low incomes and limited savings. The exact criteria for Medicaid eligibility and the benefit packages provided by Medicaid programs vary considerably from state to state. Most programs pay Medicare Part B premiums, and many pay Medicare deductibles and co-insurance costs. Most important, Medicaid pays for long-term care in nursing homes for those who qualify. Several states have begun offering fixed capitation payments to managed-care organizations that are willing to provide Medicaid and Medicare benefits to residents who are "dually eligible" (for Medicaid and Medicare).

Medigap supplemental plans fill some of the holes in the insurance coverage provided by Medicare Part A and Part B. Private insurance companies offer FFS medigap plans of ten types (A through J), classified according to the benefits they cover. For new Medicare beneficiaries at age 65, the premiums for A-level (basic) plans across the United States range from $40 to $125 per month. These policies cover a person's Part A and Part B co-insurance costs, for example, 20% of Medicare's allowed fees for durable medical equipment and physicians' services, respectively. (In Minnesota, Wisconsin, and Massachusetts, even A-level medigap policies are required by law to cover more than just the costs of Medicare Part B co-insurance.) B-level plans cover Part A and Part B co-insurance plus Part A deductibles ($792 per benefit period). Each successive level of medigap policy provides additional benefits and costs more. J-level plans cover co-insurance, deductibles, care in foreign countries, preventive services, and some of the cost of medications—at a cost of $175 to $400 per month. Consumers can obtain less expensive medigap coverage by purchasing plans that require the insured to pay high deductibles (F- and J-level plans only) or plans that cover the services of only selected physicians and hospitals ("Medicare SELECT" policies). Medigap policies do not cover long-term care, dental care, eyeglasses, hearing aids, or private-duty nursing.

Within 6 months of their initial enrollment in Medicare Part B, beneficiaries are entitled to purchase any medigap policy on the market at advertised prices. After this open enrollment period, medigap insurers can refuse to insure individual beneficiaries or charge them higher premiums because of their past or present health problems.

Medicare HMOs hold contracts with CMS specifying that, for each Medicare beneficiary they enroll, they will provide at least the standard Medicare benefits in return for fixed monthly capitation payments. In order to attract enrollees, most Medicare HMOs also cover additional benefits and charge low or no premiums, deductibles, and copayments. The HMOs achieve cost savings by managing their enrollees' use of services within their networks of providers, with whom they negotiate price discounts in return for patient volume. Each January the HMOs have the option of changing their premiums, benefits, and provider networks—or of discontinuing their Medicare plans altogether.

Each November, beneficiaries covered by Medicare Part A and Part B have the option of joining any Medicare HMO operating in their area; they cannot be denied enrollment because of any health problems except end-stage renal disease. Enrollees must continue to pay their monthly Medicare Part B premiums, and they must obtain their health care from the HMO's provider network. They have the option of leaving the HMO at any time and going back to the FFS Medicare program. The frequency at which beneficiaries may switch managed-care plans is becoming progressively more restricted.

The primary advantages and disadvantages of each of Mrs. Murat's options are outlined in Table 5.2. Additional information about all the options is available at each state's medical assistance office, at 1-800-MEDICARE (1-800-633-4227), and at http://www.medicare.gov.

Table 5.2—Advantages and Disadvantages of Four Types of Health Insurance

Type of Insurance	Primary Advantages	Primary Disadvantages
FFS Medicare (Part A and Part B)	Traditional Medicare benefits, choice of any provider that participates in the Medicare program	Cost of co-insurance, deductibles, noncovered goods and services (eg, eyeglasses, hearing aids, medications)
Medicaid	Coverage of co-insurance, deductibles, and some benefits* not covered by Medicare	Choice of providers restricted to a single network in some states
Medigap insurance	Coverage of co-insurance, deductibles, and some benefits** not covered by Medicare	Out-of-pocket monthly premiums range from $40 to $400, depending on the coverage provided by the policy purchased
Medicare Plus Choice plan (eg, HMO)	Traditional Medicare benefits plus coverage of additional goods and services**	Choice of providers restricted to a single network; potential for changes in premiums, copayments, deductibles, benefits, and providers at the discretion of the plan

NOTE: FFS = fee-for-service; HMO = health maintenance organization.

* Benefits vary from state to state.

** Benefits vary from plan to plan.

Managed Care

Mrs. Murat's provider of primary care, knowledgeable about her health and prognosis, can help her to choose the plan(s) that will cover the goods and services that she needs, both now and in the future. If she can obtain what she is likely to need from the HMO's network of providers, joining the HMO might be her best option, because it will allow her to obtain "free" eyeglasses, hearing aids, and preventive services and to avoid paying the usual Medicare premiums, deductibles, and co-insurance. Data about the quality of care or the satisfaction of other enrollees in the HMO are available at the CMS Web site, http://www.medicare.gov.

In the event that she needs health care that is not available from the HMO's network, or if she is reluctant to change providers, retaining the flexibility of her traditional Medicare coverage (which covers her use of any provider that participates in the Medicare program) might be a better choice, especially if she also qualifies for Medicaid or buys a medigap policy. Information from Medicare's information line or from http://www.medicare.gov/MGCompare would help her compare the prices and coverage of the medigap policies available in her area.

The health care provider's recommendations to Mrs. Murat are likely to be influenced by the economic realities of the different plans she is considering. For instance, if the provider is not in the HMO's service network, her enrollment in the HMO would require her to select a new primary care provider. If the provider does participate in the HMO's network, Mrs. Murat's enrollment would change the payment for her care. As shown in Table 5.3, the payments would depend on the type of HMO involved. If it is a group or independent practice association (IPA) model, the HMO may pay providers "discounted FFS," that is, less than Medicare Part B would pay for each service. Or it may pay primary providers a fixed capitation amount each month to cover specified services. If these services are limited to primary ambulatory care, the capitation amount will be relatively small. The HMO may reward primary providers with end-of-the-year bonus payments if they have limited their referrals to specialists and their admissions to hospitals. If the covered services also include specialty and inpatient care, the capitation amounts will be considerably larger, and the provider will have incentives to use these services judiciously because he or she will have to pay for them, at least in part.

Fee for Service

Under the Medicare FFS system, providers obtain the fairest possible reimbursement by understanding and following MCS's payment system, which is based on evaluation and management (E&M) codes (see Table 5.4).

For each Medicare-covered service provided, the provider submits to the regional Medicare carrier the appropriate E&M code and the international classification of disease (ICD) code that indicates the diagnosis for which the service was provided. Entries in the medical record, which are subject to audit, must document that the data collection and medical decision-making aspects of the service conform to standards established for the E&M code submitted. By providing and documenting services efficiently, providers can maximize their FFS reimbursements within the (tight) limits imposed by the Medicare fee schedules.

Regardless of the payment mechanism, the crucial question is whether the amount of payment suffices to

Table 5.3—How Medicare HMOs Pay Providers of Health Care

	Type of HMO		
	Staff Model	Group Model	IPA Model
Providers are:	Employees	One large group practice	Many small independent practices
Method of payments:	Salary	FFS or capitation*	FFS or capitation*

NOTE: FFS = fee for service; HMO = health maintenance organization; IPA = independent practice association.

* The services covered by the capitation payments range from "primary care only" in some plans to "medications and all acute care" in others.

Table 5.4—Fee-for-Service Reimbursement by Medicare, Year 2000

E&M Service	E&M code	"Allowed" Amount ($)*	80%	CMS Payment ($)**
Comprehensive office visit, new patient	99205	154.67	× 0.80 =	123.74
Intermediate office visit, established patient	99213	45.88	× 0.80 =	36.70
Intermediate office visit (mental health problem), established patient	99213	45.88	× 0.50 =	22.94
Comprehensive emergency department visit	99285	149.03	× 0.80 =	119.22
Comprehensive hospital consultation	99255	189.83	× 0.80 =	151.86
Comprehensive nursing-home visit	99313	69.70	× 0.80 =	55.76
Complex hospital admission	99223	150.32	× 0.80 =	120.26
Complex hospital visit	99233	76.50	× 0.80 =	61.20
Complex hospital discharge	99239	85.02	× 0.80 =	68.02
House call, established patient	99349	103.83	× 0.80 =	83.06
Care plan oversight (CPO)	99375	96.69	× 0.80 =	77.35

NOTE: CMS = Centers for Medicare & Medicaid Services; E&M = evaluation and management.

* For physicians who participate in Medicare; amounts vary by state.

** For eligible services provided by nurse practitioners, payment is 85% of the amount shown.

support high-quality care. If capitation rates are below the aggregate cost of the services they are intended to cover, the provider will feel pressure to take on more patients and limit the amount of service that each patient receives. Similarly, if FFS amounts are too small, the provider will feel pressure to schedule more visits and procedures and to reduce the time devoted to each patient. Each provider should, therefore, monitor carefully and continuously the many changing elements in the practice environment (eg, payment schedules, covered services, expenses, patients' and families' expectations, population demographics) to help determine the numbers and types of services that are appropriate for each older patient.

INPATIENT CARE

Four months later, Mrs. Murat awakes dysarthric and unable to feel her left hand. Her face is asymmetric, and her left arm and left leg are weak. Her husband calls 911; the ambulance rushes her to the nearest emergency department, where the physician on duty diagnoses a right hemispheric stroke and admits her to the hospital.

Managed Care

If Mrs. Murat had joined the Medicare HMO, the HMO would pay for the ambulance, emergency, and physician services; in most cases, it would pay the hospital a prenegotiated lump sum or a per diem fee to cover all of her inpatient care. The amount of this lump sum would be determined by the diagnosis-related group (DRG) of her admitting diagnosis, in this case stroke. If the admitting hospital had no contract with her HMO, Mrs. Murat would probably be transferred to a hospital in the HMO's provider network as soon as she was medically stable. Depending on the HMO's benefit package, she might be responsible for copayments and deductibles for some of these services.

Fee for Service

If Mrs. Murat had retained traditional Medicare as her only health insurance, she would have to pay Medicare's required deductibles ($100 per year under Part B for the ambulance and the emergency medical care, plus $792 under Part A for the hospital admission) and co-insurance amounts (20% of Medicare's allowed charges by physicians and the ambulance service). She would also have to pay any ambulance charges in excess of Medicare's approved fee. If she had supplemented her Medicare coverage, her Medicaid or private medigap coverage would cover some of these deductibles and co-insurance payments. She would not be transferred to another hospital for insurance reasons.

The hospital would submit its claim for emergency and inpatient care, which would be based on the DRG of her admitting diagnosis, to Medicare's regional intermediary insurance company. The involved physicians and the ambulance service would submit their E&M coded claims to Medicare's regional insurance carrier. The intermediary and the carrier would pay their shares of these costs and, if Mrs. Murat had supplemental coverage, they would forward requests for payment of the balances to the state Medicaid program or her medigap insurance company. Ultimately, CMS would reimburse the intermediary from the Medicare Part A Trust Fund and the carrier from the Medicare Part B Trust Fund.

POSTACUTE REHABILITATION

After 4 days of stabilization, evaluation, and rehabilitation, Mrs. Murat is deemed stable enough for discharge from the acute-care hospital. She has improved somewhat, but she is still mildly hemiparetic and dysarthric, and she is apathetic and easily fatigued. Because her days in the hospital are fewer than the average number of hospital days associated with the DRG of her admitting diagnosis, ie, 4.9 days, and because her admitting diagnosis is one of those listed in Table 5.5, CMS regards her "early" discharge as a "transfer." This permits CMS to reduce the amount it pays the hospital for her care. The consulting neurologist advises her and her husband that her progress

Table 5.5—Primary Admitting Diagnoses for Which "Early" Discharges From Hospitals are Regarded as "Transfers" to Postacute Care Facilities

Primary Admitting Diagnosis	DRG Number	Average Number of Days in Hospital for People with this DRG
Stroke	14	4.9
Amputation of lower extremity	113	9.8
Hip replacement	209	4.9
Other hip or femur procedures with complications	210	6.1
Other hip or femur procedures without complications	211	4.7
Fracture of hip or pelvis (no surgery)	236	4.1
Skin graft with complications	263	8.8
Skin graft without complications	264	5.4
Organic disturbances	429	5.2
Tracheostomy	483	33.9

NOTE: DRG = diagnosis-related group.

during the next few weeks will determine her potential for functional recovery. Mr. Murat asks the neurologist to recommend a rehabilitation facility for his wife.

Managed Care

If she had joined the Medicare HMO, Mrs. Murat's insurance coverage would include postacute rehabilitative care, probably at a nursing home in the HMO's provider network rather than at a rehabilitation facility. Some nursing homes concentrate such high-acuity patients in transitional (or postacute) care units and provide them with coordinated rehabilitative (physical, occupational, and speech), social, and nursing services. Most homes, lacking such units, offer only custodial care supplemented by rehabilitative services as needed. The HMO would also cover the physician's postacute services, but the Murats may be responsible for a deductible and copayments.

Fee for Service

If Mrs. Murat could tolerate 3 hours of therapy per day, Medicare Part A would pay for 20 days of postacute rehabilitation, in either a rehabilitation facility or a transitional (postacute) care unit of a nursing home. Upon her admission to either type of postacute care unit, rehabilitation professionals would evaluate Mrs. Murat's functional status, establish a plan for her care, and certify her as needing one of 26 levels of intensity of care according to the resource utilization group system (RUGS). Her RUGS category would determine the daily rate that Medicare Part A would pay the facility for the first 2 weeks of her care as long as she was demonstrating progress in rehabilitation. After 2 weeks, a nurse would reevaluate her status, update her plan of care, and adjust her RUGS category and thereby adjust Medicare's payments to the facility for the next 2 weeks. Under this prospective payment system (PPS), which CMS is introducing between 2000 and 2003, the facility would be responsible not only for Mrs. Murat's nursing, rehabilitative, and social services, but also for the costs of her medications, laboratory tests, and visits to an emergency department not resulting in admission to the hospital.

Using nursing-home rates, Medicare Part B would pay 80% of the allowed charges for the postacute medical care provided by her physician. Any postacute care related to an inpatient surgical procedure would be the responsibility of the surgeon, who would receive a "global fee" to cover the surgery and all postoperative surgical care. The Murats would need to satisfy Medicare Part B's $100 annual deductible and then make 20% co-insurance payments for the physician's care. Their out-of-pocket expenses would be reduced or eliminated by any Medicare supplements in effect, such as Medicaid, medigap, or long-term-care coverage.

More than 3 million Americans have long-term-care insurance policies, but these policies pay for less than 2% of all nursing-home care. The high premiums for these policies, combined with consumers' uncertainty about needing long-term care in the future and their doubts about the policies' ability to cover the costs of long-term care in the future, have limited the growth of the long-term-care insurance sector. Many middle-aged Americans believe they will retain good health and independence into old age; they appear to be relying on a combination of good fortune, social insurance (ie, Medicaid), and their personal assets to see them through their later years.

HOME-HEALTH CARE

During the first 10 days of rehabilitative therapy, Mrs. Murat regains her ability to speak, and her left arm becomes stronger. During the following 8 days, however, she makes few additional gains. After 18 days, she is still unable to walk, cook, bathe, or dress herself without help. Her lack of continued progress toward functional independence will probably make her ineligible for coverage of additional rehabilitative services in either the HMO or the FFS Medicare program. The Murats will have to purchase any future physical therapy or occupational therapy on their own.

To obtain long-term care for her functional deficits, they will need to choose between a home-health agency and a custodial nursing home. If she returns home, neither the HMO nor the FFS Medicare program will be likely to pay for a home-health aide unless she is homebound and requires the services of a registered nurse or rehabilitation therapist. Local community agencies, however, may be able to offer assistance.

Managed Care

If Mrs. Murat's condition made her homebound and dependent on skilled professional services, her HMO probably would pay a home-health agency a fixed fee to provide her with the services and equipment necessary to treat her primary diagnosis. The HMO would also provide her with the services of a primary care physician.

Fee for Service

In the FFS environment, if Mrs. Murat were homebound and dependent on skilled professional services, the traditional Medicare Part A would pay any Medicare-certified home-health agency a fixed fee to provide her with the services and equipment necessary to treat her primary diagnosis. Medicare Part B would pay her primary care physician 80% of the allowed charges for house calls and office visits. If her physician documents more than 30 minutes per month overseeing her care, Medicare Part B will pay an additional $100 per month for care plan oversight (CPO). The Murats would be responsible for the annual Part B annual deductible ($100) and the 20% co-insurance payments, unless they had supplemental coverage through Medicaid, a medigap policy, or a long-term-care policy. (See also "Community-Based Care," p 91.)

PACE

If a health care organization in the area had contracted with CMS and the state Medicaid agency to create a Program for All-inclusive Care of the Elderly (PACE), it could provide community-based long-term care for "dually eligibles" (people eligible for both Medicare and Medicaid) whose disabilities qualified them for custodial care in a nursing home. If she were eligible for Medicaid and she enrolled in PACE, Mrs. Murat would attend an adult day health care center several days each week and receive comprehensive outpatient, inpatient, acute, and long-term care from a salaried interdisciplinary team composed of a physician, a nurse, a social worker, and other members of the PACE staff.

NURSING-HOME CARE

Three months after Mrs. Murat returns home, Mr. Murat, now 84 years old, suffers a myocardial infarction and is no longer able to care for his wife at home. Their daughter logs on to http://www.medicare.gov to shop for a nursing home. After comparing the local facilities' nurse-to-resident ratios, results of recent quality-of-care inspections, and rates of pressure ulcers and behavior problems, she arranges for her mother to enter a high-quality nursing home in her neighborhood, at least until Mr. Murat recovers.

Managed Care

If Mrs. Murat had joined the Medicare HMO, one of the HMO's providers would provide her primary care in the nursing home. Unless she had arranged for supplemental coverage through Medicaid or a long-term-care policy, however, she and her husband would be responsible for the nursing home's per diem charges for room, board, and other basic services, usually about $100 per day. After "spending down" their savings at this rate, the Murats might become sufficiently impoverished to qualify, if they had not qualified previously, for the Medicaid program. If the Murats own their house, some states would put a lien on it in order to recover some of its payments to the nursing home when the house was eventually sold.

Fee for Service

The FFS Medicare program would pay 80% of the allowed charges submitted by her provider for visits to the nursing home. The Murats would be responsible for the annual Medicare Part B deductible ($100) and the 20% co-insurance payments. Medicare would not cover any of the nursing home's per diem charges.

HOSPICE CARE

After residing in the nursing home for 6 months, Mrs. Murat suffers a massive stroke that leaves her physiologically stable, but in a persistent vegetative state. Her husband reports that she had always said she would not want to go on living in such a condition if there were little hope of recovery. Although she is unable to swallow thin liquids, her husband says she would not want to be fed through any sort of tube. Her physician says that, with oral feeding, she is likely to live for several weeks. With the understanding that she will receive palliative care without life-prolonging interventions, her husband agrees to enroll her in a hospice program.

Enrollment in hospice would require the traditional FFS Medicare program (Part A) to pay a Medicare-certified hospice program a daily fee that would cover all care of her terminal diagnosis, including home care, medications, equipment, respite, counseling, and social services even if she had enrolled in (and remained in) the Medicare HMO.

If she had remained in the FFS Medicare program, Part B would pay her primary care provider, 80% of the allowed charges for home or office visits, plus about $100 per month for documented CPO in excess of 30 minutes per month. Mr. Murat would be responsible for the 20% co-insurance and for small copayments for outpatient prescription medications, respite care, and CPO.

CHANGES IN THE FEDERAL FINANCING OF HEALTH CARE

The complex and evolving combinations of coverage and programs create difficult choices for older Americans and powerful incentives for the providers of their health care. The U.S. Congress continues to revise the Medicare program.

The Balanced Budget Act of 1997

In 1997 Congress passed, and President Bill Clinton signed, the Balanced Budget Act (BBA 97) through which they intended to limit future growth in the cost of the Medicare program, improve the quality of the health care it provides, and expand the number and variety of managed-care plans from which Medicare beneficiaries could choose. It authorized five types of Medicare Plus Choice plans:

- Medicare HMOs (IPA, group, or staff model)—insurance companies that accept capitation payments from HCFA and provide or purchase Medicare-covered health services;

- Preferred provider organizations (PPOs)—alliances of providers that accept capitation payments and deliver Medicare-covered health services to their enrolled patients;

- Provider-sponsored organizations (PSOs) — partnerships of physician groups and hospitals that accept capitation payments and deliver Medicare-covered health services to their enrolled patients;

- Private FFS plans—plans that may charge beneficiaries a premium, pay providers more liberally than the original Medicare FFS plan does, and allow physicians to charge their patients copayments of up to 15%;

- Medical savings accounts (MSAs)—accounts into which Medicare beneficiaries can make tax-deductible contributions and out of which they can withdraw funds to purchase routine health-related goods (including medications) and services (including long-term-care insurance) from any Medicare provider. Linked to the MSA is a catastrophic insurance policy that limits the individual beneficiary's expenses for health care to $6000 per year.

Perhaps because of the risks and uncertainties involved, very few PPOs, PSOs, private FFS insurance companies, or MSA providers entered into Medicare Plus Choice contracts with HCFA. Citing inadequate capitation payments and burdensome administrative requirements, many HMOs have withdrawn from the Medicare market, constricted their service areas (eliminating many rural counties), reduced the scope of the benefits they cover, and increased the premiums, deductibles, and copayments for which their enrollees are responsible. The total number of Medicare beneficiaries enrolled in Medicare Plus Choice plans declined from 6.4 million (17%) in 1999 to 6.2 million (16%) in 2000. As a result, hundreds of thousands of older Americans have had to select new health plans and new health care providers.

Federal actuaries projected that BBA 97 would save the Medicare program $116 billion during 1998–2003 and extend the life of the Medicare Part A Trust Fund until 2023. The specific actions by which BBA 97 attempted to control costs include restricting Medicare benefits (eg, home care), reducing payments to providers (eg, hospitals and HMOs), and requiring HCFA to begin risk-adjusting the capitation rates at which it paid managed-care plans.

HCFA (now CMS) pays each managed-care plan a monthly county-specific capitation fee for each of its Medicare enrollees, an amount based on recent average adjusted per capita cost (AAPCC) for FFS Medicare beneficiaries in the county. The AAPCC amounts range from $401.61 per month in many rural counties to $814.32 per month in Richmond County, New York. Before BBA 97, the payment formulae adjusted these capitation amounts only for enrollees' age, sex, Medicaid enrollment status (yes or no), and living situation (nursing home or independent residence). BBA 97 required that HCFA also begin adjusting capitation amounts according to enrollees' risk of requiring expensive health care. This would result in higher capitation payments for high-risk enrollees and lower payments for low-risk enrollees.

Initially, this risk-adjustment method incorporated only enrollees' hospital admissions during the previous year. If an enrollee were admitted for more than 1 day during a year, HCFA would increase its capitation payments during the next year according to the principal inpatient diagnostic cost group (PIP-DCG) into which people with that diagnosis fell. For example, if an enrollee were hospitalized for congestive heart failure during 2000, HCFA would increase its capitation payments during 2001 by $1074 per month to provide the extra funds typically needed to care for people who have been hospitalized recently for congestive heart failure. In order to make the PIP-DCG risk-adjustment system cost-neutral, HCFA offsets the PIP-DCG increases in capitation payments by reducing its capitation payments for people who have not been hospitalized during the previous year. These adjustments are being incorporated gradually into the Medicare capitation schedules between 2000 and 2004. CMS has announced that it intends to expand this system soon to incorporate outpatient as well as inpatient diagnoses in adjusting its capitation payments.

BBA 97 provisions for improving the quality of health care for older Americans include:

- the Quality Improvement System for Managed Care (QISMC);

- the Healthcare Employers' Data Information System (HEDIS), which requires Medicare Plus Choice plans to monitor and report to CMS their rates of compliance with selected processes and outcomes of health care (eg, mammography and immunization against influenza);

- the Medicare Health Outcomes Survey, which requires Medicare Plus Choice plans to contract with third parties to survey a sample of their members and report information to CMS about their health status, functional ability, and satisfaction with their recent health care.

CMS summarizes the information generated by all three systems and makes it available (http://www.medicare.gov) to help older Americans make informed choices about Medicare's FFS program and its various Medicare Plus Choice options.

Balanced Budget Revision Act of 1999

Within the first 18 months of the enactment of BBA 97, the quality of health care for older Americans began to erode, and the decreases in the payments to providers proved to be steeper than projected. For example, Medicare payments for home-health care decreased by 45% between 1997 and 1999. In response, Congress passed the Balanced Budget Revision Act at the end of 1999. This legislation restored some of the budget cuts made 2 years earlier (including $4.5 billion to Medicare Plus Choice plans), and it deferred the need for Medicare Plus Choice plans to collect and report outpatient encounter data for HCFA's new system for risk-adjusting its capitation payments to these plans.

CMS is now conducting demonstration projects to test the feasibility of applying lessons learned by managed Medicare plans to the FFS sector, for example, paying provider organizations a set fee for providing case management or disease management services to FFS beneficiaries with chronic conditions such as congestive heart failure. As this edition of the *GRS* goes to press, Congress and the president are debating the merits and the costs of different approaches to adding a drug benefit to the Medicare program.

REFERENCES

- Ettinger WH Jr. The Balanced Budget Act of 1997: implications for the practice of geriatric medicine. *J Am Geriatr Soc.*1998;46(4):530–533.

- Health Care Financing Administration. *Medicare and You 2002.* Rockville, MD: US Government Printing Office;

2000. Pub. No. 10050. (Available from http://medicare.gov in regular and large print.)

■ Health Care Financing Administration. *2002 Guide to Health Insurance for People with Medicare.* Rockville, MD: US Government Printing Office; 2000. Pub. No. HCFA-02110. (Available from http://medicare.gov in regular and large print.)

■ Henton FE, Hays BJ, Walker SN, et al. Determinants of Medicare home healthcare service use among Medicare recipients. *Nurs Res.* 2002;51(6):355–362.

■ http://www.medicare.gov.

■ Yeaworth RC. Long-term care insurance. *J Gerontol Nurs.* 2002;28(11):45–51.

CHAPTER 6—PHARMACOTHERAPY

Persons aged 65 years and older are prescribed the highest proportion of medications in relation to their percentage of the U.S. population. This has been true since 1968, when those who were 65 years and older constituted 10% of the population yet purchased 25% of all prescription drugs. Currently, these figures are 13% and 33%, respectively, and they are expected to increase to 25% and 50% by the year 2040.

Drugs are the most common treatment for acute and chronic diseases. They are also used to prevent many of the diseases and disorders experienced by the older adult. Pharmacotherapy that is successful requires the correct drug at the correct dosage, for the correct disease or condition, for the correct patient. Unfortunately, achieving these goals is not simple or easy. Many other factors come into play, including the patient's other disease states, other medications, adherence, beliefs, functional status, physiologic changes due to aging and disease, and ability to afford the medication. The basic principles of prescribing for older patients—briefly, start low, go slow—are repeated often. However, even the best clinicians who religiously adhere to these principles will encounter patients who have negative outcomes from one or more of their medications.

The principles of pharmacotherapy have not changed significantly during the past 20 years, but drug treatment has become more complex. More drugs are available every year, some with a new pharmacologic profile or mechanism of action. In addition, physicians must contend with expanded indications for available agents, both those that are approved by the Food and Drug Administration and those that are off-label. Clinicians also must be responsive to frequent changes in the managed-care formulary, the scientific advances in the understanding of drug-drug interactions (ie, the cytochrome P-450 system), the change of many drugs from prescription to nonprescription, and the boom in an unregulated third class of medications called *nutriceuticals,* that is, nutritional supplements, alternative medicines, and herbal preparations. Finally, very little information is available about the use of these unregulated medications in older patients—particularly sick older patients on other medications.

AGE-ASSOCIATED CHANGES IN PHARMACOKINETICS

Pharmacokinetic studies define the time course of a drug and its metabolites throughout the body with respect to four parameters: absorption, distribution, metabolism, and elimination. The effects of aging on each parameter have been studied, and the resulting generalizations have been incorporated into the principles of prescribing for the older patient.

Absorption

Aging does not affect drug absorption to any clinically significant degree. The rate of absorption may be slowed, but the extent of absorption remains unchanged. Consequently, the peak serum concentration of a drug in the older patient may be lower and the time to reach it delayed, but the overall amount absorbed (*bioavailability*) does not differ in younger and older patients. Exceptions include drugs that undergo an extensive first-pass effect; they tend to have higher serum concentrations or increased bioavailability, since less drug is extracted by the liver as a consequence of decreased liver size and blood flow.

Factors that have a greater impact on drug absorption include the way a medication is taken, what it is taken with, and a patient's comorbid illnesses. For example, the absorption of many fluoroquinolones (eg, ciprofloxacin) is reduced when they are taken with divalent cations such as calcium, magnesium, and iron that are found in antacids, sucralfate, dairy products, or vitamins. Enteral feedings interfere with the absorption of some drugs (eg, phenytoin). An increase in gastric pH from proton pump inhibitors, H_2 antagonists, or antacids may increase the absorption of some drugs, such as nifedipine and amoxicillin, and decrease the absorption of other drugs, such as the imidazole antifungals, ampicillin, cyanocobalamin, and indinavir. Agents that promote or delay gastrointestinal motility, such as stimulant laxatives and metoclopramide, can, in theory, affect a drug's absorption by increasing or decreasing the time spent in the segment of the intestinal tract necessary for dissolution or absorption. Another mechanism that can increase or decrease drug absorption is the inhibition or induction of enzymes in the gastrointestinal tract (this is discussed below, in the section on drug interactions).

Distribution

Distribution refers to the locations in the body a drug penetrates and the time required for the drug to reach those locations. Distribution is expressed as the volume of distribution (Vd), with units of volume (eg, liters) or volume per weight (eg, L/kg).

Age-associated changes in body composition can alter drug distribution. In older patients, drugs that are water soluble (*hydrophilic*) have a lower volume of distribution, as older people have less body water and lean body mass. Drugs affected include ethanol and lithium. Digoxin, which distributes and binds to skeletal muscle, has been reported to have a reduced volume of distribution in older persons because of the reduced muscle mass of older adults. Drugs that are fat soluble (*lipophilic*) have an increased volume of distribution in older persons because they have greater fat stores than do younger persons. Thus, it takes longer for an older patient taking a lipophilic drug to reach a steady-state concentration and longer for the drug to be eliminated from the body. Examples of fat-soluble drugs include diazepam, flurazepam, thiopental, and trazodone.

The extent to which a drug is bound to plasma proteins also influences its volume of distribution. Albumin, the primary plasma protein to which drugs bind, is decreased in older patients; thus, a higher proportion of drug is unbound (free) and pharmacologically active. Drugs that bind to albumin and whose unbound fraction has been shown to be increased in older persons include ceftriaxone, diazepam, lorazepam, phenytoin, valproic acid, and warfarin. Normally, additional unbound drug is eliminated; however, age-related decreases in the organ systems of elimination may result in the accumulation of unbound drug in the body. Phenytoin provides an example of the way an increase in unbound drug can lead to an unnecessary and potentially harmful dosage increase. A patient with a low serum albumin (≤ 3 g/dL) whose phenytoin dose is increased because his or her total phenytoin concentration is subtherapeutic may, even though seizure-free, develop symptoms and signs of phenytoin toxicity after a dose increase because the concentration of free phenytoin is elevated.

α_1-Acid glycoprotein is a plasma protein that binds to drugs that are lipophilic and basic (*cationic*). In addition to being an acute-phase reactant, α_1-acid glycoprotein has been shown to increase with aging. Drugs that bind to α_1-acid glycoprotein include lidocaine, propranolol, salicylic acid, quinidine, erythromycin, amitriptyline, imipramine, and desipramine. The clinical ramifications of the age-related change in α_1-acid glycoprotein are probably not significant, but additional study is needed to confirm this conclusion.

Metabolism

The liver is the most common site of drug metabolism, but metabolic conversion also can take place in the intestinal wall, lungs, skin, kidneys, and other organs. Aging affects the liver by decreasing liver blood flow as well as decreasing liver size and mass. Consequently, in the older patient the metabolic clearance of drugs by the liver may be reduced. This is the case for drugs that are subject to the phase I pathways or reactions, which include hydroxylation, oxidation, dealkylation, and reduction. Most drugs metabolized through these pathways may be converted to metabolites of lesser, equal, or greater pharmacologic effect than the parent compound. Drugs metabolized through the phase II pathways are converted to inactive compounds through glucuronidation, conjugation, or acetylation. Medications subject to phase II metabolism are generally preferred for older patients, as their metabolites are not active and will not accumulate. One exception may be metoclopramide, which is conjugated. Its clearance is significantly lower in frail older persons than in younger persons, even though clearance in younger and in fit older persons does not differ. Neither liver volume nor bioavailability is different among the three groups. These facts suggest that in frail older patients drug clearance by conjugation pathways may be reduced.

Age and gender differences also have been reported. For example, oxazepam is metabolized faster in older men than in older women. (The reason is unknown.) Nefazodone concentrations have been reported to be 50% greater in older women, but no differences were found between older men and younger persons.

In drug metabolism, factors other than aging can exaggerate or override the effects of aging. For example, hepatic congestion due to heart failure decreases the metabolism of warfarin, resulting in an increased pharmacologic response. Smoking stimulates monooxygenase enzymes and increases the clearance of theophylline even in older patients.

Elimination

Elimination refers to a drug's final route(s) of exit from the body. For most drugs, this involves elimination by the kidney as either the parent compound or as a metabolite or metabolites. Terms used to express elimination are a drug's *half-life* and its *clearance*.

A drug's half-life is the time it takes for its plasma or serum concentration to decline by 50%, for example, from 20 mg/L to 10 mg/L. Half-life is usually expressed in hours. Steady state is reached when the amount of drug entering the systemic circulation is equal to the amount being eliminated. For a drug administered on a regular basis, 95% of steady state in the body is achieved after five half-lives of the drug.

Clearance is usually expressed as volume per unit of time (eg, L/hour or mL/min) and represents the volume of plasma or serum from which the drug is removed (ie, cleared) per unit of time. Clearance may also be expressed as volume per weight per unit of time (L/kg/hr). Half-life and clearance can also refer to metabolic elimination.

The effects of aging on renal function have been studied to a greater extent than have the effects of aging on hepatic function. Glomerular filtration declines as a consequence of a decrease in kidney size and renal blood flow and a decrease in functioning nephrons. On average, renal function begins to decline when people reach their mid-30s, with an average decline of 6 to 12 mL per minute per 1.73 m² per decade. Follow-up studies (conducted in men only) over 10 to 15 years found three normally distributed groups: those whose creatinine clearance declined to the extent that it was clinically significant; a second group whose creatinine clearance declined to the extent that it was statistically but not clinically significant; and a third group whose creatinine clearance did not change. Renal tubular secretion also declines with age.

Serum creatinine is not an accurate reflection of creatinine clearance in older adults. Because of the age-related decline in lean muscle mass, the older person's production of creatinine is reduced. The decrease in glomerular filtration rate counters the decreased production of creatinine, and serum creatinine stays within the normal range, not revealing the change in creatinine clearance.

The conservative approach in treating the older patient is to calculate the appropriate dose for renally eliminated medications as if the patient's renal function actually has declined with aging. Measuring a patient's 24-hour creatinine clearance would be the most accurate way to determine the appropriate dose, but this is time consuming and requires an accurate 24-hour urine collection. An 8-hour collection time has been shown to be accurate but has not been widely accepted.

To initially estimate a patient's creatinine clearance (CrCl), the clinician can use the Cockroft and Gault equation (see box below).

The equation is widely applied, but it has limitations. First, not all patients experience a significant age-related decline in renal function, and for them, the equation would underestimate creatinine clearance. Second, for patients whose muscle mass is reduced beyond that of normal aging, the creatinine clearance would be overestimated. This would apply to persons whose serum creatinine is less than normal, that is, < 0.7 mg/dL. It has been suggested that 1 mg/dL be substituted for a low serum creatinine. However, normalizing the serum creatinine has not been shown to be a precise estimate, and it generally underestimates the actual creatinine clearance.

In cases in which the patient's renal function may be impaired but estimates of function are uncertain, the clinician should consider the following:

- Avoid drugs that are entirely dependent on renal elimination and with which accumulation would result in toxicity (eg, imipenem).
- If the use of such an agent cannot be avoided, obtain an accurate measure of renal function (eg, a 24-hour creatinine clearance).
- Monitor serum or plasma concentrations of the drug (eg, aminoglycosides), if available, and important metabolites procainamide and N-acetyl procainamide (NAPA).

AGE-ASSOCIATED CHANGES IN PHARMACODYNAMICS

The pharmacodynamic action of a drug—that is, its time course and intensity of pharmacologic effect—may change with the increasing age of the patient. An excellent example of such pharmacodynamic changes in

$$\text{Estimated CrCl (mL/minute)} = \frac{(\text{IBW in kg})\,(140 - \text{age in years})}{(72)\,(\text{serum creatinine in mg/dL})} \times (0.85 \text{ if female})$$

For men: IBW in kg = 50 + (2.3) (each inch > 5 feet). For women: IBW in kg = 45 + (2.3) (each inch > 5 feet).

older persons has been demonstrated with the benzodiazepines. Older persons have been found to have more sedation and lower performance than younger persons on a psychomotor test following a single dose of triazolam. These differences are attributed to pharmacokinetic changes, that is, to significantly higher plasma triazolam concentrations that are due to reduced clearance in older adults. However, a different pattern has been found for nitrazepam: The pharmacokinetics of nitrazepam (an intermediate-acting benzodiazepine similar to lorazepam) were found to be no different in young and older persons after a single 10-mg dose; yet, 12 hours and 36 hours after a 10-mg dose, older persons made significantly more mistakes on a psychomotor test than when they had taken placebo. Younger persons did not demonstrate significant impairment at any time. In addition, even with short-term use, young and older patients may experience impaired balance and posture following a single dose of a benzodiazepine.

It is uncertain whether the age-associated pharmacokinetic changes of morphine account for the increased level and prolonged duration of pain relief experienced by older patients. In older adults, morphine has been shown to have a smaller volume of distribution, higher plasma concentrations, and longer clearance than in younger adults. Older patients achieve pain relief at least equivalent to younger patients at half the intramuscular dose, and they have an increased duration of pain relief. Thus, the dose or frequency, or both, of morphine given intramuscularly or by intravenous infusion should be lower, at least initially, in older patients.

Pharmacodynamic and pharmacokinetic changes, alone or together, generally result in an increased sensitivity to medications by the older adult. In some patients, particularly those who are frail, the use of lower doses, longer intervals between doses, and longer periods between changes in dose are ways to successfully manage drug therapy and decrease the chances of medication intolerance or toxicity. Disease- and drug-specific monitoring are also necessary to ensure a successful outcome.

OPTIMIZING PRESCRIBING

Optimizing drug therapy for older adults means achieving the balance between overprescribing (ie, excessive prescribing or use of inappropriate drug therapy) and underprescribing of beneficial therapies. Overprescribing of drug therapies not only refers to the use of multiple medications but also implies a lack of appropriateness in medication selection, dose, or use. One survey found that 40% of nursing-home residents had an order for at least one potentially inappropriate medication. As many as 6 million older

Americans may be exposed to potentially inappropriate medications. The causes of inappropriate prescribing include the use of multiple prescribers and multiple pharmacies, the prescription of "a pill for every ill," and the accumulation of chronic conditions that require treatment. However, simply limiting the number of medications for a given patient is not always possible or desirable. For example, a patient with congestive heart failure due to systolic dysfunction may be appropriately treated with three or four drugs: a diuretic, an angiotensin-converting enzyme inhibitor, a β-blocker, and perhaps digoxin. If this patient has hyperlipidemia and diabetes mellitus, another two or three medications could be required. Hence, such a patient would be taking five to seven indicated medications for major medical conditions alone.

The consequences of overprescribing include adverse drug events, drug-drug interactions, duplication of drug therapy, decreased quality of life, and unnecessary costs.

ADVERSE DRUG EVENTS

An adverse drug event (ADE) is defined as an injury from a medication. Preventable adverse drug events are among the most serious consequences of inappropriate drug prescribing among older adults. Adverse drug reactions (ADRs) are a type of ADE. ADEs are estimated to be responsible for 5% to 28% of acute geriatric medical admissions; the estimated annual incidence rate is 26 per 1000 beds for hospitalized patients. Annually, at least 35% of community-dwelling older adults experience an ADE. It has been estimated that in the nursing home, for every dollar spent on medications, $1.33 in health care resources is consumed in the treatment of drug-related morbidity and mortality. A cohort study of all long-term-care residents in 18 nursing homes in Massachusetts demonstrated that adverse drug events are common and often preventable in nursing homes. During the 28,839 resident-months of observations, 546 adverse drug events were identified. Overall, 51% of these adverse events were judged to have been preventable. Most of the errors occurred at the ordering and monitoring stages.

Cardiovascular, central nervous system, and musculoskeletal medications are most commonly involved in ADEs, regardless of the setting. Medications most often involved in ADEs are those used with the greatest frequency by older patients (eg, diuretics, digoxin) or that have a narrow margin of safety (eg, antiparkinson agents). The majority of ADEs ($\geq$ 95%) experienced by older patients are considered to be predictable.

Lists of potentially inappropriate medications and medication-disease pairs have been published. One list

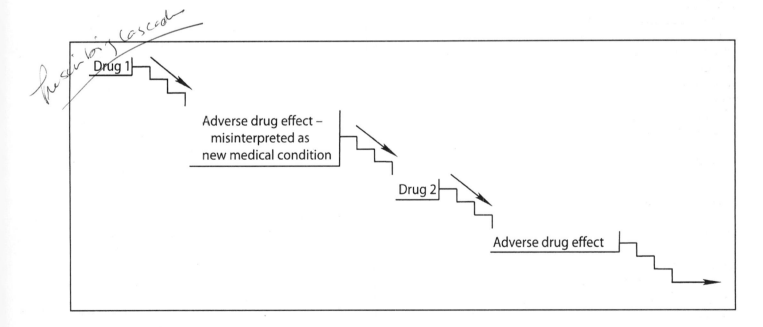

that was developed by the consensus of experts in geriatric medicine and pharmacology has been adapted by the Centers for Medicare & Medicaid Services (CMS) for identifying potentially inappropriate or unnecessary medication use by nursing-home residents. (For the current version, see the most recent edition of *Geriatrics At Your Fingertips*, published annually by the American Geriatrics Society.)

For patient characteristics that place older patients at risk for ADEs, see Table 6.1.

A common pathway for ADEs and polypharmacy has been described as the "prescribing cascade," as described in Figure 6.1. One form of this cascade occurs when a medication results in an ADE that is mistaken as a separate diagnosis and treated with more medications, which puts the patient at risk for additional ADEs and more medications. Examples that have been studied include metoclopramide-induced parkinsonism and the subsequent prescribing of antiparkinson medications, and anticholinergic agents that result in constipation and the subsequent use of laxatives.

DRUG INTERACTIONS

A drug-drug interaction (DDI) is defined as the pharmacologic or clinical response to the administration of a drug combination that differs from that anticipated from the known effects of each of the two agents when given alone. Drug-drug interactions are important because they may lead to adverse drug events. The likelihood of DDIs increases as the number of medications a patient takes increases. Among prescription drugs, cardiovascular and psychotropic drugs are most commonly involved in DDIs. A positive correlation exists between the number of potential DDIs and the number of adverse effects experienced by hospitalized older patients. The most common adverse effects are neuropsychologic (primarily confusion) or cognitive impairment, arterial hypotension, and acute renal failure. Drug combinations that are reported to result in increased risk for hospitalization for older patients are shown in Table 6.2. Risk factors associated with DDIs include the use of multiple medications, receiving care from several prescribing clinicians, and using more than one pharmacy.

Drug interactions can take many forms. For example, absorption can be enhanced or diminished (as described above), drugs with similar or opposite pharmacologic effects can result in exaggerated or impaired effects, and drug metabolism may be inhibited or induced. Research focusing on the cytochrome P-450 system has proposed or studied in vivo or in vitro numerous DDIs involving the different P-450 isozymes. The effect of aging on the cytochrome P-450 system and the clinical implications for prescribing have not been completely determined. Cross-sectional data have shown that cytochrome P-450 content declines incrementally, once in the fourth decade and again after the age 70. In vitro microsomal activity of cytochrome (CYP) 3A4 is not altered by aging, but in vivo age- and gender-related

Figure 6.1—Prescribing cascade.

SOURCE: Rochon PA, Gurwitz JH. Optimising drug treatment for elderly people: the prescribing cascade. *BMJ*. 1997;315(7115):1097. Reprinted with permission from the BMJ Publishing Group.

Table 6.1—Risk Factors for Adverse Drug Events in Older Patients

- ≥ 6 Concurrent chronic diagnoses
- ≥12 Doses of medications per day
- ≥ 9 Medications
- A prior adverse drug reaction
- Low body weight or body mass index
- Age > 85 years
- An estimated creatinine clearance < 50 mL per minute

Table 6.2—Most Common Drug-Drug Adverse Effects Identified Upon Hospitalization

Combination	Risk
ACE inhibitor + diuretic	Hypotension; hyperkalemia
ACE inhibitor + potassium	Hyperkalemia
Antiarrhythmic + diuretic	Electrolyte imbalance; arrhythmias
Benzodiazepine + antidepressant	Confusion, sedation, falls
Benzodiazepine + antipsychotic	Confusion, sedation, falls
Benzodiazepine + benzodiazepine	Confusion, sedation, falls
Calcium channel blocker + diuretic	Hypotension
Calcium channel blocker + nitrate	Hypotension
Digitalis + antiarrhythmic	Bradycardia, arrhythmias
Diuretic + digitalis	Arrhythmias
Diuretic + diuretic	Dehydration, electrolyte imbalance
Diuretic + nitrate	Hypotension
Nitrate + vasodilator	Hypotension

SOURCE: Data from Doucet J, Chassagne P, Trivalle C, et al. Drug-drug interactions related to hospital admissions in older adults: a prospective study of 1000 patients. *J Am Geriatr Soc.* 1996;44(8):944–948.

reductions in drug clearance have been found for CYP3A4 substrates erythromycin, prednisolone, verapamil, alprazolam, nifedipine, and diazepam. CYP3A4 accounts for 30% of the P-450 content in the liver and is also prominent in the intestinal tract. This isozyme is involved in the metabolism of more than 50% of drugs on the market and can be induced by drugs such as rifampin, phenytoin, and carbamazepine, and inhibited by many drugs, including the macrolide antibiotics, nefazodone, itraconazole, ketoconazole, as well as grapefruit juice. The isozyme CYP2D6 is involved in the metabolism of 25% to 30% of marketed drugs and has been associated with only minimal age-related changes. CYP2D6 is involved in the metabolism of many psychotropic drugs and can be inhibited by many agents. In addition, approximately 10% of white people are deficient in this isozyme and have reduced ability to clear and increased sensitivity to CYP2D6 substrates. Clinically, these patients and those

taking CYP2D6 inhibitors (eg, quinidine, paroxetine, fluoxetine) cannot convert codeine and tramadol to their active metabolites and have a reduced analgesic response to these agents.

P-glycoprotein has been found to function as an efflux pump in the intestinal tract. Grapefruit juice has been shown to induce P-glycoprotein and therefore may reduce the bioavailability of drugs subject to this efflux pump. It is unknown whether aging affects P-glycoprotein content or activity.

For DDIs involving herbal preparations, see "Complementary and Alternative Therapies" (p 42).

DRUG-DISEASE INTERACTIONS

Drug-disease combinations common in older patients can affect drug response and *lead to adverse drug events. Obesity and ascites alter the volumes of distribution of lipophilic and hydrophilic drugs, respectively.* Patients with dementia may have increased sensitivity or paradoxical reactions to drugs with central nervous system or anticholinergic activity. Patients with renal insufficiency or impaired hepatic function due to cirrhosis or hepatic congestion have impaired detoxification and excretion of drugs.

PRINCIPLES OF PRESCRIBING

Principles of prescribing for older patients are shown in Table 6.3. This basic approach applies primarily to medications that will be used to treat chronic conditions for which an immediate, complete therapeutic response is not necessary. A dose adjustment may still be needed for medications used to treat conditions requiring an immediate response (eg, when prescribing antibiotics for a patient with impaired renal function).

Overprescribing can be prevented by reviewing a patient's medications on a regular basis and each time a new medication is started or a dose is changed. The importance of maintaining accurate records of all medications taken by the patient cannot be overemphasized. Knowing what other prescribers have given the patient and what patients are self-prescribing, and documenting all of this in the patient's records is crucial. Many patients do not consider vitamins, herbal preparations, or over-the-counter medications (even aspirin) to be medications, so clinicians must be specific when they inquire about a patient's use of other medications. Medications that have been newly approved by the Food and Drug Administration should be used cautiously in treating older patients. Such drugs are likely to be more expensive, and information about their use in older patients is often limited.

Table 6.3—Principles of Prescribing for Older Patients

The basics:

- Start with a low dose.

- Titrate the dose upward slowly, as tolerated by the patient.

- Try not to start two drugs at the same time.

Determine the following before prescribing a new medication:

- Is the medication necessary? Are there nonpharmacologic ways to treat the condition?

- What are the therapeutic end points and how will they be assessed?

- Do the benefits outweigh the risks of the medication?

- Is one medication being used to treat the adverse effects of another?

- Is there one medication that could be prescribed to treat two conditions?

- Are there potential drug-drug or drug-disease interactions?

- Will the new medication's administration times be the same as those of existing medications?

- Do the patient and caregiver understand what the medication is for, how to take it, how long to take it, when it should start to work, possible adverse effects that it might cause, and what to do if they occur?

At least annually:

- Ask the patient to bring in all medications (prescription, over-the-counter, supplements, and herbal preparations) to the office; for new patients, conduct a detailed medication history.

- For prescription medications, determine whether the label directions and dose match those in the patient's chart; ask the patient how each medication is being taken.

- Ask about medication side effects.

- Note who else is prescribing medications for the patient, and what the medications are and their indications.

- Look for medications with duplicate therapeutic, pharmacologic, or adverse effect profiles.

- Screen for drug-drug and drug-disease interactions.

- Eliminate unnecessary medications; confer with other prescribers if necessary.

- Simplify the medication regimen; use the fewest possible number of medications and doses per day.

- Always review any changes with the patient and caregiver; provide the changes in writing.

It is best if the patient brings all medications to the review, including over-the-counter medications, vitamins, and any herbal preparations or other types of supplements (a "brown-bag" evaluation). Examining the containers and labels and asking what each medication is for and how and when it is taken can provide insight into the patient's understanding and adherence to his or her medication regimens. Discontinue any medications when there is no longer an indication for their continued use. Any new complaints or worsening of an existing condition should prompt the consider-

ation of whether it could be drug-induced (see Figure 6.1). When considering treatment for a new medical condition, always consider nonpharmacologic approaches first. If a drug therapy is still indicated, select within the class in order to minimize the risk of an adverse drug event.

When initiating therapy, the basic principle should be to start low go and go slow. Though the Food and Drug Administration requires that labeling for new drugs regarding dosing in older patients cannot be extrapolated from another patient population (eg, patients with renal impairment), it does not require that a drug be studied explicitly in older persons. Older persons are used in the studies of many new drugs for their phase I and II dose tolerability and their pharmacokinetic and pharmacodynamic actions, but the older persons chosen for these studies are usually healthy and free of concomitant illnesses. Much of what is known about medications and how to use them in sick older patients, particularly those who are frail, is learned only after a drug has been available for several years

Just as medications are prescribed in numbers or prescribed in doses greater than necessary, they also may be inappropriately omitted or underdosed. Documented examples include pain medications and angiotensin-converting enzyme inhibitors.

NONADHERENCE

Nonadherence to medications is a huge and often unrecognized problem in drug treatment. It is estimated that nonadherence among older adults may be as high as 50%. Patients may be reluctant to admit that they are not taking medications or not following directions. If nonadherence is suspected, the clinician needs to consider the patient's financial, cognitive, and functional status, as well as his or her beliefs about and understanding of medications and diseases.

Prescription drug costs have increased substantially, and supplemental prescription drug benefits plans are expensive. Some plans still may leave a patient with a copayment that he or she cannot afford or with only a fixed dollar amount for the year. Clinicians should avoid prescribing expensive new medications that have not been shown to be superior to less expensive generic alternatives.

Cognitive impairment may also cause nonadherence, as patients forget to take medications or confuse them. Simplifying the regimen and involving a caregiver to oversee medication management can be helpful approaches. Medication trays or drug calendars also may help with organization, and they are very useful for patients who have difficulty remembering when they last took a medication.

The older patient's ability to read labels, open containers, or pour medications or even a glass of water may be impaired, so functional assessment can be useful. Some patients may need additional education or reinforcement about the purpose of a medication, especially those used to treat conditions that are usually asymptomatic, such as diabetes mellitus and hypertension. Older patients also may need reassurance regarding the safety and possible adverse effects of certain medications, particularly newly prescribed medications or those associated with serious adverse events, such as warfarin.

REFERENCES

■ Beers MH. Explicit criteria for determining potentially inappropriate medication use by the elderly: an update. *Arch Intern Med.* 1997;157(14):1531–1536.

■ Devane CL, Pollock BG. Pharmacokinetic considerations of antidepressant use in the elderly. *J Clin Psychiatry.* 1999; 60(suppl 20):38–44.

■ Fulmer T, Foreman M, Zwicker D. Medication in older adults. In: Mezey M, Fulmer T, Abraham I, eds. *Geriatric Nursing Protocols for Best Practice, 2nd ed.* New York: Springer Publishing Company. (in press)

■ Gurwitz JH, Field TS, Avorn J, et al. Incidence and preventability of adverse drug events in nursing homes. *Am J Med.* 2000;109(2):87–94.

■ Hanlon JT, Shimp LA, Semla TP. Advances in geriatrics: drug-related problems in the elderly. *Ann Pharmacother.* 2000;34(3):360–365.

■ Rochon PA, Gurwitz JH. Drug therapy. *Lancet.* 1995;346(8966):32–36.

CHAPTER 7—COMPLEMENTARY AND ALTERNATIVE THERAPIES

Alternative therapies are defined by the National Center for Complementary and Alternative Medicine of the National Institutes of Health as "an unrelated group of non-orthodox therapeutic practices often with explanatory systems that do not follow conventional biomedical explanations." The term *alternative* implies that the therapy is being used in place of conventional treatment, whereas *complementary* refers to therapies used in conjunction with traditional medications, therapies, or procedures. These two terms are often combined in the acronym CAM (complementary and alternative medicine).

PATTERNS OF USE IN THE UNITED STATES

In 1998, a follow-up survey to one conducted in 1990 estimated that 42% of Americans used at least 1 of 16 alternative therapies. Since 1990, the greatest increases in use had occurred in herbal medicine, massage, megavitamins, folk remedies, self-help groups, energy healing (eg, magnets), and homeopathy. These alternative therapies were used for conditions such as back problems, neck problems, depression, anxiety, headaches, digestive problems, fatigue, and arthritis. In the survey, 58% of respondents reported using alternative therapies to prevent future illness or maintain health; 42% were using them to treat an existing illness. The typical user of complementary medicine was described as female, 35 to 49 years of age, college educated, middle class, and living in the western part of the United States. Race and age did not seem to correlate with use. Most respondents were white, so findings should not be assumed to apply to other racial or ethnic groups.

Sixty percent of survey respondents said that they had not informed their primary physician about their use. The reasons for this lack of communication probably rests with both patients and clinicians. Patients may forget or may be uncomfortable about relating this information out of fear that the physician will have a negative reaction or think that they are foolish. Physicians may feel that they do not have time to address this issue and are assuming other clinicians are asking these questions. Health care professionals may also believe that patients know more about complementary medicine than they do or that they have no reliable sources to turn to regarding safety and efficacy.

Few specific data have been published on the use of CAM by older people. The 1998 study estimated that 1 in 5 prescription medication users (15 million adults) in 1997 took their medications with herbal preparations, high-dose vitamins, or both. These people, especially those with chronic diseases and liver or kidney problems, could be at risk of adverse drug-drug interactions. Drug interactions are of particular concern in older patients because they are more likely to have these medical conditions and have pharmacokinetic and pharmacodynamic changes that could affect the way that the prescription drugs, as well as the herbal preparations and vitamins, are handled by the body. Little is known about how herbal preparations are handled by the cytochrome P-450 system in the liver, but experience with drug-drug interactions has shown that some of these interactions can be serious or life threatening. Since multiple possible combinations of drug-drug interactions may occur, it can be very difficult to anticipate such interactions when patients are taking multiple medications and herbal products. Patients and clinicians need to become aware of and monitor for adverse reactions.

The cost of CAM is high, a financial burden borne mainly by the patient. Interestingly, on the basis of the 1998 survey, the expenditures for alternative therapies were estimated at $27 billion. This figure is similar to the out-of-pocket expenditures for all U.S. physician services ($29 billion) and greater than hospital out-of-pocket expenditures ($9 billion). Although the survey had not asked about expenditures for herbal preparations in 1990, the follow-up survey found that $5 billion was spent on herbal products alone to help conditions such as allergies, insomnia, and digestive problems. Remarkably, despite these high expenditures, 80% of respondents did not have insurance coverage for herbal products. However, more health maintenance organizations and private insurance companies have begun to offer discounted herbal and vitamin products, as well as some benefits for other complementary treatments (eg, chiropractic care, self-help groups).

REASONS FOR USE OF CAM

A survey study specifically looked at why patients use alternative medicine. People reported using chiropractic care, life style changes, diet, exercise or movement training, and relaxation to help treat the most frequently cited health problems: chronic pain, anxiety, chronic fatigue syndrome, sprains or muscle strains, addictive problems, arthritis, and headaches. Herbal therapies were used most often to treat anxiety, sprains or muscle strains, arthritis, depression, and digestive problems.

The same research also identified predictors of alternative medicine use: more education, poorer health status, having a transformational experience that changes the person's world view; a commitment to environmentalism or feminism, an interest in spirituality and personal growth psychology, and having such health problems as anxiety, back pain, chronic pain, and urinary tract problems. Dissatisfaction with conventional medicine did not predict CAM use. Racial and ethnic differences, sex, and age were also not predictors of use.

CLINICAL APPROACHES TO PATIENTS' CAM USE

Clinicians caring for older adults should inquire about their use of alternative therapies. Often it is the caregivers who ask about CAM or who administer these therapies to the older patient. Asking about a patient's use of herbal preparations or dietary supplements is essential before prescribing drugs that could have clinically important drug interactions, for example, drugs such as warfarin and other agents with a narrow therapeutic window. Table 7.1 lists a selection of such medications that are commonly used in treating older patients, along with examples of herbal preparations that could interact with them and the possible effect of their interaction. (See also "Pharmacotherapy," p 35.)

HERBAL PREPARATIONS: REGULATION AND RESEARCH

Herbal products have become increasingly popular, in part because patients may feel that these products are "natural" and therefore safe, and because they are available without a prescription. Many herbal supplements have drug-like effects. In fact, several prescription medications have been derived from plant or herbal sources, including tamoxifen, digoxin, aspirin, and morphine. Studies of prescription medications reveal important dosing parameters, drug interactions, and adverse effect profiles; however, manufacturers of herbal preparations are not required to provide the same intensity of study or even to establish safety and efficacy. Thus, the information about herbal preparations that is available to clinicians and consumers alike is scanty or anecdotal.

The Food and Drug Administration (FDA) does not regulate herbal products, and no proof of their safety, efficacy, or purity is required. In the United States they can be promoted for health conditions without proof that they work or that they are safe for people to use. Without regulation, the dosing and purity of herbal products remains uncertain. Case reports have been published describing contaminated or misidentified herbal preparations. Publicity regarding adverse effects resulting from such problems has resulted, on occasion, in herbal products being voluntarily recalled.

The FDA cannot take action unless people have suffered major harm or injury from an herbal product, and even then, it must prove that the herbal product is unsafe before it can require that the product be withdrawn from the market. In much of Europe, herbal preparations are manufactured uniformly under regulations similar to those for other medications, and

Table 7.1—Possible Interactions of Drugs and Herbal Preparations

Prescription Medication	Possible Interactive Effect	Herbal Preparations
Anticoagulants, antiplatelets	Increased bleeding time	Arnica, celery, chamomile, dan-shen, dong quai, fenugreek, feverfew, garlic, ginger, ginkgo, green tea
Anticoagulants, antiplatelets	Decreased bleeding time	Ginseng
Hypoglycemic agents	Hypoglycemic effect	Chromium, fenugreek, garlic, ginseng, nettle, sage
Digoxin	Cardiac glycoside additive effect	Adonis (false hellebore, pheasant's eye), broom, dogbane, figwort, lily-of-the-valley, milkweed, motherwort, pleurisy root, purple foxglove, strophanthus, uzara root, white squill, wild ipecac, yellow foxglove
Digoxin	Falsely elevated digoxin level without toxicity in lab assays	Ginseng, kyushin
Digoxin	Hypokalemia, increased digoxin sensitivity	Licorice
Digoxin	Reduced digoxin bioavailability	St. John's wort
Diuretics	Increased diuresis	Agrimony, artichoke, boldus, broom, buchu, burdock, celery seed, cough-grass, dandelion, elder, goldenseal, guaiacum, juniper, pokeroot, shepherd's purse, squill, uva-ursi, yarrow, zea
Trazodone	Central nervous system depression, somnolence	Ginkgo

herbal preparations are sold in pharmacies as well. In the United States, however, the herbal manufacturing industry is not uniform; producers range from pharmaceutical-grade companies to home processors with unsanitary conditions who do not understand the intricacies of the production of herbal preparations.

To better educate patients and their caregivers about appropriate and inappropriate use of herbal preparations, clinicians need to educate themselves first with the most reliable information. Increasing amounts of clinical information are being released as quality research becomes available, especially with the development of the National Center for Complementary and Alternative Medicine. Very few studies to date have described the use of herbal preparations for given indications or specific pharmacokinetic information for herbal preparations used by older persons, although increasingly, randomized and controlled trials are being conducted to evaluate such therapies.

SPECIFIC HERBAL PREPARATIONS

Several herbal preparations or nutritional supplements are of particular interest to older patients: St. John's wort, kava, valerian, ginkgo, saw palmetto, and glucosamine with chondroitin.

St. John's wort is commonly used for depressed mood. The mechanism of action is unknown but is believed to result from blockage of norepinephrine and serotonergic reuptake. More than 24 studies have been published on St. John's wort, but only 9 are considered well-controlled studies using standardized doses with measurement of outcomes. Of these studies, 5 used 900 mg of an aqueous methanol extract for at least 4 weeks and measured scores on the Hamilton Depression Scale. There was a slightly greater improvement in the scores with St. John's wort versus placebo. An additional 4 studies compared efficacy and tolerability of St. John's wort (900 mg extract) with standard tricyclic antidepressants (maprotiline, imipramine, amitriptyline) for mild to moderate depression and found no statistically significant difference in response, but the study populations were small and no placebo group was included. A National Institutes of Health study of the efficacy and tolerability of St. John's wort is under way; St. John's wort is being compared with sertraline for 8 weeks in depressed patients. Side effects from St. John's wort occur infrequently (2.4% of 3000 patients); they include allergic reactions, gastrointestinal upset, dry mouth, sedation, headache, and, at higher doses than that used for depressed mood, photosensitivity.

Kava is an herbal preparation used for anxiety. Its active ingredients, kavapyrones, act as muscle relaxants, anticonvulsants, and limbic system suppressants. The exact mechanism of action is unclear; however, there is evidence of inhibition of voltage-dependent sodium channels, increased γ-aminobutyric acid (GABA) receptor densities, suppression of glutamate release, and blockade of norepinephrine reuptake. Most of the double-blind, placebo-controlled trials of kava have poorly defined, small patient populations and were very short in duration. One large study found a significant difference in the Hamilton Anxiety Scale scores after 8 weeks of therapy that continued throughout the 25 weeks of the study time period. Adverse effects include allergic reaction, yellowing or scaling of the skin, gastrointestinal upset, pupil dilation, and blurred vision.

Valerian is an herbal preparation that is used to improve sleep. Of the 100 constituents found in this plant, valerianic acids appear to cause sedation and anticonvulsant effects by affecting GABA neurons and increasing GABA concentrations in animals. At doses of 400 to 900 mg of valerian extract, sleep latency is decreased and sleep quality is improved in healthy persons only. However, the maximum effect may not occur until after 2 to 4 weeks of therapy. Adverse effects are reported as rare; they include gastrointestinal upset, contact allergies, headache, restless sleep, and mydriasis.

Ginkgo is an herbal preparation currently being used to prevent and treat memory problems. A standardized extract should contain 24% flavone glycosides (antioxidant) and 6% terpenoids. The ginkgolide B constituent of ginkgo is responsible for inhibiting platelet activation factor. Of the 40 trials published on ginkgo, all but one found it to be clinically significant in improving memory loss symptoms, concentration difficulties, fatigue, anxiety, and depression. The patient populations in most of these studies were small and ill defined, and nonstandard outcome measures were used. In 1997, an American study reported that *Ginkgo biloba* (EGb 761) 120 mg per day provided a 27% improvement, whereas placebo provided only 14% improvement on the cognitive subscale of the Alzheimer's Disease Assessment Scale. Patients with Alzheimer's disease and vascular dementia were included; however, there was a significant dropout rate. A later study from the Netherlands found no effect from ginkgo 160 to 240 mg per day after 24 weeks of use in institutionalized older patients with mild to moderate Alzheimer's disease, vascular dementia, or age-associated memory impairment. Adverse effects reported with ginkgo include headache, gastrointestinal upset, allergic skin reactions, and cerebral hemorrhage.

Saw palmetto is being used for prostate symptoms in men. The mechanism of action is unknown but may involve alteration of cholesterol metabolism, antiestrogenic, antiandrogenic, anti-inflammatory effects, and decreased concentration of sex-hormone-binding globulin. A meta-analysis of trials done with saw palmetto for moderate benign prostatic symptoms found it to be superior (74% improvement) to placebo (51% improvement) and comparable to finasteride (37% versus 40%, respectively) in improving nocturia, peak urine flow rate, residual urine volumes, and urologic symptoms. Adverse effects were reported as mild and included erectile dysfunction (1.1% saw palmetto versus 4.9% finasteride) and gastrointestinal upset. This herbal preparation is particularly attractive for patients, since it costs half as much as α_1-blockers and one fourth as much as finasteride.

Finally, glucosamine and chondroitin combinations are used for arthritic joint pain. Most of the studies reported in the literature have major methodologic flaws (inadequate allocation concealment, absence of intent-to-treat analysis, the use of varied forms of the supplement, and different outcome measures) that are associated with an exaggeration of the estimate of benefit for either ingredient in knee or hip osteoarthritis. Small effects from glucosamine or chondroitin after 1 month of therapy may suggest that there is a delayed response of 4 to 6 weeks; long-term efficacy has not been reported. New findings on the efficacy of glucosamine are promising (see the section on osteoarthritis in "Musculoskeletal Diseases and Disorders," p 261).

REFERENCES

- Astin JA. Why patients use alternative medicine: results of a national study. *JAMA.* 1998;279(19):1548–1553.

- Center for the Study of Complementary and Alternative Therapies, University of Virginia, School of Nursing. http://nursing.virginia.edu/centers/cscat/

- Corless IB, Abrams D, Nicholas PK, et al. The use of complementary and alternative therapies. *AACN Clin Issues.* 2000;11(1):4–6.

- Eisenberg DM, Davis RB, Ettner SL, et al. Trends in alternative medicine use in the United States, 1990–1997. *JAMA.* 1998;280(18):1569–1575.

- Facts and Comparisons. *Review of Natural Products.* St. Louis, MO: Facts and Comparisons; 2002.

- Miller LG. Herbal medicinals: selected clinical considerations focusing on known or potential drug-herb interactions. *Arch Intern Med.* 1998;158(20):2200–2211.

- Miller LG, Murra WJ. *Herbal Medicinals: A Clinician's Guide.* New York: Haworth Press; 1999.

- National Institutes of Health, Center for Complementary and Alternative Medicine. http://nccam.nih.gov/nccam/about/general.shtml

- O'Hara M, Kiefer D, Farrell K, et al. A review of 12 commonly used medicinal herbs. *Arch Fam Med.* 1998;7(6):523–536.

APPROACH TO THE OLDER PATIENT

CHAPTER 8—ASSESSMENT

Geriatrics focuses on function, which is broadly defined to encompass the physical, cognitive, psychologic, and social domains. These domains are often combined into a single instrument for measuring quality of life. The scope of the assessment of any individual domain depends on the site of care, the patient's level of frailty, time constraints, and the availability of a multidisciplinary team. The essential aspects of geriatric assessment should be performed routinely in all sites of care, whether the ambulatory setting, the hospital, the nursing home, or the home. Whenever possible, assessments should be performance based. An informant, ideally a caregiver or family member who lives with the patient, is often required to provide or to verify pertinent historical information about the older patient's day-to-day functioning. Geriatric assessment is a multifaceted approach with the goal of promoting wellness and independent function. One efficient approach to geriatric assessment entails rapid screening of targeted areas (See Appendix, p 418) followed by comprehensive assessment in areas of concern.

Nurses play a vital role in providing comprehensive geriatric assessment. *Try This*, a publication of The John A. Hartford Foundation Institute for Geriatric Nursing, is a series of assessment tools; each issue focuses on a topic specific to the assessment of older adults. The goal of the *Try This: Best Practices in Care to Older Adults* series is to provide knowledge of best practices in the care of older adults, to make this knowledge easily accessible, easily understood, and easily implemented; and to encourage the use of these best practices by all direct-care nurses. All the tools in the *Try This* series are downloadable from The John A. Hartford Foundation Institute for Geriatric Nursing Web site: http://www.hartfordign.org/publications/trythis/. The tools included in the series are as follows:

Issue 1: PICES: An Overall Assessment Tool of Older Adults
Issue 2: Katz Index of Independence in Activities of Daily Living (ADL)
Issue 3: The Mini-Mental State Examination (MMSE)
Issue 4: The Geriatric Depression Scale (GDS)
Issue 5: Predicting Pressure Ulcer Sore Risk
Issue 6: The Pittsburgh Sleep Quality Index (PSQI)
Issue 7: Assessing Pain In Older Adults
Issue 8: Fall Risk Assessment
Issue 9: Nutrition and Hydration Assessment
Issue 10: Sexuality Assessment
Issue 11: Urinary Incontinence Assessment
Issue 12: Hearing Screening
Issue 13: Confusion Assessment Method (CAM)
Issue 14: Caregiver Strain Index (CSI)
Issue 15: Elder Abuse and Neglect Assessment

PHYSICAL ASSESSMENT

The physical domain of function includes functional status, nutrition, and vision and hearing.

Functional Status

Functional status refers to the tasks a person can perform within the context of daily life. These tasks, usually referred to as activities of daily living (ADLs), are listed in Table 8.1. The self-care tasks or basic ADLs are considered essential to independent living. When assessing disability, clinicians should ask whether the patient requires the help of another person to complete the tasks. (See the Appendix, pp 384, 385, for formal screens.) Bathing is typically the basic ADL with the highest prevalence of disability, and disability in bathing is often the reason why older persons receive home aide services. To identify patients with "preclinical" disability, that is, those who do not yet require personal assistance but who are at risk for becoming disabled, clinicians should ask about perceived difficulty with the tasks and whether the patient has changed the way he or she completes the task because of a health-related problem or condition.

Table 8.1—Activities of Daily Living

Self-care	
Bathing	Toileting
Dressing	Grooming
Transferring from bed to chair	Feeding oneself
Instrumental	
Using the telephone	Doing laundry
Preparing meals	Doing housework
Managing household finances	Shopping
Taking medications	Managing transportation
Mobility	
Walking from room to room	
Climbing a flight of stairs	
Walking outside one's home	

NOTE: See the Appendix, pp 384, 385, for formal screens for activities of daily living and instrumental activities of daily living.

Outside of a rehabilitation setting, performance-based testing of most of the self-care and instrumental ADLs is not practical. Hence, performance-based testing of functional status should focus primarily on transfers, gait, and balance. The patient should be asked to stand from the seated position in a hard-backed chair while keeping his or her arms folded. Inability to complete this task suggests lower-extremity, or quadriceps, weakness and is highly predictive of future disability. Once standing, the patient should be observed to walk back and forth over a short distance, ideally with the usual walking aid. Abnormalities of gait include path deviation; diminished step height or length or both; trips, slips, or near falls; and difficulty with turning. The tasks of rising from the chair, walking 10 feet (3 meters), turning around and returning to the chair, turning, and then sitting back down in the chair make up the "Timed Get Up and Go" test. Persons who take longer than 10 seconds to complete this sequence of maneuvers have been shown to be at increased risk for falls (ie, those taking 10 to 19 seconds are considered to be "fairly mobile"; 20 to 29 seconds, to have "variable mobility"; and 30 seconds or more, to be "dependent" in balance and mobility).

An alternative assessment strategy is to measure gait speed as a predictor of future disability. A gait speed of 0.80 m per second allows for independent community ambulation; a speed of 0.60 m per second allows for community activity without the use of a wheelchair. These norms indicate that patients who can walk 50 feet in your office corridor in 20 seconds or less should be able to walk independently in normal activities.

Balance can be tested progressively by asking the patient to stand first with his or her feet side by side, then in semi-tandem position, and finally in tandem position. Difficulty with balance in these positions predicts an increased risk of falling. Although standardized instruments, such as the Tinetti Performance-Oriented Mobility Assessment (see the Appendix, p 426), may be used to quantify impairments in gait and balance, a qualitative assessment is usually sufficient to make recommendations about the need for an assistive device, such as a cane or walker. When assessing gait and balance, particularly among older women, clinicians should observe for the use of proper footwear, that is, flat, hard-soled shoes. (Also see the Appendix, p 391, for falls-assessment guidelines.)

Finally, clinicians can often glean useful functional information by observing their older patients complete simple tasks, such as unbuttoning and buttoning a shirt or blouse, picking up a pen and writing a sentence, taking off and putting on shoes, touching the back of the head with both hands, and climbing up and down from an examination table. Abnormalities detected during the self-reported or performance-based functional test may necessitate referral to rehabilitation specialists. (See "Rehabilitation," p 82)

Nutrition

Poor nutrition among older persons may reflect concurrent medical illness, depression, inability to shop or cook, inability to feed oneself, or financial hardship. Aside from visual inspection for signs of malnutrition, older persons should have their weight and height measured routinely. A low body mass index (ie, < 20 kg/m^2) or an unintentional weight loss of more than 10 pounds in 6 months suggests poor nutrition and should prompt further evaluation. (See "Malnutrition," p 182.)

Vision and Hearing

Although visual impairment from cataracts, glaucoma, macular degeneration, and abnormalities of accommodation usually worsens with age, older persons are often unaware of their visual deficits. Asking about difficulty with driving, watching television, or reading may uncover a problem with vision. As a brief performance-based screen, an older patient can be asked to read (using corrective lenses, if applicable) a short passage from a newspaper or magazine, with the caveat that low literacy is not an uncommon problem among older persons. Significant impairment in vision can be confirmed through the use of a Snellen chart or Jaeger card; the inability to read greater than 20/40 is the criterion standard. (See "Visual Impairment," p 169.)

The high prevalence of hearing loss among older persons and its association with depression, dissatisfaction with life, and withdrawal from social activities make it an important target for assessment. Assessment of the external auditory canal is essential, as cerumen impaction is a common cause of hearing loss in older adults. Hearing loss is usually bilateral and in the high-frequency range. Hearing should be assessed routinely during the history-taking session and can be assessed more formally using a hand-held audioscope. Inability to hear a 40-dB tone at 1000 or 2000 Hz in both ears or at either of these frequencies in one ear should be considered abnormal and, in the absence of cerumen impaction, should result in referral for formal audiometry testing. (See "Hearing Impairment," p 163.)

COGNITIVE ASSESSMENT

The prevalence of cognitive decline doubles every 5 years after the age of 65 and approaches 40% to 50% at age 90. Most patients with dementia do not complain of memory loss or even volunteer symptoms of cognitive impairment unless specifically questioned. Older persons with cognitive impairment, even in the absence of dementia, are at increased risk for accidents, delirium, medical nonadherence, and disability. Clinicians should incorporate brief cognitive screening strategies into their visits with older patients, especially those aged 75 years and older.

Because memory loss is typically the first sign of dementia, the best single screening question is recall of three words after 1 minute. Anything other than perfect recall should lead to further testing. The most commonly used instrument for formal testing of cognition is the Folstein Mini–Mental State Examination, which assesses orientation, registration and recall, attention and calculation, language, and visual-spatial skills. Although scores on the MMSE need to be interpreted in the context of educational attainment and age, scores lower than 24 warrant further evaluation for possible dementia.

An often overlooked area of cognition, which is essential for proper goal-directed behaviors, is executive control. The clock-drawing test is valuable because it assesses executive control and visual-spatial skills, two domains of cognition that are otherwise not tested or incompletely tested by the MMSE. In the clock-drawing test, the patient is asked to draw the face of a clock and to place the hands correctly to indicate 2:50 or 11:10. Another useful question to assess executive control is asking the patient to name as many four-legged animals as possible in 1 minute. Fewer than 8 to 10 animals or repetition of the same animals is abnormal and suggests the need for further evaluation.

PSYCHOLOGIC ASSESSMENT

Although the prevalence of major depression among community-dwelling older persons is only about 1% to 2%, a large number of older persons suffer from significant symptoms of depression below the severity threshold of major depression, as defined by the fourth edition of the *Diagnostic and Statistical Manual of Mental Disorders*. These subthreshold depressive symptoms have been shown to indicate an increased the risk of physical disability and slower recovery after an acute disabling event. A study, moreover, found that depressive symptoms in older persons are associated with a significant increase in the cost of medical services, even after adjusting for the severity of chronic medical illness. Hence, clinicians should have a high index of suspicion for depressive symptoms and a low threshold for treatment. The best single question to ask is, "Do you often feel sad or depressed?" An affirmative response warrants further evaluation of other depressive symptoms, perhaps through the use of a standardized instrument such as the 15-item Geriatric Depression Scale. (See the Appendix, p 390.)

Anxiety and worries are also important symptoms in older patients and are often a manifestation of an underlying depressive disorder. Finally, because older persons are particularly likely to experience the loss of a loved one, special efforts should be made to recognize and manage the consequences of bereavement. (See "Depression and Other Mood Disorders," p 211.)

SOCIAL ASSESSMENT

The social assessment consists of several elements, including the availability of a personal support system, the need for a caregiver or the nature of the caregiver's burden, the patient's economic well-being, the possibility of elder mistreatment, and the patient's advance directives. Although a comprehensive social assessment may not be feasible in a busy office practice, clinicians caring for older patients should be mindful of these special needs. Inquiring about the availability of help in case of an emergency might provide important clues to potential problems. For frail older persons, particularly those who lack social support, referral to a visiting nurse may be helpful in assessing home safety and level of personal risk. (See "Psychosocial Issues," p 13.)

QUALITY OF LIFE

During the past decade, quality of life has been embraced as a convenient catchphrase to denote important patient outcomes other than death and traditional physiologic measures of morbidity. Although a "gold standard" does not exist, most instruments designed to measure quality of life include various aspects of physical, cognitive, psychologic, and social function. Perhaps the most commonly used instrument is the Short Form-36 Health Survey (SF-36), which includes 36 items organized into eight domains—physical function; role limitations due to physical and emotional health; bodily pain; social functioning; mental health; vitality; and general health perceptions. (See Appendix, p 393.) The SF-36 has been tested extensively among community-living persons and hospitalized patients, but it may not be suitable for use among the oldest-old persons, especially those who are frail, because of floor effects and insensitivity to clinically important changes in health status.

COMPREHENSIVE GERIATRIC ASSESSMENT

Comprehensive geriatric assessment (CGA) is a diagnostic process intended to determine a patient's medical, psychosocial, and functional capabilities and limitations, with the goal of developing an overall plan for treatment and long-term follow-up. Because CGA typically requires a highly trained team of geriatric specialists in medicine, nursing, physical and occupational therapy, psychiatry, and social work, it is expensive and time consuming. Success generally requires the geriatric team to take over the direct care of the patient. An extended period of intensive team involvement with ongoing care is essential to assure the efficacy of the intervention. When the geriatric team assumes a purely consultative role (ie, without a role in implementing the recommendations), CGA is unlikely to be successful in improving patient outcomes.

CGA has had its greatest success, in terms of improving function and reducing nursing-home placement and hospital readmissions, in inpatient geriatric units that are staffed by highly trained professionals. Although an initial trial of annual in-home CGA by gerontologic nurse practitioners, in consultation with geriatricians, was found to be effective in reducing disability and nursing-home admissions, a published follow-up trial by the same set of investigators failed to demonstrate an overall benefit for this intervention. See the Appendix, p 402, for a general geriatric screen useful in primary care practice.

THE OLDER DRIVER

Evaluating the older driver presents a difficult challenge to the physician. The automobile is the most important, and often the only, source of transportation for older persons. Yet, a variety of age-related changes, chronic conditions, and medications place the older person at risk for automobile mishaps. Although the absolute number of crashes involving older drivers is low, the number of crashes per mile driven and the likelihood of serious injury or death are higher than for any age group other than those aged 16 to 24 years.

To their credit, the vast majority of older persons make prudent adjustments in their driving behaviors, by avoiding rush hour or congested thoroughfares or by not driving at night or during adverse weather conditions. Nonetheless, impaired older persons who continue to drive represent an important safety hazard, not only to themselves, but also to other drivers, passengers, and pedestrians. Although research is incomplete, pertinent risk factors include poor peripheral vision and near visual acuity (less than 20/40); dementia, particularly deficits in visual-spatial skills and visual attention; impaired neck and trunk rotation; limitations in range of motion of the shoulders, hips, and ankles; foot abnormalities; and poor motor coordination. Alcohol and medications that adversely affect alertness, such as narcotics, benzodiazepines, antihistamines, antidepressants, antipsychotics, hypnotics, and muscle relaxants, have also been shown to either increase crash risk or impair driving skills, as assessed by simulators or road tests.

Any report of an accident or moving violation should trigger an assessment of the patient's driving capacity. Clinicians should discuss their safety concerns honestly with the older driver, and ideally with a spouse or other family member, particularly when the patient lacks insight into his or her driving limitations. Alternative modes of transportation should be considered. Recommendations to stop driving, however, should not be proffered lightly, since driving cessation can lead to a decrease in activity level and an increase in depressive symptoms. Referral for a formal driving evaluation, by a skilled occupational therapist, may be helpful in confirming unsafe driving behaviors or, perhaps, in suggesting interventions, such as adaptive equipment, to correct for specific physical disabilities.

In the interest of public safety, physicians should know their state's law on reporting impaired drivers. In many states, physicians are encouraged, if not mandated, to report their concerns to the department of motor vehicles. (See also the section on driving in "Legal and Ethical Issues," p 25.)

CLINICIAN–PATIENT COMMUNICATION

Because of the demands of a busy clinical practice, the time available for office visits is often constrained. Time tends to be less important, however, than the skills of the clinician in facilitating communication with older patients. Table 8.2 lists several simple strategies that may be used to enhance communication. (See also the table on communication in "Hearing Impairment," p 167.) To accommodate the high prevalence of sensory deficits among older persons, particular attention should be given to the environment of the examination room. The use of simple, inexpensive amplification devices with lightweight earphones can be especially effective, even for the severely hearing impaired person. During the course of the interview, the clinician should go beyond the customary clinical inquiries by asking open-ended questions such as, "What would you like me to do for you?" Finding out what the patient wants can be a prime mechanism for-

Table 8.2—Effective Strategies to Enhance Communication

- Use a well-lit room and avoid backlighting.

- Minimize extraneous noise and interruptions.

- Carefully introduce yourself to establish a friendly relationship.

- Face the patient directly, sitting at eye level.

- Address the patient by his or her last name.

- Speak slowly in a deep tone.

- Inquire about hearing deficits and raise the volume of your voice accordingly.

- If necessary, write questions in large print.

- Allow sufficient time for the patient to answer.

- Touch the patient gently on the hand, arm, or shoulder during the conversation.

solving potential problems, generating trust, and improving mutual satisfaction in the clinician–patient relationship.

REFERENCES

- Boult C, Pacala JT. Care of older people at risk. In: Calkins E, Boult C, Wagner EH, et al., eds. *New Ways to Care for Older People: Building Systems Based on Evidence in Managed Care*. New York: Springer Publishing Company, 1999:65–84.

- Chodosh J, McCann RM, Frankel RM, et al. *Geriatric Assessment and the Twenty Minute Visit*. Rochester, New York: Division of Geriatrics, University of Rochester, School of Medicine and Dentistry; 1997.

- Fried LP, Guralnik JM. Disability in older adults: evidence regarding significance, etiology, and risk. *J Am Geriatr Soc*. 1997;45(1):92–100.

- Froehlich TE, Robison JT, Inouye SK. Screening for dementia in the outpatient setting: the time and change test. *J Am Geriatr Soc*. 1998;46(12):1506–1511.

- Gill TM, Robison JT, Williams CS, et al. Mismatches between the home environment and physical capabilities among community-living older persons. *J Am Geriatr Soc*. 1999;47(1):88–92.

- Saliba D, Orlando M, Wenger NS, et al. Identifying a short functional disability screen for older persons. *J Gerontol A Biol Sci Med Sci*. 2000;55(12):M750–756.

- Stuck AE, Walthert JM, Nikolaus T, et al. Risk factors for functional status decline in community-living elderly people: a systematic literature review. *Soc Sci Med*. 1999;48(4):445–469.

- Wallace M, ed. *Try This: Best Practices in Nursing Care to Older Adults*. New York: Hartford Institute for Geriatric Nursing; 1998–. Available at http://www.hartfordign.org/publications/trythis/

CHAPTER 9—ELDER MISTREATMENT

The term *elder mistreatment* generally refers to acts of omission or commission that result in harm or threatened harm to the health or welfare of an older adult, according to the *Diagnostic and Treatment Guidelines on Elder Abuse and Neglect* of the American Medical Association (AMA). Elder mistreatment (EM) is a syndrome that may manifest itself in a variety of ways. It may take the form of physical abuse, emotional abuse, intentional or unintentional neglect, financial exploitation, or abandonment, or it may be a combination of these. Research suggests that the national incidence of EM is approximately 450,000 annually, with a prevalence range of 700,000 to 1.2 million older adults, accounting for approximately 4% of those aged 65 years or older. Given these estimates, clinicians providing primary care to elderly people should routinely screen for EM.

Research conducted in the context of a longitudinal aging cohort study sought to determine the mortality of EM. In a pooled logistic regression that adjusted for demographics, chronic disease, functional status, social networks, cognitive status, and depressive symptoms, the risk of death was found to remain elevated for cohort members experiencing either EM or self-neglect. To date, no intervention studies have evaluated the impact of screening on health outcomes, and such studies are needed. However, screening for EM appears warranted, given the findings of case studies and longitudinal studies that document risk factors, as well as the information in the databases from the adult protective services organizations across the country.

RISK FACTORS AND PREVENTION

Risk factors for EM are known to include poverty, dependency of the elderly person for caregiving needs, age, race, functional disability, frailty, and cognitive impairment. Some factors may really be proxies for other variables. For example, lower socioeconomic status is often associated with fewer resources to meet caregiving demands.

Frail, debilitated older persons may need a level of care that at times exceeds caregiver ability. In particular, the demented person who exhibits disturbing behaviors, such as hitting, spitting, or screaming, poses immense challenges to caregivers. Caregiver stress may give way to any of the forms of EM, and a careful assessment of caregiver stress may identify opportunities to prevent EM. Table 9.1 lists factors that indicate

Table 9.1—Risk Factors for Inadequate or Abusive Caregiving

- Cognitive impairment in patient, caregiver, or both
- Dependency of the caregiver on the elderly patient, or vice versa
- Family conflict
- Family history of
  - abusive behavior
  - alcohol or drug misuse or abuse
  - mental illness
  - mental retardation
- Financial stress or lack of funds to meet new health demands
- Isolation of the patient or the caregiver, or both
- Living arrangements inadequate for the needs of the ill person
- Stressful events in the family, eg:
  - death of a loved one
  - loss of employment

a risk for the development of inadequate or abusive caregiving. A number of caregiver burden scales are available to help obtain the information the clinician needs to assess the potential for EM Screening for depression in the caregiver may also be appropriate. Shared living circumstances do not in themselves cause undue caregiver burden or stress.

HISTORY

An interdisciplinary approach to assessment and care planning is optimal. Comprehensive interdisciplinary geriatric assessment (see "Assessment," p 47) that includes the physical, psychosocial, and financial domains of the older adult should detect potential or any alleged EM.

The EM history, provided by both the older person and caregiver(s), should be conducted in privacy, so that the patient and the caregiver(s) can speak freely and frankly. Studies suggest that the different cultures of racial and ethnic groups define abuse and neglect very differently; thus, cultural sensitivity is important. The older patient or caregiver from a different culture than the clinician's may be offended by some EM screening questions. EM history questions should be carefully worded, in order to avoid alienating the patient or caregiver and closing down any further opportunity to help the patient and family.

Questions directed to the patient should become progressively specific if the patient's responses indicate that EM may be occurring. For example, the clinician might first ask, "Is there any difficult behavior in your family you would like to tell me about?" If the answer is positive, more specific questions to follow then might be, "Has anyone tried to hurt or hit you?" "Has anyone made you do things that you did not want to do?" "Has anyone taken your things?" Obtaining such information requires clinical interviewing skills similar to those needed when asking about sexual orientation, alcoholism, or substance abuse.

Caregivers should be interviewed privately, not necessarily to detect abusive or neglectful behavior, but in all cases to detect signs of stress, isolation, or depression, so that help for the caregiver can be provided, as needed. Caregivers may be reluctant to discuss their own problems in the presence of the person who depends on their care. Caregivers may range from registered professionals to well-intended neighbors, and it is important to know and to document the level of skill the caregiver has, as well as his or her understanding of the situation. The caregiver's level of understanding is an essential factor for evaluating the intentionality underlying any mistreatment of a dependent older person. For example, a registered nurse in a nursing home is held to a different level of accountability than a frail spouse providing care in the home setting.

Identification of shortcomings in the patient's care may be the most elusive aspect of a comprehensive assessment. The symptoms and signs of incomplete, inadequate, or neglectful caregiving may be subtle (eg, when a patient fails to do as well as expected on a given regimen), or attributable to the patient's physical or emotional disorders (eg, weight loss in a patient with a history of depression).

Effective assessment is that which detects EM without directing undue suspicion on well-meaning caregivers or undermining a family's ability to care for an older person with appropriate support and counseling.

Examples of symptoms and signs that indicate a particularly high level of risk for EM are listed in Table 9.2. Screening tools to detect EM have been developed by a number of institutions; these can be useful to clinicians as guides for their assessment of older patients for EM.

PHYSICAL ASSESSMENT

The clinician should look for physical indicators, such as bruises and welts in unusual places or in various stages of healing, that are incongruent with the patient's history. For example, bilateral bruises on the upper torso are rarely the result of falls and warrant follow-up. Other indications of possible EM include frequent, unexplained, or inconsistently explained falls and injuries, multiple emergency department visits, delays in seeking treatment, inconsistent follow-up, or constant switching among doctors. The clinician needs

Table 9.2—Signs That Raise Suspicion for Elder Mistreatment

Type of Mistreatment	Examples
Abandonment	Patient brought to clinic or emergency department by someone other than the caregiver
	Patient dropped off and abandoned at the facility by the caregiver
Abuse	Fractures or bruises in various stages of healing
	Repeated falls
	Unexplained azotemia
	Unexplained bruises, especially bilateral or on inner arms or thighs
Exploitation	Evidence that material goods are being taken in exchange for care
	Evidence that personal belongings (house, jewelry, car) are being taken over without consent or approval
	Unexplained loss of Social Security or pension checks
Neglect	Dermatitis from urine in contact with skin
	Inappropriate dress
	Listlessness, apathy
	Malnourishment
	Poor hygiene
	Pressure ulcers, especially unattended ulcers
	Reports of being left in an unsafe situation
	Reports of inability to get needed medication

to search for unusual patterns or marks, such as bruises on inner arms or thighs; cigarette, rope, chain, or chemical burns; lacerations and abrasions on the face, lips, and eyes; or marks occurring in areas of the body usually covered by clothes. The presence of head injuries, hair loss, or hemorrhages beneath the scalp as a consequence of hair pulling are significant markers. Cachectic states may be the result of malnutrition that is a consequence of neglect. Unusual discharges, bruising, bleeding, or trauma around the genitalia or rectum raise concern of possible sexual abuse, prompting gynecologic and rectal examinations to be performed.

The behavior of the patient when in the presence of the suspected abuser may be significant. An EM victim may avoid eye contact, or dart his or her eyes continuously. He or she may sit a distance away from an abusive caregiver, cringe, back off, or startle easily as if expecting to be struck. The caregiver may be nervous and fearful, or quiet and passive. The patient may defer excessively to the caregiver, who may invariably answer for the older adult or even try not to allow a private interview with or examination of the patient. Dubious explanations may be given to explain the patient's injuries.

The emergency department is an important setting for EM assessment. The emergency department may see older persons in crisis, and every effort should be made not to simply treat and release patients whose situation merits further assessment. Astute emergency personnel can identify cases where there may be serious safety problems in the caregiving situation.

PSYCHOLOGIC ASSESSMENT

EM is not invariably or entirely physical. Psychologic abuse or neglect is generally more difficult than outright physical abuse to detect and confirm, but it can be equally dangerous to the dependent older person. As mentioned above, the behavior of both the patient and the caregiver may provide important clues about the quality of their relationship and of the care the older person is receiving. Factors that suggest a poor or deteriorating social and emotional situation should be one focus of assessment for EM.

Psychologic abuse includes taunting, name-calling, the promotion of regressive behaviors by infantilization, making painful jokes at the expense of the patient, or other activities that are demeaning. The caregiver's style of communication should be observed. Impatience, irritability, and demeaning statements may indicate a pattern of verbal abuse. However, psychologic neglect or mistreatment by the caregiver may take more subtle forms. For example, failing to provide social or emotional stimulation, or restricting or preventing the patient's normal activities may result in the patient's total social isolation.

The patient's demeanor and emotional status may indicate the presence of psychologic neglect or abuse. For example, high levels of anxiety, fearfulness, and ambivalence or anger directed toward the caregiver are indications of the need for further assessment. Unexpected depression or uncharacteristic withdrawal also merits follow-up. Other high-risk behaviors include lack of adherence with treatment recommendations, frequent requests for sedating medication, or frequently canceled appointments.

Cognitive impairment and dementia are both known to be highly prevalent in older adults referred for evaluation for possible EM. When an older adult presents with cognitive impairment or dementia, the clinician should be especially alert for symptoms and signs of EM. Aggressive behaviors associated with certain stages of dementia may trigger abusive responses in caregivers. (See also "Neuropsychiatric and Behavioral Disturbances in Dementia," p 121.)

FINANCIAL ASSESSMENT

Financial mistreatment includes unauthorized use of the older adult's funds, possessions, or property. Fiscal neglect consists of the failure to use the older adult's funds and resources for his or her needs. Signs that the older patient is being mistreated financially include:

- a recent marked disparity between the patient's living conditions or appearance and his or her assets,
- a sudden inability to pay for health care or other basic needs,
- an unusual interest on the part of caregivers in the patient's assets.

SELF-NEGLECT

For some older persons, especially those who live in isolation or who choose to accept and endure mistreatment, self-neglect may be an issue. Successful management in such cases will require an assessment of the patient's capacity to understand the risks and benefits of the situation, as well as consequences of allowing circumstances to persist. (See sections on decisional capacity in "Legal and Ethical Issues," p 18.) These are complex situations, but the patient's right to autonomy and self-determination must be honored. Paternalistic viewpoints regarding what the older person "should" do need to be avoided. In self-neglect cases, the clinician may need support when coming to terms with the requirement to respect the decisionally capable older person's wishes when this involves his or her choosing to continue in an abusive or neglectful situation. (The clinical dilemma resembles that confronting clinicians who treat battered women.) Intervention contrary to the decisionally capable patient's choice is generally inappropriate, although this may be uncomfortable for the clinician. (See also the section on autonomy versus protectionism in "Legal and Ethical Issues," p 18.)

THE ROLE OF THE OLDER PERSON

The relationship of the older person with caregivers can be very complex, and dysfunctional relations between a dependent older person and a caregiver may not be the fault entirely of the caregiver. To approach such situations with the idea that the older person is inevitably the victim infantilizes the person and is unfair to caregivers. Situations in which older persons are mistreated can be arrayed along a spectrum from victimization to mutual abusiveness to relationships where the older person can be viewed as a witting cause of the mistreatment. Moreover, there are cases where the older person and his or her caregivers are making the best of a tragic situation.

The clinician must make every effort to determine the facts in a situation and fathom the motives of the people involved, to determine the best possible approach for ameliorating if not solving the problem. Consultation with social workers, psychologists, or psychiatrists may be useful. Reporting requirements are not limited in any way by these considerations. If an older man hits his son and the son strikes back, clinicians in most states are required to report the latter hitting.

INSTITUTIONAL MISTREATMENT

EM in the setting of home care by family or friends has been the focus of much of the discussion so far, but detecting and intervening to prevent EM in the institutional setting is also important. The two most common types of nursing home mistreatment are physical and sexual abuse. These are often due to negligent hiring and supervision of employees.

The Omnibus Budget Reconciliation Act of 1987 set a new standard for care in nursing homes. OBRA established a Nursing Home Bill of Rights for residents of Medicaid- and Medicare-certified facilities. The Nursing Home Bill of Rights states that residents, among other things, have the right to be free from physical and mental abuse. The Long-Term Care Ombudsman Program was created by the federal Older Americans Act in response to the need for a neutral third party to protect nursing-home residents. An ombudsman is responsible for investigating and resolving a broad range of issues or complaints regarding circumstances that adversely affect a nursing-home resident's health, safety, welfare, or rights. Adult and Elder Protective Service laws include institutional mistreatment in many states, and some states have separate institutional mistreatment statutes. Sexual abuse is also covered under state criminal statutes. (See "Nursing-Home Care," p 97.)

The clinician should be attentive to the possibility of abuse and neglect in any institutional setting and be ready to use the resources available through the institution itself or through state regulatory agencies to investigate and intervene, where appropriate. In cases of suspected institutional EM, the challenge is to balance the rights of staff members with the rights of patients. State departments of public health are usually responsible for investigating nursing-home abuse and neglect cases.

INTERVENTION

The clinician who suspects EM can use the following questions to guide intervention:

- How safe is the patient if I send him or her back to the current setting, or does he or she need to be removed to a safe environment?
- What services or resources are available locally to support the care of this older person?
- Are there any caregivers who have health problems of their own that need attention?
- Does this situation need the expertise of others (eg, in medicine, nursing, social work), and if so, who would best serve the patient's needs?

Successful intervention in cases of EM can become complex. Among the factors governing the clinician's course of action are these:

- the exact nature and degree of the EM,
- whether the patient can or will cooperate with evaluation and intervention, and
- whether the caregiver(s) can or will cooperate with evaluation and intervention.

Procedures and interventions are laid out in two algorithms developed under AMA auspices (see Figure 9.1 and Figure 9.2). Both algorithms take into account the issues highlighted above, especially the patient's safety, willingness to accept help, and capacity to understand and cooperate with the health care team.

Local resources in support of interventions for EM vary, but information is readily available. (See, eg, resources listed in the Appendix, p 418.) Consultation with the social work staff of the hospital, nursing home, or local health department may be a useful early step. Each state's Adult Protective Services will yield relevant information as well as direct assistance. In addition, the AMA Web site also provides a convenient starting point in the search for information and resources (http://www.ama-assn.org), as does the National Center on Elder Abuse (http://www.elderabusecenter.org).

THE MEDICAL-LEGAL INTERFACE

It is important to know state laws applicable to cases of EM; all 50 states and the District of Columbia have a reporting mechanism for EM, either through Adult Protective Services (APS) or state agencies associated with aging. Clinicians need to be familiar with the reporting mandates that apply in their area. In some states, neglect by others must be reported, but reports of self-neglect are not required. Adult children can be charged with neglect of the older parent if a caregiving relationship can be proven and it can also be proven that care has been precipitously withdrawn without substitute services. In states where self-neglect is reportable, this is usually the largest intake category.

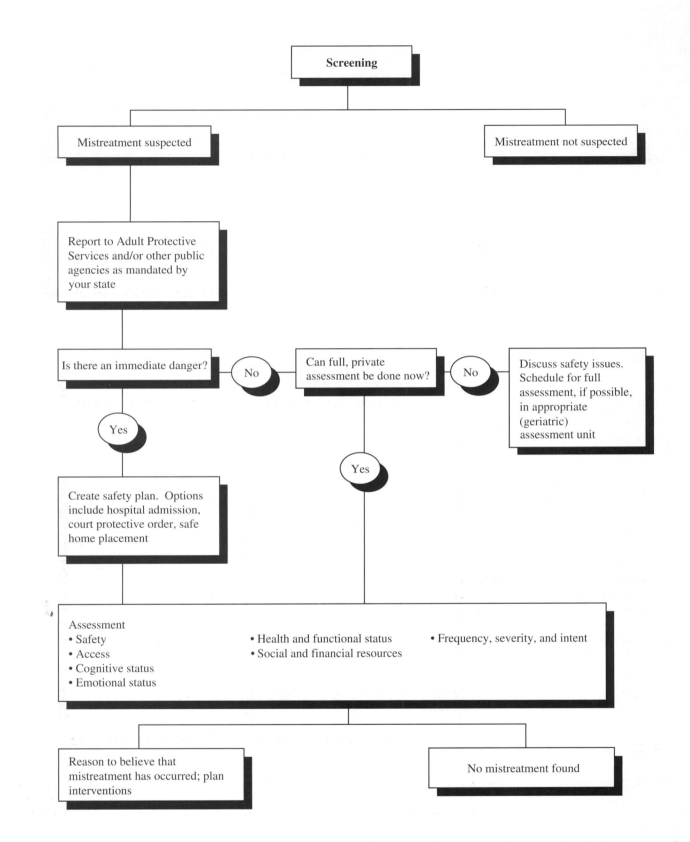

Figure 9.1—Assessment for elder mistreatment. Screening should be a routine part of the comprehensive assessment of all elderly patients.

SOURCE: Reprinted with permission from American Medical Association. *Diagnostic and Treatment Guidelines on Elder Abuse and Neglect*. Chicago, IL: American Medical Association; 1992:13.

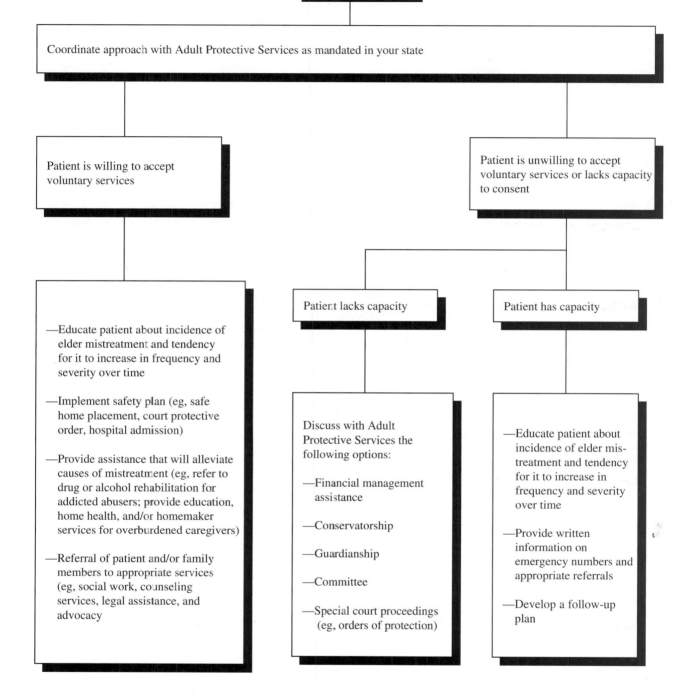

Figure 9.2—Case management in elder mistreatment. Choose the alternatives that least restrict the patient's independence and decision-making responsibilities, and that fulfill the state-mandated reporting requirements. The choice of interventions depends on the patient's cognitive status and decision-making capability and on whether the mistreatment is intentional or unintentional.

SOURCE: Reprinted with permission from American Medical Association. *Diagnostic and Treatment Guidelines on Elder Abuse and Neglect.* Chicago, IL: American Medical Association; 1992:14.

Finally, states may mandate reports for self-neglect but may not provide any services unless the older adult agrees to accept them.

Clinicians are in a key position to assess and report suspected EM, and most states require such reporting. Penalties may be assessed against a nonreporter in some regions. Reports of EM are confidential, and, as is the case with child abuse reporting, the clinical reporter is protected from litigation unless it can be proven that the report was made maliciously. The home page for the National Center on Elder Abuse (cited above) provides one means for reporting information; in addition, published articles include tables that review all 50 states and the procedures expected in each (see the references, p 58, and the resources listed in the Appendix, p 418). The AMA guidelines also provide clinical algorithms for reporting suspected EM cases (see Figure 9.1 and Figure 9.2 and the references, p 58).

Especially when a case is to be reported, photographs and body charts may be required to document the findings on physical examination. Risk management personnel can provide guidance in documentation and assist the clinician when evidence suggests there may be a need for police or court action. In any case where the clinician is called to court to discuss his or her findings, documentation is an important part of testimony. Although clinicians may be wary of acting precipitously, they should be willing to enlist the help of government agencies and the courts when EM is clearly dangerous for an older patient. EM cases are often extremely complicated, and it is likely that experts in several fields will need to work with clinicians and administrators to avoid under- or overreporting of EM and to provide the best outcomes for the victims of EM.

REFERENCES

■ Aravanis SC, Adelman RD, Breckman R, et al. *Diagnostic and Treatment Guidelines on Elder Abuse and Neglect.* Chicago, IL: American Medical Association; 1992.

■ Capezuti E, Brush BL, Lawson WT. Reporting elder mistreatment. *J Gerontol Nurs.* 1997;23(7):24–32.

■ Dyer CB, Pavlik VN, Murphy KP, et al. The high prevalence of depression and dementia in elder abuse or neglect. *J Am Geriatr Soc.* 2000;48(2):205–208.

■ Hirst SP. Defining resident abuse within the culture of long-term care institutions. *Clin Nurs Res.* 2002;11(3):267–284.

■ Lachs MS, Williams CS, O'Brien S, et al. The mortality of elder mistreatment. *JAMA.* 1998;280(5):428–432

■ The National Center on Elder Abuse at The American Public Human Services Association (Formerly the American Public Welfare Association) in Collaboration with Westat, Inc. *The National Elder Abuse Incidence Study; Final Report: September 1998.* Washington, DC: National Aging Information Center; 1998.

CHAPTER 10—PREVENTION

INTRODUCTION

As the population ages and the average active life expectancy increases, issues of primary and secondary prevention become increasingly important. The prevalence of undetected, correctable conditions and comorbid diseases is high in older adults. Moreover, a growing number of older adults are enthusiastic and highly motivated about disease prevention and health promotion. The clinician provides the information and opportunity for preventive care that helps older patients to maintain functional independence for as long as possible.

Many findings from research on preventive care and the appropriate components of periodic health examinations are inconclusive. In addition, older persons are typically not included in clinical trials of preventive strategies, which has limited the ability of geriatricians to adjust guidelines for preventive practices for patients aged 65 and older on the basis of new scientific findings. Primary care clinicians are consequently compelled to rely on clinical judgment in planning the preventive care of their older patients.

A number of factors, including age, functional status, comorbidity, patient preference, socioeconomic status, and the availability of care, affect health care decisions of the older adult. Unlike chronologic age, physiologic age may be determined by self-rated health and overall medical condition. Classifications that are based on life expectancy, physiologic age, and functional status may facilitate medical decision making with older patients. For example, the clinician might strongly recommend fecal occult blood testing (FOBT) to a healthy, functionally independent patient; discuss the potential pros and cons of FOBT and offer the test to a chronically ill, partially dependent patient; and actually recommend against FOBT for a severely frail, demented patient. It is important that the clinician consider all of the relevant issues in determining which conditions to screen for, the appropriate screening interval, and when (if ever) to discontinue screening in older patients.

Attention to the underlying principles of primary and secondary prevention is important for patients of any age. Screening measures should be systematically performed when the prevalence and morbidity or mortality of the condition outweigh both the economic cost and potential consequences of a falsely positive or negative test result. Some recommendations may be applicable only to high-risk individuals, not to the general population.

RECOMMENDED PREVENTIVE SERVICES

A number of preventive services have been shown to be effective in older persons and are widely endorsed. Table 10.1 summarizes these preventive activities, which are discussed below.

Screening

Hypertension

The prevalence of hypertension increases with advancing age. Treatment of hypertension in older adults has been associated with a reduction in morbidity and mortality from left ventricular hypertrophy, congestive heart failure, myocardial infarction, and stroke. However, older adults are more susceptible to adverse effects of antihypertensive therapy, such as hyponatremia, hypokalemia, depression, confusion, or postural hypotension. (See "Hypertension," p 256.)

Breast Cancer

It is unclear at what age, if any, mammography screening should be stopped. The U.S. Preventive Services Task Force (USPSTF) and the Canadian Task Force recommend biennial screening until age 70, the American College of Physicians recommends biennial screening until age 74, and the American Geriatrics Society supports screening every 2 to 3 years until age 85. Mammography screening at any age is more defensible if the patient has an active life expectancy of at least 3 years. Medicare provides coverage for annual screening mammograms. There is no compelling evidence that breast self-examination reduces breast cancer morbidity and mortality. (See "Oncology," p 349, and "Hormone Replacement Therapy," p 329.)

Colorectal Cancer

The USPSTF recommends annual FOBT or sigmoidoscopy every 5 years beginning at age 50. For older patients, colonoscopy every 10 years may be more cost-effective and have a more significant impact on colorectal cancer mortality than other screening programs. Medicare provides coverage for annual FOBT and biennial flexible sigmoidoscopy for all beneficiaries. As of July 1, 2001, Medicare will pay for a screening colonoscopy every 10 years for all beneficiaries. A screening barium enema may be substituted

.eventive Activity	Frequency (*year*)	Condition To Detect or Prevent
Screening		
Blood pressure	≤ 1	Hypertension
Mammography	2–3	Breast cancer
Fecal occult blood testing *and/or*	1	Colorectal cancer
flexible sigmoidoscopy *or*	5	
colonoscopy or double-contrast barium		
enema	10	
Pap smear	≤ 3*	Cervical cancer
Height and weight	≤ 1	Obesity, malnutrition
Alcoholism questionnaire	—**	Alcoholism
Depression questionnaire	1	Depression
Serum lipids in persons with prior myocardial infarction, angina	1	Recurrent CAD
Vision testing	1	Sensory deficits
Hearing ability	1	Hearing impairment
Counseling to encourage:		
Low-fat, well-balanced diet	1	Obesity, CAD
Adequate calcium intake	1	Osteoporosis
Physical activity	1	Immobility, CAD, osteoporosis
Injury prevention	1	Injurious falls, motor vehicle crashes, burns, other injuries
Smoking cessation	—†	COPD, many cancers, CAD
Regular dental visits	1	Malnutrition, oral cancers, edentulism
Immunization		
Influenza vaccination	1	Influenza
Pneumococcal vaccination	—‡	Pneumococcal disease
Tetanus booster	10	Tetanus
Chemoprophylaxis		
Discussion, implementation of hormone replacement therapy	—§	Osteoporosis
Aspirin therapy in persons with prior MI	daily	Additional MI, TIA, or stroke

NOTE: CAD = coronary artery disease; COPD = chronic obstructive pulmonary disease; MI = myocardial infarction; TIA = transient ischemic attack. For updates from the U.S. Preventive Services Task Force, see http://www.ahrg.gov/clinic/prevenix.htm

* May stop screening at age 65 if patient has had regularly normal smears up to that age; if never tested prior to age 65, may stop after two normal annual smears.

** Should be performed at initial visit and whenever problem drinking is suspected.

† Should be discussed at every visit of patients who smoke.

‡ Immunize once at age 65 for immunocompetent patients; revaccination after 7 to 10 years may be appropriate for high-risk immunocompromised patients.

§ Should be discussed at menopause and at least one more time after age 65.

for either a screening flexible sigmoidoscopy or a screening colonoscopy. "Virtual" colonoscopy, a new method using thin-section, helical computed tomography, is currently under investigation as a screening tool for colorectal cancer. Studies have refuted the concept that a low-fat, high-fiber diet plays a role in the prevention of colorectal cancer. Although epidemiologic data suggest that aspirin or nonsteroidal anti-inflammatory drugs may be protective against colorectal cancer, there is insufficient evidence to support the routine use of these medications for primary prevention. (See "Oncology," p 349.)

Cervical Cancer

Approximately 40% of new cases of invasive cervical cancer and deaths from cervical cancer occur in women aged 65 years and over. The Papanicolaou smear is most cost-effective in older patients who have previ-

ously had incomplete screening. Between 4% and 8% of cervical cancers are found in the cervical stump in women who have undergone incomplete hysterectomy. Regular Pap smears every 1 to 3 years are recommended for all women who are or have been sexually active and who have a cervix. Medicare has covered triennial screening without age limit since 1990. The appropriate cut-off age for screening remains controversial, although most experts recommend cessation of screening after age 65 if the patient has had a history of regularly normal smears. In older women never previously screened, screening can cease after two normal Pap smears are obtained 1 year apart.

Obesity or Malnutrition

Routine measurement of height and weight can be used to calculate body mass index (BMI). Obesity has been defined in men as a BMI ≥ 27.8 kg/m² and in women as a BMI $\geq 27.3 \text{ kg/m}^2$. An unintentional weight loss of 10 pounds in 6 months can indicate malnutrition or a serious occult illness. (See "Malnutrition," p 182.)

Alcoholism

All older adults should be screened for alcohol abuse at least once and whenever a drinking problem is suspected. Screening questionnaires such as the CAGE (see p 237, Table 36.1) can be useful in detecting alcohol problems. (See "Substance Abuse," p 234.)

Depression

The USPSTF recommends screening for depression when accurate diagnosis, effective treatment, and careful follow-up can be assured. Many tools to screen for depression are available. (See the Appendix p. 390.)

Dyslipidemia

There is good evidence that correcting lipid abnormalities (ie, levels of low-density lipoprotein $\geq 130 \text{ mg/dL}$, of high-density lipoprotein $\leq 35 \text{ mg/dL}$, of triglycerides $\geq 200 \text{ mg/dL}$) lowers the risk of recurrent cardiac events in older persons with prior myocardial infarction or angina. These persons should be screened for lipid abnormalities; treatment goals for those found to have dyslipidemia should be low-density lipoprotein levels of $< 100 \text{ mg/dL}$, high-density lipoprotein levels of $> 40 \text{ mg/dL}$, and triglycerides levels of $< 200 \text{ mg/dL}$. There is no evidence that screening older adults who are clinically free of coronary artery disease (CAD) or who have few cardiac risk factors for primary prevention of CAD is effective. (See "Cardiovascular Diseases and Disorders," p 243.)

Vision and Hearing Deficits

Uncorrected refractive errors, glaucoma, cataracts, and macular degeneration account for most undetected visual disorders. Routine screening with a Snellen chart is recommended by the USPSTF. Undetected hearing loss can lead to social isolation and may indicate other underlying disorders. The USPSTF recommends periodically questioning older adults about their hearing and counseling them about the availability of hearing aid devices. The evidence for routine audiometry as a screening tool is unproven. (See "Visual Impairment," p 169, and "Hearing Impairment," p 163.)

Counseling

Dietary Counseling

The importance of a well-balanced diet should be addressed routinely with older adults. An appropriate diet is high in fruits and vegetables and low in fat and salt, and has adequate calcium content. (See "Malnutrition," p 182.)

Physical Activity

Physical activity has been associated with greater mobility and lower rates of CAD and osteoporosis. Older adults should be counseled about an exercise program that balances modalities of flexibility (eg, stretching), endurance (eg, walking or cycling), strength (weight training), and balance (eg, Tai Chi or dance therapy). (See "Physical Activity," p 65.)

Injury Prevention

The USPSTF recommends counseling older persons on measures to reduce the risk of falling (see "Falls," p 143, and "Gait Disturbances," p 148, for details about preventing falls), safety-related skills and behaviors, and environmental hazard reduction. Safety-related behaviors include the regular use of seat and lap belts in automobiles, regular driving tests, and avoidance of alcohol use while driving or operating machinery. Environmental hazard reduction might include lowering hot-water temperature to prevent serious burns, installing smoke detectors, and, in homes of demented persons, installing alarms and automatic shut-off features on appliances and removing or safely storing firearms. A home safety checklist or formal environmental assessment by a physical or occupational therapist can facilitate injury prevention. (See the Appendix, p 416, for a checklist.)

Smoking Cessation

Smoking cessation at any age reduces rates of chronic obstructive pulmonary disease, many cancers, and CAD. All older adult smokers should be encouraged to and helped with smoking cessation at each office visit. (See "Substance Abuse," p 234, and "Respiratory Diseases and Disorders," p 302.)

Dental Care

Many common problems can be detected and effectively treated by regular dental visits, including malnutrition, xerostomia, and oral cancers. (See "Oral Diseases and Disorders," p 307.)

Immunizations

Medicare covers the costs of influenza, pneumococcal, and tetanus immunizations.

Influenza Vaccine

The current influenza vaccine is a killed virus that is moderately immunogenic, with estimated efficacy rates of 70% for illness and 90% for mortality. Multiple evaluations of the vaccine's efficacy reveal that, although it incompletely protects against disease, it clearly reduces rates of respiratory illness, hospitalization, and mortality in the older age group. Annual vaccine administration must be provided because of antigenic drift and the short-lived (4 to 5 months) protection provided by the vaccine. Current recommendations are that all patients aged 65 or over or those under age 65 with underlying medical illnesses be immunized annually between October and mid-November, but any time from September to the end of influenza season is appropriate. Medical personnel and caregivers for high-risk patients should also be immunized. Potential adverse effects include fever, chills, myalgias, and malaise, but these are rare. Contraindications include anaphylactic egg hypersensitivity or allergic reactions following occupational exposure to egg protein. Live, attenuated influenza vaccines have been developed, appear to be more effective, and are likely to be approved for widespread use in the near future.

In outbreak situations, chemoprophylaxis can protect against influenza during the 2 weeks immediately after immunization until the antibody response is mounted, or in persons who cannot receive the vaccine. Amantadine, rimantadine, zanamivir, and oseltamivir are all effective for influenza A, but they differ greatly with regard to cost, side effects, mechanism of action, and mode of delivery. Only the neuraminidase inhibitors zanamivir and oseltamivir have activity against influenza B. Zanamivir is administered via a disk-inhaler system; the others are taken orally.

Treatment of influenza is also possible with any of the four drugs and reduces the duration of illness by about 1 to 1.5 days, if started within 24 hours of symptom onset. Again, only the neuraminidase inhibitors can be used for treatment of influenza B. Resistance to amantadine and rimantadine can develop rapidly in many persons during the course of treatment; resistance to the neuraminidase inhibitors is less well characterized at this time.

Pneumococcal Vaccination

Pneumococcal vaccination is indicated for all persons aged 65 years or older and many persons under age 65 with comorbid conditions. If ≥ 5 years has elapsed since the first dose and the patient was vaccinated prior to the age of 65, repeat vaccination is indicated. Studies show that adverse events following revaccination are rare and mild. Thus, an unknown vaccination history should prompt administration of the pneumococcal vaccine. (*When in doubt, vaccinate!*) The vaccine does not prevent mucosal disease such as sinusitis and has unclear efficacy for preventing pneumonia. However, there is strong evidence that suggests that the vaccine reduces the risk of invasive disease (ie, bacteremia) and that it is cost-effective for older, immune, competent adults.

Although the protective efficacy of the pneumococcal vaccine is estimated to be only 60% to 70% and studies have revealed mixed results regarding benefits in high-risk older adults, all patients aged 65 years and older should receive one dose of 0.5 mg IM. Studies suggest that high-risk individuals may benefit from revaccination every 7 to 10 years. Other than local soreness, adverse effects are usually minimal.

Tetanus Vaccination

More than 60% of tetanus infections occur in persons aged 60 years of age and older. There is evidence that the absorbed tetanus and diphtheria toxoids provide long-term protection 35 years after the primary series or booster. Older adults who have never been vaccinated should receive two doses, 0.5 mg IM 1 to 2 months apart, followed by an additional dose 6 to 12 months later. The optimal interval for booster doses is not established; the USPSTF and Canadian Task Force recommend booster vaccinations every 10 years. Local pain and swelling or, rarely, hypersensitivity may accompany vaccination. A neurologic or hypersensitivity reaction to a previous dose is an absolute contraindication.

Chemoprophylaxis: Hormone Replacement Therapy

The potential risks and benefits of hormone replacement therapy should be discussed with all women who are perimenopausal and at least once after the age of 65. (See "Hormone Replacement Therapy," p 329.)

OTHER PREVENTIVE SERVICES TO CONSIDER

A number of other preventive activities are recommended by assorted specialty organizations even though the evidence for effectiveness is lacking. Some of these preventive measures are listed in Table 10.2. In the face of unproven effectiveness for each of these

Table 10.2—Potentially Beneficial Services Lacking Evidence

Preventive Activity	Condition to Detect or Prevent
Screening	
Blood glucose	Diabetic complications
Thyrotropin	Hypo- and hyperthyroidism
Mental status examination	Dementia
Depression screening questionnaire	Depression
Serum lipids in persons without apparent CAD	MI, angina
Bone densitometry	Osteoporosis
PSA *and/or* digital rectal examination	Prostate cancer
Skin inspection	Skin cancer
Chemoprophylaxis	
Aspirin therapy	Initial MI, stroke, colon cancer

NOTE: CAD = coronary artery disease; MI = myocardial infarction; PSA = prostate specific antigen.

* Serial bone densities may be helpful in determining the risk of developing osteoporosis.

procedures, clinicians must weigh the potential benefits of the preventive procedure against the potential risks of unnecessary treatment. Procedures that are particularly pertinent and controversial in the older adult population are discussed below.

Screening

Diabetes Mellitus

The increased prevalence of diabetes mellitus with age and the consequent morbidity burden warrants consideration for prevention. Routine screening of asymptomatic adults for diabetes is not recommended by the USPSTF; however, measurement of fasting glucose may be appropriate for high-risk older persons. (See "Endocrine and Metabolic Disorders," p 319.)

Thyroid Disease

The prevalence of subclinical and clinical hyperthyroidism and hypothyroidism increase with advancing age. The USPSTF does not recommend routine screening but acknowledges that screening may be performed on the basis of the high prevalence of the disease and the likelihood that its symptoms will be overlooked in older adults. The preferred test is the immunometric assay that is sensitive to thyrotropin. (See "Endocrine and Metabolic Disorders," p 319.)

Dementia

See "Dementia" (p 113).

Depression

Older patients with a positive personal or family history of depression, chronic underlying illness, recent loss, or sleep disorder are at high risk for the development of depression. The USPSTF recommends maintaining a high index of suspicion for depressive symptoms in high-risk persons. There are several reliable and valid depression screening instruments, including the Geriatric Depression Scale (see the Appendix, p 390; "Depression and Other Mood Disorders," p 211).

Osteoporosis

Although certain organizations recommend screening bone density measurements in all older women, the evidence to support routine bone mineral densitometry for the general population is lacking. The USPSTF does recommend that all older women be counseled about hormone replacement therapy, adequate calcium intake, smoking cessation, exercise, and avoidance of falls and injuries in order to prevent osteoporosis and fall-related fractures. (See "Osteoporosis and Osteomalacia," p 174.)

Prostate Cancer

Randomized, controlled trials of screening by prostate-specific antigen or digital rectal examination, currently in progress, should provide valuable information on the efficacy of these modalities. Until the results of those trials are known, however, patients should be counseled about the implications of an elevated prostate-specific antigen level or a mass detected by digital rectal examination and the potential adverse effects (surgery, incontinence, impotence) of treating false or even true positives. The American College of Physicians supports selected testing in 50- to 69-year-old men, provided that optimistic assumptions are used and the risks, benefits, and uncertainties are understood. With evidence currently available, it is difficult to justify screening in men aged 70 and over. Medicare covers the cost of prostate cancer screening. (See "Prostate Disease," p 366.)

Skin Cancer

The USPSTF recommends neither for nor against annual skin examination to detect early skin cancers because of a lack of research-proven effectiveness. However, the relatively low cost associated with annual skin examinations and the low costs and morbidity associated with treatment (eg, excision, cryotherapy) of false positives makes the decision to screen for skin cancer considerably less weighty than for prostate cancer. The USPSTF does recommend counseling high-risk patients (those who are light-skinned or with a past history of skin cancer) to avoid excess sun exposure and to use protective clothing when outdoors. (See "Dermatologic Diseases and Disorders," p 372.)

Chemoprophylaxis: Aspirin Therapy

Aspirin therapy up to 500 mg per day has not been consistently shown to reduce myocardial infarction or cardiovascular mortality. The adverse bleeding effects of aspirin increase with age, although the absolute serious side effect rate of dosages ≤ 325 mg per day is low. Older adults with risk factors for myocardial infarction or stroke may be more appropriate for prophylaxis with aspirin. (See "Cardiovascular Diseases and Disorders," p 243.)

PREVENTIVE SERVICES NOT INDICATED IN OLDER ADULTS

Table 10.3 lists services that have been shown not to be effective in preventing certain conditions or their adverse outcomes. There is mounting evidence that the general screening modality of the annual complete history and physical examination is not any more effective for improving outcomes than a more targeted approach of individual screening, counseling, immunoprophylaxis, and chemoprophylaxis. Current evidence does not support specific screening for lung, ovarian, pancreatic, bladder, or hematologic malignancies for the general population. However, promising new screening modalities, such as helical low-density computed tomography of the chest for lung cancer and homocystinemia for heart disease, are actively being developed and investigated.

DELIVERY OF PREVENTIVE SERVICES

A well-organized systems-based approach, using various personnel, sites, and communication modalities, may narrow the gap between the knowledge of age-appropriate practice recommendations and the implementation of preventive measures. Lack of time and inadequate reimbursement are only two of the barriers faced by clinicians. Overcoming these barriers commonly involves the assistance of paramedical personnel and the use of technology. Reminders may prompt clinicians to offer selected screening tests and improve adherence to recommendations. Mailed or computer-generated reminders may be used to enhance

Table 10.3—Preventive Services That Have Been Demonstrated Not To Be Beneficial

Screening for Specific Diseases
  Bladder cancer
  Lung cancer
  Hematologic malignancies
  Ovarian cancer
  Pancreatic cancer

Routine Laboratory Testing
  Annual blood chemistry panel
  Annual chest radiography
  Annual complete blood cell count
  Annual electrocardiogram

screening rates for procedures such as mammography, colorectal cancer screening, and influenza vaccination. Automated telephone technology may be useful to assess troublesome behaviors and even deliver behavioral interventions for improving medication adherence, dietary modification, and physical activity among sedentary persons. Primary and secondary preventive services may be provided at a variety of sites, including ambulatory clinics, assisted-living and long-term-care facilities, mobile vans, and supermarket-based pharmacies.

The implementation and evaluation of novel approaches for preventive practice are clearly warranted if progress is to be made in this increasingly important field. The more the primary care physician is able to rely upon others to explain and perform preventive maneuvers, the greater the likelihood that the patient adherence will improve as well.

REFERENCES

- American Geriatrics Society Clinical Practice Committee. Breast cancer screening in older women. *J Am Geriatr Soc.* 2000; 48(7):842–844.

- Christmas C, Andersen RA. Exercise and older patients: guidelines for the clinician. *J Am Geriatr Soc.* 2000; 48(3):318–324.

- Edelberg HK, Wei JY. Primary-care guidelines for community-living older persons. *Clin Geriatrics.* 1999;7:42–55.

- Humphrey LL, Helfand M, Chan BK, et al. Breast cancer screening: a summary of the evidence for the U.S. Preventive Services Task Force. *Ann Intern Med.* 2002;137(5 part 1):347–360.

- Kinsinger LS, Harris R, Woolf SH, et al. Chemoprevention of breast cancer: a summary of the evidence for the U.S.

Preventive Services Task Force. *Ann Intern Med.* 2002;137(1):59–69.

■ Pignone M, Saha S, Hoerger T, et al. Cost-effectiveness analyses of colorectal cancer screening: a systematic review for the U.S. Preventive Services Task Force. *Ann Intern Med.* 2002;137(2):96–104.

■ Resnick B. Health promotion practices of older adults: testing an individualized approach. *J Clin Nurs.* 2003;12(1):46–55; discussion 56.

■ Rowe JW. Geriatrics, prevention and the remodeling of Medicare. *N Engl J Med.* 1999;340(9):720–721.

■ Screening for osteoporosis in postmenopausal women: recommendations and rationale. *Ann Intern Med.* 2002;127(6):526–528.

■ U.S. Preventive Service Task Force. Screening for colorectal cancer: recommendation and rationale. *Ann Intern Med.* 2002;137(2):129–131.

CHAPTER 11—PHYSICAL ACTIVITY

*P*hysical activity is defined as bodily movement produced by skeletal muscles that expends energy. *Exercise* is a subset of physical activity that involves a structured program designed to improve one or more components of fitness. The level of physical activity in older adults is a major determinant of chronic disease burden, functional limitations, dependence, and mortality. The exact effects of activity depend on its type, duration, frequency, and intensity. Promoting physical activity is one of the most important and effective preventive and therapeutic interventions in older adults.

PREVENTIVE HEALTH EFFECTS

Prevention of Disease and Mortality

Regular physical activity has beneficial effects on most (if not all) organ systems, and consequently it prevents a broad range of health problems and diseases. There is longstanding scientific consensus that physical activity reduces the risk of cardiovascular disease, high blood pressure, non-insulin-dependent diabetes mellitus, obesity, osteoporosis, and colon cancer. There is substantial evidence that physical activity prevents sarcopenia, depressive illness, some lipid disorders, fall-related injuries, and stroke. Preliminary evidence links physical inactivity to an increased risk of gall stones, sleep problems, and decline in immune function. Whether inactivity might be a risk factor for breast, testicular, prostate, ovarian, endometrial, lung, and other cancers is under investigation.

Consistent with its breadth of physiologic effects, regular physical activity decreases both cardiovascular mortality and noncardiovascular mortality in older adults. The mortality benefit is large; some studies report that inactive older adults have mortality rates that are twice as high as those of active adults.

The health benefits of physical activity accrue independently of other risk factors. For example, sedentary, obese smokers will experience health benefits from increasing physical activity, even if they continue to smoke and do not lose weight.

Prevention of Functional Limitations and Dependency

Regular physical activity substantially delays the onset of functional limitations and loss of independence. A Danish study reported that inactive 75- to 80-year-old adults were more than four times more likely to be dependent at 5-year follow-up. An analysis of Established Populations for Epidemiologic Studies of the Elderly (EPESE) data reported that inactive, nonsmoking women at age 65 have 12.7 years of active life expectancy, compared with 18.4 years of active life expectancy for highly active women, and higher levels of physical activity were associated with fewer years of disability preceding death.

Randomized trials of exercise in older adults show that exercise improves functional limitations and health-related quality of life. Generally speaking, the benefits of exercise are most demonstrable in older adults with low fitness and clinically significant functional limitations. It has been more difficult to demonstrate exercise effects in relatively healthy older adults with mild functional limitations. A study of relatively healthy adults used a highly sensitive physical performance measure and reported that 6 months of endurance and strengthening exercise caused a 14% improvement in functional limitations. These results suggest that even relatively healthy older adults experience some functional gains with exercise.

Reduction of Health Care Costs

Physically active older adults have lower health care costs. The estimated health care costs due to inactivity in all age groups is about $25 billion to $100 billion per year (or 2.4% to 9.4% of all health care costs), depending upon what percentage of health care costs due to obesity are attributed to physical inactivity. The few data about the cost-effectiveness of promoting physical activity in older adults are promising. For example, a European study estimated that twice-weekly exercise classes for older adults would cost roughly $500 per life year saved—a much lower cost per life year saved than most accepted medical treatments.

AMOUNT OF PHYSICAL ACTIVITY

Recommended Amount of Activity

The 1996 U.S. Preventive Services Task Force report does not recommend a medical evaluation of healthy asymptomatic adults before increasing their level of activity. However, it is reasonable for adults with chronic illness to consult their primary care provider before substantially increasing or decreasing activity levels. The purpose of such consultation is to coordinate physical activity with medical management and possibly to do additional medical evaluation to minimize the risk of exercise injuries.

A moderate amount of physical activity has substantial health benefits and is recommended for all adults, including older adults. Current recommendations regarding physical activity are shown in Table 11.1. The definitions of a moderate amount of activity differ slightly; generally speaking, a moderate amount of activity expends about 150 to 200 kcal per day over 30 to 45 minutes on at least 5 days per week. A common example of a moderate amount of activity is 30 to 45 minutes of a brisk walk, that is, a walk at 3 to 4 mph that expends 4 to 7 kcal per minute.

In the United States, older adults are the least physically active age group. National surveillance data from the Centers for Disease Control and Prevention show that about 35% of adults aged 65 to 75 and 46% of adults 75 years and older are sedentary. About 40% to 45% of adults are insufficiently active, and only about 20% to 25% of older adults achieve the recommended moderate amount of activity. There has been no improvement in activity levels of older adults over the past decade.

Several bouts of activity as short as 10 minutes each may substitute for one 30- to 45-minute bout. Short bouts of activity can be more feasible and are preferred by older adults with symptoms that limit exercise, such as arthritis pain.

Recommendations emphasize that older adults can be sufficiently active by performing activities of daily life, such as walking as a means of transportation, gardening, and performing some household chores. It is not necessary for older adults to travel to an exercise class. Indeed, surveys show that most older adults do not prefer this option. However, exercise classes can be useful for older adults just starting to be more active, as classes provide supervision, instruction, and motivation. Some older adults prefer supervised, home-based exercise classes rather than travel to an exercise center.

Recommending that older adults attain and monitor exercise-induced sweating is questionable. Whether activity causes perspiration depends on several factors, including the duration of activity, the ambient temperature, and the person's clothing and gender. A study found that monitoring exercise-induced sweating is less reliable for monitoring activity levels in older adults. For some older adults, sweating is an unpleasant aspect of activity, and mentioning it makes counseling more difficult. Monitoring either heart rate or symp-

Table 11.1—Selected Current Recommendations on Physical Activity

Source	Recommendation
Centers for Disease Control and Prevention with the American College of Sports Medicine (1995)	"Every US adult should accumulate 30 minutes or more of moderate-intensity physical activity on most, preferably all, days of the week."
U.S. Surgeon General's Report, *Physical Activity and Health* (1996)	"Significant health benefits can be obtained by including a moderate amount of physical activity (eg, 30 minutes of brisk walking or raking leaves, 15 minutes of running, or 45 minutes of playing volleyball) on most, if not all, days of the week."
Healthy People 2010 (2000)	Objective 22-1. "Reduce the proportion of adults who engage in no leisure-time activity." Objective 22-2: "Increase the proportion of adults who engage regularly, preferably daily, in moderate physical activity for at least 30 minutes per day."

SOURCE: Data from: (1) Pate RR, Pratt M, Blair SN, et al. Physical activity and public health: a recommendation from the Centers for Disease Control and Prevention and the American College of Sports Medicine. *JAMA*. 1995;273(5):402–402. (2) US Department of Health and Human Services. *Physical Activity and Health: A Report of the Surgeon General.* Atlanta, GA: US Department of Health and Human Services, Centers for Disease Control and Prevention, National Center for Chronic Disease Prevention and Health Promotion, 1996. (3) US Department of Health and Human Services. *Tracking Healthy People 2010.* Washington, DC: US Government Printing Office, November 2000. Also available at (http://www.cdc.gov/nchs/hphome.htm)

toms with exercise can be a useful way to guide exercise intensity. In group programs, an exercise leader can help older adults "calibrate" themselves to maintain their exercising at moderate levels of intensity.

Optimal Amount of Activity

There is an incompletely characterized, nonlinear relationship between the "dose" of physical activity and the health benefits. Although a moderate amount of physical activity is sufficient to realize some benefit, achieving all possible health benefits requires higher amounts of activity. The dose-response relationship also means that low amounts of activity have important health benefits and are therefore preferable to a sedentary life style.

Although the optimal dose of activity is not known precisely, it is reasonable to encourage older adults who meet moderate activity recommendations to increase their level of activity to maximize health benefits. The most important aspect of increasing activity is to perform a mix of activities that promote endurance, strength, balance, and flexibility and that affect all aspects of fitness. When exercise is performed above a minimal threshold, the total volume of activity as measured by total kcal of energy expenditure is important. That is, the effects of lower intensity–longer duration bouts appear to be similar to those of higher intensity–shorter duration bouts, if total energy expenditure of both bouts is similar. Therefore, programs with moderate intensity–longer duration are preferred for most older adults, as moderate-intensity training has lower injury risk and better adherence. It is generally not recommended that older adults increase activity levels by running unless they are habitual runners, as studies report high rates of exercise-related injuries in older adults who start running.

SARCOPENIA AND RESISTANCE TRAINING

Sarcopenia

Age-related decreases in skeletal muscle mass and quality, termed *sarcopenia*, contribute to functional limitations and dependence in older adults. Sarcopenia is more than just disuse atrophy, as even highly trained older athletes loose muscle mass with age. The biologic mechanisms for sarcopenia are incompletely understood. Neurogenic mechanisms may involve loss of motor neurons for a variety of reasons, such as exposure to toxins (eg, heavy metals and alcohol), loss of blood supply, and mechanical damage. Denervated muscle fibers can be reinnervated by axonal sprouting of remaining motor neurons, but the process appears to be incomplete, so that cycles of denervation and reinnervation result in net loss of fibers. Myogenic mechanisms include the possibility that repair processes for contraction-induced muscle damage are impaired with aging. General mechanisms of cell damage may involve skeletal muscle. For example, skeletal muscle mitochondrial DNA and consequently oxidative function may be damaged by the free radicals produced by aerobic cells.

Prospective cohort studies suggest that regular physical activity in old age greatly reduces loss of muscle mass. For example, one study of 22 active older men found no change in fat-free mass over 6.5 years. A Finnish study reported that everyday physical activities, such as household work, walking, and gardening, were effective at maintaining skeletal muscle strength at a level adequate for independent living.

Resistance Training

Isotonic resistance training has been extensively studied and is recommended as a means of building muscle mass and counteracting sarcopenia. In contrast, there are few studies of the benefits of isokinetic and isometric resistance training. The initial enthusiasm was for optimal resistance training regimens—3 days per week of vigorous intensity training involving multiple sets per muscle group. Subsequently it was shown that lesser amounts of training have both physiologic effects on muscle function and health benefits; 2 days per week of resistance training is sufficient, and even 1 day per week has some benefits. One set of 10 to 15 repetitions for 8 to 10 exercises is sufficient. It is reasonable to recommend that older adults perform daily activities that increase muscle strength, such as heavy chores, but there are few data on how much a person's strength can be increased with this approach.

Vigorous, or high-intensity, resistance training involves a resistance that is at least 70% of the one repetition maximum (the maximum weight a person can lift just once). Resistance training of vigorous intensity produces muscular hypertrophy and large changes in muscle strength, from 30% to over 100%, with 3 to 6 months of training. Older adults gain strength steadily for many months without substantial "plateau effect." With proper supervision, vigorous training is safe even for nursing-home residents. However, it is time consuming and less practical, as vigorous resistance training essentially requires weight machines or comparable equipment. Vigorous training probably causes subclinical muscle injury and an associated inflammatory response, causing some experts to raise concerns about routinely recommending vigorous training for older adults.

In contrast, moderate-intensity resistance training programs typically use free weights such as weight cuffs or dumbbells at a lower exercise stimulus. In theory, a moderate-intensity program can be based upon the progressive overload principle and, given sufficient repetitions, strength should increase steadily. In practice, many participants in these programs do not progress steadily in weight lifted, and programs typically report 10% to 30% gains in strength over 3 to 6 months. However, randomized trials of such programs report several beneficial health effects in the exercise groups, such as improved measures of gait, balance, and overall physical function, as well as reduced fall risk. Programs are inexpensive and can be done safely with older adults in a variety of settings, such as nursing homes, senior centers, and residences.

Resistance training has become a standard component of many therapeutic exercise programs, including cardiac rehabilitation and pulmonary rehabilitation (Table 11.2). Strength training can improve glycemic control in older adults with diabetes mellitus. Resistance training is effective in improving function and joint symptoms of older adults with osteoarthritis.

OSTEOPOROSIS, FALLS, FRACTURES, AND BALANCE TRAINING

As noted by the National Institutes of Health consensus conference on osteoporosis (Table 11.2), regular physical activity by older adults probably has a modest effect in slowing age-related loss of bone mass. Some evidence indicates that resistance and high-impact exercise are the most beneficial. Weight-bearing aerobic activities also can provide the mechanical loading that maintains bone mass.

Randomized trials demonstrate that in older adults at increased risk for falls, about 25% of falls can be prevented by multicomponent interventions targeting factors such as sedative use, environmental hazards, and poor balance. Increasing physical activity is regarded as an effective component of fall prevention programs. A meta-analysis of the FICSIT (Frailty and Injury: Cooperative Studies of Intervention Techniques) studies suggests that one effect of exercises that improve balance was a reduction in fall risk. A meta-analysis of epidemiologic studies reported that physical activity was found to reduce risk of hip fracture by up to 50% and concluded that daily activities such as walking and climbing stairs reduce hip fracture risk. However, there is no experimental evidence that exercise reduces either total fractures or hip fractures.

BALANCE TRAINING

Some types of balance training, such as Tai Chi, can improve balance in older adults and reduce risk of falls.

Some programs prescribe separate balance exercises, such as standing on narrow bases of support (eg, a one-leg stand). Other programs, such as the program described in the book *Exercise: A Guide from the National Institute on Aging*, or that developed for Age Page by the American Geriatrics Society and the National Institute on Aging entitled "Exercise: Feeling Fit for Life" (http://www.nih.gov/health/agepages/exercise.htm) propose that some stretching and strengthening exercises can be done in a manner that also improves balance. Balance exercises can be graduated in difficulty, and older adults progress to more difficult exercises as training causes improved balance. For example, a tandem-walk exercise is easiest when holding onto a table and becomes progressively harder with arms in any position, arms close to the body, and arms close to the body and holding a weight.

WALKING AND AEROBIC ACTIVITIES

Walking is the core activity in most exercise plans for older adults. Walking remains, by far, the most common and popular form of physical activity for older adults. The health benefits of walking are confirmed by studies showing that walking by older adults reduces mortality, reduces risk of cardiovascular disease, and mitigates risk factors for falls. Of course, some older adults prefer other forms of aerobic activity, such as swimming, biking, dancing, and racket sports.

REDUCING SEDENTARY BEHAVIOR

Clinically significant health benefits accrue from reducing sedentary behavior, even if an older adult does not attain recommended moderate amounts of activity. For example, the Nurses Health Study reported dose-response data between physical activity and risk of coronary events. In this study, an activity level roughly equivalent to 10 minutes a day of moderate activity was found to reduce the risk of coronary events by about 23%, and an activity level roughly equivalent to 22 minutes a day reduced the risk by about 35%. Activity levels comparable to the recommended 30 to 45 minutes reduced the risk by more than 50%.

Several experimental studies report that clinically meaningful improvements in function and disability occur in exercise programs that cause only small improvements in fitness. For example, the Fitness, Arthritis, and Seniors Trial reported that 2% to 4% improvements in aerobic fitness and leg strength caused 8% to 10% improvements in functional limitations and disability. The Dunedin New Zealand falls prevention study in women aged 80 and over reported that 90 minutes of walking per week supplemented by

Table 11.2—Selected Clinical Practice Guidelines That Include Recommendations for Physical Activity

Topic	Guideline Source	Activity Recommended
Cardiovascular disease	NIH Consensus Conference on Physical Activity and Cardiovascular Health	Increased physical activity benefits adults with "clinically significant CVD, including myocardial infarction, angina pectoris, peripheral vascular disease, and congestive heart failure. Benefits include reduction in mortality, reduction in symptoms, improvement in exercise tolerance and functional capacity, and improvement in quality of life."
Cholesterol	Second Report of the Expert Panel on Detection, Evaluation, and Treatment of High Blood Cholesterol in Adults	Physical activity is regarded as an essential component of nonpharmacologic treatment of elevated cholesterol.
Chronic lung disease	American College of Chest Physicians with the American Association of Cardiovascular and Pulmonary Rehabilitation Guidelines Panel	Lower- and upper-extremity training should be included in pulmonary rehabilitation.
Diabetes mellitus	American Diabetes Association	Aerobic exercise is recommended with precautions to prevent foot injury. Moderate weight-training programs can be used for nearly all patients with diabetes.
Falls	American Geriatrics Society with the British Geriatrics Society and American Academy of Orthopaedic Surgeons	"Older people who have recurrent falls should be offered long-term exercise and balance training."
High blood pressure	Sixth Report of the Joint National Committee on Prevention, Detection, Evaluation, and Treatment of High Blood Pressure	"Blood pressure can be lowered with moderately intense physical activity (40 to 60 percent of maximum oxygen consumption), such as 30–45 minutes of brisk walking most days of the week."
Knee osteoarthritis	American College of Rheumatology	Nonpharmacologic management of knee osteoarthritis includes aerobic exercise and physical therapy, with therapy involving range-of-motion exercises and appropriate strength training of the leg.
Obesity	NHLBI Expert Panel on the Identification, Evaluation, and Treatment of Overweight and Obesity in Adults.	"Physical activity should be an integral part of weight loss therapy and weight maintenance."
Osteoporosis	NIH Consensus Conference on Osteoporosis Prevention, Diagnosis, and Therapy	"Exercise during the later years, in the presence of adequate calcium and vitamin D intake, probably has a modest effect on slowing the decline in bone mineral density." "Regular exercise, especially resistance and high impact activities, contributes to development of high peak bone mass and may reduce risk of falls in older individuals."

NOTE: CVD = cardiovascular disease; NHLBI = National Heart, Lung, and Blood Institute; NIH = National Institutes of Health.

SOURCE: Data from: (1) Physical Activity and Cardiovascular Health. NIH Consensus Statement Online. 1995 December 18–20; 13(3):1–33. (2) National Cholesterol Education Program. Second Report of the Expert Panel on Detection, Evaluation, and Treatment of High Blood Cholesterol in Adults (Adult Treatment Panel II). *Circulation*. 1994;89(3):1333–1445. (3) Pulmonary rehabilitation: joint ACCP/AACVPR evidence-based guidelines. ACCP/AACVPR Pulmonary Rehabilitation Guidelines Panel. American College of Chest Physicians. American Association of Cardiovascular and Pulmonary Rehabilitation. *Chest*. 1997;112(5):1363–1396. (4) American Diabetes Association. Diabetes mellitus and exercise. *Diabetes Care*. 2000;23 (suppl 1):S50–S54. (5) American Geriatrics Society with the British Geriatrics Society and the American Academy of Orthopaedic Surgeons. An evidence based clinical practice guidelines for the prevention of falls in older people. *J Am Geriatr Soc*. 2000; 49(5):664–672. (6) Sixth Joint National Committee on Prevention, Detection, Evaluation, and Treatment of High Blood Pressure. The sixth report of the Joint National Committee on Prevention, Detection, Evaluation, and Treatment of High Blood Pressure. *Arch Intern Med*. 1997;157:2413–2445;. (7) Hochberg MC, Altman RD, Brandt KD, et al. Guidelines for the medical management of osteoarthritis. Part II. Osteoarthritis of the knee. American College of Rheumatology. *Arthritis Rheum*. 1995;38(11):1541–1546. (8) National Institutes of Health. National Heart Lung and Blood Institute. *Clinical Guidelines on the Identification, Evaluation, and Treatment of Overweight and Obesity in Adults*. June 1998. Also available at http://www.nhlbi.nih.gov/guidelines/obesity/practgde.htm. (9) NIH Consensus Development Panel. Osteoporosis Prevention, Diagnosis, and Therapy. *JAMA*. 2000; 285(6):785–795, or http://consensus.nih.gov/111/111_intro.htm

low-intensity weight training and balance training caused more than a 50% reduction in falls and a 40% reduction in injurious falls.

PHYSICAL ACTIVITY FOR PATIENTS WITH LOW FITNESS

In aerobic activities, *intensity* is defined either in absolute terms as the amount of energy expended, or in relative terms, as the amount of energy expended in relation to a person's fitness level. The majority of adults have sufficient levels of physical fitness to expend 150 to 200 calories over 30 to 45 minutes without doing (relatively) high-intensity aerobic activity—defined as activity that exceeds 60% of heart rate reserve or 70% of maximal heart rate. However, many older adults are sufficiently unfit that they would have to perform relatively high-intensity activities to achieve this goal. High-intensity activity is associated with greater risk of cardiovascular events, greater risk of orthopedic injury, and lower adherence to activity plans.

Maximal heart rate is the highest heart rate observed during a bout of maximal exercise. Several prediction equations have been developed to estimate maximal heart rate when direct measurements of maximal heart rate are not available. It has recently been argued the most common prediction equation, max HR = 220 − age, is too conservative, and should be replaced by: max HR = 208 − 0.7 × age. However, the standard deviation of max heart rate in older adults is on the order of 15 beats/minute, limiting the accuracy of the prediction. For example, while the predicted maximum heart rate of an 80-year-old is around 150, maximum heart rate in 80-year-old adults commonly varies between 120 to 180.

Hence, a realistic, appropriate goal for unfit older adults is 30 to 45 minutes of activity a day that is relatively moderate in intensity—at 40% to 59% of heart rate reserve or 55% to 69% of maximal heart rate. In older adults with low fitness, relative intensities as low as 40% to 50% of heart rate reserve can cause a significant improvement in aerobic fitness.

Increases in activity levels should be made gradually over time, and this is particularly important for sedentary, unfit older adults. Initially, short bouts of activity are encouraged. There is no reason to discount activity that is less than 10 minutes (the shortest bout that qualifies under current activity recommendations), and no reason to specify a minimum heart rate target.

Older adults in community-based long-term-care programs and residents of nursing homes benefit from physical activity. Supervised exercise classes of a few months' duration cause improvements in measures of physical fitness and functional limitations, even in older adults who are physically frail, incontinent, or mildly demented. One study reported that increasing physical activity and removing sleep-disruptive nighttime events improves sleep and decreases agitation in nursing-home residents. Exercise programs for nursing-home residents may include high-intensity strength training, which has been shown in randomized trials to be safe, increase strength, improve functional limitations, and increase amount of spontaneous activity.

STRETCHING EXERCISES

Stretching exercises and other activities that improve flexibility in older adults are recommended, despite few data about their health effects. Flexibility can be increased in older adults, either by specific stretching exercises, by exercise programs that include stretching exercises, or by some daily activities such as walking. The extent that stretching reduces risk of injury during exercise is unknown for older adults. Current practice is to encourage stretching at the end of an activity bout, or after low-intensity warm-up activities.

THERAPEUTIC EFFECTS

Physical activity has therapeutic effects in the management of a wide variety of chronic conditions in older adults. Selected guidelines for the use of physical activity in managing common chronic diseases in older adults is shown in Table 11.2. In addition, there is substantial evidence that physical activity improves symptoms of depressive illness. One study suggested that the reduction in depressive symptoms that occurs with strength training is comparable to that seen with medication. Regular physical activity may improve sleep in older adults and should be considered as part of sleep hygiene recommendations.

PROMOTING PHYSICAL ACTIVITY

Healthy People 2010 and the 1996 U.S. Preventive Services Task Force recommend that physically inactive adults should be counseled about increasing their physical activity by their clinicians. Controlled trials show that short-term counseling can cause a short-term increase in physical activity levels in about 10% of adults counseled. Observational studies suggest that counseling can have long-term effects. Physically active older adults are more likely to report they have been counseled in the past by a clinician to increase their physical activity. Clinicians are consistently identified by older adults as a key source of advice about physical activity and exercise. See Figure 11.1 for one approach to discussing physical activity with patients.

Although more research on the ways that clinicians can effectively counsel patients about physical activity is needed, key elements of effective, brief, primary care–based interventions appear to include the following:

- Assessment of the patient's current level of physical activity;
- Collaborative goal setting between the clinician and the patient (goal setting should take into account the patient's health status, preferences, and life style); a written agreement probably increases the likelihood of behavior change;
- Problem solving with the patient about barriers to activity (barriers commonly mentioned by older adults include symptoms of disease, such as joint pain or shortness of breath; concern about neighborhood crime; being too busy for a variety of reasons, including caregiver duties; and weather);

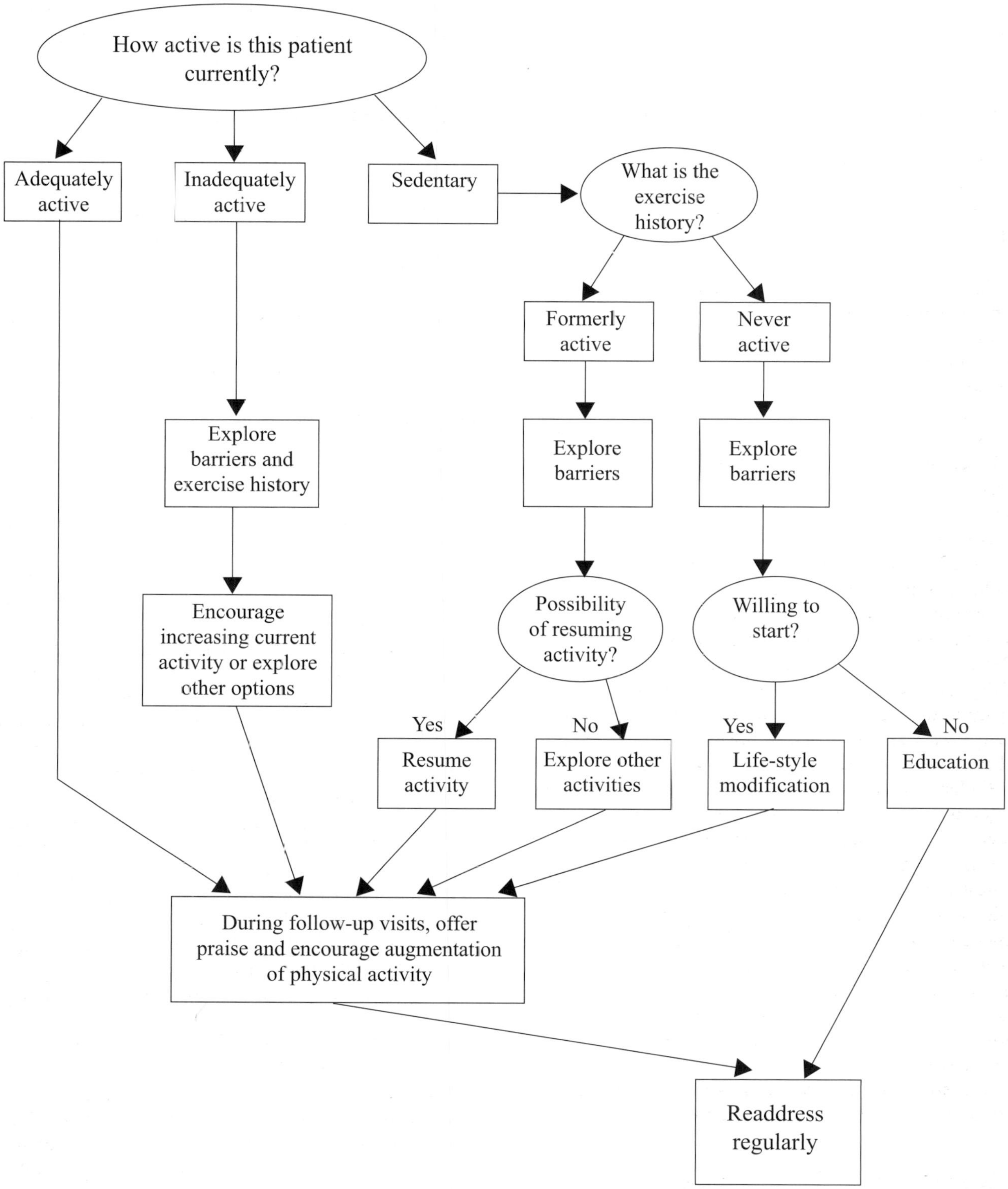

Figure 11.1—Framework for initiating discussions about physical activity with the older patient.

SOURCE: Christmas C, Andersen RA. Exercise and older patients: guidelines for the clinician. *J Am Geriatr Soc.* 2000;48(3):321. Reprinted by permission of Blackwell Science, Inc.

- Identification of supports to help the patient maintain a higher level of activity (support could include social support such as a walking partner, telephone follow-up, community programs, and Web-based programs that provide encouragement by regular email messages).
- Provision of nurse-initiated personal or automated phone calls is associated with significantly more engagement in physical activity.

Qualitative studies of failed counseling suggest that a patient becomes discouraged when a clinician makes behavior change sound too easy.

REFERENCES

- American College of Sports Medicine. Position stand: exercise and physical activity for older adults. *Med Sci Sports Exerc*. 1998;30(6):992–1008.

- Campbell AJ, Robertson MC, Gardner MM, et al. Randomised controlled trial of a general practice programme of home based exercise to prevent falls in elderly women. *BMJ*. 1997;315(7115):1065–1069.

- Chao D, Espeland MA, Farmer D, et al. Effect of voluntary weight loss on bone mineral density in older overweight women. *J Am Geriatr Soc*. 2000:48(7):753–759.

- Dubbert PM, Cooper KM, Kirchner KA, et al. Effects of nurse counseling on walking for exercise in elderly primary care patients. *J Gerontol A Biol Sci Med Sci*. 2002;57(11):M733–740.

- Gill TM, DiPietro L, Krumholz HM. Role of exercise stress testing and safety monitoring for older persons starting an exercise program. *JAMA*. 2000:284(3):342–349.

- Manson J, Hu FB, Rich-Edwards JW, et al. A prospective study of walking as compared with vigorous exercise in the prevention of coronary heart disease in women. *N Engl J Med*. 1999;341(9):650–658.

CHAPTER 12—HOSPITAL CARE

Older people are at disproportionate risk of becoming seriously ill and requiring hospital care, whether it is in an emergency department, on a medical or surgical ward, or in a critical-care unit. Persons aged 65 years or older, who make up only 13% of the U.S. population, account for 31% of acute-care hospital admissions and 45% of hospital expenditures for adults. The impact of older persons on acute hospital care will increase rapidly with the aging of the population: the proportion of the U.S. population aged 65 years or older is expected to increase to as much as 19% by 2025, with those aged 85 years or older increasing most rapidly.

GENERAL PRINCIPLES

Functional Decline in Hospitalized Patients

Once hospitalized, older patients are at high risk for loss of independence and institutionalization. Among hospitalized medical patients aged 70 years or older, approximately 10% decline during hospitalization in their ability to perform basic self-care activities of daily living (ADLs), another 10% are discharged without recovering their baseline prehospitalization abilities,

and 15% of those admitted from home are discharged to a nursing home. Loss of personal independence is often promoted by reciprocal interaction between the acute illness that led to hospitalization and underlying chronic illnesses and impairments. In addition, many older patients have lost their "bounce"—their ability to adapt and maintain the homeostasis of their physiologic, psychologic, and social systems in the face of the acute insults to these systems by illness and hospitalization. Functional decline during hospitalization and failure to recover baseline function has been independently associated with increasing age, lower preadmission function in instrumental activities of daily living (IADLs), and several admission characteristics, including cognitive impairment, symptoms of depression, and malnutrition. Optimal care for the hospitalized older patient requires an interdisciplinary approach to simultaneously manage acute illness and intervene where necessary to promote or maintain independent functioning.

Patient Preferences Regarding Hospital Care

It is often assumed that older persons would prefer to be treated for acute illness at home rather than in the hospital whenever possible. The safety and feasibility of this approach for acutely ill older persons who would usually be hospitalized has been demonstrated. This approach, sometimes called the "home hospital," requires intensive resources for medical and nursing care at home that are not yet widely available.

Older persons' preferences for home rather than hospital care vary widely. In a study of community-dwelling older persons, virtually all preferred care in the site that would provide the higher probability of survival. When home care and hospital care provide equivalent probabilities of survival, roughly half of patients prefer care in each site, with those preferring home care being more likely to be white, better educated, living with a spouse, deeply religious, and dependent in two or more ADLS. The major difference perceived by older persons between home care and hospital care was feeling safer in the hospital than at home.

There is also wide variability among seriously ill older persons in preferences for life-sustaining treatments. On the basis of findings of the large Study to Understand Prognoses and Preferences for Outcomes and Risks of Treatments (SUPPORT), it has been recognized that even though fewer older patients prefer aggressive care than do younger patients, many older patients want cardiopulmonary resuscitation and care that is focused on life extension. Moreover, patients' families and clinicians commonly underestimate older patients' desire for aggressive care. Thus, in providing care for acutely ill older persons, it is essential to determine individual preferences for the site of care and major goals of care.

Variation in Patterns of Hospital Care Practices

Hospital use rates for Medicare beneficiaries with many illnesses and surgical procedures vary as much as threefold among different parts of the United States, without evidence that these differences in practice patterns are explained by differences in disease rates. Hospital use and the use of hospital resources is much lower among patients enrolled in capitated insurance plans than among those enrolled in fee-for-service plans; this difference in resource use has not been systematically linked to differences in patient outcomes.

During hospitalization, older patients tend to receive less costly care than do younger patients. In SUPPORT, for example, seriously ill patients in their 80s were found to have received fewer invasive procedures and less resource-intensive, less costly hospital care than similar younger patients received. This preferential allocation of hospital services to younger patients was not based on differences in patients' severity of illness or general preferences for life-extending care, and such preferential allocation of hospital resources is

consistent with evidence of the preferential allocation of outpatient care to younger patients with specific diseases. Differences in the aggressiveness of care have not been shown to explain differences between older and younger patients in survival or other outcomes. Clinicians caring for hospitalized older persons should tailor their management to patients' preferences and clinical condition largely without regard for their age.

Nurses Improving Care for Health System Elders

Recognizing the need to improve the care of older adults in hospitals, leaders in geriatric nursing created the Nurses Improving Care for Health System Elders (NICHE) program in 1992. NICHE has evolved into a national geriatric nursing program encompassing 55 health systems comprising 105 hospitals nationally. A program of The John A. Hartford Foundation Institute for Geriatric Nursing at New York University, the goal of NICHE is to achieve systematic nursing change that will benefit hospitalized older patients. The focus of NICHE is on programs and protocols that are dominantly under the control of nursing practice, in other words, areas where nursing interventions have a substantive and positive impact on patient care.

NICHE is unlike other programs in that it does not prescribe how institutions should modify geriatric care; rather, it provides the materials and services necessary to stimulate and support the planning and implementation process. NICHE enables an institution to assess staff perceptions and knowledge regarding quality of geriatric care and the gaps and needs in this area; modify nursing care practice to better meet the needs of older patients, particularly the gaps identified; and evaluate the effectiveness of the interventions. Upon implementation of NICHE, hospitals report enhanced nursing knowledge and skills regarding treatment of common geriatric syndromes, greater patient satisfaction, decreased length of stay for older patients, reductions in readmission rates, increases in the length of time between readmissions, and reductions in costs associated with hospital care for older patients.

In conjunction with a team of nationally recognized geriatric nursing leaders, NICHE has created a variety of tools to improve geriatric care. In order to assess a hospital's readiness for NICHE, each hospital is asked to complete a "NICHE Ready Sheet" (see the Appendix, p 409). Once an institution is committed to the NICHE model of improving care, a comprehensive assessment process is then conducted to determine what nurses working in the hospitals know about basic principles of caring for older adults and whether these principles are used in practice.

One instrument, the Geriatric Institutional Assessment Profile (GIAP), was designed to help hospitals define how well they incorporate best practice standards of care. The GIAP addresses six major dimensions: knowledge of institutional policies, institutional obstacles to best practice, conflict over appropriate care, clinical knowledge of selected content matter, personal liability for inadequate practice, and perceptions of support in the workplace. GIAP results help guide a hospital's performance improvement. Items for each of the six dimensions in the GIAP focus on the management of four geriatric syndromes that commonly affect older hospitalized patients: pressure ulcers, incontinence, confusion, and sleep disturbances. These geriatric syndromes are benchmarks for best practice and provide a baseline from which a hospital can assess current practice and measure subsequent improvement in care for older adults. Once the GIAP is completed, the data are analyzed and gauged against a standard for best practice. Such benchmarking against other NICHE institutions nationally helps to provide an empirical basis for mentoring and improving care at the institutional level. Once the data has been analyzed, an institution selects a specific model to guide their program.

The Geriatric Resource Nurse Model

The Geriatric Resource Nurse (GRN) model originally began at Beth Israel Hospital in Boston and was further developed at Yale–New Haven Hospital. The GRN model is based on the following beliefs:

- Primary nurses know the most about the patterns and problems of older patients who are admitted to their units.
- Primary nurses serving as GRNs are more likely to integrate new behaviors into practice because of the unit-based visibility and regular feedback available.
- A GRN program can recognize nursing expertise, which later maybe reflected in a clinical ladder program for primary nurses.

Geriatric Resource Nurses are unit-based RNs who gain enhanced skills in care of older adults through a continued education program developed in the NICHE hospital by an advanced practice geriatric nurse. GRNs carry a usual caseload of patients while serving as the unit's resource on geriatric best practices. A geriatric advanced practice nurse works closely with the GRNs through clinical rounds and through activities such as geriatric nursing interest group conferences. Where possible, the GRN model uses a geriatrician to consult on complex geriatric care problems. Alternatively, when a geriatrician is unavailable, primary care and internal medicine physicians are invited to consult. This highly popular model has been adopted in numerous NICHE sites.

The Geriatric Syndrome Management Model

The Geriatric Syndrome Management model was developed at the University of Chicago Hospitals and provides for consultation and education by a Gerontological Nurse Specialist (GNS) to improve nurses' accuracy and speed in detecting and managing common geriatric syndromes such as falls, urinary incontinence, and sleep disturbance in hospitalized older patients. As one example, in the initial focus on delirium, nurses learned:

- the use and interpretation of simple bedside tests for assessing cognition;
- the clinical features that distinguish delirium, dementia, and depression;
- common causes of delirium in older patients;
- independent, interdependent, and dependent strategies for preventing and managing delirium;
- when and how to communicate patients' symptoms to physicians; and
- how to document findings in the medical record.

Strategies used to address a syndrome include receiving initial and repeated direct instruction on all NICHE units and on every shift. Printed assessment forms and a large poster that summarize all instrumental components of the approach are commonly placed in a prominent position in each nursing station. This model uses a target condition to open the way for improving geriatric care comprehensively.

The Quality Cost Model of Transitional Care

The Discharge Planning Model was developed at the University of Pennsylvania School of Nursing. It contains a discharge planning protocol developed specifically for the hospitalized older adult and is implemented by Gerontological Nurse Specialists (GNS) (geriatric nurse practitioners and clinical specialists).

The assumption is made that the GNS has advanced knowledge and skill in caring for high-risk older adults and their caregivers; therefore, the GNS provides care under a general protocol and adapts this protocol to the specific needs of the older adults. The GNS assesses patients soon after admission and at least every 48 hours during the course of the patient's hospital stay. Initially, the GNS was accessible to patients and family members by telephone 7 days a week and worked with unit staff to customize care. Recently, the GNS has followed patients at home to coordinate a plan of care in the critical period following discharge. By coordinating care of multiple health care providers involved in discharge planning, the GNS becomes the one person to whom patients and families can consistently turn to during and soon after hospitalization.

Evaluating the effectiveness of this model as compared to the hospital's general discharge planning procedures indicates that this intervention has lengthened improved outcomes and significantly lengthened the time between rehospitalizations for patients in the experimental group.

For additional information about the NICHE model, see http://www.hartfordign.org.

SYSTEMATIC ASSESSMENT OF THE HOSPITALIZED PATIENT

A systematic approach to the hospitalized older patient incorporates an assessment of function at the level of the organ system, the whole person, and the person's environment. This assessment can identify needs for which targeted interventions may improve function or reduce risk for adverse outcomes. This approach complements the traditional medical assessment by highlighting problems that are common in hospitalized older persons, but it is similar in concept to comprehensive geriatric assessment conducted in other settings. (See "Assessment," p 47.)

Table 12.1 summarizes a suggested systematic assessment of 10 common problems that are commonly overlooked in older hospitalized patients. Each problem highlights the importance of the continuity of care before and after hospitalization. These problems were selected on the basis of their importance in relation to other problems, the quality of relevant evidence, and their specificity to older persons. Other important problems (eg, prevention of perioperative venous thrombosis, use of alcohol or tobacco, pain, and advance directives) are not specific to older persons, and some problems specific to older persons (eg, age-related decline in renal function) are widely recognized. (See also "Substance Abuse," p 234, "Palliative Care," p 103, "Legal and Ethical Issues," p 18, "Renal Diseases and Disorders," p 357.)

Two types of evidence suggest that these interventions are good investments. First, for each problem, there is compelling evidence (cited below) supporting the proposed intervention, either because the efficacy of the intervention is well established (eg, warfarin to prevent stroke associated with atrial fibrillation), or because the associated problem is common, often overlooked, and ameliorable with a safe and inexpensive intervention. Second, systematic approaches to the evaluation and management of acutely ill older persons

Table 12.1—The Systematic Assessment of Hospitalized Older Patients: A Framework Highlighting 10 Common Problems

Problem	Assessment Methods	Illustrative Interventions
Assessment at the Level of Organ Systems		
Atrial fibrillation	Take pulse, ECG	Warfarin or treatment to maintain sinus rhythm, or both
Malnutrition	Use subjective global assessment	Supplementation of water, calorie, protein intake; assessment of social environment
Influenza and pneumonia	Ask about vaccination	Vaccination against influenza or pneumococcus, or both
Cognitive impairment	Use screen: SPMSQ or MMSE	Evaluation for dementia or delirium; assessment of social environment
Immobility and falls	Ask about difficulty walking and falls	Avoidance of restraints and tethers; prescription of walking and physical therapy
Sensory impairment	Assess vision and hearing	Glasses, hearing aids
Depression	Use depression screen	Use of cognitive therapy, pharmacotherapy
Assessment at the Level of the Whole Person		
Disability	Ask about help needed	Use of physical or occupational therapy; assessment of social environment
Suboptimal drug use	Assess indications for therapy, dosing, potential interactions	Modification of prescriptions
Assessment at the Level of the Environment		
Mistreatment	Ask about level of social support and perceived freedom, safety	Early involvement of family and social services in planning to go home

NOTE: ECG = electrocardiogram; MMSE = Mini–Mental State Examination; SPMSQ = Short Portable Mental Status Examination.

SOURCE: Adapted from Landefeld CS, Johnston CB, Johnson MA. Approach to the hospitalized older patient. In: Wachter RM, Goldman L, Hollander H, eds. _Hospital Medicine._ New York: Lippincott Williams and Wilkins; 2000:62. Reprinted with permission.

can improve patient outcomes and reduce hospital costs.

Assessment at the Level of Organ Systems

Atrial Fibrillation

Nonvalvular atrial fibrillation is present in 5% or more of hospitalized older persons, often as an incidental finding. Consistent and compelling evidence from randomized trials shows that the risk of stroke in persons with atrial fibrillation can be reduced approximately two thirds by treatment with warfarin (eg, from 4.5% per year to 1.4% per year). Moreover, the beneficial effect of warfarin is maintained in persons aged 75 years or older and in those with other risk factors for stroke. Alternatively, cardioversion and pharmacologic maintenance of sinus rhythm may attain comparable benefits. Nonetheless, many older patients with atrial fibrillation are discharged from hospital without warfarin therapy, even when warfarin is indicated. Failure to prescribe warfarin is likely due to underestimation of the benefit of therapy, overestimation of its potential risk, and the difficulty of implementing, monitoring, and modifying therapy to minimize adverse effects.

Every hospitalized older patient should be assessed for the presence of chronic nonvalvular atrial fibrillation. When atrial fibrillation is diagnosed, valvular disease and hyperthyroidism should be excluded. In the absence of a strong contraindication, treatment should be instituted to prevent stroke, usually with warfarin (see the section below on prevention of venous thromboembolism, p 80). Attaining and maintaining sinus rhythm may have benefits comparable to those of warfarin treatment. (See also the section on atrial fibrillation in "Cardiovascular Diseases and Disorders," p 262.)

Malnutrition

Serious deficiencies of macronutrients and micronutrients are common in hospitalized older patients. Key macronutrients are protein, calories, salt, water, and fiber. On admission, severe protein-calorie malnutrition is present in approximately 15% of patients aged 70 years or older, and moderate malnutrition is present in another 25%. Moreover, 25% of older patients suffer further nutritional depletion during hospitalization. Even after controlling for the underlying illness, its severity, and comorbid illnesses, malnutrition is associated with increased risk for death, dependence, and institutionalization.

In addition to other deficiencies of vitamins and electrolytes that may develop with protein-calorie malnutrition, vitamin D deficiency is especially common among older hospitalized patients. In one large hospital, nearly two thirds of medical inpatients aged 65 years or older were found to be vitamin D deficient; vitamin D deficiency was nearly as common in inpatients without a risk factor for vitamin D deficiency and in those taking multivitamins as in other patients. These data regarding the high prevalence of vitamin D deficiency in hospitalized older persons complement evidence that vitamin D and calcium supplementation reduce by half the incidence of nonvertebral fractures in men and women aged 65 years or older.

The efficacy of interventions to detect, prevent, or correct malnutrition in hospitalized older persons has not been demonstrated. When malnutrition is identified, remediable contributing factors should be sought and corrected, such as difficulty chewing or insufficient time or encouragement to eat. It remains unclear whether the benefits of invasive alimentation (alimentary or parenteral) outweigh their risks. (See "Eating and Feeding Problems," p 191.) Long-term supplementation with vitamin D (1000 IU daily) and calcium (1000 mg daily) should be considered. (See "Malnutrition," p 182.)

Influenza and Pneumococcus

All persons aged 65 years or older should be asked at the time of admission to the hospital whether they have received influenza or pneumococcal vaccination. During the fall and winter months, influenza vaccination should be administered to those who have not already received it. Pneumococcal vaccination should be administered to older hospitalized patients who do not recall having received it in the past 10 years. (See also "Prevention," p 59.)

Cognitive Impairment

Underlying cognitive impairment consistent with dementia is present on admission in 20% to 40% of hospitalized older persons, and it commonly goes undetected. Preexisting cognitive impairment is a risk factor for delirium, falls, use of restraints, and nonadherence with therapy. Also, there is intrinsic value in identifying previously undiagnosed dementia so that appropriate evaluation and management strategies can be implemented after discharge. Tests of mental status are sensitive and specific tests for dementia; for example, in one study of hospitalized older persons, three or more errors on the 10-item Short Portable Mental Status Questionnaire (SPMSQ) was 87% sensitive and 99% specific for a diagnosis of dementia. Mental status should be assessed by the use of an established test of cognitive function, such as the SPMSQ or the 30-item Mini–Mental State Examination. The diagnosis of dementia should be considered in those with three or more errors on the SPMSQ or a score of 24 or less on the MMSE. When dementia is a possibility, the patient should be assessed to exclude reversible causes and to identify those for whom pharmacologic therapy and family-oriented interventions are warranted. (See "Dementia," p 113.)

Delirium is present in 10% to 15% of hospitalized older persons on admission and develops in up to 30% during the course of hospitalization. Delirium is associated with increased rates of in-hospital death, nursing-home placement, and prolonged length of stay, and it may worsen chronic cognitive impairment. Roughly one third of cases of delirium can be prevented by managing six risk factors for delirium appropriately: cognitive impairment, sleep deprivation, immobility, visual impairment, hearing impairment, and dehydration. The diagnosis of delirium should be considered when any of the following is observed: fluctuation in mental status or behavior, inattention, disorganized thinking, and altered consciousness. Prudent measures to prevent or ameliorate delirium include avoiding medicines associated with delirium whenever possible, treating infection and fever, detecting and correcting metabolic abnormalities, frequently orienting patients with cognitive or sensory impairment, and avoiding excessive bed rest. (See "Delirium," p 127.)

Immobility and Falls

Walking facilitates the performance of virtually all ADLs and IADLs. The ability to walk briskly and the habit of regularly walking 1 mile or more daily are associated with prolonged survival. Immobility during hospitalization, however, leads rapidly to deconditioning and subsequent difficulty walking. The major risk for deconditioned hospital patients of walking is falling, which can lead to serious injury. Falls and fall-related injuries in hospitalized patients are associated with cognitive impairment, new medications and polypharmacy, environmental factors in the hospital, and abnormalities of cognition, gait, balance, and the lower extremities, as well as with multiple chronic medical conditions and depression.

The patient's gait, balance, lower-extremity strength, ability to get up from bed, cognition, and mood should be assessed during the initial physical examination. Persons able to walk independently should be encouraged to do so frequently during hospitalization. Those able to walk but unable to do so safely and independently should receive assistance from hospital staff while walking several times daily. Formal

physical therapy may yield additional benefits. A patient's risk for falls should be assessed by inquiring about a history of falls and by examination. Adopting interventions that reduce falls in other settings may also prevent falls in the hospital. Prudent preventive strategies include avoiding restraints, providing walking assistance for those who walk with difficulty, and physical therapy for those with weakness or gait abnormalities. Soft-tissue and bony abnormalities of the feet should receive appropriate podiatric care. (See "Falls," p 143; "Gait Disturbances," p 148; "Physical Activity," p 65; "Rehabilitation," p 82; and "Diseases and Disorders of the Foot," p 275.)

Sensory Impairment

Most hospitalized older persons have impaired vision or hearing, and these sensory impairments are risk factors for falls, incontinence, and functional dependence. Although most visual and hearing impairments are readily corrected by glasses or hearing aids, these appliances are often forgotten in the hospital.

Hospitalized older persons should be routinely asked if they have difficulty with seeing or hearing and whether they use glasses or hearing aids. Physical examination should include a test of visual acuity (eg, with a pocket card of the Jaeger eye test) and the whisper test of hearing, in which a short, easily answered question is whispered in each ear. In people with visual or hearing impairments, glasses or hearing aids should be provided (ideally brought from home), and staff should be informed that patients may need to use appliances to communicate effectively. (See "Hearing Impairment," p 163, and "Visual Impairment," p 169.)

Depression

Depressive symptoms in hospitalized older persons are common, prognostically important, and potentially ameliorable. Major or minor depression occurs in roughly one third of hospitalized patients aged 65 years or older but is often undiagnosed. The presence of depressive symptoms is associated with increased risk for dependence in ADLs, nursing-home placement, and shortened long-term survival, even after controlling for baseline function and the severity of acute and chronic illness.

The possibility of depression should be considered in hospitalized older patients, who should be asked whether they feel down, depressed, or hopeless, or whether they have lost interest or pleasure in doing things. A positive response to any one of these questions is likely sensitive to the diagnosis of depression (based on evidence from outpatients) and should trigger a formal assessment for an affective disorder. In hospitalized older persons, the presence of 3 or more of 11 depressive symptoms has been found to be 83% sensitive and 77% specific for a diagnosis of major depression.

Detection is the first and most important step in the management of depression. Psychotherapeutic interventions (environmental, behavioral, cognitive, and family) are safe and often effective, and they should be initiated for all patients with suspected depression. It is rarely necessary to begin pharmacotherapy during hospitalization for a medical or surgical condition, but follow-up shortly after discharge is critical. If pharmacotherapy is initiated, selective serotonin reuptake inhibitors are often preferred because approximately 50% of older hospitalized patients have a contraindication to tricyclic antidepressants. (See "Depression and Other Mood Disorders," p 211.)

Assessment at the Level of the Whole Person

Disability

The ability to perform ADLs and IADLs is necessary if the older person is to live independently, and functional dependence is independently associated with worse quality-of-life outcomes, shortened survival, and increased resource use. The older patient's ability to perform ADLs and IADLs should be determined at the time of admission. The causes of functional dependence should be determined (eg, dependence in IADLs is often associated with dementia), and strategies to maintain and improve functional capacity should be considered (eg, physical and occupational therapy). These strategies may be best implemented effectively for many patients by nurses without consultation or referral. Social work consultation and early involvement of family or other caregivers is often necessary to plan postdischarge care for those older patients who are functionally dependent. (See also "Rehabilitation," p 82; "Psychosocial Issues," p 13.)

Suboptimal Pharmacotherapy

The number of drugs prescribed to hospitalized patients is directly proportional to their age. Moreover, hospitalization is a period of rapid turnover in drug therapies for older patients: One study found that 40% of drugs prescribed before admission were discontinued during hospitalization and 45% of drugs prescribed at discharge were started during hospitalization. Although older patients are at increased risk for inappropriate drug therapy, adverse drug effects, and drug-drug interactions, they may also be undertreated when effective therapies are not used or are used in inadequate doses. Thus, hospitalization is an opportunity for a thorough review of each older patient's medications and adjustments, as needed. In one study 88% of older hospitalized patients were found to have had at least one or more clinically significant drug problems, and 22%, at least one potentially serious and life-threatening problem. Consultation by clinical pharmacists can improve appropriate prescribing and improve the older patient's adherence to prescribed therapy.

Each patient's medications should be reviewed on admission, and those that are unnecessary or have low therapeutic indices (eg, sedative hypnotics) should be discontinued. During hospitalization and at discharge, medications should be reviewed to identify prescribing in six common categories: inappropriate choice of therapy, dosage, schedule, drug-drug interactions, therapeutic duplication, and allergy. (See "Pharmacotherapy," p 35.)

Assessment at the Level of the Environment: Mistreatment and Social Support

Hospitalization of older persons is sometimes precipitated by mistreatment, which includes physical or psychologic abuse, neglect, self-neglect, exploitation, and abandonment. Elder mistreatment was not recognized in the medical literature until 1975; it is now estimated to affect 700,000 to 1.2 million Americans annually. In a large prospective cohort study, the annual incidence of referral to protective services for mistreatment was found to be approximately 1% among persons aged 65 years or older. Those referred for abuse, neglect, or exploitation were found to have a lower rate of survival over 13 years of follow-up (9%) than those referred for self-neglect (17%) and those not referred (40%). Most older persons referred to protective services because of physical abuse have been seen in hospital emergency departments, and many emergency visits lead to hospitalization.

Universal screening for mistreatment has been recommended and can be implemented by asking each older patient, "Do you feel safe returning where you live?" (The sensitivity and specificity of this and other screening approaches are unknown.) Further questions can explore the living situation and specific settings or aspects of mistreatment. The diagnosis of mistreatment should be considered when there are physical or psychologic stigmata, such as unexplained injury, dehydration, malnutrition, social withdrawal, or recalcitrant depression or anxiety. When mistreatment is suspected, Adult Protective Services or the equivalent state agency should be contacted; this is required in most states. (See "Elder Mistreatment," p 52.)

Strategies for Managing the Hospitalized Patient

Resuscitation: Approaches and Outcomes

Principles of Resuscitation

The maintenance of physiologic function of individual organ systems may be especially important in acutely ill older persons because of their commonly diminished physiologic reserve and ability to maintain homeostasis. For example, even brief periods of hypotension related to bacteremia or hypovolemia may lead to acute and sometimes persistent damage to the heart, brain, and kidney in acutely ill older persons. Conversely, excessive fluid resuscitation aimed at averting this damage may cause pulmonary edema in such a patient, who may have left ventricular diastolic dysfunction and mild renal insufficiency with a normal serum creatinine. Thus, in situations in which prolonging survival and function is a primary goal of therapy, careful attention to the function of each major organ system is needed.

Hospitalized older persons are at higher risk than younger persons for cardiopulmonary arrest. Moreover, among hospitalized persons in whom resuscitation is attempted after cardiopulmonary arrest, survival is less likely among older patients. Thus, it is especially important to establish whether prolonged survival is a primary goal of therapy for each older hospitalized patient and, if it is, whether the benefit of cardiopulmonary resuscitation is felt to outweigh the possibility that it will prolong life only briefly while contributing to pain and suffering. These questions are best addressed by a direct conversation with the patient because such conversations frequently reveal a discrepancy between the patient's goals and preferences and the views of the physician and family about his or her goals and preferences.

Fluid Management

The maintenance of water and electrolyte balance requires special attention in older persons during and after resuscitation because of their decreased capacity to achieve and maintain homeostasis. Initial efforts should be directed toward achieving normovolemia and correcting electrolyte abnormalities. Subsequent efforts to maintain fluid and electrolyte balance should be based on estimates of daily metabolic requirements. The intracellular volume is about 25% to 30% of body weight for men aged 65 to 85 years weighing between 40 and 80 kg (90 to 176 lb) and about 20% to 25% of body weight for women in the same age and weight ranges. The daily metabolic requirements, as a propor-

tion of intracellular volume, can be estimated as follows: water in L, 10%; energy in 1000 kcal, 10%; protein in g, 0.3%; sodium in mmol, 0.3%; and potassium in mmol, 0.2%. Thus, for a 75-year-old woman weighing 60 kg (intracellular volume 12 to 15 L), the daily maintenance requirements are 1.2 to 1.5 L of water and nutrients providing 1200 to 1500 kcal, 36 to 45 mmol of sodium, and 24 to 30 mmol of potassium. Administration of fluids and electrolytes should be adjusted on the basis of daily physical examination and of serum values of electrolytes and renal function, as needed.

Perioperative Care

Optimal perioperative care for older persons involves risk assessment, the use of strategies shown to prevent pulmonary and thromboembolic complications, management of abnormalities of physiologic function, prevention and early detection of delirium, and pain management. Increased risk of cardiac complications of noncardiac surgery is associated with emergency surgery, aortic and other major vascular procedures, large fluid losses or shifts, unstable coronary disease, arrhythmias, severe valvular heart disease, and decompensated congestive heart failure. The potential benefits of surgery should be weighed against these and other risks, with surgery being postponed or avoided when the risks outweigh the benefits. Strategies shown to prevent pulmonary complications in high-risk patients with chronic lung disease include smoking cessation 6 weeks or more before surgery, antibiotic therapy of bronchitis, perioperative bronchodilator therapy, postural drainage, chest physiotherapy, and inhalation of humidified gases. Various regimens have been shown to reduce the incidence of deep-vein thrombosis and pulmonary embolism in patients undergoing orthopedic, abdominal, gynecologic, or urologic surgery (see next section).

Although strategies to manage hypertension and optimize cardiac function have not been shown to improve outcomes of noncardiac surgery, they are reasonable. Antihypertensive medicines should be given on the day of surgery and started as soon as practical postoperatively. Preoperative diastolic blood pressure of 110 mm Hg or greater is a contraindication for surgery. Acute postoperative elevations of blood pressure require immediate evaluation for pulmonary insufficiency, bladder distention, and uncontrolled pain. In the absence of a secondary cause of the acute elevation, treatment may be undertaken with β-blockers or calcium antagonists; potent vasodilators may be hazardous without close monitoring. (See "Hypertension," p 256.) Standard treatment of congestive heart failure, including angiotensin-converting enzyme inhibitors, β-blockers, and diuretics, should be initiated and stabilized preoperatively. Intraoperative and perioperative monitoring with Swan-Ganz catheters or intraesophageal echocardiography is widely used and may be useful; these modalities have not been shown to improve patient outcomes, however. (See "Cardiovascular Diseases and Disorders," p 243.)

Delirium occurs in 15% to 25% of postoperative older patients and in higher proportions of those with either underlying cognitive impairment or alcohol abuse. A multicomponent strategy that addresses cognitive impairment, sleep deprivation, immobility, visual impairment, hearing impairment, and dehydration has been shown to reduce the frequency of delirium in medical patients and may also be effective in postoperative patients. (See "Delirium," p 127.)

Pain is common in hospitalized older patients and is almost universal during the postoperative period. All postoperative patients should be monitored frequently for pain by the use of a standard rating scale (see "Palliative Care," p 107, for pain intensity scales in common use). Ineffective or an absent verbal expression of pain by cognitively-impaired patients may necessitate the observation of behavioral indicators such as facial expressions, verbalizations, vocalizations, body movements, change in interpersonal interactions, or changes in activity patterns or routines. The cause of pain should be determined in patients with moderate or severe pain, and reversible causes of pain should be eliminated. Therapeutic maneuvers should be initiated in all patients with moderate or more severe pain and include nonpharmacologic approaches as well as medicines. Nonpharmacologic approaches include physical agents (such as heat, cold, massage, and immobilization) and cognitive-behavioral approaches (such as relaxation, imagery, distraction, education, music, and biofeedback). Opioids are effective in adequate doses in most situations, and the risk of addiction in acute treatment is virtually nonexistent. Acetaminophen is effective for mild pain and may potentiate the analgesic effect of other agents; hepatic toxicity can be avoided by restricting the daily dose to 4 g or less in patients with normal liver function. Nonsteroidal anti-inflammatory agents are also effective but are frequently avoided postoperatively because of their toxicity. (See "Palliative Care," p 103; pain medication table in the Appendix, p 411.)

Prevention of Venous Thromboembolism

Deep-vein thrombosis and pulmonary embolism are prevented by postoperative subcutaneous administration of unfractionated heparin (5000 units two or three times a day) to patients undergoing abdominal, gynecologic, or urologic surgery or elective neurosurgery without excess bleeding risk. Low-molecular-weight heparins have been shown to be as effective as unfractionated heparin, and in certain groups of patients at high risk of venous thromboembolism (eg, patients undergoing total hip or knee replacement or hip fracture repair), they are more effective. Several low-molecular-weight heparins are approved for this purpose, and it is unknown whether they differ in efficacy or side effects. In patients in whom the risk of bleeding related to even low doses of heparin must be avoided, pneumatic compression stockings should be used. (See anticoagulation guidelines in the Appendix, p 387.)

In patients undergoing total hip replacement, a meta-analysis found that the best prophylactic agent in terms of both efficacy and safety was warfarin, followed by pneumatic compression, then low-molecular-weight heparin; the least effective and safe was low-dose heparin. Aspirin further reduces the risk of pulmonary embolism and deep-vein thrombosis by at least a third in patients undergoing surgery for hip fracture or replacement. In patients undergoing hip replacement, desirudin, a recombinant hirudin that directly inhibits thrombin, has been shown to be more effective than either unfractionated or low-molecular-weight heparin in preventing venous thromboembolism. In patients undergoing total knee replacement, a meta-analysis found that intermittent pneumatic compression devices and low-molecular-weight heparins were significantly better than warfarin ($P < 0.0001$) or aspirin ($P < 0.0001$) in preventing deep-vein thrombosis.

Several studies have provided compelling evidence that heparins prevent venous thromboembolism in acutely ill medical patients as well. In a meta-analysis of seven trials comparing a prophylactic heparin treatment to a control (15,095 patients), a significant decrease in deep-vein thrombosis and in clinical pulmonary embolism was observed with heparins as compared with control (risk reductions, 56% and 58%, respectively; $P < 0.001$ in both cases), without significant difference in the incidence of major bleedings or deaths. In nine trials comparing a low-molecular-weight heparin to unfractionated heparin (4669 patients), no significant difference was observed in the rates of deep-vein thrombosis, clinical pulmonary embolism, or mortality, but low-molecular-weight heparin reduced by 52% the risk of major hemorrhage ($P = 0.049$). The benefits of low-molecular-weight heparins in medical patients may be dose dependent: In a randomized trial, treatment with 40 mg (but not 20 mg) of enoxaparin subcutaneously per day was found to reduce the risk of venous thromboembolism.

Systematic Approaches

Two systematic approaches have been demonstrated in controlled trials to improve hospital care of older persons. Both approaches involve comprehensive, multicomponent interventions implemented on specified general medical units.

The first approach involves a system of care designed to help acutely ill older patients to maintain or achieve independence in ADLs and IADLs; this system has been called Acute Care for Elders (ACE) and has been implemented on a specific unit in several major hospitals. The four components of this intervention are as follows:

- a prepared environment to promote mobility and orientation (eg, with carpeting, raised toilet seats, low beds, clocks, calendars, and pictures to promote orientation);
- patient-centered care with nursing-initiated protocols for independent self-care, nutrition, sleep hygiene, skin care, mood, and cognition;
- planning to go home with early social work intervention to mobilize family and other resources at home; and
- medical care review to promote optimal prescribing.

In a randomized trial involving 651 medical patients aged 70 years or older in a university teaching hospital, ACE was found to be associated with greater independence in ADLs at discharge, less frequent nursing-home discharge, and somewhat shorter and less expensive hospitalization. In a second randomized trial involving 1531 community-dwelling persons aged 70 years or older in a community teaching hospital, ACE was found to be associated with substantial differences in the satisfaction of patients, family members, physicians, and nurses but with only modest differences ADL function. These findings demonstrate that ACE is a promising approach to improving outcomes and reducing hospital costs for acutely ill older general medical patients, but the effects of ACE on patient outcomes are likely sensitive to factors dependent on the function of the interdisciplinary team.

The second approach involves a multicomponent intervention to prevent delirium in hospitalized older patients; the intervention consists of protocols to manage six risk factors for delirium: cognitive impairment, sleep deprivation, immobility, visual impairment, hearing impairment, and dehydration. In a prospective controlled study, the incidence of delirium was reduced by one third, from 15.0% to 9.9%. The intervention was also associated with significant improvement in the degree of cognitive impairment among patients with cognitive impairment at admission and a reduction in the rate of use of sleep medications among all patients. Among the other risk factors, there were trends toward improvement in immobility, visual impairment, and hearing impairment. The intervention was not associated with a reduction in the severity, duration, or recurrence of delirium, and the effects of the intervention on other outcomes have not yet been reported. Nonetheless, these findings suggest that primary prevention of delirium is probably the most effective treatment strategy.

REFERENCES

- Brass LM, Krumholz HM, Scinto JD, et al. Warfarin use following ischemic stroke among Medicare patients with atrial fibrillation. *Arch Intern Med*. 1998;158(19):2093–2100.

- Counsell SR, Holder CM, Liebenauer LL, et al. Effects of a multicomponent intervention on functional outcomes and process of care in hospitalized older patients: a randomized controlled trial of Acute Care for Elders (ACE) in a community hospital. *J Am Geriatr Soc*. 2000; 48(12):1572–1581.

- Covinsky KE, Kahana E, Chin MH, et al. Depressive symptoms and three-year mortality in older hospitalized medical patients. *Ann Intern Med*.1999;130(7):563–569.

- Fulmer T, Mezey M, Bottrell M, et al. Nurses Improving Care for Healthsystem Elders (NICHE): using outcomes and benchmarks for evidenced-based practice. *Geriatr Nurs*. 2002;23(3):121–127.

- Inouye SK, Bogardus ST Jr, Charpentier PA, et al. A multicomponent intervention to prevent delirium in hospitalized older patients. *N Engl J Med*. 1999;340(19):669–676.

- Mismetti P, Laporte-Simitsidis S, Tardy B, et al. Prevention of venous thromboembolism in internal medicine with unfractionated or low-molecular-weight heparins: a meta-analysis of randomised clinical trials. *Thromb Haemost*. 2000;83(1):14–19.

- Prevention of pulmonary embolism and deep vein thrombosis with low dose aspirin: Pulmonary Embolism Prevention (PEP) trial. *Lancet*. 2000; 355(9212):1295–1302.

- Samama MM, Cohen AT, Darmon JY, et al. A comparison of enoxaparin with placebo for the prevention of venous thromboembolism in acutely ill medical patients: Prophylaxis in Medical Patients with Enoxaparin Study Group. *N Engl J Med*. 1999;341(11):793–800.

- Siegler EL, Mirafzali S, Foust JB. *An Introduction to Hospitals and Inpatient Care*. New York: Springer Publishig Company; 2003.

CHAPTER 13—REHABILITATION

Rehabilitation is a critical component of geriatric health care, because disabling conditions, which are common among older adults, profoundly affect their quality of life and are amenable to treatment. In older adults chronic disease almost always underlies disability; for example, stroke occurs most commonly in people with other vascular diseases, and hip fractures occur most commonly in people with osteoporosis and gait disorders. Worsening disability also occurs in progressive chronic diseases, such as osteoarthritis, Parkinson's disease, and amyotrophic lateral sclerosis, or in the context of deconditioning from inactivity during acute illness. In order to provide the best functional recovery possible, those providing geriatric rehabilitation must

- use systematic approaches to assess the causes of disability,
- be familiar with the advantages and disadvantages of the various sites of rehabilitative care,
- understand the role of multidisciplinary teams and care plans,

- adapt care to other diseases and disabilities, and
- be familiar with the basic requirements for rehabilitation of common geriatric conditions.

CONCEPTUAL MODELS FOR GERIATRIC REHABILITATION

Geriatric rehabilitation services can be organized on the basis of a conceptual model of disability that allows optimum assessment of the status and needs of the patient, an appropriate match of treatments with specific conditions, and evaluation of rehabilitation outcomes. The revised *International Classification of Impairments, Disabilities, and Handicaps* (ICIDH-2) of the World Health Organization (WHO) offers a useful framework (Figure 13.1). The ICIDH-2 framework has two main parts: functioning and disability, and contextual factors. Functioning and disability include the activities and participation components. The body component is considered to have both structures

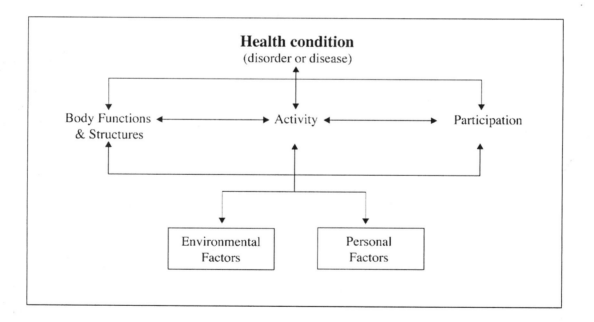

Figure 13.1—Current understanding of interactions among the components of the disability model of ICIDH-2.

The new edition of the *International Classification of Functioning, Disability and Health* (ICIDH-2) differs substantially from the 1980 version of ICIDH in the depiction of the interrelations between functioning and disability. It should be noted that any diagram is likely to be incomplete and prone to misrepresentation because of the complexity of interactions in a multidimensional model. The model is drawn to illustrate the multiple interactions. Other depictions indicating other important foci in the process are certainly possible. Interpretations of interactions among different components and constructs may also vary (eg, the impact of environmental factors on body functions certainly differs from their impact on participation).

SOURCE: World Health Organization, *International Classification of Functioning, Disability and Health–ICIDH-2 Final Draft 2001*. Geneva: World Health Organization; 2001:16. Reprinted with permission.

such as organs and limbs and physiologic functions. Impairments are defined as problems in body function or structure, such as a significant deviation or loss. The activities and participation components address functioning from both an individual and a societal perspective. Activity is defined as the execution of a task or action by an individual and participation is defined as involvement in a life situation. Participation restrictions are problems a person experiences in his or her involvement in work, leisure, and social activities.

The second part of the WHO framework is the context, including environmental and personal factors. Environmental factors have an impact on all components of functioning and disability; they range from an individual's immediate environment to the general environment. Personal factors include age, race, gender, educational background, personality, fitness, and life style.

In the WHO model, interventions can be designed to modify impairments, limitations in activities, or restrictions in participation. For example, a treatment plan may be developed to improve strength (impairment level), but the significance of this intervention is due to its effect on physical mobility (activity) and ultimately the ability to return to social or physical roles (participation). The effect of gains in strength and physical mobility on participation could be modified by the person's motivation or social support. If a person improves in strength and balance but family and friends continue to do everything for him or her and thus discourage independent function, the person may remain dependent.

The physical environment is another powerful modifier. Even if a person achieves improved function, he or she cannot regain prior public and personal roles if physical barriers to access are not removed with such facilities as ramps or modified bathrooms.

In summary, the interaction of disease and disability is particularly complex in older adults. The ICIDH-2 model is useful for structuring organized approaches to assessment, treatment, and evaluation of outcomes.

SITES OF REHABILITATION CARE

Rehabilitation services are offered in both inpatient and community-based sites. Inpatient care may be provided in rehabilitation centers (freestanding hospitals or units attached to acute hospitals), or nursing facilities. Outpatient rehabilitation services can be provided in hospital-based or independent clinics, in day hospital settings, or in the home. Eligibility requirements, the services provided, and costs vary across sites of care. These factors influence the balance of advantages and disadvantages for the individual patient and in turn influence the recommendations of the clinician.

An inpatient rehabilitation hospital program that is Medicare certified must demonstrate that 75% of the patients have at least one of ten conditions (nine are related to neurologic and musculoskeletal disorders; the tenth, to burns), and that at least 75% of patients receive 3 hours of therapy per day. Patients must be seen by a physician on a daily basis, have 24-hour rehabilitation nursing care, and be managed by a multidisciplinary team of skilled nurses and therapists. Medicare reimbursement is dependent on documented patient progress as a result of therapy. The maximum length of stay is 90 days per illness. The Medicare-approved skilled nursing facility must provide 24-hour nursing care. Dietary, pharmaceutical, dental, medical, and social services must also be available. Physicians must supervise patient care; they may visit the patient infrequently but must be available 24 hours a day for emergencies. Therapeutic services are available, but multidisciplinary coordination may not occur. In this setting, the maintenance of function without progress may be the goal of care. The amount of reimbursable therapy services provided is allocated on the basis of patient assessments by the use of the Minimum Data Set (MDS). Medicare limits reimbursement for rehabilitation therapy to 750 minutes per week. Current eligibility for Medicare skilled nursing benefits is restricted to persons who have had a hospital stay of at least 3 days in the past 30-day period. The length of Medicare coverage for rehabilitation in nursing homes is limited.

Subacute care is a cross between the hospital and the nursing facility, addressing the medical and rehabilitative needs of those who are adequately stabilized to no longer require acute care services but are too complex for treatment in a conventional nursing home. The number of providers of subacute care has risen sharply in the last decade. It is provided in freestanding facilities or units within a hospital or nursing home, although more than three quarters is offered in nursing homes. Older adults are the primary users of subacute care. Such care can be provided in rehabilitation hospitals; however, most Medicare recipients receive rehabilitation in subacute units if they can only tolerate only 90 minutes of therapy per day.

Rehabilitation subacute care refers to conditions requiring intense rehabilitative therapies (physical, occupational, speech) for specific conditions (stroke, hip fracture, amputation surgery) or general deconditioning following lack of mobilization associated with hospitalization or a medical condition. Although better patient outcomes following stroke are associated with post-acute care provided in a rehabilitation hospital than with subacute nursing-home units, subacute nursing-home units have demonstrated better outcomes following stroke than traditional nursing-home units. No differences have been found in patient outcomes following hip surgery for care in the sub-acute unit versus care in the rehabilitation hospital.

Medicare provides home-health benefits to patients who require intermittent or part-time skilled nursing care and therapy services and who are homebound, defined flexibly to include individuals who "occasionally leave the home." There is no prior hospitalization requirement or limit on the number of visits a person may receive. Home-health services provide skilled nursing and home-health aides, therapeutic services, medical and social services, and supplies. Even though primary care providers must certify the patient for services, they are rarely involved in the supervision of care, and multidisciplinary coordination of care may not be available. On October 1, 2000, Medicare began paying all home-health agencies under a prospective payment system. Payment rates are based on relevant data from patient assessments conducted by clinicians using the Outcome and Assessment Information Set (OASIS). The OASIS, originally developed to assess quality of care in home health, encompasses sociodemographic, environmental, support system, health status, and functional status attributes.

Inpatient rehabilitation facilities are also reimbursed by Medicare by the use of a prospective payment system. The system uses information from a patient assessment instrument, a functional independence measure, to develop Function Related Groups (FRGs), which supports classification of patients by case-mix groups.

The effect of site of care on rehabilitation outcomes is not well established. One study of outcomes among persons with stroke and hip fracture compared rates of discharge to home and recovery of function of those receiving inpatient or nursing rehabilitation services. The study, which controlled for case-mix differences, found that stroke but not hip-fracture patients were more likely to be discharged home and to recover activities of daily living (ADLs) if treated in an inpatient rehabilitation setting. Nursing homes with a high volume of Medicare patients were found to influence stroke outcomes more than did traditional nursing homes. Overall, there were no differences in outcomes for hip fracture patients by site of care. In a comparison of stroke patients treated under fee-for-service and managed care, the managed-care patients were found to be more likely to receive rehabilitation in skilled nursing facilities than in inpatient rehabilitation hospitals. Patients in fee-for-service care improved more in ADLs, during the treatment phase, but there were no differences in ADLs between groups 1 year later. However, at the 1-year follow-up, the patients in managed care were found to be 2.4 times more likely to reside in nursing homes. The effect of site of rehabilitation care outcomes for a more broad range of conditions has also been studied.

Consecutive patients enrolled from 52 hospitals in three cities and having one of five targeted conditions (chronic obstructive pulmonary disease, congestive heart failure, hip procedures, hip fractures, stroke) were assessed. Researchers, using case-mix adjustment models, found that, in general, patients discharged to nursing homes fared the worst, and that those sent home with home-health services or to rehabilitation hospitals did best. Despite statistical adjusting, concerns remain about using observational data to assess the effects of site of care on outcomes, since patients with better prognoses may go to inpatient or home-health settings, whereas those with poorer prognoses for functional recovery go to nursing homes. Nevertheless, it appears that site of care might well be an important factor in recovery. The clinician may improve the older patient's outcomes in rehabilitation by selecting site of rehabilitation with care.

From the patient's perspective, each site of care has advantages and disadvantages. Inpatient care is the most intense but may not be possible for frail older patients, since it requires 3 hours per day of active (and fatiguing) therapy. Skilled nursing offers 24-hour care for those who cannot care for themselves or do not have a full-time caregiver. Outpatient services have clear advantages and disadvantages. Patients often prefer to return to their own homes but may not have the caregiving they need. Participation in a day hospital or outpatient clinic requires transportation, which can be costly and time consuming.

In summary, clinicians must be familiar with the services provided in a wide range of rehabilitation settings and with the advantages and disadvantages of each type of setting. The clinician is responsible for recommending the best match between patient needs and program services. However, in reality, under certain plans such as managed care, the choice of settings and services may be determined by costs. Systematic evaluation of rehabilitation outcomes in various settings is needed. The Centers for Medicare & Medicaid Services (CMS) is currently funding initiatives to monitor the quality of patient care by the use of data from patient assessments in the MDS and OASIS.

MULTIDISCIPLINARY TEAMS

For many older adults, health professionals in several fields are required if their rehabilitation needs are to be met. The primary goal of multidisciplinary team management is to ensure that patients receive comprehensive assessments and interventions for the disabling illness and for associated comorbid conditions. All health professionals who work with older adults should have a basic understanding of the roles and functions of various rehabilitation team members. An effective team establishes common goals and a cohesive treatment plan for each patient. The patient's and family's expectations and preferences must be integrated into care planning. Unlike many other interventions, rehabilitation treatments require active patient participation. A patient-centered decision-making framework makes sense, given the chronic nature of many disabilities of older adults, for example, arthritis, diabetes mellitus, hypertension, and congestive heart failure. Patient self-management incorporates self-monitoring, education about the disease, and personal control over many prevention and management practices.

IMPACTS OF COMORBIDITIES

Comorbidities often require adaptations in the rehabilitation care plan and may even prevent, interrupt, or delay treatment. Many illnesses that can interfere with the rehabilitation of the older patient are predictable in this high-risk population and are potentially preventable. A systematic approach to the assessment, prevention, and management of comorbidities can improve the patient's chance of receiving maximal benefit from rehabilitation services.

One of the most common complications of inactivity is thromboembolisms; their prevention should be a routine part of rehabilitation care for older patients (see the Appendix, pp 387–388). Bladder problems due to detrusor hyperactivity, obstruction, or neurogenic bladder are also prevalent among older patients. Indwelling catheters increase the risk of infection and are rarely appropriate. The assessment and treatment of bladder problems should be a basic component of any rehabilitation service (see "Urinary Incontinence," p 134, and "Renal Diseases and Disorders," p 357). The risk of pneumonia is increased by inactivity and disordered swallowing. Prevention includes increasing ventilation through mobilization and incentive spirometry, especially in persons with obstructive lung disease. The prevention of aspiration pneumonia poses difficult tradeoffs: Routine radiologic screening for aspiration has precipitated a marked increased awareness of this problem, but the clinical relevance of modest amounts of aspiration detected radiologically are unknown. (See "Eating and Feeding Problems," p 191.)

Cognitive functioning is critical for rehabilitation, which depends on the patient's ability to follow directions and to learn. Older adults who have been acutely ill or who are newly disabled should be screened for delirium, dementia, and depression. (See "Delirium," p 127, "Dementia," p 113, and "Depression and Other Mood Disorders," p 211.)

Conditions that do not prevent or delay rehabilitation may nonetheless require ongoing modifications of the rehabilitation care plan (Table 13.1). Since activity level is a powerful factor in glucose metabolism,

Table 13.1—Conditions That Require Modification of the Rehabilitation Plan

Condition	Adaptations
Coronary artery disease	Adjust anti-anginal agent doses on the basis of expected increased myocardial oxygen demand resulting from increased activity and energy inefficiency of new disability; monitor for side effects of medications
Diabetes mellitus	Adjust insulin or oral agent doses: requirements may be reduced because of increased activity, increased if calorie intake increases; resolve any infection
Musculoskeletal disorders	Anticipate higher risk of overuse syndrome; monitor musculoskeletal status; incorporate planned rests in program; adapt assistive devices, as needed; treat any problems with heat, medications, injections
Peripheral vascular disease	Monitor for skin breakdown with weight bearing; modify plan for insensitive feet; treat painful peripheral neuropathies
Sensory disorders	Screen for vision and hearing impairments; adapt teaching approach, as needed

Source: Studenski S, Duncan P, Maino J. In: Hazzard WR, Blass JP, Ettinger WH Jr, et al., eds. *Principles of Geriatric Medicine and Gerontology.* 4th ed. New York: McGraw-Hill; 1999:440. © The McGraw-Hill Companies, Inc. Reprinted with permission.

diabetic patients are likely to experience changes in glucose levels and medication requirements during rehabilitation. Increased caloric intake during recovery may also affect medication needs. Since most abnormal gaits increase the energy requirements of walking, coronary artery disease symptoms may worsen, and persons with poor cardiac output may have extreme exercise limitations. Medication adjustments for heart disease may be necessary but can cause side effects of their own, such as orthostasis. Patients with one vascular disease often have others; peripheral vascular disease is common, often associated with insensitive or painful feet and a high risk of skin breakdown. Treatment of painful peripheral neuropathy may foster increased activity. Immobility or altered weight bearing can precipitate pressure ulcers that heal poorly. The clinician should monitor pressure and weight-bearing areas and be prepared to modify footwear, wheelchairs, and bedding, as needed.

REHABILITATION STRATEGIES: AN OVERVIEW

The primary goals of rehabilitation are restitution of function, compensation or adaptation to functional losses, and prevention of secondary complications. Rehabilitation should maximize the older person's potential for participation in social, leisure, or work activities. Rehabilitation should not be defined simply as improving independence in ADLs but also as a program to prevent disability. A wide variety of strategies can be used to achieve these goals.

Restitution of physical function usually depends on therapeutic exercises to improve flexibility, strength, motor control, and cardiovascular endurance. Although exercise has been shown to improve strength and motor control in well-defined populations of disabled older adults, there is still uncertainty about whether these gains translate into changes in mobility, ADLs, participation, or risk of falling.

Speech and language therapy can be used to treat aphasia in stroke patients, and cognitive rehabilitation can be used to improve their alertness and attention. As yet, however, there is no clear evidence that speech and language therapy or cognitive rehabilitation improves functional deficits.

Massage, heat, cold, and ultrasound are used to decrease pain and muscle spasm. These and other pain management strategies may contribute to increased function and tolerance for further rehabilitation. There is little evidence supporting objective benefits from these modalities, but patients commonly report symptomatic relief.

Equipment such as mobility aides, orthotic and prosthetic devices and splints, and dressing and bathroom aids can augment or replace the function of impaired body parts and thereby reduce limitations in activities and participation. For example, an ankle orthosis can prevent foot drop and improve safety and speed of walking.

Repeated practice of task-specific activities, such as bed mobility, transfers, and walking, can improve functional mobility. Upper-extremity function can also be improved with specific functional training activities, such as grasps, reaches, and fine manipulations. Balance training may reduce the risk of falls. (See "Falls," p 143.) Many older adults benefit from retraining in instrumental activities of daily living (IADLs), such as cooking, managing finances, or driving a car.

Contextual factors, both environmental and personal, need to be addressed in rehabilitation to minimize restrictions on the older person's activities and participation. Environmental modifications such as grab bars and raised toilet seats in the home or curb cutouts on public streets may be required to optimize the older person's independence in the home and the community.

A collaborative approach to goal setting, good patient and family education, and support groups may be used to address such personal factors as motivation. Each patient must be encouraged to accept responsibility for managing his or her condition and well-being.

ASSESSMENT AND REHABILITATION PLANNING

Comprehensive assessment of each patient is necessary for appropriate clinical management and evaluation of outcomes. The treatment plan should be guided by the results of the assessment. The primary components of any assessment include patient demographics, social support, place of residence prior to illness, medical comorbidities, severity of current illness, and patient's prior functional status. Impairments such as deficits in range of motion and flexibility, strength, sensory functions, balance, cognition, and mood should always be assessed. In conditions such as stroke there should also be an evaluation of swallowing and language function. The patient's functional status should be assessed with standardized measures of ADLs (eg, the Functional Independence Measure, the Barthel ADL Index), and of IADLs. The patient's participation or quality of life should also be assessed. (For specific screens, see the Appendix, pp 384–385.)

STROKE

Natural History

Stroke is a major cause of mortality and morbidity in the United States, particularly among persons aged 55 years and older. Acute stroke occurs in more than 700,000 persons each year, and more than 80% of them are likely to survive, many with residual neurologic difficulties. Stroke-related deficits are severe in approximately one third of the survivors and moderate or mild in the other two thirds. Many patients with mild and moderate stroke become independent in ADLs, but other more complex dimensions of health status may be affected. Rehabilitation programs must address a broad range of stroke-related disabilities, including not only deficits in the patient's basic ADLS but also deficits in IADLS and in the ability to participate fully in social activities.

Assessment and Management

The overall goals of rehabilitation for the stroke patient are restitution of function, compensation for or adaptation to functional losses, and prevention of secondary complications. The specific objectives of stroke rehabilitation include:

- preventing, recognizing, and managing comorbid illness and medical complications;
- assessing the patient's status comprehensively, using standardized instruments,
- matching the rehabilitation program to the patient's needs and capabilities;

- maximizing the patient's independence in ADLs and IADLs;

- facilitating the patient's and the family's psychosocial coping and adaptation;

- preventing recurrent stroke and other vascular conditions, such as myocardial infarction; and

- assisting the patient in reintegrating into the community.

Rehabilitation for older stroke patients is complex because of the heterogeneity of causes and residual symptoms of stroke, site and size of the brain lesions, and prestroke status of older patients. The most common type of neurologic deficit is hemiparesis; other residual symptoms may include sensory deficits, aphasia, dysarthria, cognitive deficits, motor incoordination, hemianopsia, visual-perceptual deficits, depression, dysphagia, and bowel and bladder incontinence. The patient's degree of initial recovery and the time he or she needs to reach maximal recovery is affected by the number of deficits. For example, those who have hemiparesis, hemianopsia, and sensory deficits are less likely to ambulate independently and will require a longer time to regain skills than do those with hemiparesis only.

Stroke patients usually experience the most dramatic recovery in the first 30 days but may continue to improve more gradually for months. The Framingham study showed that improvement in motor function and self-care slowed 3 months after stroke but continued at a reduced pace throughout the first year. Language and visual-spatial function recovered over 12 months, but cognitive function improved only during the first 3 months.

In 1995 the Agency for Health Care Policy and Research (now the Agency for Healthcare Research and Quality) convened a multidisciplinary panel of stroke experts to review the evidence for stroke rehabilitation practice and make recommendations (Table 13.2). A considerable body of evidence indicates that better clinical outcomes are achieved when patients with acute stroke are treated in a setting that provides coordinated, multidisciplinary stroke-related evaluation and services. Coordinated care has been shown to reduce 1-year mortality and improve functional independence. The apparent benefits are not restricted to any particular subgroup of patients. There is less evidence to support specific therapeutic interventions for stroke. Treatment approaches based on theories of proprioceptive neuromuscular facilitation have been most commonly used for restitution of motor control. A new approach introduced in the late 1980s incorporates active practice of motor tasks with appropriate feedback and promotion of motor learning and recovery. Studies have compared techniques, but there is no

Table 13.2—AHCPR Rehabilitation Recommendations for Stroke

- When possible, treat the acute stroke patient in a setting that provides coordinated, multidisciplinary stroke-related evaluation and services.

- Fully document the patient's condition and clinical course in the medical record; evaluate the patient at key stages throughout acute care and rehabilitation.

- Screen the patient for formal rehabilitation during the acute hospitalization; begin rehabilitation care immediately, and increase the patient's activity as soon as medically feasible during the acute phase.

- Manage general health functions and take steps to prevent complications throughout all stages of treatment.

- Recommend whether the patient should receive further individual or multidisciplinary rehabilitation; if interdisciplinary rehabilitation is recommended, choose an appropriate program in consultation with the patient and family.

- Perform a baseline assessment on admission to rehabilitation, using well-validated standardized measures for assessment.

- Develop explicit rehabilitation goals and a plan for achieving them with the patient and family.

- Provide remedial treatment for sensorimotor deficits and compensatory training for disabilities; identify and treat cognitive and perceptual deficits as well as speech and language disorders.

- Maintain a high index of suspicion for depression and provide treatment.

- Educate the patient, family, and caregivers.

- Provide support and assistance to caregivers.

NOTE: AHCPR = Agency for Health Care Policy and Research (now, Agency for Healthcare Research and Quality).

SOURCE: Adapted from Greshem GE, Duncan PW, Stason WB, et al. *Post-Stroke Rehabilitation: Clinical Practice Guideline, No. 16*. Rockville, MD: US Department of Health and Human Services, Public Health Service, Agency for Health Care Policy and Research. May 1995. AHCPR Pub. No. 95-0662.

convincing evidence that one technique is superior. In the past few years several new therapeutic interventions for restitution of motor function have been introduced. Constraint-induced movement therapy discourages the use of the unaffected extremity and encourages active use of the hemiparetic extremity, with the goal of improving motor recovery. The early results from several studies suggest that this technique may be useful. A national multisite randomized clinical trial is currently under way to compare the functional outcomes of two groups of patients who are 3 to 6 months post-stroke, one group receiving constraint of the better upper arm for 2 weeks and the other receiving customary care. Walking on a treadmill with body-weight support using a harness connected to an overhead support is a new method of training for walking. Several randomized clinical trials and several case studies of this method suggest that gait velocity, balance, and motor recovery may be enhanced with this therapy.

Speech and language therapy are often provided for stroke patients with aphasia. However, there is no universally accepted treatment, and analysis of evidence from studies of speech and language therapy for stroke survivors indicates that this therapy has not been shown to be either effective or ineffective.

Tertiary Prevention

The patient who has had a stroke is at very high risk for recurrence, at a rate of 7% to 10% annually. The rehabilitation phase is an appropriate time to assure that assessment and treatment for stroke prevention has occurred. Assessments for significant carotid stenosis and for atrial fibrillation should be completed. Indications for carotid endarterectomy and anticoagulation with warfarin should be reviewed. The use of aspirin or other antiplatelet agents should be considered. Other risk factors to be targeted include hypertension, diabetes mellitus, hyperlipidemia, and smoking.

HIP FRACTURE

Natural History

Currently, more than 250,000 people fracture a hip each year in the United States. Risk of fracture is higher with older age and among women, nursing-home residents, and persons with dementia. Mortality is about 5% during the initial hospitalization but up to 20% in the year following fracture. Recovery to the prior level of function is achieved by about 75% of survivors, but overall mobility is limited, requiring assistive devices in half of survivors. Up to 50% of patients have an initial decline requiring temporary long-term care, and about 25% remain in long-term care 1 year later.

About one third of hip fractures involve the femoral neck and about two thirds are intertrochanteric. Fractures can be displaced or nondisplaced, affecting surgical approach. Traditionally, displaced femoral neck fractures are treated with a prosthetic femoral head. Nondisplaced femoral neck fractures are often treated by internal fixation with pins or nails, and intertrochanteric fractures are often treated with open reduction and internal fixation with compression screws or sliding nails.

Assessment and Management

Initial assessment includes prior mobility and functional status, comorbid conditions, cognitive status, and social support. Other information includes type of injury and repair as well as pain status. Mobility performance should be systematically assessed.

Rehabilitation of hip fracture consists of mobilization, pain management, prevention of complications, and functional adaptation. Coordinated inpatient care has shown a modest benefit (about 10%) in the reduction of pooled outcomes such as death, worsened function, and institutionalization. Organized rehabilitation is beneficial for those older patients with mild to moderate dementia. Factors that influence recovery include the timing of mobilization and the frequency of therapy. Delay in mobilization is often driven by surgical recommendation. Some surgeons prescribe limited or no weight bearing for up to 6 weeks after surgery in order to maximize healing and stabilization. Partial weight bearing may be difficult for many older patients to achieve, although they will spontaneously shift weight in response to discomfort. Prolonged inactivity is clearly associated with poorer functional outcomes, and early weight bearing as tolerated has been shown to be associated with low rates of surgical failure.

Tertiary Prevention

Persons who have had a hip fracture are often osteoporotic and unstable. They are at increased risk for further fractures. Efforts to treat osteoporosis, improve balance, and reduce injury risk are a key part of treatment planning during rehabilitation. Hip protectors have been shown to reduce hip fracture rates, although adherence may be a barrier to use.

AMPUTATION

Natural History

Approximately 50,000 people have a lower-extremity amputation each year in the United States. Most have widespread vascular disease, with or without diabetes mellitus. Many have other manifestations of systemic vascular disease, such as cardiac or cerebrovascular deficits. Diabetic patients often have other end organ disease, such as blindness, end-stage renal disease, and peripheral neuropathy. Mortality rates of those with amputations secondary to peripheral vascular disease is high: 50% at 2 years and 70% at 5 years. Up to 20% lose the other extremity within the first 2 years after an initial amputation. Most amputees with peripheral vascular disease have so much comorbid disease that limited mobility for transfers and ambulation within the home are the major goals of prosthetic use.

Assessment and Management

Initial assessment includes prior functional status, status of comorbid conditions, mental status, status of the stump and the other lower extremity, and function of the upper extremities. Predictors of functional ambulation with a prosthesis include prior independent ambulation, weight-bearing ability of the contralateral leg, medical stability, and mental status. Blindness and end-stage renal disease do not necessarily preclude rehabilitation.

The rehabilitation phase should start promptly after surgery, starting with teaching about the recovery process and exercises for strength and flexibility of the lower and upper extremities. Amputation of the lower extremity generally aims to preserve the knee, since the below-the-knee amputee has a much lower energy requirement for walking than does the above-the-knee amputee. This decision must be weighed against risks of poor wound healing with more distal amputation.

Postoperative rehabilitation focuses on mobilization, wound healing, and shaping of the stump. Poor wound healing delays rehabilitation in about 25% of cases. A rigid removable dressing can facilitate early weight bearing without increasing wound breakdown and allows direct monitoring of the healing tissues. Prostheses vary in weight, socket type, style of foot, and type of suspension; the older amputee does better with prostheses of low weight, stability, and ease of use. Prostheses may also need to be adapted to other medical conditions. For example, the patient with frequent changes in stump volume due to edema from heart or kidney disease must have a prosthesis that is adaptable to wide swings in the size of the stump. Rehabilitation for patients with amputations includes teaching the patients and their caregivers about prosthesis and stump care and self-monitoring for stump injury.

Tertiary Prevention

Since the amputee's risk of contralateral amputation reaches 20% at 2 years, the monitoring and care of the other lower extremity is important. Vascular risk reduction includes smoking cessation, cholesterol reduction, and glucose control. Programs of endurance exercise can improve function and reduce claudication. Daily monitoring for infection and skin breakdown are essential.

ASSISTIVE DEVICES, ADAPTIVE TECHNIQUES, AND ENVIRONMENTAL MODIFICATIONS

Assistive devices and adaptive techniques are effective for patients with disabilities and handicaps. It is impor-
tant to identify the underlying causes of disability before prescribing a device because medical or surgical treatment for individual diseases and impairments may be more effective or may enhance the usefulness of these devices.

Mobility Aids

Canes typically support 15% to 20% of the body weight. The tips, handles, materials, and lengths of canes vary. As the number of tips increases, the degree of support also increases, but the cane becomes heavier and more awkward to use. The cane tip is fitted with a 5-cm diameter rubber tip with a concentric ring to prevent slipping. The handle of the cane may be curved or have a pistol grip; the pistol grip offers more support but is less aesthetically pleasing to some people. Canes can be made of a variety of materials, but most are made of wood or light-weight aluminum. The length of the cane is important for stability. Some canes are adjustable, but wooden canes must be cut to size. One of three methods may be used to evaluate the proper cane length: measuring the distance from the distal wrist crease to the ground when the patient is standing erect, measuring the distance from the greater trochanter to the ground, or measuring the distance between the ground 15 cm in front of and to the side of the tip of the shoe and the elbow flexed at 30 degrees. The first method is preferred.

Crutches can support full body weight but are seldom used with older persons. Problems with crutches include the large amount of arm strength required, the risk of brachial plexus injury, and the necessity to use an unnatural gait pattern.

A walker is prescribed when a cane does not offer sufficient stability. A walker can completely support one lower extremity but cannot support full body weight. Walker types include pick-up and wheeled walkers. The pick-up walker is lifted and moved forward by the patient, who then advances before lifting the walker again; the result is a slow, staggering gait. It requires strength to repeatedly pick up the walker and cognitive ability to learn the necessary coordination. A wheeled walker allows for a smoother, coordinated, and faster gait and takes advantage of overlearned gait patterns. It is more likely to be correctly used by persons with cognitive impairment. The most commonly used type is the two-wheeled walker, which brakes automatically with increased downward pressure. Four-wheeled walkers are rarely used because they are less stable and more difficult to control, although they are occasionally useful for persons with Parkinson's disease. Three-wheeled walkers may offer some advantages in ease of turning but are not yet in common use. The Merry Walker© Ambulation Device has a seat and bars all the way around. It is the same size as a wheelchair and is best reserved for those with severe balance problems.

Patients who cannot safely use or are unable to ambulate with an assistive device will require a wheelchair. A wheelchair must be fitted according to the patient's body build, weight, disability, and prognosis. Incorrect fit may result in poor posture, joint deformity, reduced mobility, pressure sores, circulatory compromise, and discomfort. For the older patient with only one functional arm, the wheelchair may be lowered to allow for foot propulsion. Patients with lower-extremity amputations may have the wheels set posteriorly to compensate for a change in the center of gravity. Motorized wheelchairs may be used by mentally alert persons with bilateral upper-extremity weakness or severe cardiopulmonary disease who lack the endurance to push a wheelchair. Motorized scooters offer less trunk support than motorized wheelchairs but are more acceptable to some people. Motorized scooters and wheelchairs increase patients' mobility but increase their risk of deconditioning, as they might otherwise push a wheelchair or ambulate. The use of a wheelchair commonly requires home modifications, including ramps and widened doorways. Cars may need to be adapted with lifts.

Orthotics, Adaptive Methods, and Assistive Devices

Orthotics are exoskeletons designed to assist, resist, align, and stimulate function. Orthotics are named by the use of letters for each joint that the device involves in its structure. Thus, an AFO is an ankle and foot orthotic device used to support weak calf or pretibial muscles (eg, for a stroke patient with lower-extremity weakness).

Adaptations to facilitate dressing may be necessary for patients with problems such as frequent soiling or diminished flexibility, coordination, and endurance. Their clothing should be easy to clean, and tops should fit easily over the head or fasten in the front and allow for freedom of movement. Fastening clothes is frequently a problem for older persons. Hooks and loops are usually easier to use than buttons, and they may be sewn on to replace buttons and zippers. When buttons are necessary, button hooks with customized grips may be used, or the buttons can be sewn on with elastic thread, which may eliminate the need to unbutton the buttons. Donning shoes and socks is particularly difficult for older persons with decreased agility. Longer,

looser socks (eg, tubular socks) are easier to don. For patients who find that reaching the feet to put on shoes is a problem, a long-handled shoehorn may be useful. Elastic shoelaces eliminate the need for tying and untying.

Environmental modifications can have a major impact on the older person's ability to function independently or with minimal assistance at home. A variety of assistive devices, such as reachers, special utensils, and adapted telephone, can reduce the difficulty of performing daily tasks and have a significant impact on a person's quality of life.

The bathroom is a common place for falls. Any older person with impaired balance or lower-extremity weakness should have bars installed near the toilet and tub or shower. Raised toilet seats and bathtub benches are available to assist those with lower-extremity weakness. These are also useful for persons with arthritis of the hips or knees because they reduce biomechanical stress on the joint. Long-handled bath brushes, hand-held shower, and "soap on a rope" may be helpful for persons with upper-extremity impairment.

REFERENCES

■ Greshem GE, Duncan PW, Stason WB, et al. *Post-Stroke Rehabilitation: Assessment, Referral and Patient Management. Clinical Practice Guideline. Quick Reference Guide for Clinicians, No. 16.* Rockville, MD: US Department of Health and Human Services, Public Health Service, Agency for Health Care Policy and Research. May 1995. AHCPR Pub. No. 95-0663.

■ Johnson MF, Kramer AM, Lin MK, et al. Outcomes of older persons receiving rehabilitation for medical and surgical conditions compared with hip fracture and stroke. *J Am Geriatr Soc.* 2000;48(11):1389–1397.

■ Jorgensen HS, Nakayama H, Pedersen PM, et al. Outcome and time course of recovery in stroke: part II: time course of recovery. The Copenhagen Stroke Study. *Arch Phys Med Rehabil.* 1995;76(5):406–412.

■ Kramer AM, Kowalsky JC, Lin M, et al. Outcome and utilization differences for older persons with stroke in HMO and fee-for-service systems. *J Am Geriatr Soc.* 2000;48(7):726–734.

■ Rawl SM, Easton KL, Kwiatkowski S, et al. Effectiveness of a nurse-managed follow-up program for rehabilitation patients after discharge. *Rehabil Nurs.* 1998; 23(4):204–209.

CHAPTER 14—COMMUNITY-BASED CARE

HOME CARE

Home-health care grew tremendously starting in the mid-1980s and through the 1990s, mainly as a result of the shift toward earlier hospital discharge because of the trend toward prospective hospital payment and the expansion of managed care. Further, Medicare reimbursement was lucrative for many home-health agencies and led to further growth. Although the evidence is not overwhelming, a few studies have shown that home care can reduce hospital days, readmission to the hospital, and nursing-home placement. Home-care models shown to be successful include interdisciplinary home care, postacute hospital home care, home rehabilitation, home geriatric assessment, and the home hospital.

The Balanced Budget Act of 1997 (BBA) considerably reduced payments for home care. Following implementation of the BBA, the number of Medicare home-health beneficiaries dropped from 3.6 million to 3 million, and a considerable number of home-health agencies closed. An interim payment system was in effect until October 2000, at which time a prospective payment system (PPS) became operative. Under prospective payment, Medicare will pay a set fee for Home Health Related Groups (HHRGs) that are based on the Outcome and Assessment Information Set (OASIS). OASIS is a broadly based assessment, which is completed by the home-health-care agency and focuses on a variety of areas, including function, need for services, and therapy needs. On the basis of the OASIS, home-health agencies will be reimbursed according to a specific HHRG, adjusted for clinical severity, functional status, and location. Initially, the BBA was scheduled to reduce home-health prospective payments by another 15% in October 2000. However, the Balanced Budget Refinement Act of 1999 delayed the 15% reduction until after October 2001, though the PPS still went into effect in October 2000.

The Primary Care Provider's Role in Home Care

The primary care provider's role in home care is to serve as a member of an interdisciplinary team that generally includes nurses, therapists (speech, physical, occupational, and respiratory), social workers, personal care aides, home medical equipment suppliers, and, most importantly, informal caregivers. A physician is, by law, responsible for the patient's care plan. The primary care provider determines the patient's health care needs and should confer regularly with team members to address patient care issues and to handle documentation and other administrative matters.

Physicians and other primary care practitioners are reimbursed for care plan oversight of complex cases in skilled home care and hospice if they document the specific activities performed (eg, paperwork, telephone calls with other professionals) and the total time in a month exceeds 30 minutes. The documentation requirements for billing allow activities over multiple days in a month to be combined.

House calls can add an important dimension to the practitioner's knowledge of the patient's circumstances and environment. Home evaluation can identify additional problems not readily apparent in office-based assessment. Barriers to maximum functioning can be identified and addressed. House calls have the additional benefit of reducing the burden of transportation for patients who have difficulty getting outside of the home. Changes in Medicare have increased reimbursement for home visits, making home visits more financially feasible.

Patient Assessment

Homebound patients generally have significant impairment in at least one dimension and frequently more. Comprehensive geriatric assessment is particularly valuable in this setting to establish a baseline, monitor the course of illness, and evaluate effects of intervention. However, assessment in the home has some important differences from office-based assessment.

During a home visit, an assessment of the patient's actual environment can be performed to determine whether the home is safe and supportive in the context of the particular patient's abilities and disabilities. Performance-based functional assessment can focus on the practical aspects of performing activities of daily living (ADLs) by direct observation of the environment for bathing, dressing, and transferring. Difficulties can be identified, and the assessor can evaluate the caregiver's abilities to address the patient's needs. The caregiver's needs for counseling, training, support, and education can also be identified and addressed.

Environmental modifications can be recommended to improve function. For example, modifications of the bathtub, a hand-held shower, a shower seat, grab-bars, and a bedside commode can improve the patient's quality of life and functioning. Barriers to wheelchairs and walkers such as door sills can be identified and removed. Chair lifts and outdoor ramps can help patients circumvent stairs. Occupational therapy consultation can be particularly useful in identifying other personal care and assistive devices for performing ADLs and housekeeping chores. A number of home safety checklists are available to help a reviewer assess the home (see the Appendix, p 400, for one such list). Additional technological additions to improve home safety, including necklace or wrist radio devices to call for help, can be considered.

Health care providers are finding that home diagnostics, including radiology and electrocardiography, are available in most areas, and hand-held laboratory devices are becoming more common. These home diagnostics allow for a much more comprehensive medical evaluation to take place in the home.

Developing an Office-Based House-Call Program

Medical care in the home may be provided as part of an ongoing office-based program, as an extension of hospitalization through a postacute care program, or as a freestanding entity. Regardless of the method chosen, it is important that the organization of the home-care program be well conceived to maximize effectiveness and efficiency and to remain financially viable. Current regulations allow house calls to be provided by physicians, nurse practitioners, and physician assistants. Regardless of the primary care provider, appropriate links to other providers of home-based services are necessary to develop an interdisciplinary team. Consistency and familiarity with other members of the interdisciplinary team are essential to a smoothly functioning house-call program.

Choosing the Right Patients

To qualify for Medicare home-care benefits, a patient must meet two criteria to establish homebound status. First, the patient must be absent from the home for reasons other than obtaining medical treatment infrequently ($\leq$ three times per month) or for short periods of time. Second, leaving home must require considerable and taxing effort on the part of the patient or the caregiver, or both, such as if the patient is bedbound or has a severe mobility impairment.

Patients who are likely to be good candidates for house calls are those with mobility impairments that make transportation to the office difficult; those with disruptive behaviors; patients with terminal illnesses; and patients with multiple medical, psychiatric, and social problems. House calls are needed for some patients a limited amount of time, but others require house visits on an ongoing basis. Home visits may be particularly useful for patients who are either not responding to adequate therapy or responding inconsistently. A diagnostic home visit may reveal caregiver burnout, elder mistreatment, or the use of medications

from other sources that may be interfering with the expected response. (See also "Pharmacotherapy," p 35; "Elder Mistreatment," p 52.)

Equipment for House Calls

Table 14.1 lists suggested equipment and drugs for house calls. A small bag with key equipment will be particularly useful. A supply of forms needed for common diagnostic tests and orders, educational material for common problems, and community referral information are also useful.

Caregiver Support

Family caregivers provide most of the care received by patients in the community. In the United States, three out of four caregivers are women, either wives or daughters. Caregiving is often intense, time consuming, and stressful. The caregiver's physical and emotional health may be affected, resulting in depression and a worsening of his or her own health problems. Attention to caregiver support and issues are essential to help the patients continue to provide care. Caregiver support groups may be particularly helpful (see the resources listed in the Appendix, p 418).

For discussions of specific issues concerning caregiving, see "Psychosocial Issues" (p 13), "Dementia" (p 113), "Neuropsychiatric and Behavioral Disturbances in Dementia" (p 121), "Elder Mistreatment" (p 52), and "Depression and Other Mood Disorders" (p 211).

Table 14.1—Suggested Equipment and Supplies for House Calls

Basic equipment and supplies	
Cerumen curette	Sphygmomanometer
Cotton tip applicators	Stethoscope
Gloves	Stool guaiac cards and
Intravenous starting kit and	developer
fluid	Tape measure
Lubricating jelly	Toenail clippers
Oto-ophthalmoscope	Tongue depressors
Phlebotomy equipment	Tuning fork
Reflex hammer	Urine dipsticks
Snellen chart	

Additional supplies	
Emergency medications	Specimen cups
(protect from heat and cold)	Wound debridement kit
Foley and coudé catheter	Wound dressing materials
Genitourinary syringe	
Nasogastric tube	

Also consider	
Audioscope	Portable oxygen
Glucometer with lancets in strips	Pulse oximeter
Portable electrocardiograph	Voice amplifier
machine	

Case Management

Case management refers to the organization of health care services and social services provided to the older person. Case managers are often registered nurses but may also be from other disciplines, including social work and public health. The role of the case manager is to follow, organize, and coordinate health care for the older person.

The current health care system is fragmented. Numerous physicians, health care professionals, and social service providers care for the older person. Coordinating this multitude is a challenge that often cannot be met by the patients or their caregivers. Hence, the role of the case manager is to assist in arranging and following the patient's social (and occasionally medical) problems. Case managers have become more common, especially in managed-care settings, where they are felt to improve efficiency and cost-effectiveness.

Primary care providers should work closely with case managers to optimize care for their older patients. However, in some cases an established interdisciplinary team already provides case management, and adding another member will not necessarily help and may actually confuse the situation.

Most managed-care plans provide case management, though many case managers are paid privately.

The Aging Network

The Older Americans Act (OAA) in 1965 established the "aging network," including the Administration of Aging. The latter is responsible for grant authorization in community planning and service programs and demonstration projects in the field of gerontology. Each state has one or more state unit on aging that directs money from the federal government to various OAA programs in the state. Each state has one or more area agencies on aging that are often referred to as "Triple As," that provide various programs and services. The six core services that are funded by the OAA are: supportive services; nutrition services; preventive health services; The National Family Caregiver Support Program (NFSCP); services that protect the rights of vulnerable older persons; services to Native Americans; and Eldercare Locator. Examples of supportive services enable local communities to provide transportation to medical appointments, errands, small chores, and personal care services. Under the OAA Nutritional Program, meals are provided for at-risk older adults. The services provided by a local area agency on aging depends on additional funds provided by local/state taxes, lottery funds or private foundations or donations. The primary service provided by every area agency on aging is information and referral to local aging services.

Limitations of Home Care

Most elderly persons would prefer to remain in their own home, but certain situations and conditions arise that make institutional care a more appropriate choice than in-home care. For example, caregivers may not be available to adequately address the needs of the patient. Relatively unstable medical situations requiring frequent laboratory testing, respiratory interventions, or intravenous medications may make institutional care a better choice than home care for some patients. Caregiver burnout and caregiver stress may prevent continued safe care for the patient in the home.

Further, the home environment itself may be a barrier to continuing in-home care. Unsafe neighborhoods, ongoing household social disruptions from alcohol or drug use, and inadequate room for equipment or environmental modifications may prohibit in-home care.

Finally, home care may be prohibitively expensive. It is not always the least expensive alternative, and out-of-pocket expenses may prohibit ongoing home care. Insurance coverage is more likely to cover care that is rendered in a nursing facility or other institutional setting.

Liability and Legal Issues

Malpractice suits related to home care are relatively uncommon. It is important that appropriate documentation be maintained for medical purposes and also to support providers' compensation.

Ethics and Decisions about Institutionalization

Two ethical themes arise commonly in home care. The first is the balance between patient autonomy and patient safety. The second involves issues surrounding elder mistreatment and neglect.

Respect for patient autonomy often dictates that the patient remain in the home as a result of the patient's (or surrogate decision maker's) choice. Conflict arises when a patient's medical care or safety cannot be adequately maintained in the home, yet the patient insists on staying at home. It is difficult to balance respect for patient autonomy with the desire to prevent patient neglect. In some situations, the outcome is likely to be terminal, regardless of whether the patient is maintained at home or in an institution. In such situations, a hospice referral may help provide additional services in the home and support for both the patient and family. In situations where there is a clearly neglectful or abusive situation, Adult Protective Services should be contacted (see "Elder Mistreatment," p 52, and "Legal and Ethical Issues," p 18).

COMMUNITY-BASED SERVICES NOT REQUIRING A CHANGE IN RESIDENCE

Adult Day Care

Adult day care is a community-based option that provides a wide range of social and support services in a congregate setting. Adult day care has become increasingly common. Providers of adult day care may offer a variety of services, ranging from simple nonskilled custodial care to more advanced skilled services. The availability of a registered nurse allows for on-site health services, clinical assessment and monitoring, and assistance with medication management. Adult day care is used commonly for patients with dementia who need supervision and assistance with their ADLs while primary caregivers work. Adult day care may also serve as a form of respite for caregivers. Most adult day care centers are community based, either in churches or community centers. In general, custodial adult day care is not covered by Medicare, though some costs may be covered by Medicaid or other insurers.

Day Hospitals

Day hospitals provide a broad range of skilled nursing care services, including parenteral antibiotics, chemotherapy, and intensive rehabilitation. The majority of programs are housed in chronic care hospitals or rehabilitation centers. This arrangement allows for the provider to take advantage of in-house professional expertise and resources, while allowing the patient to return to his or her own home or alternative living site after day treatment is complete. Services are covered under Medicare, with similar requirements to those surrounding home-health care.

Day hospitals are most often used for two groups of patients: those needing multidisciplinary rehabilitation and those with psychiatric illnesses. A systematic review of day hospital care found that there are no significant differences between day hospitals and alternative sources of care with respect to death, disability, or use of health services, but that among those receiving care in a day hospital there is a trend toward less functional decline and less hospital and institutional care.

Program of All-Inclusive Care for the Elderly

The Program of All-Inclusive Care for the Elderly (PACE) is a capitated model of care that pools funds from Medicare and Medicaid to provide acute and long-term care to frail older people. (See also "Financing, Coverage, and Costs of Health Care," p 26.) Participants in the PACE program must meet state-defined requirements regarding their need for a nursing-home level of care. The goal of the program is to keep the participant in the community for as long as it is medically, socially, and financially feasible. The system, designed to be seamless, uses an interdisciplinary team of health care providers who know the patient and caregivers well and who provide care across the spectrum of hospital, home, alternative living situations, and institutional care. Integrated financing allows the program to provide traditional coverage of acute, rehabilitative, home, and institutional care. It also allows for adult day care, respite care, transportation, medication coverage, rehabilitation including maintenance physical and occupational therapy, hearing aids, eyeglasses, and a variety of other benefits. The program, at the discretion of the interdisciplinary team, has the flexibility to pay for nonmedical costs in unusual circumstances (eg, paying a person's electric or gas bill). Care by the interdisciplinary team provides for the complex social as well as the medical needs of the participant. PACE has been described as one of the few truly integrated systems of care in the United States. Although the effectiveness of PACE has not been directly tested by a randomized, controlled trial, research has shown that PACE provides a high standard of quality, albeit with significant site-to-site variation.

In 1997, legislation was passed that changed the status of PACE from a demonstration program to a permanent provider under Medicare. PACE is an optional program under state Medicaid. As of May 2001, 26 programs in 13 states are operational, and 40 more are in various stages of development. It is anticipated that the program will continue to expand.

Capitated financing for PACE is provided through Medicare and, in participating states, Medicaid. The Medicare rate-setting method for PACE has traditionally been based on the average cost of providing care to Medicare beneficiaries in a given geographic area, which is multiplied by a frailty adjuster. This method is likely to change in the near future. Each state determines the Medicaid rate of capitation.

Additional information can be found at http://www.medicare.gov/nursing/alternatives/pace.asp and http://www.natlpaceassn.org.

Social Health Maintenance Organizations

The first generation Social Health Maintenance Organization (SHMO) project started in the middle 1980s with the intention of developing innovative, integrated, acute, and long-term care for Medicare beneficiaries. The four initial sites offered a variety of services and a system of care that focused on assessment and case management and that offered additional home and community-based services. Unlike the PACE program, the SHMOs serve not only low-income frail seniors but also the healthier, more affluent, nondisabled Medicare recipients. The first round of the SHMO demonstration found outcomes that were similar to controls without any clear cost savings. One of the original four sites elected to drop out of the demonstration in 1994; an additional six sites for the second generation (SHMO II) were approved in 1996. It is hoped that SHMO II will provide a greater degree of effectiveness and integration through a variety of modifications to SHMO I, including more emphasis on personnel with geriatrics expertise, geriatric practice guidelines, and education of nongeriatrician practitioners on the essentials of geriatric care. Changes in financing for SHMO II allow for reimbursement for patients who are at higher risk.

Telemedicine

The role of telemedicine in home care is evolving. It may have particular applicability in rural settings or other areas where access to physicians and other health care providers is limited. Telemedicine involves the transmission of data to the primary care provider, who can then evaluate and make decisions regarding the patient's health care. Systems vary considerably. For example, some systems are relatively disease specific. One example is an automated scale, blood pressure cuff, and heart rate monitor for patients with congestive heart failure. More elaborate telemedicine systems allow for audio and video two-way communication, distance electrocardiography, distance auscultation through the use of an onsite stethoscope that can transmit breath, heart, and abdominal sounds, and camera lenses that allow for detailed examination of the skin and eyes. System costs vary considerably, ranging from approximately $1500 for simple audio and video systems to $20,000. In the future they are likely to become more affordable. In certain situations telemedicine is Medicare reimbursable in rural areas. Some states are providing coverage through Medicaid.

Home Hospital

The home hospital focuses on providing more complex care at home to older people who would have been hospitalized for an acute care need. Patients receiving home hospital care have access to nurses and physicians on a regular basis and for episodic care through an on-call system that allows problems to be addressed promptly. The concept may be viewed as an evolution of home care, which it resembles, though it is more intense. Studies conducted outside of the United States suggest that care is comparable for selected patients and that patient satisfaction is high.

COMMUNITY-BASED SERVICES REQUIRING A CHANGE OF RESIDENCE

Assisted Living

There has been tremendous growth in the number of assisted-living facilities (ALFs) during the late 1990s. It is estimated that between 40,000 and 65,000 ALFs were operating in the United States in 1997. State definitions of assisted-living services vary considerably, and the terminology used is not consistent among states. The common features of ALFs include care management and living services. Typically, services include meals, housekeeping, maintenance and laundry service, and some level of assistance with ADLs, transportation, structured activities, and recreation. Health care coordination, medication monitoring or administration or both, and some limited health care are also provided. Residents have a wide range of choices, ranging from smaller, simple home-like environments, to larger, more elaborate (and even luxurious) accommodations. The tremendous variability in types of ALFs allows people to choose a home that best suits their needs, tastes, and financial situation. Special care units focusing on Alzheimer's disease and other forms of dementia are becoming more common.

Services provided under assisted living vary considerably. Different licensing requirements in individual states make cross-state comparison difficult. For example, depending on licensing requirements, medication administration and management may be directed by nonskilled, skilled, or fully licensed nursing staff. In areas where regulations do not require skilled care, home-health skilled care is often provided in the ALFs. Thus, the boundary between ALFs and skilled nursing facilities often becomes blurred.

Reimbursement for assisted living is largely out of pocket, though some states provide funding through Medicaid. Generally, care in an ALF is less expensive than in similar nursing-home units. Part of this difference in cost is due to the fact that less service is provided and less overhead is thus incurred. In addition, ALFs generally have fewer regulations to observe than nursing homes do and are therefore able to operate more economically.

Group Homes

Group homes (including domiciliary care, single-room occupancy residences, board-and-care homes, and some congregate living situations) are houses or apartments in which two or more unrelated people live together. Group homes vary in types of residents and often serve patients with chronic mental illness or dementia. Residents share a living room, dining room, and kitchen but usually have their own bedrooms. Advantages of this arrangement include a lower cost of living and socialization with peers. Independence and functional status are supported through the interdependence and relationships of the residents. Resident-to-staff ratios may be higher than in other supported living environments. Opportunities for socialization are increased, reducing social isolation. Most group homes are run as for-profit businesses, and some states require licensing.

Adult Foster Care

Foster care homes generally provide room, board, and some assistance with ADLs by the sponsoring family or by paid caregivers, who customarily live on the premises. Perhaps the longest experience with adult foster care is in the state of Oregon, where it is used as an alternative to long-term care and institutionalization. Adult foster care has the advantages of maintaining frail older adults in a more home-like environment. Regulations for foster care vary by state, and some states require licensing. Some states provide coverage of adult foster care through their Medicaid programs.

Sheltered Housing

Sheltered housing is funded through the Older Americans Act and is offered as an option for housing subsidized through section 8, Housing and Urban Development programs for older adults and disabled residents. Often these arrangements are sheltered homes offering personal care assistance, housekeeping services, and meals. Programs may be supplemented by social work services and activities coordinators. Charges to clients are based on a sliding scale, which may cost up to 30% of income.

Continuing Care Retirement Communities

More affluent seniors may choose a continuing-care retirement community (CCRC). CCRCs usually have a variety of living options, ranging from apartments or condominiums, to assisted living, and skilled nursing-home care. Often, residents enter the more independent living areas and progress through assisted living and into skilled care as they age.

Three financial models are common: the all-inclusive model, which provides total health care coverage, including long-term care; the fee-for-service model in which payments match the level of care; and the modified coverage model, which covers long-term care to a predetermined maximum. Most CCRCs require an entry fee, which may or may not be refundable, plus a variable monthly fee to pay for rent and supportive services. Monthly fees vary, depending upon the level of care being provided. Funding is largely private, though some facilities have Medicare- or Medicaid-funded beds for skilled care.

See also "Financing, Coverage, and Costs of Health Care" (p 26).

REFERENCES

■ Bodenheimer T. Long-term care for frail elderly people—the On Lok model. *N Engl J Med*. 1999;341(17):1324–1328.

■ Boult C, Pacala JT. Integrating healthcare for older populations. *Am J Managed Care*. 1999;5:45–52.

■ Burton LC, Leff B, Harper M, et al. Acceptability to patients of a home hospital. *J Am Geriatr Soc*. 1998;46(5):605–609.

■ Caplan GA, Ward JA, Brennan NJ, et al. Hospital in the home: a randomised controlled trial. *Med J Aust*. 1999;170(4):156–160.

■ Forster A, Young J, Langhorne P. Systematic review of day hospital for elderly people: the Day Hospital Group. *BMJ*. 1999;318(7187):837–841.

■ Hughes SL, Ulasevich A, Weaver FM, et al. Impact of home care on hospital days: a meta-analysis. *Health Serv Res*. 1997;32(4):415–432.

■ Hedrick SC, Koepsell TD, Inui T. Meta-analysis of home-care effects on mortality and nursing home placement. *Med Care*. 1989;27(11):1025–1026.

■ Pacala JT, Kane RL, Atherly AJ, et al. Using structured implicit review to assess quality of care in the Program of All-inclusive Care for the Elderly (PACE). *J Am Geriatr Soc*. 2000;48(8):903–910.

■ Pierce CA. Program of All-inclusive Care for the Elderly in 2002. *Geriatr Nurs*. 2002;23(3):173–174.

■ Saliba D, Elliott M, Rubenstein LZ, et al. The Vulnerable Elders Survey: a tool for identifying vulnerable older people in the community. *J Am Geriatr Soc*. 2001;49(12):1691–1699.

CHAPTER 15—NURSING-HOME CARE

Nursing homes have evolved dramatically over the past several years, responding to a variety of government and market-driven forces. The almshouse, common at the turn of the century, has been transformed into a highly regulated institution for persons with severe physical and mental disabilities. Nursing homes, more than ever, present the clinician with a set of unique and complex care issues, many of which are best understood in the context of population needs, government policy, and reimbursement and staffing patterns.

THE NURSING-HOME POPULATION

The average nursing-home resident is characterized by significant impairments in physical and instrumental activities of daily living (ADLs). Overall, the level of disability in the nursing home has increased over the past decade and exceeds that found in persons receiving home care. Among nursing-home residents, 22.3% require assistance with one or two ADLs, and 74.9% require assistance with three or more. In addition to impairments of ADLs, 81% of nursing-home residents are impaired in their ability to make daily decisions; two thirds have orientation difficulties or memory problems, or both, and over half (54%) have either bowel or bladder incontinence. Hearing and visual impairments are found in 36% and 39% of residents, respectively. Dementia remains the most commonly occurring condition in the nursing home, with estimates ranging from 50% to 70%. Behavioral problems, understandably, are also common, occurring in at least one third of nursing-home residents. Such behaviors include verbal and physical abuse, social inappropriateness, resistance to care, and wandering. Communication problems are noted in 60% of residents; 44% have difficulty with both being understood and understanding others. Depression is diagnosed in 20% of nursing-home residents.

Almost half of all nursing-home residents are aged 85 years or over, with less than 9% under the age of 65. The majority are women (72%), white (89%), and unmarried (60% widowed) with limited social supports. The percentage of black residents in U.S. nursing homes has increased in recent years (9%), approaching national population norms. In fact, black Americans 65 to 74 years of age are more likely than white Americans to be admitted to a nursing home. Nonetheless, other nonwhite populations, such as Hispanic Americans, Asian Americans, and Native Americans, are underrepresented in nursing homes despite even higher disability rates in these groups. Older adults with developmental disabilities constitute another unique population that is requiring increasing nursing-home care as their older parents die (see "Mental Retardation," p 240). These persons often require specialized care that many nursing homes have difficulty providing.

NURSING-HOME AVAILABILITY AND FINANCING

Currently there are 17,000 nursing homes with 1.8 million beds, 1.6 million residents, and 2.4 million discharges (ie, to home, hospital, or secondary to death). Of these facilities, 65% are proprietary (for-profit), with voluntary nonprofit (25%) and government nursing homes (10%) accounting for the remainder. The average nursing home operates 107 beds, and a minority (8%) have more than 200 beds. A little more than half of all nursing homes (56%) are part of a chain.

By age 65 a person's risk of nursing-home admission before death is estimated at 43%; one third have lifetime risk of nursing-home stays of 90 days or less. The risk of nursing-home admission rises steeply with age; approximately 20% of persons aged 85 years and over reside in nursing homes versus 1.4% of those 65 to 74 years of age. Interestingly, the occupancy rates in nursing homes nationally have declined over the past several years and now stand at 88%. This decline has generally been attributed to the availability of other long-term-care options, such as assisted living, but there are likely other causal social and financial variables that have yet to be articulated. The availability and use of home-care services for Medicare-eligible patients have not been found to reduce nursing-home admissions.

Postacute care is increasingly being offered in nursing-home settings, a response to higher care needs of older persons occurring in conjunction with declining lengths of hospital stays. Though the types of postacute services and programs vary significantly from one locale to another (ie, dialysis, orthopedic, ventilator, postoperative, rehabilitative, or wound care), they remain distinct from the standard nursing-home services by integrating the features of acute medical, long-term-care nursing, and rehabilitative settings. The challenge in postacute care is that of accommodating to patients with varying degrees of disease severity, functional dependence, and comorbidities. Some limited studies suggest that, for selected patient populations, postacute care in the nursing home achieves outcomes equal to or better than postacute care in acute hospitals. Definitions as to what constitutes postacute care, however, vary widely, as do regulatory standards, thus making comparison studies difficult.

Despite the significant disability associated with most nursing-home residents, this population remains quite heterogeneous. Short stayers (3 months or less) currently account for 25% of all nursing-home admissions; 50% will spend at least 1 year in the nursing home, and 21% will reside in the nursing home almost 5 years. Many short-stay residents are admitted for rehabilitation, and some enter nursing homes for terminal care. Interestingly, improvement in function for the longer-stay nursing-home residents is quite common, which reflects the heterogeneity of this population. The number of nursing-home admissions has risen since 1994, reflecting the dynamic nature of this sector of the long-term-care continuum.

Nursing-home expenditures currently total $90 billion and are projected to increase to $150 billion by 2007. Public expenditures constitute 62% of all nursing-home spending (Medicaid 48%; Medicare 12%; other 2%), with private spending constituting 38% of the total (31% out of pocket; 5% health insurance; 2% other private funds). Under the new prospective payment system enacted as part of the Balanced Budget Act of 1997, Medicare payments to skilled nursing facilities are no longer cost-based, but are predicated on functional needs and rehabilitative potential. Although the prospective payment system has not conclusively limited access to skilled nursing care for Medicare beneficiaries, it has definitely forced nursing homes to be more diligent with regard to their admission policies. Not unexpectedly, physical, occupational, and speech therapies are commonly prescribed in the nursing home, with half of all nursing-home admissions receiving at least 90 minutes of these rehabilitation services, according to one study. The prospective payment system requires nursing-home staff to carefully document gains in function to ensure reimbursement. (See "Financing, Coverage, and Costs of Health Care," p 26.)

STAFFING PATTERNS

It is generally conceded that the current nursing-home population is "sicker" and more disabled than nursing-home residents were in the past. Studies have confirmed the correlation between the provision of quality care to total nursing hours and to the ratio of professional nurses (ie, registered nurses) to nonprofessional nursing staff. An Institute of Medicine report in 1996 recommended increasing nurse staffing levels to enhance the quality of nursing-home care and has spurred Congress to debate the merits of mandatory

minimum staffing ratios. Even if significantly higher staffing ratios eventually are mandated, the financial resources to achieve them remain elusive. Recruiting and retaining staff, particularly nursing assistants who constitute the bulk of the nursing-home workforce, also continues to be difficult. Turnover rates for registered nurses and licensed practical nurses also are very high, at more than 50% per year.

Staffing issues are also pertinent to physicians practicing in nursing homes. Currently, 20% of primary care physicians spend 2 hours or more per week in a nursing facility. Although the resident's choice of physicians may be limited with closed medical staffs, evidence now suggests that the closed staff model delivers a higher intensity and quality of care.

FACTORS ASSOCIATED WITH NURSING-HOME PLACEMENT

Although there is a significant chance of being admitted to a nursing home with increasing age, other factors, such as low income, poor family supports (especially lack of spouse and children), and low social activity have been associated with institutionalization. Cognitive and functional impairments have also predicted nursing-home placement, often permanently. Interestingly, for patients with dementia, education and caregiver support have been shown to delay the need for nursing-home placement for up to 1 year. Not surprisingly, older adults with more positive attitudes toward nursing homes are more likely to use skilled nursing facilities than are adults with less favorable dispositions. The range of long-term-care services that are now available (ie, skilled nursing, home care, assisted living) further increases the complexity of placement decisions, as the relative value and merits of available options have not been empirically tested. The use of formal (ie, paid-for) community services does not necessarily reduce the likelihood of nursing-home placement for patients with severe disabilities.

THE INTERFACE OF ACUTE AND LONG-TERM CARE

The majority of nursing-home admissions derive from acute-care hospitals. Conversely, nursing-home residents have high rates of hospitalization, ranging upward of 549 admissions per 1000 nursing-home beds per year. Infection is the most common reason for transfer of nursing-home residents to short-stay hospitals, accounting for one quarter of all such admissions. Studies have noted that increased physician and nurse practitioner or physician assistant involvement and the availability of special care units in the nursing home mitigates transfers to the hospital.

QUALITY ISSUES

Extensive nursing-home reforms enacted in 1987 (in the Omnibus Budget Reconciliation Act of 1987) significantly changed the landscape of long-term care. In addition to setting training guidelines and minimum staffing requirements and bolstering residents' rights, including limiting the use of restraints and psychoactive medications, the law required a periodic comprehensive assessment of all nursing-home residents. This assessment, known as the Minimum Data Set, focuses specifically on clinical issues with relevance to quality care. If any real or potential problems are identified with any of these issues, the health care team must review accompanying resident assessment protocols that outline standard diagnostic and therapeutic approaches to the specific problems in question. The protocols are, in essence, practice guidelines that the team, including the primary care clinician, is encouraged to use. In addition to comprehensive assessments, the clinician must also clearly document the need for all medications, particularly psychoactive agents. Unnecessary drugs are defined as those that are given in excessive doses, for excessive periods of time, without adequate monitoring, without adequate indications for use, or in the presence of adverse consequences that indicate the need for dose reduction or discontinuation. In addition to these generic instructions, specific types of drugs have been banned (ie, usage will warrant a citation from the state survey inspection team unless a clear rationale is documented in the chart) from use in the nursing home on the basis of criteria developed by a group of experts. Although some evidence exists to suggest that the 1987 act and subsequent mandates have resulted in a decreased prevalence of pressure ulcers and reduced use of restraints, their impact on quality of care overall has been difficult to quantify. A new set of quality indicators based on Minimum Data Set items has been instituted nationally in an effort to hasten quality improvement efforts. With this system, nursing facilities are able to compare their individual performance with regional and national norms to help guide their efforts to improve the quality of care.

A host of variables interact in nursing homes to determine the level of quality achieved. These include staffing levels, reimbursement rates, and processes of care extant in the nursing home. Repeal of the Boren Amendment, however, has raised concern that states will eventually cut back nursing-home funding and further jeopardize care. The Boren Amendment had required that state Medicaid payments match the needs of the nursing-home population in order to maintain all relevant quality and safety standards.

MEDICAL CARE ISSUES

The care of nursing-home residents has become more complex over the past several years, commensurate with an increasing level of medical acuity in an environment continually constrained by lack of adequate resources. Comprehensive, ongoing assessment within an interdisciplinary framework provides the practitioner the opportunity to restore function, whenever possible, and almost always to enhance quality of life.

Clinical challenges abound in the nursing home, created, in part, by the atypical and subtle presentation of illness so characteristic of patients with profound physical and psychologic frailty. In addition, limited access to biotechnology, frequent dependence on nonphysicians such as nurses and nurse assistants for patient evaluation, and the high prevalence of cognitive impairment in a setting of intense regulatory oversight all complicate the medical decision-making process. Families of nursing-home residents often remain an integral part of the overall care plan and may require specific educational and psychosocial supports. Ethical and legal concerns are also very common, particularly regarding end-of-life, feeding, hydration, and resident rights issues. (See "Legal and Ethical Issues," p 18.) Finally, the heterogeneity among nursing-home residents precludes a uniform care plan, but rather demands an individualized, thoughtful, and reasoned approach to each person in the nursing-home setting.

Problems in nursing homes that commonly require unique diagnostic and treatment strategies include infections and nutrition. Treatment of infection and maintenance of infection control programs are among the most difficult issues encountered in nursing homes. The treatment of feeding disorders and poor nutrition also raises problems. For example, determining the risks and benefits of tube feedings for frail nursing-home patients must be predicated not only on underlying illness but also on the resident's and the family's value system, the resources available in the nursing facility, and staff acceptance of the intervention. Given that the evidence for and against enteral feeding in nursing-home patients is controversial (ie, benefits are not well established, with up to one fourth of residents with chewing and swallowing problems able to have their feeding tubes removed), the practitioner must continue to individualize therapy. (See "Eating and Feeding Problems," p 191.)

PHYSICIAN PRACTICE IN THE NURSING HOME

Physicians have traditionally had limited involvement in nursing homes. Perceptions of excessive regulations, paperwork, and limited reimbursement raise further disincentives to nursing-home practice. In reality, the medical care of nursing-home residents is both challenging and fulfilling, requiring excellent clinical skills as well as sensitivity to a variety of ethical, legal, and interdisciplinary issues. Medical interventions, whether they be curative, preventive, or palliative, demand an individualized approach that recognizes the complex interplay among resident, family, and staff needs. Further, the evidence upon which to base treatment may be nonexistent.

The comorbidity present in most nursing-home residents commonly creates the need for multiple drug therapies, with attendant complications. Even though residents receiving more than nine medications are flagged by state survey teams as reflecting potential quality concerns, the use of multiple medications cannot always be avoided. The most common health conditions found in the nursing home for persons aged 65 years and older, following dementia, are heart disease, hypertension, arthritis, and stroke. The approaches to these and other illnesses have evolved dramatically in recent years and complicate treatment decisions where cost-effectiveness is increasingly looked upon as a desirable goal. Clear documentation of the rationale for a given medication or intervention is the best way to protect against potential scrutiny; frequent discussion with the facility's consultant pharmacist is also helpful. Physicians who schedule and structure their visits to the nursing home will benefit from the resultant efficiencies and secondarily will be more fully integrated into the health care team (see Table 15.1). Nurse practitioners and physician assistants have become increasingly involved in the primary care of nursing-home residents. Studies suggest that nurse practitioners and physician assistants who act in concert with the primary care physician as a coordinated team provide more intensive care to the nursing-home resident and may decrease hospitalization rates while maintaining cost neutrality. Information regarding physician responsibilities and Omnibus Budget Reconciliation Act mandates can be found at the Web site of the American Medical Directors Association (http://www.amda.com).

Several studies have documented misdiagnoses, inappropriate interventions, and poor preventive care practices in nursing homes. In an often-cited study of Maryland nursing homes, for example, only 11% of patients with four common types of infection were found to have received even a minimal evaluation (eg, failure to obtain a urine sample when treated for a urinary tract infection). In a study of nursing-home patients with nonmalignant pain, 25% were found to be receiving no analgesics.

Certain care strategies that have been developed may enhance care quality. The commonly employed special care units, though conceptually attractive, have

Table 15.1—Role of the Attending Physician in the Nursing Home

- Comprehensively assess each resident and coordinate all aspects of medical care. Implement specific treatments and services to enhance or maintain physical and psychosocial function.

- Participate in the development of individual care plans and review and revise such plans periodically with the health care team.

- Review progress of each resident in individualized therapy (ie, speech, occupational therapy, speech therapy) and, in concert with appropriate therapists, approve continued use.

- Evaluate the need for rehabilitative services. Order appropriate measures and assistive devices to reduce the risk of accidents.

- Evaluate the need for restraints, minimizing their use whenever possible.

- Periodically review all medications and monitor for both continued need and adverse drug reactions. Respond appropriately to periodic review and recommendations of the consultant pharmacist.

- Physically attend to each resident in a timely fashion according to established state and federal guidelines. Document progress and changes in care plans.

- Respond in a timely fashion to medical emergencies.

- Facilitate information transfer when possible and appropriate between acute and long-term-care facilities.

- Inform residents of their health status and, whenever possible, optimize each resident's decision-making capacity while assisting in establishing advance directives.

SOURCE: Katz PR, Feather J. Medical practice in the nursing home. In: Calkins E, Ford AB, Katz PR, eds *Practice of Geriatrics.* 2nd ed. Philadelphia: W.B. Saunders; 1992:87. Reprinted with permission.

not consistently been shown to enhance quality of care apart from the involvement of individual professionals. Specific consultation services in the nursing home, however, may improve care practices and patient outcomes, as shown by a randomized, controlled trial of an effort to reduce falls in a group of Tennessee nursing-home residents. In addition, interactive educational programs for physicians and nursing staff may improve practice, as has been demonstrated in programs to promote appropriate psychoactive drug use.

Understanding each nursing-home resident's preference for care in the context of his or her underlying value system will undoubtedly improve overall quality. Interestingly, fewer than one in eight nursing-home residents have discussed preferences with their health care providers. In addition, there is often a lack of follow-up of do-not-resuscitate discussions in the hospital when the patient is subsequently admitted to the nursing home. Sixty percent of nursing-home residents have orders for cardiopulmonary resuscitation, and almost 90% desire hospitalization for acute illness. When ethical dilemmas do present themselves, the availability of institutional ethics committees can provide important guidance. The multidisciplinary nature of these committees ensures a spectrum of opinion and insight critical for nursing-home residents, and they are particularly relevant to end-of-life issues.

THE ROLE OF THE NURSE PRACTITIONER

The increasing numbers of nurse practitioners (NPs) in health care in the United States has brought exciting change to the practice setting. Geriatric nurse practitioners (GNP's) are a vital, albeit small, component of the nurse practitioner movement. The estimated 3500 GNP's in the country make up about 5% of all nurse practitioners, the largest percentage of whom operate in the adult and family nurse practitioner role.

The utilization of GNP's in nursing homes is more popular than ever, as studies have repeatedly demonstrated the efficacy and quality of care provided. There are numerous ways in which a physician, NP, and long-term care facility can choose to organize their operations. The model selected will determine how the relationship between these three entities will function, including the division of responsibility, division of power, method of payment, and method of reimbursement. Each model is associated with its own profile of advantages and disadvantages.

The Nurse Practitioner as Nursing-Home Employee

Some institutions choose to retain NPs as full-time employees, paying them a regular salary to serve as a complement to regular physician care. The physician is paid on a fee-for-service basis. This arrangement increases the influence the nursing facility has on the NP, connecting him or her more to the facility than to the physician with whom he or she works. This has its positives and negatives; it allows the two individuals to work more as equals without dealing with financial matters, but it also introduces a third party to their relationship to cause complications where they do not exist in other arrangements.

The Teaching Nursing Home

This model uses both fee-for-service and full-time, salaried NPs. Regardless of how the NP is paid, however, he or she will receive joint appointments to a school of nursing and to the teaching nursing home. The key element of this model is that the NP is expected to do a great deal of active in-service training of other staff members. In fact, in some cases, the NP will spend up to 50% of his or her time performing training activities and participating in specialized team functions (eg, wound care, pain management). However, it is important to note that most of these activities are nonreimbursable under Medicare, so it is vital under this model to clearly define the role of the NP and the amount of nonreimbursable activity that he or she is to perform.

The Private Practice Model

The most popular model is one in which the NP is salaried by the physician; NPs provide care to nursing facilities on a fee-for-service basis. In some cases, the NP works with a group of physicians, while in others, the NP is the direct employee of an individual. This method has the advantage of simplicity and ease of communication, eliminating the third party from the physician–NP relationship.

Other Models

Most other models involve health maintenance organizations and other forms of managed care. Under this format, either the physician and the NP work in a team of two, or the NP provides primary care while the physician provides follow-up.

Financial Considerations

The most important financial issue regarding the use of NPs also applies to the payment of physicians: striking a balance between productivity and effective care. If a nursing facility hires a physician or NP, then the facility obviously will have somewhat more control over the operations of its employees. However, a direct salary payment schedule reduces the incentive for a physician or NP to see as many patients as possible. The facility can therefore be hurt, because a certain number of visits per day is required in order to receive reimbursement for the employee's salary.

For this reason, many long-term-care facilities choose to employ physicians and NPs on a fee-for-service basis, accepting a separate bill for each patient treated. The problem is that such a payment system can lead to troubles of its own, such as "blitzes of service," where a physician and nurse practitioner claim to see 50 or more patients in a single day. In such cases, patients are clearly not receiving an appropriate level of care. Moreover, the nursing home may suffer financially from such acts; Medicare will often recognize these blitzes for what they are and deny reimbursement. Therefore, it is vital that the nursing facility find the right balance between productivity and adequate care.

Other Medicare reimbursement issues are especially significant in the case of nurse practitioners. Because the role of the NP is often vaguely defined and varies among different institutions, there is a tendency for the

NP to accumulate considerable hours in nonreimbursable activities, including in-service training of other staff members. Administrators and other staff members commonly view an NP as a kind of clinical expert, able to dispense knowledge and resources about any condition or problem that might arise. The end result is that the facility must be prepared to absorb the cost of all this assistance, which is not reimbursable under Medicare.

In addition, Medicare provides a stringent set of regulations that must be strictly observed in order for nursing facilities to receive reimbursement for care provided. Personal visits after the initial visit must alternate between the NP and the physician, and the physician must sign all rehabilitation orders. In fact, all NP orders must be countersigned by the physician within 24 hours in order to be eligible for reimbursement. Unfortunately, this can cause a number of handicaps for the NP and for the nursing facility interested in providing effective care. Additional state regulations may further complicate this process; in New York State, NPs may not perform an initial assessment of a patient, and the physician must conduct a "meaningful review" of each patient's records every 3 months. Constant and systematic communication between the NP and the physician is the surest way of overcoming these restrictions.

The Collaborative Practice Agreement

The best way to avoid many of these difficulties is for the physician and the NP to agree upon and sign a collaborative practice agreement at the outset of their professional relationship, spelling out the specifics of that relationship in a way that both parties are comfortable with. A collaborative practice agreement should document responsibilities of both individuals relating to charting, coverage agreements, and peer review, and should provide a system for resolving disputes. Many administrators and physicians prefer to begin with a restrictive agreement in the beginning, to be altered and made more liberal as the NP earns a greater degree of trust. Finally, a collaborative practice agreement should enumerate in the most detailed fashion possible the duties and assigned role of the nurse practitioner. This will avoid confusion on the part of the physician, NP, and nursing facility, and allow all concerned to provide the most effective and efficient care possible.

THE ROLE OF THE MEDICAL DIRECTOR

The quality of physician practice in the nursing home is, in many ways, determined by the medical director. The medical director, in concert with the medical staff, sets quality standards for the nursing home and operationalizes these through specific policies and procedures. The medical director must ensure compliance with all relevant state and federal guidelines and work with the nursing-home administrator and director of nursing to foster effective team care and continuing staff education. The medical director of a nursing home works closely with all disciplines and must be constantly cognizant of the unique interplay between laws, regulations, organization, and delivery of medical care. Certification for medical directors following completion of a formal course is now offered through the American Medical Directors Association.

REFERENCES

- Bishop CE. Where are the missing elders? The decline in nursing home use, 1985 and 1995. *Health Aff.* 1999;18(4):146–155.

- Harrington C, Kovner C, Mezey M, et al. Experts recommend minimum nurse staffing standards for nursing facilities in the United States. *Gerontologist.* 2000;40(1):5–16.

- Katz PR, Kane RL, Mezey MD, eds. *Emerging Systems in Long-Term Care. Volume IV in Long-Term Care.* New York: Springer Publishing Company; 1999.

- Ouslander JG, Osterweil D, Morley J, eds. *Medical Care in the Nursing Home.* 2nd ed. New York: McGraw-Hill, Inc; 1997.

- Saliba D, Kington R, Buchanan J, et al. Appropriateness of the decision to transfer nursing facility residents to the hospital. *J Am Geriatr Soc.* 2000;48:154–163.

CHAPTER 16—PALLIATIVE CARE

In the United States the overwhelming majority of deaths occur among older adults. Older persons typically die slowly of chronic diseases, with multiple coexisting problems, progressive dependency on others, and heavy care needs that are met mostly by family members. Many of these deaths become protracted processes that must be negotiated by clinicians, patients, and family members, who must make difficult decisions about the use or discontinuation of life-prolonging treatments. There is abundant evidence that the quality of life during the dying process is often poor. For many older persons, dying is characterized by inadequately treated physical distress, fragmented care systems, poor to absent communication among doctors, patients and families, and enormous strains on family caregiver and support systems.

Terminally ill people spend the majority of their final months at home, but in most parts of the country their deaths actually occur in the hospital or nursing home. The experience of dying, however, varies greatly from one part of the nation to another. In Portland, Oregon, for example, only 35% of adult deaths occur in hospitals, but in New York City more than 80% occur in hospitals, a difference associated in part with differences in regional hospital bed supply and the availability of community supports for the dying. Social and medical differences also account for some patterns. The need for institutionalization or paid caregivers in the last months of life is much higher among poor people and women. Similarly, older persons suffering from cognitive impairment and dementia are much more likely than cognitively intact older persons to spend their last days in a nursing home.

PALLIATIVE CARE AND HOSPICE

Palliative care seeks to prevent, relieve, reduce, or soothe the symptoms of disease or disorder without effecting cure. It attends closely to the emotional, spiritual, and practical needs and goals of patients and of those close to them. Palliative care is generally restricted to those who are at imminent risk of dying but is also important to those who are extremely ill or who are living with serious complications at the end stages of chronic disease.

The term *hospice* has at least four somewhat different uses in the United States. A hospice may be a site of care for dying patients, such as a free-standing institution or a unit within a hospital or nursing home. Second, the term may refer to an organization that provides care for dying patients in a variety of settings, most commonly at home. Third, it may describe an approach to care that is commonly thought to be synonymous with palliative care but is not: all patients in hospice care are dying, whereas patients in palliative care may not be terminal. Finally, it may refer to a benefit available to Medicare beneficiaries with an expected prognosis of 6 months or less who are willing to forgo standard Medicare-reimbursed services in favor of hospice care. The following services are covered under the Medicare hospice benefit: physician services related to the hospice diagnosis, nursing care, medical equipment and supplies, medications, short-term inpatient care for symptom management or family respite, physical and occupational therapy, bereavement services, and an average of 4 hours per day of home-health-aide services. (See "Financing, Coverage, and Costs of Health Care," p 26, for details.)

Despite a steady growth in the number of agencies providing hospice services in the United States, fewer than 20% of Americans are enrolled in hospice prior to death. A number of reasons account for the limited use of this benefit. Access to hospice is limited for patients living in rural areas and inner cities because of a paucity of programs in these areas. Additionally, because the hospice benefit provides only 4 hours of custodial home-health services on average, the family of a hospice patient needs to be able to provide the remaining coverage. Many families cannot meet this time or financial obligation (ie, to hire paid help). Many physicians and families do not consider hospice an option in the earlier stages of life-threatening illnesses, so that referrals are made when patients are actively dying and cannot avail themselves of all of the services that hospice has to offer. In 1998 the median length of stay in hospice prior to death was only 20 days. Finally, the difficulty of determining a 6-month prognosis in dying patients is often a barrier and inhibits physician referrals. A task force from the National Hospice and Palliative Care Organization has published guidelines to aid physicians in determining the appropriate timing of hospice referral.

COMMUNICATING BAD NEWS

The vast majority of Americans (> 90%) want to be told if they have a life-threatening illness. The ability to deliver bad news in an effective manner is an essential skill for clinicians. However, clinicians receive little formal training in communication skills, and as a result they may feel unprepared to deliver bad news. Others may fear that the news will adversely affect the patient and the family or the provider-patient relationship. A systematic approach to delivering bad news can foster collaboration among the patient, the family, and clinicians. Effective discussions can improve the patient's and the family's ability to plan for the future, set realistic goals, and support one another emotionally.

A six-step framework for communicating bad news can be used as a guide for these difficult conversations.

Step 1: Preparation

Discussions of bad news require careful preparation. Before delivering bad news to a patient, plan what will be discussed, ensure the medical facts, and ensure that all needed confirmation is available. Establishing the proper physical context is also important. Ideally, bad news should be delivered in person in a private area in which there will be no interruptions. Allot adequate time for discussions, minimize interruptions, and determine whether any support staff, family, or friends that the patient may want on hand are available.

Step 2: Establishing the Patient's Understanding

Begin the discussion by exploring the patient's knowledge of the illness. Patients with a thorough understanding of their illness require a different approach than an uninformed or less sophisticated patient. Useful questions to elicit this information include the following: "What do you understand about your illness?" "When you first had symptom *x*, what did you think it might be?" "What have you been told about your condition or procedures that you have had?"

Step 3: What the Patient Wants to Know

Although the majority of Americans say they want to be fully informed about their illnesses, a substantial minority may not want to know the full details or may prefer to have another family member informed. Data suggests that this may be particularly true for certain ethnic groups. Just as patients have the right to be told the truth, they also have the right to decline to learn unwanted information. Thus, it is crucial to establish how much each patient wants to know. Helpful questions to ask include the following: "If this condition turns out to be something serious, do you want to know?" "Would you like me to tell you the full details of your condition? If not, is there somebody else you would like me to talk to?"

Step 4: Telling the Patient

Once the clinician has established the patient's understanding of the illness and willingness to hear bad news, it is time to tell the patient. Deliver information in a sensitive, straightforward manner, avoiding technical language or euphemisms. Frequently check for understanding and clarify difficult concepts and terms. Phrasing that includes a "warning shot" helps brace and prepare patients for the bad news. For example: "Mr. X, I feel bad to have to tell you this, but the growth turned out to be cancer." "The report is back, and it's not as we had hoped. It showed that there is cancer in your colon."

Step 5: Responding to Feelings

The responses of patients and families are both unpredictable and diverse. Active listening, encouraging the expression of emotion, and acknowledging patient's emotions are all important and helpful. Useful probes to help elicit an understanding of the patient's emotions include the following: "What does this news mean to you?" "What worries you the most?" "You appear angry. Can you tell me what you are feeling?" "Tell me more about how you are feeling about what I just said."

Step 6: Planning and Follow-Up

Finally, the clinician should organize an immediate therapeutic plan that includes specific references to the patient's concerns and incorporates the patient's agenda. The plan should include an appointment for a follow-up visit; a discussion of additional tests, referrals, and sources of support; and information as to how you can be reached if additional questions arise. The clinician also needs to ensure that the patient will be safe when he or she leaves the office.

PAIN

Pain is the most common medical problem associated with both advanced and acute illness, and it is the most feared symptom by patients and families alike. The word *pain* is originally derived from the Latin *poena*, which means "punishment." Pain is defined as an unpleasant sensory and emotional experience associated with actual or potential tissue damage, or sometimes it is defined in terms of such damage. Pain can be conceptualized as either nociceptive or neuropathic. Nociceptive pain results from direct tissue damage to normally functioning nerves. Common examples of this type of pain are arthritic, acute postoperative, and posttraumatic pain. Nociceptive pain can be further divided into somatic or visceral pain. Somatic pain (eg, pain located in skin, soft tissue, muscle, and bone) is generally well localized and described as stabbing, aching, or throbbing. Visceral pain (eg, cardiac, lung, or gastrointestinal pain) is generally dull, crampy, and poorly localized; patients find this pain difficult to describe. Visceral pain responds well to opioids or coanalgesics, or both. Neuropathic pain is thought to result from disordered function of the peripheral or central nervous system in the absence of ongoing tissue damage. Examples include peripheral processes (eg, painful neuroma), central nervous system processes (eg, phantom pain), and complex pain syndromes like reflex sympathetic dystrophies. Patients describe this type of pain as burning, tingling, numbness, shooting, or stabbing. Although neuropathic pain is responsive to opioids, adjuvant agents are often required to achieve adequate pain control. Data suggest that gabapentin may be a particularly effective agent for the treatment of a variety of neuropathic pain syndromes, including diabetic and herpetic neuralgias. Pain can be adequately controlled in up to 90% of patients by the use of noninvasive therapies, although barriers to good pain control that are profession related, patient related, and system related result in inadequate pain control in as many as half of all older cancer patients.

Appropriate pain management begins with an assessment directed at understanding the causes and clinical characteristics of the patient's pain. Pain should be assessed at regular intervals after treatment is initiated, at each new pain report, and at suitable intervals after dosing (eg, 15 to 30 minutes after parenteral dosing). The mainstay of pain assessment is patient self-report; clinicians should believe the patient's description of pain. Visual analog scales or other rating scales can be used (see Figure 16.1). It is not necessary to delay treatment until investigation or treatment of the underlying disease is complete. Untreated pain may lead to increased pain as well as to reduced responsiveness to treatment and can significantly add to the patient's and the family's burden and suffering.

The importance of pain assessment in the care of older adults cannot be underestimated. Nurses play a vital role in the assessment and management of pain. Therefore, nurses need to have the knowledge to provide the most appropriate pain assessment to their patients. *Try This*, a publication of The John A. Hartford Foundation Institute for Geriatric Nursing, is a series of assessment tools. Each issue focuses on a topic specific to the assessment of older adults. The *Try This* issue on pain assessment provides easily accessible, easily understood, and easily implemented pain assessment tools for geriatric nurses. This and all the other issues in the *Try This* series are all downloadable from The John A. Hartford Foundation Institute for Geriatric Nursing Web site at http://hartfordign.org/publications/trythis/.

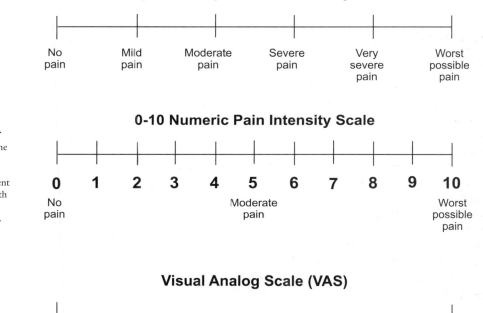

Figure 16.1—Pain intensity scales.

SOURCE: Acute Pain Management Guideline Panel. *Acute Pain Management in Adults: Operative Procedures. Quick Reference Guide for Clinicians.* Rockville, MD: US Department of Health and Human Services, Public Health Service, Agency for Health Care Policy and Research. February 1992. AHCPR Pub. No. 92-0019.

PAIN MANAGEMENT

The American Geriatrics Society has published guidelines on the management of persistent pain in older persons. These include discussion and specific recommendations for pain assessment, medications, and nonpharmacologic strategies for managing pain. An update to incorporate new pharmacologic information and research on pain management is under way. See the Appendix (pp 411–412) for a pain medication table from the guidelines.

Nonpharmacologic Interventions

Patients should be encouraged to be as active as possible and participate in self-care if they are able. Noninvasive physical and psychologic modalities can be used concurrently with drugs to manage pain. Some physical modalities that have been shown to be effective are heat, cold, massage, acupuncture, and transcutaneous electrical nerve stimulation. Cognitive-behavioral interventions include relaxation and imagery, psychotherapy, and structured support. Patient education can also be efficacious when combined with pharmacologic therapy.

Pharmacologic Interventions

There is worldwide consensus favoring the use of the World Health Organization three-step analgesic ladder, a simple, validated, and effective method of ensuring pain relief in patients with cancer. The same basic principles have been empirically accepted for pharmacologic treatment of persistent pain of non-cancer etiologies. (Figure 16.2).

Step 1: Mild Pain

All analgesics in the step 1 category have a ceiling effect to their analgesia (ie, a maximum dose past which no further analgesia can be expected). Acetaminophen and nonsteroidal anti-inflammatory drugs (NSAIDs) have an opioid dose-sparing effect that helps reduce side effects when given with opioids for moderate to severe pain. Doses greater than 4.0 g per 24 hours of acetaminophen should not be used, because they could cause hepatotoxicity.

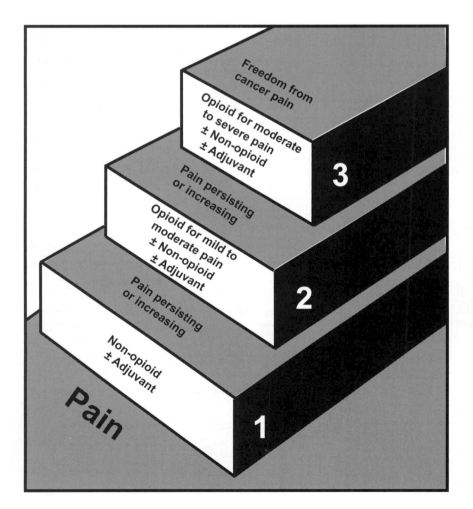

Figure 16.2—WHO three-step analgesic ladder.

SOURCE: World Health Organization. Technical Report Series No. 804, Figure 2. Geneva: World Health Organization; 1990 Reprinted with permission.

NSAIDs, including aspirin, can also be used in combination. Some patients respond better to one class of NSAIDs than to another, so that serial trials with different agents can also be used. NSAIDs are relatively contraindicated in anyone with significant renal insufficiency, and they can have side effects, including gastropathy, renal failure, inhibition of platelet aggregation, and central nervous system changes. Misoprostol or omeprazole should be employed in patients with significant risk of gastropathy. The role of COX-2 selective inhibitors is unclear, but these drugs are thought by many clinicians to be safer.

Steps 2 and 3: Moderate and Severe Pain

Opioids (eg, codeine, hydromorphone, morphine, hydrocodone, oxycodone, fentanyl) are the standard agents for the treatment of moderate to severe pain. Meperidine, although widely used, particularly for surgical patients, is poorly absorbed orally and has a short half-life (3 hours). Its principal metabolite, normeperidine, has no analgesic properties, has a longer half-life than the parent compound (6 hours), and produces significant adverse effects when it accumulates. Older patients, at risk for reduced renal clearance, and all patients with decreased renal function, will accumulate potentially toxic metabolites of merperidine and morphine. Tremulousness, dysphoria, myoclonus, and seizures result from normeperidine toxicity. There is rarely, if ever, an indication for meperidine for the treatment of pain. All opioids behave similarly pharmacologically and follow first-order kinetics. Peak plasma concentration is reached approximately 60 to 90 minutes after oral dosing, 30 minutes after subcutaneous or intramuscular dosing, and 6 minutes after intravenous injection. Irrespective of dose, opioids are conjugated in the liver and then excreted by the kidneys. When renal clearance is normal, codeine, hydrocodone, hydromorphone, morphine, oxycodone, and their metabolites all have effective half-lives of approximately 3 to 4 hours.

For routine oral dosing in patients with continuous pain and normal renal function, opioids can be administered every 3 to 4 hours. When dehydration or renal failure impairs clearance, doses must be decreased or the dosing interval increased, or both. In cases of oliguria or anuria, opioids should be administered on an as-needed basis. Steady state is typically reached within 24 hours. If pain remains uncontrolled after 24 hours, doses should be increased by 25% to 50% for mild to moderate pain and by 50% to 100% for severe pain.

Currently available extended release or sustained release opioids are formulated to release medicine over 12 to 24 hours. They should be taken whole and not crushed or chewed, although Kadian©, a capsule with beads, can be opened and sprinkled on food or administered via G-tube without alteration in absorption pharmacokinetics. Best pain control is usually achieved within 2 to 4 days, once steady state is reached. Fentanyl is available as a transdermal patch, which provides continuous pain relief for 48 to 72 hours. Maximum pain relief is typically achieved within 8 to 24 hours, and steady state is reached between 48 and 72 hours.

As a part of a standing pain regimen, "rescue" analgesia should be available for breakthrough pain or acute pain flares. Rescue doses are calculated at 5% to 15% of the 24-hour dose. These doses can be offered every hour if administered orally, every 30 minutes if administered subcutaneously or intramuscularly, or every 10 to 15 minutes if offered intravenously. Transmucosal fentanyl, commercially available as a lozenge on a stick, provides more rapid relief of breakthrough pain than oral opioid preparations.

Side Effects of Opioids

Constipation is an inevitable side effect of long-term opioid use, and it should be treated prophylactically with regularly scheduled doses of mild laxatives. (For details, see the section below on constipation.)

Nausea and vomiting are also common side effects. Opioids can cause gastrointestinal symptoms by slowing gut motility, activating the chemoreceptor trigger zone of the vomiting center, and irritating the vestibular system. Patients who develop symptoms after eating should be encouraged to consume frequent, small meals. Such patients also benefit from promotility agents, such as metoclopramide. Patients whose symptoms develop soon after taking the medication may respond better to either serotonergic (eg, ondansetron, granisetron) or dopaminergic blockade (eg, haloperidol, metoclopramide, prochlorperazine). Finally, patients who develop nausea with head movement, reading, watching television, riding in a vehicle, or changes in position may benefit from H_1 blockers, such as meclizine or scopolamine if they can tolerate the sedating effects of these drugs.

Central nervous system side effects (sedation and delirium) are common in older adults. If patients develop symptoms and pain control is adequate, decreasing the medication dose by 25% may eliminate the problem. Additionally, changing to a different opioid preparation (eg, changing from morphine to hydromorphone) may help alleviate symptoms. For patients in whom this is not effective, small doses of psychostimulants (eg, 2.5 to 5.0 mg of methylphenidate or dextroamphetamine) can be used to treat excessive somnolence. Low doses of nonsedating antipsychotics (eg, haloperidol, risperidone) are often effective in managing delirium. Finally, targeted delivery of medication (eg, epidural opioid infusions, neurolytic blockade) may be effective if central nervous system side effects using systemic medications are intolerable.

Respiratory depression rarely occurs in patients on long-term opioids because tolerance to the respiratory depressant effects of these agents develops rapidly (within 48 to 72 hours). Respiratory depression can develop in opioid-naive patients and in patients whose opioid dose is rapidly escalated, and it is usually preceded by slowly progressive somnolence. Respiratory depression should be treated with low-dose naloxone, and the naloxone should be titrated slowly (eg, 1 ml/min of a 1:10 dilution [40 mgm/ml]) until the breathing pattern returns to normal. Continuous monitoring and repeated administration of naloxone may be required because naloxone metabolism and clearance may be faster than that of the opioid agonist(s). Other infrequent side effects of opioids include dry mouth, urinary retention, myoclonus, and hypnagogic hallucinations.

Addiction, Pseudoaddiction, Tolerance, and Dependence on Opioids

The hallmarks of true *addiction* are a psychologic dependence on drugs and a behavioral syndrome characterized by compulsive drug use and continued use, despite harm to self and others. Addiction is a complex disorder, triggered and maintained by genetic and environmental conditions. True iatrogenic addiction, although uncommon, and a fear that has led to insufficient pain management when opioids are indicated, is still an important concern. Like other low-incidence but significant adverse effects of drug therapies, a risk-assessment should precede prescribing, and an ongoing monitoring program should run concurrently with other principles of prescribing. One must not confuse addiction with *pseudoaddiction*, which occurs in the context of undertreatment of pain, or behavioral, family, or psychologic dysfunction. Opioid pseudoaddiction consists of a set of behaviors that are reminiscent of addiction but that are driven by untreated or undertreated pain and that disappear once pain control is adequate.

Tolerance refers to reduced effects of a given dose of medication over time. Tolerance to unwanted side effects is observed and is desired. Tolerance to opioid analgesics is less common than has been conventionally thought, and doses can often remain unchanged when the pain stimulus is relative stable. Disease progression, not tolerance, should be suspected when increasing doses are required for pain control.

Physical dependence is a property of opioids and is defined as the development of a withdrawal syndrome if opioids are abruptly discontinued or the dose is rapidly decreased. It is not equivalent to addiction. Dependence results from neurophysiologic changes that occur in the presence of exogenous opioids. Dependence rarely causes a clinical problem unless opioids are withdrawn abruptly or the dose is rapidly reduced. Such action will lead to an abstinence syndrome characterized by nausea and vomiting, diarrhea, body aches, abdominal pain, psychosis, and hallucinations, although there is great inter-individual variation in how abstinence manifests. If the pain stimulus lessens or disappears, doses should be reduced by 50% every 2 to 3 days.

Pain Assessment in Persons with Cognitive Impairment

Pain assessment in older adults is often complicated by the coexistence of cognitive impairment. The assessment and management of pain in cognitively impaired patients presents special challenges to the clinician. The cognitively impaired patient is often unable to express pain adequately, request analgesics, or operate patient-controlled delivery systems for analgesia medications and thus may be at substantial risk for undertreatment of pain. The fear of exacerbating a delirious episode or precipitating delirium in an otherwise stable older patient by employing opioids in the management of pain may also lead to inadequate pain management.

As with the cognitively intact patient, the initial step in the assessment of pain in the demented patient is to ask him or her about the pain. Although patients with severe dementia may be incapable of communicating, many patients with moderate degrees of impairment can accurately localize and grade the severity of their pain, and their self-reports should be regarded as valid.

In the noncommunicative patient, alternative means of assessment are needed. Pain assessment of these patients is of particular importance, given tentative evidence that suggests that physicians undertreat pain in patients with cognitive impairment, and that pain is aggravated in the presence of cognitive deficits. Untreated pain can result in agitation or disruptive behavior, and it may precipitate or worsen a delirious episode.

The best means of assessing pain in the noncommunicative patient is probably through the interpretation of nonverbal cues, such as the patient's facial expressions (grimacing, frowning) and motor behavior (bracing, restlessness, agitation), as well as verbal cues, such as groaning, screaming, or moaning. Data from studies of cognitively intact persons suggest that these nonverbal behaviors correlate with self-reported pain in nondemented patients recovering from surgery. Pharmacologic therapy should be titrated upward in small increments until the behavior disappears or side effects become apparent. This approach is particularly useful in the treatment of the agitated postoperative patient whose agitation may stem from untreated or undertreated pain. The risk of undertreating severe pain is generally more concerning, both medically and ethically, than the risk of worsening delirium with medications.

PALLIATION OF NONPAIN SYMPTOMS

Constipation

Constipation is one of the most common and distressing symptoms seen in terminally ill patients. Constipation is a universal side effect of opioids, and it is exacerbated by the immobility and poor fluid intake that accompanies most serious and life-threatening illnesses. Other unwanted side effects of opioids generally diminish over time, but constipation can be expected to persist, requiring ongoing bowel management as long as opioid therapy is used. Patients on opioids should receive prophylactic laxatives consisting of either a stool softener (eg, docusate sodium) or a bulking agent (eg, methylcellulose or psyllium). If these measures fail, then an osmotic laxative (eg, sorbitol, lactulose) should be added. Any time there has been no bowel movement within 4 or more days, an enema should be administered. Patients presenting with constipation should be evaluated for bowel ob-

struction or fecal impaction. If impaction is present, the patient should be disimpacted manually or with enemas before laxative therapy is initiated.

Nausea and Vomiting

The incidence of nausea and vomiting is estimated to be between 40% and 70% in patients with advanced cancer. Symptoms may be caused by disease or its treatment, so it is first important to clarify the cause of the nausea and vomiting. Emesis is mediated centrally by the chemoreceptor trigger zone in the area postrema, in the floor of the fourth ventricle. Peripherally, emesis is mediated in the gut and in the vestibular apparatus. Various receptors are involved in the mediation of emesis (eg, serotonin [5-hydroxytryptamine or 5-HT], dopamine, histamine, acetylcholine), and the selection of an appropriate antiemetic agent should therefore seek to identify the likely cause, the pathway that is mediating symptoms, and the neurotransmitters involved (see Table 16.1).

Dopamine antagonists like haloperidol, metoclopramide, or domperidone act primarily on the chemoreceptor trigger zone. Serotonin antagonists such as ondansetron or granisetron act in synergy with dopaminergic antagonists in the chemoreceptor trigger zone and additionally act peripherally in the gut. Muscarinic blockers such as scopolamine or meclizine are useful for patients with disturbed vestibular function. Prokinetic agents like metoclopramide can potentiate cholinergic activity in the gastrointestinal tract and

Table 16.1—Treatment of Nausea and Vomiting

Site	Involved Receptors	Common Causes	Medications
Chemoreceptor trigger zone in the vomiting center	Dopamine Serotonin H_1	Drugs: opioids, digoxin, estrogen, cefotaxime Biochemical disorders: hypercalcemia, uremia Toxins: tumor-produced peptides, infection, radiotherapy, abnormal metabolites	Butyrophenones, phenothiazines: haloperidol, prochlorperazine Prokinetic agents: metoclopramide, domperidone Serotonergic antagonists: ondansetron, granisetron
Gut	Serotonin H_1	Gastric irritation (eg, drugs: alcohol, iron, mucolytics, expectorants; blood), tumors (external compression, intestinal obstruction), constipation, liver capsule stretch, peritoneal inflammation, gastric distension, stasis (eg, opioids), upper bowel, genitourinary, and biliary stasis	Serotonin antagonists, antihistamines, motility agents (eg, metoclopramide) for stasis
Vestibular apparatus	Muscarine Acetylcholine H_1	Toxic action of drugs: ASA, opioids Motion sickness Ménière's disease, labyrinthitis Local tumors: acoustic neuroma, brain tumors, bone metastases to base of skull	Scopolamine, hydrobromide, meclizine
Cerebral cortex		Raised intracranial pressure	Dexamethasone

NOTE: ASA = acetylsalicylic acid; H_1 = histamine receptor type I.

are useful if the cause is gastroparesis. Antihistamines (eg, hydroxyzine, dimenhydrinate) may be useful adjuvant agents when combined with either serotonergic or dopaminergic agents, although their side effects (eg, sedation, urinary retention, delirium) may limit their use in frail older adults. It is believed that these agents act on H_1 receptors in the vomiting center, vestibular afferents, and the gut. Serotonin-receptor blockers, including ondansetron, granisetron, and tropisetron, are extremely effective for radiotherapy- or chemotherapy-induced emesis. They do not reverse nausea mediated by dopamine pathways (eg, those that are opioid induced). Finally, corticosteroids possess intrinsic antiemetic properties and enhance the effect of other antiemetics. Corticosteroids are also useful for nausea and vomiting associated with increased intracranial pressure.

Diarrhea

Diarrhea is defined as the passage of more than three unformed stools within a 24-hour period. Diarrhea, a relatively uncommon complaint of terminally ill patients, affects 7% to 10% of patients with cancer being admitted to hospice. The clinician should be alert to the possibility of fecal impaction that presents as watery diarrhea, particularly in immobile older adults on opioids. Treatment should be initiated with manual disimpaction and tapwater enemas, followed if unsuccessful by high colonic enemas. Laxatives should not be administered until the impaction is cleared because of the risk of bowel perforation. Untreated fecal impaction can be life threatening. Another common cause of diarrhea in palliative medicine is an imbalance in laxative therapy, especially after laxatives doses have been increased to clear an impaction. This will respond to temporary cessation of laxatives and reintroduction at a lower dosage. Radiotherapy involving the abdomen and pelvis causes diarrhea, peaking during the second or third week of therapy. This typically responds to cholestyramine 4 to 12 g three times a day. Diarrhea caused by fat malabsorption (eg, pancreatic insufficiency or small bowel disease) will respond to pancreatic enzymes such as pancreatin. Diarrhea following ileal resection also responds to cholestyramine.

Anorexia and Cachexia

Loss of appetite is almost a universal symptom of patients with serious and life-threatening illness. Anorexia in patients who are actively dying and who do not express a desire to eat should not be treated. Symptoms of dry mouth can be alleviated with ice chips, popsicles, moist compresses, or artificial saliva. Lemon glycerin swabs should not be used, because they irritate dry and cracked mucosa. Patients with anorexia who are in an early stage of illness may benefit from appetite stimulants. Megestrol acetate and corticosteroids have been found to enhance appetite, cause weight gain, and improve quality of life. These agents, however, have not been found to prolong survival. In addition to pharmacologic therapy, patients should be encouraged to eat whatever is most appealing without regard to dietary restrictions.

Delirium

Delirium, agitation, and confusion are common in older terminally ill patients and are often distressing to both patients and family members. Initial efforts should be directed at identifying potentially reversible causes (eg, infection, impaction, uncontrolled pain, urinary retention, hypoxia). Dehydration is another reversible cause of delirium in some dying patients, though there is much controversy over automatic use of parenteral hydration. However, it is worth considering in those few patients who are suffering symptoms such as confusion or opioid toxicity. Antipsychotics like haloperidol or risperidone in low doses are effective treatments for both hypoactive and hyperactive delirium. Actively dying patients who are nonambulatory and who experience terminal delirium often benefit from sedating antipsychotics, such as chlorpromazine. Benzodiazepines are often associated with paradoxical agitation and a worsening of the delirium in older adults, and they should be avoided. (See also "Delirium," p 127.)

Depression

Depression is under-recognized and undertreated both in older adults and terminally ill patients. It may be underdiagnosed because of the clinician's mistaken belief that it is either a normal consequence of aging or appropriate in the context of a terminal illness. Because of the underlying illness, standard vegetative symptoms described in the fourth edition of the *Diagnostic and Statistical Manual of Mental Disorders* (insomnia, anorexia, weight change) are often not reliable indicators. Instead, the clinician should watch for change in mood, loss of interest, and suicidal ideation. Suicidal ideation should be openly discussed, including any symptoms that are contributing to the patient's suffering, which may be influencing his or her consideration of suicide. Aggressive treatment of symptoms, antidepressant therapy, and psychiatric consultation are all appropriate initial responses. Continued discussion with the patient about the wish to die often reveals a change of mind as time passes.

Standard antidepressant therapy is effective, but most agents have a delayed onset of 2 to 6 weeks.

Psychostimulants (methylphenidate, dextroamphetamine) are well tolerated, safe, and effective treatments for medically ill depressed persons. Additionally, they have a rapid onset and beneficial effect on energy, mood, appetite, and mental alertness. Methylphenidate can be started at 2.5 mg in the early morning hours, can be given concurrently with standard antidepressants, and should be avoided in the evening hours. Finally, electroconvulsive therapy is an effective, safe method of rapidly treating depression and should be used for those who are severely depressed. The American Psychiatric Task Force Report states clearly that electroconvulsive therapy be considered a first-line therapy when rapid response is needed. Space-occupying central nervous system lesions are an important contraindication. (See also "Depression and Other Mood Disorders," p 211.)

Dyspnea

Dyspnea, the subjective experience of breathlessness, is one of the most distressing symptoms experienced by dying patients. Patient self-report is the only reliable measure of dyspnea, as respiratory rates and laboratory tests often do not correlate with breathlessness. Physicians may mistakenly fear that treating dyspnea in patients close to the end of life is associated with unacceptably high risks, leading some to withhold treatment and others to dose medications inadequately, which only increases the patient's suffering.

There can be many causes of breathlessness (eg, anxiety, airway obstruction, bronchospasm, hypoxemia, pneumonia), so symptomatic management should begin immediately, while the underlying cause is being sought. Treatment should not be delayed in the pursuit of disease-modifying interventions. Like pain, dyspnea is mediated through the interaction of complex pathophysiologic processes with poorly defined psychologic factors. At a physiologic level, dyspnea results from the interplay of chemoreceptors in the respiratory tract and central nervous system, upper airway receptors that sense the mechanical effect of airflow or the temperature changes that accompany it, stretch receptors in chest wall skeletal muscles, irritant receptors in the airway epithelium, and C fibers located in the alveolar wall and blood vessels. The experience of dyspnea, however, depends on the modulation of these physiologic events by psychologic factors, and as a consequence, the patient's perception of dyspnea may not correlate well with objective signs, such as respiratory rate, pulmonary congestion, hypoxia, or hypercarbia.

The optimal therapy for dyspnea is to treat its underlying cause. When this is not possible, one of a number of agents that have been evaluated for the treatment of intractable dyspnea might be used. Oxygen is considered by many to be an important component of any regimen, although caution must be used for patients retaining carbon dioxide. Although oxygen is usually considered beneficial only when oxygen saturation falls below 90%, there are some circumstances when oxygen may reduce dyspnea when this saturation value is exceeded. Cool air moving across the face (eg, from fans or an open window) may also treat dyspnea by stimulating the second branch of the fifth cranial nerve (V2), which has a central inhibitory effect on the sensation of breathlessness.

In addition to oxygen, several centrally acting agents have been evaluated for the treatment of intractable dyspnea. Benzodiazepines may be beneficial in controlling the anxiety associated with dyspnea, but these agents have not been found to improve breathlessness in randomized, controlled trials involving nonanxious persons with chronic obstructive pulmonary disease. The fact that respiratory depression can occur following the administration of benzodiazepines in normal adults suggests that these medications should be used only in breathless patients with an accompanying component of anxiety. Studies with phenothiazines, and the phenothiazine antihistamine promethazine, have shown mild improvement in dyspnea with their use. However, anticholinergic and sedative side effects may limit the use of these agents in older patients.

The most widely used centrally active agents for the treatment of dyspnea are opioids. Opioids are believed to act via a number of different mechanisms, although their predominant effect appears to be a reduction in the central respiratory responsiveness to carbon dioxide, resulting in a decrease in respiratory drive. The increase in Pco_2 that often accompanies this respiratory suppression can occasionally limit this approach in dyspnea management because of somnolence induced by the hypercarbia and by a decreased respiratory response to hypoxia. Opioids also appear to act centrally by decreasing the perception of dyspnea and peripherally on opioid receptors in the lung, perhaps by decreasing ventilatory response to, and oxygen cost of, exercise without affecting respiratory drive. Randomized, controlled trials have shown both oral and parenteral formulations to be effective. Anecdotal evidence supports the use of nebulized morphine (2.5–5 mg) or fentanyl (10–25 µg) for intractable dyspnea. Opioids have been found to inhibit the activation of pulmonary-irritant receptors and C fibers in animal models, and opioid receptors have been found throughout the pulmonary airways. The advantages of nebulized morphine include the avoidance of systemic absorption and the resulting constipation, hypotension, sedation, respiratory depression, and hypercapnia; rapid and efficient absorption because of the large surface area of the lung parenchyma; and the ease of administration. Randomized, controlled trials employing nebulized morphine have not demonstrated consistent benefit, and this route of administration should be reserved for patients who experience intolerable side effects from opioids administered by other routes.

Cough

Cough is a common symptom whose prevalence has been reported in the palliative care literature as ranging from 29% to 83%. Normal cough maintains the patency and cleanliness of the airways. Cough can be caused by the production of excessive amounts of fluids (eg, blood, mucus), inhalation of foreign material, or stimulation of irritant receptors in the airway. Additionally, patients with neuromuscular disorders may be unable to swallow saliva because of the involvement of bulbar cranial nerves, with the result that saliva causes coughing as it trickles into the larynx or trachea.

Underlying causes of cough should be sought and treated (eg, furosemide for congestive heart failure, antibiotics for infection, anticholinergics for aspiration of saliva resulting from motor neuron disease); however, resolution of the underlying cause may be impossible. Opioids can be useful in these situations.

Dextromethorphan is structurally related to opioids and has central cough-suppressant action with few sedative effects. Codeine and dihydrocodeine, usually in the form of elixirs, are also good first-line choices. Methadone syrup may also be helpful when taken as a single dose because of its longer duration of action.

Cough due to an irritated pharynx because of local infection or malignancy may be helped by nebulized anesthetics. Nebulized lidocaine up to four times daily has been reported, anecdotally, to offer relief.

LATEST DEVELOPMENTS

The Hospitalized Elderly Longitudinal Project (HELP) attempted to characterize the last 6 months of life and dying in very old persons. It used a prospective study design, providing a retrospective characterization of the last 6 months of the lives of 1266 patients aged 80 and older. Results showed that patients tended to overestimate their chances of survival near the end of life. Patients who died within 1 year of enrollment had significant functional impairment in activities of daily living and expressed strong preferences for not being resuscitated and for comfort care. The number of patients reporting severe pain increased toward the end of life, with one in three reporting severe pain within 3 months of death. These results highlight the need for physicians to talk with their patients early about their preferences, as well as to provide better symptom control and palliative measures at the end of life.

REFERENCES

■ AGS Panel on Persistent Pain in Older Persons. The management of persistent pain in older persons. *J Am Geriatr Soc.* 2002;50(6 suppl):5205–5224.

■ Buckman R. *How to Break Bad News: A Guide for Health Care Professionals.* Baltimore, MD: The John Hopkins University Press; 1992.

■ Doyle D, Hanks GWC, Macdonald N, eds. *Oxford Textbook of Palliative Medicine.* 2nd ed. Oxford, England: Oxford University Press; 1998.

■ The EPEC Project (Education for Physicians on End-of-Life Care) http://www.epec.net

■ Field M.J, Cassel CK. *Approaching Death: Improving Care at the End of Life.* Washington, DC: National Academy Press for the Institute of Medicine; 1997.

■ Fried TR, van Doorn C, O'Leary JR, et al. Older persons' preferences for site of terminal care. *Ann Intern Med.* 1999;131(2):109–112.

■ Gloth FM 3rd. Pain management in older adults: prevention and treatment. *J Am Geriatr Soc.* 2001; 49(2):188–199.

■ Growth House, Inc. *(resources for end-of-life care)* http://www.growthhouse.org

■ The *Internet Journal of Pain, Symptom Control and Palliative Care* http://www.ispub.com

■ Jacox A, Carr DB, Payne R, et al. *Management of Cancer Pain. Clinical Practice Guideline No. 9.* Rockville, MD: US Department of Health and Human Services, Public Health Service, Agency for Health Care Policy and Research. March 1994. AHCPR Pub. No. 94-0592/3.

■ Phillips RS, Hamel MB, Covinsky KE, et al. Findings from SUPPORT and HELP: Study to Understand Prognoses and Preferences for Outcomes and Risks of Treatment; Hospitalized Elderly Longitudinal Project. *J Am Geriatr Soc.* 2000;48 (suppl 5):S1–S233

■ Standards and Accreditation Committee, Medical Guidelines Task Force. *Medical Guidelines for Determining Prognosis in Selected Non-Cancer Diseases.* 2nd ed. Arlington, VA: National Hospice Organization; 1996.

■ SUPPORT Principal Investigators. A controlled trial to improve care for seriously ill hospitalized patients: The Study to Understand Prognoses and Preferences for Outcomes and Risks of Treatment (SUPPORT). *JAMA.* 1995;274(20):1591–1598.

GERIATRIC SYNDROMES

CHAPTER 17—DEMENTIA

Dementia is a general term used to describe significant decline in two or more areas of cognitive functioning. It is the most common cause of mental decline in old age. Of those who suffer from dementia, most have Alzheimer's disease (AD), which affects an estimated 4 million people in the United States. Epidemiologic projections estimate that by 2040 approximately 14 million Americans will suffer from AD. The pain and anguish of the disorder also afflicts millions more caregivers and relatives, who must cope with the patient's progressive and irreversible decline in cognition, functioning, and behavior. Both caregivers and patients may misinterpret initial symptoms of AD as normal age-related cognitive losses, and physicians may not recognize early signs or may misdiagnose them. However, dementia and aging are not synonymous. As people age, they usually experience such memory changes as slowing in information processing, but these kinds of changes are benign. By contrast, dementia is progressive and disabling and not an inherent aspect of aging. (See Table 17.1.)

Diagnostic and treatment advances have benefited many patients. Early and accurate diagnosis of AD may minimize costly medical resource use and give patients and their relatives time to anticipate future medical, financial, and legal needs. Reversal of the progressive cognitive decline of AD is not currently possible, but pharmacologic and psychosocial treatments may improve such associated conditions as depression, psychosis, and agitation. Medications are available that may produce cognitive improvement in many patients. (See also "Psychosocial Issues," p 13, "Legal and Ethical Issues," p 18, "Financing, Coverage, and Costs of Health Care," p 26.)

EPIDEMIOLOGY AND SOCIETAL IMPACT

Dementia is a disease of late life, generally beginning after age 60 years, although in rare cases AD may begin as early as age 30. AD has a gradual onset and continuous progression, and on average patients live from 8 to 10 years after the symptoms begin. The prevalence of AD varies, depending on the age of persons sampled, the particular diagnostic definition for cases, and the methods used to assess patients. For the age group 65 years and older, the prevalence of AD approximates 6% to 8%. The disease prevalence doubles every 5 years after age 60; an estimated 30% or more of those who are aged 85 or older have AD.

Table 17.1—Normal Cognitive Lapses Versus Symptoms of Dementing Illness

Domain	Examples of Occasional Normal Lapses	Examples of a Symptom of Dementia*
Memory in daily tasks	Forgetting an acquaintance's name	Unexplained confusion in familiar situations, settings
Performance of familiar tasks	Leaving the kettle on the boil	Forgetting to serve a meal just prepared
Language	Finding the right word	Forgetting simple words; substituting inappropriate words
Orientation	Forgetting the day or date	Getting lost in own neighborhood, inability to find the way home
Judgment	Choosing to wear a light sweater on a cold night	Wearing a bathrobe to the store; wearing two blouses at once
Abstract thinking	Having trouble balancing the checkbook	Not recognizing numbers, inability to do basic calculations
Misplacing objects	Losing car keys, glasses	Putting the iron in the freezer, wristwatch in the sugar bowl
Mood and behavior	Getting the blues in a sad situation	Rapid mood swings for no apparent reason
Personality	Gradual perceptible change with age, changing circumstances	Sudden, dramatic change from, eg, easy-going to suspicious
Initiative	Getting tired of housework, social obligations at times	Sustained lack of interest, involvement in usual pursuits

* Persons who exhibit several of these symptoms should see the physician for a complete evaluation.

SOURCE: Data from Alzheimer's Association, "What are the warning signs?" Available at: http://www.alz.org. Accessed September 1998.

In one study of primary care physicians' knowledge of dementia, only 40% knew that the most common cause of dementia in older persons is AD. Prevalence studies of community samples also detect many undiagnosed cases. Clinicians often apply a dementia diagnosis incorrectly by diagnosing the condition when it is not present or overlooking it when it is. Such errors may result from a lack of attention to cognitive functioning during medical screening examinations or a lack of knowledge about the normal aging process.

Dementia has a major impact on society. The total costs approach $100 billion annually if the costs of medical and long-term care, home care, and lost productivity for caregivers are included. Much of the direct cost is paid by Medicare, Medicaid, and private insurance, but families caring for patients with dementia must bear the greatest burden of expense.

The financial costs of dementia are only one aspect of the total burden. The emotional toll is immense for both patients and their families. Nearly half of primary caregivers of patients with dementia experience psychologic distress, particularly depression. An accurate economic assessment of the problem underestimates the true cost of the disease to society unless the quality of life of both patients and caregivers is included in the analysis.

GENETIC AND OTHER RISK FACTORS

The two greatest risk factors for AD are age and family history. Studies that account for death from other causes suggest that by age 90 years, nearly half of persons with first-degree relatives (ie, parents, siblings) with AD develop the disease themselves. For the rare forms of familial AD beginning before age 60, genetic mutations on chromosomes 1, 14, and 21 are the cause. More commonly, AD begins late in life; for such late-onset cases, the apolipoprotein E gene (*APOE*) on chromosome 19 influences risk.

The *APOE* gene has three alleles, *APOE*2*, *APOE*3*, and *APOE*4*. Everyone inherits one allele from each parent, so that six common genotypes are possible (2/2, 2/3, 3/3, 2/4, 3/4, and 4/4). Approximately 3% of the general population has the 4/4 genotype, 20% has the 3/4 genotype, and most persons have the 3/3 genotype. The *APOE*4* allele increases risk and decreases dementia onset age in a dose-related fashion, whereas the *APOE*2* allele may have a protective effect. Thus, the 2/3 genotype has a lower risk for AD than the 3/4 genotype; the AD risk is higher for the 3/4 genotype, and highest for the 4/4 genotype. The *APOE*4* allele may be less common in black Americans.

Using *APOE* genotyping as a prognostic test for asymptomatic persons is not recommended until results from further studies are available. *APOE*4* is neither necessary nor sufficient to cause AD, and cognitively normal centenarians who are homozygous for *APOE*4* have been reported. The asymptomatic person who learns that his or her genotype is 3/3 or 2/3 may be falsely reassured, whereas the person who learns that his or her genotype is 3/4 may be falsely alarmed. *APOE* genotyping may be useful in increasing the likelihood of a diagnosis of AD if a patient already has dementia.

Other genetic risk factors are likely since familial aggregation is present in families without *APOE*4*. Other reported risk factors include a previous head injury, female sex, and fewer years of educational achievement. Possible protective factors include the use of estrogen replacement therapy after menopause and nonsteroidal anti-inflammatory drugs. Table 17.2 lists both risk and protective factors for AD.

DIFFERENTIAL DIAGNOSIS OF DEMENTIA

Dementia can be defined as an acquired syndrome of decline in memory and other cognitive functions sufficient to affect daily life in an alert patient. AD accounts for approximately two thirds of all cases, and vascular dementia causes an estimated 15% to 25%. In recent years dementia associated with Lewy bodies (DLB) has received increased attention. For a diagnosis of DLB, both dementia and at least one of the following must be present: detailed visual hallucinations, parkinsonian signs, and alterations of alertness or attention. A diagnosis of DLB may overlap with AD and the dementia associated with Parkinson's disease.

AD is characterized by gradual onset and progressive decline in cognitive functioning; motor and sensory functions are spared until late stages. Memory impairment is a core symptom of any dementia, and in

Table 17.2—Risk Factors and Protective Factors for Alzheimer's Disease

Definite	
Protective Factors	**Risk Factors**
Unknown	Age
	Family history
	*APOE*4* allele
	Down syndrome

Possible	
Protective Factors	**Risk Factors**
Estrogen	Other genes
Nonsteroidal anti-inflammatory drugs	Head trauma
Antioxidants	Lower educational achievement
	Depression

AD it is present in the earliest stages. Typically, AD patients demonstrate difficulty learning new information and retaining it for more than a few minutes. In later disease stages their ability to learn shows even greater compromise, and patients are unable to access older, more distant memories. Aphasia, apraxia, disorientation, visuospatial dysfunction, and impaired judgment and executive functioning are also present. (See Table 17.3 for the *DSM-IV* diagnostic criteria.)

The cognitive impairment of dementia eventually has a profound effect on the patient's daily life. Difficulties in planning meals, managing finances or medications, using a telephone, and driving without getting lost are not uncommon. Such functional impairments may first alert others that a problem is emerging. Numerous functions are maintained in patients with AD of mild to moderate severity, including such activities of daily living as eating, bathing, and grooming. Many patients remain socially appropriate during the early disease stages.

Behavior and mood changes are common, including personality alterations, irritability, anxiety, or depression. During the middle and late stages of the disease, delusions, hallucinations, aggression, and wandering may develop. These behaviors are extremely troubling to caregivers and often result in family distress and nursing-home placement. Although the course of AD is variable, the progression of AD often follows a sequential clinical and functional pattern of decline (see Table 17.4).

Dementia recognition may be complicated by the presence of either delirium or depression. Delirium has been defined as a syndrome of acquired impairment of attention, alertness, and perception. Delirium and dementia are in some ways similar: both are characterized by global cognitive impairment. Delirium can be distinguished by an acute onset, cognitive fluctuations throughout the course of a day, impaired consciousness and attention, and altered sleep cycles. In hospitalized patients, delirium and dementia often occur together. The presence of dementia increases the risk for delirium and accounts in part for the high rate of delirium in elderly patients. A delirium episode in an older person, therefore, should alert the clinician to search for dementia once the delirium clears, if cognitive impairment persists. (See also "Delirium," p 127.)

Symptoms of depression and dementia often overlap, presenting additional diagnostic challenges. Patients with primary dementia commonly experience symptoms of depression, and such patients may minimize cognitive losses. By contrast, patients with primary depression may demonstrate decreased motivation during the cognitive examination and express cognitive complaints that exceed objectively measured deficits. Patients with primary depression, moreover, usually have intact language and motor skills, whereas patients with primary dementia may show impairment in these domains. As many as half of older patients who present with reversible dementia and depression become progressively demented within 5 years. (See also "Depression and Other Mood Disorders," p 211.)

Table 17.3—Diagnostic Criteria for Dementia of the Alzheimer's Type (*DSM-IV*)

A. The development of multiple cognitive deficits manifested by both
    (1) memory impairment (impaired ability to learn new information or to recall previously learned information)
    (2) one (or more) of the following cognitive disturbances:
        (a) aphasia (language disturbance)
        (b) apraxia (impaired ability to carry out motor activities despite intact motor function)
        (c) agnosia (failure to recognize or identify objects despite intact sensory function)
        (d) disturbance in executive functioning (ie, planning, organizing, sequencing, abstracting)

B. The cognitive deficits in Criteria A1 and A2 each cause significant impairment in social or occupational functioning and represent a significant decline from a previous level of functioning.

C. The course is characterized by gradual onset and continuing cognitive decline.

D. The cognitive deficits in Criteria A1 and A2 are not due to any of the following:
    (1) other central nervous system conditions that cause progressive deficits in memory and cognition (eg, cerebrovascular disease, Parkinson's disease, Huntington's disease, subdural hematoma, normal-pressure hydrocephalus, brain tumor)
    (2) systemic conditions that are known to cause dementia (eg, hypothyroidism, vitamin B_{12} or folic acid deficiency, niacin deficiency, hypercalcemia, neurosyphilis, HIV infection)
    (3) substance-induced conditions

E. The deficits do no occur exclusively during the course of a delirium.

F. The disturbance is not better accounted for by another Axis I disorder (eg, Major Depressive Disorder, Schizophrenia).

SOURCE: Reprinted with permission from the *Diagnostic and Statistical Manual of Mental Disorders*. 4th ed., text revision. Washington, DC: American Psychiatric Association; 1994:142–143. © American Psychiatric Association.

Table 17.4—The Progression of Alzheimer's Disease

Mild Impairment

Disorientation for date	Decreased insight
Naming difficulties (anomia)	Social withdrawal
Recent recall problems	Irritability, mood change
Mild difficulty copying figures	Problems managing finances

Moderate Impairment

Disoriented to date, place	Delusions, agitation, aggression
Comprehension difficulties (aphasia)	Not cooking, shopping, banking
Impaired new learning	Restless, anxious, depressed
Getting lost in familiar areas	Problems with dressing, grooming
Impaired calculating skills	

Severe Impairment

Nearly unintelligible verbal output	No longer grooming or dressing
Remote memory gone	Incontinent
Unable to copy or write	

ASSESSMENT METHODS

Consensus guidelines maintain that the diagnosis of AD must be primarily one of inclusion, not exclusion, as is often supposed. Most cases of AD can be diagnosed on the basis of a general medical and psychiatric evaluation. It is important for primary care clinicians to be alert to early symptoms of AD. If a patient or family member expresses concerns about cognitive decline, a mental status assessment and probably a dementia evaluation are indicated.

The informant interview and office-based clinical assessment are the most important diagnostic tools for dementia. Both the patient and a reliable informant should be interviewed to determine the patient's current condition, medical and medication history, patterns of alcohol use, and living arrangements. Useful informant-based instruments, such as the Functional Activities Questionnaire (see the Appendix, p 385), can help determine lapses in memory and language use, the ability to learn and retain new information, handle complex tasks, and demonstrate sound judgment. Any changes should be compared with previous performance, since functional decline and multiple cognitive deficits confirm the diagnosis.

A comprehensive physical examination should include a brief neurologic and mental status evaluation. Brief quantified screening tests of cognitive function, such as Folstein's Mini–Mental State Examination, and a laboratory evaluation, generally including a complete blood cell count, blood chemistries, liver function tests, a serologic test for syphilis, and thyrotropin and vitamin B_{12} levels, are also recommended. In addition, the history or physical examination may indicate the need for other laboratory tests.

Although brain imaging studies are optional, they are commonly recommended by specialists (Table 17.5). They should be ordered if

- onset occurs at an age below 65 years;

- the condition is postacute, that is, symptoms have occurred for less than 2 years;

- neurologic signs are asymmetric; or

- the clinical picture suggests normal-pressure hydrocephalus, that is, if onset has occurred within 1 year, gait disorder is present, unexplained incontinence is present.

In general, a noncontrast computed tomography head scan is adequate to exclude space-occupying lesions and hydrocephalus. If vascular dementia is suspected, magnetic resonance imaging (MRI) is often performed, but white matter changes revealed by T2 weighted MRI images generally are not related to dementia and should not be overinterpreted. In cases of unclear diagnosis, a repeat assessment in 6 months will confirm the presence or absence of progressive cognitive decline. Functional brain imaging studies such as positron emission tomography often show the characteristic parietal and temporal deficits in AD or the widespread irregular deficits in vascular dementia and may be useful when the diagnosis is uncertain after routine testing.

The MMSE is influenced by prior educational level, wherein affected patients with greater years of educational achievement may show normal scores. By contrast, older adults with lower levels of educational achievement may have low MMSE scores and no decline in function. The practical utility of cognitive measures is that they provide a quantitative baseline against which to compare future assessments. Neuropsychologic testing is sometimes helpful in distinguishing normal aging from dementia, as well as identifying deficits that point to a specific diagnosis, and it is recommended when the diagnosis is unclear.

Clinicians should avoid overreliance on and overinterpretation of laboratory findings, particularly

Table 17.5—Dementia Assessment: Brain Imaging Techniques

Structural (computed tomography, magnetic resonance imaging) scans may show:

- Atrophy

- Space-occupying lesions

- Vascular disease

- White matter disease

Functional (positron emission tomography) scans may show:

- Alzheimer's disease (parietal and temporal deficits)

- Depression (frontal or global deficits)

- Parkinson's disease with dementia (parietal deficits)

- Vascular dementia (focal, asymmetric, cortical, or subcortical deficits) computed tomography and MRI results. In general, the diagnosis of dementia is a clinical one, and the laboratory assessment is used to identify uncommon treatable causes and common treatable comorbid conditions.

Patients with AD commonly suffer from physical illnesses, but such illnesses rarely cause dementia. However, treatment of coexisting medical problems often improves quality of functioning. Vascular dementia is probably overdiagnosed. A history of "small strokes," unless accompanied by a clear demonstration of focal signs of motor or sensory impairment, is commonly not vascular dementia, which becomes clear when such patients are followed to autopsy. Cerebrovascular disease, however, does appear to contribute to the severity of cognitive symptoms in AD. Dementias that are potentially reversible are rare.

The initial stages of AD are characterized by normal motor, sensory, and cerebellar functioning. If focal motor or sensory signs, except fluent aphasia and apraxia, are present, a diagnosis of vascular dementia or mixed vascular dementia with AD is likely. Parkinsonian signs, particularly a "pill rolling" tremor that develops prior to cognitive impairment, generally indicate Parkinson's disease rather than AD. When parkinsonian rigidity and bradykinesia are present during the onset of dementia, a diagnosis of DLB should be considered.

AGITATION

Demented patients with agitation need to be evaluated for undiagnosed medical problems, pain, depression, anxiety, sleep loss, or delirium. Other factors that may contribute to agitation include interpersonal or emotional issues. Addressing such issues, treating underlying medical conditions, providing reassurance, and attending to the possible need for changes in the patient's environment may reduce agitation. (See "Neuropsychiatric and Behavioral Disturbances in Dementia," p 121.)

TREATMENT AND MANAGEMENT

The primary treatment goals for patients with dementia are to enhance quality of life and maximize functional performance by improving cognition, mood, and behavior. Both pharmacologic and nonpharmacologic treatments are available, and the latter should be emphasized. The use of pharmacologic treatments for behavioral problems is recommended only after nonpharmacologic ones prove ineffective, or there is an emergent need for them (eg, risk of danger, extreme patient distress).

Nonpharmacologic

Cognitive Enhancement

Reality orientation and memory retraining have been proposed as possible psychotherapeutic techniques to restore cognitive impairment. Although memory retraining may provide modest, transient benefit, it can also cause frustration for both patients and caregivers.

Individual and Group Therapy

Emotion-oriented psychotherapy, such as "pleasant events" and "reminiscence" therapy, and stimulation-oriented treatment, including art and other expressive recreational or social therapies, exercise, and dance, are examples of psychosocial treatments that may influence depressive symptoms. Patient support groups may be helpful, but only when patients are mildly impaired. Well-controlled trials have not demonstrated efficacy for these approaches, but preliminary studies and clinical experience suggest their usefulness for some behavioral and mood symptoms in patients and family members.

Regular Appointments

One approach to ensuring optimal health care for patients with dementia is to schedule regular patient surveillance and health maintenance visits every 3 to 6 months. During such visits the clinician should address and treat comorbid conditions, evaluate ongoing medications, and consider initiating drug-free periods. In addition, it is useful to check for sleep disturbances and provide guidance on proper sleep hygiene.

Communication with Family and Caregivers

Working closely with family members and caregivers will establish an alliance that facilitates management. Relatives are often helpful sources of information about cognitive and behavioral changes, and generally they take the primary responsibility for implementing and monitoring treatment. Areas to pursue with family include medical and legal advance directives (also called *advance care plans* in some contexts). It is often best for a trusted relative to cosign important financial transactions and attend to paying bills. (See "Legal and Ethical Issues," p 18.)

Discussion about long-term-care placement options should be initiated early rather than late, to provide family members time to complete the arrangements and begin to adjust emotionally. Eventually, almost 75% of patients with dementia need admission to a long-term-care facility and remain for a long time. Caregivers often express concern about their own memory lapses, which should be addressed with counseling or neuropsychologic assessment. Caregiver distress is often reduced with support-group participation, which may relieve common feelings of anger, frustration, and guilt. Respite care is another community resource that offers caregivers relief. Psychosocial support may enhance quality of life for patients and family and even delay nursing-home placement. (See the resources section in the Appendix, p 418.)

Environmental Modification

Patients with dementia can be extremely sensitive to their environment; in general, a moderate level of stimulation is best. When they experience overstimulation, increased confusion or agitation may result, whereas too little stimulation may cause withdrawal. Familiar surroundings will maximize existing cognitive functions, and predictability through daily routines is often reassuring. Other helpful orientation and memory measures include conspicuous displays of clocks, calendars, and to-do lists. Links to the outside world through newspapers, radio, and television may benefit some mildly impaired patients. Simple sentence structure and repeated reminders about conversation content also may enhance communication.

Attention to Safety

Door locks or electronic guards prevent wandering, and many families benefit from registering with Safe Return through the Alzheimer's Association. (See the resources section in the Appendix, p 418.) Using patient name tags and medical-alert bracelets will assist in locating lost patients.

Cognitive impairment affects driving skills, and the visuospatial and planning disabilities of many even mildly demented patients may make them unsafe drivers. Discussions about driving are best initiated early in treatment. In California and some other states, clinicians must report patients with AD to the health department, which forwards the information to the motor vehicle department for further assessment. Clinicians agree that patients with advanced dementia definitely should not drive, but many disagree on whether mildly demented patients should drive. Certainly, when a patient has a history of traffic accidents or significant spatial and executive dysfunction, driving abilities should be carefully scrutinized. (See also the section on the older driver in "Assessment," p 50.)

Pharmacologic

Age-Related Issues

When prescribing medications for older patients with dementia, the clinician should consider several factors. Patients in the upper age groups vary in their response, so that treatments need to be individualized. In addition, age is associated with decreased renal clearance and slowed hepatic metabolism. Older patients often take several medications simultaneously, so drug interactions and side effects are likely. Drugs with anticholinergic effects present a particular problem for patients with dementia because they may worsen cognitive impairment and lead to delirium. Another group of problem drugs that may worsen cognition include those causing central nervous system sedation. In light of such factors, clinicians should start with low doses and increase dosing gradually ("start low and go slow"). The goal is to identify the lowest effective dose, thus minimizing side effects; however, subtherapeutic dosing should be avoided. Prior to initiating any treatment, the clinician should conduct a thorough medical examination to identify and treat any underlying medical conditions that might impair cognition.

Cholinesterase Inhibitors

The primary treatments available for improving cognitive function in AD are cholinesterase inhibitors. The two most commonly used drugs are donepezil and rivastigmine. These agents may improve cognitive functioning or even delay cognitive decline. Clinical trials also show that these drugs may improve clinician and family assessments and activities of daily living functioning in patients with AD of mild to moderate severity. Extended cholinergic therapy also may delay nursing-home placement, but the long-term benefits and length of time that treatment should be continued are unknown. Data on the effects of cholinesterase inhibitors on more severely impaired patients or in patients with dementing disorders other than AD are not available. When these agents are prescribed, serial ratings of cognition from standardized mental tests (eg, MMSE) and of functional status are suggested so that the drug's effectiveness can be monitored. Long-term controlled trials have not been performed. Short-term trials demonstrate that when cholinesterase inhibitors are discontinued, the cognitive function of the treated patients returns to the levels of placebo-treated patients.

Donepezil is the most widely prescribed cholinesterase inhibitor. Donepezil has a longer duration of action than does tacrine, as well as higher specificity for brain tissue. Double-blind, placebo-controlled trials show that donepezil has significantly greater cognitive effects than placebo. The recommended starting dosage is 5 mg per day; after 1 month of treatment, an increase to 10 mg daily is recommended. Rivastigmine is started at 1.5 mg twice daily and increased to a maximum of 6 mg twice daily. Although the higher doses are more efficacious for both agents, they are more likely to cause such cholinergic effects as nausea, diarrhea, and insomnia, especially if the dose is increased too rapidly. Such side effects also may worsen the patient's behavior.

Several other cholinesterase inhibitors and cholinergic receptor antagonists are currently under development and will likely become available soon. Direct comparisons among them have not been conducted, and their degree of efficacy appears similar. Cholinergic drugs that have been studied include galantamine, metrifonate, M_1 agonists, nicotinic agonists, and eptastigmine, a physostigmine derivative with a long duration of action. Such direct cholinergic agonists as bethanechol, oxotremorine, pilocarpine, and arecoline do not show meaningful benefit and have significant cholinergic side effects.

Treating patients with cholinergic stimulation in the long term may have effects beyond symptomatic cognitive and behavioral improvement, including influences on neuronal function and survival. For example, both muscarinic agonists and cholinesterase inhibitors stimulate M_1 receptors, and such stimulation may enhance amyloid precursor protein derivative secretion and decrease tau phosphorylation. Thus, drugs that stimulate the M_1 receptor may delay AD progression, but controlled long-term studies are needed to determine any disease-modifying effects. The burdens and benefits of a cholinesterase inhibitor trial should be discussed with all patients with mild to moderate AD.

Other Cognitive Enhancers

Ongoing studies are assessing a variety of other agents that may improve cognitive functioning, including estrogen, nonsteroidal anti-inflammatory agents, and such botanical agents as *Ginkgo biloba*. In a trial including over 300 patients with moderately severe AD, treatment with vitamin E (α-tocopherol) or the selective monoamine oxidase-B inhibitor selegiline (approved for Parkinson's disease treatment) was found to lower rates of functional decline. The use of these agents, however, was not associated with evidence of cognitive improvement. Unfortunately, any clinical benefit for various treatments has been inconclusive thus far. Many patients also use over-the-counter preparations, which physicians should ask about routinely.

Extract from the leaf of the ginkgo tree has been promoted in China and the Orient for memory enhancement. One 52-week double-blind, placebo-controlled study of ginkgo leaf extract in treating AD seemed to show small but statistically significant improvement in cognitive measures. However, global measures did not improve in the small, limited study. Uncommonly, *Ginkgo biloba* has been linked to increased bleeding diathesis. More research is needed before ginkgo can be recommended.

Antidepressants

Antidepressant drug treatment is generally considered for AD patients with depressive symptoms, including depressed mood, appetite loss, insomnia, fatigue, irritability, and agitation. (See "Depression and Other Mood Disorders," p 211.)

"Sundowning"

In people with mild dementia who appear relatively normal in the day, "sundowning" takes the form of confusion in the late afternoon or evening. In more severely demented people who appear relatively calm during the day, sundowning takes the form of agitated, restless, or aggressive behavior during the night.

Sundowning is probably a nonspecific reaction to an assortment of causes. It has been suggested that sometimes a lack of clues from light and dark cycles may precipitate sundowning. Other factors that have been implicated include sensory deprivation, lack of structure in daily routine, and reaction to novel environments. In some cases sundowning may reflect disruptive behaviors that occur with similar frequency throughout the day and night but that have a different impact on nursing staff or the caregiver at night. The sudden onset of sundowning may also indicate the presence of some occult medical problem, such as a urinary tract infection, pulmonary infection, a disturbance in blood chemistry, or the introduction of a new medication. Table 17.6 gives strategies for reducing sundowning.

Other Resources

Most primary care providers should be able to successfully treat and manage many patients with dementia, but specialist or specialty referral is sometimes necessary. When the presentation or history is atypical or complex, particularly when the onset begins before age 60, consultation with a specialist with experience in treating dementia patients (eg, geriatric psychiatrist, neurologist) can be useful. Geriatric specialists with psychology or psychiatry training can assist with behavioral management, particularly when patients are agitated, psychotic, or violent. They are also helpful when

Table 17.6—Checklist for Reducing "Sundowning"

- Provide orientation cues.
- Give adequate daytime stimulation.
- Evaluate for delirium.
- Maintain adequate levels of light.
- Establish bedtime routine and ritual.
- Allow the same people to care for the patient every day.
- Investigate environmental factors that might keep the patient awake.
- Encourage exercise that expends energy to help the body feel more fatigued at bedtime.
- Avoid drinking any stimulant (eg, coffee) or smoking close to bedtime.
- Give diuretics and laxatives early in the day to prevent elimination at night.
- Provide care (baths, meals, activities) at the same time every day.
- Be sure the patient has glasses and functioning hearing aids in place.
- Place familiar objects at bedside or on the bed to help assure the patient of his or her safety.
- Monitor the amount of sensory stimulation in the environment.
- Consider exposure to bright light in the late afternoon.
- Avoid the use of as-needed sedative hypnotic medication.
- Establish a regular dose of medication for disturbing behavior.
- Assist the caregiver in obtaining respite help.

patients are suicidal or suffer from major depression or when individual or family therapy is indicated for patients or caregivers.

Organizations providing information and referral for dementia patients and families are listed in the resources section of the Appendix (p 418).

REFERENCES

- Gifford DR, Holloway RG, Frankel MR, et al. Improving adherence to dementia guidelines through education and opinion leaders: a randomized, controlled trial. *Ann Intern Med.* 1999;131(4):237–246.

- Petersen RC, Smith GE, Waring SC, et al. Mild cognitive impairment: clinical characteristics and outcome. *Arch Neurol.* 1999;56(3):303-308.

- Royall DR, Chiodo LK, Polk MJ. Correlates of disability among elderly retirees with "subclinical" cognitive impairment. *J Gerontol A Biol Sci Med Sci.* 2000;55(9):M541–M546.

- Small GW. Treatment of Alzheimer's disease: current approaches and promising developments. *Am J Med.* 1998;104(4A):32S–38S.

- Small GW, Rabins PV, Barry PP, et al. Diagnosis and treatment of Alzheimer disease and related disorders: consensus statement of the American Association for Geriatric Psychiatry, the Alzheimer's Association, and the American Geriatrics Society. *JAMA.* 1997;278(16):1363–1371.

CHAPTER 18—NEUROPSYCHIATRIC AND BEHAVIORAL DISTURBANCES IN DEMENTIA

Most dementias are associated with a range of neuropsychiatric and behavioral disturbances, with as many as 80% to 90% of demented patients developing such a disturbance at some point over the course of their illness. Neuropsychiatric disturbances of dementia, such as depression, agitation, anxiety, fearfulness, delusions, and apathy, increase the morbidity of the patient and adversely affect others, especially caregivers. Additionally, they are associated with a greater likelihood of nursing-home placement for the patient. Because these disturbances are potentially treatable, clinicians must anticipate them, recognize them early, differentiate among the different types, evaluate patients for contributing causes, and develop and implement appropriate interventions.

Although this discussion draws from empirical evidence as much as possible, there is a dearth of such evidence, particularly with regard to treatment effectiveness. Thus, many of the treatment suggestions are based primarily on clinical experience.

PRESENTATIONS

Table 18.1 lists common presentations of behavioral disturbances in dementia. They are usually brought to the clinician's attention by a family member or a caregiver. The complaints from family caregivers and professional caregivers in a nursing home or assisted-living facility are commonly different. Because a neuropsychiatric disturbance may be the first indication of dementia in an older person, clinicians should consider conducting an evaluation for dementia in any older patient who newly exhibits one of these disturbances.

Agitation is the most common presentation. Because caregivers may use the word *agitation* to describe various behaviors, the clinician should consider agitation to be a nonspecific complaint and pursue further history of the problem. Excess reactions to stressors are also common. Patients may develop rather marked emotional distress at a particular time of day or in response to having a limit set on them. Difficult behaviors may also present in clusters. Less often, the presenting complaint relates to a symptom of the patient's mental state or to a disturbance of a basic drive.

ASSESSMENT AND DIFFERENTIAL DIAGNOSIS

The first step in assessment is to obtain a history both from the patient and from an informant or other collateral sources. Information should include a clear description of the behavior: its temporal onset, course, associated circumstances, and relationship to key environmental factors, such as caregiver status and recent stressors. The problem behaviors and symptoms should be then considered in the context of the patient's family, past, personal, social, and medical history.

History taking is followed by a careful physical and neurologic examination. The mental status of the patient must also be assessed. Important domains to include are assessment of appearance and behavior, speech, mood, thoughts and perceptions, and cognitive function. Laboratory studies should be used to exclude metabolic or other precipitants of the disturbance. Generally speaking, a complete blood cell count and metabolic panel should be considered in all cases. Other tests, such as brain imaging, chest radiography, urinalysis, sedimentation rate, and electrocardiography, should be obtained "for cause."

A differential diagnosis of the disturbance should proceed on the basis of the findings (see Figure 18.1). The first step is to decide whether the disturbance is a symptom of a new or preexisting medical condition or a medication side effect. Disturbances that are new, acute in onset, or evolving rapidly are most often due to a general medical condition or medication toxicity.

A full-blown delirium or isolated and atypical neuropsychiatric presentations can be the *sole* present-

---

Table 18.1—Presenting Complaints for Neuropsychiatric Disturbances in Dementia

Agitation

Disturbances of the drives
- Anorexia (decreased appetite, not always with weight loss)
- Hyperphagia
- Hypersexuality
- Hypersomnia
- Insomnia
- Sleep-cycle disruption
- Weight loss

Excessive reaction to a stressor
Mental symptoms
- Delusions
- Depression
- Emotional distress
- Hallucinations
- Irritability, labile moods, moodiness
- Sadness
- Suspiciousness, paranoia

Problem behaviors
- Apathy and disinterest
- Combativeness
- Hoarding of objects
- Physical aggression
- Recurrent calling out
- Refusal of redirection
- Repetitive behaviors
- Social withdrawal
- Uncooperativeness
- Verbal aggression
- Walking away
- Wandering

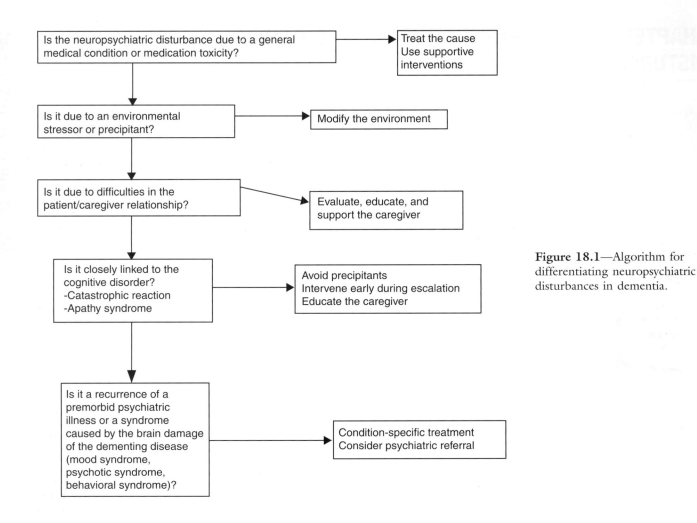

Figure 18.1—Algorithm for differentiating neuropsychiatric disturbances in dementia.

The boxes in the figure read:

Is the neuropsychiatric disturbance due to a general medical condition or medication toxicity? → Treat the cause / Use supportive interventions

Is it due to an environmental stressor or precipitant? → Modify the environment

Is it due to difficulties in the patient/caregiver relationship? → Evaluate, educate, and support the caregiver

Is it closely linked to the cognitive disorder?
-Catastrophic reaction
-Apathy syndrome
→ Avoid precipitants / Intervene early during escalation / Educate the caregiver

Is it a recurrence of a premorbid psychiatric illness or a syndrome caused by the brain damage of the dementing disease (mood syndrome, psychotic syndrome, behavioral syndrome)? → Condition-specific treatment / Consider psychiatric referral

ing symptoms for acute conditions such as pneumonia, urinary tract infection, arthritis, pain, angina, constipation, or poorly controlled diabetes mellitus. Additionally, neglect of basic physical needs (leading to hunger, sleepiness, thirst, boredom, or fatigue), which the patient cannot adequately communicate, might be a cause of neuropsychiatric disturbance. Medication toxicity due to new or existing medications might also present as neuropsychiatric symptoms alone. Treatment or stabilization of the cause can be sufficient to resolve the disturbance. Older patients with dementia may require several weeks longer to recover from routine medical problems than do those without dementia.

The second step is to consider whether a neuropsychiatric disturbance is related to an environmental precipitant; examples include disruptions in routine, time change (such as with daylight savings time or travel across time zones), changes in the caregiving environment, new caregivers, residence moves, or a life stressor (eg, death of a spouse). Other common environmental precipitants include overstimulation (too much noise or too many people around), understimulation (relative absence of people around, with the patient spending much time alone), and other patients. For some disturbances, correcting an environmental precipitant or riding out the effects of a stressor will often suffice as treatment.

Another consideration is whether the disturbance results from difficulty in the patient-caregiver relationship. Caring for dementia patients is difficult and requires a degree of sophistication that most caregivers are capable of acquiring with proper guidance. However, inexperienced caregivers or caregivers who themselves are impaired by medical or psychiatric disturbances may exacerbate or cause a neuropsychiatric disturbance. Most such problems occur in long-term care, but many occur in private homes. Interventions to improve the patient-caregiver relationship or to provide the patient with routines and activity may suffice.

After medical, environmental, and caregiving causes are excluded, it might be concluded that the primary cause is the dementia itself. Neuropsychiatric disturbances that are closely linked to the dementia syndrome take on the form of a catastrophic reaction. A catastrophic reaction is an acute behavioral, physical, or verbal reaction to seemingly minor stressors. The reaction might include anger, emotional lability, or aggression when the patient is confronted with a deficit, such as the inability to find a word, or confusion about where she is or what she is supposed to do. Catastrophic reactions are best treated by avoiding their precipitants, by providing routines and activities, and by recognizing early signs of the impending catastrophic reaction so that the patient can be distracted and supported before exploding.

If the disturbance is none of the above, a relapse of a longstanding psychiatric illness that preceded the onset of the dementia should be considered. Patients with chronic mental illness such as schizophrenia and bipolar disorder are at risk for dementia, and they may develop relapses of their illness after cognitive decline. The same is true for patients with premorbid mood and anxiety disorders such as major depression, obsessive compulsive disorder, or posttraumatic stress disorder. If such relapse is suspected, evaluation by a specialist is critical to help disentangle the origins of the neuropsychiatric symptoms and to guide appropriate treatment.

Finally, if the disturbance is not related to any of these causes, it may be a consequence of brain damage from the underlying disease causing the dementia. Disturbances with a more insidious onset or that are persistent are more likely to be symptoms of the underlying disease. Epidemiologic and clinical studies suggest that such disturbances fall into three groups: affective, psychotic, and specific behaviors. There is overlap in the symptoms of these groups. Thus, the clinician must first decide whether the predominant symptom of a polysymptomatic disturbance is a psychosis (delusions or hallucinations), a mood disorder (dysphoria, sadness, irritability, lability), or other behaviors and then target treatment to them.

Other characteristic behavior problems associated with dementia are seen usually in more severe dementia and are associated with widespread brain damage or loss of inhibitory control. These include inappropriate social behavior, pacing, wandering, or perseveration. Such behaviors may be related to damage to specific frontal lobe and basal ganglia areas. Another syndrome consists of exploratory curiosity with hyperphagia and hypersexuality. In animals this has been termed the Klüver-Bucy syndrome and is associated with damage to the temporal poles and the amygdala. Brain damage involving disturbed (usually increased) noradrenergic or dopaminergic neurotransmission has been associated with unprovoked aggression. Repetitive or compulsive behaviors have been associated with brain injury to orbitofrontal areas and the cingulum. Finally, disturbances of the basic drives, namely, sleep, sex, and feeding, may present as the dementing disease spreads to relevant brain areas.

The treatment of these disturbances is complex and may require several interventions at once. Specialists should be consulted in refractory cases. In general, treatment begins with appropriate environmental and caregiver interventions, depending on the situation. Table 18.2 provides a list of key nonbiologic interventions that might ameliorate neuropsychiatric symptoms in patients with dementia. The implementation of a daily routine and of activities is a central part of these. However, if the disturbances persist despite best efforts, specific or empirical biologic interventions targeted at particular disturbances are necessary. These include psychotropic medications, electroconvulsive therapy, or bright-light therapies. Their disorder-specific use, in conjunction with nonbiologic therapies, is discussed in the next section.

TREATMENTS FOR SPECIFIC DISTURBANCES

Symptoms Due to Medical Illnesses or Medications

At the core of treatment is the identification and removal or stabilization of the underlying cause. Environmental modifications can improve patient orientation. Good lighting, one-on-one attention, supportive care, and attention to personal needs and wants are

Table 18.2—Nonbiologic Interventions

Treat underlying medical precipitants

Remove offending medications

Modify environment on basis of results of assessment

Provide regular daily activities and structure (consider adult day care)

Monitor for new medical problems

Attend to patient's sleep and eating patterns

Install safety measures to prevent accidents

Ensure that the caregiver has adequate respite

Educate caregivers about practical aspects of dementia care and about behavioral disturbances

Teach caregivers the skills of caregiving: activities, behavior management, ADL support

Provide access to experienced professionals and community resources

Refer family, patient to local Alzheimer's Association

Consult in-house caregiving professionals, such as geriatric case managers also important aspects of treatment. If there is sleep-cycle disturbance, efforts should be made to stabilize the sleep cycle through the use of bright lights or medications (see the sleep section, below).

Pharmacologic intervention becomes warranted if patients are aggressive, engaging in other dangerous behaviors, or suffering from delusions or hallucinations. Antipsychotic medications are preferred (see Table 18.3). Haloperidol (0.25 to 0.5 mg before bed) is a first-line treatment option. This can be given orally or intramuscularly. Alternatives are risperidone (0.25 to 0.5 mg) or olanzapine (1.25 to 2.5 mg before bed). Dosing frequency might be increased to control aggression, delusions, or hallucination. Patients should be monitored carefully for side effects. Benzodiazepines, such as lorazepam (0.25 to 0.5 mg one to three times per day), should be used infrequently and in extreme situations. Some clinicians prefer a low dose of a long half-life drug; clonazepam, 0.25 to 0.5 mg at bedtime; is an example, but this drug increases the risks of falls, as do benzodiazepines and other psychotropics.

Mood Disturbances

All patients with depressed, irritable, manic-like, and anxious states should be provided with routines, distraction, and predictability in their environment. Physi-

cal health status should be optimized. Sustained depression warrants treatment with antidepressant medications. First-line agents are the selective serotonin-reuptake inhibitors, preferred for their lower side-effect profiles. Some clinicians believe sertraline or citalopram are the best starting agents, given their shorter half-life in comparison with fluoxetine and because they are less likely than paroxetine to have anticholinergic side effects, but whether this has clinical significance is not known. Also, these two medications are the best studied in the context of dementia. Table 18.4 lists the antidepressants most commonly used to treat depressive symptoms in dementia, with starting doses, titration rates, and peak doses beyond which additional benefits are unlikely.

The treatment of depression requires persistence. If a first agent has failed an adequate therapeutic dose for 6 to 8 weeks, an alternative agent should be tried. Venlafaxine, bupropion, nefazodone, the tricyclics desipramine and nortriptyline, and the monoamine oxidase inhibitors might be considered. Tricyclics should be avoided if a bundle branch block rhythm disturbance is present. For patients who are partial responders to an antidepressant, boosting strategies might be considered; use an antipsychotic agent such as risperidone (0.25 to 1.0 mg a day), or thyroid hormone augmentation such as thyroxin (50 to 100 μg

Table 18.3—Drugs to Treat "Psychotic" and Other Neuropsychiatric Disturbances in Dementia

Antipsychotic Medication	Starting Dosage	Weekly Titration	Peak Effective Dosage
Clozapine	12.5–25 mg twice daily	12.5–25 mg twice daily	100 mg daily
Haloperidol	0.25 mg at bedtime	0.25 mg daily	3–5 mg daily
Olanzapine	1.25–2.5 mg at bedtime	1.25–2.5 mg daily	5 mg daily
Risperidone	0.25–0.5 mg at bedtime	0.25–0.5 mg daily	1–1.5 mg daily

Table 18.4—Drugs to Treat Depressive and Other Neuropsychiatric Disturbances in Dementia

Antidepressant	Starting Dosage	Weekly Titration	Usual Maximum Dose
Selective serotonin-reuptake inhibitors			
Citalopram	10 mg in AM	10–20 mg/day	40 mg daily
Fluoxetine	10 mg in AM	10 mg/day	60–80 mg daily
Paroxetine	10 mg at bedtime	10 mg/day	30–40 mg daily
Sertraline	25 mg in AM	25 mg/day	125–150 mg daily
Tricyclics			
Desipramine	10 mg at bedtime	10 mg/day	therapeutic range 125–200 ng/mL
Nortriptyline	10 mg at bedtime	10 mg/day	therapeutic range 5–140 ng/dL
Other agents			
Bupropion SR	100 mg daily	100 mg daily	400 mg daily
Nefazodone	50 mg daily	50 mg twice daily	500 mg daily
Venlafaxine XR	37.5 mg daily	37.5 mg daily	225 mg daily
Mirtazapine	7.5 mg at bedtime	7.5 mg daily	45 mg daily

NOTE: SR = sustained release; XR = extended release.

a day). The advantage of boosting strategies is that the patient may respond within a week or two. If the patient does not improve, the booster should be discontinued. If a patient continues to be depressed after several antidepressant trials, particularly if he or she is in danger, as with serious weight loss or suicidal ideas, electroconvulsive therapy should be considered. This is the most efficacious and rapidly effective treatment for major depression and has a favorable safety profile in dementia, despite the stigma associated with it.

Treatment of manic-like states, emotional lability, or irritability typically begins with the use of mood-stabilizing agents such as valproic acid, followed by antipsychotics. Given its low side-effect profile, divalproex sodium is preferred over lithium carbonate. In dementia patients, the starting dosage of divalproex is 125 mg twice a day. The dose should be titrated upward slowly to a blood level as close to 100 ng/dL as possible. To prevent rare but serious side effects on liver or bone marrow, transaminase levels and a complete blood cell count should be monitored during the first week of therapy, rechecked monthly during the first 3 months of treatment, and quarterly thereafter. Alternatives to divalproex sodium are carbamazepine or one of the antipsychotics with lower side-effect profiles in Table 18.3. Carbamazepine starting at 100 mg twice a day and increasing to a blood level between 8 and 10 ng/dL if tolerated (monitoring with liver tests and complete blood cell counts) is an acceptable alternative for mania, manic-like states, lability, or irritability in dementia. The same monitoring schedule described for divalproex sodium must be pursued.

Combination therapies of antipsychotics and mood stabilizers, or combinations of mood stabilizers, might also be considered (Table 18.3), but these regimens are best used by experienced clinicians. Side effects of mood stabilizers include tremor, gait instability, falls, sleep disturbance, slurred speech, cerebellar signs, bone marrow suppression, and hepatotoxicity.

"Psychotic" Disturbances: Delusions and Hallucinations

Delusions or hallucinations, whether occurring independently or in association with mood syndromes, typically require specific pharmacologic treatment if the patient is disturbed by these experiences, or if the experiences lead to disruptions in the patient's environment that cannot otherwise be controlled. The preferred antipsychotic drugs are listed in Table 18.3. Lower potency agents, such as thioridazine, are more likely to cause sedation, orthostatic hypertension, constipation, urinary retention, and other anticholinergic side effects than higher potency antipsychotics, such as

haloperidol. The latter are more likely to cause extrapyramidal side effects, such as parkinsonism, akathisia, and dystonia. All antipsychotics have been associated with neuroleptic malignant syndrome and with tardive dyskinesia. Tardive dyskinesia is more likely to occur in patients who are brain injured, female, or aged 65 years or older. Given their equal efficacy to other antipsychotics and their lower side-effect profile, one of the atypical antipsychotics such as risperidone or olanzapine is the agent of choice. Alternatives include low-dose haloperidol or thioridazine (see Table 18.3 for dosing). There is some evidence that cholinomimetic agents such as donepezil, galantamine, or rivastigmine may ameliorate the delusions and hallucinations of Alzheimer's disease.

Disturbances of Sleep and Hypersexuality

Treatment of insomnia and sleep-wake cycle disturbance should begin with improvement of sleep hygiene. This consists of efforts to get the patient to go to sleep late every day, around 10:00 or 11:00 PM, while keeping him or her in a dark room for as long as possible into the next morning. Attempts should also be made to provide daytime activity and to prevent patients from falling asleep during the day. If the sleep disturbance is associated with depression, suspiciousness, or delusions, then those conditions should be treated.

For primary sleep disturbances when bright-light therapy or good sleep hygiene are not successful, trazodone (25 to 150 mg at bedtime), nefazodone (100 to 500 mg per day), or zolpidem (5 to 10 mg a day) might be used as hypnotics. Benzodiazepines or antihistamines, such as diphenhydramine, should be avoided, since they carry a high risk for addiction, disinhibition, or cognitive disturbance when prescribed chronically in patients with dementia.

If hypersexuality occurs in association with another recognizable syndrome such as a mania-like state, treatment of the specific syndrome should be attempted. In men with dementia who are dangerously hypersexual or aggressive, a trial of an antiandrogen might be attempted to reduce the sexual drive. Patients may be tried on progesterone 5 mg orally a day at first. The dose should be adjusted to suppress serum testosterone well below normal. If they respond well behaviorally, then they might be treated with 10 mg of depot intramuscular progesterone every week to maintain a reduction of sexual drive. An alternative treatment to reduce sexual drive is leuprolide acetate (5 to 10 mg intramuscularly every month), also an anti-androgen.

Aggression or Agitation

Behavioral interventions for aggression, such as distraction, supervision, routine, and structure, should be tried first. Behavior modification using token economies, rewards, and other contingencies have been reported to reduce some aggressive behaviors. If unprovoked aggression is infrequent (events occurring once a week or less often), it becomes very difficult to develop and implement a consistent and sustained behavior-modification plan. Pharmacologic interventions are sometimes indicated. Sequential trials of the following should be considered for unprovoked aggression: antipsychotics, antidepressants (trazodone, selective serotonin-reuptake inhibitors), mood stabilizers (divalproex sodium, carbamazepine, lithium, gabapentin), buspirone, β-blockers, and benzodiazepines.

Restraint in any form should be avoided if at all possible. If restraining measures are necessary, careful supportive care should be provided to patients. Over time, it is usually possible to reduce or eliminate the amount of restraint. (See the section on quality issues in "Nursing-Home Care," p 99, and the section on restraints in the nursing home in "Legal and Ethical Issues," p 24.)

REFERENCES

- American Psychiatric Association. Practice guideline for the treatment of Alzheimer's disease and other dementias of later life. *Am J Psychiatry*. 1997; 154(5 suppl):1–39.

- Behavioral and Psychological Signs and Symptoms of Dementia: Implications for Research and Treatment. Proceedings of an international consensus conference. Lansdowne, Virginia, April 1996. *Int Psychogeriatr*. 1996; 8 (suppl 3):215–552.

- Heard K, Watson TS. Reducing wandering by persons with dementia using differential reinforcement. *J Appl Behav Anal*. 1999; 32(3):381–384.

- Lyketsos CG, Sheppard JM, Steele CD, et al. Randomized, placebo-controlled, double-blind clinical trial of sertraline in the treatment of depression complicating Alzheimer's disease: initial results for the Depression in Alzheimer's Disease study. *Am J Psychiatry*. 2000;157(10):1686–1689.

- Lyketsos CG, Steinberg M, Tschantz J, et al. Mental and behavioral disturbances in dementia: findings from the Cache County Study on Memory in Aging. *Am J Psychiatry*. 2000; 157 (5):708–714.

- Patterson CJ, Gauthier S, Bergman H, et al. The recognition, assessment and management of dementing disorders: conclusions from the Canadian Consensus Conference on Dementia. *CMAJ*. 1999; 160(Suppl): S1–15.

- Rabins PV, Lyketsos CG, Steele CD. *Practical Dementia Care*. New York: Oxford University Press; 1999.

- Webster J, Grossberg GT. Late-life onset of psychotic symptoms. *Am J Geriatr Psychiatry*. 1998; 6(3):196–202.

CHAPTER 19—DELIRIUM

Delirium has been described in the medical literature for more than two thousand years. Despite this, it remains underrecognized and often inappropriately evaluated and managed. Clinicians call delirium by many different names: up to 30 synonyms exist in the peer-reviewed literature, and far more in common medical parlance. *Acute confusional state* is the most common synonym, and the term still preferred today by many neurologists. Other synonyms for delirium range from the frequently used *acute mental status change*, *altered mental status*, *organic brain syndrome*, *reversible dementia*, and *toxic* or *metabolic encephalopathy* to the arcane *dysergastic reaction* and *subacute befuddlement*. The current definition of delirium in the *DSM-IV* is shown in Table 19.1.

INCIDENCE AND PROGNOSIS

Delirium is common and associated with substantial morbidity. Approximately one third of patients aged 70 or older admitted to the general medical service experience delirium: one half of these are delirious on admission to the hospital; the other half develop delirium in the hospital. One third of older patients presenting to the emergency department are delirious. The prevalence and incidence in other settings, including postacute facilities where acutely ill older persons are increasingly being sent to recuperate, is not yet determined.

Although delirium is traditionally viewed as a transient phenomenon, there is increasing evidence that it may persist for weeks to months in a substantial portion of affected persons. A study of very old hospitalized medical and surgical patients found that approximately one third of those with incident delirium still met full criteria 3 and 6 months later. Subsequent studies performed in somewhat younger groups have found slightly lower but substantial persistence rates weeks to months after acute hospitalization.

There is mounting evidence that delirium is strongly and independently associated with poor patient outcomes. Delirium has been associated with a tenfold increased risk of death in the hospital and three- to fivefold increased risk of nosocomial complications, prolonged hospital length of stay, and greater need for postacute nursing-home placement. Studies that have incorporated postdischarge follow-up have found that delirium is associated with poor functional recovery and increased risk of death up to 2 years after hospital discharge. Most of these associations persist after adjustment for factors such as patient age, preexisting dementia, and severity of illness. There is evidence that patients still delirious 1 month after hip fracture had worse functional recovery than those whose delirium cleared, suggesting that persistence of delirium may play an important role in poor long-term outcomes.

DIAGNOSIS AND DIFFERENTIAL DIAGNOSIS

Underrecognition of delirium is a major problem. Nurses recognize and document fewer than 50% of cases; physicians recognize and document only 20%. The *DSM-IV* criteria, although precise, may be difficult to apply in clinical practice. More clinically useful is the Confusion Assessment Method (CAM), which was derived from *DSM-III-R* but is equally compatible with *DSM-IV*. The CAM requires a brief but structured assessment of the patient. By judging the presence or absence of the four key elements shown in Table 19.2, the clinician can establish the diagnosis of delirium. With appropriate training, general physicians, nurses, and lay interviewers using the CAM can achieve better than 95% sensitivity and specificity diagnosing delirium, even in groups with a high prevalence of underlying dementia. A study demonstrated that frequent screening by primary care professionals in the hospital using the CAM had greater sensitivity for picking up cases of delirium than did a systematic one-time surveillance by a psychiatrist. In the absence of a formal evaluation or when there is doubt, any

---

Table 19.1—*DSM-IV* Diagnostic Criteria for Delirium Due to a General Medical Condition

- Disturbance of consciousness (ie, reduced clarity of awareness of the environment) with reduced ability to focus, sustain, or shift attention

- A change in cognition (such as memory deficit, disorientation, language disturbance) or the development of a perceptual disturbance that is not better accounted for by a preexisting, established, or evolving dementia

- The disturbance develops over a short period of time (usually hours to days) and tends to fluctuate during the course of the day

- There is evidence from the history, physical examination, or laboratory findings that the disturbance is caused by the direct physiological consequences of a general medical condition

NOTE: *DSM-IV* distinguishes between delirium due to a general medical condition, delirium due to a drug or toxic ingestion, and delirium due to mixed causes. In practice, the cause is often not known at the time of diagnosis and may ultimately prove to be multiple interacting factors.

SOURCE: Reprinted with permission from the *Diagnostic and Statistical Manual of Mental Disorders*, 4th ed, text revision. Washington, DC: American Psychiatric Association; 2000:143. © American Psychiatric Association.

Table 19.2—The Confusion Assessment Method

The diagnosis of delirium requires the presence of features 1 and 2 and either 3 or 4.

1. Acute change in mental status and fluctuating course

   —Is there evidence of an acute change in cognition from the patient's baseline?

   —Does the abnormal behavior fluctuate during the day, ie, tend to come and go, or increase and decrease in severity?

2. Inattention

   —Does the patient have difficulty focusing attention, eg, being easily distractible, or having difficulty keeping track of what was being said?

3. Disorganized thinking

   —Is the patient's thinking disorganized or incoherent, eg, rambling or irrelevant conversation, unclear or illogical flow of ideas, or unpredictable switching from subject to subject?

4. Altered level of consciousness

   —Is the patient's mental status anything besides alert, ie, vigilant (hyperalert), lethargic (drowsy, easily aroused), stuporous (difficult to arouse), or comatose (unarousable)?

SOURCE: Inouye SK, van Dyck CH, Alessi CA, et al. Clarifying confusion: The Confusion Assessment Method. *Ann Intern Med.* 1990;113(12):941–948. Reprinted with permission.

older patient with acute change in mental status should be considered delirious, and evaluated and managed as described below.

The differential diagnosis of delirium includes dementia, depression, and acute psychiatric syndromes. In many cases, it is not truly a "differential" diagnosis, since these syndromes can coexist and indeed are risk factors for one another. Instead, it is better thought of as a series of independent questions: Does this patient have delirium? . . . dementia? . . . depression? The most common diagnostic issue is whether a newly presenting confused patient has dementia, delirium, or both. To make this determination, the clinician must know the patient's baseline status. In the absence of baseline data, information from family members, caregivers, or others who know the patient is essential. An acute change in mental status from baseline is not consistent with dementia and suggests delirium. In addition, a rapidly fluctuating course (over minutes to hours) and an abnormal level of consciousness are also highly suggestive of delirium. Depression may also be confused with hypoactive delirium. A study of psychiatric consultations for depression in the acute-care setting found that at least one third of these patients actually had hypoactive delirium. Finally, certain acute psychiatric syndromes, such as mania, can present similarly to hyperactive delirium. In the absence of known bipolar disease, it is best initially to evaluate and manage these patients as if they have delirium rather than attributing the presentation to psychiatric disease and missing a serious underlying medical disorder.

THE SPECTRUM OF DELIRIUM

The classic presentation of delirium is thought to be the wildly agitated patient. However, studies have demonstrated that agitated or hyperactive delirium represents only 25% of all cases. More common is hypoactive or "quiet" delirium, or delirium with mixed features. Hypoactive delirium has no better prognosis than hyperactive delirium; it is recognized and appropriately treated less frequently. Special case-finding efforts are necessary to detect quiet delirium among high-risk older patients. If agitation is present, behavioral control measures may be necessary (see below), but such measures alone are not adequate treatment for delirium, and in some cases they may exacerbate or prolong the delirium.

In addition to psychomotor variability, evidence supports the heterogeneous nature of the symptoms and timing of delirium. A study of 717 very old patients (mean age = 85 years) in a variety of settings found that 77% of patients with delirium had emotional symptoms, and 43% had pronounced psychotic symptoms. Although neither of these symptoms is required to make the diagnosis of delirium, either one can complicate its management. In addition, this study found the time of onset of delirium to be highly variable. Classically, mental status is thought to worsen in the evening hours ("sundowning"); however, more of these patients demonstrated delirium in the morning (47%) than in the afternoon, evening, or night (37%).

Though we often speak of delirium as being either present or absent, it is important to recognize that the number and severity of symptoms varies widely. To more completely describe delirium, several severity scales have been validated and published: the Memorial Delirium Assessment Scale, Confusional State Evaluation, and the Delirium Severity Scale are among these; the Delirium Rating Scale is older. When patients with delirium are stratified according to these scales, it is found that those with severe delirium have worse outcomes than those with mild delirium. Moreover, patients who do not fulfill all CAM or *DSM* criteria for delirium but who still demonstrate significant delirium symptoms have worse outcomes than patients with no symptoms of delirium. It is likely that a gradient of worsening outcomes over the spectrum of delirium exists.

THE NEUROPATHOPHYSIOLOGY OF DELIRIUM

Recent years have seen significant progress in understanding several neural mechanisms for delirium. This research also suggests that delirium may have a number of different underlying mechanisms that pertain in different situations. Unfortunately, this work has not yet progressed to the point that it has an impact on the management of most delirious patients. One of the best-documented mechanisms for delirium is cholinergic deficiency. This is seen classically in overdoses of anticholinergic drugs such as atropine, which in severe cases can be reversed by the administration of physostigmine. In addition, many drugs not classified as anticholinergic (antihistamines, certain opioids, and antidepressants) have substantial anticholinergic activity and may also precipitate delirium. Delirium has been associated with increased serum anticholinergic activity measured by bioassay in both medical and surgical patients. Moreover, significant anticholinergic activity has been found in the serum of patients who were taking no drugs with anticholinergic properties, which suggests that there may be endogenous activity predisposing certain patients to the development of delirium.

A second potential mechanism for delirium is an alteration in the ratio of amino acids important in neurotransmitter production. Serotonin, a key central nervous system neurotransmitter, is dependent on the transport of tryptophan across the blood-brain barrier. Tryptophan competes with other large neutral amino acids, most notably phenylalanine, for transport into the central nervous system. Alterations in the tryptophan-to-phenylalanine ratio may result in serotonin excess or deficiency, which in turn may result in delirium. In fact, high levels of phenylalanine (common in postoperative or posttraumatic catabolic states) and low tryptophan-to-phenylalanine ratios have been associated with delirium in several medical and surgical cohorts.

Other mechanisms for delirium may be important in other settings. In patients with infections or cancer, delirium may be mediated through cytokines, particularly interleukin-2 and tumor necrosis factor. Other neurotransmitter systems, including γ-aminobutyric acid and dopamine, are also involved in some cases of delirium. The evidence for most of these mechanisms is based on cross-sectional comparisons of patients with and without delirium. Better longitudinal data, in which blood samples are examined at several time points in the same patient, are a crucial next step. In addition, more research is necessary to determine what mechanisms are most important in which patient populations, to begin to design targeted, pathophysiologically based preventive or treatment strategies.

RISK FACTORS

In the absence of a clear neuropathophysiologic basis for delirium, the cornerstone of its management focuses on the assessment and treatment of modifiable risk factors. Fortunately, research has identified several consistent risk factors for delirium (see Table 19.3), which have been nicely summarized in a review. These risk factors classify into two groups: baseline factors that predispose patients to delirium, and acute factors that precipitate delirium. Among the predisposing factors, advanced age, preexisting dementia, preexisting functional impairment in activities of daily living, and high medical comorbidity are consistent risk factors. Male gender, sensory impairment (poor vision and hearing), and history of alcohol abuse have also been reported by some studies. Among acute precipitating factors, medications, especially those that are psychoactive or highly anticholinergic, uncontrolled pain, low hematocrit level, bed rest, and use of certain indwelling devices and restraints have been associated with the development of delirium. A proposed model suggests that delirium is precipitated when the sum of predisposing and precipitating factors crosses a certain threshold. In such a model, the greater the predisposing factors, the fewer the precipitating factors that would be required to initiate delirium. This would explain why older, frail persons develop delirium in the face of much less severe stressors than younger, healthy persons.

Table 19.3—Risk Factors for Delirium

Predisposing factors
- Advanced age
- Dementia
- Functional impairment in activities of daily living
- High medical comorbidity
- History of alcohol abuse
- Male gender
- Sensory impairment (blindness, deafness)

Precipitating factors
- Acute cardiac events: myocardial infarction, congestive heart failure exacerbation, arrhythmia
- Acute pulmonary events: asthma or chronic obstructive pulmonary disease exacerbation, pulmonary embolism, hypoxemia, hypercarbia
- Bed rest
- Drug withdrawal (sedatives, alcohol)
- Fluid or electrolyte disturbances, including dehydration, hyponatremia, hypernatremia
- Infections (especially respiratory, urinary)
- Intracranial events (stroke, bleeding, infection)*
- Medications (see Table 19.5)
- Severe anemia (hematocrit < 30%)
- Uncontrolled pain
- Urinary retention, fecal impaction
- Use of indwelling devices, such as urinary catheters
- Use of restraints

*Intracranial factors are rare and should be considered only when all other factors have been excluded or if there are new focal neurologic signs.

SOURCE: Adapted from Marcantonio ER. Delirium. In: Rakel RE, Bope ET. *Conn's Current Therapy, 2001: Latest Methods of Treatment for the Practicing Physician.* Philadelphia, PA: W.B. Saunders Company; 2001:1145. Adapted with permission.

POSTOPERATIVE DELIRIUM

Delirium may be the most common complication after surgery in older persons. There is a 15% incidence after elective noncardiac surgery, and the incidence may exceed 50% after emergency procedures such as hip-fracture repair. A prospectively validated clinical prediction rule for delirium after elective noncardiac surgery described seven risk factors that can be identified preoperatively: advanced age, cognitive impairment, physical functional impairment, history of alcohol abuse, markedly abnormal serum chemistries, intrathoracic surgery, and aortic aneurysm surgery. Patients with none of these risk factors had a 2% risk of delirium, those with one or two risk factors had a 10% risk, and those with three or more risk factors had a 50% risk.

In addition to baseline risk factors, postoperative management plays an important role in the development of delirium. Contrary to popular belief, the peak incidence of delirium is not immediately upon emergence from anesthesia, but on the second postoperative day. The stress of surgery and anesthesia are not likely to be the sole precipitants of most cases of postoperative delirium.

Several studies have demonstrated that the route of intraoperative anesthesia, whether general, spinal, epidural, or other, has little impact on the risk of delirium. Postoperative medication management plays a much more important role. Postoperative use of benzodiazepines and certain opioids, especially meperidine, is strongly associated with the development of delirium. Although pain medications can cause delirium, adequate pain management is also important, because high levels of postoperative pain have also been associated with delirium. Strategies to provide adequate analgesia with minimum doses of opioids should be employed. These include use of scheduled rather than as-needed dosing, patient-controlled or regional analgesia, and opioid-sparing analgesics such as acetaminophen or nonsteroidal anti-inflammatory drugs. Low postoperative hematocrit level (< 30%) has also been associated with postoperative delirium. Appropriate transfusion of high-risk patients should be considered, especially after elective procedures for which autologous blood is available.

The presumed relationship between delirium and long-term cognitive dysfunction following surgery is increasingly being appreciated. A large study found that more than 25% of patients aged 60 or older had significant cognitive dysfunction (defined as a decline from baseline) 1 week after surgery, and nearly 10% still had cognitive dysfunction 3 months after surgery. Surprisingly, neither hypotension nor hypoxemia was associated with cognitive dysfunction at 1 week or 3 months. Increased age, duration of anesthesia, low education, a second operation, postoperative infection, and respiratory complications were risk factors for cognitive dysfunction at 1 week. Only advanced age was a risk factor for cognitive dysfunction at 3 months. Unfortunately, these investigators did not assess delirium, so the association between delirium and long-term cognitive dysfunction remains unclear.

EVALUATION

All patients with newly diagnosed delirium require a careful history, physical examination, and targeted laboratory testing. Most of the treatable causes for delirium lie outside the central nervous system, and these should be investigated first (see the precipitating factors listed in Table 19.3). Moreover, multiple contributing factors are often present, so the work-up should not be terminated because a single "cause" is identified.

The history should focus on the time course of the changes in mental status and their association with other symptoms or events (eg, fever, shortness of breath, medication change). Because medications are the most common and treatable cause of delirium, a careful medication history, using the nursing administration sheets in the hospital or a "brown-bag" review in the outpatient setting, is imperative. In the outpatient setting, it is also important to review the patient's use of over-the-counter drugs and alcohol. The physical examination should include vital signs and oxygen saturation, a careful general medical examination, and a neurologic and mental status examination. The emphasis should be on identifying acute medical problems or exacerbations of chronic medical problems that might be contributing to delirium. Laboratory tests should be selected on the basis of history and examination findings. Most patients require at least a complete blood cell count, electrolytes, and renal function tests. Urinalysis, tests for liver function, serum drug levels, and arterial blood gases, as well as chest radiograms, electrocardiogram, and appropriate cultures are helpful in selected situations. Cerebral imaging is often performed but is rarely helpful, except in cases of head trauma or new focal neurologic findings. In the absence of seizure activity or signs of meningitis, electroencephalograms and cerebrospinal fluid analysis rarely yield helpful results.

MANAGEMENT

Delirious hospitalized patients are particularly vulnerable to complications and poor outcomes and must be given special care. This requires an interdisciplinary effort by physicians, nurses, family members, and others involved in the care of the patient. A multifactorial approach is the most successful since many factors contribute to delirium; thus, multiple interventions, even if individually small, may yield marked clinical improvement. Failure to diagnose and manage delirium properly may result in costly and life-threatening complications and long-term loss of function.

Modifying the risk factors that contribute to delirium is critically important. Some factors, such as age and prior cognitive impairment, cannot be modified. Common reversible contributors are listed under precipitating risk factors in Table 19.3. However, even some predisposing factors, such as sensory impairment, may be modifiable through proper use of eyeglasses and hearing aids. Drugs are the most common reversible causes of delirium. High-risk drugs such as anticholinergics, H_2-blockers, benzodiazepines, opioids, and antipsychotic medications should be replaced with drugs that have no central effects. For example, H_2-blockers may be replaced by sucralfate, and regular dosing of 1 g of acetaminophen three to four times daily may reduce or eliminate the need for opioids in many patients (see Table 19.4).

The delirious patient is susceptible to a wide range of iatrogenic complications, and careful surveillance is critical. Bowel and bladder function should be monitored closely, but urinary catheters, which can lead to urinary tract infection, are to be avoided unless absolutely required for monitoring fluids or treating urinary retention. Laxatives can be used to prevent obstipation, particularly in those who are concomitantly using opioids. Complete bed rest should be avoided, as it may lead to increasing disability through disuse of muscles and the development of pressure ulcers and atelectasis in the lungs. Exercise and ambulation prevent the deconditioning often associated with hospitalization. Malnutrition can be avoided through the use of nutritional supplements and careful attention to intake of food and fluids. Some delirious patients may need assistance in feeding.

Managing behavioral problems while ensuring both the comfort and safety of the patient can be challenging. The patient should be placed in a room near the nursing station for close observation. Nonpharmacologic behavioral measures provide orientation and a feeling of safety. Orienting items such as clocks, calendars, and even a window view should be made available. Patients should be encouraged to wear their eyeglasses and hearing aids. Although physical restraint use has not been well studied in the hospital, evidence from long-term care suggests that such restraints probably do not decrease the rate of falls by confused ambulatory patients, and they may actually increase the risk of fall-related injury. Restraints, though objectionable, may be required because of violent behavior or to prevent the removal of important devices, such as endotracheal tubes, intra-arterial

devices, and catheters. Even for persons with these devices, the calm reassurance provided by a sitter or family member may be much more effective than the use of physical restraints or drugs. Whenever restraints are used, the indicators for use should be frequently reassessed, and the restraints should be removed as soon as possible.

When drugs are used as restraints to "save staff time," they extract a costly toll in accidents, side effects, and loss of mobility, and they should be avoided if possible. Pharmacologic intervention may be necessary for symptoms such as delusions or hallucinations that are frightening to the patient when verbal comfort and reassurance are not successful. Some delirious patients display behavior that is dangerous to themselves or others and cannot be calmed by the provision of a sitter or family companionship. However, the mere presence of delirium is not an indication for pharmacologic intervention. Indications for such interventions should be clearly identified, documented, and constantly reassessed.

When medications are used, high-potency antipsychotics are preferred because of their low anticholinergic potency and minimal hypotensive effects. However, these medications must be used cautiously, as they may actually prolong delirium and may increase the risk of complications by converting a hyperactive, confused patient into a stuporous one whose risk of a fall or aspiration is increased. In older patients with mild delirium, low doses of haloperidol (0.25 to 0.50 mg orally or 0.125 to 0.25 mg parenterally) should be used initially, with careful reassessment prior to additional dosing. In more severe delirium, somewhat higher doses may be used initially (0.5 to 2 mg parenterally), with additional dosing every 60 minutes as required for symptom management. One must be careful to assess for akathisia (motor restlessness), which may be a side effect of high-potency antipsychotic medications and can be confused with worsening delirium. The treatment for akathisia is less, not more antipsychotic medication. Because of extrapyramidal effects, haloperidol should be avoided in older persons with parkinsonism, and a benzodiazepine such as lorazepam may be substituted. Low doses of the atypical antipsychotic agent risperidone may be effective in delirium, as well.

Sleep-wake cycle alterations during delirium may be of concern to patients, their families, and the medical team. One study of 27 postcardiotomy patients found that insomnia in the immediate postoperative period correlated best with confusion during the prior day, suggesting that the sleep disturbance resulted from the delirium, and not vice versa. Sedative-hypnotic drugs are high risk for precipitating or prolonging delirium and should be avoided if possible. On the other hand, environmental and behavioral approaches

Table 19.4—Drugs to Reduce or Eliminate in the Management of Delirium

Agent	Mechanism of Action	Possible Substitute	Notes
Alcohol	CNS sedation, withdrawal syndrome	If history of heavy intake, careful monitoring and benzodiazepines if withdrawal symptoms	Alcohol history is imperative
Antibiotics (ciprofloxacin, penicillin)	Neurotoxic (specific mechanisms unknown)	Adjust dose or use other antibiotics	
Anticholinergics: oxybutynin, benztropine	Anticholinergic toxicity	Lower dose, employ behavioral measures	Rare at low doses
Anticonvulsants, esp. phenytoin	Unknown	Consider need for agent; lower dosage; use alternative agent	Toxic reactions can occur despite "therapeutic" drug levels
Antidepressants, esp. the tertiary amine tricyclic agents: amitriptyline, imipramine, doxepin	Anticholinergic toxicity	Secondary amine tricyclics: nortriptyline, desipramine; SSRIs or other agents	Secondary amines as good as tertiary for adjuvant treatment of chronic pain
Antihistamines, including diphenhydramine	Anticholinergic toxicity	Nonpharmacologic protocol for sleep; pseudoephedrine for colds	Must take OTC history
Antiparkinsonian agents: levodopa-carbidopa, dopamine agonists, amantadine	Dopaminergic toxicity	Lower dose; adjust dosing schedule	Usually with end-stage disease and high doses
Antipsychotics: esp. low-potency anticholinergic agents and atypical agents (clozapine)	Anticholinergic toxicity, CNS sedation	Eliminate, or if necessary use low-dose, high-potency agents	
Barbiturates	Severe withdrawal syndrome	Avoid inadvertent discontinuation, or substitute benzodiazepine	
Benzodiazepines, esp. long-acting, including diazepam, flurazepam, chlordiazepoxide	CNS sedation	Nonpharmacologic sleep management, intermediate agents (lorazepam, temazepam)	Associated with delirium in medical and surgical patients
Benzodiazepines, ultra-short-acting, including triazolam, alprazolam	CNS sedation and withdrawal	Nonpharmacologic sleep management, intermediate agents (lorazepam, temazepam)	Associated with delirium in case reports and series
Choral hydrate	CNS sedation	Nonpharmacologic sleep protocol	No better for delirium than benzodiazepines
H_2-blocking agents	Possible anticholinergic toxicity	Lower dosage; consider antacids or proton pump inhibitors	
Agent	Mechanism of Action	Possible Substitute	Notes
Lithium	Electrolyte imbalance, CNS activation, or sedation	Adjust dose, use other mood stabilizers, correct electrolyte imbalance	Risks of toxicity increased if used with diuretics
Opioid analgesics: esp. meperidine	Anticholinergic toxicity, CNS sedation, fecal	Use local measures and nonpsychoactive pain drugs round-the-clock; save opioids for breakthrough severe pain	Higher risk in patients with renal insufficiency; must titrate risks from drugs vs risks from pain
Almost any medication if time course is appropriate		Consider risks vs benefits of all medications in older patients	

NOTE: CNS = central nervous system; OTC = over-the-counter [drugs]; SSRIs = selective serotonin-reuptake inhibitors.

SOURCE: Adapted with permission from Marcantonio E. Delirium. In: *Physician's Information and Education Resource*. Philadelphia, PA: American College of Physicians–American Society of Internal Medicine; 2001.

to make the hospital more conducive to sleep are certainly beneficial (see below).

It is important to stress to family members that delirium is usually not a permanent condition, but rather that it improves over time. Unfortunately, persistence of delirium is common. Thus, when counseling families, it is important to point out that many cognitive deficits associated with the delirium syndrome can continue, abating only weeks and even months following the illness. Careful monitoring of mental status and provision of adequate functional supports during this period are crucial, to give the patient the maximum chance of returning to his or her baseline level. Family members can play an important role in the hospital and postacute setting by providing appropriate orientation, support, and functional assistance. Hospitals are increasingly making provisions for family members to sleep overnight with relatives who are already delirious or at high risk for developing delirium.

PREVENTION

Finally, it should be stated that the most effective way to manage delirium is to prevent it from developing in the first place. A study demonstrated that a unit-based proactive multifactorial intervention can reduce the incidence of delirium among older hospitalized patients aged 70 or older by more than one third (adjusted odds ratio = 0.60, 95% confidence interval [0.39, 0.92]). Six intervention components were used selectively on the basis of patient-specific risk factors determined at an admission assessment. These included interventions for cognitive impairment, sleep deprivation, immobility, visual impairment, hearing impairment, and dehydration. Among these, the most creative and successful was a nonpharmacologic sleep protocol that involved trained volunteers offering patients warm milk, back rubs, and soothing music at bedtime; this intervention substantially reduced the use of sedative-hypnotic medication. Interestingly, this program seemed to have no impact on delirium once it developed, so prevention is its key contribution. Similar programs to prevent and treat delirium should be developed and implemented in hospitals and other settings that care for acutely ill older patients.

Although a unit-based intervention can be highly successful, it may be difficult to apply in all settings, especially in surgical patients. A randomized trial demonstrated that proactive geriatrics consultation can reduce the incidence of delirium in older patients undergoing hip fracture repair. Consultation began in most cases preoperatively and continued throughout the duration of hospitalization. Daily recommendations were based on a structured protocol that covered key elements in delirium prevention, such as limitation of psychoactive medications; 77% adherence was achieved.

The geriatrics consultation group achieved a reduction in the incidence of delirium (32% versus 50% usual care, $P < .05$) of similar magnitude to the unit-based protocol described above. Geriatrics consultation, if performed proactively and intensively, may be an important strategy for preventing delirium in high-risk surgical patients.

REFERENCES

- American Psychiatric Association. Practice guideline for the treatment of patients with delirium. *Am J Psychiatry.* 1999;156(5 Suppl):1–20.

- Breitbart W, Rosenfeld B, Roth A, et al. The Memorial Delirium Assessment Scale. *J Pain Symptom Manage.* 1997;13(3):128–137.

- Elie M, Cole MG, Primeau FJ, et al. Delirium risk factors in elderly hospitalized patients. *J Gen Intern Med.* 1998;13(3):204–212.

- Flacker JM, Lipsitz LA. Neural mechanisms of delirium: current hypotheses and evolving concepts. *J Gerontol A Biol Sci Med Sci.* 1999;54(6):B239–B246.

- Inouye SK, Bogardus ST, Charpentier PA, et al. A multicomponent intervention to prevent delirium in hospitalized older patients. *N Engl J Med.* 1999;340(9):669–676.

- Marcantonio ER, Flacker JM, Wright RJ, et al. Reducing delirium after hip fracture: a randomized trial. *J Am Geriatr Soc.* 2001;49(5):516–522.

- Marcantonio ER, Goldman L, Orav EJ, et al. The association of intraoperative factors with the development of postoperative delirium. *Am J Med.* 1998;105(5):380–384.

- McDowell JA, Mion LC, Lydon TJ, et al. A nonpharmacologic sleep protocol for hospitalized older patients. *J Am Geriatr Soc.* 1998;46(6):700–705.

CHAPTER 20—URINARY INCONTINENCE

Urinary incontinence (UI) is a multifactorial syndrome produced by a combination of genitourinary pathology, age-related changes, and comorbid conditions that impair normal micturition or the functional ability to toilet oneself, or both.

PREVALENCE AND IMPACT

The prevalence of UI increases with age and affects women more than men (2:1) until age 80, after which men and women are equally affected. Of persons aged 65 years and over, 15% to 30% in the community and at least 50% in long-term care are incontinent. UI can cause morbidity, including cellulitis, pressure ulcers, urinary tract infections, falls with fractures, sleep deprivation, social withdrawal, depression, and sexual dysfunction. UI is not associated with increased mortality. UI impairs quality of life, affecting the older person's emotional well-being, social function, and general health. Incontinent persons often manage to maintain their activities, but with an increased burden of coping, embarrassment, and poor self-perception. Caregiver burden is higher with incontinent older persons, which can contribute to decisions to institutionalize. Estimated annual UI-related costs total more than $36 billion.

THE PATHOPHYSIOLOGY OF INCONTINENCE

Normal Micturition

For older persons in particular, continence requires mobility, manual dexterity, the cognitive ability to recognize and react to bladder filling, and the motivation to stay dry.

Bladder smooth muscle (the detrusor) contracts via parasympathetic nerves from spinal cord levels S2 to S4. Urethral sphincter mechanisms include proximal urethral smooth muscle (which contracts with sympathetic stimulation from spinal levels T11 to L2), distal urethral striated muscle (which contracts via cholinergic somatic stimulation from cord levels S2 to S4), and musculofascial urethral supports. In women, these supports form a two-layered "hammock" that supports and compresses the urethra when abdominal pressure increases. Micturition is coordinated by the central nervous system: Parietal lobes and thalamus receive and coordinate detrusor afferent stimuli; frontal lobes and basal ganglia provide signals to inhibit voiding; and the pontine micturition center integrates these inputs into socially appropriate voiding with coordinated urethral

relaxation and detrusor contraction until the bladder is empty. Urine storage is under sympathetic control (inhibiting detrusor contraction and increasing sphincter tone), and voiding is parasympathetic (detrusor contractor and relaxation of sphincter tone).

Age-Related Changes

Age-related changes in the lower urinary tract and micturition (Table 20.1) are found in both continent and incontinent older persons. Why some older persons develop UI and others do not remains unclear; differences in lower urinary tract (LUT) and non-LUT compensatory mechanisms may play a role.

Risk Factors

Any condition, medication, or factor that affects lower urinary tract function, volume status and urine excretion, or the ability to toilet can predispose a person to UI. Causation is suggested by temporal links between such factors and the development or worsening of UI. Risk factors in community-dwelling older persons include advanced age, parity, depression, transient ischemic attacks and stroke, congestive heart failure, fecal incontinence and constipation, obesity, chronic obstructive lung disease, chronic cough, diabetes mellitus, impaired mobility, and impaired activities of daily living. Among institutionalized older persons, UI is associated with impaired mobility, depression, stroke, diabetes mellitus, and Parkinson's disease; at least one third have multiple conditions. Table 20.2 lists the mechanisms by which these conditions may impair

Table 20.1—Age-Related Changes Affecting Micturition

Change	Predisposes to
Detrusor overactivity (-20% of healthy, continent persons)	Frequency, urgency, nocturia, UI
Benign prostatic hyperplasia	Outlet obstruction with frequency, urgency, nocturia, urge or overflow UI
More urine output later in the day	Nocturia, nocturnal UI
Atrophic vaginitis and urethritis	Decreased urethral mucosal seal, irritation, urge and stress UI, UTIs
Increased postvoid residual	Frequency, nocturia, UI
Decreased ability to postpone voiding	Frequency, urgency, nocturia, UI
Decreased total bladder capacity	Frequency, urgency, nocturia, UI
Decreased detrusor contractility	Decreased flow rate, elevated postvoid residual, hesitancy, UI

NOTE: UI = urinary incontinence; UTI = urinary tract infection.

Table 20.2—Common Medical Conditions Associated With Incontinence

Condition	Effect on continence
Neurologic disease	
Cerebrovascular disease; stroke	DO from damage to upper motor neurons; impaired sensation to void from interruption of subcortical pathways; impaired function and cognition
Delirium	Impaired function and cognition
Dementia	DO from damage to upper motor neurons; impaired function and cognition
Multiple sclerosis	DO, areflexia, or sphincter dyssynergia (dependent on level of synergy)
Multisystem atrophy	Detrusor and sphincter areflexia from damage to spinal intermediolateral tracts
Normal-pressure hydrocephalus	DO from compression of frontal inhibitory centers; impaired function and cognition
Parkinson's disease	DO from loss of inhibitory inputs to pontine micturition center; impaired function and cognition; retention and overflow from constipation
Spinal cord injury	DO, areflexia, or sphincter dyssynergia (dependent on level of injury)
Spinal stenosis	DO from damage to detrusor upper motor neurons (cervical stenosis); DO or areflexia (lumbar stenosis)
Metabolic disease	
Diabetes mellitus	Detrusor underactivity due to neuropathy, DO, osmotic diuresis; altered mental status from hyper- or hypoglycemia; retention and overflow from constipation
Hypercalcemia	Diuresis; altered mental status
Vitamin B_{12} deficiency	Impaired bladder sensation and detrusor underactivity from peripheral neuropathy
Infectious disease	
Herpes zoster	Urinary retention if sacral dermatomes involved; outlet obstruction from viral prostatitis in men; retention and overflow UI from constipation
Human immunodeficiency virus	DO, areflexia, or sphincter dyssynergia
Neurosyphilis	DO, areflexia, or sphincter dyssynergia
Tuberculosis	Inanition and functional impairments (sterile pyuria found in $\leq$ 50% of genitourinary TB cases)
Psychiatric disease	
Affective and anxiety disorders	Decreased motivation
Alcoholism	Functional and cognitive impairment; rapid diuresis and retention in acute intoxication
Psychosis	Functional and cognitive impairment; decreased motivation
Cardiovascular disease	
Arteriovascular disease	Detrusor underactivity or areflexia from ischemic myopathy or neuropathy
Congestive heart failure	Nocturnal diuresis
Other organ system diseases	
Gastrointestinal disease	Retention and overflow UI from constipation
Musculoskeletal disease	Mobility impairment; DO from cervical myelopathy in rheumatoid arthritis and osteoarthritis
Peripheral venous insufficiency	Nocturnal diuresis
Pulmonary disease	Exacerbation of stress UI by chronic cough

NOTE: DO = detrusor overactivity; TB = tuberculosis; UI = urinary incontinence.

SOURCE: Adapted with permission from DuBeau CE. Interpreting the effect of common medical conditions on voiding dysfunction in the elderly. *Urol Clin North Am.* 1996;23(1):11–18.

continence. Although moderate to severe dementia is associated with UI, even severely demented persons remain continent if they have mobility for transfers. Thus, UI in demented persons may not be caused by dementia, but may be a multifactorial epiphenomenon with treatable causes.

CLINICAL TYPES OF INCONTINENCE

Incontinence can be classified into diagnostic clinical types that are useful in planning evaluation and treatment.

Transient Incontinence

UI precipitated by remediable factors is called *transient incontinence.* Transient UI affects approximately one third of community-dwelling older persons and accounts for one half of the incontinence among hospitalized older persons. The causes of transient incontinence are summarized in Table 20.3. Although transient UI is more likely in persons with lower urinary tract abnormalities, correction of the precipitating factor remains effective without abolishing the specific abnormality.

Urge Incontinence

Urge UI is the most common type of UI in older persons. It is characterized by abrupt urgency, frequency, and nocturia; the volume of leakage may be small or large. The term *overactive bladder* refers to a condition with frequency, nocturia, and urgency or urge UI, or both. Urge UI is associated with detrusor overactivity (DO) that may be age-related, idiopathic,

Table 20.3—Causes of Transient Incontinence

Cause	Comment
Delirium, confusional state	UI resolves once underlying cause(s) treated
Urinary infection	UI may be only symptom of infection; antibiotic trial warranted in asymptomatic persons only on initial evaluation and with new onset/exacerbation of UI
Atrophic urethritis, vaginitis	Aggravates stress or urge UI; agitation can be presenting symptom in demented patients
Medications	Any agent that impairs cognition, mobility, fluid balance, bladder contractility, or sphincter function; many agents impair several functions
Psychiatric disorders	Severe depression or psychosis
Increased urine output	Frequency or nocturia; causes: excessive fluid intake, diuretics, hyperglycemia, hypercalcemia, volume overload (congestive heart failure, venous insufficiency, hypothyroidism, hypoalbuminemia, and drug-induced peripheral edema)
Restricted mobility	Treat underlying cause; provide a urinal or bedside commode
Stool impaction	Urge or overflow UI; fecal incontinence common

NOTE: UI = urinary incontinence.

SOURCE: Data from Resnick NM. Urinary incontinence in the elderly. *Medical Grand Rounds.* 1984;3:281–290.

secondary to lesions in central inhibitory pathways (eg, stroke, cervical stenosis), or due to local bladder irritation (infection, bladder stones, inflammation, tumors). Because DO is found in healthy, continent older persons, failure of lower urinary tract and functional compensatory mechanisms may play an important role in UI. Distinctions between detrusor hyperreflexia (DO associated with central nervous system lesions) and detrusor instability (DO without such lesions) are frequently blurred in the older persons. Less common causes of urge UI are interstitial cystitis (urge UI with otherwise unexplained pelvic pain) and spinal cord injury, which results in impaired detrusor compliance (excessive pressure response to filling) or detrusor-sphincter dyssynergia (concomitant detrusor and sphincter contraction), or both.

DO may coexist with impaired detrusor contractility (detrusor hyperactivity with impaired contractility, or DHIC), with an elevated postvoid residual volume (PVR) in the absence of outlet obstruction. DHIC accounts for most established UI in frail older persons. Women can be misdiagnosed with stress UI if weak DHIC contractions are not detected, and men can be misdiagnosed with outlet obstruction because of the similarity of the symptoms (urgency, frequency, weak flow rate, and elevated residual urine). Persons with DHIC may be at increased risk for urinary retention if treated with bladder-relaxant drugs.

Stress Incontinence

Stress UI, the second most common type of UI in older women, results from failure of the sphincter mechanism(s) to preserve outlet closure during bladder filling. Stress UI occurs coincident with increased intra-abdominal pressure, in the absence of a bladder contraction. Leakage is due to impaired pelvic supports or, less commonly, failure of urethral closure; the latter intrinsic sphincter deficiency occurs with trauma and scarring from anti-incontinence surgery in women and prostatectomy in men, or with severe urethral atrophy. Unlike the episodic leakage of genuine stress UI, this leakage is typically continual and can occur while the person is sitting or standing quietly. Stress maneuvers may trigger DO; with such stress-related urge UI, leakage occurs after a several-second delay following the stress maneuver.

Overflow Incontinence

Overflow UI results from detrusor underactivity, bladder outlet obstruction, or both. Leakage is small in volume but continual. The PVR is elevated, and symptoms include dribbling, weak urinary stream, intermittency, hesitancy, frequency, and nocturia. Associated urge and stress leakage may occur. Rarely, continual leakage is due to extraurethral incontinence (eg, cystovaginal fistula).

Outlet obstruction is the second most common cause of UI in older men; most obstructed men, however, are not incontinent. Causes include benign prostatic hyperplasia, prostate cancer, and urethral stricture. In women, obstruction is uncommon and usually due to previous anti-incontinence surgery or a large cystocele that kinks the urethra.

Detrusor underactivity causing urinary retention and overflow UI occurs in only 5% to 10% of older persons. Intrinsic causes are replacement of detrusor smooth muscle by fibrosis and connective tissue (eg, with chronic outlet obstruction). Neurologic causes include peripheral neuropathy (from diabetes mellitus, pernicious anemia, Parkinson's disease, alcoholism) or mechanical damage to the spinal detrusor afferents by disc herniation, spinal stenosis, or tumor.

ASSESSMENT OF URINARY INCONTINENCE

The multifactorial nature of UI in older persons requires a comprehensive diagnostic evaluation, with a careful search for all possible causes and precipitants beyond a focus on specific genitourinary diagnoses. Table 20.4 lists the key points in the evaluation of UI in older persons. The evaluation must determine the cause(s) of UI and exclude serious conditions.

Routine urodynamic testing is optional and usually is not needed. Precise diagnosis is most important when surgical treatment is being considered for stress UI or outlet obstruction, because surgery is ineffective for DO, DHIC, and detrusor weakness that present with similar symptoms. Geriatric UI is multifactorial, and lower urinary tract pathology is rarely the only cause. A focus on urodynamic diagnosis detracts from more relevant precipitants. Moreover, some treatments are effective for several types of UI (see below). Thus, urodynamics should be considered only before surgical intervention, if the diagnosis is unclear, or when empiric therapy has failed. Cystometry determines only bladder proprioception, capacity, detrusor stability, and contractility; carbon dioxide cystometry may be unreliable. Simultaneous measurement of abdominal pressure is necessary to exclude abdominal straining and detect DHIC. Fluoroscopic monitoring, abdominal leak-point pressure, or profilometry tests detect and quantify stress UI. Pressure-flow studies detect obstruction. Peak urine flow rates ≥ 12 mL per second (without straining for voids of at least 150 to 200 mL) reliably exclude obstruction. Low flow rates are nondiagnostic, and precise diagnosis requires urodynamic evaluation.

Bedside cystometry may detect DO and measure bladder capacity. The PVR is measured by catheterization; then the bladder is filled through a syringe attached to the catheter. DO is identified by a rise in fluid level in the syringe column. Although bedside cystometry has moderate sensitivity and specificity for DO in ambulatory older persons, its true utility is unclear. Among community-dwelling older persons, its benefit over history and physical examination is unknown. When it is used in long-term-care patients, low-pressure DHIC contractions can be missed, and it may be difficult to differentiate DO from abdominal straining.

MANAGEMENT

Overview

Because age-related changes render older persons more vulnerable to developing UI from factors such as medical illnesses and medications, correction of those factors alone often improves continence. Relieving the most bothersome aspects of UI for the patient is key. A stepped strategy moving from least to more invasive treatments should be used, with behavioral methods tried before medication, and both tried before surgery. Treatment that simply decreases the number of UI episodes may not be sufficient for persons most bothered by the timing of UI, nocturia, or leakage with exercise. Cure often requires multiple visits. Evidence for the efficacy of UI treatment is summarized in Table 20.5, Table 20.6, and Table 20.7.

General Measures

Fluid management includes avoiding caffeinated beverages and alcohol, and minimizing evening intake if nocturnal UI is bothersome. Constipation should be reduced. If pads and protective garments are used, they should be chosen on the basis of gender and the type and volume of UI. Because these products are expensive, some patients may not change pads frequently enough. Medical supply companies and patient advocacy groups publish illustrated catalogs for product selection.

Urge Incontinence

Behavioral treatment for urge UI employs two principles: frequent voluntary voiding to keep bladder volume low, and retraining of central nervous system and pelvic mechanisms to inhibit detrusor contractions and leakage. Cognitively intact persons can use bladder retraining, with timed voiding while awake and suppression of precipitant urges by relaxation techniques. The initial toileting frequency (based on a voiding record) uses the shortest interval between voids. When a precipitant urge occurs, patients are instructed to stand still or sit down and concentrate on making the urge decrease and pass: to take a deep breath and let it out slowly, or to visualize the urge as a wave that peaks and then falls. Once in control of the urge, they should walk slowly to a bathroom and void. After 2 days without leakage, the time between scheduled voids is increased by 30 to 60 minutes until the person voids every 3 to 4 hours without leakage. Although its marginal benefit is unproven, many experts find biofeedback an important adjunct to improve teaching and execution of pelvic muscle exercises to control urge UI. Successful bladder retraining usually takes several weeks; patients need reassurance to proceed despite any initial failure. (See the Appendix, p 403, for an example of patient instructions for bladder retraining and bladder urge control.)

Table 20.4—Evaluating Incontinence

Components	Comments
History	
Provider initiation	50% of affected persons do not report UI; many assume UI is normal with age
Specific symptoms	Diagnostic value varies with symptom definition, age and gender, underlying pathology
	Precipitant urgency suggests DO; precipitants include running water, handwashing, cold temperatures, sight of garage or front door
	UI with coughing, laughing, bending, etc., is sensitive for stress UI; delay between maneuver and UI or urge before leakage suggests stress-induced urge UI; leakage with minimal maneuvers or continual urine dripping suggests ISD
	Frequency, nocturia, slow urine stream, hesitancy, interrupted voiding, straining, and terminal dribbling are common with DO, DHIC, BOO, detrusor underactivity, many medical conditions, volume overload
	Voiding symptom scores (eg, AUA BPH symptom score; see the Appendix, p 389) useful as severity measure but lack specificity, are not diagnostic
UI characteristics	Onset, frequency, volume, timing, and precipitants (eg, medications, caffeine, alcohol, physical activity, cough)
Associated factors	Bowel and sexual function; medical conditions and medications with temporal relation to UI (see Table 20.3)
Quality of life	Inquire how patient and caregiver are affected, ie, activities of daily living, social, emotional, interpersonal (eg, sexual) relations, self-concept, and general health perception; most bothersome aspect
Physical examination	
General	Orthostatic vital signs, alertness, cognition, functional status
Cardiovascular	Volume overload, peripheral edema, congestive heart failure
Abdominal, rectal	Bladder by palpation (insensitive); rectal masses and impaction; rectal tone
Back	Dimpling or hair tuft at spine base suggests incomplete spina bifida
Musculoskeletal	Mobility and manual dexterity
Neurologic	Cervical disease suggested by limited lateral rotation and lateral flexion, interossei wasting, and Hoffman's or Babinski's sign
	Sacral root integrity: perineal sensation; anal sphincter tone (rest and volitional); anal "wink" and bulbocavernosus reflex
Genitourinary	Men: prostate exam (see "Prostate Disease," p 366); if uncircumcised, check for phimosis, paraphimosis, and balanitis
	Women: vaginal mucosa for atrophy and pelvic support (see "Gynecologic Diseases and Disorders," p 334)
Testing	

Components	Comments
Voiding record	48-hour record establishes baseline severity; timing and circumstances of UI and continent voids; voided volume; voiding frequency; total day and nocturnal urine output*; UI-associated activities (eg, coffee drinking, exercise). In institutions, staff record patient continence status (dry, damp, soaked) every 2 hours. If nocturnal diuresis, seek causes (eg, pedal edema, CHF, or alcohol "nightcap"); UI occurrence at a typical time of day suggests association with medication, beverages, or activity
Clinical stress test	Best if bladder full, patient relaxes perineum, and single vigorous cough used; specific for stress UI if leakage instantaneous with cough; insensitive if patient cannot cooperate, is inhibited, or if bladder volume low; several-second delay before UI suggests stress-induced DO
Urine flow rate	Peak flow $\geq$ 12 mL/sec for voided volume $\geq$ 200 mL excludes BOO; low flow rate not specific
Postvoid residual	Done by catheterization or ultrasound; repeated measures possibly needed; PVR > 50 mL can contribute to frequency or nocturia, exacerbate urge and stress UI; PVR > 200 mL suggests detrusor weakness or BOO, and in men hydronephrosis should be excluded (rare in older women)
Laboratory tests	Renal function; glucose, calcium, vitamin B_{12} levels, urinalysis and culture; urine cytology and cystoscopy only if hematuria or pelvic pain present; PSA in men, if cancer screening appropriate or desirable

*Example: if nocturnal output (volume voided during hours of sleep, plus first morning void) = 800 mL and modal volume voided (proxy for functional bladder volume) = 200 mL, then patient must void 3 to 4 times per night (800 ÷ 200 = 4), and decreasing output will decrease voiding or UI.

NOTE: AUA = American Urological Association; BOO = bladder outlet obstruction; BPH = benign prostatic hyperplasia; CHF = congestive heart failure; DHIC = detrusor hyperactivity with impaired contractility; DO = detrusor overactivity; ISD = intrinsic sphincter deficiency; PSA = prostate-specific antigen; PVR = postvoid residual volume; UI = urinary incontinence.

SOURCE: Data from DuBeau CE. Problems in voiding and diseases of the prostate. In: Wei JY, Sheehan MN, eds. *Geriatric Medicine: A Case-Based Manual.* New York: Oxford University Press; 1997:155.

Table 20.5—Efficacy of Behavioral and Pharmacologic Treatments for Urge Incontinence

Treatment	Target Population	Efficacy	Evidence
Behavioral			
Bladder retraining	Cognitively intact	≥ 50% decrease in episodes in 75% of women	A
Prompted voiding	Dependent, cognitively impaired	Average reduction 0.8–1.8 episodes daily	A
Habit training	Voiding record available	≥ 25% decrease in episodes in one third of patients	B
Scheduling toileting	Unable to toilet independently	30%–80% decrease in episodes	C
Pelvic muscle exercises	Women only	Up to 80% decrease in episodes; motivated patients	A
Pharmacologic			
Oxybutynin	Unresponsive to behavioral treatment alone	15%–60% decrease in episodes over placebo; side effects common but decreased with extended release	A
Tolterodine	Unresponsive to behavioral treatment alone	12%–18% decrease in episodes over placebo; side effects about 20% less than with maximum dose oxybutynin, less with extended release	A

NOTE: NH = nursing home; NSAIDs = nonsteroidal anti-inflammatory drugs. Evidence strength: A = randomized, controlled studies; B = case-control studies; C = case descriptions or expert opinion.

SOURCE: Data from Fantl JA, Newman DK, Colling J, et al. *Urinary Incontinence in Adults: Acute and Chronic Management. Clinical Practice Guideline No. 2*, 1996 Update. Rockville, MD: US Department of Health and Human Services, Public Health Service, Agency for Health Care Policy and Research; March 1996. AHCPR Pub. No. 96-0682, and 2nd International Consultation on Incontinence, Paris, 2001.

Table 20.6—Efficacy of Behavioral and Pharmacologic Treatments for Stress and for Mixed Urge and Stress Incontinence

Treatment	Target Population	Efficacy	Evidence
Behavioral			
PME	Women	56%–95% decrease in episodes; efficacy dependent on program intensity	A
PME and biofeedback	Women	50%–87% improvement	A
	Men, postprostatectomy	Limited data	C
PME and vaginal cones	Women	68%–80% cured or greatly improved, no data on postmenopausal women	B
Electrical stimulation	Women, stress +/– urge UI	50%–94% cured or improved	B
Bladder retraining	Mixed UI, cognitively intact	≥ 50% decrease in episodes in 75% of patients	A
Prompted voiding	Mixed UI, dependent, cognitively impaired	Average reduction 0.8–1.8 episodes daily	A
Habit training	Mixed UI, voiding record available	≥ 25% decrease in episodes in one third of patients	B
Scheduled toileting	Mixed UI, unable to toilet independently	30%–80% decrease in episodes	C
Pharmacologic			
Estrogens	Women	30% decrease in episodes over placebo; other systemic benefits may exist	B

NOTE: PME = pelvic muscle exercises; UI = urinary incontinence. Evidence strength: A = randomized, controlled studies; B = case-control studies; C = case descriptions or expert opinion.

SOURCE: Data from Fantl JA, Newman DK, Colling J, et al. *Urinary Incontinence in Adults: Acute and Chronic Management. Clinical Practice Guideline No. 2*, 1996 Update. Rockville, MD: US Department of Health and Human Services, Public Health Service, Agency for Health Care Policy and Research; March 1996. AHCPR Pub. No. 96-0682, and 2nd International Consultation on Incontinence, Paris, 2001.

Table 20.7—Efficacy of Surgical Treatments for Stress Incontinence

Treatment	Target Population	Efficacy	Evidence
Retropubic suspension	Women	Cure 79%, cure or improvement 84%*; complications 18% (range 6%–57%)	A–B
Needle suspension	Women	Not effective	A
Anterior vaginal repair (colporrhaphy)	Women	Cure 66% (range 30%–90%), cure or improvement 74%*	A
Vaginal sling	Women with ISD, hypermobility	Cure 80%*; complications less likely with fascial than with synthetic slings	C
Marshall-Marchetti-Krantz	Women	Success rate 88%	C
Periurethral bulking injections	Women with ISD	Cure 50% (range 8%–100%), cure or improvement 67%	B
	Men with ISD	Cure 20% (range 0%–66%), cure or improvement 42% (range 0%–80%)	B
Artificial sphincter	Women with ISD	Cure 77%, cure or improvement 80%; high complication rate	B
	Men with ISD	Cure 66% (range 33%–88%), cure or improvement 85% (range 75%–95%); high complication rate	B

* Subjective cure may be less because of persistent or de novo urge incontinence or voiding difficulty.

NOTE: ISD = intrinsic sphincter deficiency.

SOURCE: Data from Fantl JA, Newman DK, Colling J, et al. *Urinary Incontinence in Adults: Acute and Chronic Management. Clinical Practice Guideline No. 2,* 1996 Update. Rockville, MD: US Department of Health and Human Services, Public Health Service, Agency for Health Care Policy and Research; March 1996. AHCPR Pub. No. 96-0682, and 2nd International Consultation on Incontinence, Paris, 2001.

For cognitively impaired patients, behavioral methods include habit training (timed voiding, with the interval based on a person's usual voiding schedule), scheduled voiding (timed voiding usually every 2 to 3 hours), and prompted voiding. Prompted voiding has three components: regular monitoring with encouragement to report continence status, prompting to toilet on a scheduled basis, and praise and positive feedback when the person is continent and attempts to toilet. Persons most likely to respond to prompted voiding are those with who void fewer than four times every 12 hours during the day and those who toilet correctly over 75% of the time in an initial trial. These methods require training, motivation, and continued effort by patients and caregivers; special attention and staff reinforcement is needed in institutionalized settings to ensure continued treatment success.

When behavioral methods alone are unsuccessful, bladder-suppressant medications can be added. Although medications usually do not abate DO, they can improve UI and frequency. Drug choice is based on efficacy, side effects, and comorbid conditions (eg, avoiding anticholinergic effects for a person with constipation). Lack of response to one agent does not preclude response to another, and low-dose combinations may work when side effects occur with higher doses of single agents. Oxybutynin has both antimuscarinic and musculotropic action; the initial dosage is 2.5 mg two to three times daily (5 mg once daily for extended release), followed by titration as needed up to 20 mg per day. Quick onset of action makes regular release useful when protection is needed at specific times. Extended-release oxybutynin (5 to 20 mg once daily) allows once-daily dosing and fewer side effects. Anticholinergic side effects can be limiting; constipation and compensatory fluid intake for xerostomia may exacerbate UI, and xerostomia predisposes a person to caries. The PVR should be monitored if UI worsens, as it may indicate retention that requires lowering the dose. Tolterodine (2 mg twice daily) has similar efficacy and possibly decreased xerostomia, especially with extended release (4 mg daily). One case report suggests that it may increase the international normalized ratio in persons on warfarin. The dose of tolterodine should not exceed 2 mg daily if the patient is taking medications that inhibit cytochrome P-450 3A4 (eg, erythromycin, ketoconazole).

Other agents including propantheline, dicyclomine, imipramine, hyoscyamine, calcium channel blockers, and nonsteroidal anti-inflammatory agents have scant efficacy data. Flavoxate is ineffective. Vasopressin was found to decrease nocturnal voids in a small randomized trial in healthy older persons, yet its expense and risks of congestive failure and hyponatremia argue against routine use.

In patients with DHIC on bladder-suppressant medications, careful monitoring for urinary retention is crucial. Double voiding (waiting and trying to void again before leaving the toilet), Valsalva's maneuver, or Credé's maneuver (pressure applied to the bladder) may improve bladder emptying. Constipation should be treated. If acceptable to the patient, retention may be induced with medication and the bladder emptied by intermittent clean catheterization several times daily.

Sacral nerve neuromodulation by an implanted S3 electrode may decrease severe refractory DO, but reimplantation is required in one third of patients. Augmentation cystoplasty surgery has high morbidity and is reserved for patients with profound DO (usually younger persons with poorly compliant bladders from neurologic disease).

Stress Incontinence

Pelvic muscle exercises (PME) strengthen the muscular components of urethral supports and are the cornerstone of noninvasive treatment for stress UI. PME, like strength training, employs a small number of isometric repetitions at maximal exertion. Unfortunately, there is much professional and lay misinformation about PME; persons who report failing PME trials may have used inadequate methods. PME requires motivated patients and careful instruction and monitoring by health professionals; poor adherence may occur even with close monitoring. PME instruction should focus on isolation of pelvic muscles; avoidance of buttock, abdomen, or thigh muscle contraction; moderate repetitions of the strongest contraction possible (3 sets of 8 to 10 contractions held for 6 to 8 seconds 3 to 4 times a week); and contraction for progressively longer times (up to 10 seconds, if possible). (See the Appendix, p 419, for an example of PME instructions for patients.) Biofeedback may help patients perform correct muscle contraction and monitor progress. The efficacy of other adjuncts—such as electrical or magnetic stimulation of pelvic muscle contractions, and progressively weighted cones retained in the vagina during ambulation—is less clear. Pessaries may benefit women with stress UI exacerbated by bladder or uterine prolapse. (See "Gynecologic Diseases and Disorders," p 334.)

Systemic or topical estrogen may reduce stress and urge UI in some patients with atrophic vaginitis and urethritis. Several epidemiologic and intervention studies, however, have not found estrogen to be beneficial for stress UI. Topical agents (estrogen creams, vaginal tablets, or slow-release rings) may be preferable. α-Adrenergic agonists stimulate urethral smooth muscle contraction; however, no pure α-agonists are currently available. Estrogen increases α-receptor responsiveness and may potentiate α-adrenergic agonists. Imipramine's α-agonist and anticholinergic actions have been used in women with mixed stress and urge UI, but if the PVR increases, stress leakage may worsen, and efficacy data is scant.

Surgical correction offers the highest cure rates for stress UI at a cost of some increased morbidity. The surgical approach depends on the underlying defect and coexistent prolapse. For urethral hypermobility (genuine stress UI), bladder neck suspension procedures that repair urethra support defects are preferred (eg, transvaginal colposuspension). Complications include urinary retention and vaginal wall prolapse. The Marshall-Marchetti-Krantz abdominal procedure has greater morbidity. Anterior colporrhaphy and needle suspensions are less effective and not recommended. For intrinsic sphincter deficiency, sling procedures using autologous or synthetic material to support the urethra, and periurethral bulking injections with collagen or autologous fat are preferred. Increasingly, slings also are used for genuine stress UI (urethral hypermobility).

Treatment for men with postprostatectomy stress UI often is difficult. For milder cases PME and bulking injections can be helpful, whereas severe cases often require management with protective garments or catheters. Artificial sphincter replacement can be effective but has high reoperation rates (up to 40%), even with experienced surgeons.

Overflow Incontinence

Treatment of overflow incontinence depends on its cause. For outflow obstruction from benign prostatic hyperplasia, a range of medical and surgical alternatives are available (see "Prostate Disease," p 366). Outlet obstruction should be considered in women with previous vaginal or urethral surgery; treatment by unilateral suture removal or urethrolysis (remobilization of adhesions) can restore continence.

For detrusor underactivity, treatment is supportive. Drugs that impair detrusor contractility and increase urethral tone should be decreased or stopped, and constipation treated. Bethanechol chloride is ineffective except possibly for patients with overflow UI who must remain on anticholinergic agents (eg, antidepressant or antipsychotic medications). Intermittent clean catheterization can provide effective management; sterile intermittent catheterization is preferred for frailer patients and those in institutionalized settings. Bladder emptying may improve with Credé's or Valsalva's maneuvers during voiding, double voiding, or simply unhurried voiding.

Catheters and Catheter Care

Indwelling catheters cause significant morbidity, including polymicrobial bacteriuria (universal by 30 days), febrile episodes (1 per 100 patient days), nephrolithiasis, bladder stones, epididymitis, and chronic renal inflammation and pyelonephritis. External collection devices also cause bacteriuria, infection, penile cellulitis and necrosis, and urinary retention and hydronephrosis if the condom twists or its external band is too tight.

Indwelling catheters should be reserved for short-term decompression of acute retention: when retention cannot be managed surgically or medically, when wounds need to be kept clean of urine, when a terminally ill or severely impaired patient cannot tolerate garment changes, or when there is persistent patient preference for catheter management despite risks. The passage of the 1990 Omnibus Budget Reconciliation Act has resulted in more appropriate and decreased catheter use in long-term care but with an increased prevalence of UI.

Several general principles guide safe and effective catheter care. Bacteriuria and infection are reduced by closed drainage systems. Topical meatal antimicrobials, catheters with antimicrobial coating, collection bag disinfectants, and antimicrobial irrigation are not effective. Although antibiotics decrease bacteriuria and infection, routine use induces resistant organisms and secondary infections such as *Clostridium difficile* colitis. Bacteriuria is universal in catheterized patients and should not be treated unless there are clear symptoms. Routine cultures should not be done because of the changing flora and failure to predict infection. In symptomatic patients, cultures should be done after the old catheter is removed and a new catheter is placed. Institutionalized patients with catheters should be kept in separate rooms to decrease cross-infection.

With acute urinary retention, decompression should continue at least 7 days, followed by a voiding trial after catheter removal (never clamping). Prophylactic antibiotics are recommended only with short-term catheterization in high-risk patients (eg, those with prosthetic heart valves). For men with chronic obstruction, intraurethral stents may be preferred to indwelling catheters.

Risk factors for catheter blockage include alkaline urine, female gender, poor mobility, calciuria, proteinuria, copious mucin, *Proteus* colonization, and preexistent bladder stones. Changing the catheter every 7 to 10 days may decrease blockage in such patients. In the absence of risk factors for blockage, catheters need not be changed routinely as long as monitoring is adequate. If patients cannot be monitored, changing catheters every 30 days is reasonable. Persistent leakage around the catheter can be caused by irritation by a large Foley balloon, catheter diameter that is too large, bacteriuria, constipation or impaction, improper catheter positioning, or catheter materials.

Clean intermittent catheterization is an alternative for willing patients with sufficient dexterity. Strict sterility is not necessary, although good handwashing and regular decontamination of the catheters is needed. Bacteriuria can be minimized by a frequency of catheterization that keeps bladder volume < 400 mL. Stiffer catheters are easier to insert.

Resources, including Web site addresses, of use to clinicians treating patients with UI are listed in the Appendix (p 427).

REFERENCES

■ *Am J Med Sci.* 1997;314(4):214–272.

■ Berghmans LC, Hendriks HJ, Bo K, et al. Conservative treatment of stress urinary incontinence in women: a systematic review of randomized controlled trials. *Br J Urol.* 1998;82(2):181–191.

■ Burgio KL, Locher JL, Goode PS, et al. Behavioral vs drug treatment for urge urinary incontinence in older women: a randomized controlled trial. *JAMA.* 1998;280(23):1995–2000.

■ Burgio KL, Locher JL, Goode PS. Combined behavioral and drug therapy for urge incontinence in older women. *J Am Geriatr Soc.* 2000;48(4):370–374.

■ Hay-Smith EJ, Bo Berghmans LC, Hendriks HJ, et al. Pelvic floor muscle training for urinary incontinence. *Cochrane Database Syst Rev.* 2001;(2):CD001407.

■ Roe B, Williams K, Palmer M. Bladder training for urinary incontinence in adults. *Cochrane Database Syst Rev.* 2000;(2):CD001308.

■ Schulz JA, Drutz HP. The surgical management of recurrent stress urinary incontinence. *Curr Opin Obstet Gynecol.* 1999;11(5):489–494.

■ Scientific Committee of the First International Consultation on Incontinence. Assessment and treatment of urinary incontinence. *Lancet.* 2000;355(9221):2153–2158.

CHAPTER 21—FALLS

PREVALENCE AND MORBIDITY

Falls are one of the most common geriatric syndromes threatening the independence of older persons. A fall is considered to have occurred when a person comes to rest inadvertently on the ground or a lower level. Most discussions in the literature of falls by older persons do not include falls associated with loss of consciousness (eg, syncope, seizure) or associated with overwhelming trauma. The majority of falls are not associated with syncope.

The incidence of falls increases with age and varies according to living status. Between 30% and 40% of community-dwelling persons aged 65 years and older fall each year. Among those with a history of a fall in the previous year, the annual incidence of falls is close to 60%. In the long-term-care setting, about half of all persons fall each year.

Complications resulting from falls are the leading cause of death from injury in men and women aged 65 and older. The death rate attributable to falls increases with age, with white men aged 85 years and older having the highest death rate (> 180 deaths per 100,000 population). Most falls result in an injury of some type, usually minor soft-tissue injuries, such as bruises and scrapes; however, 10% to 15% result in fracture or other serious injury. In general, falls are associated with subsequent declines in functional status, greater likelihood of nursing-home placement, increased use of medical services, and the development of a fear of falling. Of those older persons who fall, only half are able to get up without help, thus experiencing the "long lie." Long lies are associated with lasting declines in functional status.

The true cost of falls in health care dollars is difficult to ascertain. It has been estimated that in the United States the lifetime costs of fall-related injuries for persons aged 65 and older is $12.6 billion. Since many falls result in injury, there is a significant use of emergency department facilities among fallers. Studies from the early 1990s indicate that almost 8% of persons aged 70 and older go to emergency departments each year because of a fall-related injury, and close to a third of these people are admitted to the hospital for a median length of stay of 8 days. A population-based study conducted in Washington State identified 149,504 hospital stays for patients aged 65 years of age and older discharged from the state's hospitals in 1989. Of these, 7873 (5.3%) of the stays were for injuries from falls. Of the $995,499,233 in hospital charges in 1989 for persons in Washington aged 65 and older, $53,346,191 (5% to 6%) were attributable to hospitalizations of patients with fall-related trauma.

CAUSES

Falls, incontinence, delirium, and other geriatric syndromes result from the accumulated effect of impairments in multiple domains. The falls of older people are rarely due to a single cause. Rather, there is often a complex interaction among factors intrinsic to the individual (age-related declines, chronic disease, acute illness, medications), challenges to postural control (environment, changing positions, normal activities), and mediating factors (risk-taking behaviors, underlying mobility level).

At least five community-based prospective cohort studies of risk factors for falls have been published over the past decade. The risk factors for falls identified in three of the five studies reviewed were age and cognitive impairment; those identified in two studies were female gender, past history of a fall, lower-extremity weakness, balance problems, psychotropic drug use, and arthritis. These studies differed significantly in the types of risk factors evaluated, the types of population studied (eg, past fall history was sometimes an entry criterion), and the outcome (one fall, two or more falls, injurious falls). The fact that as many as 25 different risk factors were found across five studies highlights the multifactorial nature of falls and suggests the existence of other circumstances surrounding falls that are not accounted for in studies of this type. In general, the risk of falling increases with the number of risk factors, although some persons with no risk factors experience falls.

Successful falls prevention begins with a knowledge of the age-related changes that increase the risk of falls. The ability to maintain upright posture depends on sensory input from the visual, proprioceptive, and vestibular systems. With aging, there are declines in all three systems. For example, the visual system demonstrates reductions in visual acuity, depth perception, contrast sensitivity, and dark adaptation. The proprioceptive system loses sensitivity in the lower extremities. The vestibular system demonstrates a loss of labyrinthine hair cells, vestibular ganglion cells, and nerve fibers.

Despite these age-related changes in sensory systems, it has been difficult to quantify the age-related changes in postural control that are independent of disease. In general, when postural stability is tested in young and old persons with no apparent musculoskeletal or neurologic impairment, age-related differences in measured sway are found to be most pronounced when moderately severe perturbations of stance are administered, such as changing the support surface, changing body position, altering the visual input, or moving the support surface horizontally or rotationally. This occurs because these perturbations stress the redundancy of the sensory systems in their ability to maintain postural stability. In addition, there may be other age-related changes in the central nervous system that affect postural control, including loss of neurons and dendrites, and depletion of neurotransmitters, such as dopamine, within the basal ganglia.

Since it is difficult to find older persons without at least subtle neurologic findings, studies have been unable to determine whether some of the young-old differences may be due to these factors. Some of the most striking postural control differences between young and old persons relate to the order or grouping of muscle activation patterns. Thus, in response to perturbations of the support surface, older persons tend to activate the proximal muscles, such as the quadriceps, before the more distal muscles, such as the tibialis anterior. This strategy may not be an efficient way to maintain postural stability. Similarly, in the older person there may be greater co-contraction of antagonistic muscles, and the onset of the muscle activation and associated joint torque may be delayed. Finally, the ability to recover balance upon a postural disturbance may be compromised by an age-related decline in the ability to rapidly develop joint torque by using muscles of the lower extremity. All of these strategies potentially undermine upright posture.

Another important physiologic contributor to the successful maintenance of upright posture is the regulation of systemic blood pressure. The failure to perfuse the brain, which accompanies hypotension, increases the risk of a fall, usually in association with syncope. In addition to the age-related declines in baroreflex sensitivity to hypotensive stimuli manifested as a failure to cardio-accelerate, everyday stresses such as changing posture, eating a meal, or suffering an acute illness may result in hypotension. Since many older adults have a resting cerebral perfusion that is compromised by vascular disease, even slight reductions in blood pressure may produce cerebral ischemic symptoms, such as falls. Finally, with aging, there is a reduction in total body water, which places older persons at increased risk of dehydration with acute illness, diuretic use, or hot weather. Since there is a progressive decrease in basal and stimulated renin levels, as well as a decrease in aldosterone production with aging, dehydrating stresses may lead to orthostatic hypotension and a fall.

A number of age-related chronic conditions deserve special mention because of their association with fall risk. Parkinson's disease, in particular, increases the risk of falls through several mechanisms, including the rigidity of lower-extremity musculature, the inability to correct sway trajectory because of the slowness in initiating movement, hypotensive drug effects, and, in some cases, cognitive impairment. Another common disease contributing to falls is osteoarthritis. When present in the knee, osteoarthritis may affect mobility, the ability to step over objects and maneuver, and the tendency to avoid complete weight bearing on a painful joint.

One of the most easily modified risk factors for falls that has been repeatedly demonstrated in observational studies is medication use. Individual classes of medications, such as the benzodiazepines, antidepressants, and antipsychotic drugs, have been associated with an increased risk of hip fracture. An increased risk of falling has also been found to be associated with recent changes in the dose of a medication and the total number of prescriptions.

The relative importance of environmental factors to the risk of falling has not been well-quantified because they so frequently interact with risk factors intrinsic to the individual. Well-designed intervention studies have focused on improving the risk-factor profile of the person or have combined individual interventions with environmental manipulation, making it difficult to isolate the contributions of the environmental factors. Nevertheless, attention to safety hazards in the home environment would appear to be worthwhile, and one intervention study targeting environmental factors was successful in reducing falls.

DIAGNOSTIC APPROACH

History and Physical Examination

Many falls never come to clinical attention for a variety of reasons: The patient may never mention the event, there is no injury at the time of the fall, the clinician may fail to ask the patient about a history of falls, or the patient or the clinician may make the invalid assumption that falls are an inevitable part of the aging process. Treatment of injuries resulting from falls commonly fails to include an investigation of the cause of the fall.

In the clinical evaluation of the geriatric patient who is not specifically being seen for a problem with falling, it is still important that an assessment of fall risk be integrated into the history and physical examination. (See Figure 21.1 for an overview of falls assessment and management in all older persons.) The most important point in the history is the previous history of a fall, since this is a strong risk factor for future falls. For patients presenting with a fall, important components of the history include the activity of the faller at the time of the incident, the occurrence of

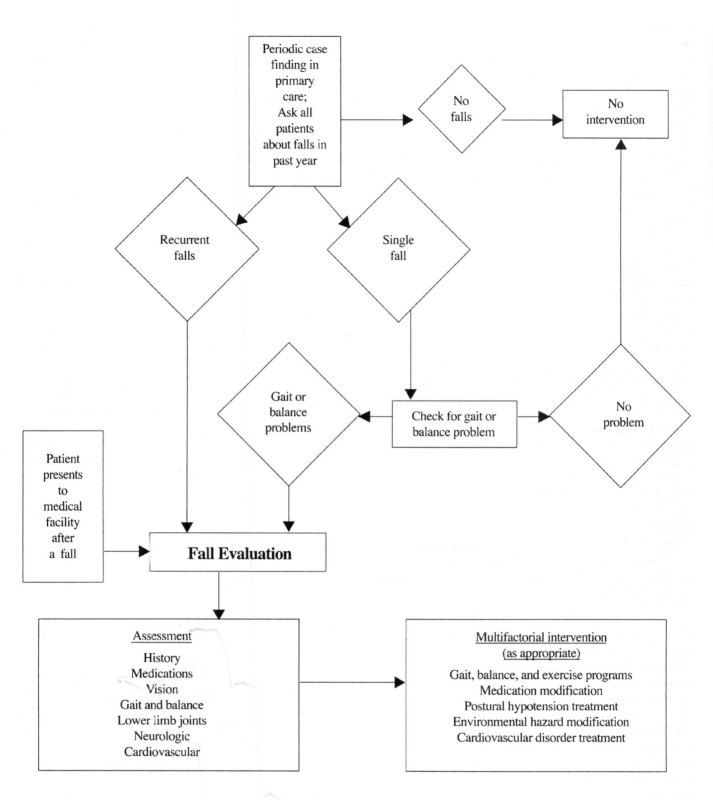

Figure 21.1—Algorithm summarizing the assessment and management of falls.

SOURCE: American Geriatrics Society, British Geriatrics Society, and American Academy of Orthopaedic Surgeons Panel on Falls Prevention. Guideline for the prevention of falls in older persons. *J Am Geriatr Soc.* 2001;49(5):666. Reprinted by permission of Blackwell Science, Inc.

prodromal symptoms (lightheadedness, imbalance, dizziness), the location of the fall, and the time of the fall. Loss of consciousness is associated with injurious falls and should raise important considerations, such as orthostatic hypotension or cardiac or neurologic disease. (See "Syncope," p 159.) Information on previous falls should be collected to identify patterns that may help target strategies to reduce risk factors. A complete medication history should focus specifically on vasodilators, diuretics, and sedative hypnotic drug use because these agents have been associated with increased risk of falls. In addition to inquiring about the circumstances surrounding the fall, the clinician taking the history should attempt to identify environmental factors that may have contributed. Thus, information on lighting, floor covering, door thresholds, railings, and furniture may add important clues.

The physical examination of the person who has fallen should focus on risk factors. Much of the examination duplicates that of a gait assessment (see "Gait Disturbances," p 148.) Footwear may also be an important factor to consider. In one small study to test the effect of various shoe types on balance in older men, shoes with thin, hard soles were found to produce the best results, even though they were perceived as less comfortable than thick, soft, mid-soled shoes, such as running shoes.

Probably the most important part of the physical examination is an assessment of integrated musculoskeletal function, which can be accomplished by performing one or more tests of postural stability. (See "Gait Disturbances," p 148.)

A simple maneuver called the "functional reach" test is a practical way to test the integrated neuromuscular base of support and has predictive validity for falls by older men. This test is performed with a leveled yardstick secured to a wall at the height of the acromion. The person being tested assumes a comfortable stance without shoes or socks and stands so that his or her shoulders are perpendicular to the yardstick. He or she makes a fist and extends the arm forward as far as possible along the wall without taking a step or losing balance. The total reach is measured along the yardstick and recorded. Inability to reach 6 inches or more is cause for concern and merits further evaluation. In its initial description, the functional reach correlated with other physical performance measures, such as walking speed ($r = 0.71$), tandem walk using an ordinal scale ($r = 0.67$), and standing on one foot measured as number of seconds that a one-footed stance could be maintained ($r = 0.64$).

Laboratory and Diagnostic Tests

There is no standard diagnostic evaluation of a person with a history of falls or with a high risk of falls.

Obviously, laboratory tests for hemoglobin, serum urea nitrogen, creatinine, or glucose levels can help to exclude such causes of falling as anemia, dehydration, or hyperglycemia with hyperosmolar dehydration. There is no proven value of routinely performing Holter monitoring of persons who have fallen. Because data demonstrate that carotid sinus hypersensitivity contributes to falls and even hip fracture, some have advocated performing carotid sinus massage with continuous heart rate and phasic blood-pressure measurement in persons with unexplained falls. Similarly, the decision to perform echocardiography, brain imaging, or radiographic studies of the spine should be driven by the findings of the history and physical examination. Echocardiography should be reserved for those with heart murmurs believed to contribute to the maintenance of blood flow to the brain. Spine radiographs or magnetic resonance imaging may be useful in patients with gait disorders, abnormalities on neurologic examination, lower-extremity spasticity, or hyperreflexia to exclude cervical spondylosis or lumbar stenosis as a cause of falls.

TREATMENT AND PREVENTION

Multiple studies of preventive interventions have been conducted over the past decade, including programs to improve strength or balance, educational programs, optimization of medications, and environmental modifications in homes or institutions. Some interventions have targeted single risk factors; others have attempted to address multiple factors.

A Cochrane Collaboration systematic review of interventions to reduce the incidence of falling in older adults was performed. This review considered only studies that included older persons randomized to an intervention versus control, or into one of two interventions. As of May 1997, 18 individual study reports meeting the inclusion criteria and one planned meta-analysis were identified. The meta-analysis came from the group of studies called the FICSIT trials (Frailty and Injuries: Cooperative Studies of Intervention Techniques) and was not included in the review. Three of the studies that were part of the FICSIT group, however, were individually included. Of the 18 studies, 14 reported the effect of interventions in persons living in the community, two were set in long-term-care institutions, and two were hospital-based, either in a rehabilitation hospital or an acute geriatric assessment and treatment unit. Five of the studies compared a physical exercise intervention with an attention control visit, education only, or no intervention. One also included a cognitive intervention, and another compared a more intense exercise program with a lower-intensity program. In nine of the studies the intervention was targeted to risk factors identified on an initial assessment, including intrinsic risk factors and environmental factors. The other studies employed a variety of interventions, including physician referrals with or without a formal recommendation; health visitor assessments of nutrition, medical conditions, environmental hazards, and physical fitness; multifactorial interventions based on geriatric assessment; targeted risk factor intervention; counseling; and even hormone replacement therapy. The hospital-based studies evaluated the effectiveness of a bed alarm system and the use of blue identification bracelets for the prevention of falls by high-risk older inpatients.

The results of this systematic review revealed that neither an untargeted exercise intervention alone, nor an untargeted exercise and health education or health education alone significantly reduced the risk of falls when compared with usual care. Behavioral interventions targeting risk factors might reduce the risk of falls. The most favorable results were observed in studies in which health screening was followed by targeted interventions. Pooling of the data from five studies suggested that a targeted intervention in which older people are assessed by a clinician trained to identify intrinsic and environmental risk factors is likely to reduce the fall rate (odds ratio = 0.79; 95% confidence interval 0.65–0.96). The costs of implementing such a program with a multidimensional health assessment followed by targeted interventions have been explored in one of the five studies to investigate such an approach. The results of that study indicate that targeted intervention is apparently cost-effective.

Since the release of this systematic review of interventions, several additional randomized, controlled trials have been published. In one of the FICSIT studies, the effect in older adults of strength and endurance training on gait, balance, physical health status, fall risk, and health services use was examined. This single-blinded, randomized, controlled trial enrolled 105 older persons with at least mild deficits in strength and balance. There were three exercise groups (strength training using weight machines, endurance training using bicycles, and strength and endurance training) and a control group. After 6 months of the intervention, with all exercise groups combined versus the control group, a significant beneficial effect of exercise on time to the first fall (relative hazard = 0.53, 95% confidence interval 0.30–0.91) was found, despite the fact that there was virtually no effect on intermediate outcomes such as gait and balance. The fall rate among those in the control group (0.81 falls per year) was significantly higher than the rate among those in the exercise groups (0.49 falls per year) (relative risk = 0.61, 95% confidence interval 0.39–0.93). In contrast to the Cochrane review, which did not find exercise to be effective in reducing falls, these findings support the overall FICSIT meta-analysis results that found positive effects of strength and endurance training on fall risk. Of course, it is possible that only some endurance and strength training protocols are effective and possibly effective only in certain subgroups. All these studies highlight the need for clarification of the effect of exercise on groups of older persons with differing functional status.

The efficacy of an interdisciplinary approach to falls prevention was confirmed by a study of patients aged 65 and older who presented to an emergency department with a fall. Patients randomly assigned to an intervention group, who had a detailed medical and occupational therapy assessment with referral to relevant services, if needed, had fewer falls (183) than the control group assigned to usual care (510). The odds ratio of falling for the intervention group was 0.39. In another randomized study of 530 persons aged 65 and over who were recruited prior to discharge from hospitals, a home visit by an experienced occupational therapist to address specific home modifications was found to result in a 19% reduction in the risk of falling in the next 12 months over that of a control group not receiving the home visit. The intervention reduced falls by 36% among participants who had a history of a fall in the year prior to enrollment. The success of this intervention may have been due to a combination of home modification and changes in behavior, but it suggests that simple, cost-effective interventions are available to prevent falls among vulnerable older persons.

CLINICAL GUIDELINES

For older patients who have sustained a fall, a multifactorial approach that is based on data about risk factors and a multidimensional assessment of the patient and that targets interventions on the basis of these findings is appropriate. For older persons who have no history of falling, it is reasonable to use traditional multidimensional geriatric assessment with targeted interventions as risk factors are identified. For a summary of the recommendations of the expert panel on falls prevention assembled by the American Geriatrics Society, the British Geriatrics Society, and the American Academy of Orthopaedic Surgeons, see the Appendix (p 391).

REFERENCES

■ American Geriatrics Society, British Geriatrics Society, and American Academy of Orthopaedic Surgeons Panel on Falls Prevention. Guidelines for the prevention of falls in older persons. *J Am Geriatr Soc.* 2001;49(5):664–672.

- Close J, Ellis M, Hooper R, et al. Prevention of falls in the elderly trial (PROFET): a randomised controlled trial. *Lancet*. 1999:353(9147):93–97.

- Cumming RG, Thomas M, Szonyi G, et al. Home visits by an occupational therapist for assessment and modification of environmental hazards: a randomized trial of falls prevention. *J Am Geriatr Soc*. 1999;47(12):1397–1402.

- Gillespie LD, Gillespie WJ, Cumming R, et al. Interventions for preventing falls in the elderly. *Cochrane Database Syst Rev*. 2000;2:CD000340.

- Robertson MC, Devlin N, Gardner MM, et al. Effectiveness of economic evaluation of a nurse delivered home exercise programme to prevent falls. 1: randomised controlled trial. *BMJ*. 2001;322(7288):697.

- Robertson MC, Gardner MM, Devlin N, et al. Effectiveness of economic evaluation of a nurse delivered home exercise programme to prevent falls. 2: controlled trial in multiple centres. *BMJ*. 2001;322(7288):701.

- Rubenstein L. Approaching falls in older persons. *Annals of Long-Term Care*. 2000;8(8):61–64.

CHAPTER 22—GAIT DISTURBANCES

Limitations in walking increase with age. From 8% to 19% of noninstitutionalized older adults admit to walking difficulty or require the assistance of another person or special equipment to walk. In some samples of noninstitutionalized older adults aged 85 and over, the incidence is as high as 40%, and among older adult nursing-home residents, it reaches 60% or higher. Although age-related gait changes (eg, slower speed) are most apparent past age 75 or 80, most gait disorders appear in connection with underlying diseases, particularly as disease severity increases. Attributing a gait disorder to one disease in older adults is particularly difficult because so many diseases cause similar gait abnormalities.

GAIT ASSESSMENT

Technological assessments of gait disorders of older adults involving kinematic and kinetic analyses have not been applied clinically. Clinical gait assessments use a battery of items either timed or scored semi-quantitatively; most evaluate whether a person is able to perform the task and, if able, how normal or abnormal the performance was. Batteries that focus primarily on gait include:

- the Dynamic Gait Index, which rates the patient's performance of a series of tasks, including turning, walking while turning the head, clearing obstacles, and using stairs;

- the Emory Functional Ambulation Profile, a battery of timed tasks, including walking on a hard floor, walking on a carpeted surface, stepping over an obstacle, and walking up and down four stairs;

- the Functional Ambulation Classification scale, rating the patient's use of assistive devices, the degree of human assistance (either manual or verbal) needed, the distance the patient can walk, and the types of surfaces the patient can negotiate;

- the Functional Obstacle Course, a timed test of the patient's negotiation of different floor textures, graded surfaces, stairs, and simultaneous functional activities while walking (such as opening and closing doors);

- the Timed Get Up and Go test, which times the patient's rising from a hard-backed chair, walking 10 feet (3 meters), turning, returning to the chair, and sitting down (see "Assessment," p 47, for discussion of scoring);

- the Modified Gait Abnormality Rating scale, modified to score the patient's gait variability, guardedness, staggering, foot contact, hip range of motion, shoulder extension, and arm-heel synchrony; and

- the Performance Oriented Balance and Mobility Assessment (POMA; see the Appendix, p 407) gait subsection, which rates the patient's gait initiation, turning, step length and height, step symmetry and continuity, path deviation, and trunk sway.

These scales have been used reliably in smaller, selected published samples, although perhaps less reliably in larger epidemiologic studies. (See references, p 152, for complete source information.) Two of the screening instruments have been validated for use with elderly patients. The Timed Get Up and Go test evaluates general functional mobility; most adults can complete the task in 10 seconds, and most frail older persons, in 11 to 20 seconds. Those requiring more than 20 seconds should be referred for comprehensive evaluation. A strong association exists between performance on this test and a person's functional independence in activities of daily living (ADLs).

Comfortable gait speed has become a powerful assessment and outcome measure. Gait speed measured as part of a timed walk for a short distance (eg, 8 feet) or as distance walked over time (eg, 6 minutes) predicts disease activity (eg, in arthritis), cardiac and pulmonary function (particularly in congestive heart failure), and ultimately mobility disability and ADL disability, institutionalization, and mortality.

CONDITIONS CONTRIBUTING TO GAIT DISORDERS

Patients in primary care settings consider pain, stiffness, dizziness, numbness, weakness, and sensations of abnormal movement to be the most common contributors to their walking difficulties. The most common conditions found in a primary care setting that are thought to contribute to gait disorders are degenerative joint disease, acquired musculoskeletal deformities, intermittent claudication, impairments following orthopedic surgery and stroke, and postural hypotension. Usually, more than one contributing condition is found. Dementia and fear of falling also contribute to gait disorders. The conditions found in a neurologic referral population include frontal gait disorders (usually related to normal-pressure hydrocephalus and cerebrovascular processes), sensory disorders (also involving vestibular and visual function), myelopathy, previously undiagnosed Parkinson's disease or parkinsonian syndromes, and cerebellar disease. Known conditions causing severe impairment, such as hemiplegia, Parkinson's disease, and severe hip or knee disease, are commonly not referred to a neurologist. Thus, many gait disorders, particularly those that are classical and discrete (eg, those related to stroke and osteoarthritis) and those that are mild or may relate to irreversible disease (eg, multi-infarct dementia), are presumably diagnosed in a primary care setting and treated without a referral to a neurologist. Other less common contributors to gait disorders include metabolic disorders (related to renal or hepatic disease), central nervous system tumors or subdural hematoma, depression, and psychotropic medications. Case reports also document reversible gait disorders that are due to clinically overt hypo- or hyperthyroidism and vitamin B_{12} and folate deficiency.

Though older adults may maintain a relatively normal gait pattern well into their 80s, some slowing occurs, and decreased stride length thus becomes a common feature described in older adult gait disorders. Some authors have proposed the emergence of an age-related gait disorder without accompanying clinical abnormalities, that is, essential "senile" gait disorder.

This gait pattern is described as broad-based with small steps, diminished arm swing, stooped posture, flexion of the hips and knees, uncertainty and stiffness in turning, occasional difficulty initiating steps, and a tendency to fall. These and other nonspecific findings (eg, the inability to perform tandem gait) are similar to gait patterns found in a number of other diseases, and yet the clinical abnormalities are insufficient to make a specific diagnosis. This "disorder" may be a precursor to an undiagnosed disease (eg, one related to subtle extrapyramidal signs) and is likely to be a manifestation of concurrent, progressive cognitive impairment (eg, Alzheimer's disease or vascular dementia). "Senile" gait disorder thus potentially reflects a number of potential diseases and is generally not useful in labeling gait disorders in older adults.

CLASSIFICATION OF GAIT DISORDERS

In one approach to classification, gait disorders are divided into predominantly low, middle, and high sensorimotor levels (Table 22.1). These levels may overlap when certain disorders involve multiple levels. For example, Parkinson's disease involves high (cortical) and middle (subcortical) structures; drug-metabolic causes (eg, phenothiazine) can cause high- (sedation) and middle- (extrapyramidal) level effects.

Diseases that are considered part of the low sensorimotor level can be divided into peripheral sensory and peripheral motor dysfunction, including musculoskeletal (arthritic) and myopathic or neuropathic disorders that cause weakness. These disorders are generally distal to the central nervous system. With peripheral sensory impairment, unsteady and tentative gait is commonly caused by vestibular disorders, peripheral neuropathy, posterior column (proprioceptive) deficits, or visual impairment. With peripheral motor impairment, a number of classical gait patterns emerge, including obvious compensatory maneuvers (eg, Trendelenburg gait, antalgic gait, and foot drop). These conditions involve extremity (both body segment and joint) deformities, painful weight bearing, and focal myopathic and neuropathic weakness. Note that if the gait disorder is limited to this low sensorimotor level (ie, the central nervous system is intact), the person adapts well to the gait disorder, compensating with an assistive device or learning to negotiate the environment safely.

At the middle level, the execution of centrally selected postural and locomotor responses is faulty, and the sensory and motor modulation of gait is disrupted. Gait may be initiated normally, but stepping patterns are abnormal. Examples include diseases causing spasticity (eg, those related to myelopathy, B_{12} defi-

Table 22.1—Gait Disorders Classified by Sensorimotor Level

Sensorimotor Level	Condition (pathology, symptoms, signs)	Typical Gait Findings
Low		
Peripheral sensory	Sensory ataxia (posterior column, peripheral nerves)	Unsteady, uncoordinated
	Vestibular ataxia	Unsteady, weaving ("drunken")
	Visual ataxia	Tentative, uncertain
Peripheral motor	Arthritic (antalgic, joint deformity)	Avoids weight bearing on affected side, shortened stance phase
		Painful hip may produce Trendelenburg's sign (trunk shift over affected side)
		Painful knee is flexed
		Painful spine produces short, slow steps and decreased lumbar lordosis
		Other non-antalgic features: contractures, deformity-limited motion, buckling with weight bearing
		Kyphosis and ankylosing spondylosis produce stooped posture
		Unequal leg length can produce trunk and pelvic motion abnormalities (including Trendelenburg's sign)
	Myopathic and neuropathic (weakness)	Pelvic girdle weakness produces exaggerated lumbar lordosis and lateral trunk flexion (Trendelenburg's sign and waddling gait)
		Proximal motor neuropathy produces waddling gait and foot slap
		Distal motor neuropathy produces distal weakness (especially ankle dorsiflexion, or foot drop), which may lead to exaggerated hip flexion or foot lifting (steppage gait) and foot slap
Middle		
Spasticity	Hemiplegia, hemiparesis	Leg swings outward and in semi-circle from hip (circumduction); knee may hyperextend (genu recurvatum), and ankle may excessively plantar flex and invert (talipes equinovarus); with less paresis, some may only lose arm swing and only drag or scrape the foot
	Paraplegia, paraparesis	Both legs circumduct, steps are short shuffling and scraping, and when severe, hip adducts so that knees cross in front of each other (scissoring)
Parkinsonism		Small shuffling steps, hesitation, acceleration (festination), falling forward (propulsion), falling backward (retropulsion), moving the whole body while turning (turning en bloc), absent arm swing
Cerebellar ataxia		Wide-based with increased trunk sway, irregular stepping, especially on turns
High		
Cautious gait		Fear of falling with appropriate postural responses, normal to widened base, shortened stride, decreased velocity, and en bloc turns
Frontal-related gait disorders	Cerebrovascular, normal-pressure hydrocephalus	Proposed spectrum ranges from gait ignition failure to frontal gait disorder to frontal disequilibrium; may also have cognitive, pyramidal, and urinary disturbances
		Gait ignition failure: difficulty initiating gait, short shuffling gait, may freeze with diversion of attention or turning
		Frontal gait disorder: similar to Parkinson's disease
		Frontal disequilibrium: cannot stand unsupported

SOURCE: Alexander NB. Differential diagnosis of gait disorders in older adults. *Clin Geriatr Med.* 1996;12(4):697–698. Reprinted with permission.

ciency, and stroke), parkinsonism (idiopathic as well as drug-induced), and cerebellar disease (eg, alcohol-induced). Classical gait patterns appear when the spasticity is sufficient to cause leg circumduction and fixed deformities (eg, equinovarus), when the Parkinson's disease produces shuffling steps and reduced arm swing, and when the cerebellar ataxia increases trunk sway sufficiently to require a broad base of gait support.

At the high level, the gait characteristics become more nonspecific, and cognitive dysfunction and slowed cognitive processing become more prominent. Behavioral aspects such as fear of falling are also important, particularly in cautious gait. Frontal-related gait disorders often have a cerebrovascular component and are not merely the result of frontal masses and normal-pressure hydrocephalus. The severity of the frontal-related disorders run a spectrum from gait ignition failure (ie, difficulty with initiation) to frontal dysequilibrium, where unsupported stance is not possible. Cognitive, pyramidal, and urinary disturbances may also accompany the gait disorder. Gait disorders that might fall in this category have been given a number of overlapping descriptions, including gait apraxia, marche à petits pas, and arteriosclerotic parkinsonism. Cerebral white matter changes on either computed tomography scan or on magnetic resonance imaging are associated with gait disorders.

EVALUATION AND TREATMENT

Because there are no clearly accepted standards for "normal" gait in older adults, particularly for those of advanced age, an abnormal gait may simply be one that appears aesthetically abnormal or that suggests residual disability. Such a gait pattern may still provide the older adult with a safe, independent gait pattern. The use of standard functional, clinical, and radiologic methods to evaluate a gait disorder parallels the evaluation of fall risk (see the section on diagnostic approaches in "Falls," p 150). Emphasis should be placed on assessing the cardiovascular, visual, vestibular, musculoskeletal, and neurologic systems, as well as assessing medication use. Blood pressure should be measured with the patient both supine and standing to exclude orthostatic hypotension. Vision screening, at least for acuity, is essential. Examining the cardiovascular system helps exclude arrhythmia, valvular heart disease, and heart failure. The neck, spine, extremities, and feet should be evaluated for deformities and for pain or limitations in range of motion. A formal neurologic assessment is critical, to include assessment of strength and tone, sensation (including proprioception), coordination (including cerebellar function), and station and gait. With regard to the latter, the Romberg test screens for simple postural control and indicates whether the proprioceptive and vestibular systems are functional. A number of other tests have been proposed to establish high-level balance function: one-legged stance and tandem gait; a one-legged stance for up to 30 seconds (eyes open), and an accurate 10-foot tandem gait suggest minimal intrinsic postural control deficit. Other screening for vestibular function may include the Dix-Hallpike test, where subjective and objective responses to head motion from sitting to lying may provide evidence of positional vertigo. (See "Dizziness," p 153) Given the importance of cognition as a risk factor, screening for mental status, by using a tool such as the Folstein Mini–Mental State Examination, is also indicated.

Depending upon the history and physical examination, further laboratory and diagnostic evaluation may be warranted. Electrocardiograms and echocardiograms, Holter monitors, or tests for cardiac enzymes are not routinely recommended unless a cardiac source is suspected. Similarly, a complete blood cell count, serum chemistries, and tests of stool for occult blood are useful only where acute systemic disease is suspected. Head or spine imaging, including radiography, computed tomography, or magnetic resonance imaging, are of unclear use unless neurologic abnormalities are indicated by history and physical examination, either prior to or of recent onset in relation to the gait disorder. The sensitivity, specificity, and cost-effectiveness of these evaluations and age-specific guidelines for their use remain to be determined.

Even if a diagnosable condition is found on evaluation, many conditions causing a gait disorder are, at best, only partially treatable. The patient is often left with at least some residual disability. However, other functional outcomes, such as reduction in weight-bearing pain, may justify treatment. Achievement of premorbid gait patterns may be an unrealistic goal, and improvement in measures such as gait speed may be reasonable expectations as long as gait remains safe. Comorbidity, disease severity, and overall health status strongly influence treatment outcome.

Many of the studies of treatment and rehabilitation of gait disorders in older adults are retrospective chart reviews and case studies. Gait disorders presumably secondary to vitamin B_{12} deficiency, folate deficiency, hypothyroidism, hyperthyroidism, knee osteoarthritis, Parkinson's disease, and inflammatory polyneuropathy show improvement as a result of medical therapy. A variety of modes of physical therapy for diseases such as Parkinson's disease, knee osteoarthritis, and stroke also result in modest improvements but continued residual disability. Studies also suggest the use of special apparatus for rehabilitation of gait, such as body weight support and a treadmill to enhance poststroke gait retraining.

Modest improvement and residual disability are also the result of surgical treatment for compressive cervical myelopathy, lumbar stenosis, and normal-pressure hydrocephalus. Few controlled prospective studies and virtually no randomized studies address the outcome of surgical treatment for these conditions. A number of problems plague the available series: outcomes such as pain and walking disability are not reported separately, the source of the outcome rating is not clearly identified or blinded, the criteria for classifying outcomes differ, the follow-up intervals are variable, the selection factors for conservative versus surgical treatment between studies differ or are unspecified, and there is publication bias (only positive results are published). Most of the surgical series include all ages, although the mean age is usually above 60 years. Many older adults experience reduction in pain and improvement in maximal walking distance following laminectomies and lumbar fusion surgery, although they have continued residual disability. A few studies document equivalent surgical outcomes with conservative, nonsurgical treatment. Finally, it is unclear how much of the initial postoperative gains are maintained over the long term, particularly in normal-pressure hydrocephalus.

Assessments of outcomes for hip- and knee-replacement surgery for osteoarthritis indicate that they are better, although some of the same study methodologic problems exist. Other than pain relief, sizable gains in gait speed and joint motion occur, although residual walking disability continues for a number of reasons, including residual pathology on the operated side and symptoms on the nonoperated side.

Patients with gait abnormalities should be referred to physical therapy for gait training and should be assessed for appropriate assistive devices. (See "Rehabilitation," p 82.)

REFERENCES

- Alexander NB. Gait disorders in older adults. *J Am Geriatr Soc.* 1996;44(4):434–451.

- Dynamic Gait Index: In: Shumway-Cook A, Woollacott MH, eds. *Motor Control: Theory and Practical Applications.* 1st ed. Baltimore, MD: Williams and Wilkins; 1995.

- Emory Functional Ambulation Profile: Wolf SL, Catlin PA, Gage K, et al. Establishing the reliability and validity of measurements of walking time using the Emory Functional Ambulation Profile. *Phys Ther.* 1999;79(12):1122–1133.

- Functional Ambulation Classification: Holden MK, Gill KM, Magliozzi MR. Gait assessment for neurologically impaired patients: standards for outcome assessment. *Phys Ther.* 1986;66(10):1530–1539.

- Functional Obstacle Course: Means KM, Rodell DE, O'Sullivan PS, et al. Comparison of a functional obstacle course with an index of clinical gait and balance and postural sway. *J Gerontol A Biol Sci Med Sci.* 1998;53(5):M331–M335.

- Health J, Stuart MR. Prescribing Exercise for Frail Elders. *J Am Board Family Practice.* 2002;15(3):218–228.

- Modified Gait Abnormality Rating Scale: VanSwearingen JM, Paschal KA, Bonino P, et al. Assessing recurrent fall risk of community-dwelling frail older veterans using specific tests of mobility and the physical performance test of function. *J Gerontol A Biol Sci Med Sci.* 1998;53(6):M457–M464.

- Performance Oriented Mobility Assessment: Tinetti ME. Performance-oriented assessment of mobility problems in elderly patients. *J Am Geriatr Soc.* 1986;34(2):119–126.

- Schwendimann RN. Assessing gait abnormalities in the elderly. *Patient Care for the Nurse Practitioner.* 1999; 2(4):26–34.

- Timed Get Up and Go Test: Posiadlo D, Richardson S. The timed "Up & Go": a test of basic functional mobility for frail elderly persons. *J Am Geriatr Soc.* 1991;39(2):142–148.

- Visintin M, Barbeau H, Korner-Bitensky N, et al. A new approach to retrain gait in stroke patients through body weight support and treadmill stimulation. *Stroke.* 1998;29(6):1122–1128.

CHAPTER 23—DIZZINESS

Dizziness accounts for an estimated 7 million clinic visits in the United States each year and is one of the most common symptoms of patients referred to neurology and otolaryngology practices. Among older persons, the reported prevalence ranges from 13% to 38%. Several factors make dizziness a challenging symptom to evaluate and manage. First, precise classification of the cause is often difficult. Second, patients and clinicians alike may worry about a serious cardiac or neurologic cause. Third, specific therapy is not available for many patients with dizziness. Fourth, like other geriatric syndromes such as delirium and falls, dizziness may be related to multiple potentially causative factors at least half of the time.

CLASSIFICATION

Drachman popularized a symptom-oriented approach, classifying dizziness as vertigo (rotational sensation), presyncope (impending faint), disequilibrium (loss of balance without head sensation), or lightheadedness (ill-defined, not otherwise classifiable). Although some sensations correspond more often than not to at least a general etiologic category (eg, vertigo suggests vestibular dysfunction at least 80% to 90% of the time), these four sensations remain nonspecific, occurring with many different disorders. Following is a brief delineation of the sensations and the most common corresponding causes.

Vertigo

The three most common specific peripheral vestibular disorders are benign positional vertigo, labyrinthitis, and Ménière's disease. Benign positional vertigo (BPV) is episodic and aggravated or brought on by changes in position, such as turning, rolling over or getting in and out of bed, or bending over. BPV spells are often brief (5 to 15 seconds) and milder than the severe vertiginous attacks seen with disorders such as labyrinthitis and Ménière's disease. Labyrinthitis (sometimes called *vestibular neuronitis*) occurs acutely, lasts for several days, and resolves spontaneously. Ménière's disease is characterized by repeated episodes of tinnitus, fluctuating hearing loss, and severe vertigo accompanied eventually by a progressive sensorineural hearing loss. The frequency and severity of vertigo may improve as hearing impairment worsens.

Central vestibular disorders account for a minority of cases of vertigo; these include cerebrovascular disease, brain tumors, multiple sclerosis, and rarer central causes. In vertigo of vascular origin, dizziness has been reported as the presenting symptom less than 20% of the time. Much more commonly, it is preceded or accompanied by other neurologic deficits in the distribution of the posterior circulation. Indeed, verifying a transient ischemic attack as the cause of vertigo can be difficult in the absence of other neurologic deficits, since isolated vertigo is nonspecific and there is no good noninvasive diagnostic test of the vertebrobasilar circulation.

Tumors are found in less than 1% of dizzy patients and are slightly more prevalent (2% to 3%) in older patients referred to neurologists. The most common tumor associated with dizziness is an acoustic neuroma, for which cochlear symptoms (tinnitus and hearing loss) rather than dizziness predominate. Unilateral cochlear symptoms would be one marker, since bilateral symptoms in older persons typically represent presbyacusis rather than a tumor.

Nonvertiginous Dizziness

Presyncope is the sensation of near fainting. This chapter does not deal with full loss of consciousness or syncope, which requires a different diagnostic approach. (See "Syncope," p 159.) Presyncope reflects diminished cerebral perfusion. Cardiac causes of presyncope can be electrical (tachy- or bradyarrhythmias) or structural (especially aortic outflow obstruction). Vascular causes of syncope are typically not ischemic events but are less serious, reversible conditions, such as orthostatic hypotension or temporary reactions due to vagal stimulation. Most presyncopal patients presenting with dizziness have symptoms attributable to postural change (with or without orthostatic hypotension) rather than more serious cardiac causes. Postural symptoms without orthostatic blood-pressure changes are particularly common in older persons. Likewise, orthostatic blood-pressure changes in the absence of symptoms are also quite common.

Disequilibrium is a sensation of being unsteady when standing or, in particular, walking. Balance depends not only on the vestibular system but also on the visual and somatosensory systems. Thus, multiple factors can contribute to imbalance, including chronic vestibulopathies, visual problems (eg, errors of refraction, cataract, loss of binocular vision, macular degeneration), musculoskeletal disorders (eg, arthritis, muscle weaknesses), and somatosensory or gait deficits (eg, neuropathies, previous strokes, cerebellar disease, Parkinson's disease, dementia).

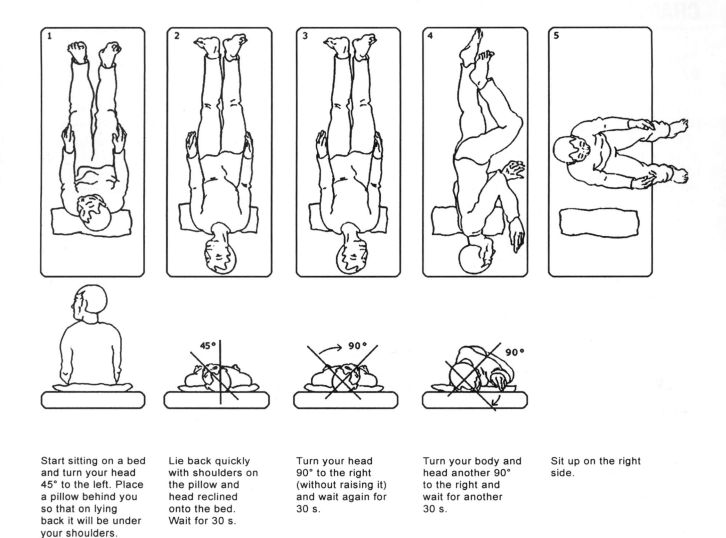

Start sitting on a bed and turn your head 45° to the left. Place a pillow behind you so that on lying back it will be under your shoulders.	Lie back quickly with shoulders on the pillow and head reclined onto the bed. Wait for 30 s.	Turn your head 90° to the right (without raising it) and wait again for 30 s.	Turn your body and head another 90° to the right and wait for another 30 s.	Sit up on the right side.

Figure 23.1—The Epley's maneuver for self-treatment of benign positional vertigo (right ear affected). This maneuver should be carried out three times a day. Repeat daily until free from positional vertigo for 24 hours. For use, see Table 23.2.

SOURCE: Radtke A, Neuhauser H, von Brevern M, et al. A modified Epley's procedure for self-treatment of benign paroxysmal positional vertigo. *Neurology.* 1999;53(6):1358–1360. Reprinted with permission by Lippincott Williams & Wilkins.

Lightheadedness is a vaguer sensation best reserved as a descriptor for patients who do not experience one of the three more discrete types of dizziness sensations—vertigo, presyncope, or disequilibrium. In the vernacular of patients, these latter three sensations may be experienced as "spinning," "fainting," or "falling." Although any cause of dizziness may occasionally produce a nondescript "lightheaded" type of sensation, the two most prominent considerations are psychiatric (primarily depressive, anxiety, or somatoform disorders) or idiopathic causes, which together account for up to a third of all cases of dizziness.

Among other causes, prescription drug toxicity is an important contributing factor to dizziness in older patients. The use of five or more medications is a risk factor for dizziness among older adults, as are drugs that cause orthostatic hypotension, most commonly cardiovascular, antihypertensive, and psychotropic drugs, as well as diuretics. Three purported causes particularly germane to older patients—cervical arthritis, visual disorders, and carotid sinus hypersensitivity—are seldom reported as causes in published series of dizzy patients. In part, this may be due to their common occurrence among older persons

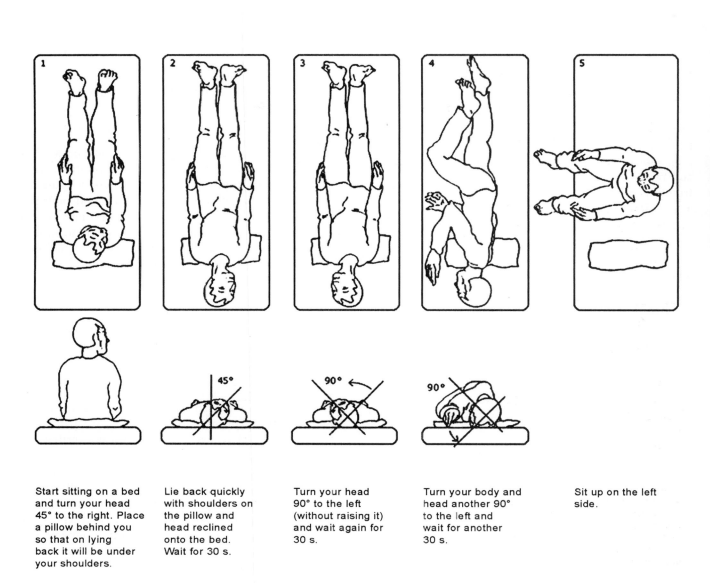

Start sitting on a bed and turn your head 45° to the right. Place a pillow behind you so that on lying back it will be under your shoulders.	Lie back quickly with shoulders on the pillow and head reclined onto the bed. Wait for 30 s.	Turn your head 90° to the left (without raising it) and wait again for 30 s.	Turn your body and head another 90° to the left and wait for another 30 s.	Sit up on the left side.

Figure 23.2—The Epley's maneuver for self-treatment of benign positional vertigo (left ear affected). This maneuver should be carried out three times a day. Repeat daily until free from positional vertigo for 24 hours. For use, see Table 23.2.

SOURCE: Radtke A, Neuhauser H, von Brevern M, et al. A modified Epley's procedure for self-treatment of benign paroxysmal positional vertigo. *Neurology.* 1999;53(6):1358-1360. Reprinted with permission by Lippincott Williams & Wilkins.

without dizziness as well as the fact that confirming these factors as the actual cause of dizziness can be difficult.

PROGNOSIS

Dizziness usually resolves within days to several months, but about one fourth of patients may experience chronic or recurrent symptoms. A 1-year prospective study of 102 patients found that dizziness due to psychiatric disorders, disequilibrium, or a vestibulopathy other than BPV or labyrinthitis was more likely to persist. Among 1087 community-dwelling older persons, the 261 (24%) individuals with dizziness lasting a month or longer were more likely to have anxiety or depressive symptoms, hearing loss, impaired balance, postural hypotension, past myocardial infarction, or to be on five or more medications.

Dizziness has not been shown to predict mortality, hospitalization, or severe disability, as measured by decrements in activities of daily living or nursing-home placement. However, persistent dizziness in older persons is associated with an increased risk of falls and possibly syncope, as well as psychologic distress and diminished social activities.

EVALUATION

A brief, focused evaluation coupled with simple follow-up rather than initial diagnostic testing or referral is warranted in most patients. As mentioned, symptoms gradually improve in most patients. Moreover, specialized testing only occasionally reveals unsuspected diagnoses. More than 75% of the cases in which a diagnosis can be established are diagnosed by history and physical examination alone, with the history contributing most of these diagnoses. Table 23.1 outlines a practical office-based approach to evaluating the dizzy patient.

History

As with many common symptoms, history is the single most useful part of the evaluation. The clinician must establish early on whether dizziness stems from a

serious or benign cause. Although it is best to elicit the patient's own description of the event without prompting, three questions are particularly helpful:

- Is the dizziness one of 3 key sensations: spinning, fainting, or falling?
- Is there a positional effect on symptoms?

With BPV, the effect is almost always one of transient dizziness with change of head position, lying down, or sitting up. The most common cause of presyncope is an orthostatic change in blood pressure, in which case the patient reports that dizziness occurs on assuming a more upright position (supine to sitting, or sitting to standing). Disequilibrium is manifested only when the patient is walking or standing.

- What other symptoms are associated with dizziness?

Syncope is a particularly important symptom to inquire about, since actual loss of consciousness targets that very small subset of dizzy patients in whom early cardiac evaluation may be contemplated. Tinnitus or hearing changes, or both, are associated with certain vestibular disorders such as Ménière's disease or the rare acoustic neuroma. Nausea and, in particular, vomiting suggests vertigo rather than a nonvertiginous cause of dizziness. A central cause would not commonly present with isolated dizziness but instead would be expected to produce "neighboring" neurologic symptoms as well. Psychogenic causes, such as depression, anxiety, or somatoform disorders, typically have fatigue, insomnia, pain, or other physical and emotional symptoms in addition to dizziness.

Physical Examination

A focused physical examination would include the following steps.

- Measure the blood pressure and pulse while the patient is supine and again after standing for 1 to 2 minutes to detect orthostatic changes.
- Perform the head-hanging (Dix-Hallpike) test (described below).
- Auscultate the heart.
- Watch the patient walk and turn (looking for balance or gait difficulties).

Dizziness correlates best with postural hypotension when the latter is defined as a drop (eg, 20% decrease) in mean blood pressure, which is one third systolic plus two thirds diastolic, rather than a drop in systolic pressure only.

A screening vestibular examination is warranted in cases in which the cause of dizziness is not obvious. The four elements of a brief vestibular examination can

---

Table 23.1—Practical Approach to Evaluating the Dizzy Patient

Initial office evaluation
  History
    Clarify sensation (spinning, fainting, falling)
    Positional effects: Does dizziness worsen with head movements (eg, benign positional vertigo), standing up (eg, orthostatic hypotension), or ambulating (eg, disequilibrium)?
    Associated symptoms (syncope, nausea or vomiting, hearing or ear symptoms, ataxia or focal neurologic deficits, multiple somatic complaints)
    Medications (especially ones initiated around the time of onset of dizziness symptoms)

  Physical examination
    Orthostatic blood pressure and pulse
    Nystagmus exam: gaze, Dix-Hallpike test, head shaking
    Brief cardiovascular (murmurs, abnormal rhythm) and neurologic (cerebellar or focal deficits) examinations

Early diagnostic testing or referral
  Certain "red flags" (present in only an occasional dizzy patient) would prompt an earlier work-up
  If true syncope, follow guidelines for syncope evaluation
  If other cardiovascular abnormalities, consider selected testing (eg, a suspicious murmur may warrant an echocardiogram; an abnormal cardiac rhythm, an electrocardiogram and, if indicated, further dysrhythmia evaluation)
  If vertical-beating nystagmus or neurologic abnormalities, consider neuroimaging or neurology or otolaryngology referral, or both

Later diagnostic testing or referral
  In the minority of patients who have persistent (> 4 to 6 weeks) unexplained dizziness, further testing is sometimes needed for diagnostic reasons and patient reassurance
  Reconsider psychiatric causes, especially depressive, anxiety, and somatoform disorders
  Referral for formal vestibular testing (eg, electronystagmography)

SOURCE: Adapted with permission from Kroenke K, Hoffman RM, Einstadter D. How common are various causes of dizziness? A critical review. *South Med J.* 2000;93(2):160–167.

be performed in about a minute and have in common the detection of nystagmus:

- Primary position. Have the patient look straight ahead and look for nystagmus.

- Gaze-evoked. Have the patient look to the right, left, up, and down, holding each position for 5 to 10 seconds. Deviations of 30 to 45 degrees of eye movement are sufficient to detect pathologic nystagmus; extreme gaze may accentuate physiologic nystagmus. More than three to five beats of nystagmus is abnormal.

- Dix-Hallpike test. With the patient seated on the examination table, help him or her lie down quickly with one ear turned toward the table. Help the patient up to a sitting position and repeat the maneuver with the other ear facing the table. Although hyperextending the patient's neck over the edge of the table has traditionally been recommended, this is not always possible and may not be necessary in many patients. The Dix-Hallpike test is positive in about half of patients with BPV—usually those with symptoms of recent onset. The occurrence of nystagmus (and often vertigo), which lasts 10 to 30 seconds after a few seconds of latency, indicates a positive response.

- Head-shaking. Have the patient close his or her eyes, rapidly shake the head back and forth for 10 seconds, and then open his or her eyes. Look for nystagmus.

Nystagmus due to peripheral causes usually beats horizontally. Vertical nystagmus (ie, upward or downward beating) is uncommon and should prompt early evaluation for central causes (eg, neuroimaging, formal vestibular testing, neurology or otolaryngology referral).

Diagnostic Testing

Simple laboratory tests, including complete blood cell counts, electrolytes, glucose level, serum creatinine, thyroid functions, and serologic tests for syphilis, have a very low yield. Audiometry may be helpful in the patient with cochlear symptoms, such as tinnitus or asymmetric hearing loss. Abnormal audiograms may indicate Ménière's disease or, rarely, a cerebellopontine angle tumor such as acoustic neuroma. However, the most common abnormal audiometric finding in older patients is high-frequency hearing loss due to presbyacusis; this represents a coincidental finding rather than a diagnostic explanation of dizziness.

Vestibular testing most commonly involves electronystagmography (ENG), which has important limitations. Sensitivity is variable, and it cannot readily distinguish between central and peripheral causes. In a community-based study of older persons, 80% of dizzy persons and 79% of persons in the control group were found to have at least two ENG abnormalities. Other tests include brain stem auditory evoked responses, rotatory chair, and dynamic posturography. The latter two tests may substitute for or augment ENG in special situations, but testing for brain stem auditory evoked responses is occasionally indicated if clinical evaluation, audiometry, or ENG suggest a central vestibulopathy.

Neuroimaging is occasionally warranted in the evaluation of the dizzy patient. Although a computed tomography scan is the procedure of choice for strokes (because of cost and availability), magnetic resonance imaging is better able to image posterior fossa structures and should be considered in the occasional case of vertigo associated with neurologic deficits. A community-based controlled study examining 149 dizzy and 97 asymptomatic older persons found that the prevalence of abnormalities on magnetic resonance imaging was high in both groups. Electroencephalography is typically not useful, and noninvasive carotid studies would be warranted only if other neurologic symptoms suggest transient ischemic attacks.

An electrocardiogram is commonly obtained in older patients with cardiovascular risk factors but has a low diagnostic value in patients with a normal cardiac examination and nonsyncopal dizziness. Other tests helpful in evaluating syncope, ischemia, or valvular disease (Holter and event monitors, echocardiography, stress testing, tilt-tables, and electrophysiologic studies) have not been shown to be useful in evaluating isolated dizziness.

Psychiatric disorders should be considered when the dizziness is nondescript (eg, lightheadedness), persistent and unexplained, or associated with multiple other somatic or emotional symptoms. Although brief case-finding instruments for depression are available, a single question about depressed mood has a sensitivity of 85% to 90% for detecting major depression. (See "Depression and Other Mood Disorders," p 211.)

MANAGEMENT

Although well-proven therapies for dizziness are limited, the natural history is nonetheless often favorable. In up to half of patients, dizziness spontaneously resolves or substantially improves within 2 weeks. In some cases, dizziness is an associated symptom of viral or other self-limited illnesses. Other times, it results from dehydration or a medication adverse effect. The two most common causes of peripheral vertigo—labyrinthitis and BPV—typically resolve within days or weeks, respectively. Types of dizziness for which specific management strategies may be helpful in some patients are delineated in Table 23.2.

Finally, when managing a patient with dizziness, it is important to remember that approximately half of patients may have two or more potential causative or contributory factors for their symptoms. For example, an older patient may have a complex type of dizziness variably described as feeling faint when standing, unsteadiness when walking, and a nagging lightheadedness unrelated to position. Upon evaluation, the patient is found to have orthostatic hypotension, depression, and disequilibrium due to a peripheral neuropathy and macular degeneration. Identifying and targeting factors that may be remediable, such as the orthostasis and depression, may ameliorate at least some of the symptoms.

Table 23.2—Management of Potentially Treatable Causes of Dizziness

Acute vertigo attacks that occur with peripheral vestibular disorders such as labyrinthitis and Ménière's disease may benefit from meclizine and, if needed, a benzodiazepine. However, meclizine probably is overprescribed for chronic vestibulopathies and nonvertiginous dizziness.

Benign positional vertigo usually can be treated with simple reassurance, since symptoms are typically mild and usually improve within weeks to several months. For severe or persistent symptoms, the patient may be educated about home habituation exercises, or the canalolith repositioning procedure (Epley's maneuver) may be attempted in the office (see Figure 23.1 and Figure 23.2).

Ménière's disease in which attacks are frequent or disabling may benefit from prophylactic treatment with salt restriction or diuretic therapy, or both. Occasional patients may require referral to otolaryngology for consideration of surgery.

Orthostatic hypotension: Correct reversible causes.

Disequilibrium: For the older patient with chronic disequilibrium, take measures to prevent falls, including the use of a cane, walker, or other assistive device, if necessary.

Psychogenic dizziness related to depressive or certain anxiety (eg, panic) disorders: Consider a trial of antidepressants. Newer antidepressants (eg, selective serotonin-reuptake inhibitors, nefazodone, bupropion) may be preferable to tricyclic antidepressants, which sometimes cause orthostatic hypotension.

Chronic vestibulopathy: Vestibular rehabilitation (a type of physical therapy exercise program) may be beneficial in persons with persistent dizziness.

SOURCE: Adapted from Khan A, Kroenke K. Diagnosis and treatment of the dizzy patient. *Prim Care Case Rev.* 1999;2(1):9. Reprinted with permission from Lippincott Williams & Wilkins.

REFERENCES

■ Drachman DA. A 69-year-old man with chronic dizziness. *JAMA.* 1998;280:2111–2118.

■ Felisati G, Battaglia A, Grazia Papini M, et al, on behalf of the Nicergoline Dizziness Study Group. Nicergoline in balance alterations in adult and elderly patients: a double-blind, placebo-controlled study. *Clin Drug Invest.* 2002;22(11):731–740.

■ Frishman WH, Azer V, Sica D. Drug treatment of orthostatic hypotension and vasovagal snycope. *Heart Disease.* 2003;5(1):49–64.

■ Hoffman R, Einstadter D, Kroenke K. Evaluating dizziness. *Am J Med.* 1999;107:468–478.

■ Hotson JR, Baloh RW. Acute vestibular syndromes. *N Engl J Med.* 1998;339;680–685.

■ Kahn A, Kroenke K. Diagnosis and treatment of the dizzy patient. *Primary Care Reviews.* 1999;2:3–11.

■ Tinetti ME, Williams CS, Gill TM. Dizziness among older adults: a possible geriatric syndrome. *Ann Intern Med.* 2000;132:337–344.

CHAPTER 24—SYNCOPE

yncope—a sudden, transient loss of postural tone and consciousness not due to trauma and with spontaneous full recovery—is common. Annually it accounts for approximately 3% of emergency department visits and 2% to 6% of hospital admissions. Approximately 80% of the patients hospitalized for syncope are aged 65 or older. Syncope is a clinically important condition that is commonly difficult to evaluate. Its potential causes range from those that are benign and self-limited to those that are life threatening. In older adults the causes of syncope may also be multifactorial, adding to the diagnostic difficulty. Because it encompasses a wide range of potential causes (Table 24.1), the diagnostic evaluation of syncope can be complex and expensive. Although a wide variety of diagnostic tools can be employed, in many cases the patient's history provide the best clues to the cause and help direct the work-up.

NATURAL HISTORY

Syncope is generally caused by a reduction in cerebral perfusion. Hemodynamic disturbances that can decrease cerebral perfusion include alterations in systemic blood pressure or an increase in cerebral vascular resistance. Common causes of transient decreases in blood pressure include:

- Cardiac arrhythmias, such as atrial fibrillation with a rapid ventricular response, ventricular tachycardia, sick sinus syndrome with sinus pauses, and atrioventricular block.

- Alterations in the peripheral vasculature due to arterial vasodilation or increased venous pooling.

- Cardiopulmonary obstruction, such as that due to pulmonary emboli, aortic stenosis, hypertrophic obstructive cardiomyopathy, and atrial myxoma.

Syncope can also occur as a consequence of an increase in cerebrovascular resistance. In hyperventilation syndrome and panic attacks, cerebrovascular vasoconstriction can occur without a change in systemic vascular resistance. In this situation, syncope can occur as a result of the relative decrease in cerebral blood flow without systemic hypotension. In rare instances localized atherosclerotic disease can predispose a person to syncope by decreasing cerebral perfusion without a decrease in systemic blood pressure (vertebral basilar insufficiency and subclavian steal).

Syncope occurs most commonly while a person is standing. The effects of gravity cause up to a third of

Table 24.1—Causes of Syncope

Cardiac
- Aortic stenosis
- Atrial myxoma
- Atrioventricular block
- Hypertrophic cardiomyopathy
- Mitral stenosis
- Myocardial infarction
- Pulmonary embolism
- Pulmonary hypertension
- Pulmonary stenosis
- Sick sinus syndrome
- Supraventricular tachycardia
- Ventricular tachycardia

Drugs
- Antiarrhythmics
- Anticonvulsants
- Antihypertensives
- Antipsychotics
- β-Blockers
- Digitalis
- Diuretics
- Narcotics
- Nitrates
- Tricyclic antidepressants

Miscellaneous
- Hyperventilation
- Hypoglycemia
- Hypoxia
- Thyroid disease

Neurally mediated disturbance of blood-pressure control
- Carotid sinus
- Cough
- Gastrointestinal events (defecation, swallow, postprandial hypotension)
- Micturition
- Psychogenic causes
- Vasovagal faint

Neurologic and psychiatric
- Anxiety disorder
- Cerebrovascular spasm
- Depression
- Migraine
- Narcolepsy
- Panic attacks
- Seizure
- Subclavian steal
- Vertebrobasilar ischemia

Orthostasis
- Drugs (see above)
- Autonomic insufficiency
- Venous pooling
- Intravascular volume depletion

the blood volume to pool in the lower extremities when a person assumes the standing position. Unopposed, this reduces cardiac output by reducing venous return and cerebral blood pressure. A number of reflex pathways involving the autonomic and endocrine systems are responsible for rapid compensation of the gravitational effects of standing. The baroreceptor reflex is triggered by carotid and aortic baroreceptors, which act to increase autonomic sympathetic tone, resulting in peripheral vasoconstriction and an increase in heart rate. Increased sympathetic activity of the renal nerve leads to stimulation of renin release from the juxtaglomerular apparatus. The activation of the renin-angiotensin system leads to direct vasoconstriction by the action of angiotensin II and the secretion of aldosterone from the adrenal cortex to retain sodium, thereby raising the extracellual fluid volume. A postural change to a standing position also rapidly reduces the level of atrial natriuretic factor, which is a vasodilator and inhibitor of the renin-angiotensin system. The reduction in atrial natriuretic factor facilitates vasoconstriction, and the activity of the volume effects of the renin-angiotensin contributes to vasoconstriction.

In aging, many of these reflex mechanisms are less responsive. The cardiac response to β-adrenergic stimulation (cardiac acceleration and increased contractility) decreases with advancing age. As a result of this and perhaps other mechanisms, the baroreflex (increasing heart rate and vasoconstriction) is also less effective with advancing age. In addition, comorbid conditions that can affect postural responses, such as diabetes mellitus, are prevalent among older persons. Medications such as α-blockers, β-blockers, and tricyclic antidepressants may also impair postural reflexes. The effects of age-related decline in adaptive reflexes, comorbid conditions, and medications may combine, becoming factors in syncopal events experienced by the older person. Because older persons have a decreased ability to increase heart rate in response to sympathetic stimulation, blood volume maintenance and vasoconstriction become more important in maintaining postural blood pressure. Thus, the older person may be particularly sensitive to the effects of dehydration and vasodilator drugs.

The prognosis of syncope depends on the underlying cause. The major issue is whether a cardiac cause is responsible. The 1-year mortality for patients with cardiac causes for syncope averages 18% to 33% (deaths are due to underlying disease, not syncope), whereas syncope due to noncardiac causes has a much more favorable prognosis, a 1-year mortality of approximately 6%. In one third to one half of syncopal patients, no cause can be found. The prognosis for these patients is the same as for those with noncardiac syncope.

EVALUATION OF THE PATIENT WITH SYNCOPE

A large number of conditions can affect systemic blood pressure and cerebral blood flow, and thus cause syncope. Rarely, some metabolic disorders may result in syncope. In the older person, age-related decline in compensatory sympathetic reflexes may make it necessary for the clinician to consider multiple causes.

History

The clinical history obtained from the patient and, if possible, from witnesses to the event, may provide a diagnosis in up to 50% of cases in which a diagnosis can be established. First, it is important to establish whether the patient suffered a true syncopal event, as opposed to dizziness (disequilibrium) or lightheadedness. Key elements to obtain from the history follow:

- Was there a precipitant? Could the patient's activities around the time of the event have triggered it? Such activities include eating, urinating, coughing, using medication, and experiencing emotional stress. Syncope occurring during physical exertion should raise the possibility of myocardial ischemia or aortic stenosis. A history of syncope after turning motions of the head should raise the possibility of carotid sinus hypersensitivity.

- Were there prodromal symptoms before the event? Symptoms of chest pain, palpitations, or shortness of breath suggest a cardiac or pulmonary cause. Gastrointestinal symptoms, such as nausea or vomiting, can be associated with vasovagal syncope. Sudden onset of syncope with less than 5 seconds of warning is characteristic of syncope due to a cardiac arrhythmia.

- What medications are being used? It is important to establish how medications were taken with relationship to meals and other activities, and whether there have been recent changes in the medication regimen. Specifics about dosage times should be obtained.

- What did witnesses observe? They should be queried about the duration of the event and the appearance of the patient during the event. Patients with cardiac causes of syncope are generally flaccid in tone and motionless while unconscious, unless the event lasts for more than 15 seconds, when myoclonic jerks and truncal extension may be seen. In contrast, increased body tone and motion occur more rapidly with most seizure activity.

- Are there significant comorbid conditions? A history of coronary artery disease or its associated symptoms is particularly important. Approximately 5% of myocardial infarctions present as syncope. Sustained ventricular tachycardia resulting in syncope is most common in patients with prior myocardial infarction. Patients with diabetes mellitus are at increased risk for coronary atherosclerosis as well as autonomic dysfunction predisposing to syncope.

Table 24.2 summarizes the characteristics of three classes of syncope.

Physical Examination

A physical examination should focus on elements raised by the history. It is estimated that of those patients in whom a cause of syncope can be established, 20% are identified by features found during physical examina-

Table 24.2—Characteristics of Three Classes of Syncope

Phase	Cardiac Arrhythmia	Vasovagal	Seizure
Prior to event	Occurs in any position	Aborted if person lies flat	Any position
	Less than 5 seconds' warning	—	No warning or prodrome
	Precipitant absent	Precipitant present	—
	Palpitations rare	—	—
	—	Nausea, diaphoresis common	—
	—	Visual changes	—
During event	Flaccid tone	Motionless, relaxed tone	Rigid tone
	Pulse absent, faint	Slow, faint pulse	Rapid pulse, elevated blood pressure
	Blue, ashen	Pale color	—
	Incontinence rare	—	—
	—	Dilated, reactive pupils	Tonic eye deviation common
	—	—	Frothing at mouth
Recovery	Rapid and complete	Fatigue common after event	Slow, incomplete recovery
	—	No retrograde amnesia	Disorientation
	—	Diaphoresis and nausea common	—
	—	—	Focal neurologic findings

tion. The blood pressure should be measured in both arms, as well as postural changes in the blood pressure. The pulse should be taken with the patient in the supine and standing positions. Blood pressure with the patient in the standing position should be obtained after 1 minute of standing and repeated after the patient has been standing for 3 minutes. Although any definition of postural hypotension is arbitrary, a decrease in systolic blood pressure of more than 200 mm Hg is the definition used most frequently.

The character of the carotid pulse should also be assessed for the delayed upstroke and low volume characteristic of significant aortic stenosis. The presence of a carotid bruit, a history of cerebrovascular disease, and recent myocardial infarction are relative contraindications to carotid sinus massage. Even in the absence of contraindications, carotid sinus massage should be performed only under continuous electrocardiographic monitoring (to detect induced AV block or other arrhythmias) in a setting where resuscitation equipment is available.

The physical examination of the patient with syncope should include cardiac examination for evidence of murmurs characteristic of valvular abnormalities or extra heart sounds suggestive of cardiomyopathy. Examination of the stool for occult blood and neurologic examination for focal deficits are also important.

An electrocardiogram (ECG) is indicated for all patients presenting with syncope. Though ECG establishes a diagnosis in only 5% of those with syncope, approximately 50% have an abnormal ECG. Abnormalities on an ECG may provide clues for further cardiovascular evaluation; a normal ECG is associated with a more favorable prognosis. Key features to assess on an ECG include evidence of acute or remote myocardial infarction. Conduction abnormalities, espe-

cially block in the AV node or below, and pre-excitation, such as Wolff-Parkinson-White, may be detected as well; inappropriate sinus bradycardia may also be found. A prolonged QT interval can predispose a person to ventricular arrhythmias, including torsade de pointes.

Ambulatory Electrocardiographic Monitoring

An ambulatory ECG recording can establish or exclude many causes of syncope if the patient experiences syncopal or presyncopal symptoms during the recording. Unfortunately, the occurrence of symptoms during ambulatory ECG monitoring is relatively rare in most patients with syncope that remains unexplained after a history, physical examination, and ECG. On average, studies examining the diagnostic yield of ambulatory ECG report an arrhythmia correlating with symptoms in approximately 4% of patients. In another 15% of patients, an arrhythmia was excluded by the presence of symptoms during the recording, but without evidence of an arrhythmia. In approximately 14% of patients, arrhythmias were present but without concomitant symptoms. These patients may represent a diagnostic dilemma. However, certain arrhythmias, even asymptomatic ones, such as nonsustained ventricular tachycardia, second- and third-degree AV block, and sinus pauses in excess of 3 seconds, are rare in persons without heart disease. Their presence, even if asymptomatic, in a patient with a history of syncope indicates the need for further evaluation.

Ambulatory loop recorders that may be worn for a many days or weeks at a time are commonly used to capture ECG recordings of symptoms that occur infrequently. These devices constantly record an ECG tracing on a 5- to 10-minute loop; the patient presses a button to stop the recording after an event has occurred and then transmits this by telephone to a monitoring center. Among patients who are able operate the recorder, the diagnostic yield is approximately 25%. However, many older patients are unable or unwilling to capture and transmit these recordings. Subcutaneous implantable loop recorders have been developed; these have long-term memories that do not require patient intervention to store recordings and thus may have a role in some situations.

Echocardiography

Two-dimensional echocardiography has a low yield in the absence of features suggestive of heart disease by history, physical examination, or ECG. It is most useful in confirming a specific diagnosis suspected by other assessment. However, unsuspected findings on echocardiography are reported in approximately 5% to 10% of unselected patients. Thus, echocardiography has been advocated for the evaluation of syncope. Occult coronary artery disease is also prevalent among older persons, and stress testing is often employed to screen for this. In some patients, particularly those without the suggestion of structural cardiac abnormalities by physical examination or ECG, it is efficient to perform stress echocardiography as a single procedure.

Tilt-Table Testing

Head-up tilt-table testing results in pooling of blood in the lower extremities and, in susceptible individuals, may trigger syncope mediated by neurocardiogenic mechanisms. Tilt-table testing is useful for patients suspected of having vasovagal syncope and those with unexplained syncope who are not suspected of having a cardiac cause. The sensitivity and specificity of tilt-table testing vary considerably, depending on the protocol used and the patient population. A positive tilt-table result occurs in approximately 11% of normal older persons. Thus, a positive tilt-table result alone does not ensure that a vasovagal event was the cause. It is generally recommended that men over the age of 45 and women over the age of 55 have stress testing prior to tilt-table testing.

Electrophysiologic Studies

Guidelines suggest that invasive electrophysiologic (EP) testing should be employed in the evaluation of patients with structural heart disease with unexplained syncope. There is also agreement that EP testing should not be employed in situations where the results of the test would not influence subsequent treatment or in which a cause of the syncope has been established. The role of EP testing in patients with recurrent syncope with no structural heart disease and negative tilt-table studies remains undefined. EP testing is most sensitive for detecting ventricular arrhythmias in the setting of ischemic heart disease and is less sensitive for the detection of ventricular arrhythmias in dilated nonischemic cardiomyopathies. The sensitivity of EP testing for detecting most bradyarrhythmias is also low.

Neurologic Testing

Neurologic testing, including imaging of the head by computed tomography or magnetic resonance imaging and electroencephalographic recording, is appropriate in situations when focal neurologic signs or symptoms are present.

TREATMENT

The treatment of syncope depends on the underlying cause. When a single underlying cause is established, that is where therapeutic interventions should be concentrated. This is particularly important for cardiac causes. Myocardial ischemia causing syncope may require revascularization (percutaneous or surgical) or aggressive medical therapy. Valvular heart disease causing syncope, particularly aortic stenosis, is typically managed surgically. Treatment of malignant arrhythmias, such as ventricular tachycardia, may involve antiarrhythmic drug therapy, but increasingly defibrillators are used for this purpose, particularly in the presence of coronary artery disease. Most bradyarrhythmias causing syncope require pacemakers, unless drug side effects or metabolic disturbances are the principal factors.

Orthostatic hypotension often responds to modifications in drug regimens. In particular, avoidance of vasodilator drugs may help. Ensure that patients have adequate volume by reducing or discontinuing diuretics and, if necessary, liberalizing salt intake. If autonomic dysfunction is present and hypertension, heart failure, and hypokalemia are not concerns, then low-dose fludrocortisone may be effective.

When vasovagal syncope occurs as the result of a specific trigger (eg, sights, smells), avoidance is best if this is feasible. A number of pharmacologic therapies have been proposed, including β-blockers, paroxetine, midodrine, and others. The pharmacologic approach to the treatment of vasovagal syncope remains somewhat controversial and may require sequential trials of several agents.

Carotid sinus hypersensitivity is best treated by avoiding stimulating factors (tight collars or rapid neck motions). If these measures are ineffective, pacemaker implantation may be useful.

Postprandial hypotension may be improved by avoidance of alcohol and large carbohydrate meals. Caffeine consumption and remaining recumbent following meals may also help.

When syncope in the geriatric patient has several causes, addressing a single factor in isolation may be only partially effective, and a broader approach addressing several contributing causes is required. Careful review of medications, as well as discontinuation of medications that increase the risk of syncope, is always an early step.

For patients with recurrent syncope without an identifiable cause, care must be taken to help them avoid harming themselves or others if they remain at risk for syncope. The issue of driving may need to be addressed. Guidelines from the American Heart Association recommend that driving be restricted for several months and that, if the patient remains recurrence free, driving be resumed. However, physicians should be aware that many states have laws regarding driving with a history of syncope.

REFERENCES

■ Colgan J. Syncope: a fall from grace. *Prog Cardiovasc Nurs.* 2002;17(2):66–71.

■ Linzer MD, Yang EH, Estes M, et al. Diagnosing syncope: part 1: value of history, physical examination and electrocardiography. *Ann Intern Med.* 1997;126:989–996.

■ Linzer MD, Yang EH, Estes M, et al. Diagnosing syncope: part 2: unexplained syncope. *Ann Intern Med.* 1997;127:76–86.

■ Youde J, Ruse C, Parker S, et al. A high diagnostic rate in older patients attending an integrated syncope clinic. *J Am Geriatr Soc.* 2000;48:783–787.

CHAPTER 25—HEARING IMPAIRMENT

Hearing loss is the fourth most common chronic disease among older persons. Hearing impairment is often assumed to be benign, but it has been shown to have profound effects on quality of life. The psychologic effects of hearing loss include family discord, social isolation, loss of self-esteem, anger, and depression. Epidemiologic studies suggest an association between hearing loss and cognitive impairment, and between hearing loss and reduced mobility. Hearing loss can also affect an older person's interaction with clinicians, making history taking and patient education difficult. Treatment of hearing loss and attention to communication strategies can improve the hearing-impaired person's quality of life by facilitating interaction with family, friends, and caregivers. Studies indicate that hearing aid use can relieve symptoms of depression associated with hearing loss.

NORMAL HEARING AND AGE-RELATED CHANGES IN THE AUDITORY SYSTEM

The normal ear is an efficient transducer of sound energy into nerve impulses. Sound energy is transmitted through the external ear to the tympanic membrane and the auditory ossicles. The malleus, incus, and stapes in series transmit vibrations to the oval window of the cochlea. Fluid waves within the cochlea stimulate the outer hair cells of the scala tympani. These cells stimulate the inner hair cells, which generate sensory potential. In turn, an excitatory postsynaptic potential is generated. When threshold is reached, impulses are sent via cochlear neurons to the cochlear nuclei and thence to auditory pathways elsewhere in the brain.

Age-related changes in the auditory system can interfere with its function. The walls of the external ear canal become thin. Cerumen becomes drier and more tenacious, increasing the likelihood of cerumen impaction. The eardrum becomes thicker and appears duller than in younger persons. Degenerative changes of the ossicular joints occur but generally do not interfere with sound transmission to the cochlea. Cochlear changes include loss of sensory hair cells and fibrocytes in the organ of Corti, stiffening of the basilar membrane, calcification of auditory structures, and cochlear neuronal loss. Changes in the stria vascularis include thickening of capillaries, decreased production of endolymph, and decreased Na+ K+ ATPase activity. These degenerative changes occur to varying degrees in different individuals. It currently is not possible to fully correlate the degree of hearing loss with histologic changes in the aging ear.

Changes in central auditory processing also occur with aging. One study found that when competing speech stimuli are presented to each ear, the right ear has a 5% to 10% advantage over the left ear in younger persons. (The effect of right- and left-handedness was not assessed; all the participants were right-handed.) In persons aged 80 to 89 years, this difference increases to more than 40%. This difference may be related to a loss of efficiency of interhemispheric transfer of auditory information through the corpus callosum.

EPIDEMIOLOGY OF HEARING LOSS

The prevalence of hearing loss increases with age. Ten percent of adults between the ages of 65 and 75 and 25% of those older than 75 years have hearing loss. In nursing homes, estimates of prevalence vary from 50% to 100%, depending on the criteria used to define hearing loss.

Hearing loss can be caused by pathology in the external ear canal, the middle ear, the inner ear, the auditory nerve, central auditory pathways, or a combination of these. Conductive hearing loss is due to disease in the external ear, such as ceruminosis or foreign body in the canal, or to middle-ear pathology such as otosclerosis, cholesteatoma, tympanic membrane perforation, or middle-ear effusion.

Sensorineural hearing loss is most often caused by cochlear disease. Noise is the most common factor in cochlear damage. Hearing loss is less common among persons in quiet rural environments than among people in industrialized communities. Other causes of hearing loss include ototoxic medications, genotype, vascular disease, and, rarely, occupational and environmental chemical exposures. Smokers have higher rates of hearing loss than nonsmokers. Autoimmune disease and auditory nerve tumors are rare causes of sensorineural hearing loss. Neuronal loss can affect the brain stem and cortical ascending auditory pathways, including the cochlear nuclei, superior olivary complex, lateral lemniscus, inferior colliculi, and medial geniculate complex. The resulting deficits in central auditory processing can affect perception of sound and the ability to understand speech.

PRESBYCUSIS

The majority of hearing loss in older persons is categorized as presbycusis (literally, "older hearing"). Presbycusis is a sensorineural, usually symmetrical hearing loss that may have central components. Presbycusis can be classified as sensory, neural, strial, cochlear conductive, combined, or indeterminate, depending on cochlear pathology. Many persons with presbycusis can be helped by amplification.

Sensory presbycusis results in a steeply sloping audiogram. It is often slowly progressive, beginning with the higher frequencies of 8000 Hz, 6000 Hz, and 4000 Hz. It may involve the 3000 and 2000 Hz range, which is the higher portion of the range of frequencies in human speech. Persons with this type of hearing loss often have trouble hearing in the presence of background noise but will be able to hear adequately in quiet settings. Amplification often helps these patients, since speech discrimination is satisfactory. This loss of auditory acuity can begin as early as the 20s but may not become clinically evident until later decades. Sensory presbycusis is attributed to a loss of sensory hair cells in the basal end of the cochlea.

Strial presbycusis is considered a metabolic form of hearing loss. The stria vascularis maintains high potassium concentrations in the endolymph. Strial presbycusis, pathologically defined as atrophy of 30% or more of the stria vascularis, is a form of cochlear dysfunction. This disorder has onset in the 20s to 50s and is characterized by mild to moderate hearing loss in most frequencies. Persons with strial presbycusis usually have good speech discrimination and do well with amplification.

Neural presbycusis is due to a cochlear neuronal loss of 50% or more compared with the normal number in neonates. Despite preserved pure-tone thresholds, which are not affected until more than 90% of cochlear neurons have been lost, patients with neural presbycusis show very poor speech discrimination. Successful use of amplification is difficult for this form of presbycusis. Cochlear conductive presbycusis is caused by changes in cochlear mechanics produced by mass or stiffness changes or spiral ligament atrophy. It has a unique audiogram, which gradually descends over at least five octaves with no more than a 25-dB difference between any two adjacent frequencies. Speech discrimination may also be impaired. Pathologically, this form is defined by the absence of histologic changes seen in the other forms of presbycusis.

Most presbycusis is probably a mixture of these forms. The shape of the audiogram and speech discrimination scores depends on the extent of injury to various components of the cochlea. (See Figure 25.1 for typical audiograms for the forms of hearing loss.)

DIAGNOSIS OF HEARING LOSS

Due in part to the slowly progressive nature of hearing loss, many older persons are unaware of their hearing deficit. In some cases, the stigma of wearing a hearing aid causes the patient to deny the problem. The hearing loss may be brought to medical attention by family members, who complain that the patient does not hear them or plays the television or radio too loud. Clinicians may notice that the patient does not respond when spoken to out of his or her field of view, or seems to misunderstand questions. Hearing loss can also masquerade as cognitive impairment. Caregivers and clinicians commonly do not recognize the presence

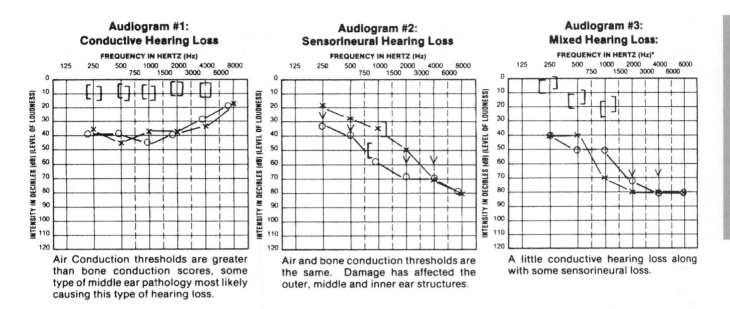

Audiogram #1:
Conductive Hearing Loss

Air Conduction thresholds are greater than bone conduction scores, some type of middle ear pathology most likely causing this type of hearing loss.

Audiogram #2:
Sensorineural Hearing Loss

Air and bone conduction thresholds are the same. Damage has affected the outer, middle and inner ear structures.

Audiogram #3:
Mixed Hearing Loss:

A little conductive hearing loss along with some sensorineural loss.

Figure 25.1—Audiograms for conductive, sensorineural, and mixed hearing loss, with instructions for interpretation. Key: [= right bone conduction (masked);] = left bone conduction (masked); V = forehead placement of bone conductor; o = right air conduction; x = left air conduction.

SOURCE: Mansour-Shousher R, Mansour WN. Nonsurgical management of hearing loss. *Clin Geriatr Med*. 1999;15(1):171. Reprinted with permission.

of hearing loss or may assume it is a benign component of aging.

A handheld otoscope with a tone generator, the Welch-Allyn pure-tone audioscope, can be used by primary care providers to screen for the presence of hearing loss at selected frequencies (0.5, 1, 2, and 4 KHz) and two loudness levels (25 and 40 dB HL). This device should be used in a quiet environment. When set at 40 dB HL, testing at 1 and 2 KHz has a sensitivity of 94% and a specificity between 82% and 90% for detecting hearing loss. A screening questionnaire such as the Hearing Handicap Inventory for the Elderly—Screening Version is useful to determine the impact that hearing loss has on a patient's daily activities (see the Appendix, p 399). A patient who fails one of these screening methods should be referred to an audiologist and an otolaryngologist. The patient's ear canals should be examined before referral to exclude the presence of obstruction. Cerumen impaction can cause a clinically significant hearing loss, as much as 40 dB.

The otolaryngologist will further evaluate the hearing loss and identify treatable causes. An asymmetrical hearing loss demands thorough investigation. Auditory nerve tumors are rare, but tumors of the posterior pharynx can obstruct the eustachian tube, causing a middle-ear effusion with conductive hearing loss.

The audiologist will assess hearing to determine the presence and the type of hearing loss. A comprehensive audiologic assessment consists of pure-tone thresholds for both air and bone conduction, speech-recognition thresholds, speech discrimination, and middle-ear function. This information, along with the medical evaluation, will be used to determine treatment for the patient. Audiologists recommend and fit hearing aids and provide auditory rehabilitation.

TREATMENT OF HEARING LOSS

Some causes of hearing loss are amenable to medical or surgical treatment. Paget's disease of the bone can affect the middle ear, causing conductive loss, or the inner ear, leading to sensorineural loss. This loss sometimes responds to bisphosphonates. Otosclerosis or tympanosclerosis may be correctable with surgery. Sudden hearing loss may be autoimmune in nature and sometimes responds to corticosteroids or immune-suppressant therapy. The majority of hearing loss cases, however, must be treated with amplification or communication strategies, or both. Hearing aids often improve ability to understand speech, particularly soft speech and conversational loud speech.

Hearing Aids

Hearing aids are the most common form of amplification. Many factors need to be considered in deciding whether to fit the patient with a hearing aid. In addition to the nature and degree of hearing loss, the patient's motivation, ability to adapt to its use and to physically manipulate the aid, the degree of social support, and financial issues must be considered (Table 25.1).

In general, two hearing aids are more beneficial than one. The first aid provides the most gain; the second one helps with speech discrimination and with localizing where sounds are coming from. However, the presence of asymmetrical hearing loss or significant difficulty in understanding competing speech stimuli may mean that the use of a single hearing aid is more appropriate.

Not everyone benefits from a hearing aid. The pattern of sensorineural damage may be such that speech discrimination is poor even with amplification. Some patients are unable to tolerate the presence of the hearing aid in the ear. Patients with dementia may remove the aid and dispose of it in the wastebasket or the toilet. It is important to be sure that the aid can be returned during an initial trial period, usually 30 days, without having to pay the full cost of the aid. It is equally important not to give up on the aid too soon, since the audiologist often can adjust it to improve

comfort and sound quality, and should provide counseling for its optimum use.

Many different styles of hearing aids are available (Table 25.2). Behind-the-ear aids hang behind the ear and are connected directly to an earmold. The earmold is custom made to fit each patient's ear. Some behind-the-ear aids can be connected to assistive listening devices via a "boot," which fits over the end of the aid to provide direct audio input. Body aids are worn on the belt or in a pocket or a harness, and are connected to a custom-made earmold by a wire. These are rarely used. All-in-the ear aids and canal aids have cases that are custom fit to the user. The smaller hearing aids may have remote controls. Selection of aid style for each individual depends on the degree of hearing loss, available features, and the dexterity and motivation of the wearer.

The telecoil is an induction coupling coil that can be built into the hearing aid. It detects the magnetic field produced by telephones compatible with hearing aids. The telecoil is used to listen to the telephone with less distraction from noise in the same room. It can also be used with many assistive listening devices.

Table 25.1—Effects and Rehabilitation of Hearing Loss, by Level of Loss

Level of Loss	Description	Effect	Need for Hearing Aid
25 to 40 dB HL	Mild	Difficulty understanding normal speech	Needed in specific situations
41 to 55 dB HL	Moderate	Difficulty understanding loud speech	Frequent need
56 to 80 dB HL	Severe	Can understand only amplified speech	Need for all communication
81 dB HL or more	Profound	Difficulty understanding amplified speech	May need to supplement with speech-reading, aural rehabilitation, or sign language

SOURCE: *A Report on Hearing Aids: User Perspectives and Concerns.* Washington, DC: American Association of Retired Persons; 1993:2. Copyright 1993, American Association of Retired Persons Reprinted with permission.

Table 25.2—Advantages and Disadvantages of Hearing Aid Styles

Style	Degree of Hearing Loss	Advantages	Disadvantages
CIC	Mild to moderate	Almost invisible Less occlusion of ear canal allows more natural sound Easier to use with headphones and telephone	Dexterity may be a problem Small size may limit available features May cost more than canal or ITE aids Shorter battery life
Canal	Mild to moderate	More cosmetic than larger aids Telecoil available in some models May be able to use with headphones	Dexterity may be a problem Small size may limit available features
ITE	Mild to severe	Ease of handling Comfortable fit Available options: telecoil, directional microphone More power than CIC or canal aid	More conspicuous than CIC or canal aid May be difficult to use with headphones
BTE	Mild to profound	Greatest power Available options: telecoil, direct audio input, directional microphone Earmold can be changed separately	More conspicuous May be more difficult to insert than ITE Difficult to use with headphones
Body aid	Severe to profound	Greatest separation of microphone from receiver reduces feedback	Most conspicuous

NOTE: BTE = behind the ear; CIC = completely in the canal; ITE = in the ear.

The amount of coupling, and therefore the volume of the signal, depends on the angle of the telecoil with respect to the magnetic field. Users may need to experiment to find the right angle. Strongly magnetic devices such as computer monitors often produce interference, which is also dependent on the angle and the distance of the telecoil from the device. These drawbacks aside, the telecoil is a useful feature and can be added to hearing aids at a relatively small cost. Consumers with moderate to severe hearing loss should be encouraged to consider purchasing an aid with a telecoil.

The choice of analog or digital hearing aids depends on the individual consumer. Analog aids are less expensive than digital aids and may provide acceptable sound quality. However, newer digital technology has allowed improved sound quality, reduced size, and increased ability to customize the amplification of the aid to the needs of the user. Programmable aids are adjusted for each individual while he or she is wearing the aid. Often, two or more programs are available within a single aid. Using a computer, the audiologist makes adjustments to gain, response in different frequency ranges, and loudness balance for each program. One program may be most useful in the presence of background noise, whereas another works better in a quiet environment, and a third works with a telecoil. Persons with Ménière's disease can have their aids reprogrammed to accommodate fluctuating hearing loss. Some hearing aids automatically adjust the volume to increase amplification of soft sounds while avoiding uncomfortable loudness, reducing the need for the user to manipulate the aid. A study comparing different methods of limiting loudness suggested that consumers with mild to moderate hearing loss were more likely to prefer compression-limiting or wide dynamic range compression circuitry to peak-clipping circuitry, though the absolute differences in consumer preference and speech comprehension between these methods was small.

The use of multiple microphones in the hearing aid, combined with digital signal processing, can decrease background noise. This can significantly improve the wearer's ability to understand speech and increase consumer satisfaction with the aid.

Strategies to Enhance Communication

Hearing-impaired persons should be encouraged to let others know about their hearing loss and to suggest strategies that will help them communicate more easily (Table 25.3). In addition to using these strategies, clinicians should provide options for patients with hearing loss, such as sign language interpreters, the use of pen and paper, or assistive devices. Office and

Table 25.3—Strategies to Improve Communication With Hearing-Impaired Persons

Obtain the listener's attention before speaking.

Eliminate background noise as much as possible.

Be sure the listener can see the speaker's lips.
  Speak face to face in the same room.
  Do not obscure the lips with hands, mustaches, or other objects.
  Make certain that light shines directly on the speaker's face, not from behind the speaker.

Speak slowly and clearly, but avoid shouting.

Speak toward the better ear, if applicable.

Use alternate phrasing if the speaker is not understood.

Spell words out, use gestures, or write them down.

Have the listener repeat back what he or she heard

hospital staff should be alerted to a patient's hearing loss. Background noise from the environment can interfere with hearing and should be reduced as much as possible.

Lipreading can be a useful adjunct to listening, but it requires thoughtfulness on the part of the speaker. When speaking to a hearing-impaired person who lip-reads, it is important to face him or her and obtain the person's attention before speaking; a gentle touch on the hand or arm will usually suffice. Speak each word clearly and distinctly. Shouting not only distorts lip movements so they are harder to read, but the speaker may sound angry even when not. Use complete sentences. Single words are hard to lip-read because the listener often needs cues from context to identify meaning. It is helpful to make certain the person knows the topic of conversation. Use appropriate language for the listener's educational level. Unlike deaf persons who have been deaf all or most of their lives, most older persons with hearing loss do not know sign language. Sometimes amplification and lip-reading are not enough. Gestures can aid communication even with cognitively impaired patients.

For patients with hearing impairment, it can also be helpful to write words down. For those with both hearing and visual impairment, large printing with a marker pen or a laptop computer screen with magnified print may be necessary. These patients may benefit from correction of the visual problem, if possible (eg, cataract removal or use of eyeglasses). In any case, providing written instructions improves understanding and retention of important information.

Be alert to misunderstandings. If a reply does not make sense, try repeating what was said, using different words. Have the patient repeat what he or she heard, since misunderstandings are common.

Assistive Listening Devices

For some persons with hearing impairment, a personal amplifier may be more useful than hearing aids. These pocket-sized devices are considerably less expensive, can be used for different people, and are harder to misplace. Headphones stay on the head better than earbuds and provide sound to both ears. The volume and microphone placement of the amplifier should be adjusted to find the best combination for a given user. Every health care facility should have at least one or two of these devices available.

Adaptive equipment can facilitate telephone use. State agencies for deaf and hard-of-hearing persons may provide amplified telephones, vibrating and flashing ringer alert devices, and text telephones (TTY) at no cost to hearing-impaired persons. This equipment is available from electronics and telephone equipment stores.

Many other assistive devices are available. Television listening devices can spare others from overly loud volume levels. FM loop systems can be used for groups of people with FM receivers or telecoil switches in their hearing aids. Wireless FM transmitters and receivers are also available for indoor or outdoor use. Infrared group listening devices are primarily useful indoors. Vibrating and flashing devices such as alarm clocks and timers, smoke alarms, doorbell alerts, and motion sensors can improve the hearing-impaired person's convenience and safety.

Cochlear Implants

For persons with severe to profound hearing loss who gain little or no benefit from hearing aids yet who are motivated to participate in the hearing world, cochlear implants can provide useful hearing. A cochlear implant is an electronic device that bypasses the function of damaged or absent cochlear hair cells by providing electrical stimulation to cochlear nerve fibers. A receiver-stimulator and an intracochlear electrode array are surgically implanted. A headset is worn behind the ear. The headset microphone transmits signals to the speech processor, which filters and digitizes the sound into coded signals. The coded signals are sent to the cochlear implant, which then stimulates auditory nerve fibers in the cochlea. Nerve signals are then sent through the auditory system to the brain. Patients must be able to tolerate general anesthesia and to participate in extensive pre-implant testing and post-implant training. The procedure is covered by most Medicare carriers and insurance companies. In general, outcomes of cochlear implantation in persons 65 and older have been comparable to those of younger adults, with patients obtaining excellent results by both audiologic and quality-of-life measures.

REFERENCES

■ American Academy of Audiology: Consumer Resources. Frequently Asked Questions About Hearing Aids. http://www.audiology.org/consumer/guides/hafaq.php

■ Buchman CA, Fucci MJ, Luxford WM. Cochlear implants in the geriatric population: benefits outweigh risks. *Ear Nose Throat J.* 1999;78(7):489–494.

■ Cohn ES. Hearing loss with aging. *Clin Geriatr Med.* 1999;15(1):145–161.

■ Department of Otolaryngology–Head and Neck Surgery, University of Washington Medical Center. Patient Care: Cochlear Implants. http://depts.washington.edu/otoweb/patients/pts_specialties/pts_hear-n-bal/pts_hear-n-bal_cochlear_implant.htm

■ Eliopoulos C. Sensory deficits. In: Epiopoulos C. *Gerontological Nursing, 5th ed.* Philadelphia, PA: Lippincott Williams & Williams; 2001:283–299.

■ Larson VD, Willam DW, Henderson WA. Efficacy of 3 commonly used hearing aid circuits: a crossover trial. *JAMA.* 2000;284:1806–1813.

■ Loovis CF, Schall DG, Teter DL. The role of assistive devices in the rehabilitation of hearing impairment. *Otolaryngologic Clin North Am.* 1997;30(5):803–847.

■ Mansour-Shousher R, Mansour WN. Nonsurgical management of hearing loss. *Clin Geriatr Med.* 1999;15(1):163–177.

CHAPTER 26—VISUAL IMPAIRMENT

Visual impairment, defined as visual acuity less than 20/40, increases exponentially with age such that 20% to 30% of the population aged 75 years or older is so affected. Blindness, visual acuity of 20/200 or worse, affects 2% of the population aged 75 years and older. Those aged 65 and over make up 12% of the total U.S. population, but 50% of the blind population. Refractive error, cataract, age-related macular degeneration, diabetic retinopathy, and glaucoma are the most common causes of blindness. The respective order of importance varies according to the region and race surveyed. As the baby boomers age, the older population will increase by 75% by the year 2030, and the prevalence of these conditions will surge.

Visual impairment has considerable impact on the medical system and the older population. Chronic eye conditions represent one of the most common reasons for office-based visits to the physician among the population aged 65 and over. Of all office visits by older persons, 14% are to ophthalmologists, one of the highest rates of all specialty visits. Falls and car crashes, each associated with impaired vision in older persons, consume considerable medical resources. Moreover, impaired vision has been linked to a significant deterioration in the quality of life and the activities of daily living of older persons.

The American Academy of Ophthalmology recommends a comprehensive eye examination every 1 to 2 years for persons aged 65 and over. The U.S. Preventive Services Task Force recommends annual vision testing. Prophylactic and therapeutic ocular management can effectively alter the course of various conditions causing visual impairment. About one third of all new cases of blindness can be avoided with effective use of available ophthalmological services.

REFRACTIVE ERROR AND CATARACT

The leading cause of visual impairment worldwide is refractive error and cataract, for which eyeglasses and surgical cataract extraction, respectively, are mainstays of treatment. Despite the considerable successes of these therapeutic options, many populations do not receive adequate treatment for these problems.

Refractive error may be categorized as emmetropia (neutral refraction), ametropia, or presbyopia. Three forms of ametropia exist: myopia (nearsightedness), hyperopia (farsightedness), and astigmatism. Typically, older patients demonstrate increasing hyperopia, unless a cataract is present, which can induce a myopic shift. Although contact lens wear and laser refractive surgery are available for myopic and hyperopic refractive errors, these alternative forms of treatment traditionally have been used more by younger persons. After the age of approximately 40, emmetropes begin to develop progressive presbyopia, impaired ability to focus at near objects, caused by gradual hardening of the lens and decreased muscular effectiveness of the ciliary body. Reading glasses or bifocal eyeglasses may be prescribed.

Approximately 20% of persons aged 65 years and over and 50% aged 75 years and over have a cataract, a vision-reducing lens opacity. Cataracts may be associated with increased glare, decreased contrast sensitivity, and decreased visual acuity. Several risk factors have been reported: decreased vitamin intake, light (ultraviolet B) exposure, smoking, alcohol use, long-term corticosteroid use, and diabetes mellitus. The most important risk factor is increased age.

Cataract extraction is one the most successful surgeries in medicine (90% of patients achieve vision of 20/40 or better). Approximately 1.5 million cataract procedures are performed each year in the United States alone. In inner cities and underdeveloped countries such as India, the demand for surgery has surpassed available resources.

Cataract extraction is a technically demanding operation requiring superior fine motor skills and extensive surgical experience. In the hands of a seasoned surgeon, however, the procedure is very safe and can be completed in less than 15 minutes under local or topical anesthesia. The surgery involves the sonographic breakdown and aspiration of the lens (phacoemulsification). An artificial implant (intraocular lens) is placed in the capsular bag that is the only remnant of the native lens retained. A secondary laser procedure (capsulotomy) may be necessary to ablate subsequent capsular opacification that may develop in 15% or more of patients.

AGE-RELATED MACULAR DEGENERATION

Age-related macular degeneration (ARMD) is the most common cause of blindness in older persons throughout the developed world. Increased age is the most important risk factor, although a genetic predisposition also contributes. Other risk factors include smoking and hypertension. Fair-skinned persons are at greater risk of developing this disease than those who are black, in whom pigment may serve as a protective element.

An international committee of retinologists have developed standards for the definition of ARMD or age-related maculopathy (ARM). These criteria are important in differentiating those with ARM who are at risk of visual loss from those with typical aging changes in the macula who are not at risk for visual loss. The committee proposed that early ARM be defined as the presence of drusen of significant size or confluence. Geographic atrophy or choroidal neovascularization (Figure 26.1) characterize late ARM. Only 10% of ARM patients have the late variety. By contrast, almost 100% of ARM patients with severe visual loss have late ARM.

Numerous genetic conditions resulting in premature macular degeneration exist for which the mutated sequence has been cloned and the protein product isolated. Mutations in ABC-R (ATP-binding cassette protein of the retina), a photoreceptor protein involved in molecular transport and exchange, leads to the development of Stargardt's disease, in which patients classically develop macular flecks and atrophy associated with central visual loss by the second or third decade of life. Stargardt's macular dystrophy has been found to have perhaps some association with ARM. Certain populations of ARM patients have been found to have an increased incidence of the heterozygous form of this mutation; other data has been conflicting. Sorsby's fundus dystrophy is associated with many of the features of ARM. Visual loss however, typically develops before the age of 50. The affected gene has been sequenced and codes for a protein involved in extracellular remodeling, TIMP-3 (tissue-inhibitor of metalloprotease). Genetic studies have failed to uncover an association of this mutation with ARM.

Vitamin and antioxidant supplementation to prevent ARM is controversial. Although associations have been made between dietary intake and serum levels of vitamins and antioxidants with the presence of ARM,

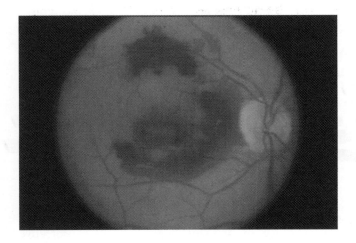

Figure 26.1—Choroidal neovascularization in a patient with late age-related maculopathy demonstrating a gray-green membrane associated with subretinal hemorrhage.

no reliable cause-and-effect data exist. The results of a nationally sponsored, prospective study of the effects of antioxidant supplementation such as oral zinc on the course of ARMD are still pending. Prophylactic laser therapy for those patients with drusen who are at high risk of developing neovascularization does not prevent visual loss. Laser therapy for choroidal neovascular membranes has been beneficial but only under very special circumstances, when membranes are well defined (ie, the margins of the lesion are clearly delineated) and extra- or juxtafoveal. Photodynamic therapy using porphyrin-derived dyes has been shown to be useful in those patients with subfoveal choroidal neovascular membranes in whom conventional laser therapy will destroy the fovea. According to the Treatment of Age-related Macular Degeneration with Photodynamic Therapy (TAP) Study Group, 43% of patients receiving photodynamic therapy sustained moderate visual loss (> 15 letters from baseline) after 1 year follow-up versus 57% of patients not receiving the photoactivated dye laser treatment. Moreover, 16% of those receiving photoactivated dye laser sustained an improvement in visual acuity, but only 7% in the placebo group showed improvement. Although the benefits are not overwhelming, photodynamic therapy is a relatively safe alternative that is the most effective procedure available for delaying visual loss in patients with ARM-related subfoveal choroidal neovascularization.

DIABETIC RETINOPATHY

Duration of disease and control of blood sugar represent the most important variables in the development and progression of diabetic retinopathy. After 10 years, 70% of those with type 2 diabetes demonstrate some form of retinopathy, and nearly 10% show proliferative disease. Diet control, exercise, and proper glucose management with frequent daily glucose testing and the use of oral hypoglycemics or insulin, or both, are crucial in maintaining glycosylated hemoglobin levels lower than 7%. The Diabetic Control and Complications Trial demonstrated that tight blood-sugar control in those with type 1 diabetes resulted in a decreased rate of development and progression of diabetic retinopathy. The United Kingdom Prospective Diabetic Study validated these results in the older population with type 2 diabetes. Tight blood-pressure control ($\leq$ 140/80) with either β-blockers or angiotensin-converting enzyme (ACE) inhibitors was also found to be an important factor in decreasing microvascular (and macrovascular) complications, such as the need for retinal laser therapy.

Background diabetic retinopathy or nonproliferative diabetic retinopathy, the earliest stage of retinopathy, may first be manifested by retinal microaneurysms, best appreciated with fluorescein angiography. Intraretinal hemorrhages and exudates, with or without associated edema, may ensue. Progressive ischemia characterized by increasing hemorrhages, venous caliber changes, intraretinal microvascular abnormalities, and capillary nonperfusion characterize the preproliferative stage of diabetic retinopathy. About 40% of patients with preproliferative retinopathy develop proliferative diabetic retinopathy (PDR) within 1 to 2 years, characterized by neovascularization, or new blood vessel growth of the retina or disc, or both.

Visual loss in the setting of diabetic retinopathy may occur as a result of macular nonperfusion or macular edema. The Early Treatment Diabetic Retinopathy Study demonstrated the benefit of focal or grid laser photocoagulation in stabilizing and improving vision in diabetics with clinically significant macular edema (Figure 26.2). Neovascularization (Figure 26.3) may cause severe visual loss in the setting of PDR as a result of vitreous hemorrhage or tractional retinal detachment. PDR is amenable to treatment by panretinal laser photocoagulation to inhibit the growth stimulus for neovascularization. The Diabetic Retinopathy Study demonstrated an 11% incidence of severe visual loss in patients treated with panretinal photocoagulation but a 26% incidence in those who did not receive laser during a 2-year follow-up. Nonclearing vitreous hemorrhage or tractional macular detachment may be addressed surgically by pars plana vitrectomy, membrane peeling, and endolaser.

GLAUCOMA

Glaucoma is the second most common cause of blindness worldwide and, in the United States, the most common cause of blindness in black Americans.

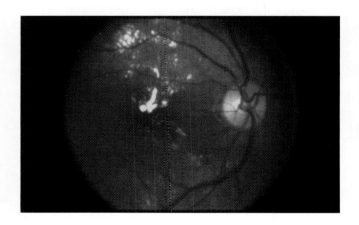

Figure 26.2—Intraretinal edema and exudate in the superior macular region consistent with clinically significant macular edema in a patient with type 2 diabetes mellitus.

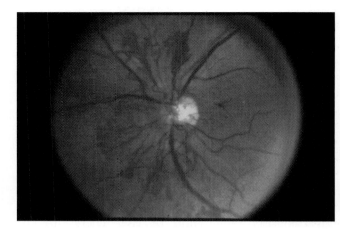

Figure 26.3—Florid neovascularization of the disc in a patient with high-risk proliferative diabetic retinopathy.

It affects more than 2.25 million Americans aged 40 years or over and results in more than 3 million office visits each year. The financial burden is considerable because of the prevalence and chronicity of this disease and the debilitation that results. Federal costs are reported to reach as high as $1 billion for glaucoma-related Medicare and Medicaid payments and disability.

The definition of glaucoma, now defined as characteristic optic nerve head damage and visual field loss, has undergone a considerable evolution. Elevated intraocular pressure (IOP) is no longer considered an absolute criterion, although it is a very important risk factor. There are many different types of glaucoma, of which primary open-angle glaucoma (POAG) is the most common.

POAG is a chronic disease most commonly affecting older patients. Aqueous may access the filtration site, but the network is "clogged," resulting in impaired passage out of the angle. Slow aqueous drainage leads to chronically elevated IOPs. This is in contrast to acute angle-closure glaucoma, in which the entry site is suddenly blocked off, IOP rises precipitously, and the patient presents with considerable pain and discomfort. The IOP rise in POAG is slow and much less severe. Patients with POAG are asymptomatic and may suffer substantial field loss before consulting an ophthalmologist.

Development of POAG is most likely multifactorial and polygenic. Initial pedigrees were found to demonstrate linkage to the 1q locus. Subsequent investigations have more precisely defined the GLC1A gene that encodes for myocillin, the trabecular meshwork-induced glucocorticoid response protein. Several other chromosomal loci, including those mapped to chromosomes 2, 3, 7, and 10, have also been found to be associated with the development of glaucoma.

Management of POAG may be approached in a stepwise manner. A variety of IOP-lowering medications, both local and systemic, exist. Mechanisms of action include decreased aqueous production or increased aqueous outflow. Various eyedrop formulations are available; latanoprost, a prostaglandin analog which increases uveal-scleral outflow, and brimonidine, an α_2-adrenergic agonist that decreases aqueous production, are two relatively new and effective drugs. In the face of visual field progression despite maximal medications or intolerance to medications, argon laser trabeculoplasty (application of laser energy to the trabecular meshwork) can be effective in lowering IOP in approximately 50% of patients for 3 to 5 years after treatment. Intraocular surgery involves the creation of a fistula or filtration site to allow an alternative route of aqueous egress (trabeculectomy). Adjunctive antimetabolite use with 5-fluorouracil or mitomycin-C has increased the success of this procedure in those patients at high risk of failure because of fibrosis and scarring of the filtration site. Alternative surgeries for glaucoma include drainage devices or aqueous shunts. Drainage devices, which are made of a foreign material such as plastic, shunt fluid from the anterior chamber to the subconjunctival space. Ciliary body destructive procedures with cryotherapy or laser (cyclocryoablation or cyclophotocoagulation) may be used in eyes with a poor visual prognosis.

ANTERIOR ISCHEMIC OPTIC NEUROPATHY

Anterior ischemic optic neuropathy (Figure 26.4) may result in acute vision or field loss. Microvascular

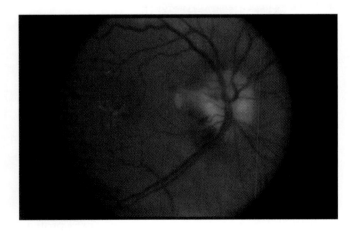

Figure 26.4—Pallid swelling of the optic nerve head in a patient with anterior ischemic optic neuropathy.

occlusion of the blood supply to the optic nerve may be attributed to atherosclerotic vascular disease or inflammation in the setting of giant cell (or temporal) arteritis. The former, the nonarteritic form, typically affects patients with vasculopathic risk factors such as diabetes mellitus and hypertension; the latter, the arteritic form, tends to occur in older patients with a history of myalgias, headaches, and weight loss. An elevated Westergren erythrocyte sedimentation rate and a positive temporal artery biopsy are diagnostic. Systemic corticosteroid treatment is crucial to avoid visual loss in the other eye.

MISCELLANEOUS

Tears serve several important functions, including corneal lubrication, debris clearance, and immune protection. With age, tear production decreases, and older patients are prone to develop dry eye syndrome or keratitis sicca, characterized by redness, foreign body sensation, and reflex tearing. Management includes tear replacement with artificial tears during the day and an ointment at bedtime. Temporary and permanent punctal plugs may be employed to retard tear egress through the nasolacrimal drainage system in more severe cases. Keratitis sicca may be associated with autoimmune disease; conditions such as Sjögren's syndrome should be excluded.

Lid abnormalities are a common problem for older persons. Because of the gradual loss of elasticity and tensile strength that develops with age, secondary degenerative changes may take place. Blepharochalasis (drooping of the brow) and blepharoptosis (drooping of the eyelid) may cause cosmetic deformity and, if severe, may impair vision. Lid ectropion or entropion, eversion and inversion of the lid margins, respectively, can disrupt the ocular surface and cause discomfort for the patient. Various surgical procedures are available to address these problems.

Herpes zoster ophthalmicus, or shingles, is a painful reactivation of varicella zoster virus that not uncommonly affects older persons. Dermatomal distribution of weeping vesicles affecting the ophthalmic division of the trigeminal nerve is the classic presentation. Ocular involvement may be signaled by lesions on the tip of the nose (Hutchinson's sign) and may include dendritic keratopathy or uveitis. Oral acyclovir may shorten the course of disease. Post-herpetic neuralgia may be quite debilitating; various local ointments (eg, capsaicin, lidocaine) or systemic medications (eg, corticosteroids, tricyclic antidepressants) may be helpful. (See also "Dermatologic Diseases and Disorders," p 372.)

LOW-VISION REHABILITATION

Despite considerable advancements in the medical treatment of ocular conditions, many patients, especially those with late ARM, may ultimately sustain permanent visual loss. Visual training and the provision of visual aids are indispensable services available to the patient with low vision (visual acuity < 20/60).

Patients with low vision may develop useful adaptive skills with proper instruction. Eccentric viewing uses the principle of off-center fixation in ARM patients with central macular pathology. The patient can benefit from formal training to find and use the most effective eccentric viewing points. Instruction in scanning and tracking and other skills may help the patient integrate his or her visual environment.

Various low-vision aids are available to improve one's ability to see both near and far. The fine detail required for reading is the most common indication for visual aids. Improved lighting is a simple modification that can enhance visualization of print. Selection of reading material using bold, enlarged fonts and accentuated black-on-white contrast may also be helpful. Magnification also is commonly employed. Various devices such as high-plus spectacles, hand-held magnifiers, stand magnifiers, and closed-circuit television can also enhance reading. Distance magnification may be achieved with the use of telescopic devices that can be hand-held for spot viewing or spectacle mounted for continuous viewing. Talking devices, which are computers used to create voice synthesis such as those used at stoplights, or Braille may be especially helpful for those who have lost vision altogether.

REFERENCES

- Bird AC, Bressler NM, Bressler SB, et al. An international classification and grading system for age-related maculopathy and age-related macular degeneration: The International ARM Epidemiological Study Group. *Survey Ophthalmol.* 1995;39(5):367–374.

- Eliopoulos C. Sensory deficits. In: Eliopoulos C. *Gerontological Nursing*, 5th ed. Philadelphia, PA: Lippincott, Williams & Williams; 2002:283–299.

- Ferris FL 3rd, David MD, Aiello LM. Treatment of diabetic retinopathy. *N Engl J Med.* 1999;341(9):667–678.

- Treatment of Age-related Macular Degeneration With Photodynamic Therapy (TAP) Study Group. Photodynamic therapy of subfoveal choroidal neovascularization in age-related macular degeneration with verteporfin: one-year results of 2 randomized clinical trials—TAP Report 1. *Arch Ophthalmol.* 1999; 117(10):1329–1345.

- U.K. Prospective Diabetes Study Group. Efficacy of atenolol and captopril in reducing risk of macrovascular and microvascular complications in type 2 diabetes: UKPDS 39. *BMJ.* 1998;317(7160):713–720.

- U.K. Prospective Diabetes Study Group. Intensive blood glucose control with sulfonylureas or insulin compared with conventional treatment and risk of complications in patients with type 2 diabetes (UKPDS 33). *Lancet.* 1998; 352(9131):837–853.

CHAPTER 27—OSTEOPOROSIS AND OSTEOMALACIA

Osteoporosis develops in older adults when the normal processes of bone formation and resorption become uncoupled or unbalanced, resulting in bone loss. Fractures are the result of decreased bone mass and strength, and, in the case of wrist and hip fractures, they usually involve a fall. Osteoporosis prevention and treatment programs should therefore focus on strategies that minimize bone resorption and maximize bone formation, as well as on strategies that reduce falls. Optimal treatment and prevention of osteoporosis require modification of risk factors, particularly smoking, physical activity, and diet, in addition to pharmacologic intervention. Osteomalacia, a less common disorder, occurs when bone is inadequately mineralized; the result is a syndrome of bone loss accompanied by bone pain, myopathy, fatigue, and fractures.

DEFINITION OF OSTEOPOROSIS

Osteoporosis was defined previously by a consensus panel as a "disease characterized by low bone mass and microarchitectural deterioration of bone tissue leading to enhanced bone fragility and a consequent increase in fracture incidence." According to this definition, the diagnosis of osteoporosis requires the presence of a fracture. The World Health Organization now defines osteoporosis by bone mineral density (BMD) measurement, which allows diagnosis and treatment of osteoporosis prior to incident fracture. If a woman has BMD measurement at any site < 2.5 standard deviations below the young adult standard (a T score of < −2.5), the diagnosis of osteoporosis can be made. Further, women with osteopenia (low bone mass, with a T score of ≥ −2.5 but < −1) and normal bone mass (with a T score of ≥ −1) can also be identified. Thus, the clinician can make the diagnosis of osteoporosis and begin the appropriate therapy prior to fracture in older adults. In addition, women with osteopenia can be placed on a preventive regimen and then followed carefully for further bone loss. Specific standards for definitions of osteoporosis have not been established for men or for racial and ethnic groups other than white persons, although it appears that similar standards apply to men and to Hispanic women.

THE EPIDEMIOLOGY AND CONSEQUENCES OF OSTEOPOROSIS

Ten million Americans already have osteoporosis, and 18 million more have low bone mass. Moreover, one out of two American women and one in every eight American men will experience an osteoporosis-related fracture in his or her lifetime. In the United States the estimated numbers of hip and vertebral fractures are more than 300,000 and 700,000, respectively, per year. To this number must be added fragility fractures in men, which occur at about one third the rate seen in women. Thus, approximately 1 million Americans suffer fragility fractures each year, at a cost of more than $14 billion. The consequences of osteoporosis include diminished quality of life, decreased independence, and increased morbidity and mortality. The pain and kyphosis, height loss, and other changes in body habitus that occur as a result of vertebral compression fractures erode quality of life for both women and men. In addition, the functional status of patients who have had vertebral crush fractures may also decrease. These patients may be unable to bathe, dress, or ambulate independently. Increased mortality is related primarily to hip fractures; 20% excess mortality occurs in older persons in the year following hip fracture. In addition, approximately 50% of women do not fully recover prior function after hip fracture. Thus, in older adults, it is important to prevent as many fractures as possible.

REVIEW OF BONE REMODELING

Bone is able to repair itself by actively remodeling, a coupled process (also called *bone turnover*) of bone resorption followed by bone formation; bone remodeling continues throughout life. Local signals, not yet fully understood, bring osteoclasts to specific areas of bone where resorption is initiated and resorption cavities are formed. Once osteoclasts have completed the resorption process, osteoblasts move into the area and begin to lay down osteoid and, later, to calcify the matrix. Under optimal conditions, once bone remodeling is completed in a specific area, the resorption spaces are completely filled with new bone. However, after menopause in women, and with aging in men and women, the remodeling cycle becomes unbalanced, and bone resorption increases more than formation does, resulting in net bone loss. The majority of treatments for osteoporosis act to inhibit bone resorption rather than to increase bone formation.

BONE LOSS

Bone mass changes over the life span of an individual. In women, bone mass increases rapidly from the time of puberty until approximately the mid-20s to mid-30s, at which time peak bone mass is reached. Once women reach peak bone mass, a few years of stability are followed by a slow rate of bone loss, beginning well before the onset of menopause. After menopause, the rate of bone loss is quite rapid—as much as 7% per year—for up to 7 years, as a consequence of estrogen deficiency. In later life bone loss continues, albeit at a slower rate, generally 1% to 2% per year; however, some older women may lose bone density at a higher rate. Data strongly suggest that terminating bone loss at any time will decrease fracture risk. It has been estimated that a 14% increase in bone density in 80-year-old women would halve hip-fracture risk. This 14% increase would also be realized if bone loss were prevented in 70-year-old women. Although studies thus far have focused mostly on women, it is well documented that men lose bone with age. Cross-sectional studies have detected a slower rate of bone loss in men than in women, but, in a longitudinal study, rates of bone loss in men were found to equal those of older women, although men start from a higher bone mass. It is estimated that men aged 30 to 90 years lose approximately 1% per year in the radius and spine; some men with risk factors lose as much as 6% per year. These data suggest that older men lose bone at rates similar to those of older women; however, vertebral fracture rates in men are lower. Both men and women lose predominantly cancellous bone, which is concentrated in the vertebral spine. Cortical bone accounts for 45% to 75% of the mechanical resistance to compression of the vertebral spine, and men actually gain cortical bone through periosteal bone deposition. Men also increase the cross-sectional area of their vertebrae by 15% to 20%, increasing maximum load levels until the age of 75. The increased bone strength seems to be reversed by thinning of the cortical ring by age 75, the age at which men begin to present with vertebral fractures. Although bone loss at the hip has not been extensively studied in men, in cross-sectional analyses healthy men were found to lose 40% of femoral neck BMD between the ages of 20 and 90 years.

PATHOGENESIS OF OSTEOPOROSIS

Estrogen Deficiency in Women

The pathogenesis of osteoporosis in women is complex. Factors that affect the level of peak bone mass, the rate of bone resorption, and the rate of bone formation need to be considered. Peak bone mass appears to be 75% to 80% genetically determined, although which genes are involved is not clear. A number of candidate genes that may be important to osteoporosis are being explored currently: vitamin D receptor, estrogen receptor, transforming growth factor, interleukin-6, interleukin-1 receptor 2, type I collagen genes, and collagenases. Several factors may work to increase bone resorption in older women. After menopause, and with estrogen deficiency, a variety of factors that act locally on bone may lead to increased bone resorption. Factors thought to play a role in the bone loss of estrogen deficiency include interleukin-1, interleukin-1 receptor antagonist, interleukin-6, and tumor necrosis factor, as well as their binding proteins and receptors. (For hormone replacement therapy regimens, see Table 49.1, p 330.)

Calcium Deficiency and Secondary Hyperparathyroidism

The mechanism by which older men and women continue to lose bone is likely related to calcium deficiency, which produces secondary hyperparathyroidism. Parathyroid hormone (PTH) is a potent stimulator of bone resorption when chronically elevated. Aging skin and decreased exposure to sunlight reduce the conversion of 7-dehydrocholesterol to cholecalciferol (vitamin D_3) by ultraviolet light, and the result is vitamin-D insufficiency in older adults. Vitamin-D insufficiency, in turn, reduces the absorption of calcium. Further, older adults tend to ingest inadequate amounts of vitamin D and calcium. As a result of decreased serum levels of calcium, PTH—acting to maintain serum levels of calcium—increases, which leads to increased bone resorption. In one study, older women (mean age 79 years) hospitalized with a hip fracture were found to have lower 25(OH)D levels and higher PTH, higher bone resorption, and lower bone formation than women in the control group (mean age 77 years). Further, data from the Study of Osteoporotic Fractures indicate that women with low fractional absorption of calcium are at increased risk for hip fracture. (See also p 322 for more on disorders of calcium metabolism.)

Androgens in Men

Androgens are important determinants for peak bone mass in men. Bone accretion is closely related to sexual maturity, and men who have abnormal puberty or delayed puberty have reduced bone mass. In addition, men with estrogen deficiency or resistance have decreased bone mass and failure of epiphyseal closure. Several studies have demonstrated that late-onset hypogonadism can also play a role in osteoporosis in men. Although it is evident that severe male hypogonadism can cause osteoporosis, the effect of moderate decreases in testosterone levels in aging men on rates of bone loss is uncertain. One study found that more than 60% of men presenting with hip fracture had low testosterone levels, compared with about 20% of those in the control group.

Changes in Bone Formation

In men and women, osteoblast activity appears to decrease with aging, compounding the bone loss that results from increased resorption seen with aging and, for women, with menopause. Growth factors, such as transforming growth factor B and insulin-like growth factor 1, may be impaired with estrogen deficiency or with aging, resulting in decreased osteoblast function.

DIAGNOSIS OF OSTEOPOROSIS AND PREDICTION OF FRACTURE

Risk Factors

Risk factors for osteoporosis and osteoporotic fracture have been identified and have been used to determine who should be placed on preventive or therapeutic regimens. Risk factors, however, are mediocre predictors of low bone density and fractures, and it is more useful to identify modifiable risk factors and to implement change as part of a treatment or preventive program. Table 27.1 lists modifications of risk factors of osteoporosis; all of these risk factors should be addressed by the clinician as part of the routine care of an older adult. Risk factors can also be used to identify women < 65 years of age who should have BMD screening.

Secondary Causes

The diagnosis of idiopathic or primary osteoporosis is made by bone density measurement prior to fracture or by incident fracture. Exclusion of other diseases that may present as fracture or with low bone mass is important in the evaluation of women and men with osteoporosis, since different treatment would be required. The major secondary causes of osteoporosis are listed in Table 27.2, along with laboratory tests used to exclude each disease. These laboratory tests should be considered for persons who present with acute compression fracture or who present with a diagnosis of osteoporosis by BMD measurement. The most common causes of secondary osteoporosis in women are primary hyperparathyroidism and glucocorticoid use. Men are more likely to have a secondary cause of osteoporosis than women; as many as 50% of osteoporotic men may have a secondary cause. The most commonly reported secondary causes of osteoporosis in men include hypogonadism and malabsorption syndromes, including gastrectomy. Medications that might have a detrimental effect on bone should be given with adjusted doses or discontinued. Medications that have been shown to adversely affect BMD include glucocorticoids, excess thyroid supplement, anticonvulsants, methotrexate, cyclosporine, and heparin. In older adults, glucocorticoids and thyroid hormone are used quite commonly; accordingly, clinicians should consider the effects these medications may have on the already increased risk of fracture when prescribing them for older adults.

Glucocorticoids result in bone loss primarily through the direct suppression of bone formation, although they also further reduce sex hormone levels and cause secondary hyperparathyroidism through their effects on intestinal calcium absorption. The prevalence of vertebral fractures in persons taking glucocorticoids for 1 year is estimated to be 11%. The rate of trabecular bone loss is dose dependent and generally

---

Table 27.1—Modifications to Reduce the Risk of Osteoporosis

Exercise: Encourage regular, weight-bearing exercise

Nutrition: Encourage

- adequate calcium and vitamin D intake
- lower animal protein intake

Medications that may increase risk of osteoporosis—use with caution:

- anticonvulsants
- cyclosporine
- glucocorticoids
- long-term heparin
- methotrexate
- thyroid hormone replacement (dose dependent)

Smoking cessation

Table 27.2—Screening for Secondary Osteoporosis*

Disease	Recommended Laboratory Tests
Cushing's disease	**Electrolytes**, 24-hour urinary cortisol
Hyperthyroidism	**TSH, T_4**
Hypogonadism (men only)	**Bioavailable testosterone**
Multiple myeloma	**Complete blood cell count, serum electrophoresis**, urine electrophoresis
Osteomalacia	**Alkaline phosphatase, 25(OH)D**
Paget's disease	**Alkaline phosphatase**
Primary hyperparathyroidism	**Calcium, PTH**

NOTE: PTH = parathyroid hormone level; TSH = thyroid-stimulating hormone; T_4 = thyroxine.

* Bolded items are recommended routinely.

occurs in the first 6 months of therapy. Although inhaled corticosteroids have not been as well studied, high doses of high-potency inhaled steroids may also result in bone loss. The best strategy for older persons who require long-term glucocorticoid therapy is to maximize bone health by a variety of interventions. It is important to use the lowest possible dose of glucocorticoids, to assure adequate calcium and vitamin D intake (see the treatment section, below), and to provide appropriate replacement of sex hormones in men (testosterone) and women (estrogen). Further, alendronate and intermittent etidronate have been shown to successfully prevent bone loss that is due to glucocorticoid therapy when they are initiated at the same time as the steroids (see the treatment section, below).

Bone Density Measurement

BMD, or bone mass measurement, is the best predictor of fracture. In fact, it is a better predictor of fracture than cholesterol level is a predictor of coronary heart disease. The relative risk of fracture is 10 times greater in women in the lowest quartile of BMD than in women whose BMD is in the highest quartile.

Bone density of the hip, spine, wrist, or calcaneus may be measured by a variety of techniques. The preferred method of BMD measurement is dual-energy radiographic absorptiometry. BMD of the hip, anterior-posterior spine, lateral spine, and wrist can be measured with this technology. The National Osteoporosis Foundation, in conjunction with numerous specialty organizations, recommends BMD testing for all women aged 65 years and over, regardless of risk-factor status. The U.S. Preventive Services Task Force also recommends that women aged 65 and over be screened routinely for osteoporosis and that routine screening begin at age 60 for women at high increased risk for osteoporotic fractures. The National Osteoporosis Foundation, in conjunction with numerous specialty organizations, recommends BMD testing for all women aged 65 years and over, regardless of risk-factor status. On the other hand, the U.S. Preventive Services Task Force states that there is insufficient evidence to recommend for or against BMD screening. Indications for BMD testing are listed in Table 27.3. BMD testing may also be used to establish the diagnosis and severity of osteoporosis in men, and it should be considered for men with low-trauma fracture, radiographic criteria consistent with low bone mass, or diseases known to place a person at risk for osteoporosis. Data relating BMD to fracture risk are derived from studies of women, but data suggest that similar associations may be valid for men.

Table 27.3—Indications for Bone Mineral Density Testing*

- Postmenopausal women with multiple risk factors** for osteoporosis

- Postmenopausal women who present with fractures

- Men with conditions*** indicating high risk for osteoporosis

- Women and men with osteoporosis who have been on treatment for prolonged periods

- All women ≥ 65 years old regardless of additional risk factors****

* In persons who would consider treatment for osteoporosis.

** Early menopause, white or Asian race, sedentary, smoking, small frame, alcohol abuse, primary hyperparathyroidism, hyperthyroidism, glucocorticoid use.

*** Hypogonadism and glucocorticoid use are the two most common.

**** Recommended by the National Osteoporosis Foundation, the U.S. Preventive Services Task Force, and numerous specialty organizations.

Biochemical Markers of Bone Turnover

Serum and urine biochemical markers can estimate the rate of bone turnover (remodeling) and may provide additional information to assist the clinician. A number of markers have been developed that reflect collagen breakdown (or bone resorption) and bone formation. Several markers have been associated with increased hip-fracture risk, decreased bone density, and bone loss in older adults. In addition, markers of bone resorption and formation decrease in response to antiresorptive treatment. The use of markers in clinical practice, however, is controversial because of the substantial overlap of marker values in women with high and low bone density or rate of bone loss. Further, few studies have compared the response of a particular marker (or combination of markers) and bone density with therapy in order to determine the magnitude of decrease of a biochemical marker necessary to prevent bone loss or, more importantly, fracture. Two markers of bone resorption, deoxypyridinoline cross-links and cross-linked N-telopeptides of type I collagen, and one formation marker, bone alkaline phosphatase, may be used in clinical practice to provide an early assessment of treatment efficacy. A decrease from baseline levels in the level of these markers after 3 to 6 months of therapy would indicate successful treatment.

PREVENTION AND TREATMENT OF OSTEOPOROSIS

The Role of Exercise

Exercise is an important component of osteoporosis treatment and prevention, although exercise alone is not adequate to prevent the rapid bone loss associated with estrogen deficiency in early menopause. Among exercisers in the Rancho Bernardo cohort, those who reported strenuous or moderate exercise had higher BMD at the hip than did those who reported mild or less-than-mild exercise. Similar associations were seen for lifelong regular exercisers and hip BMD. In a randomized study of women ≥ 10 years postmenopausal, the group receiving calcium supplementation plus exercise had less bone loss at the hip than did those assigned to calcium alone. Further, the effectiveness of high-intensity strength training in maintaining femoral neck BMD as well as in improving muscle mass, strength, and balance in postmenopausal women has been demonstrated, suggesting that resistance training would be useful to help maintain BMD and to reduce the risk of falls among older adults.

Marked decrease in physical activity or immobilization results in a decline in bone mass; accordingly, it is important to encourage older adults to be as active as possible. Weight-bearing exercise, such as walking, can be recommended for all adults. Older persons should be encouraged to start slowly and gradually increase both the number of days as well as the time spent walking each day. (See "Physical Activity," p 65.)

Calcium and Vitamin D

Calcium and vitamin D are required for bone health at all ages. In order to maintain a positive calcium balance, the current recommendations for calcium intake for postmenopausal women and men aged 65 years and older is at least 1200 mg per day of elemental calcium. The amount of vitamin D required is between 400 and 800 IU per day. In older adults, regardless of climate or exposure to sunlight, a daily supplement of ≥ 400 IU per day of vitamin D is recommended because skin changes that occur with aging result in less efficient use of ultraviolet light by the skin to synthesize vitamin-D precursors. Calcium plus vitamin D at different doses have been shown to increase or maintain bone density in postmenopausal women and to prevent hip as well as all nonvertebral fractures in older adults. The dietary intake of calcium for postmenopausal women in the United States averages 500 to 700 mg per day; thus, most American women require calcium supplementation to ensure adequate intake.

Pharmacologic Options

Estrogen Replacement Therapy

Estrogen replacement therapy (ERT) remains an important choice for the prevention of osteoporosis. In addition to the beneficial effect on bone, epidemiologic observations suggest that estrogen pre-

vents cardiovascular disease and may also reduce the incidence of Alzheimer's disease. In case-control and cohort studies, ERT is associated with a 30% to 70% reduction in hip-fracture incidence. Multiple studies have demonstrated that postmenopausal estrogen use prevents bone loss at the hip and spine when initiated within 10 years of menopause. However, in a cross-sectional study, BMD in women who initiated hormone replacement therapy (HRT) after age 60 years was found not to be significantly different from women who initiated HRT within 2 years of menopause. In the Postmenopausal Estrogen/Progestin Intervention trial, older women, women with low initial BMD, and women who had not previously used HRT were found to gain more bone than did young women, women with higher baseline BMD, and those who had previously used HRT. In the only prospective study of fracture prevention with estrogen, a decrease in incident vertebral fractures was seen in postmenopausal women using a transdermal preparation. The bone of women older than 70 years continues to be responsive to ERT, and data suggest that lower-than-usual doses of estrogen, when given with adequate calcium and vitamin D, are effective in reducing bone turnover and bone loss in older women. In a randomized, controlled study, women treated with 0.3 mg per day of conjugated equine estrogen plus 2.5 mg per day of medroxyprogesterone acetate were found to gain spine and hip BMD, whereas women treated with placebo showed no change. From the Study of Osteoporotic Fractures, separate analyses identified current estrogen use as a protective factor against hip fracture and demonstrated an increased risk of hip and vertebral fractures in women with undetectable serum estradiol levels. Thus, estrogen is useful for treatment of osteoporosis in older women, although it appears that lower doses can be recommended (see Table 27.4 and Table 49.1, p 330).

In osteoporosis management, patients who do not respond to treatment may be identified either by BMD (> 4% per year loss at any site) or by fracture that occurs ≥ 3 months after initiation of treatment. If this situation arises in women who are taking ERT, then combination therapy with alendronate and ERT is indicated, unless the patient is not tolerating ERT. In two studies, ERT and alendronate have been shown to have an additive effect on BMD in comparison with either agent alone, although fracture data for combination therapy are not available.

Although estrogen can benefit several organ systems, its use by postmenopausal women has been limited by side effects and concerns about increased endometrial and breast cancer risk, and an unclear effect on cardiovascular disease risk (see "Hormone Replacement Therapy," p 329).

Table 27.4—Medications Used to Prevent and Treat Osteoporosis

Medication	Dosage	Cost	Special Considerations
Estrogen (see Table 49.1)			
Selective estrogen receptor modulator			
Raloxifene	60 mg/d	$$$$$	May prevent breast cancer
Bisphosphonates			
Alendronate	10 mg/d or 70 mg/week; 5 mg/d for prevention	$$$$$	Adherence to dosing instructions required (Table 27.5); used in men and women to prevent glucocorticoid-induced osteoporosis
Etidronate	400 mg/day for 2 weeks every 3 months	$$	May be used in men and women to prevent glucocorticoid-induced osteoporosis; use for idiopathic osteoporosis only if all other treatments are not tolerated or effective
Risedronate	5 mg/d	$$$$$	Adherence to dosing instructions required (see Table 27.5)
Calcitonin			
nasal spray	200 IU/d	$$$$$	Metered spray; 1 spray gives daily dose; alternate nostrils each day to reduce side effects
injectable (subcutaneously or intramuscularly)	50–100 IU 3 to 5 times/ week		Injectable still useful, depending on patient

NOTE: $ = approximately $10 per month.

Bisphosphonates

Alendronate has been approved for osteoporosis prevention and treatment. Women with osteoporosis who were treated with alendronate and compared with women on placebo were found to have increased bone density of the spine and hip, as well as decreased vertebral fracture rate. The Fracture Intervention Trial examined the effect of alendronate on postmenopausal women with severe osteoporosis, with or without vertebral fracture at baseline. Regardless of the presence of vertebral fractures at baseline, alendronate decreased vertebral fracture rate. In addition, alendronate resulted in a 50% reduction in hip fractures. A study in women aged 60 to 85 years indicated that an even lower dose of alendronate might be effective in older women. Further, data indicate that once-weekly dosing with alendronate (70 mg) is as effective in increasing spine BMD over 1 year as is daily dosing (10 mg) in postmenopausal women with osteoporosis (age range 42 to 95 years). Alendronate has also been approved for the prevention of osteoporosis in early postmenopausal women. The daily dose for prevention is lower—5 mg—than that given for the treatment of osteoporosis—10 mg. If treatment with alendronate alone is not effective, combining ERT with alendronate, which has an additive effect on bone density, may be indicated. In women with lesser degrees of osteoporosis, alendronate has not been shown to prevent hip fracture. Although alendronate has not been recommended for use in men, preliminary data from a prospective trial indicate that 10 mg per day increases bone mass in men, even those with low testosterone levels. Further, alendronate also prevents bone loss in men and women on glucocorticoids when it is initiated at the same time as the glucocorticoids.

The major side effects of alendronate are gastrointestinal, including abdominal pain, dyspepsia, esophagitis, nausea, vomiting, and diarrhea. Musculoskeletal pain may also occur. Esophagitis, particularly erosive esophagitis, may be seen most commonly in patients who do not take the medication properly. The absorption of oral bisphosphonates is very poor; thus, it is extremely important to provide specific and detailed instructions for patients receiving any bisphosphonate therapy (Table 27.5).

Risedronate, another bisphosphonate, has been approved for prevention and treatment of osteoporosis. In a 3-year study of postmenopausal women with ≥ 1 vertebral fracture at baseline, the cumulative incidence of new vertebral fractures was reduced by 41% (95% CI, 18% to 58%) in the group receiving risedronate (5 mg per day) rather than placebo. In addition, the incidence of nonvertebral fractures also decreased by 39% (95% CI, 6% to 61%) in the treatment group.

Table 27.5—Instructions for Administration of Bisphosphonates

- Take first thing in the morning before eating or drinking anything else
- Take with at least 8 oz of plain tap water
- Take while upright in a chair or standing, and remain upright after ingestion
- Do not eat or drink anything for one half hour after taking the medication

BMD of the hip and spine increased significantly in the risedronate group. In the same study, 2.5 mg per day of risedronate was found to be ineffective and was discontinued after the first year of the study. Withdrawals because of side effects and any upper gastrointestinal adverse events were similar in the risedronate and placebo groups.

Etidronate was shown to increase spinal bone mass and decrease vertebral fractures in two studies in the early 1990s, and a 5-year follow-up study demonstrated continued benefit. Etidronate was given intermittently—400 mg per day orally for 14 days, and then stopped for 2.5 months—in these studies because continuous high doses can impair mineralization and produce osteomalacia. However, etidronate is not approved for use in treating osteoporosis because the data supporting fracture reduction were not sufficient. A separate study indicated a role for etidronate in preventing bone loss in patients who require long-term glucocorticoids.

Selective Estrogen Receptor Modulators

The selective estrogen receptor modulators are agents that act as estrogen agonists in bone and heart, but act as estrogen antagonists in breast and uterine tissue. These medications have the potential to prevent osteoporosis or cardiovascular disease without the increased risk of breast or uterine cancer. Tamoxifen, an agent used to treat breast cancer, has beneficial effects on bone, as reported in several studies, but it also has stimulatory effects on the uterus. Thus, tamoxifen is not indicated for osteoporosis treatment or prevention.

Raloxifene has been approved for the treatment and prevention of osteoporosis in postmenopausal women. Comparison of raloxifene with placebo in postmenopausal women with osteoporosis found that raloxifene decreased bone turnover and maintained hip and total body bone density. There were no differences between groups in breast abnormalities or endometrial thickness. Most importantly, data demonstrate that raloxifene (60 mg per day) reduces incident vertebral fractures by about 60%, despite only modest increases in bone density. Raloxifene was not found to significantly reduce nonvertebral, hip, or wrist fractures in this study. Reported side effects with raloxifene include flu-like symptoms, hot flushes, leg cramps, and peripheral edema.

Another important finding with raloxifene was a reduction in breast cancer in women who participated in the Multiple Outcomes of Raloxifene Trial. When women receiving raloxifene were compared with women receiving placebo, the relative risk for women receiving raloxifene of developing breast cancer was found to be 0.24 (95% CI, 0.13 to 0.44). In the same study, raloxifene was not found to increase the risk of

endometrial cancer but was found to increase the risk of venous thromboembolic disease. In other studies, raloxifene was found to decrease total and low-density lipoprotein cholesterol and lipoprotein(a) levels without affecting high-density lipoprotein cholesterol or triglyceride levels. Thus, in clinical trials to date, raloxifene appears to be beneficial to several organ systems, although further study is required with regard to cardiovascular diseases and breast cancer prevention.

Calcitonin

Calcitonin is a hormonal inhibitor of bone resorption used to treat osteoporosis. It is available as a subcutaneous injection and as a nasal spray. The nasal spray has fewer reported side effects and greater patient acceptance, but it may be less effective. Calcitonin has been shown to increase bone density in the spine and reduce vertebral fractures. In epidemiologic studies, calcitonin has been shown to reduce hip fractures, although in clinical trials, hip bone density has not been found to increase. Preliminary analysis of a 5-year study demonstrated that the incidence of vertebral fractures in women receiving 200 IU per day of nasal spray calcitonin was lower than that of women on placebo. The reduction in hip-fracture incidence was not statistically significant in the group receiving calcitonin in comparison with the placebo group. Doses of 100 and 400 IU per day were studied as well, but they did not reduce incidence of vertebral fractures. In the same study, BMD changes at 3 years and changes in markers of bone turnover in the treatment and placebo groups were found not to be significantly different. Although there are no direct comparisons, calcitonin appears to be less effective than other antiresorptive drugs. There is some evidence that calcitonin produces an analgesic effect in some women with painful vertebral compression fractures.

Investigational Agents

Other bisphosphonates currently under investigation for the treatment and prevention of osteoporosis include pamidronate and zoledronic acid. New selective estrogen receptor modulators are also being tested for use in osteoporosis treatment.

PTH, although leading to increased bone resorption when continuously elevated, can increase bone mass, trabecular connectivity, and mechanical strength when administered intermittently. PTH has been shown to increase spinal BMD in osteoporotic men and women. In a 3-year randomized study of postmenopausal women with osteoporosis, the group receiving estrogen plus intermittent PTH was found to have continuous increase in spinal bone mass over the study period, as well as decreased vertebral fracture rate. Bone mass of the hip and total body also increased significantly in the estrogen-plus-PTH group, in comparison with the group on estrogen alone.

The use of fluoride to treat osteporosis is appealing because fluoride results in a large increase in spine bone density; however, the increase in BMD has not been found to be consistently associated with a decrease in vertebral fractures. In fact, in one study, the group receiving fluoride therapy was found to have a higher rate of appendicular fractures. Slow-release fluoride therapy has been found to be associated with an increase in spine BMD, as well as decreased incidence of vertebral fractures. Further studies are required before slow-release fluoride can be recommended for the treatment of osteoporosis.

The use of 3-hydroxy-3-methylglutaryl coenzyme A reductase inhibitors (statins) may also affect bone. This class of medication is commonly prescribed for the management of hypercholesterolemia and has been shown to stimulate bone formation in animals. Preliminary epidemiologic data suggest that the use of statins is associated with decreased incidence of fracture. Further information is required before these agents can be recommended for osteoporosis management.

Working With the Patient

Establishing and maintaining an optimal regimen usually requires considerable discussion with individual patients and is much easier if patients are well informed. The use of educational materials can be quite helpful, as can the efforts of a nurse or other office personnel. Effective prevention and treatment of osteoporosis is possible, if the patient and clinician work together in a sustained fashion.

The osteoporosis patient's adherence to the medication regimen is important. Baseline and follow-up BMD measurements (every 1 to 2 years) are important to assess response to therapy; these measurements may also improve adherence by providing visual information regarding the effectiveness of the therapy. Another way to inform patients about their response to therapy is to measure markers of bone resorption. In particular, adequate estrogen and bisphosphonate therapy will almost certainly decrease the levels of urine or serum markers of bone resorption within 3 to 6 months.

Management of Vertebral Fractures

Most vertebral fractures are asymptomatic and are diagnosed by spinal radiographs. Over time, one may notice decreased height, increased kyphosis, or simply the fact that clothes no longer fit the person properly. Many older adults have chronic back pain due to the changes in the spine that occur with vertebral compres-

sion. In the case of symptomatic vertebral compression fractures, adequate pain control is essential. The pain usually lasts 2 to 4 weeks and can be quite debilitating. Nonsteroidal anti-inflammatory drugs and calcitonin can be tried; narcotics are commonly required to control the pain. Physical therapy is an important part of osteoporosis treatment programs for management of acute and chronic pain, as well as for patient education. The physical therapist can provide postural exercises, alternative modalities for pain reduction, and information on changes in body mechanics that may help prevent future fractures. Support groups for patients with osteoporosis are also important.

Osteomalacia

Osteomalacia, an impairment of bone mineralization, is much less common than osteoporosis and can be definitively diagnosed only by bone biopsy. The clinical syndrome associated with osteomalacia consists of pain, myopathy, and fracture. The most common cause of osteomalacia in older adults is vitamin-D deficiency as a result of inadequate intake. In addition, excessive use of phosphate-binding antacids, chronic use of anticonvulsants, chronic renal failure, hepatobiliary disease, and malabsorption syndromes may also result in osteomalacia. The use of high-dose etidronate and fluoride may cause osteomalacia, albeit rarely. The symptoms of osteomalacia may be subtle, and thus the diagnosis may be delayed. Patients typically complain of diffuse bone pain and tenderness, proximal muscle weakness, and generalized fatigue. A characteristic waddling gait may result from the hip pain and thigh weakness. Laboratory studies typically demonstrate an elevated alkaline phosphatase, low phosphate, low or normal calcium, and low 25(OH)D levels. Plain radiographic films may show osteopenia or characteristic pseudofractures, most commonly seen in the proximal femur.

Osteomalacia is managed by treating the underlying cause. If vitamin-D deficiency is diagnosed, repletion can be accomplished with oral vitamin D, 1000 IU per day. Hypophosphatemia is corrected by the use of neutral phosphate salts, 500 mg four times daily. Patients on long-term anticonvulsant therapy may be supplemented with 400 to 800 IU of vitamin D daily. Osteomalacia due to hepatobiliary disease or chronic renal failure is managed with supplemental 25(OH)D and 1,25(OH)$_2$D, respectively.

References

- Bone HG, Greenspan SL, McKeever C, et al. Alendronate effects in postmenopausal women with low bone mineral density: Alendronate/Estrogen Study Group. *J Clin Endocrinol Metab.* 2000;85(2):720–726.

- Cummings SR, Browner WS, Bauer D, et al. Endogenous hormones and the risk of hip and vertebral fractures among older women: Study of Osteoporotic Fractures Research Group. *N Engl J Med.* 1998;339(11):733–738.

- Dore RK. Osteoporosis: fractures and key risk factors. *Female Patient.* 2002; March Supplement.

- Ettinger B, Black DM, Mitlak BH, et al. Reduction of vertebral fracture risk in postmenopausal women with osteoporosis treated with raloxifene: results from a 3-year randomized clinical trial. Multiple Outcomes of Raloxifene Evaluation (MORE) Investigators. *JAMA.* 1999;282(7):637–645.

- Harris ST, Watts NB, Genant HK, et al. Effects of risedronate treatment on vertebral and nonvertebral fractures in women with postmenopausal osteoporosis: a randomized controlled trial. *JAMA.* 1999;282(14):1344–1352.

- Lindsay R, Cosman F, Lobo RA, et al. Addition of alendronate to ongoing hormone replacement therapy in the treatment of osteoporosis: a randomized, controlled clinical trial. *J Clin Endocrinol Metab.* 1999;84(9):307–3081.

- Orwoll E, Ettinger M, Weiss S, et al. Alendronate treatment of osteoporosis in men. *N Engl J* 2000;343:604–610.

- Prestwood KM, Thompson DL, Kenny AM, et al. Low dose estrogen and calcium have an additive effect on bone resorption in older women. *J Clin Endocrinol Metab.* 1999;84(1):179–183.

- Recker RR, Davies KM, Dowd RM, et al. The effect of low-dose continuous estrogen and progesterone therapy with calcium and vitamin D on bone in elderly women: a randomized, controlled trial. *Ann Intern Med.* 1999;130(11):897–904.

- Schnitzer T, Bone HG, Crepaldi G, et al. Therapeutic equivalence of alendronate 70 mg once-weekly and alendronate 10 mg daily in the treatment of osteoporosis. *Aging (Milano).* 2000;12(1):1–12.

CHAPTER 28—MALNUTRITION

Older persons suffer a burden of malnutrition that spans the spectrum from under- to overnutrition. Nutrition concerns impact many of the chronic disease processes that afflict older persons. Moreover, age-related changes in physiology, metabolism, and function alter the older person's nutritional requirements. Better understanding among clinicians of the aging process and of nutritional screening, assessment, and interventions can improve the health and independence of older persons.

AGE-RELATED CHANGES

Body Composition

Aging is associated with notable changes in body composition: bone mass, lean mass, and water content decrease, while fat mass increases. The increase in total body fat is commonly accompanied by greater intra-abdominal fat stores. The consequence is that well-standardized nutrient requirements for younger or middle-aged adults cannot be generalized to older persons. The aging process also affects organ functions, although the degree of change observed is highly variable among individuals. Decline in organ functions may affect nutritional assessment and intervention.

Energy Requirements

Reduced basal metabolic rate in older persons reflects loss of muscle mass. The basal metabolic rate is the principal determinant of total energy expenditure; energy expenditure in relation to physical activity is the most variable component. The Harris-Benedict equations may be used to predict basal energy expenditure. A simple method for estimating the total daily energy needs of the older patient is based on body weight alone (Table 28.1). In any determination of energy needs for older persons, care must be taken to avoid overfeeding while still meeting basal requirements.

Macronutrient Needs

Modified food guide pyramids for older persons based upon the U.S. Department of Agriculture food guide pyramid have been released (see Figure 28.1). The food selections are more relevant to the target audience, and appropriate intakes of water, fiber, and supplements of calcium, vitamin D, and vitamin B$_{12}$ are highlighted.

The protein needs of healthy older persons may be somewhat higher than was formerly thought. The federal recommended dietary allowance (RDA) for protein for persons aged 51 years and older is 0.8 g

Table 28.1—Nutritional Requirement Calculations

Estimation of energy needs on basis of body weight
25–30 kcal/kg body weight /day
For the obese individual, use a reduced compromise body weight that approximates 120% of ideal.

Estimation of energy needs using the Harris-Benedict equation for basal energy expenditure (BEE)
Male BEE = 66 + (13.7 x weight in kg) + (5 x height in cm) – (6.8 x age)
Female BEE = 655 + (9.6 x weight in kg) + (1.8 x height in cm) – (4.7 x age)
Adjust BEE with empiric stress factors (1.00 for nonstressed and 1.5 for stressed) to estimate total energy expenditure of ill older patients.

Estimation of protein needs on basis of body weight
Protein = (0.8 to 1.5) g/kg body weight / day
For the obese individual, use ideal body weight.

per kg of body weight per day, but current recommendations are 1.0 g per kg of body weight per day or higher. With stress or injury, protein requirements are typically estimated at 1.5 g per kg of body weight per day, but underlying renal or hepatic insufficiency may warrant protein restriction (Table 28.1).

The Dietary Guidelines for Americans do not make specific recommendations for older persons but suggest a dietary intake of no more than 30% of total energy from fat for any age group. Fat, in addition to providing insulation and protection, serves as a source of energy and essential fatty acids, as well as for the transport of fat-soluble vitamins. Carbohydrates are a major source of energy for the body and also provide fiber in the diet. Energy obtained from carbohydrates should approximate 55% to 60% of total kcal per day, and complex carbohydrates are preferred over simple sugars.

Micronutrient Requirements

Revisions of the Dietary Reference Intakes include RDAs with more specific guidelines for older persons; those for the group aged 71 years and older are shown in Table 28.2. Recommendations for selected nutrients have been adjusted in view of new research findings.

Fluid Needs

Dehydration is the most common fluid or electrolyte disturbance in older persons. Normal aging is associated with decreased perception of thirst, impaired response to serum osmolarity, and reduced ability to concentrate urine following fluid deprivation. A decline in fluid intake can also result from disease states that cause a reduction in mental or physical ability to recognize or express thirst, or result in decreased access to water. In general, fluid needs of older persons can be met with 30 mL per kg of body weight per day or 1 mL per kcal ingested. Fluid needs may be altered during episodes of fever or infection, as well as with diuretic or laxative therapy. Common signs of dehydration are decreased urine output, elevated body temperature, constipation, mucosal dryness, skin turgor changes, and confusion. Altered fluid status (overhydration or underhydration) may affect anthropometric and biochemical measures, resulting in inaccurate assessments.

NUTRITION SCREENING AND ASSESSMENT

Anthropometrics

Anthropometric measurements are a mainstay of nutritional assessment of older persons. A weight loss of 10 pounds in the preceding 6 months is a useful indicator of nutritional risk and morbidity. This degree of weight loss is predictive of functional limitations, health care charges, and need for hospitalization. The Minimum Data Set (MDS) used by Medicare-certified nursing homes defines weight loss as 5% or greater in the past month or 10% or greater in the past 6 months. Body mass index (BMI)—weight (kg)/ height (m^2)—has received increasing attention. National Institutes of Health guidelines regarding body size classification have been released (Table 28.3). BMI is a useful measure of body size and indirect measure of body fatness that does not require the use of a reference table of ideal weights. The risk threshold for low BMI is set at 18.5 kg/m^2. Other anthropometric tools include skin-fold and circumference measurements, but these have had limited practical application because of the difficulty of training personnel to achieve acceptable reliability. High-technology body composition assessments that are impractical for routine clinical use include water displacement, bioelectrical impedance, dual energy radiographic absorptiometry, computed tomography, nuclear magnetic resonance imaging, and total body counting of the naturally occurring potassium isotope (^{40}K).

Nutritional Intake

Generally, inadequate nutritional intake has been defined as average or usual intake of servings of food groups, nutrients, or energy below a threshold level of the RDA. The limited reliability of accurately assessing dietary intake measures is well known, so thresholds of 25% to 50% below the RDA have generally been

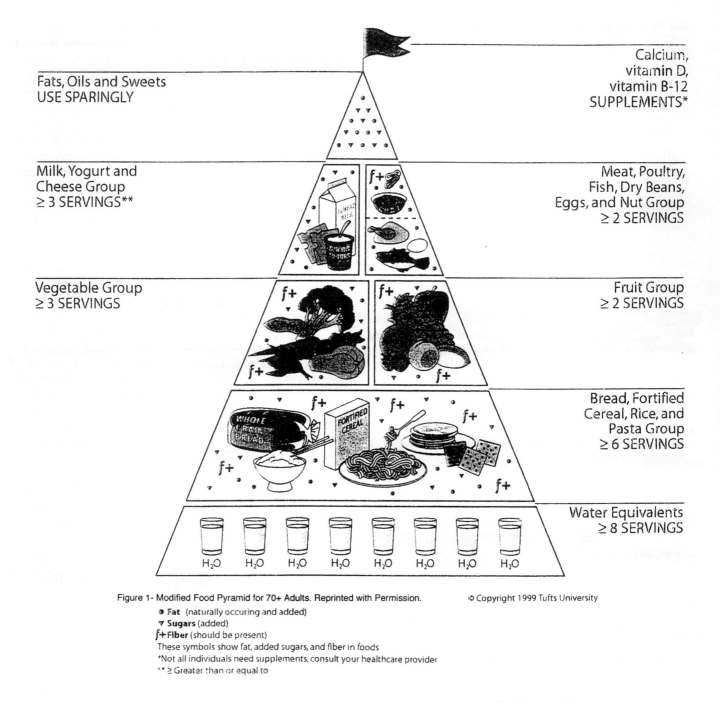

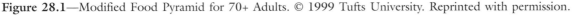

Figure 1- Modified Food Pyramid for 70+ Adults. Reprinted with Permission. © Copyright 1999 Tufts University

- **Fat** (naturally occuring and added)
- **Sugars** (added)
- **Fiber** (should be present)

These symbols show fat, added sugars, and fiber in foods

*Not all individuals need supplements, consult your healthcare provider

** ≥ Greater than or equal to

Figure 28.1—Modified Food Pyramid for 70+ Adults. © 1999 Tufts University. Reprinted with permission.

selected. A study found reduced energy intake (less than 50% of calculated maintenance energy requirements) in 21% of a sample of hospitalized older persons. This subset of patients had higher rates of in-hospital mortality and 90-day mortality than did those above the threshold of energy intake. The MDS uses a different measure: less than 75% of food provided is the threshold to trigger nutrition assessment in nursing homes. Surveys of nutritional status conducted among chronically institutionalized older persons suggest that 5% to 18% of nursing-home residents have energy intakes below their recommended average energy expenditure.

Energy intakes of men and women aged 65 to 98 years have been estimated in a nationwide food consumption survey. Investigators report that 37% to 40% of the men and women studied had energy intakes lower than two thirds of the RDA, and many reported skipping at least one meal each day. Estimated intakes by consumption surveys, however, may be unreliable because some studies suggest that older persons underreport energy intakes by 20% to 30%.

Table 28.2—Recommended Dietary Allowances for Persons Aged 71 and Older

Nutrient	Men	Women
Calcium (mg)*	1200	1200
Phosphorus (mg)	700	700
Magnesium (mg)	420	320
Vitamin D (μg)*	15	15
Fluoride (mg)*	4	3
Thiamin (mg)	1.2	1.1
Riboflavin (mg)	1.3	1.1
Niacin (mg)	16	14
Vitamin B$_6$ (mg)	1.7	1.5
Folate (μg)	400	400
Vitamin B$_{12}$ (μg)	2.4	2.4
Pantothenic acid (mg)*	5	5
Biotin (μg)*	30	30
Choline (mg)*	550	425
Vitamin C (mg)	90	75
α-Tocopherol (mg)	15	15
Selenium (μg)	55	55

*Adequate intakes, not recommended dietary allowances.

SOURCE: Data from: Standing Committee on the Scientific Evaluation of Dietary Reference Intakes, Food and Nutrition Board, Institute of Medicine, *Dietary Reference Intakes for Calcium, Phosphorus, Magnesium, Vitamin D, and Fluoride*. Washington, DC: National Academy Press; 1997. Standing Committee on the Scientific Evaluation of Dietary Reference Intakes, Institute of Medicine, *Dietary Reference Intakes for Thiamin, Riboflavin, Niacin, Vitamin B6, Folate, Vitamin B12, Pantothenic Acid, Biotin, and Choline*. Washington, DC: National Academy Press; 1999. Standing Committee on the Scientific Evaluation of Dietary Reference Intakes, Food and Nutrition Board, *Dietary Reference Intakes for Vitamin C, Vitamin E, Selenium, and Beta Carotene, and Other Carotenoids*. Washington, DC: National Academy Press; 2000.

Table 28.3—Body Size Classification

Body Size	Body Mass Index (kg/m^2)
Underweight	< 18.5
Normal weight	18.5–24.9
Overweight	25–29.9
Obesity	≥ 30
Extreme obesity	≥ 40

SOURCE: Data from: NHLBI Obesity Education Initiative Expert Panel. *Clinical Guidelines on the Identification, Evaluation, and Treatment of Overweight and Obesity in Adults: The Evidence Report*. Bethesda, MD: National Institutes of Health, National Heart, Lung and Blood Institute; September 1998: xiv. Pub. No. 98-4083.

Laboratory Tests: Albumin, Prealbumin, Cholesterol

Serum albumin has been recognized as a risk indicator for morbidity and mortality. Hypoalbuminemia lacks specificity and sensitivity as an indicator of malnutrition; however, it may be associated with injury, disease, or inflammatory conditions. As a negative acute phase reactant, it is subject to cytokine-mediated decline in synthesis and to increased degradation and transcapillary leakage. It is thought that albumin synthesis does not decrease with age; however, longitudinal studies of serum albumin suggest a modest decline in levels with aging that may be independent of disease. A value of 3.8 g/dL or less appears to be useful as a screening indicator among older persons. The prognostic value of hypoalbuminemia may be largely due to its utility as a proxy measure for injury, disease, or inflammation. In the community setting, hypoalbuminemia has been associated with functional limitation, sarcopenia, increased health care use, and mortality. In the hospital setting, it has also been associated with increased length of hospital stay, complications, readmissions, and mortality. Other protein markers of nutritional status are being investigated. Prealbumin has received the most attention, as it has a considerably shorter half-life than albumin and may therefore more adequately reflect short-term changes in protein status. Unfortunately, prealbumin otherwise appears to suffer the same limitations as albumin as an indicator of nutritional status.

Serum cholesterol has also been linked to nutritional status. Low cholesterol levels (< 160 mg/dL) are often detected in persons with serious underlying disease, such as malignancy. Poor clinical outcomes have been observed among hospitalized and institutionalized older persons with hypocholesterolemia. A study of community-dwelling older persons found that those in the lowest quartile of serum cholesterol did not differ from others in their nutrient intakes. It appears likely, again, that acquired hypocholesterolemia is a nonspecific feature of poor health status that is independent of nutrient or energy intakes, and that it may better reflect a proinflammatory condition. Of interest is the observation that community-dwelling older persons with both hypoalbuminemia and hypocholesterolemia exhibit the highest rates for adverse functional and mortality outcomes in comparison with those with hypoalbuminemia or hypocholesterolemia alone.

Drug-Nutrient Interactions

Drugs may modify the nutrient needs and metabolism of older persons. Certain drugs, such as theophylline and digoxin, even at therapeutic levels, can cause anorexia in the older person. Many drugs are known to reduce the availability of specific nutrients (Table 28.4).

Multi-Item Tools for Nutrition Screening

The nutritional status of the older person can be influenced by a variety of factors (Table 28.5). The absence of single assessment measures that are valid indicators of comprehensive nutritional status has prompted the development of multi-item tools. Older

Table 28.4—Drug-Nutrient Interactions

Drug	Reduced Nutrient Availability
Alcohol	Zinc, vitamins A, B_1, B_2, B_6, folate, vitamin B_{12}
Antacids	Vitamin B_{12}, folate, iron, total kcal
Antibiotics, broad-spectrum	Vitamin K
Colchicine	Vitamin B_{12}
Digoxin	Zinc, total kcal
Diuretics	Zinc, magnesium, vitamin B_6, potassium, copper
Isoniazid	Vitamin B_6, niacin
Levodopa	Vitamin B_6
Laxatives	Calcium, vitamins A, B_2, B_{12}, D, E, K
Lipid-binding resins	Vitamins A, D, E, K
Metformin	Vitamin B_{12}, total kcal
Mineral oil	Vitamins A, D, E, K
Phenytoin	Vitamin D, folate
Salicylates	Vitamin C, folate
SSRIs	Total kcal
Theophylline	Total kcal
Trimethoprim	Folate

NOTE: SSRI = selective serotonin-reuptake inhibitor.

SOURCE: Modified from Silver AJ. Malnutrition. In: Beck JC, ed. *Geriatric Review Syllabus: A Core Curriculum in Geriatric Medicine.* 1st ed. New York: American Geriatrics Society; 1989:100.

Table 28.5—Risk Factors for Poor Nutritional Status

Alcohol or substance abuse
Cognitive dysfunction
Decreased exercise
Depression, poor mental health
Functional limitations
Inadequate funds
Limited education
Limited mobility, transportation
Medical problems, chronic diseases
Medications
Poor dentition
Restricted diet, poor eating habits
Social isolation

persons in acute or chronic care facilities have been extensively studied to identify indicators and predictors of nutritional status, but those in the community setting have been subject to less investigation. Nutrition screening tools for older persons have been widely disseminated, and health professionals are beginning to use such tools for a variety of purposes. Their effectiveness remains to be demonstrated; specifically, we need to learn whether these tools can identify undernourished individuals whose problems are amenable to intervention.

The Nutrition Screening Initiative is a collaborative effort of the American Dietetic Association, the American Academy of Family Practitioners, and the National Council on Aging, Inc. Three interdisciplinary nutrition risk-screening tools were developed by the Nutrition Screening Initiative to aid in the evaluation of the nutritional status of older persons. The DETERMINE checklist was created to raise public awareness about the importance of nutrition to the health of older persons (see the Appendix, p 410). This self-report questionnaire is composed of 10 items and is intended to identify potential risks, but not to diagnose malnutrition. The Level I screen, intended for use by health care professionals, incorporates additional assessment items regarding dietary habits, functional status, living environment, and weight change, as well as measures of height and weight. The Level II screen, for use by more highly trained medical and nutrition professionals and suggested for use in the diagnosis of malnutrition, contains all the items from Level I with additional biochemical and anthropometric measures, as well as provision for more detailed evaluation of depression and mental status, as indicated.

The Mini Nutritional Assessment was developed to evaluate the risk of malnutrition among frail older persons and identify those who may benefit from early intervention. More extensive cross-validation studies among healthy older persons have since been completed. This assessment tool requires administration by a trained professional and is composed of 18 items. The assessment includes questions about body mass index, mid-arm and calf circumferences, weight loss, living environment, medications use, dietary habits, clinical global assessment, and self-perception of health and nutrition status. A shortened screening version that contains only 6 items is being evaluated.

NUTRITION SYNDROMES

Sarcopenia

Age-related loss of skeletal muscle mass is called *sarcopenia*. Biopsy studies reveal a reduction in the number and size of type II muscle fibers with aging, while type I fibers are spared. The relationship between sarcopenia and functional limitation is unknown. It is not evident whether sarcopenia is an inexorable part of aging or is more a reflection of sedentary life style or unrecognized factors. Possible causes include age-related accelerated muscle loss or changes in muscle accretion or responsiveness to trophic hormonal or neurologic factors. Decline in endogenous growth hormone production, altered cytokine regulation, decreased androgen and estrogen production, and loss of alpha motor neurons in the spinal column have been suggested as factors. Changes in dietary intake, protein metabolism, or disuse atrophy resulting from a sedentary life style may also be contributors. Current research has focused on testing trophic factors like growth hormone and testosterone and the use of resistance strength training. The role of undernutrition in the development of sarcopenia has not been established, and the role, if any, of nutritional intervention awaits further study.

Cachexia and Wasting

Although the terms *cachexia* and *wasting* have often been used interchangeably in the clinical setting to describe patients with severe weight loss and diminished nutritional intake, distinct definitions have been suggested for these syndromes on the basis of the presence (cachexia) or absence (wasting) of cytokine-mediated response to injury or disease. This conceptual approach is useful, even though patients commonly exhibit components of both inflammatory response and semistarvation. The inflammatory cytokines (tumor necrosis factor, interleukin-1, and interleukin-6) are believed to play key roles in triggering the acute-phase metabolic response to inflammation. Manifestations of this response may include elevation in resting energy expenditure, a net export of amino acids from muscle to liver, an increase in gluconeogenesis, a shift toward the production of positive acute-phase proteins, and a decline in the synthesis of albumin. Despite erosion of body cell mass, observable weight loss may not be apparent because of an increase in the extracellular fluid compartment. Although the acute-phase metabolic response may be an appropriate adaptive response in the setting of acute inflammation, it can be associated with increased complications and mortality if severe or protracted. Diseases or injury states characteristic of cachexia include rheumatoid arthritis, congestive heart failure, chronic obstructive pulmonary disease, human immunodeficiency virus infection without serious opportunistic infection, and critical injury with adequate nutrition support. Anticytokine agents and anabolic agents offer the potential to modulate response to inflammation, but they have seen only limited clinical application to date. Nutrition support interventions may serve to blunt semistarvation and associated wasting.

Semistarvation without cytokine-mediated inflammation results in wasting of body cell mass without manifestations of the acute-phase metabolic response. In pure wasting syndrome, resting energy expenditure commonly is reduced, and visceral proteins are preserved. Increased extracellular fluid is generally not observed. The common feature of wasting conditions is poor dietary intake that results in obvious weight loss. Typical wasting disorders include marasmus, cancer, advanced acquired immune deficiency syndrome (AIDS) with opportunistic infection, critical illness without nutrition support, and chronic organ failure syndromes (eg, renal, hepatic, lung). Many patients with these disorders may also have evidence of active inflammation, so the distinction between wasting and cachexia is often blurred. Marasmus is the classic syndrome of semistarvation with manifest loss of subcutaneous fat and skeletal muscle. Among cancer, AIDS, and organ failure syndrome patients, observed weight loss associated with wasting portends an ominous prognosis. Interventions for wasting syndromes have generally focused on nutritional supplementation and administration of appetite-stimulating agents, but patient outcome and ability to accrue body cell mass appear to be determined largely by the underlying disease process.

Protein–Energy Undernutrition

Protein–energy undernutrition (PEU) has been defined by the presence of both clinical (physical signs such as wasting, low BMI) and biochemical (albumin or other protein) evidence of insufficient intake. In acute and chronic health care settings the most commonly used threshold to define PEU has been albumin < 3.5 g/dL. The prevalence rate for PEU among older persons in the hospital is greater than one third, while prevalence rates for nursing homes and other long-term-care facilities also approach one third or greater. Community-dwelling older persons have a lower prevalence, generally less than 10%. Many hospitalized patients with PEU have evidence of active or recent inflammatory response, so it is likely that components of both inadequate nutritional intake and cytokine-mediated inflammation are manifest. Approaches to treatment of PEU have generally focused on nutritional support, but identification and treatment of any underlying disease process or injury must be a priority.

Failure to Thrive

Although the term *failure to thrive* was originally used to describe infants who did not achieve height, weight, or behavioral milestones established by population-based normative data, it has also been used to describe older persons who lose weight, exhibit decline in physical or cognitive function or both, and demonstrate signs of hopelessness and helplessness. The National Institute on Aging has described failure to thrive as "a syndrome of weight loss, decreased appetite and poor nutrition, and inactivity, often accompanied by dehydration, depressive symptoms, impaired immune function, and low cholesterol." Since it is not clear that failure to thrive is a discrete clinical entity, some have advocated abandoning this disease construct in favor of targeting four potentially treatable contributing domains: impaired physical functioning, undernutrition, depression, and cognitive impairment. Prevalence estimates for failure to thrive are not available, and nutritional or other treatments have not been systematically tested.

Obesity

Excess body weight and modest weight gain ($\geq$ 5 kg) in middle age may be associated with medical comorbidities in later life that include hypertension, diabetes mellitus, cardiovascular disease, and osteoarthritis. Adverse outcomes associated with obesity include impaired functional status, increased health care resource use, and increased mortality. Change (increase or decrease) in body weight may be even more strongly correlated with mortality and comorbid conditions like cardiovascular disease or functional limitation. The growing prevalence of obesity in America extends to older persons in their 60s and 70s. The prevalence of obesity (BMI $\geq$ 30 kg/m^2) has climbed from NHANES I (14.1%) to NHANES II (14.5%) to NHANES III (22.5 %). Trends were similar for all age, gender, and racial or ethnic groups. A notable 33% of a rural Pennsylvania sample of Medicare risk participants met this obesity threshold. The National Institutes of Health has suggested: "Age alone should not preclude weight loss treatment for older adults. A careful evaluation of potential risks and benefits in the individual patient should guide management." The focus must be on achieving a more healthful weight to promote improved health, function, and quality of life. A combination of prudent diet, behavior modification, and activity or exercise may be appropriate for selected candidates.

NUTRITIONAL INTERVENTIONS

Oral Nutrition and Supplements

Preventing undernutrition is much easier than treating it. Vigilant attention to nutrition and hydration is required to identify and correct deficiencies in frail individuals. Food intake can be enhanced by catering to food preferences as much as possible and avoiding therapeutic diets unless their clinical value is certain. Patients should be prepared for meals with appropriate hand and mouth care, and they should be comfortably situated for eating. Those needing assistance with eating should be helped. Placing two or more patients together for meals can increase sociability and food intake. Foods should be of appropriate consistency, prepared with attention to color, texture, temperature, and arrangement. The use of herbs, spices, and hot foods helps to compensate for loss of the sense of smell often accompanying old age and to avoid the excessive use of salt and sugar. Hard-to-open individual packages should be avoided. Adequate time should be taken for leisurely meals. Title III C of the Older Americans Act has provided for congregate and home-delivered meals for older persons, regardless of economic status. This service is available in most parts of the country, although in some locations there is a waiting list.

Another approach that may result in improved nutrient intake for older persons who can eat is to use dietary supplements. Food intake is often decreased by the use of such supplements, but there is usually an increase in overall nutritional intake owing to the nutrient quality and density of the supplements.

There is also growing interest in the use of nutritional supplements in health promotion. A wide variety of vitamin and mineral supplements are now commonly available in supermarkets and drugstores. New recommendations for older persons include higher intake of calcium and vitamin D to prevent osteoporosis (see Table 28.2). Folic acid, B$_6$, and B$_{12}$ can lower homocysteine levels, possibly reducing the risk of coronary artery disease and helping to prevent the decline in the cognitive function associated with aging. Immune function may be improved by supplementation of protein, vitamin E, zinc, and other micronutrients. Whether the effects of antioxidants are beneficial is the subject of controversy; it has been suggested that they may help in preventing age-related cataracts and macular degeneration and reduce cardiovascular disease and mortality. Vitamin E has also been thought to slow the progression of Alzheimer's disease. Since approximately 50% of older persons may also take self-prescribed dietary supplements, it is imperative that the clinician obtain information about the older patient's use of all supplements. The appropriateness and safety of each supplement should be evaluated, since consumers are often unaware of potential risks and side effects of many over-the-counter supplements.

Tube Feeding

For patients who are unable to eat enough to sustain adequate nutrition, tube feeding may be appropriate. A video fluoroscopic study may be indicated to identify swallowing disorders for those patients at risk for aspiration. Feedings can be provided through several different access routes to the gastrointestinal tract. Nasoenteric tubes (8 or 10 French) are often used for short-term enteral feedings. For patients who require support over the longer term or who are at risk for accidental tube displacement or removal, gastrostomy tubes may be considered. A percutaneous endoscopic gastrostomy offers a less invasive alternative to a surgical gastrostomy without requiring general anesthesia. Jejunostomy feedings deliver nutrients into the jejunum and may be appropriate for patients with gastric dysfunction. Tube feeding requires a high level of care and may necessitate institutionalization. The patient's manual dexterity and cognitive ability may limit his or her ability to provide routine self-care with enteral feeding tubes.

Selection of enteral feeding formula should take into consideration the estimated duration of tube feeding, the location of the feeding tube, the energy and protein requirements of the patient, the ability of the patient to digest and absorb nutrients, and the expense and availability of the product to be used. Many patients on long-term feeding can be supported with standard polymeric 1 kcal/mL formula that provides RDA levels or greater for nutrients. Pancreatic or biliary insufficiency and alterations in intestinal absorptive function may warrant the use of specialized elemental formulations that contain medium-chain triglycerides. Disease-specific formulas may also be considered for selected patients. Fluid constraints may dictate the use of more concentrated solutions of 1.5 to 2 kcal/mL, but these also carry greater risk for dehydration. Most older persons require 1500 to 2400 mL of 1.0 kcal/mL over a 24-hour period to meet their calculated energy requirements. Free water can be added by the use of a bolus regimen throughout the day to meet fluid requirements. Tube feedings should be started at full strength at low rates, increasing gradually in volume to allow accommodation of the gastrointestinal system. Intermittent gastric residuals should be monitored while feedings are being advanced and tolerance is being established. It is often possible to bolus feed by the gastric route such that feedings are delivered several times daily over 20 to 30 minutes, allowing for greater freedom and eliminating the requirement for infusion pumps.

Diarrhea is frequently associated with tube feedings, occurring in 5% to 30% of tube-fed older persons. Medications and their vehicles (eg, sorbitol) are the leading cause for diarrhea and warrant thorough review. Bacterial contamination and formula osmolarity are also frequently cited causes of diarrhea. A trial of a fiber-enriched formulation is a consideration when other interventions have failed. Aspiration, the most serious common complication of enteral feeding, may occur in 23% to 58% of patients receiving gastric feedings. (See also "Eating and Feeding Problems," p 191.)

Parenteral Nutrition

Parenteral nutrition should be considered only when the gastrointestinal tract cannot be used for an extended period. Indications for use include a nonfunctional gastrointestinal tract, obstruction of the gastrointestinal tract, prolonged ileus, severe gastrointestinal hemorrhage, severe malabsorption, intractable vomiting, fistulas with high output (> 500 mL per day), severe enterocolitis, severe pancreatitis, mesenteric ischemia, or peritonitis. There has been little published research concerning the use of parenteral nutrition for older persons, so there are many unanswered questions.

Standard solutions for parenteral nutrition containing dextrose and amino acids are generally used for older patients. Modified amino acid profiles may be considered to meet requirements of selected disease states, as in renal disease. Lipid emulsions are added to provide a concentrated source of energy and essential fatty acids, and electrolytes, minerals, and vitamins in the solution may be adjusted to meet patient needs.

Older persons appear to tolerate parenteral nutrition well; however, fluid issues and dextrose tolerance may be concerns. It is not appropriate to exclude potential candidates for parenteral nutrition on the basis of age alone. Older persons do not appear to be at any greater risk than younger adults for complications. Older and younger persons are susceptible to the same complications of parenteral nutrition, including those of catheter insertion, as well as those of deep-vein thrombosis and sepsis.

Refeeding

A refeeding syndrome has been described in severely undernourished persons who are subject to overzealous enteral or parenteral feedings early in the course of resuscitation. The syndrome is characterized by severe electrolyte abnormalities and fluid retention. Hypokalemia, hypophosphatemia, and hypomagnesemia are commonly observed, probably resulting from extracellular-intracellular compartment shifting due to nutrient transport. These difficulties may be avoided by cautious advance to feeding goals over several days, with close monitoring of fluid and electrolyte status during this period. (See also "Eating and Feeding Problems," p 191.)

ETHICAL AND LEGAL ISSUES

In the nursing home unacceptable weight loss, as defined by the Omnibus Budget Reconciliation Act of 1987, is any loss greater than or equal to 5% in the past month or 10% in the past 6 months. The MDS is a functionally based assessment tool performed on admissions to long-term care facilities that are receiving payments from the Centers for Medicare & Medicaid Services. Sections of the MDS that are related to nutritional status include those assessing cognitive function, mood and behavior, physical function, health condition, oral and nutritional status, dental status, skin condition, and special treatments and procedures, including restorative care for eating and swallowing. Resident Assessment Protocols ensure prompt identification of problems focused on by the MDS. Standards of care dictate that

- a resident maintain acceptable parameters of nutritional status such as body weight and protein levels, unless the resident's clinical condition demonstrates that this is not possible, and
- a resident receive a therapeutic diet when there is a problem.

Adequate nutrition and hydration should always be provided to the older patient unless

- a fully competent older person refuses invasive nutritional support after having been fully apprised of the potential consequences and states this in written form with witnesses, or
- the terminally ill older person has executed a legally binding living will or medical directive that precludes artificial feeding in the event of terminal illness or impending death.

Standards of care and ethical principles also maintain that artificial feeding may be withheld or terminated in accordance with a patient's advance directive (known as "advance care plan" in some contexts), with careful consideration of additional comorbidities and futility. Appropriate counseling of the patient and surrogate regarding the consequences of withholding feeding is obligatory. After total cessation of nutrition, several weeks may ensue before death. In this setting, palliative care, including emotional support, is extremely important and complex (see "Palliative Care," p 103).

REFERENCES

- Calle EE, Thun MJ, Petrelli JM, et al. Body-mass index and mortality in a prospective cohort of U.S. adults. *N Engl J Med*. 1999;341(15):1097–1105.

- Jensen GL, Kita K, Fish J, et al. Nutritional risk screening characteristics of rural older persons: relation to functional limitations and health care charges. *Am J Clin Nutr*. 1997; 66(4):819–828.

- Kitler DP. Cachexia. *Ann Intern Med*. 2000;133:622–634.

- Morley JE. Anorexia of aging: physiologic and pathologic. *Am J Clin Nutr*. 1997;66(4):760–773.

- Reuben DB, Greendale GA, Harrison GG. Nutrition screening in older persons. *J Am Geriatr Soc*. 1995;43(4):415–425.

- Russell RM. New views on the RDAs for older adults. *J Am Diet Assoc*. 1997;97(5):515–518.

- Sheiman SL. Nutritional problems. In: Cotter VT, Strumpf NE. *Advanced Practice Nursing with Older Adults*. New York: Mc-Graw Hill Company; 2002:285–308.

Swallowing is an important and complex task that can be affected by both normal aging and by diseases that are common in older persons. Treatment of eating and feeding problems varies, depending on the identified cause or causes and contributing factors.

SWALLOWING IN HEALTH AND DISEASE

Swallowing and Aging

Swallowing can be divided into three phases on the basis of anatomy. First is the preparatory or oral phase, which includes the complex activities of mastication and propelling the food bolus to the back of the mouth toward the pharynx. This stage is under voluntary control. The second or pharyngeal phase is involuntary and involves the initiation of the swallow reflex with propulsion of the food bolus past the laryngeal vestibule and into the esophagus. Execution of the oral and pharyngeal phases of swallowing require the complex coordination of five cranial nerves and a large number of small muscles in the head and neck, with regulation from cortical input to the medullary swallow center, all in the appropriate sequence, usually within 1 second. The third stage of swallowing is the esophageal phase, during which food is propelled down the esophagus by the action of skeletal muscle proximally and smooth muscle distally; this phase is regulated by its own intrinsic innervation.

Normal aging is associated with several alterations in eating. With advanced age, there is a diminution of the taste sensation, but not of taste discrimination (an older person may be able to distinguish sweet from salty but may need to add more salt to food to taste it sufficiently). Further, olfactory function declines with advancing age, further impairing taste sensation. Salivary function is not clearly reduced with aging, but xerostomia is a common complaint of older persons, usually owing to the adverse effects of medication. Loss of teeth greatly reduces chewing efficiency (ie, the need to chew for a longer period of time and with more chewing strokes to achieve the same level of food maceration), which is only partly ameliorated with dental prostheses. Sarcopenia, or age-related loss of lean muscle mass, may contribute to loss in chewing efficiency and to pharyngeal muscle weakness demonstrated on videofluoroscopic deglutition examination of asymptomatic older persons. Whether aging alone contributes to esophageal dysmotility (so-called *presbyesophagus*) remains a subject of debate.

Esophageal function is probably well preserved, except, perhaps, in very advanced age. In total, these changes result in a prolonged duration of each swallow with age. Further, many diseases that produce dysphagia are more common in older persons.

Dysphagia

Dysphagia, or difficulty swallowing, can occur when a disease affects any level of swallowing function. Dysphagia is usually classified as oral, pharyngeal, or esophageal. Oral dysphagia occurs when there is difficulty with the voluntary transfer of food from the mouth to the pharynx. This might be diagnosed, for example, when scrambled eggs are discovered in the cheeks of a demented patient shortly before lunch. The most common cause of oral dysphagia is dementia. In pharyngeal dysphagia, reflexive transfer of the food bolus from the pharynx to initiate the involuntary esophageal phase of swallowing while simultaneously protecting the airway from misdirection of food is difficult. The affected person may note coughing, choking, or nasal regurgitation while eating, and localize the symptoms to the throat. The most common cause of pharyngeal dysphagia is stroke, but any disease that impairs the swallowing center in the brain stem or the cranial nerves involved (eg, Parkinson's disease, central nervous system tumor), the oropharyngeal striated muscle (eg, myasthenia gravis, amyotrophic lateral sclerosis), or the local structures involved (eg, retropharyngeal abscess, tumor) may lead to pharyngeal dysphagia. Treatment of both oral and pharyngeal dysphagia involves treatment of the underlying disorder and devising an individualized, often labor-intensive, feeding program.

Esophageal dysphagia presents with the sensation that food has gotten "stuck" after a swallow. Dysphagia for both solids and liquids suggests an esophageal motility disorder (eg, achalasia, scleroderma), whereas progressive dysphagia for solids suggests a mechanical obstruction (eg, cancer, esophageal ring, stricture from mucosal irritation). None of these diseases is unique to the geriatric population, though older persons tend to take more medications and are therefore more likely to experience medication-induced esophagitis (which presents as odynophagia initially, followed by dysphagia). Common causes of medication-induced esophagitis in older persons are potassium, nonsteroidal anti-inflammatory agents, alendronate, and tetracycline-related antibiotics.

Aspiration

The misdirection of pharyngeal contents into the airway is termed *aspiration*. Despite this relatively straightforward definition, however, controversy persists over the definition of *aspiration pneumonia*. Aspiration pneumonia is believed to occur when bacteria arrive in the lungs from the pharynx in a large enough inoculum to overcome host defenses. Generally, there are two major sources of aspiration: oropharyngeal flora or gastric contents. Pneumococcal pneumonia arises from aspiration of this organism from a colonized oropharynx, however, and is usually not considered an aspiration pneumonia. Aspiration of gastric contents, or Mendelson's syndrome, usually results in a chemical pneumonitis, and the usefulness of antibiotics in this situation is questionable. Most often, local host defense mechanisms clear the lung of the offending aspirate, without serious clinical impact.

Aspiration of neither contaminated oral contents nor gastric contents is prevented by placement of a feeding tube. Tube feeding is universally cited as a risk factor for major aspiration, and some patients who have never previously aspirated begin to do so after placement of a feeding tube. A 1996 review found no evidence that tube feeding of any sort reduced the risk of aspiration pneumonia. A common misconception is that jejunostomy tube feeding has lower rates of associated aspiration of gastric contents than gastrostomy does; however, there is no evidence to support this misconception. A single nonrandomized prospective observation found that in patients with oropharyngeal aspiration, hand feeding (personal assistance with oral intake) resulted in lower rates of pneumonia than did tube feeding. No prospective randomized trials comparing hand feeding with tube feeding to reduce aspiration have been published.

Assessment of Oropharyngeal Dysphagia

Several tools may be used to assess swallowing function when oropharyngeal dysphagia is clinically suspected. The most common are the full bedside evaluation, of which there are many variations, and the videofluoroscopic deglutition examination (VDE), a variant of the modified barium swallow. There is considerable controversy regarding the relative efficacy of these tools.

VDE is usually performed by a speech-language pathologist who videotapes the patient swallowing several consistencies of barium-impregnated foods while the patient maintains various head positions. This may permit identification of the food consistency or compensatory mechanisms that minimize fluoroscopic evidence of aspiration. Depending on the results of the VDE, the therapist may recommend swallow therapy or diet modifications, or both. Swallow therapy may be compensatory (eg, turn head toward weaker side while swallowing), indirect (eg, exercises to improve the strength of the involved muscles), or direct (ie, exercises to perform while swallowing, such as swallowing multiple times per bolus). Dietary recommendations generally consist of altering bolus size or consistency of food or of restricting foods of certain consistencies.

Data are conflicting regarding the usefulness of VDE and subsequent treatment recommendations and derive from small historically controlled studies rather than larger prospective randomized trials. A systematic review of studies of dysphagia secondary to stroke published by the Agency for Health Care Policy and Research (now the Agency for Healthcare Research and Quality) concluded that evidence was insufficient to recommend one type of swallowing study over another and that data correlating specific findings from any type of examination with clinically meaningful outcomes are lacking.

FEEDING

When an older person experiences difficulty eating, the two main therapeutic approaches are careful feeding by hand or tube feeding. The first requires extraordinary patience and is labor intensive; the latter is an invasive intervention associated with its own risks. Data about either approach are limited, and randomized comparisons have not been done. The role of dietary supplements, if any, in augmenting the caloric intake of hand-fed persons has not been clearly defined. (See Table 29.1 for details about the composition of specific feeding solutions.)

The number of percutaneous endoscopic gastrostomy (PEG) feeding tubes placed in patients aged 65 years and older has grown at an astonishing rate over the past decade. Low procedure-related complication rates are often cited; however, long-term studies reveal substantial mortality among tube-fed patients. Despite the popularity of feeding tubes, a review of the literature from 1966 to 1999 found no studies demonstrating improved survival, reduced incidence of pneumonia or other infections, improved symptoms or function, or reduced pressure ulcers with the use of feeding tubes of any type in demented persons who have eating difficulties. Median survival after placement of a feeding tube is well under a year, but it is unknown whether this results from tube feeding or if the need for tube feeding is a marker that death is near.

Complications described with feeding tubes are numerous and include an increased risk of aspiration

Table 29.1—Composition of Commonly Used Tube-Feeding Solutions

Trade Name	Calories (*kCal/mL*)	Protein (*g/L*)	Carbohydrate (*g/L*)	Sodium (*mEq/L*)	Osmolarity (*mOsm/kg*)	Comments
Ensure HP	0.95	50	150	53	610	Useful when caloric requirements are less
Ensure Plus HN	1.50	63	199	52	650	Useful for fluid-restricted patients
Jevity Plus	1.20	56	175	59	450	Good source of fiber
Nepro	2.00	70	215		635	Designed for patients with renal failure
Osmolite	1.06	37	151	28	300	Standard feeding solution
Pulmocare	1.50	63	106	57	475	Designed to reduce CO_2 production
Two Cal HN	2.00	84	217	57	690	Useful for fluid-restricted patients

pneumonia, metabolic disturbances, diarrhea, and local cellulitis. Monitoring for these complications should be meticulous. A study employing a large administrative data set found that 1-year mortality was higher in 5266 nursing-home residents with chewing or swallowing difficulties who were fed with a tube than in those who were not, even when statistically accounting for potential confounding variables. A second study of 1386 nursing-home residents with recent progression to severe cognitive impairment by the same authors found no improvement in 2-year survival in the group who were tube fed, again adjusting for potential confounders. No prospective randomized studies comparing the tube and hand feeding have been published, and information on quality-of-life outcomes is sorely needed.

Not all feeding problems, of course, are related to dysphagia, and many contributing factors are quite amenable to therapy. Other approaches to consider in older persons who demonstrate eating or feeding problems are evaluation for depression, elimination of unduly restrictive diets, consideration of individual food preferences, consideration of the environment in which the person eats to improve socialization and reduce disruptive stimuli, examination of the condition of the oral cavity, determination of the needs for personal assistance with feeding, and reduction or elimination of medications that may cause inattention, xerostomia, movement disorders, or anorexia.

REFERENCES

■ Feinberg MJ, Knebl J, Tully J. Prandial aspiration and pneumonia in an elderly population followed over 3 years. *Dysphagia.* 1996;11(2):104–109.

■ Finucane TE, Christmas C, Travis K. Tube feeding in patients with advanced dementia. *JAMA.* 1999;282(14):1365–1370.

■ Grant MD, Rudberg MA, Brody JA. Gastrostomy placement and mortality among hospitalized Medicare beneficiaries. *JAMA.* 1998;279(24):1973–1976.

■ Mitchell SL, Kiely DK, Lipsitz LA. Does artificial enteral nutrition prolong the survival of institutionalized elders with chewing and swallowing problems? *J Gerontol A Biol Sci Med Sci.* 1998;53(3):M207–M213.

■ Sheiman SL. Nutritional problems. In: Cotter VT, Strumpf NE. *Advanced Practice Nursing with Older Adults.* New York: Mc-Graw Hill Company; 2002:285–308.

CHAPTER 30—PRESSURE ULCERS

Pressure ulcers are a serious and common problem for older persons, affecting approximately 1 million adults in the United States. As the population ages, pressure ulcers will continue as a major health care problem. The surgeon general's Healthy People 2010 document has identified pressure ulcers as a national health issue for long-term care, and the Centers for Medicare & Medicaid Services (CMS) has designated pressure ulcers as one of three sentinel events for long-term care. The prevention and healing of pressure ulcers requires the cooperation and skills of the entire interdisciplinary health care team.

EPIDEMIOLOGY

A pressure ulcer can be defined as any lesion caused by unrelieved pressure that results in damage to underlying soft tissue when the tissue is compressed between a bony prominence and external surface over a prolonged period of time. With aging, local blood supply to the skin decreases, epithelial layers flatten and thin, subcutaneous fat decreases, and collagen fibers lose elasticity. These changes in aging skin and the resultant lowered tolerance to hypoxia may enhance pressure-ulcer development in older persons. Since pressure is the major physiologic factor that leads to soft-tissue destruction, the term *pressure ulcer* is most widely used and preferred over *decubitus ulcer* or *bedsore*.

The incidence and prevalence of pressure ulcers vary greatly, depending on the setting. In the hospital, incidence rates have ranged from 1% to 30%. Higher rates are noted in intensive care units, where patients are less mobile and have severe systemic illnesses. The Fourth National Pressure Ulcer Prevalence Survey found an annual hospital prevalence rate of 10.1%. In the long-term-care setting, incidence and prevalence rates have ranged from 3% to 30%. Less is known about pressure ulcers in home care, but studies have reported incidence rates of 4% to 15% and prevalence rates of 5% to 15%.

The incidence of pressure ulcers not only differs by health care setting but also by stage of ulceration. The stage I pressure ulcer (persistent erythema) occurs most frequently, accounting for 47% of all pressure ulcers. The stage II pressure ulcers (partial thickness loss involving only the epidermal and dermal layers) are second, at 33%. Stage III (full-thickness skin loss involving subcutaneous tissue) and stage IV (full thickness involving muscle or bone or supporting structures) pressure ulcers make up the remaining 20%. Several studies have noted that the incidence of pressure ulcers among black Americans and among white Americans may differ. Blacks tend to have a greater incidence of stage III and stage IV pressure ulcers than whites have. Whether this can be attributed to structural skin changes or socioeconomic factors is unknown because of the paucity of pressure-ulcer research among patients in U.S. minority groups.

COMPLICATIONS FROM PRESSURE ULCERS

The development of pressure ulcers can lead to several complications. Probably the most serious complication is sepsis. When a pressure ulcer is present and there is aerobic or anaerobic bacteremia, or both, the pressure ulcer is most often the primary source of the infection. Additional complications of pressure ulcers include localized infection, cellulitis, and osteomyelitis. Quite often, a nonhealing pressure ulcer may indicate underlying osteomyelitis. Mortality can also be associated with pressure-ulcer development. Several studies have noted the association of pressure-ulcer development and mortality in both the hospital and nursing-home settings. In fact, the mortality rate has been noted to be as high as 60% for those older persons who develop a pressure ulcer within 1 year of hospital discharge. Thus, careful assessment of a pressure ulcer is essential. Finally, other complications of pressure ulcers include pain and depression. Both pain and depression have been associated with decreased wound healing.

RISK FACTORS AND RISK-ASSESSMENT SCALES

The literature abounds with lists of risk factors associated with pressure-ulcer development. However, any disease process that renders an older person immobile for an extended period of time will increase the risk for pressure-ulcer development. There are intrinsic factors and extrinsic factors that determine the tolerance of soft tissue to the adverse affects of pressure. Intrinsic risk factors are physiologic factors or disease states that increase the risk for pressure-ulcer development (eg, age, nutritional status, and decreased arteriolar blood pressure). Extrinsic factors are external factors that damage the skin (eg, friction and shear, moisture, and urinary or fecal incontinence, or both). Variables that appear to be predictors of pressure-ulcer development include age $\geq$ 70 years, impaired mobility, current smoking history, low body mass index, altered mental status (eg, confusion), urinary and fecal incontinence, malnutrition, restraints, malignancy, diabetes mellitus, stroke, pneumonia, congestive heart failure, fever, sepsis, hypotension, renal failure, dry and scaly skin, history of pressure ulcers, anemia, lymphopenia, and hypoalbuminemia.

Because of the myriad of risk factors associated with pressure-ulcer development, various scales have been developed to quantify a person's risk by identifying the presence of factors in several categories. The Braden Scale (see the Appendix, p 413) and the Norton Scale are probably the most widely used tools for identifying older patients who are at risk for developing pressure ulcers. Both tools are recommended by the Agency of Health Care Policy and Research (AHCPR, renamed the Agency for Healthcare Research and Quality). The Braden Scale has a sensitivity of 83% to 100% and a specificity of 64% to 77%; the Norton Scale has a sensitivity of 73% to 92% and a specificity of 61% to 94%.

Guidelines recommend that bed- and chairbound patients or those with impaired ability to be repositioned should be assessed upon admission to the hospital or the nursing home for additional factors that increase the risk for developing pressure ulcers. A systematic risk assessment can be accomplished by use of a validated risk-assessment tool, such as the Braden Scale or the Norton Scale. Pressure-ulcer risk should also be reassessed at periodic intervals and when there is a change in level of activity or mobility. Studies have demonstrated that the incorporation of systematic risk-assessment tools has significantly reduced the incidence of pressure ulcers. To date, the Braden Scale is the only tool to be validated in nonwhite populations. It is important to note that the use of risk-assessment tools will not guarantee that all older persons at risk for pressure ulcers will be identified.

PREVENTION

The AHCPR sponsored the development of recommendations for the prevention of pressure ulcers in adults. These clinical practice guidelines (*Pressure Ulcers in Adults: Prediction and Prevention*, published in May 1992) provide an excellent approach to evidenced-based pressure-ulcer prevention.

Skin Care

There is limited evidence on skin care to prevent pressure ulcers. Most recommendations are based on expert opinions. The goal of skin care after identifying the older person at risk for pressure ulcers is to maintain and improve tissue tolerance to pressure in order to prevent injury.

All older persons at risk should have a systematic skin inspection at least once a day, with emphasis on the bony prominences. The skin should be cleansed with warm water and a mild cleansing agent to minimize irritation and dryness of the skin. Every effort should be made to minimize environmental factors leading to skin drying, such as low humidity (less than 40%) and exposure to cold. Decreased skin hydration has been found to result in decreased pliability, and severely dry skin has been noted to damage the stratum corneum. Dry skin should be managed with moisturizers.

Massaging over bony prominences should be avoided. Previously, it was believed that massaging the bony prominences promoted circulation. However, postmortem biopsies found degenerated tissue in those areas exposed to massage but no degenerated tissue on those areas that were not massaged. All efforts to avoid exposing the skin to urine and fecal matter resulting from incontinence, to perspiration, and to wound drainage should be undertaken. When disposable briefs are used to manage incontinence, the patient must be checked and changed frequently, since perineal dermatitis can develop quickly. The use of disposable underpads to control excessive moisture and perspiration may help wick moisture away from skin. The use of moisturizers and moisture barriers should also be considered to protect the skin.

Minimizing friction and shear is also important. This can be accomplished through proper repositioning, transferring, and turning techniques. The use of lubricants (eg, cornstarch and creams), protective films (eg, transparent film dressings and skin sealants), protective dressings (eg, hydrocolloids), and protective padding may be used to reduce the possibility of friction and shear. Malnutrition should be anticipated and treated promptly. Maintaining or improving mobility is also important. There are benefits of both active and passive range-of-motion exercises to decrease pressure on bony prominences.

Mechanical Loading

Older persons who are at risk for developing pressure ulcers should be repositioned at least every 2 hours. Bed-positioning devices such as pillows or foam wedges should be used to keep bony prominences from direct contact with one another. The head of the bed should be at the lowest degree of elevation consistent with medical conditions. The use of lifting devices, such as trapezes or bed linen, to move the person in bed will also decrease the potential for friction and shear forces. The heel is quite vulnerable to pressure-ulcer development. Studies suggest that approximately 20% of all pressure-ulcer development occurs at the heels. This may be attributed to the limited amount of soft tissue over the heel. Specific clinical interventions to prevent heel pressure ulcers have been developed (see Table 30.1).

Patients seated in a chair should be assessed for good postural alignment, distribution of weight, and balance. They should be taught or reminded to shift weight every 15 minutes. The use of doughnuts as seating cushions are contraindicated since they may cause pressure ulcers.

Support Surfaces

Any older person identified as being at risk for developing pressure ulcers should be placed on a pressure-reducing device. Two types exist: static (foam, static air, gel or water, or combination) or dynamic (alternating air, low air loss, or air fluidized). Most static devices are less expensive than dynamic surfaces. Table 30.2 provides details about the various types of support surfaces that can guide selection for particular situations. Most experts would agree that for

pressure-ulcer prevention, the use of static devices is appropriate. Two conditions warrant consideration of a dynamic surface:

- bottoming out occurs (the static surface is compressed to less than 1 inch), and
- the patient is at high risk for pressure ulcers and reactive hyperemia is noted on a bony prominence despite the use of a static support surface.

Although effective at reducing pressure, dynamic airflow beds have several potential adverse effects, including dehydration, sensory deprivation, loss of muscle strength, and difficulty with mobilization.

MANAGEMENT

The AHCPR developed evidence-based guidelines on the management of pressure ulcers. This guideline, *Treatment of Pressure Ulcers*, published in December 1994, reviews the foundation for providing evidence-based pressure-ulcer management.

General Assessment

The pressure ulcer will not heal unless the underlying causes are effectively managed. A general assessment should include identifying and effectively managing the medical diseases, health problems (eg, urinary incontinence), nutritional status, pain level, and psychosocial health issues that may have placed the older person at risk for pressure-ulcer development. Unless these areas are effectively addressed, the probability that the pressure ulcers will heal is low.

Ulcer Assessment

When a pressure ulcer has developed, a comprehensive evaluation is necessary. Table 30.3 presents a systematic approach to assessment and documentation when a pressure ulcer develops.

Table 30.1—Prevention of Heel Pressure Ulcers

- Assess the heels of patients at high risk for pressure ulcers every day.
- Use moisturizer on the heels (do not massage) twice a day.
- Apply transparent film dressings to the heels of older persons prone to friction problems (eg, stroke patients).
- Apply hydrocolloid dressing (either single or extra-thick) to the heels of older persons with reactive hyperemia (pre-stage I).
- Have older persons wear socks to help prevent friction (remove at bedtime).
- Have older persons in wheelchairs wear properly fitting padded sneakers or shoes.
- Place pillow vertically under the person's legs (without hyperextending them) to support heels off the bed surface.
- Place heel cushions to prevent pressure (check for excessive moisture).
- Turn the person every 2 hours, repositioning heels.

Table 30.2—Support Surfaces for Persons at Risk for Pressure Ulcers

Type	Examples	Support area	Low moisture retention	Reduced heat accumulation	Shear reduction	Pressure reduction	Cost per day
Static surfaces	Foam	Yes	No	No	No	Yes	Low
	Standard mattress	No	No	No	No	No	Low
	Static flotation—air or water	Yes	No	No	Yes	Yes	Low
Dynamic surfaces	Air fluidized	Yes	Yes	Yes	Yes	Yes	High
	Low-air-loss	Yes	Yes	Yes	?	Yes	High
	Alternating air	Yes	No	No	Yes	Yes	Moderate

SOURCE: Adapted from Bergstrom N, Bennett MA, Carlson CE, et al. *Treatment of Pressure Ulcers. Clinical Practice Guideline No. 15.* Rockville, MD: US Department of Health and Human Services, Public Health Service, Agency for Health Care Policy and Research. December 1994:38. AHCPR Pub. No. 95-0652.

Table 30.3—A Systematic Approach to the Management of Pressure Ulcers

Evaluate and Document:	Consider These Strategies:
Location	Examine other high-risk sites; develop targeted pressure-relieving strategies (eg, positioning and repositioning, padding, seat cushions, and heel elevation); limit shearing forces by special attention to positioning when the head of bed is elevated; lift rather than slide the patient; cleanse and dry regularly if wetted frequently.
Stage	Differentiate between minor stage I lesions (nonblanchable erythema related to extravasation of red blood cells into the interstitium) and deep tissue injuries that can progress to full-thickness lesions; discuss with caregivers and families the possibility of significant pressure-ulcer development when deep tissue injury is identified.
Area	Record diameter for circular lesions; record lengths of largest perpendiculars for irregular lesions.
Depth	Measure depth from plane of skin; probe and measure extent of undermining or depth of sinus tracts.
Drainage	Estimate amount; identify degree of odor and purulence; monitor hematocrit if more than minor blood loss with dressing changes occurs; monitor serum albumin if volume of ulcer drainage is large.
Necrosis	Consider simple blunt debridement of small amounts of necrotic tissue; involve general or plastic surgeons for extensive debridement; monitor damage to healthy tissue whenever using blunt, enzymatic, or wet-to-dry dressings for debridement; monitor use of pressure dressings (which can cause necrosis) after blunt debridement.
Granulation	Identify granulation as an indication that wound healing is occurring; look for regression when other infections (eg, urinary tract infection or pneumonia) occur; develop strategies to protect and enhance growth of granulation tissue (eg, nourishment, vitamins, and minerals; use of dressings to ensure moist wound surfaces); avoid damage with dressing changes.
Cellulitis	Differentiate from a thin rim of erythema surrounding most healing wounds; look for tender, warm redness, particularly if there is progression; consider treatment with systemic antibiotics active against gram-positive cocci.

SOURCE: Bennett RG. Pressure ulcers. In: Cobbs EL, Duthie EH Jr, Murphy JB. *Geriatrics Review Syllabus: A Core Curriculum in Geriatric Medicine*, 4th ed. Dubuque, Iowa: Kendall Hunt Publishing Company for the American Geriatrics Society; 1996:155.

There is no universal agreement on a single system for classifying pressure ulcers. Most experts do agree that the stage of an ulcer determines the appropriate treatment plan. It should be noted that staging alone does not determine the seriousness of the ulcer. Most systems use four stages to classify ulceration. Table 30.4 describes one staging system. When eschar, a thick brown or black devitalized tissue, is covering the ulcer, the ulcer cannot be accurately staged.

The challenge for most staging systems occurs in the definition of the stage I pressure ulcer. There is more variability in attempts to classify the first stage of ulcer development than in any other stage. Most systems define the stage I pressure ulcer as nonblanchable erythema of intact skin; both the AHCPR prediction and prevention guidelines and the CMS Minimum Data Set (required for all patients in long-term-care facilities) refer to stage I pressure ulcer in these terms. However, it is difficult (at best) to blanch the skin of persons with darkly pigmented skin. To address this concern, the National Pressure Ulcer Advisory Panel (NPUAP) revised its definition of a stage I pressure ulcer to encompass the skin alterations that might be seen in stage I pressure ulcers regardless of skin pigmentation. This system defines a stage I ulcer as an observable pressure-related alteration of intact skin whose indicators, as compared with an adjacent or opposite area on the body, may include changes in one or more of the following: skin temperature (warmth or coolness), tissue consistency (firm or boggy feel), or sensation (pain, itching). The NPUAP definition further states that the pressure ulcer appears as a defined area of persistent redness in lightly pigmented skin, whereas in darker skin tones, the pressure ulcer may appear with persistent erythema, or blue or purple hues. Although this definition is cumbersome, it is the only definition that includes patients with darkly pigmented skin.

Monitoring Healing

Monitoring the healing of pressure ulcers can pose a challenge to the practitioner. The accurate measurements of a pressure ulcer can inform the practitioner about the effectiveness of ulcer treatment. However, the use of traditional measurements (rulers and tracing paper) produces highly variable results among raters. In the past 8 years, two instruments to measure healing of pressure ulcers with some level of validity and reliability have been developed. The Pressure Sore Status Tool and the Pressure Ulcer Scale for Healing (PUSH; see the Appendix, p 415) are excellent tools for monitoring pressure-ulcer healing. The use of high-frequency portable ultrasound to measure wound healing has been introduced. The use of this technology, which can capture three-dimensional measurements, has been shown to be quite beneficial in objectively monitoring healing. Moreover, because ultrasound is "color blind," it can detect stage I pressure ulcers in darkly pigmented skin.

Table 30.4—Staging System for Pressure Ulcers

Stage I	Persistent erythema of intact skin
Stage II	Partial-thickness skin loss involving epidermis or dermis, or both. The ulcer is superficial and presents clinically as an abrasion, blister, or shallow crater.
Stage III	Full-thickness skin loss involving damage or necrosis of subcutaneous tissue that may extend down to, but not through, underlying fascia.
Stage IV	Full-thickness skin loss with extensive destruction, tissue necrosis, or damage to muscle, bone, or supporting structures (eg, tendon or joint capsule). Undermining and sinus tracts may also be associated with stage IV pressure ulcers.

SOURCE: Adapted from definitions by the Agency for Health Care Policy and Research. See Bergstrom N, Bennett MA, Carlson CE, et al. *Treatment of Pressure Ulcers. Clinical Practice Guideline No. 15.* Rockville, MD: US Department of Health and Human Services, Public Health Service, Agency for Health Care Policy and Research. December 1994:47–49. AHCPR Pub. No. 95-0652.

There has been considerable debate regarding the use of reverse staging of pressure ulcers to monitor healing. Staging of pressure ulcers is appropriate only for defining the maximum anatomic depth of tissue damage. Since pressure ulcers heal to a progressively more shallow depth, they do not replace lost muscle, subcutaneous fat, or dermis before they re-epithelialize. Instead, pressure ulcers are filled with granulation (scar) tissue composed primarily of endothelial cells, fibroblasts, collagen, and extracellular matrix. A stage IV pressure ulcer cannot become a stage III, stage II, and then stage I; reverse staging does not accurately characterize what is physiologically occurring as the pressure ulcer heals. When a stage IV pressure ulcer has healed, it should be classified as a healed stage IV pressure ulcer, not a stage 0. The progress of healing can be documented only by describing ulcer characteristics or measuring wound characteristics with a validated tool.

Control of Infections

All pressure ulcers will become colonized with both aerobic and anaerobic bacteria, and superficial, swab cultures of the wounds have not been shown to be helpful in management. Wound cleansing and dressing changes are two of the most important methods for minimizing the amount of bacterial colonization. Increasing the frequency of wound cleansing and dressing changes is an important first step when purulent or foul-smelling drainage is observed on the ulcer. When ulcers are not healing or have persistent exudate after 2 weeks of optimal cleansing and dressing changes, it is reasonable to consider a 2-week trial of topical antibiotics (eg, silver sulfadiazine, triple antibiotic), monitoring carefully for allergic reactions. The use of topical antiseptics (eg, povidone iodine, iodophor, sodium hypochlorite, hydrogen peroxide, and acetic acid) is not recommended because of their tissue toxicity.

When ulcers fail to heal despite these treatments, it is reasonable to consider the possibility of cellulitis or osteomyelitis. Biopsy of the ulcer for quantitative bacterial cultures or of the underlying bone can be used to establish these diagnoses. The presence of cellulitis, osteomyelitis, bacteremia and sepsis are all indications for the use of systemic antibiotics.

Ulcer Care

Ulcer care should be evaluated for healing progress on a weekly basis. There are no standard healing rates for pressure ulcers. Review of the literature suggests that a majority of stage I pressure ulcers heal within 1 day to 1 week; stage II, within 5 days to 3 months; stage III, within 1 month to 6 months; and stage IV, within 6 months to 1 year. Clearly, some full-thickness pressure ulcers may never heal, depending on comorbidity; however, no clear guidelines exist to determine when a pressure ulcer can be truly defined as recalcitrant nor what characteristics must be present to predict that an ulcer will never heal.

Debridement

The presence of necrotic, devitalized tissue supports the growth of pathologic organisms and prevents healing. Because devitalized tissue is avascular, the use of topical antibiotics is not recommended. There are four types of debridement methods: mechanical, enzymatic, autolytic, and sharp (Table 30.5). The debridement method should be selected on the basis of the patient's health condition, the ulcer presentation, the presence or absence of infection, and the patient's ability to tolerate the procedure.

Dressings

Numerous dressings are used in the healing of pressure ulcers. The use of gauze wet-to-dry has been discouraged by experts, since this technique can damage the tissue matrix and prolong healing. Many experts advocate the use of hydrocolloid dressings. These dressings,

Table 30.5—Methods of Debridement

Type	Description	Advantages, Disadvantages
Mechanical	Use of physical forces to remove devitalized tissues; methods include wet-to-dry irrigation (using 19-gauge needle with 35-cc syringe), hydrotherapy, and dextranomer	May remove both devitalized and vitalized tissues; may cause pain
Surgical, Sharp	Use of scalpel, scissors, and forceps to remove the devitalized tissue; laser debridement is also under this category	Quick, effective if performed by skilled professional; should be used when infection is suspected; pain management is needed
Enzymatic	Use of topical debriding agent to dissolve the devitalized tissue (chemical force)	Appropriate when there are no signs or symptoms of local infection; some may damage surrounding skin
Autolytic	Use of synthetic dressings to allow the devitalized tissue to self-digest from the enzymes found in the ulcer fluids (natural force)	Recommended when the older person cannot tolerate other forms of debridement and when infection is not suspected; may take a long time to be effective

SOURCE: Data from Bergstrom N, Bennett MA, Carlson CE, et al. *Treatment of Pressure Ulcers. Clinical Practice Guideline No. 15.* Rockville, MD: US Department of Health and Human Services, Public Health Service, Agency for Health Care Policy and Research. December 1994:47–49. AHCPR Pub. No. 95-0652.

when compared with gauze, have been found to significantly speed the healing process. This is most likely because hydrocolloids require fewer dressing changes (inflicting less trauma), block bacteria from penetrating the wound bed, and maintain a moist wound environment (facilitating increases in the growth factors needed in the healing process). It is essential to select an appropriate dressing, not on the basis of the stage of the pressure ulcer, but rather on the amount of wound exudate maximizing the moist wound environment. Table 30.6 identifies some of the most common dressings and the indications for their use.

Nutrition

An association has been observed between pressure ulcers and malnutrition, and several studies have identified malnutrition as a risk factor for pressure-ulcer formation. Ensuring an adequate diet to prevent malnutrition, to the extent compatible with an individual's wishes, is a reasonable strategy to reduce the risk of ulcer formation. If a patient with a pressure ulcer is malnourished, the importance of diet and dietary supplements is more controversial. The AHCPR guideline rates the strength of the evidence as "C," the weakest rating, for nutritional support that achieves approximately 30 to 35 calories/kg/day and 1.25 to 1.50 g of protein/kg/day. Evidence to support the use of supplemental vitamins and minerals is equally weak.

Adjunctive Therapy

Throughout the years a myriad of treatments have been advocated for the healing of pressure ulcers without sufficient data to support their various claims. Data on the therapeutic efficacy of hyperbaric oxygen, low-energy laser irradiation, and therapeutic ultrasound have not been established. However, areas of great promise include the use of recombinant platelet-derived growth factors to stimulate healing and skin equivalents that may prove to heal stage III and stage IV pressure ulcers. Preliminary data on the uses of electrical stimulation, vacuum-assisted closures, and warm-up therapy, which increases the basal temperature of the ulcer to promote healing, are promising.

Surgical Repair

The use of surgical repair of a pressure ulcer remains a viable option for stage III and stage IV pressure ulcers. However, since many stage III and stage IV pressure ulcers eventually heal over a long period of time with the use of modern wound-healing principles, and since the rate of recurrence of surgically closed pressure ulcers is high, the practitioner must carefully weigh the benefits of the surgery. When the surgical option is exercised, the most common type of surgical repairs include direct closure, skin grafting, skin flaps, musculocutaneous flaps, and free flaps.

Table 30.6—Common Dressings for Treating Pressure Ulcers

Dressing	Indication	Contraindications	Example
Transparent film	Stage I ulcer Protection from friction Superficial scrape Autolytic debridement of slough Apply skin prep to intact skin to protect from adhesive	Draining ulcers Suspected skin infection or fungus	Bioclusive Tegaderm Opiate
Foam island	Stage II, III Low to moderate exudate Can apply as window to secure transparent film	Excessive exudate Dry, crusted wound	Alleyn Lyofoam
Hydrocolloids	Stage II, III Low to moderate drainage Good peri-wound skin integrity Autolytic debridement of slough Left in place 3–5 days Can apply as window to secure transparent film Can apply over alginate to control drainage Must control maceration Apply skin prep to intact skin to protect from adhesive	Poor skin integrity Infected ulcers Wound needs packing	Duoderm Extrathin film Duoderm Tegasorb RepliCare Comfed
Alginate	Stage II, III, IV Excessive drainage Apply dressing within wound borders Requires secondary dressing Must use skin prep Must control for maceration	Dry or minimally draining wound Superficial wounds with maceration	Sorbsan Kaltostat Algosteril AlgiDerm
Hydrogel (amorphous gels)	Stage II, III, IV Needs to be combined with gauze dressing Stays moist longer than saline gauze Changed 1–2 times/day Used as alternative to saline gauze for packing deep wounds with tunnels, undermining Reduces adherence of gauze to wound Must control for maceration	Macerated areas Wounds with excess exudate	Intrasite gel Solosite gel Restore gel
(gel sheet)	Stage II Skin tears Needs to be held in place with topper dressing	Macerated areas Wounds with moderate to heavy exudate	Vigilon Restore Impregnated Gauze
Gauze packing (moistened with saline)	Stage III, IV Wounds with depth, especially those with tunnels, undermining Must be remoistened often to maintain moist wound environment		square 2X2s, 4X4s Fluffed Kerlix Plain Nugauze

SOURCE: Copyright © 1999 by Rita Frantz. Reprinted from Reuben DB, Herr K, Pacala JT, et al. *Geriatrics At Your Fingertips.* 2003 ed. Malden, MA: Blackwell Science, Inc., for the American Geriatrics Society; 2003: 130–131. Reprinted with permission.

REFERENCES

■ Allman RM, Goode PS, Patrick MM, et al. Pressure ulcer risk factors among hospitalized patients with activity limitation. *JAMA* 1995;273(11):865–870.

■ Beitz JM, van Rijswijk L. Using wound care algorithms: a content validation study. *JWOCN.* 1999;26(5):236–249.

■ Bergstrom N, Bennett MA, Carlson CE, et al. *Treatment of Pressure Ulcers. Clinical Practice Guidelines No. 15.* Rockville, MD: US Department of Health and Human Services, Public Health Service, Agency for Health Care Policy and Research. December 1994. AHCPR Pub. No. 95-0652.

■ Berlowitz DR, Bezerra HQ, Brandeis GH, et al. Are we improving the quality of nursing home care: the case of pressure ulcers. *J Am Geriatr Soc.* 2000;48(1):59–62.

■ Lyder CH. Exploring pressure ulcer prevention and management. *Annual Review of Nursing Research.* 2002;20:35–61.

■ Lyder CH. Pressure ulcer prevention and management. *JAMA.* 2003;289(2):223–226.

EMIOLOGY

studies have documented a high prevalence of sleeping problems among older people. In one representative sample, the most common sleeping complaints among community-dwelling older people were found to include difficulty falling asleep (37% of the sample), nighttime awakening (29%), and early morning awakening (19%). Daytime sleepiness is also common, with 20% of noninstitutionalized Americans reporting that they are "usually sleepy in the daytime." In addition, at least one half of community-dwelling older persons use either over-the-counter or prescription sleeping medications.

Three large epidemiologic studies of older adults found an association between sleep complaints and risk factors for sleep disturbance (eg, chronic illness, mood disturbance, less physical activity, and physical disability) but little association with older age, suggesting that these risk factors, rather than aging per se, accounts for insomnia in the majority of those studied. However, some primary sleep disorders, such as sleep apnea and periodic limb movements in sleep, increase in prevalence with age. Although some studies have shown an increased risk of sleep complaints in women, others have not. Two studies have shown that self-reported sleeping difficulties are more common in older black Americans, particularly women and those with depression and chronic illness.

Unfortunately, late-life insomnia is commonly a chronic problem. A study of older people in Britain found that 36% of those with insomnia at baseline reported severely disrupted sleep 4 years later. Of those who reported use of prescription hypnotics at baseline, 32% were still using these agents 4 years later. Another study of a volunteer sample of urban women aged 85 years and older found that all had health problems and sleeping difficulties, and the majority regularly used alcohol, an over-the-counter sleeping medication, or both, in an effort to improve their sleep. Previous research has suggested that insomnia is a predictor of death and nursing-home placement in older men, but not in older women.

CHANGES IN SLEEP WITH INCREASED AGE

Older people have a decreased sleep efficiency (time asleep divided by time in bed), a similar or decreased total sleep time, and an increased sleep latency (time to fall asleep). Older people also report an earlier bedtime and earlier morning awakening, more arousals during the night, and more daytime napping. Notable age-related changes in sleep structure as measured by polysomnography include a decrease in stage 3 and stage 4 sleep (the deeper stages of sleep). Stages 1 and 2 (the lighter stages of sleep) increase or remain the same. The decline in deep sleep seems to begin in early adulthood and progresses throughout life. In persons over age 90 years, stages 3 and 4 may disappear completely. Other common findings include an earlier onset of rapid-eye-movement (REM) sleep in the night and decreased total REM sleep but no change or a decrease in percentage of REM sleep. Older people have more equal distribution of REM sleep throughout the night, whereas younger people have longer periods of REM sleep as the night progresses. Older persons also have a decrease in spindles and K complexes on electroencephalogram during sleep.

The significance of these changes in sleep is unclear. There is some evidence that older people need less sleep, although establishing need for sleep is difficult. After a period of sleep deprivation, older people do show less daytime sleepiness, less evidence of decline in performance measures, and a quicker recovery of normal sleep structure than younger people show. Although older people do have more sleep disturbance with jet lag and shift work, this may reflect physiologic changes in circadian rhythm with age. In addition, it is not clear to what extent changes in sleep are due to changes of normal aging or to pathologic changes from other processes. In studies comparing good sleepers with poor sleepers, poor sleepers were found to take more medications, make more physician visits, and have poorer self-ratings of health. In addition, chronologic age per se does not seem to correlate with higher prevalence of poor sleep.

EVALUATION OF SLEEP

To aid in screening older patients for sleep problems, the National Institutes of Health Consensus Statement on the Treatment of Sleep Disorders of Older People suggests that clinicians ask three simple questions:

- Is the person satisfied with his or her sleep?
- Does sleep or fatigue interfere with daytime activities?
- Does the bed partner or others complain of unusual behavior during sleep, such as snoring, interrupted breathing, or leg movements?

Transient sleep problems (eg, those lasting less than 2 to 3 weeks) are usually situational; persistent sleep problems are likely to be more serious and require more detailed evaluation.

The initial and subsequent office evaluations of a patient with sleep complaints can be rather lengthy. To obtain a careful description of the sleep complaint, it may be helpful to have the patient keep a sleep log, recording each morning the time spent in bed, the estimated amount of sleep, the number of awakenings, the time of morning awakening, and any symptoms that occurred during the night. This should be supplemented by information from the spouse, bed partner, or others who may have observed unusual symptoms during the night. The focused physical examination depends on evidence from the history. For example, reports of painful joints should be followed by a careful examination of the affected areas. Reports of nocturia that disrupts sleep should be followed by evaluation for cardiac, renal, or prostatic disease, or diabetes mellitus. Careful mental status testing is also indicated. The history and physical examination should guide laboratory testing.

Polysomnography is indicated when the clinician suspects a primary sleep disorder, such as sleep apnea or periodic limb movements of sleep. Even when symptoms of these conditions are not evident, polysomnography may be advisable before embarking on chronic treatment of insomnia with sleeping medications in older persons, in whom primary sleep disorders are so common. Methods to measure sleep other than traditional polysomnography in a sleep laboratory have been developed and are being used more extensively in studies of sleep in older people. For example, a wrist-activity monitor estimates sleep versus wakefulness on the basis of the person's nighttime wrist activity. In fact, one study demonstrated that the wrist monitor is sensitive enough to assess the efficacy of treatment for insomnia in older persons. Another nonintrusive measure of sleep for home sleep monitoring is a pressure-sensitive pad that reports signals from respiration and movement. An observational tool for detecting sleep problems and sleep-related breathing disorders has been used for research in nursing-home residents. Ambulatory monitoring devices that measure pulse oximetry, heart rate, respirations, and nasal airflow are being used extensively in both clinical and research settings.

COMMON SLEEP DISORDERS

Insomnia (ie, difficulty in initiating or maintaining sleep) is usually due to psychiatric, medical, or neurologic illness; excessive daytime sleepiness is usually due to a primary sleep disorder, such as sleep apnea. However, there is significant overlap among these symptoms. In one large study of patients of all ages referred to sleep disorders centers, insomnia was found

to be most commonly due to psychiatric illness, psychophysiologic problems, drug and alcohol dependence, and restless legs syndrome; excessive daytime sleepiness was found to be most commonly due to sleep apnea, periodic limb movements of sleep, or narcolepsy. However, patients referred to sleep centers are a select population, and the most common causes of excessive sleepiness in the community are probably chronic insufficient sleep (either voluntarily or due to work schedules), or sleep-disruptive, medical, and environmental conditions. Thus, the clinician should not exclude a primary sleep disorder in the patient presenting with insomnia and likewise should probably not refer every patient with daytime sleepiness to a sleep laboratory.

Psychiatric Disorders and Psychosocial Problems

Many studies report that psychiatric disorders are the cause of sleep problems in more than half of all patients presenting with insomnia. Depression is a particularly common cause. Early morning awakening is a common pattern, although increased sleep latency and more nighttime wakefulness are also seen. However, these changes may not be present or may be less marked in depressed persons who do not seek medical care. Conversely, sleep disturbance in older people who are not currently depressed may be an important predictor of future depression. In depressed older patients with sleep disturbance, treatment of depression may also improve the sleep abnormalities. Several studies using electroencephalography have found that sleep takes on a more normal structure with antidepressant medications, leading some authors to suggest that antidepressant drug efficacy may depend to some extent on regulation of sleep and changes in REM-sleep regulation. (See also "Depression and Other Mood Disorders," p 211.)

Bereavement can also affect sleep. Bereavement without major depression is not associated with significant changes in sleep measures, but people with bereavement and depression and those with major depression have identical sleep patterns. These sleep abnormalities improve with treatment of depression. Anxiety and stress can also be associated with sleeping difficulty, usually difficulty with initiating sleep or perhaps early awakening. Patients may have difficulty falling asleep because of excessive worrying at bedtime. (See also "Anxiety Disorders," p 220.) Research has found that older caregivers report more sleep complaints than do similarly aged healthy adults. In one study, nearly 40% of older women who were family caregivers of adults with dementia reported using a sleeping medication for themselves in the past month. (See also the sections on caregiving in "Psychosocial

Issues," p 13; "Community-Based Care," p 91; and "Elder Mistreatment," p 52.)

Drug and Alcohol Dependency

Drug and alcohol use account for 10% to 15% of cases of insomnia. Chronic use of sedatives may cause light, fragmented sleep. Most sleeping medications, when used chronically, lead to tolerance and the potential for increasing doses. When chronic hypnotic use is suddenly stopped, rebound insomnia may occur, and the person may start taking the medication again.

Alcohol abuse is often associated with lighter sleep of shorter duration. In addition, some persons try to treat their sleeping difficulties with alcohol. Older persons with poor sleep should be instructed to avoid nighttime alcohol, because although alcohol causes an initial drowsiness, it can impair sleep later in the night. Finally, it is important to remember that sedatives and alcohol can worsen sleep apnea; the use of these respiratory depressants should be avoided in older persons with documented or suspected sleep apnea. (See also "Substance Abuse," p 234.)

Medical Problems

Examples of treatable medical problems that may contribute to sleep difficulty in older people include pain from arthritis and other conditions, paresthesias, cough, dyspnea from cardiac or pulmonary illness, gastroesophageal reflux, and nighttime urination. In patients with sleeping difficulties who describe pain at night, assessment and management of the painful condition is the appropriate approach. Nighttime urination may be associated with sleep disorder, poorer quality of sleep, nighttime thirst, and increased fatigue in the daytime.

Sleep can be impaired by diuretics or stimulating agents (eg, caffeine, sympathomimetics, and bronchodilators) taken near bedtime. Some antidepressants, antiparkinson agents, and antihypertensives (eg, propranolol) can induce nightmares and impair sleep. Required medications that are sedating (eg, antihistamines, anticholinergics, and sedating antidepressants) should be given at bedtime if possible.

Sleep Apnea and Snoring

See the section on sleep-disordered breathing (sleep apnea) in "Respiratory Diseases and Disorders" (p 304).

Periodic Leg Movements During Sleep and Restless Legs Syndrome

Periodic leg movements during sleep (PLMS) is a condition of debilitating, repetitive, stereotypic leg movements that occur in non-REM sleep. The leg movements occur every 20 to 40 seconds and can last hours or even much of the night, and each movement may be associated with an arousal. The occurrence of PLMS seems to increase with age. One study found evidence of PLMS in over one third of community-dwelling older persons. Correlates of PLMS included dissatisfaction with sleep, sleeping alone, and reported kicking at night. Some authors have suggested that the high prevalence of PLMS with age is associated with delayed motor and sensory latencies noted on nerve conduction testing. PLMS may present as difficulty maintaining sleep or excessive daytime sleepiness. A bed partner may be aware of the leg movements, or these movements may remain occult until identified in a sleep laboratory.

The restless legs syndrome is a condition of an uncontrollable urge to move one's legs at night. The symptoms can also involve the arms. The diagnosis is based on the patient's description of symptoms, and the patient's complaint is usually of difficulty in initiating sleep. There may be a family history of the condition and, in some cases, an underlying medical disorder (eg, anemia, renal, or neurologic disease). The prevalence of restless legs syndrome also increases with age. Many patients with the condition also have PLMS. In older patients with PLMS or restless legs syndrome, dopaminergic agents are the initial agent of choice (eg, an evening dose of controlled-release carbidopa-levodopa or pergolide). Some patients may describe a shift of their symptoms to daytime hours with successful treatment of symptoms at night. Benzodiazepines, anticonvulsants, and narcotics have also been used for these conditions but likely have more side effects than carbidopa-levodopa in older people.

Disturbances in the Sleep-Wake Cycle

Disturbances in the sleep-wake cycle may be transient, as in jet lag, or associated with an obvious cause (eg, shift work). Some patients have persistent disturbance, with either a delayed sleep phase (fall asleep late and awaken late) or an advanced sleep phase (fall asleep early and awaken early). The advanced sleep phase is particularly common in older people. Some patients have persistent sleep-phase disturbance, in which circadian rhythms and sleeping period have become completely desynchronized (eg, persons who are always asleep during the day and awake at night), or sleep-wake cycles are irregular and sleep habits are very disjointed. It is unclear to what degree, if any, changes in sleep pattern in older people (such as increased daytime napping and disrupted nighttime sleep) are due to alterations in the circadian rhythm. Although results are mixed, several studies have shown age-related decreases in hormonal levels and evidence of earlier circadian rises in certain hormones, suggesting the existence of age-related alteration in circadian rhythm. Problems related to an advanced sleep phase may respond to appropriately timed exposure to bright light (see the section on nonpharmacologic interventions, p 207). Patients with a significant sleep-phase cycle disturbance should be referred to a sleep laboratory for evaluation. Dementia and delirium may also cause sleep-wake disturbance, frequent nighttime awakenings, nighttime wandering, and nighttime agitation.

REM Sleep Behavior Disorder

REM sleep behavior disorder is characterized by excessive motor activities during sleep and a pathologic absence of the normal muscle atonia during REM sleep. The presenting symptoms are usually vigorous sleep behaviors associated with vivid dreams. These behaviors may result in injury (to the patient or bed partner). The condition may be acute or chronic, and it is more common in older men. There may be a family predisposition. Transient REM sleep behavior disorder has been associated with toxic-metabolic abnormalities, primarily drug or alcohol withdrawal or intoxication. The chronic form of the disorder is usually idiopathic, or associated with a neurologic abnormality (eg, drug intoxication, vascular disease, tumor, infection, degenerative disorder, or trauma). Polysomnography is recommended to establish the diagnosis. Clonazepam is reported to be highly effective for the treatment of REM sleep behavior disorder, with little evidence of tolerance or abuse over long periods of treatment. Environmental safety interventions are also indicated, such as removing dangerous objects from the bedroom, putting cushions on the floor around the bed, protecting windows, and, in some cases, putting the mattress on the floor.

CHANGES IN SLEEP WITH DEMENTIA

Most studies of sleep in dementia have focused on Alzheimer's disease. Unfortunately, the baseline slowing of electroencephalographic activity often seen with dementia can cloud the distinction between sleep and wakefulness and between the various stages of non-REM sleep in the sleep laboratory. Older patients with dementia have more sleep disruption and arousals, lower sleep efficiency, a higher percentage of stage 1 sleep, and decreases in stage 3 and 4 sleep than do nondemented older people. Some authors have noted a decreased percentage of sleep spent in REM, but this has not been reported in all studies. Of interest, some studies suggest that older persons with dementia have

less sleep disturbance than older depressed persons. In fact, some suggest that sleep disturbance may be an indicator of depression as the diagnosis in persons with cognitive impairment and therefore recommend sleep electroencephalography as a diagnostic tool for distinguishing major depression from dementia. Disturbances of the sleep-wake cycle are common with dementia, resulting in daytime sleep and nighttime wakefulness.

SLEEP IN THE NURSING HOME

Studies of sleep in nursing-home residents have demonstrated prevalent disruptions in sleep with frequent nighttime arousals. In addition, sleep-related problems are a common reason for institutionalization. For example, up to 70% of caregivers report that nighttime difficulties played a significant role in their decision to institutionalize, often because the sleep of the caregiver was being disrupted. Once in the nursing home, many residents sleep during much of the day and have frequent awakenings during the night. One study found that 65% of residents reported problems with their sleep and that hypnotic use was common, but no association was found between the use of sedative hypnotics and the presence, absence, or change in sleep complaints after 6 months of follow-up. Another study found the average duration of sleep episodes during the night in nursing-home residents to be only 20 minutes. Common conditions in nursing-home residents that may contribute to these sleep difficulties include multiple physical illnesses, the use of psychoactive medications, debility and inactivity, increased prevalence of sleep disorders, as well as environmental factors such as nighttime noise, light, and disruptive nursing care. The lack of exposure to bright light during the day may also be a factor.

MANAGEMENT OF SLEEP PROBLEMS

The appropriate treatment of sleep problems must be guided by knowledge of likely causes and potential contributing factors. It is not appropriate to start an older patient with sleep complaints on a sedative hypnotic agent without a careful clinical assessment to identify the cause. Sedative hypnotics have a documented association with falls, hip fracture, and daytime carryover symptoms in older patients. If the initial history and physical examination do not suggest a serious underlying cause for the sleep problem, a trial of improved sleep hygiene is usually the best first approach (see Table 31.1). If the patient takes daytime naps, it is important to determine whether these are needed rest periods or due to inactivity, boredom, or

Table 31.1—Measures to Improve Sleep Hygiene

- Maintain a regular rising time.

- Maintain a regular sleeping time, but do not go to bed unless sleepy.

- Decrease or eliminate naps, unless necessary part of sleeping schedule.

- Exercise daily, but not immediately before bedtime.

- Do not use bed for reading or watching television.

- Relax mentally before going to sleep; do not use bedtime as worry time.

- If hungry, have a light snack (except with symptoms of gastroesophageal reflux or medical contraindications), but avoid heavy meals at bedtime.

- Limit or eliminate alcohol, caffeine, and nicotine, especially before bedtime.

- Wind down before bedtime, and maintain a routine period of preparation for bed, eg, washing up, going to the bathroom.

- Control the nighttime environment with comfortable temperature, quiet, and darkness.

- Try a familiar background noise, eg, a fan or other "white noise" machine.

- Wear comfortable bed clothing.

- If unable to fall asleep within 30 minutes, get out of bed and perform soothing activity such as listening to soft music or light reading (but avoid exposure to bright light).

- Get adequate exposure to bright light during the day.

sedating medications. It is important to explain to the person that daytime naps will decrease nighttime sleep.

Short-term hypnotic therapy may be appropriate in conjunction with improved sleep hygiene in some cases of transient, situational insomnia, particularly during bereavement, acute hospitalization, and other periods of temporary acute stress. The clinician should not withhold sedative hypnotic medication treatment in situations where it is clearly indicated. However, in the patient with chronic insomnia, sedative hypnotic agents should avoided because of the complications associated with their long-term use (see the section on chronic hypnotic use, p 206). The chronic use of benzodiazepines can lead to dependence or cognitive impairment. In chronic insomnia, it is imperative that the clinician exclude primary sleep disorders and review medications and other medical conditions that may be contributory.

Pharmacotherapy

Some commonly used sleeping medications are listed in Table 31.2, with special consideration given to the use of these agents in older people. Benzodiazepines and related agents remain the most commonly suggested agents for sleep, and several new agents have

become available. These medications should be used as briefly as possible, not to exceed 2 to 3 weeks of therapy; if used longer, they should be used for only 2 or 3 nights per week. Extreme care should be taken with these medications to avoid dependence, since continued use results in tolerance with most of these agents and may result in increasing dosages.

Short-acting agents are recommended for problems initiating sleep, and intermediate-acting agents are recommended for problems with sleep maintenance. Short-acting agents have lower associations with falls and hip fractures. However, agents with rapid elimination in general also produce the most pronounced rebound and withdrawal syndromes after discontinuation. Rebound insomnia after cessation of short-acting agents is dose dependent and can be reduced by tapering the dosage prior to discontinuing the drug. Triazolam is a short-acting benzodiazepine that is not listed in Table 31.2 because it has been associated with nocturnal amnesia and confusion and is generally not recommended for older persons.

Intermediate-acting agents have less association with daytime drowsiness than long-acting agents. If the patient also has difficulty falling asleep, these agents should be given 30 minutes before bedtime. Temazepam has an intermediate half-life and no known active metabolites, and its metabolism is not thought to be affected by aging. However, daytime sedation may occur with this agent. Estazolam is a benzodiazepine with rapid onset and intermediate duration of action, so it may be effective in both initiating and maintaining sleep. This agent has slightly active metabolites, and some accumulation may occur. The most common adverse effects are somnolence and hypokinesia. Estazolam is thought to have little effect on daytime psychomotor performance and may not result in tolerance. Long-acting agents such as quazepam and flurazepam (which has an active metabolite with a half-life of more than 100 hours in the older person) should not be prescribed for older people because of daytime sedation, lethargy, ataxia, falls, and cognitive and psychomotor impairment. The use of shorter-acting agents greatly reduces the frequency of these effects.

Zolpidem and zaleplon are two newer short-acting nonbenzodiazepine hypnotics. Both agents are structurally unrelated to the benzodiazepines, but they share some of the pharmacologic properties of benzodiazepines and have been shown to interact with the central nervous system γ-aminobutyric acid (GABA) receptor complex at benzodiazepine (GABA-BZ) receptors. The selectivity of these newer agents to the GABA-BZ receptor may account for their decreased muscle-relaxant, anxiolytic, and anticonvulsant effects in comparison with benzodiazepines in some studies. Zolpidem is a nonbenzodiazepine

Table 31.2—Prescription Sleeping Medications Commonly Used for Treating Older People

Class, Drug	Starting Dose	Usual Dose	Half-Life (hours)	Comments
Intermediate-acting benzodiazepines				
Estazolam	0.5–1.0 mg	0.5–2.0 mg	12–18	Rapidly absorbed; effective in initiating and maintaining sleep; slightly active metabolites
Lorazepam	0.25 mg	0.25–2.0 mg	10–16	Available in tablet or injectable form; associated with falls, memory loss, irritability
Temazepam	15 mg	15–30 mg	8–10 (can be as long as 20–30 in older persons)	Daytime drowsiness may occur with repeated use; effective for sleep maintenance
Short-acting nonbenzodiazepines				
Zaleplon (a pyrazolopyrimidine)	5 mg	5–10 mg	1 (reported unchanged in older persons)	Action similar to that of zolpidem
Zolpidem (an imidazopyridine)	5 mg	5–10 mg	1.5–4.5 (3 in older persons, 10 in hepatic cirrhosis)	Action similar to that of triazolam; reportedly little daytime carryover, tolerance, or rebound insomnia
Sedating antidepressants				
Nefazodone	50 mg	50–200 mg	2–4	Reportedly less GI upset and hypotension than with trazodone; anti-anxiety effect; risk of serotonin syndrome if used with MAOIs
Trazodone	25–50 mg	25–150 mg	Reportedly 6 ± 2; prolonged in older and obese persons	Moderate orthostatic effects; reportedly effective for insomnia with depression; administration after food minimizes sedation and postural hypotension; overdose safer than many other antidepressants; risk of serotonin syndrome if used with MAOIs

NOTE: GI = gastrointestinal; MAOIs = monoamine oxidase inhibitors.

imidazopyridine that has been studied in older insomniacs. In older patients, studies suggest that zolpidem does not produce rebound insomnia, agitation, or anxiety with cessation; does not seem to produce impaired daytime performance on cognitive and psychomotor performance tests; and may have a therapeutic effect that outlasts the period of drug treatment. Zaleplon is a nonbenzodiazepine hypnotic from the pyrazolopyrimidine class, which has also been studied for short-term use by older persons with insomnia. Because of their rapid onset of action, zolpidem and zaleplon should be taken only immediately before bedtime or after the patient has gone to bed and has been unable to fall asleep. Despite evidence of effectiveness with long-term administration, zolpidem or zaleplon, like benzodiazepines, are recommended for short-term use only (2 to 3 weeks) and, if used longer, for use only 2 or 3 nights per week.

Low doses of sedating antidepressants such as trazodone or nefazodone at bedtime may be used as a sleeping aid, particularly for patients with depression. These agents have been suggested for use as a nighttime adjuvant for sleep in depressed patients receiving another antidepressant at therapeutic doses during the daytime. However, side effects may limit their usefulness.

Chloral hydrate is a nonbarbiturate, nonbenzodiazepine central nervous system depressant that may cause gastrointestinal discomfort, and it can have interactions with medications such as warfarin and phenytoin. It is contraindicated for patients with marked liver or kidney impairment. Use of chloral hydrate medication has also been associated with confusion in nursing-home residents, so it is generally not recommended for use in older people.

Chronic Hypnotic Use

Two European studies have reported the prevalence of regular (eg, daily) benzodiazepine use in older people to be at least 5%, with greater use among older women than among older men. One Finnish study found chronic use of these agents to be even higher, with habitual use reported by 8% of older men and 25% of older women; the prevalence of use increased with age for both genders. There is strong evidence for increased morbidity and mortality with chronic use. Use of prescription sleeping pills 30 times in the past month (ie, nightly use) is associated with an increased mortality that is similar to the mortality hazard of smoking one to two packs of cigarettes per day. In addition, after tolerance to hypnotics develops, long-term use of these agents may actually make sleep worse. In data reported from a longitudinal study of older people in Germany, those who took sleeping medications had a higher rate of sleep-related complaints than those who did not take a medication for sleep.

Several studies have shown that the bulk of prescription sleeping medication use is occurring among chronic users, and not those with transient sleeping difficulties. A cross-sectional study in Spain found that 88% of prescription hypnotic users reported daily use of the drug, and 72% of people reported use for more than 3 months. Long-term use was two to three times more common in older than in middle-aged respondents. Likewise, studies in Canada and France have shown that sleep-promoting medications were prescribed for a year or longer in more than two thirds of people who were taking these medications. Studies in the United States have also demonstrated more benzodiazepine use by older persons and by women, with chronic use being more common in older people. The association between long-acting benzodiazepines and falls in older people has been known for some time. A prospective, population-based Finnish study found this association to be particularly true in older people with physical disability, but not in independent older persons.

It is important for the clinician to help older chronic hypnotic users to reduce or eliminate their use of these agents. This can be difficult to achieve, but telling patients that their age predisposes them to developing the side effects of forgetfulness and falls can help. One small controlled trial in older women found that decreasing hypnotic dose by one-half for 2 weeks, followed by full withdrawal (perhaps with use of a substitute pill to maintain the ritual of nightly pill taking) was effective (over short-term follow-up) in eliminating hypnotic use without adverse effects on nighttime sleep, depressive symptoms, or daytime sleepiness. Another small controlled trial involving tapering benzodiazepine use to complete withdrawal over as many as 6 weeks found better success in those persons randomized to receive a nightly dose of 2 mg of controlled-release melatonin rather than placebo. At follow-up 6 months later, nearly 80% of persons who successfully discontinued benzodiazepines continued to report good sleep quality.

Nonprescription Sleeping Agents

Nearly half of older people report using nonprescription sleeping products. The most frequently used products are sedating antihistamines, acetaminophen, alcohol, and melatonin. Sedating antihistamines (eg, diphenhydramine) are common ingredients in over-the-counter sleeping agents as well as in combination analgesic-sleeping agents that are marketed for nighttime use. Diphenhydramine has potent anticholinergic effects, and tolerance to its sedating effects develops after several weeks, so it is generally not recommended for older people. Patients with mild discomfort and sleeping difficulties may have adequate relief with a simple pain reliever (eg, acetaminophen) at bedtime and thus avoid risking the side effects of the combination agent. Although alcohol causes some initial drowsiness, it can interfere with sleep later in the night and may actually worsen sleeping difficulties. Evidence is mixed regarding the effectiveness of melatonin as a treatment for insomnia. There is some evidence in older people with insomnia that melatonin administration decreases sleep latency (time to fall asleep) and wake time after sleep onset, and increases sleep efficiency (time asleep over time in bed). However, a small trial in which persons aged 55 years and older with sleep-maintenance insomnia were treated with either 0.5 mg of transbuccal melatonin or placebo for 4 days at a time did not find polysomnographic evidence of improved sleep. Because of these mixed results and the lack of regulative control in the currently available melatonin products, it is difficult for the clinician to recommend use of these products. The exception may be chronic hypnotic users, for whom there is some evidence for success in withdrawal of the hypnotic with concomitant use of melatonin.

Nonpharmacologic Interventions

Trials have shown that nonpharmacologic interventions can be quite effective in improving sleep in older people (see Table 31.3 for a summary of such interventions). A review of more than 12 studies of behavioral interventions in community-dwelling older people with insomnia concluded that these interventions produce reliable and durable therapeutic benefits, including improved sleep efficiency, sleep continuity, and satisfaction with sleep; treatment is also helpful in reducing chronic hypnotic use. Stimulus control and sleep restriction, which focus on poor sleep habits, seem to be especially helpful for older insomniacs. Cognitive and educational interventions are also important in changing inaccurate beliefs and attitudes about

Table 31.3—Examples of Nonpharmacologic Interventions to Improve Sleep

Intervention	Goal	Description
Stimulus control	To recondition maladaptive sleep-related behaviors	Patient instructed to go to bed only when sleepy, not use the bed for eating or watching television, get out of bed if unable to fall asleep, return to bed only when sleepy, get up at the same time each morning, not take naps during the day.
Sleep restriction	To improve sleep efficiency (time asleep over time in bed) by causing sleep deprivation	Patient first collects a 2-week sleep diary to determine average total daily sleep time, then stays in bed only that duration plus 15 minutes, gets up at same time each morning, takes no naps in the daytime, gradually increases time allowed in bed as sleep efficiency improves.
Cognitive interventions	To change misunderstandings and false beliefs regarding sleep	Patient's dysfunctional beliefs and attitudes about sleep are identified; patient is educated to change these false beliefs and attitudes, including normal changes in sleep with increased age and changes that are pathologic.
Relaxation techniques	To recognize and relieve tension and anxiety	In progressive muscle relaxation, patient is taught to tense and relax each muscle group. In electromyographic biofeedback, the patient is given feedback regarding muscle tension and learns techniques to relieve it. Meditation or imagery techniques are taught to relieve racing thoughts or anxiety.
Bright light	To correct circadian rhythm causes of sleeping difficulty (ie, sleep-phase problems)	The patient is exposed to sunlight or a light box. Best evidence is from treatment of seasonal affective disorder (from 2500 lux for 2 hours/day to 10,000 lux for 30 minutes/day). For delayed sleep phase, 2 hours early morning light at 2500 lux. For advanced sleep phase, 2 hours evening light at 2500 lux. Shorter durations may be as effective. Routine eye examination is recommended before treatment; avoid light boxes with ultraviolet exposure.

sleep. However, relaxation-based interventions seem less effective for older persons. One large randomized trial of insomniacs with a mean age of 65 years compared cognitive behavior therapy (stimulus control, sleep restriction, sleep hygiene, and cognitive therapy), pharmacotherapy (with temazepam), both cognitive therapy and pharmacotherapy, and placebo. All three active treatments were found to be effective in short-term follow-up in improving sleep, as indicated by sleep diaries and polysomnography. However, people reported more satisfaction with the behavioral treatment, and sleep improvements were found to be better sustained over time (up to 2 years) with behavioral treatment.

Several small studies have also tested the effectiveness of exposure to bright light (either natural sunlight or with light boxes) on the sleep of older insomniacs. Positive effects on sleep have been demonstrated with light exposure of various intensities for various durations and at various times during the day. Evening exposure seems to be particularly useful in the older person with an advanced sleep phase. One author recommends that older persons with sleep-maintenance insomnia be treated with 2 hours of bright light exposure equal to the amount of outdoor light found at mid-day or artificial bright light of at least 2500 lux. However, even short durations of bright light in the morning have been shown to improve sleep complaints in healthy older people. One trial reported on the beneficial effects in a small sample of women aged 65

years and over of a visor that provided 2000 lux to each eye and was worn for only 30 minutes in the evening.

Bathing before sleep has been demonstrated to enhance the quality of sleep in older people, perhaps because of the increase in body temperature with bathing. Moderate-intensity exercise has also been shown to improve sleep in healthy, sedentary people aged 50 and older who reported moderate sleep complaints at baseline. However, strenuous exercise should not be performed immediately before bedtime.

Nonpharmacologic interventions have also been studied in institutional settings. A study of institutionalized demented residents with sleep and behavior problems found that morning exposure to bright light was associated with better nighttime sleep and less daytime agitation. Another study of residents with dementia and behavioral problems found that a program of social interaction with nurses was effective in reducing behavioral problems and sleep-wake rhythm disorders in 30% of the residents. Another small trial of incontinent nursing-home residents demonstrated increased nighttime sleep and less agitation among those randomized to receive a combined daytime physical activity program plus nighttime intervention to decrease noise and light disruption. Another trial combined an enforced schedule of structured social and physical activity for 2 weeks in a small sample of assisted-living residents and found that treated residents had enhanced slow-wave sleep and improved performance in memory-oriented tasks.

Nonpharmacologic interventions may also be important in the acute hospital. A large study testing the feasibility of a nonpharmacologic sleep protocol for hospitalized older patients (consisting of a back rub, warm drink, and relaxation tapes) administered by nursing personnel was successful in reducing sedative hypnotic drug use; the sleep protocol was found to have a stronger association than sedative-hypnotic drugs with improved quality of sleep.

REFERENCES

- Alessi CA, Schnelle JF. Approach to sleep disorders in the nursing home setting. *Sleep Medicine Reviews.* 2000;4:45–56. Also available at http://www.harcourt-international.com/journals.

- Ancoli-Israel S. Insomnia in the elderly: a review for the primary care practitioner. *Sleep.* 2000;23 (suppl 1):S23–S30; discussion S36–S38.

- Foley DJ, Monjan A, Simonsick EM, et al. Incidence and remission of insomnia among elderly adults: an epidemiologic study of 6,800 persons over three years. *Sleep.* 1999;22 (suppl 2):S366–S372.

- Jensen DP, Herr KA. Sleeplessness. *Nurs Clin North Am.* 1993;28(2):385–405.

- Kripke DF. Chronic hypnotic use: deadly risks, doubtful benefit. *Sleep Medicine Reviews.* 2000;4:5–20. Also available at http://www.harcourt-international.com/journals.

GERIATRIC PSYCHIATRY

CHAPTER 32—DEPRESSION AND OTHER MOOD DISORDERS

EPIDEMIOLOGY

Prevalence studies of community residents demonstrate surprisingly low rates of depressive disorders among those aged 65 years and older. Only 1% to 2% of women and fewer than 1% of men interviewed by the use of standardized instruments and diagnostic criteria have been found to be suffering from a current major depression. Paradoxically, both current and lifetime prevalence rates for older persons are lower than those for middle-aged persons; furthermore, these relatively low rates persist after accounting for possible premature death and institutionalization, both of which may be associated with depression. Similarly, the incidence of first-episode major depression has been found to decrease after age 65. Data demonstrating that older persons are less likely to recognize depression and to endorse depressed mood offers an explanation for the lower prevalence and incidence of depressive syndromes among older community residents.

The prevalence of depression that does not meet the threshold for a clinical diagnosis is substantial in older persons, with most studies reporting rates in the range of 15%. These subsyndromal states are not inconsequential. "Minor" or subsyndromal depression has been associated with increased consumption of health services, excess disability, and poor health outcomes, including higher mortality rates. Although rates of dysthymia (2%), a minor depression that has lasted ≥ 2 years, and of adjustment disorder with depressed mood (4%) are somewhat higher than for major depression, the prevalence of these states is also lower in older adults than in persons under age 65. Similarly, the prevalence of bipolar disorder decreases across the age spectrum, from a prevalence approximating 1.5% in young adulthood, the period of peak incidence, down to 0.1% among persons aged 65 and over. This decrease occurs despite evidence that bipolar disorder does not "burn out." That is, longitudinal studies carried out before the introduction of lithium carbonate demonstrated that the length of time between bipolar episodes decreases as patients age.

The prevalence rates of both major and subsyndromal depression are related to the setting in which older persons are seen and methods used to identify cases. Thus, major depression has been identified in 6% to 10% of older persons in ambulatory primary care clinics and 12% to 20% of nursing-home residents. More varied rates of 11% up to 45% have been reported among older patients requiring inpatient

medical care. The reported prevalence rates of minor depression in outpatient medical settings have been varied as well, with rates from 8% to over 40% reported. As noted below, studies that count symptoms due to physical illness toward a diagnosis of depression may contribute to inflated prevalence rates among medical patients because of symptomatic overlap. Major depression is the most common disorder among older patients seen in psychiatric settings and accounts for more than 40% of outpatient and inpatient admissions. Similarly, bipolar disorder is common among older psychiatric patients, representing between 3% and 10% of admissions of older adults.

CLINICAL PRESENTATION AND DIAGNOSIS

Depression

Criteria from the fourth edition of the American Psychiatric Association's *Diagnostic and Statistical Manual of Mental Disorders* (*DSM-IV*) are generally used for diagnosis in the United States. Criteria required to diagnose major depression are described in Table 32.1. In contrast to previous diagnostic schema, a *DSM-IV* diagnosis is not hierarchical; that is, having one diagnosis does not exclude the presence of another. Thus, an older person with a major depression may also meet criteria for a comorbid anxiety disorder.

Table 32.1—*DSM-IV* Diagnostic Criteria for Major Depression

Depressed mood*
Loss of interest or pleasure*
Appetite change or weight loss
Insomnia or hypersomnia
Psychomotor agitation or retardation
Loss of energy
Feelings of worthlessness or guilt
Difficulties with concentration or decision making
Recurrent thoughts of death or suicide

* "Gateway" symptoms, at least one of which must be present for a diagnosis of major depression.

NOTE: The diagnosis requires that the patient have at least one "gateway" symptom and that symptoms have occurred nearly every day for most of the day for at least 2 weeks. Also, the symptoms must be causing significant distress or impaired functioning and must not be due to a direct physiologic cause.

SOURCE: Data from the American Psychiatric Association. *Diagnostic and Statistical Manual of Mental Disorders.* 4th ed. Washington, DC: American Psychiatric Association; 1994.

For assessment of depression, See also "Assessment," p 47. and the Geriatric Depression Scale (GDS) in the Appendix, p 390.

Although aging does not appear to markedly affect the overall phenomenology of major depression, some differences between younger and older depressed patients have been reported. Older patients are more preoccupied with somatic symptoms and report depressed mood and guilty preoccupations less frequently. This tendency contributes to the syndrome of masked depression, in which a major depression may be hidden because of a patient's greater preoccupation with physical health concerns rather than with feelings of sadness. Among patients who do not acknowledge sustained feelings of sadness, the demonstration of the second gateway symptom, a persistent loss of pleasure and interest in previously enjoyable activities (*anhedonia*), is necessary for a diagnosis of major depression. The gateway symptoms are particularly important in primary care settings and have been found to identify most medically ill patients who also meet full diagnostic criteria. Furthermore, the gateway symptoms are less likely to overlap with those of a medical illness.

The diagnosis of major depression in older persons is complicated by the overlap among symptoms of major depression with those of physical illness. Examples of this and other complicating factors are listed in Table 32.2. Furthermore, patients with serious medical illness may be preoccupied with thoughts about death or feel worthless because of concomitant disability. The *DSM-IV* criteria require that the symptoms are not direct physiologic effects of a general medication condition or medication used to treat it, but this distinction based on cause may be difficult to make reliably. Alternative diagnostic criteria have been suggested for medical patients, including an inclusive approach that counts all symptoms regardless of cause. Inclusive approaches result in the highest prevalence rates. Furthermore, a depressed person's thoughts about death and worthlessness appear to differ from those of a patient with a serious medical illness. In depression, these thoughts are not based on a realistic assessment of prognosis or overall self-worth. The self-assessment of depressed patients is influenced by the feelings of sadness or guilt that accompany the disordered mood. The alternative diagnosis of mood disorder due to a general medical condition should be used for patients with depression that appears to result directly from a specific medical condition, such as hypothyroidism.

The recognition of psychotic depression has particular relevance to primary care clinicians. Patients with psychotic depression have sustained irrational beliefs in association with their depression. Although this severe form of major depression is most common among older patients requiring inpatient psychiatric admission, patients with psychotic depression may be seen in primary care settings when the irrational belief focuses on somatic symptoms or an imagined physical condition.

Bipolar Disorder

A diagnosis of mania requires a distinct period of persistently elevated mood lasting for 1 or more weeks and three additional symptoms that may include inflated self-esteem or grandiosity, hypersexuality, increased activity, decreased need for sleep, pressured speech, racing thoughts or flight of ideas, and distractibility. Grandiose or paranoid delusions may be present. Although the criteria for diagnosing bipolar disorder in geriatric patients are identical to those for younger adults, some differences in phenomenology have been noted. Older patients with bipolar disorder are more likely to have an admixture of depression that may present as irritability. Pressured speech that tends to go off on tangents is common, although the severity of thinking disturbance is less pronounced than in young adults and flight of ideas is less common. Hypersexuality and grandiosity may be present but are less prominent as well.

Older patients with bipolar disorder may also suffer from the depressive phase of this cycling illness. Although there have been few studies of late-life bipolar depression, the presentation of late-life bipolar depression is similar to that of unipolar major depression.

Table 32.2—Factors That Complicate Diagnosing Depression in Medical Settings

Overlap of symptoms of medical illness and those of depression (eg, fatigue, disturbed sleep, diminished appetite)

Tendency of seriously ill persons to be preoccupied with thoughts of death or worthlessness from disability

Tendency of older persons with depression to emphasize physical symptoms

Tendency of older persons to minimize emotional symptoms

Presence of side effects of medications used to treat medical illness

DIFFERENTIAL DIAGNOSIS

Approximately 50% of patients with late-life depression are having recurrences of episodes that began in early adulthood; in such cases a history of prior depressions assists patients and clinicians to recognize the diagnosis. However, 50% of older depressed patients are suffering their first episode. Despite the associations between late-onset depression and chronic medical illness, disability, and psychosocial stresses, most episodes develop without an identifiable precipitant. Because late-onset depression is less likely to run in families than typical recurrent depression, a positive family history is less useful for establishing a diagnosis. Awareness that late-onset depression commonly develops "out of the blue" requires that clinicians rely on diagnostic criteria. Clinicians should include as part of their management an explanation to patients that new-onset depression may occur without an identifiable cause.

Differentiation From Medical Illness

Medical disorders that may imitate depression are particularly important to consider in older patients because of the increased vulnerability of this population to physical illnesses. Hyperthyroidism merits special consideration, because older hyperthyroid patients may present atypically with apathy and diminished energy that may mimic depression. Apathy may accompany other medical conditions as well. Apathy is experienced as an absence of feeling or of not caring and differs from having feelings of sadness. Although apathy may be commonly associated with the gateway symptom of anhedonia, apathy may also occur in persons who retain a capacity for experiencing pleasure. The distinction of apathy from true depression becomes particularly important among patients with Parkinson's disease, carcinoma of the pancreas, and dementia, because depressive syndromes that occur commonly in these disorders are responsive to conventional antidepressants.

Depression Associated With Structural Brain Disease

Major depression may be prodromal for a progressive dementia such as Alzheimer's disease or may develop after the onset of cognitive decline. Differentiation may be confounded because depression is commonly accompanied by symptoms of impaired concentration, lack of motivation, and somatic preoccupations that are also associated with dementia. An older person with depression may both report symptoms of memory loss and poor concentration and be unable to perform simple cognitive tests without having a progressive dementia. Differentiation from dementia requires evidence that the cognitive impairment is not present consistently, developed concurrently with the onset of depression, and reverses with improvement in mood. Conversely, patients with true dementia may have symptoms that imitate depression. These include loss of interest, apathy, psychomotor retardation, and dis-

rupted sleep. A diagnosis of major depression requires the presence of at least one gateway symptom and the persistence of symptoms for at least 2 weeks; approximately 20% of patients with early Alzheimer's disease meet these criteria

Studies have described a syndrome of "vascular" or "executive dysfunction" depression that is associated commonly with anhedonia and the absence of guilty preoccupations. The syndrome is thought to result from prefrontal and subcortical lesions due to microinfarcts and should be distinguished from the more classical poststroke depression. These patients tend to have a late age of onset, risk factors for vascular disease, prefrontal or subcortical white matter hyperintensities on T2 weighted magnetic resonance imaging, and evidence of neuropsychologic deficits in functions requiring initiation. Execution of tasks requiring planning and shifting cognitive sets is impaired. Patients with vascular or executive dysfunction depression meet the full *DSM-IV* criteria but may have a diminished response to standard pharmacotherapies.

Bereavement

Bereavement following the loss of a spouse or another close relationship is common among older persons. The most disturbing symptoms of bereavement are generally time-limited and resolve within 2 months. Feelings of sadness, disturbed sleep, and diminished appetite are common in uncomplicated bereavement. Fourteen percent of bereaved persons develop a major depression within 2 years of the loss. However, bereaved older persons appear to develop depressive syndromes or full major depression at lower rates than do younger bereaved adults.

Symptoms indicating that bereavement has evolved into a full major depression include morbid preoccupations with guilt or death beyond transient thoughts that would be expected in association with the loss. Also, bereavement is not associated with marked functional impairment.

COURSE

Outcomes associated with depression in older persons are listed in Table 32.3. Major depression is a recurrent disorder in both younger and older adults. Evidence

Table 32.3—Outcomes of Depression

Recurrence; partial recovery and chronicity
Increased disability
Increased use of health care resources
Increased morbidity and mortality
Suicide

from observational studies in which treatment is not provided systematically indicate that up to one third of patients run a chronic course and another third have incomplete recovery associated with residual disability. Patients who suffer their first episode in later life take longer to recover fully from a depressive episode. Depressed older adults also use health services far more than do nondepressed older persons. Services used at increased rates include outpatient visits, specialist consultations, and laboratory assessments.

Comorbid medical illness is associated with a poorer course of late-life depression, and medical morbidity and mortality are themselves increased in patients who have suffered a depressive episode. The relationship between depression and increased mortality rates from cardiovascular causes is particularly striking. Depressed patients have an increased risk of cardiovascular mortality generally, and the development of depression in patients following a myocardial infarction, congestive heart failure, or cardiac bypass surgery has been shown to increase mortality from cardiovascular events.

Old age is associated with an increased risk for suicide. Persons aged 65 and over represent less than 13% of the population but account for 25% of suicides. The likelihood that an attempt will be successful approximates 25%, a rate that is far greater than in young adults. "Psychologic autopsy" studies that use interviews with relatives and physicians to reconstruct a suicide victim's premorbid psychiatric state have demonstrated that more than 75% of older adults who commit suicide were suffering from a major depression. The vast majority had seen a primary care physician within 1 month of the act. In addition to depression, risk factors for late-life suicide include a comorbid physical illness, living alone, male gender, and alcoholism. Older men and women commit suicide violently, with firearms and hanging being the methods most commonly used, despite the potential for overdosing on prescribed medications. More men than women use guns to commit suicide.

TREATMENT

Overview

The treatment stages for major depression can be conceptualized as follows: acute treatment to reverse the current episode, continuation treatment to prevent a relapse of that episode, and prophylaxis or maintenance treatment to prevent a future recurrence. Continuation treatment to stabilize the recovery involves continuing antidepressant therapy for an additional 6 months. Maintenance treatment is provided to patients with recurrent depression for 3 years or longer. The duration of maintenance therapy should be based on the frequency and severity of previous episodes. Psychotherapy, pharmacotherapy with antidepressants, and electroconvulsive therapy (ECT) are effective treatments for depression in older persons.

Initiatives have been developed to increase the likelihood that patients with major depression treated in primary care settings will receive antidepressant treatment that is adequate in dose and duration. The increased attention to this problems results from findings that most older patients prefer being treated for their depressions by their primary care physicians, even though depression has been underrecognized and undertreated in this setting. Also, studies have shown that the majority of patients who are prescribed antidepressants by their primary care physicians do not obtain refills of their initial prescription. Educational programs and the use of depression nurse specialists have been developed to increase recognition and treatment intensity. Of note, primary care patients have been shown to demonstrate response rates to antidepressant treatment that are comparable to those of patients seen in mental health settings.

Psychotherapy

Research demonstrating the efficacy of psychotherapy for major depression in older adults has relied on treatments that are both individualized and standardized, including cognitive-behavioral therapy, interpersonal psychotherapy, and, most recently, problem-solving therapy. The latter was developed in primary care settings. Problem-solving therapy involves working with the patient to identify real life difficulties that are causing distress and providing guidance to help the patient address them. The treatment is delivered generally in six to eight meetings spaced 1 to 2 weeks apart. Cognitive and interpersonal psychotherapy are also time-limited and highly structured. Ongoing research using psychotherapy for the treatment of minor depression has been promising, with efficacy demonstrated particularly in persons who have suffered a loss. Also, caregivers of older persons may develop minor or major depressive syndromes that benefit from psychotherapy. Psychotherapy may be combined with an antidepressant, and the combination has been associated with a longer period of remission following recovery from the acute episode. Research with younger adults suggests that the effectiveness of psychotherapy alone may be limited to patients with mild to moderately severe forms of major depression.

Antidepressants

All approved antidepressants are effective treatments of major depression in older adults. The choice of agents depends, therefore, on a particular patient's comorbid medical conditions and both the side-effect profile of the antidepressant and the individual patient's sensitivity to these effects. Potential interactions with other medications a patient is taking should be considered. Table 32.4 provides guidelines for selection from among approved antidepressants; the guidelines are based on the discussion of specific therapies in the sections that follow.

Although methylphenidate and other psychostimulants have been used to treat major depression for

Table 32.4—Guidelines for Selecting Antidepressants

Secondary amine tricyclic antidepressants (nortriptyline, desipramine)

- Severe depression with melancholic features (eg, marked weight loss, diurnal mood variation, retarded motor movement or agitation)
- Absence of conduction disturbance
- Absence of significant heart disease
- Ability to tolerate anticholinergic side effects

Selective serotonin-reuptake inhibitors (eg, citalopram, fluoxetine, paroxetine, sertraline)

- Mild to moderately severe depression
- Contraindication to or inability to tolerate a tricyclic antidepressant

Bupropion

- Psychomotor retardation and lack of energy
- A history of mania

Venlafaxine

- Presence of a comorbid generalized anxiety disorder or pronounced anxiety
- Presence of melancholia and a contraindication to tricyclic antidepressants

Nefazodone

- Pronounced sleep disturbance without melancholia
- Prominent anxiety
- Sensitivity to developing sexual side effects

Mirtazapine

- Prominent insomnia and anorexia

Monamine oxidase inhibitors (eg, phenelzine, tranylcypromine)

- "Atypical" depression with increased sleep and appetite
- Resistance to other classes of antidepressants
- Ability to adhere to dietary restrictions

Electroconvulsive therapy

- Psychotic depression
- High suicidal risk
- Life-threatening poor intake
- Failure to respond to multiple medication trials

decades, controlled data demonstrating their efficacy are lacking. However, these agents may have a role in reversing the apathy and lack of energy seen in some patients with dementia or disabling medical conditions. Benzodiazepines may be useful temporary adjuncts to treat anxiety symptoms associated with a major depression, but older persons are particularly sensitive to the adverse cognitive effects of these medications, and prolonged use may lead to dependency.

Tricyclic Antidepressants

Nortriptyline and desipramine, the secondary amine metabolites of imipramine and amitriptyline, are the most appropriate tricyclic antidepressants for use in older persons. These medications are effective in the most severe forms of depression but are associated with greater side effects and potential risks than newer classes of medications. Tricyclics are unique among the antidepressants in that relationships between concentrations and efficacy have been clearly established. For nortriptyline, therapeutic response is associated with blood levels between 50 and 150 ng/mL and for desipramine, levels above 120 ng/mL. Over 60% of patients with nonpsychotic major depression or with depression that is not associated with dementia respond within 6 weeks to levels in these ranges. Of interest, relationships of blood level to response are more variable in patients who have depression that occurs in the context of dementia. Although 5% of the population requires lower dosing because of the absence of the enzyme required to metabolize secondary amine tricyclics, most patients achieve target concentrations at doses of 50 to 75 mg per day of nortriptyline and 100 to 150 mg per day of desipramine.

The potential for side effects due to the anticholinergic and sedative properties of tricyclics limits their use in older patients. These medications are particularly inappropriate for patients who are sensitive to constipation, who have conditions or treatments that cause orthostatic hypotension, and for men with benign prostatic hyperplasia. Also, tricyclic antidepressants have a quinidine-like effect that delays ventricular conduction. Among patients with a pretreatment first-degree heart block, 10% may develop a second-degree block during treatment. Patients with a bundle branch blocked or prolonged QT_c interval are at risk for developing a ventricular arrhythmia. Also, patients with ischemic heart disease are more likely to develop cardiovascular side effects during treatment with nortriptyline than with a selective serotonin-reuptake inhibitor (SSRI).

Selective Serotonin-Reuptake Inhibitors

SSRIs and tricyclic antidepressants are comparably effective for treating mild to moderate major depression, but SSRIs are better tolerated. Controversy continues about whether the most severe melancholic form of depression that generally requires treatment in a psychiatric hospital responds better to a secondary amine tricyclic antidepressant. Melancholic patients typically suffer from marked appetite and weight loss, diurnal mood variation that is worse in the morning, early morning awakening, and either retardation of motor movement or agitation.

Recommended doses for older adults are 10 to 40 mg of citalopram, fluoxetine, or paroxetine. These doses are somewhat lower than those used for younger adults because of the somewhat decreased metabolism associated with aging. The recommended target dose for sertraline ranges from 50 to 100 mg in most cases.

Although the SSRIs are generally free of severe side effects, a small proportion of older patients develop hyponatremia due to the syndrome of inappropriate antidiuretic hormone secretion during SSRI treatment, particularly at higher doses. Some patients may be unable to tolerate SSRIs because of a tendency to become highly anxious or agitated. This reaction appears to be more common in older persons. Beginning at lower doses may reduce the incidence of anxiety with activating SSRIs such as fluoxetine and may decrease the gastrointestinal side effects of nausea or diarrhea that occur with other SSRIs. Sexual side effects occur commonly with all SSRIs, and many older patients prefer treatment with another medication to avoid them. Although SSRIs have been associated with mild weight loss initially, long-term use with many of these medications has been associated with weight gain. Pseudoparkinsonism and other movement disorders may occur, particularly if these medications are used in combination with other drugs that block dopamine (eg, metoclopramide).

Much has been written about potential drug interactions with SSRIs. These medications inhibit various P-450 hepatic cytochrome isoenzymes that metabolize most medications. Fluoxetine and paroxetine are potent inhibitors of the P-450 2D6 isoenzyme responsible for the metabolism of most psychiatric medications, in addition to dextromethorphan, codeine, and metoprolol. Sertraline is a weak inhibitor of both the 2D6 and 3A4 isoenzymes. Thus, downward dose adjustment of medications such as tricyclic antidepressants and risperidone is appropriate if used with these SSRIs. Inhibition of 2D6 can decrease the analgesic effects of codeine (and related compounds) and tramadol by preventing their conversion to their active metabolites, morphine and O-desmethyltramadol. Evidence for a clinically significant effect due to inhibition of 2D6 metabolism of metoprolol metabolism is lacking. Nefazodone is a potent inhibitor of the P-450 3A4 isoenzyme that metabolizes medications such as alprazolam, astemi-

zole, cyclosporin, and erythromycin. Fluvoxamine, an SSRI used to treat obsessive-compulsive disorder, is approved as an antidepressant in Europe. Fluvoxamine inhibits both the 3A4 and 1A2 systems. Because P-450 1A2 is required to metabolize theophylline, olanzapine, and phenacetin, concurrent use of fluvoxamine may result in marked increases in marked concentrations of these medications.

SSRIs are known to be tightly protein bound. For this reason, they may displace warfarin from binding sites and increase the anticoagulant effects of this medication. Careful monitoring of prothrombin times or another suitable index of blood clotting is indicated following the introduction of an SSRI to patients being treated with warfarin.

SSRIs have been considered particularly safe for older persons to use because these antidepressants do not cause orthostatic hypotension, arrhythmias, or marked sedation. However, evidence indicates that nursing-home residents treated with SSRIs are at increased risk for falling and suffering hip fractures. It is not clear whether these findings are due to patient selection in that patients considered at greatest risk for falling may be treated with SSRIs preferentially. Alternatively, SSRIs may contribute to falls by causing a subtle balance disturbance or pseudoparkinsonism in vulnerable patients.

Other Antidepressants

Bupropion is generally safe and well tolerated when used at recommended doses. Bupropion has been associated with a 0.4% risk of seizures, which is much higher when recommended doses are exceeded. Although the precise mechanism of action is unknown, bupropion appears to act through increasing the activity of dopamine and norepinephrine. This mechanism may explain the activating property of bupropion and the recommendation that dosing of the short-acting form be completed by mid-afternoon to avoid insomnia. Long-acting bupropion has a smaller seizure risk and is less likely to cause insomnia. Doses are increased gradually by the use of a twice-a-day regimen to achieve target doses of 150 to 300 mg of the short-acting form, although doses as high as 450 mg are used in young adults. The dose range of sustained-release bupropion is between 200 and 300 mg per day, and doses below 300 mg can be given as a single daily dose. Although systematically obtained data are unavailable, older patients may be more vulnerable to developing anxiety, a tremor, or myoclonus at doses at the high end of the approved therapeutic range.

Venlafaxine acts as an SSRI at lower doses while also inhibiting the reuptake of norepinephrine at the high end of the therapeutic range of 75 to 225 mg per day. Venlafaxine is available in short-acting and extended-release forms. Venlafaxine is effective for both generalized anxiety and major depression and may treat both effectively at doses between 75 and 150 mg per day. A dose-response relationship for severe depression has been demonstrated, and patients with melancholia may require doses of 225 mg per day or greater. Initial dosing should use gradual increases to minimize the early side effect of nausea. The noradrenergic properties of higher doses may explain the association between doses of 225 mg and higher with hypertension. Patients requiring doses at the high end of the therapeutic range should have blood-pressure monitoring. Paradoxically, this side effect does not occur in patients with preexisting hypertension that is being controlled by treatment with a β-blocker. Venlafaxine, like other SSRIs, has been associated with decreased sexual functioning. Venlafaxine should be discontinued by gradual tapering to avoid the risk of flu-like discontinuation symptoms.

Nefazodone has SSRI properties as well as being a 5-HT$_2$ antagonist. In addition to being approved as an antidepressant, nefazodone is thought to reduce anxiety. In young adults, the antidepressant response to nefazodone has been shown to be dose related, with greatest response rates occurring in the range of 300 to 500 mg per day given by twice-a-day dosing. However, older persons may have difficulty tolerating the sedative side effects of nefazodone at this dose range. As described above, nefazodone is a potent inhibitor of the P-450 3A4 system and must be used cautiously in patients being treated with other medications metabolized by this isoenzyme. Nefazodone treatment is not associated with sexual side effects or insomnia.

Mirtazapine is a norepinephrine, 5-HT$_2$, and 5HT$_3$ antagonist. The total daily dosage is 15 to 45 mg. Mirtazapine may be given as a single bedtime dose and is available in sublingual form, which may be useful for patients who have difficulty swallowing. Bedtime administration uses the sedative side effects of mirtazapine to help patients sleep. Mirtazapine is also associated with increased appetite and weight gain. This side-effect profile has contributed to the use of mirtazapine before bed in nursing-home residents with depression and dementia who demonstrate nighttime agitation and weight loss. Paradoxically, weight gain may be less severe at higher doses.

The monamine oxidase inhibitors (MAOIs) are effective antidepressants that have been in use for nearly half a century. Phenelzine, used at target doses of 30 to 45 mg per day, tranylcypromine, used at doses of 30 to 40 mg per day, and isocarboxazid at 30 mg per day, are the three MAOIs currently available in the United States. Orthostatic hypotension is a common side effect of MAOIs and may increase the risk of falling among older patients. Ingestion of a food product rich in tyramine or taking a pressor amine such as one used in over-the-counter cold remedies during MAOI therapy can cause a life-threatening hypertensive crisis. Use of MAOIs with an SSRI or meperidine can cause a fatal serotonin syndrome associated with delirium and hyperthermia.

Electroconvulsive Therapy for Managing Psychotic Depression

Psychotic depression is generally resistant to standard antidepressant regimens. Aggressive pharmacotherapy is required, with best results obtained in young adults when high doses of antidepressants and antipsychotic medications are combined. However, the effectiveness of combination treatment for older patients with psychotic depression remains uncertain. Available evidence suggests that most older patients who have depression with pronounced psychotic features either cannot tolerate adequate doses of conventional medications or do not respond to them. Therefore, ECT has become the standard treatment for late-life psychotic depression. (See also the discussion of ECT in the section on mania, p 218.)

Management of Nonresponders

Approximately 60% of patients with major depression demonstrate a robust response to treatment within 6 weeks. An additional 15% to 25% of patients who have begun to improve achieve remission if treatment is continued for an additional 4 to 6 weeks. Older patients may take longer than young adults to respond to SSRIs and perhaps to other antidepressants. Some published studies using SSRIs have reported 6-week response rates of 40% that increase to more than 60% when treatment is extended to 12 weeks. As in the treatment of young adults, improvement at 2 to 4 weeks is indicative of whether a particular patient will respond fully.

Lithium carbonate, methylphenidate, or triiodothyronine combined with a secondary amine tricyclic has been used to treat patients who fail to respond to one of the monotherapies. However, empirical data supporting these combinations are scant, particularly in older persons. Consideration should be given initially to whether another diagnosis is present. The options of switching to an antidepressant from another class or consulting with a geriatric psychiatrist are more appropriate than initiating combination treatments that have not been studied systematically.

PHARMACOTHERAPY OF MANIA: MOOD STABILIZERS

Lithium Carbonate

Lithium carbonate is highly effective for the acute and maintenance treatment of classical manic episodes. Target plasma levels in the range of 0.8 to 1.2 mEq/L are used to treat acute mania, and levels of 0.6 to 0.8 mEq/L are used for prophylaxis in young adults. The use of lithium for treating older patients is complicated by the 30% decrease in renal functioning that accompanies normal aging and the increased sensitivity of older persons to neurologic side effects from this medication, particularly if structural brain disease is present. Lithium treatment is further complicated by the potential for pharmacokinetic interactions with medications used to treat physical illnesses.

The decreased renal clearance of lithium is addressed simply by reducing the total daily dose. Furthermore, lower concentrations may be adequate in older adults, with some patients responding acutely to levels in the range of 0.6 to 0.8 mEq/L or less. Levels below 0.6 mEq/L may provide effective prophylaxis. Also, older persons develop neurologic side effects at concentrations that are well tolerated in young adults. A fine resting tremor, myoclonus, an intention tremor, or pseudoparkinsonism may develop with levels in the standard therapeutic range. Sensitivity to these effects and to increased confusion is greatly increased among patients with dementia and when lithium is coadministered with an antipsychotic medication. In the absence of empirically driven guidelines, clinicians are advised to balance the therapeutic effects of a concentration at the low end of the usual target range against side effects that develop in a particular patient. Consideration should be given to a time lag of 1 to 2 weeks that may occur between achieving a steady-state dose and either therapeutic efficacy or the development of neurologic side effects.

Drugs that inhibit lithium excretion may raise concentrations by up to 50% and result in toxicity if the lithium dose is not decreased. Many of the nonsteroidal anti-inflammatory agents, including ibuprofen, have this effect. Thiazide and potassium-sparing diuretics raise lithium levels as well. The effect of furosemide is less clear, but lithium levels should be checked a few days after this diuretic is added in a patient receiving lithium. Both dehydration and salt depletion are known to raise lithium levels. Bipolar patients who have benefited from lithium should not be deprived of this medication because of aging, but dosage adjustments may be required.

Anticonvulsants

Valproic acid (valproate, divalproex) has been approved for the treatment of bipolar disorder and is comparable in efficacy to lithium. Although the concentrations of valproic acid necessary for anti-manic effects have not been clearly established in either young adults or older persons, the target concentrations of 50 to 100 μg/mL used to treat seizure disorders appear to be appropriate. Divalproex has been used effectively to treat agitation in patients with dementia and may be particularly useful for the treatment of behavior disturbance associated with mood lability. Placebo-controlled trials for this indication are ongoing. However, upward titration in the frail older person must be carried out carefully because dementia patients may be particularly sensitive to developing excessive sedation during valproic acid treatment. As with other antiepileptics used to treat mania, valproic acid is associated with allergic skin rashes in 5% to 10% of patients. Decreased platelet counts occur at higher doses, and platelet functioning may be diminished. Patients with hepatic disease may develop liver toxicity during valproic acid treatment.

Carbamazepine is another antiepileptic medication that has been used to treat mania. Mild bone-marrow suppression with leukopenia and thrombocytopenia occurs in 5% to 10% of patients within the first 2 weeks of treatment. However, life-threatening agranulocytosis and aplastic anemia may occur rarely. Other antiepileptics such as lamotrigine and gabapentin have been reported to be effective for bipolar disorder in young adults, although evidence for their efficacy as a sole therapeutic agent is limited. Lamotrigine has been associated with the development of Stevens-Johnson syndrome.

Electroconvulsive Therapy

ECT is highly effective for the treatment of major depression and mania, with response rates exceeding 70% in older adults. ECT is the first-line treatment for patients at serious risk for suicide or life-threatening poor intake due to a major depression. Older patients who suffer delusions in association with depression are generally quite impaired and more likely to be suicidal. Patients with delusional depression may demonstrate paranoia about their food or caregivers, precluding pharmacologic treatment. Also, delusional depression is less responsive to standard medication regimens. Therefore, ECT is generally the first-line treatment for these patients and is associated with response rates that approximate 80%.

The cognitive side effects of ECT are the principal factor limiting its acceptance. Anterograde amnesia or the inability to learn new information may be pronounced initially, particularly during bilateral treatment, but it improves rapidly following completion of treatment. Retrograde amnesia is more persistent, and the recall of events that immediately preceded ECT may be lost irretrievably. Although patients may complain that ECT has had a long-term effect on their memory, longitudinal studies have failed to demonstrate lasting cognitive effects; furthermore, improved memory, perhaps owing to recovery from depression, has been reported. There are few absolute medical contraindications other than the presence of increased intracranial pressure. Patients with coronary artery disease or cerebral vascular disease may be administered ECT safely by the use of appropriate pharmacologic management to decrease the autonomic responses that may occur during treatment. Nevertheless, a recent myocardial infarction or cerebral vascular event and unstable coronary artery disease increases the risk of complications. Right unilateral treatment produces less severe, fewer cognitive side effects than bilateral treatment but is less effective unless doses markedly exceeding a patient's seizure threshold are used. Machines that can deliver high-dose right unilateral ECT are not available at many hospitals. Also, high-dose unilateral ECT adversely affects memory more than low-dose unilateral treatment does.

The selection of ECT over aggressive pharmacotherapy is generally made by weighing the risk of waiting for a medication to work against the inconvenience of hospital treatment, the memory effects of ECT, and patient biases against this treatment. Patients with ECT should be treated with continuation pharmacotherapy following recovery. Patients who have failed intensive antidepressant treatment before receiving ECT have lower acute response rates and are more likely to relapse subsequently, even when antidepressant continuation treatment with a new medication is provided. Although maintenance ECT is sometimes used to prevent relapse, the burden that maintenance ECT places on patients and their families may limit its usefulness for the long-term management of late-life major depression.

REFERENCES

- Alexopoulos GS, Meyers BS, Young RC, et al. Executive dysfunction and long-term outcomes of geriatric depression. *Arch Gen Psychiatry.* 2000;57(3):285–290.

- Beekman ATF, Copeland JRM, Prince MJ. Review of community prevalence of depression in later life. *Br J Psychiatry.* 1999; 174:307–311.

- Denihan A, Kirby M, Bruce I, et al. Three-year prognosis of depression in the community-dwelling elderly. *Br J Psychiatry.* 2000;176(5):453–357.

- Gallo JJ, Rabins PV, Lyketsos CG. Depression without sadness: functional outcomes of nondysphoric depression in later life. *J Am Geriatr Soc.* 1997; 45(5):570–588.

- Kroenke K. A 75-year old man with depression. *JAMA.* 2002;287(12):1568–1576.

- Kurlowicz LH. Delirium and depression. In: Cotter VT, Strumpf NE, eds. *Advanced Practice Nursing with Older Adults: Clinical Guidelines.* New York: McGraw-Hill; 2001:141–162.

- Reynolds CF, Frank E, Perel J, et al. Nortriptyline and interpersonal psychotherapy as maintenance therapies for recurrent major depression: a randomized controlled trial in patients older than 59 years. *JAMA.* 1999; 281(1):39–45.

- Roose SP, Laghrissi-Thode F, Kennedy JS, et al. Comparison of paroxetine and nortriptyline in depressed patients with ischemic heart disease. *JAMA.* 1998; 279(4):287–291.

- Shulman KI, Hermann N. The nature and management of mania in old age. *The Psychiatric Clinics of North America.* 1999; 22(3):649–665.

- Tew JD, Mulsant BH, Haskett RF, et al. Acute efficacy of ECT in the treatment of major depression in the old-old. *Am J Psychiatry.* 1999;156(12):1865–1870.

CHAPTER 33—ANXIETY DISORDERS

Older adults suffer from the entire range of anxiety disorders. The clinician treating older persons therefore needs to be familiar with the hallmarks and available treatments for each type of anxiety disorder. Since the published literature on anxiety in older patients is relatively sparse, some of the characterizations and treatment strategies described here are based on research carried out in younger populations. They have been modified to take into account the physiologic and psychologic differences between older and younger adults.

Familiarity with the various diagnostic criteria, along with the skill to conduct a thorough psychologic assessment, is crucial in determining the most appropriate treatment for anxiety. Clinicians need to be aware of difficulties in proper assessment of geriatric anxiety; these include medical comorbidity, the difficulty of differentiating anxiety from depression, falsely high scores on anxiety rating scales resulting from overemphasis of cardiac and respiratory problems, and the tendency of older cohorts to resist psychiatric evaluation.

Anxiety assessment begins with a clinical interview to determine the course and nature of symptoms, along with the nature of the patient's mental status and external support. Supplemental rating scales, which aid in comparing a patient's level of difficulties with that of others and assessing difficulties over time, along with laboratory investigations can result in an accurate clinical picture and the ability to formulate an effective management plan. Even though anxiety disorders are less prevalent among older than among younger adults, the ability to recognize and effectively treat such disorders in older persons is important, given the debilitating effects that an unhealthy level of anxiety can have in this vulnerable population.

CLASSES OF ANXIETY DISORDERS

The types of anxiety disorders as currently defined in the fourth edition of the *Diagnostic and Statistical Manual of Mental Disorder* (*DSM-IV*) are listed in Table 33.1.

Panic Disorder

Panic attacks are acute, discrete episodes of intense anxiety that result as a reaction to some perceived threat (eg, emotional, environmental). The term *panic attack* is used when a person experiences an intense and acute reaction to an internal or external cue; it lasts between a few minutes and a half hour. The physiologic symptoms may include trembling, acceler-

Table 33.1—Types of Anxiety Disorders Defined in *DSM-IV*

Panic disorder without agoraphobia

Panic disorder with agoraphobia

Agoraphobia without history of panic disorder

Specific phobias
    Animal type
    Natural environment type
    Blood-injection-injury type
    Situational type
    Other type

Social phobia

Obsessive-compulsive disorder

Posttraumatic stress disorder

Acute stress disorder

Generalized anxiety disorder

Anxiety disorder due to a general medical condition

Substance-induced anxiety disorder

Anxiety disorder not otherwise specified

Source: Data from *Diagnostic and Statistical Manual of Mental Disorders*. 4th ed. Washington, DC: American Psychiatric Association; 1994.

ated heart rate, sweating, shortness of breath, chest pain, dizziness, nausea, and the sense that one is somehow detached from the surroundings. For example, a person might have a fear of being trapped on an elevator and report feeling dizzy and nauseated when entering one. Another might report high levels of acute anxiety at the mere sight of elevator doors. A clinically significant degree of panic symptoms exist if a review of the patient's history reveals that recurrent and unpredictable panic attacks have occurred for at least 1 month and time is being spent in worried anticipation of possible reoccurrence. Diagnostically, one needs also to consider whether agoraphobia related to the panic attacks is present. In such cases, agoraphobia involves the persistent fear of situations that result in a panic attack, as when a patient reports remaining at home in order to avoid an attack. Common examples of feared situations include being caught in a crowd or trapped in traffic. Comparison of young and older adults with panic disorder indicates that age of onset can effect the clinical presentation. Patients with late-onset panic disorder (at or after age 55) report fewer panic symptoms and less avoidance, and they score lower on somatization measures than do those with early-onset panic disorder.

Phobic Disorders

Phobias include several distinct disorders, categorized as specific phobia and social phobia. A specific phobia involves a distinct trigger, such as a specific person, animal, place, object, event, or situation, that results in symptoms of anxiety. Commonly, the person's anxiety level increases instantly when the feared trigger is encountered. Interestingly, the patient is able to identify this fear as unrealistic and unsupported, even though the cognitive and physiologic responses persist. Specific phobias often involve a great amount of anticipatory anxiety (thoughts of just the possibility of encountering the feared stimulus), and avoidance behaviors are likely to be reported. The consequence of such a clinical profile is that the person experiences a variety of personal difficulties as a result of the anxiety. These behaviors interfere with work and daily routines, and they decrease the person's opportunities to experience pleasurable situations (for fear that a trigger might be present). They may also contribute to secondary symptoms, such as frustration, hopelessness, and a sense that one lacks control in one's life. The level of anxiety or fear usually varies as a function of both the degree of proximity to the phobic stimuli and the degree to which escape is limited. Examples of common phobias include fear of specific animals, closed spaces, flying, or heights. Frequently, specific phobias occur with panic disorder, with or without agoraphobia. Among older persons, especially in urban settings, fear of crime seems to be particularly prevalent, despite the fact that older people are in the group least likely to be victimized.

Persons with social phobia suffer from fears that they will behave in a manner that is inept, mortifying, and embarrassing. Commonly, the fear is that of trembling, blushing, or sweating profusely in social situations. Other common feared situations involve giving public speeches, going on dates, or simply socializing with others at a function or party. Again, as with specific phobias, social phobia is often accompanied with a significant degree of anticipatory anxiety or avoidance, or both. Though systematic studies of this disorder in older persons are lacking, epidemiologic data indicate that this disorder is chronic and persistent in old age. Common manifestations in old age include the inability to eat food in the presence of strangers, and, especially in men, being unable to urinate in public lavatories.

Obsessive-Compulsive Disorder

Obsessive-compulsive disorder involves persistent thoughts (obsessions) and behaviors (compulsions) that are performed in an effort to decrease the anxiety experienced as a result of the thoughts. Obsessions are thoughts or ideas that come to a person's mind, commonly while completing a specific task or during a particular type of situation. For example, a person may wash his hands repeatedly, for hours at a time, after shaking a stranger's hand; the unwanted thought is that he may have exposed himself to a serious disease. The act of washing in this example is the compulsion. Obsessive-compulsive disorder is chronic and often disabling. Depression and other symptoms of anxiety may also occur.

Posttraumatic Stress Disorder

The distinctive feature of posttraumatic stress disorder is that the person has experienced, either as a witness or a victim, a traumatic event to which he or she has reacted with feelings of fear and helplessness. Examples of such events include those that involve actual or threatened death or serious injury, other threats to one's integrity, witnessing an event that involves death or serious injury of another, or even hearing about death or serious injury to a family member or close associate. Commonly observed symptoms include the reexperiencing of the traumatic event, avoidance (both cognitively and behaviorally) of stimuli associated with the event, psychologic numbing, and increased physiologic arousal. Symptoms of hyperarousal include difficulty falling or staying asleep, hypervigilance, and exaggerated startle response. Disorders frequently found to occur with posttraumatic stress disorder include depression, panic disorder, and substance-use disorders. Symptoms must be present for at least 1 month and cause clinically significant distress or impairment in social, occupational, or other important areas of functioning. In the short term, that is between 2 days and 1 month after the traumatic event, a diagnosis of acute stress disorder is given; thereafter one must consider a diagnosis of posttraumatic stress disorder.

Generalized Anxiety Disorder

The distinctive symptoms of generalized anxiety disorder include feeling easily tired and experiencing other physical symptoms, such as muscle tension, having trouble sleeping through the night, having difficulty concentrating on a task, and feeling irritable or on edge. These symptoms need to have occurred for at least 6 months and must be accompanied by the sense that one cannot control the feelings of anxiety. In addition, these feelings of intense worry must be a result of more than one stressor. For example, intense worry over financial matters or a medical illness alone, even with all the associated symptoms, in and of itself does not qualify a person for a diagnosis of generalized anxiety disorder. Because many older patients with this disorder also present with features of depression, the clinician must distinguish between the two diagnoses.

COMORBIDITY

Mixed Anxiety and Depression

Mixed anxiety and depression is a presentation that is included in the *DSM-IV* "Criteria for Further Study." The essential features of this proposed disorder are dysphoric mood for at least 1 month composed of at least four anxious or depressive symptoms, such as irritability, worry, sleep disturbance, anticipating the worst, concentration or memory difficulties, and hopelessness. Clinicians working with older persons have long observed the significant overlap in symptoms of anxiety and depression. In fact, it is quite common to see individuals with a combination of anxiety and depression, although one or both disorders might only be present at subsyndromal levels.

Anxiety and Agitation in Dementia

Patients with dementia, whether living at home or in a long-term-care institution, commonly display behaviors described as agitation. Agitation takes the form of verbal or motor activity that is either appropriate behavior but repeated frequently or inappropriate behavior that suggests lack of judgment. As many as 85% of dementia patients eventually develop disruptive, agitated behavior. Early identification of triggers, including environmental stimuli, medication side effects, and uncommunicated internal needs, can result in effective treatment and relief for already overburdened caregivers. See "Dementia" (p 113) and "Neuropsychiatric and Behavioral Disturbances in Dementia" (p 121) for details on diagnosing and managing disruptive, agitated behavior.

Anxiety and Medical Disorders

It is common to encounter patients with comorbid anxiety and medical disorders. This could be due to longstanding anxiety disorder, which coincidentally occurs alongside a medical illness, or there could be interplay between the two. There are conditions exacerbated by anxiety, such as the common cold or influenza, and also those that are precipitated by high levels of anxiety, such as angina pectoris or myocardial infarction. Other medical illnesses that commonly accompany an anxiety disorder include cardiovascular illnesses, pulmonary disorders, drug side effects (thyroid hormone replacements, antipsychotics, caffeine, theophylline, selective serotonin-reuptake inhibitors [SSRIs]) or interactions, and hyperthyroidism. Given the complicated clinical picture that results when anxiety and medical disorders coexist, a thorough assessment, including a clinical history, is imperative before treatment begins.

PHARMACOLOGIC MANAGEMENT

Numerous compounds have been used over the years as anxiolytics: alcohol, barbiturates, antihistamines, benzodiazepines, antipsychotic medications, and β-blockers. Although empirical studies of the use of anxiolytics in treating older persons are lacking, the efficacy of these medications is inferred from clinical practice with younger patients, and their use is modified by age-appropriate dosing. A brief description of the various classes of compounds currently favored as anxiolytics follows. Table 33.2 summarizes the findings of controlled trials about the efficacy of several classes of drugs in the treatment of specific anxiety disorders.

Antidepressants

Antidepressants are efficacious in the treatment of panic disorder, obsessive-compulsive disorder, generalized anxiety disorder, and posttraumatic stress disorder in younger patients. Given their relatively favorable side-effect profile, the SSRIs should now be considered the drugs of choice for these disorders. Further, SSRIs should also be considered treatments of choice for treating mixed anxiety and depression. Compounds such as venlafaxine and nefazodone should be considered as alternatives for those patients who do not respond to SSRIs or who develop adverse effects. Case

Table 33.2—Pharmacologic Treatment of Anxiety Disorders: Results of Controlled Trials

	TCAs	SSRIs	MAOIs	Benzodiazepines	Buspirone
Panic disorder	■	■	■	■	
Generalized anxiety disorder	■	■		■	■
Obsessive-compulsive disorder	■	■			
Posttraumatic stress disorder	■	■	■		
Social phobia		■	■	■	

NOTE: MAOIs = monoamine oxidase inhibitors; SSRIs = selective serotonin-reuptake inhibitors; TCAs = tricyclic antidepressants; ■ = established efficacy.

SOURCE: Flint AJ. Anxiety disorders. In: Cobbs EL, Duthie EH, Murphy JB, eds. *Geriatrics Review Syllabus: A Core Curriculum in Geriatric Medicine*. 4th ed. Dubuque, Iowa: Kendall/Hunt Publishing Company for the American Geriatrics Society; 1999:178.

reports, open-label trials, and, more recently, controlled trials of serotonergic antidepressants like trazodone and SSRIs have also suggested a modest degree of efficacy in the management of behavioral disturbances of dementia, particularly when patients are not psychotic and comorbid depression is a strong possibility. (See also "Neuropsychiatric and Behavioral Disturbances in Dementia," p 121.)

Benzodiazepines

Over the past three decades benzodiazepines have been the most commonly prescribed anxiolytics for both young and older patients, but their use is now discouraged. When needed because symptoms are severe, benzodiazepines with a short half-life, such as lorazepam and oxazepam, are preferable in treating older patients because they are metabolized by direct conjugation, a process relatively unaffected by aging. However, it is preferable to limit the use of even short-acting benzodiazepines to less than 6 months because long-term use is fraught with multiple complications, such as motor incoordination and falls, cognitive impairment, depression, and the potential for abuse and dependence.

Buspirone, Antihistamines, and Atypical Antipsychotics

Several studies have suggested that buspirone, an anxiolytic medication with some serotonin-agonist properties, is efficacious in the treatment in patients with generalized anxiety disorder, although clinical experience is less positive. Buspirone appears to be a safer choice than benzodiazepines for patients taking several other medications or needing to be treated for longer periods of time. One drawback of buspirone is the amount of time required to see a clinical response (approximately 4 weeks). This suggests that concomitant use of a short-acting benzodiazepine in the initial stage of treatment would be useful for some patients. Buspirone may also be efficacious in reducing symptoms of anxiety and agitation in patients with dementia. Antihistamines such as hydroxyzine and diphenhydramine are sometimes used to manage mild anxiety, but there are few data that demonstrate efficacy. Given the anticholinergic side effects of antihistamines in older adults, these drugs are discouraged.

Finally, atypical antipsychotics, such as risperidone, olanzapine, and quetiapine, are increasingly being used to manage agitation associated with dementia, particularly when an underlying psychosis may be present.

PSYCHOLOGIC MANAGEMENT

Although pharmacotherapy is frequently the first-line treatment for late-life anxiety disorders, psychologic treatments are often adequate, either alone or as adjuncts to medication. Techniques generally fall into three categories. Relaxation training can be employed with the use of music, visual imagery, aromatherapy, or instruction in relaxation techniques. Cognitive restructuring helps the patient identify triggers and stimuli that maintain anxiety and helps him or her to slowly gain more control over the effect of such stimuli and develop a range of coping strategies and tools. Finally, exposure, with response prevention, has been shown to be particularly effective with both panic disorder and obsessive-compulsive disorder. Treatment of the older person typically includes a combination of these behavioral approaches. Their success depends on the appropriateness of the patient for psychotherapy; the patient's support system, intellectual functioning, and motivation level; the degree of coordination of care with health care professionals; and the nature of the disorder. Consultation with a mental health professional can assist in determining the appropriateness of a referral.

REFERENCES

- Flint AJ, Rifat SL. Two-year outcome of elderly patients with anxious depression. *Psychiatry Res.* 1997;66(1):23–31.

- Palmer BW, Jeste DV, Sheikh JI. Anxiety disorders in the elderly: DSM-IV and other barriers to diagnosis and treatment. *J Affect Disorders.* 1997;46(3):183–190.

- Sadavoy J. Survivors: a review of the late-life effects of prior psychological trauma. *Am J Geriatric Psychiatry.* 1997;5(4):287–301.

- Sheikh JI, Swales PJ. Treatment of panic disorder in older adults: a pilot study comparison of alprazolam, imipramine and placebo. *Int J Psychiatry Med.* 1999;29(1):107–117.

CHAPTER 34—PSYCHOTIC DISORDERS

Psychotic is an imprecise term; although its definition has changed over the years, it is widely used and can be useful if specifically defined. Psychotic symptoms are defined here as either *hallucinations*, that is, perceptions without stimuli, or *delusions*, that is, fixed, false, idiosyncratic ideas. Hallucinations can be in any of the five sensory modalities (auditory, visual, tactile, olfactory, gustatory); delusions can be suspicious ("paranoid"), grandiose, somatic, self-blaming, or hopeless. This chapter focuses on conditions in which psychotic symptoms are prominent and central to making the diagnosis. It only briefly discusses other disorders, such as dementia, delirium, and the mood disorders, in which psychotic symptoms can occur but whose defining features are in the cognitive or mood realms.

Hallucinations and delusions occur in a variety of disorders. The evaluation of a person with hallucinations and delusions (Figure 34.1) should first exclude neurologic diseases such as dementia, stroke, or Parkinson's disease. An acute onset of altered level of consciousness suggests delirium. Next, a primary mood disorder should be considered. Only after other causes are excluded should the diagnosis of a schizophrenia-like state be made.

SCHIZOPHRENIA AND SCHIZOPHRENIA-LIKE SYNDROMES

Schizophrenia is defined as a chronic psychiatric disorder characterized by positive symptoms—hallucinations, delusions, and thought disorder—and negative symptoms—social dilapidation and apathy. Mood disorder and cognitive disorder should be excluded. In men, schizophrenia has a modal onset at age 18; onset after age 45 years is uncommon. In women, on the other hand, modal age of onset is 28, and 20% to 30% of cases begin after age 45. Ten percent to 15% of cases of schizophrenia first come to clinical attention after patients have reached 59 years of age.

In older persons, schizophrenia-like conditions are characterized by onset after age 44, prominent persecutory (paranoid) delusions, and multi-modal hallucinations. For example, patients commonly complain that items are being stolen or report that they are being persecuted unjustly. Hallucinations often manifest in complaints, for example, that a neighbor is persistently banging on walls or the roof, that someone is pumping gas under the door, or that electrical sensations are being sent through the walls of the person's home and into his or her body. A schizophrenia-like psychosis can be diagnosed only when cognitive disorder, mood disorder, or other explanatory medical conditions such as delirium or focal brain pathology have been excluded (Figure 34.1).

The schizophrenia-like psychoses of late life differ from schizophrenia beginning in early life in two ways. First, thought disorder, a sign described as speech in which a series of thoughts are not connected to one another in a logical fashion, is much less common in older patients, being seen in only 5% of cases. In early-onset schizophrenia, thought disorder is present in approximately 50% of cases. A second significant difference is the rarity of social deterioration and dilapidation among older patients. Thus, personality is often intact in late-onset cases. However, there is a dearth of long-term follow-up studies, so it is unknown whether social deterioration and personality changes occur after many years of symptoms.

Epidemiology and Risk Factors

Late-onset schizophrenia is more common among women. The population-based frequency of late-onset schizophrenia is unknown, but the lifetime prevalence of schizophrenia is 1% among both men and women.

Late-onset schizophrenia-like psychoses affect predominantly women, with the female:male ratio ranging from 5:1 to 10:1. It has been speculated that later onset is due to decreasing natural estrogen levels, but there is little evidence to support this hypothesis. Other reported risk factors include hearing impairment, social isolation, never having been married, or having a childless marriage. However, there is controversy about each of these risk factors. Some studies suggest that the association with high rates of hearing impairment result from a lack of access to treatment of hearing disorder, and not from its being etiologic. Likewise, some researchers have suggested that premorbid social isolation and single marital status reflect early symptoms of the disorder rather than risk factors. Many persons with late-onset schizophrenia-like psychosis have been able to hold responsible jobs and work efficiently, but premorbid isolation and "schizoid" (socially isolated personality) traits are common. Studies report greater degrees of brain white matter hyperintensities on magnetic resonance imaging scans in late-onset schizophrenia, a finding that suggests that brain vascular disease is a risk factor. However, this finding has not been adequately replicated, and other causes of white matter hyperintensities are plausible.

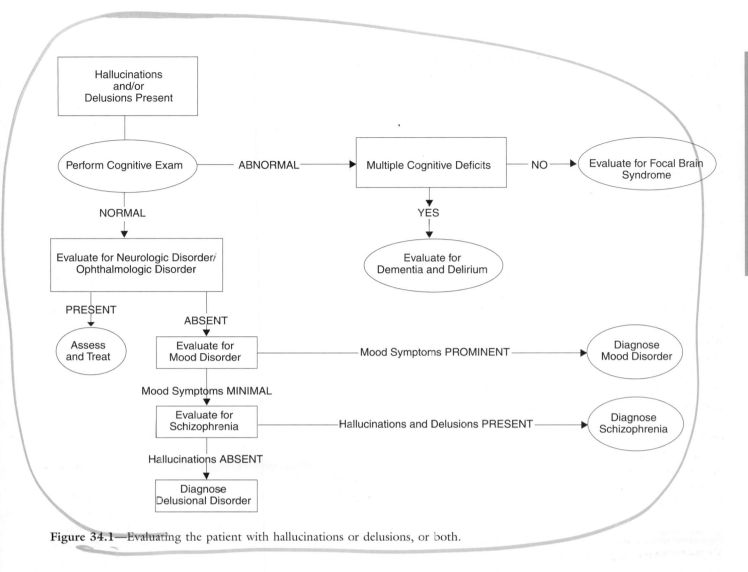

Figure 34.1—Evaluating the patient with hallucinations or delusions, or both.

Treatment and Management

Nonpharmacologic

Because suspiciousness and paranoid delusions are commonly the most prominent symptoms, the clinician's first task in treating late-onset psychosis is often to establish a trusting therapeutic relationship with the patient. On occasion, the suspicious ideas are plausible (eg, the claim that the patient is being financially abused by a relative), but usually the delusions are bizarre and implausible; very often, prominent hallucinations clarify that there is no basis in truth to the complaints. Because of the fixed, unchanging, and vivid nature of the symptoms, it is rarely effective to confront the patient with the unreality or implausibility of his or her ideas. The patient is more likely to respond positively if the clinician empathizes with the distress that the symptoms cause ("I can see how upset you are by all of this"). If patients ask whether the clinician "believes" them, a response such as, "I don't hear anything like that, but I appreciate the fact that you do" is both honest and empathic. The symptoms

are usually frightening and distressing to the patients and can lead to unusual behaviors. For example, patients who develop concerns that their food is being poisoned may exhibit unusual eating habits or food avoidance. Furthermore, suspiciousness can isolate the patient from friends and family. Therefore, encouraging patients to maintain important relationships and seeking their permission to discuss the source of symptoms with close family members or friends may help these patients maintain important, supportive relationships.

Pharmacologic

Clinical experience and descriptive case series suggest that antipsychotic drugs are as effective in late-onset schizophrenia as in early-onset cases. Most specialists recommend the newer atypical antipsychotic drugs because they have fewer side effects, are better tolerated, and are less likely to cause tardive dyskinesia, a side effect for which older age is a predisposing factor. Doses should be increased at semi-weekly or weekly intervals, as needed. While doses are being titrated, patients should be monitored for the emergence of extrapyramidal side effects (parkinsonian tremor, rigidity, dystonia) and other movement disorders. These should be treated by lowering dosage or using anticholinergic medications such as trihexyphenidyl 1 to 2 mg orally twice a day. The more common side effects with quetiapine are sedation and orthostatic hypotension; with risperidone, extrapyramidal symptoms; and with olanzapine, weight gain and extrapyramidal symptoms (Table 34.1).

No studies are available to guide the length of treatment. Clinical experience suggests that patients who respond to antipsychotic medications should be continued on the minimal effective dose for at least 6 months. For patients who relapse on treatment or when the dosage is lowered, longer term maintenance (at least 1 to 2 years) is recommended. Patients should be monitored for the emergence of tardive dyskinesia, a syndrome characterized by repetitive involuntary movements of the oral and limb musculature. If tardive dyskinesia develops, the dosage of the antipsychotic agent should be lowered, if possible. At the time antipsychotic drugs are initiated or as soon as symptoms improve enough so that the patient can understand the risk, he or she should be informed of the risk of tardive dyskinesia and the possibility that it can be irreversible.

PSYCHOTIC SYMPTOMS IN DELIRIUM

Hallucinations, particularly visual hallucinations, can be a symptom of delirium, even when it is mild. The onset of delirium is usually acute, and there is often an identifiable metabolic or infectious cause. The mental status examination reveals multiple cognitive impairments and a diminished level of consciousness. (See "Delirium," p 127.)

PSYCHOTIC SYMPTOMS IN MOOD DISORDER

Delusions can be seen in major depression and in the manic phase of bipolar disorder. These delusions are described as "mood congruent." That is, in patients with depression, the delusional content usually reflects self-deprecation, self-blame, hopelessness, or the conviction of ill health. A patient may complain that she has no blood or that her intestines are not working, for example; another patient may believe that he has caused a terrible wrong and deserves to be punished (a self-blaming delusion). Some patients become convinced that they are dying and that nothing can be done to help them when there is no physiologic evidence of this. Other common depressive delusions are the conviction that one has no insurance, no clothing, or no money when this is not true (delusion of poverty). Delusions congruent with mania are grandiose. Examples include the person's belief that that he or she is infallible, can do impossible physical or intellectual activities, has skills and abilities that no other human being has, or is a special personage such as Jesus Christ. (See "Depression and Other Mood Disorders," p 211.)

PSYCHOTIC SYMPTOMS IN DEMENTIA

Patients with dementia experience both hallucinations and delusions. These are usually less complex than the delusions seen in schizophrenia or mood disorder. Common delusions in dementia are the belief that one's belongings have been stolen or moved, or the conviction that one is being punished. (See "Dementia," p 113.)

ISOLATED SUSPICIOUSNESS

Suspiciousness can be viewed as a personality trait, that is, an aspect of all human beings that varies among people in its degree of prominence. One epidemiologic study has found that suspiciousness becomes more common in older Americans and affects 4% of those aged 65 and over. It is distinguished from psychotic disorders by the understandable nature of the ideas (for

Table 34.1—Commonly Used Antipsychotic Medications

Agent	Starting Daily Dose (*mg*)	Maximum Daily Dose (*mg*)	Common Side Effects*		
			EPS**	Drowsiness	Weight Gain
Clozapine	12.5	75	1	3	3
Haloperidol	0.5–1	8	3	2	1
Olanzapine	2.5	10	2	1	2
Quetiapine	25	200	1	3	2
Risperidone	0.5–1	4	2	1	1

* Key: 1 = uncommon to 3 = common.

** EPS = extrapyramidal side effects: rigidity, parkinsonian tremor, dystonia.

example, excessive worry about safety) and the absence of other psychotic symptoms.

SYNDROMES OF ISOLATED HALLUCINATIONS

Charles Bonnet Syndrome

Between 10% and 13% of patients with significant visual impairment (bilateral acuity worse than 20/60) experience visual hallucinations. These can take the form of shapes such as diamonds or rectangles but more commonly consist of complex hallucinations such as small children, multiple animals, or a vivid scene such as one would see in a movie. This condition, first described more than 200 years ago, goes by the eponym *Charles Bonnet syndrome*. The criteria for this syndrome are as follows:

- visual hallucinations,
- partially or fully intact insight (the patient is aware that the perceptions cannot be real but still reports that they appear absolutely real and vivid),
- visual impairment, and
- lack of evidence of brain disease or other psychiatric disorder.

It has been suggested that this syndrome is a concomitant of the phantom limb syndrome caused by retinal lesions. However, visual hallucinations have also been reported in persons with field defects due to cortical lesions of the visual pathways.

The best treatment of the Charles Bonnet syndrome is information and support. Patients should be told that the hallucinations are a sign of eye disease, not mental illness. An occasional patient has partial insight or loses insight and becomes very distressed by this symptom. When this distress is significant or leads to dangerous behavior, a cautious trial of low doses of an atypical antipsychotic medication is occasionally beneficial.

Organic Hallucinosis

Patients with Parkinson's disease, stroke, and other brain disorders occasionally experience delusions and hallucinations without prominent cognitive impairment or other evidence of psychiatric disorder. Delirium due to a superimposed condition should be excluded. In patients with Parkinson's disease, the symptoms may be secondary to prescribed dopaminergic agent, but some patients experience visual hallucinations prior to the onset of any pharmacotherapy. Education and support should be offered to all patients with these symptoms. If the patients experience significant emotional distress or the symptoms lead to dangerous or upsetting behavior, a cautious use of an antipsychotic medication is appropriate. For patients with Parkinson's disease and hallucinations, quetiapine 12.5 to 75 mg or olanzapine 2.5 to 5.0 mg daily may be beneficial. Some patients require clozapine 12.5 to 75.0 mg daily. However, clozapine requires a complete blood cell count once a week for 6 months and then biweekly thereafter because of the risk of granulocytopenia.

REFERENCES

- Howard R, Rabins PV, Castle DJ, eds. *Late Onset Schizophrenia*. Petersfield, UK: Wrightson Biomedical Publishing Ltd., 1999.

- Marsh L. Neuropsychiatric aspects of Parkinson's disease. *Psychosomatics*. 2000; 14:15–23.

- Sachdev P, Brodaty H, Rose N, et al. Schizophrenia with onset after 50 years of age: 2: neurological, neuropsychological and MRI investigation. *Br J Psychiatry*. 1999; 175:416–421.

- Teunisse RJ, Cruysberg JR, Hoefnageos WH, et al. Visual hallucinations in psychologically normal people: Charles Bonnet's syndrome. *Lancet*. 1996; 347:794–797.

CHAPTER 35—PERSONALITY AND SOMATOFORM DISORDERS

PERSONALITY DISORDERS

Personality disorders are defined in the fourth edition of the *Diagnostic and Statistical Manual of Mental Disorders* (*DSM-IV*) by the presence of chronic and pervasive patterns of inflexible and maladaptive inner experiences and behaviors. These patterns lead to significant disruptions in several spheres of function: cognitive perception and interpretation, affective expression, interpersonal relations, and impulse control. People with personality disorders are often distinguished by repeated episodes of disruptive or noxious behaviors, and as a result they often receive pejorative labels, depending on their form: difficult, hateful, strange, dramatic, overbearing, to name just a few. The developmental roots of personality disorders are believed to lie in childhood and adolescence, but their features can present clinically at any age; both genetic and environmental influences are involved.

The *DSM-IV* describes ten personality disorders, grouped into three broad clusters that are based on common phenomenology. Depressive and passive-aggressive personality disorders are two additional categories, but they are considered provisional since they appear to lack the empirical support of the other ten diagnoses. Brief definitions and late-life features of all twelve personality disorders are listed in Table 35.1. Mixed diagnoses and those that do not fit into any existing category are labeled "personality disorder, not otherwise specified" (NOS). Many older persons with personality disorders can easily become overwhelmed by age-associated losses and stresses, largely because they lack appropriate coping skills and the personal, social, or financial resources to buffer their losses. In particular, admission to a hospital or long-term-care setting poses a unique stress on all personality disorders in late life. The loss of a familiar environment, personal items, privacy, and the control over one's schedule can lead to a sense of disorganization and displacement. Conflict in an institutional setting begins when patients with personality disorders try to cope with the stresses from their new environment by exaggerating their maladaptive behaviors. An obsessive-compulsive person may attempt to maintain a sense of control by demanding rigid adherence to schedules and rules of hygiene. Dependent persons may feel helpless and panicked without enough attention to their needs, and they respond with clinging behaviors and excessive questions or requests for assistance. Paranoid, antisocial, and borderline patients may irritate staff by refusing to cooperate with treatment plans or institutional rules.

Epidemiology

Prevalence rates of late-life personality disorders in the community range from 5% to 10%, which is a slightly lower range than the 10% to 18% prevalence estimates for persons of all ages in the community. Prevalence rates in inpatient settings and with comorbid depression are much higher, ranging from 10% to over 50%, depending on the method of diagnosis. The most common personality disorders in late life are dependent, obsessive-compulsive, paranoid, and NOS. Although most research has demonstrated fewer diagnoses in older age groups, it is unclear whether this represents an actual difference in prevalence or merely reflects the fact that it is more difficult to make a diagnosis in late life. Some researchers have suggested that prevalence rates may be influenced by increased mortality among those with personality traits that are associated with higher rates of reckless, impulsive, and self-injurious behaviors.

Diagnostic Challenges

Establishing a diagnosis of personality disorder in the older patient can be especially challenging, because it requires a detailed, longitudinal psychiatric and psychosocial history. Older adults and their informants are not always able to provide sufficient history, especially when it may span 50 years or more. The history may be distorted by recall bias (the tendency to present more socially desirable traits), memory impairment, or the very personality disorder in question. For example, schizotypal and paranoid persons may be reluctant to engage in clinical interviews and share personal history, and antisocial and narcissistic persons who lack insight into their problems may refuse to divulge relevant experiences. Records often do not provide sufficient information to determine prior personality dynamics. Older diagnoses cannot be easily correlated with current ones because the diagnoses of personality disorder have changed significantly in the past 50 years. As a result of all of these limitations, clinicians are often forced to defer a diagnosis, or to make judgments that are based on insufficient information.

A further diagnostic challenge for clinicians is the need to isolate lifelong personality characteristics amidst a multitude of comorbid problems. Acute and chronic episodes of major depression, psychosis, and

Table 35.1—Features of Personality Disorders

Cluster, Disorder	General Features*	Specific Features in Geriatric Patients
Cluster A: Odd or Eccentric Behaviors		
Paranoid	Suspicious, distrustful of others; often irritable and hostile	May present with transient agitation and paranoid psychosis
Schizoid	Lack of desire for social relations, isolated, and odd appearance	Difficulty forming relationships with caregivers
Schizotypal	Odd, inappropriate beliefs and behaviors; aloof demeanor	May become overtly psychotic and more socially isolated
Cluster B: Dramatic, Emotional, or Erratic Behaviors		
Antisocial	Lack of conscience, disregard for social norms; reckless and criminal behavior; substance abuse common	May become less aggressive and impulsive
Borderline	Unstable interpersonal relations, poor control of affect, impulsive and self-injurious behaviors	May be less impulsive and self-injurious, but demonstrate persistent emotional lability and disruptive relationships
Histrionic	Extroverted, seductive, and provocative behaviors, but shallow emotions	May appear disinhibited or manic
Narcissistic	Self-entitled, arrogant, grandiose, often demanding and hostile	May present as rageful, paranoid, or depressed
Cluster C: Anxious or Fearful Behaviors		
Avoidant	Fearful of rejection, timid and inhibited demeanor, isolative, with deep sense of inadequacy	Have limited social contacts
Dependent	Excessively reliant on others for decisions and support, unable to function independently	May appear demanding or clinging if dependency needs not met; depression common
Obsessive-Compulsive	Preoccupation with orderliness and cleanliness, perfectionistic, rigid and controlling; may become more inflexible and indecisive under stress	May exaggerate these traits even more to maintain control over somatic and environmental changes
Provisional Personality Disorders		
Passive-Aggressive	Pattern of resistance to demands and authority, critical and resentful attitudes, and procrastination	Older and younger persons alike
Depressive	Gloomy, pessimistic, critical outlook on life and others, guilt-prone, and poor self-esteem	Often seen with major depression in late life

* Descriptions of the clusters and of the disorders in each cluster are based on the *Diagnostic and Statistical Manual of Mental Disorders.* 4th ed. Washington, DC: American Psychiatric Association; 1994. The provisional disorders are described in the *DSM-IV* appendix.

SOURCE: Adapted with permission from Agronin ME. Personality and psychopathology in late life. *Geriatrics.* 1998;53(supp 1):S39. © 2001 Advanstar Communications Inc. Advanstar Communications Inc. retains all rights to this material.

other major psychiatric disorders can distort personality features considerably, perhaps making it impossible to adequately assess personality at the time. Even the current diagnostic nomenclature might serve to handicap late-life diagnosis, since it is not age-adjusted, and many criteria fail to apply in late life. A final barrier to diagnosis may be present if the clinician erroneously considers all older patients to have disruptive personality features as a normal function of age.

Differential Diagnosis

In clinical settings, it is important to remember that not every older person with prominent or troubling personality features has a personality disorder. Those who demonstrate rigid and maladaptive personality traits but without the pervasiveness or severity as represented by *DSM-IV* criteria are better described as suffering from personality dysfunction or neurosis. An adjustment disorder might best characterize previously healthy and well-adjusted persons who demonstrate acute changes in personality as a result of severe stresses. For example, physical pain and disability can lead to dependent or avoidant behaviors that resemble those seen in personality disorders, but without the pervasive pattern and degree of maladaptiveness. There is also considerable overlap between symptoms of major psychiatric disorders and those of personality disorders, and without longitudinal history it can be difficult to distinguish between them. For example, the odd thinking and unusual perceptual experiences seen in psychotic disorders may resemble behaviors seen in schizotypal personality disorder. The emotional lability of bipolar states can mimic behaviors of borderline and histrionic diagnoses, and depressive symptoms from dysthymic and depressive disorders can be almost indistinguishable from depressive personality traits. Diagnosis of a personality disorder becomes more certain when seemingly acute behaviors emerge as enduring and pervasive personality traits. This process depends on the opportunity to observe a person over time and in multiple settings or situations.

Personality disorders as described in *DSM-IV* must also be differentiated from the diagnosis of personality change due to a specific medical condition. Marked personality change can also be seen after a catastrophic experience or a psychiatric illness. When personality change is a direct result of brain damage, it has classically been described within the context of an organic personality disorder. In general, manifestations of organic personalities are characterized by impaired control of affect and impulses. Alzheimer's disease and other dementias are often associated with personality changes, including apathy, egocentricity, and impulsivity. Frontal lobe injury is associated with two syndromes, one characterized by affective lability, lack of judgment, and disinhibition, and a second characterized by apathy, behavioral slowing, and lack of affective range and spontaneity. Temporal lobe epilepsy has been associated with personality change, including emotional deepening, verbosity, hypergraphia, hyposexuality, and preoccupation with religious, moral, and cosmic issues. The terms *sticky* or *viscous personality*, *interictal personality disorder*, and *Geschwind syndrome* have all been used for personality change associated with temporal lobe epilepsy.

Long-Term Course

Personality disorders may follow one of four possible courses: they persist unchanged, evolve into a different form or major psychiatric disorder (eg, depression), improve, or remit. Few disorders have actually been studied over time, and rarely into late life. Several studies have suggested that personality disorders may enter a period of relative quiescence in middle age, with fewer and less intense symptoms and increased adaptation. However, this period may precede their reemergence in late life, but with more age-appropriate symptoms. Other researchers have proposed that personality disorders characterized by emotional and behavioral lability, including antisocial, borderline, histrionic, narcissistic, and dependent, tend to improve over time, although patients remain vulnerable to depression. Personality disorders characterized by an overcontrol of affect and impulses, including paranoid, schizoid, schizotypal, and obsessive-compulsive personality disorders, are thought to either remain stable or to worsen in late life.

Only antisocial and borderline personality disorders have been looked at longitudinally, and both have shown symptom improvement and even remittance

into middle and later life for a significant percentage of patients. At the same time, there can be persistent psychopathology that is not recognized within the context of existing antisocial or borderline diagnostic criteria. In other words, longstanding personality dynamics may manifest in new behaviors. For example, those with antisocial personality disorders demonstrate less aggressiveness, violence, and criminal acts as they age, but still have antisocial tendencies expressed through substance abuse, disregard for safety, and noncompliance with institutional rules. Older borderline patients display less impulsivity, self-mutilation, and risk-taking, but more age-appropriate symptoms, such as anorexia, use of multiple medications, and nonadherence with treatment.

Treatment

The treatment of personality disorders in late life is complicated, often with limited success. Given the chronic and pervasive nature of personality disorders, the overall goal of treatment in late life is not to cure the disorder, but to decrease the frequency and intensity of disruptive behaviors. The first step should always be to clarify the diagnosis, and then to identify recent stressors that may account for the current presentation. The resultant formulation will guide the selection of realistic target symptoms and therapeutic approaches and will allow a treatment team to anticipate future stressors. Treatment of personality disorders in late life uses the same basic approaches as with younger patients, but clinicians must incorporate a much broader understanding of the impact of age-related stressors and comorbid disorders. All forms of psychotherapy have been used to treat personality disorders in older adults, ranging from intensive and long-term insight-oriented approaches to equally intensive but more focused cognitive-behavioral models. In late life, however, there may be more limitations on time and intensity of therapy, and as a result treatment must focus more on short-term, cognitive-behavioral, and pharmacologic approaches. Studies in adults generally find that comorbid personality disorders complicate the treatment of psychiatric illness, but that with consistent treatment the prognosis is often favorable. The prognosis in late life is more guarded, especially for persons with comorbid major depression. One study of older persons with major depression found that those with a concomitant personality disorder were less likely to benefit from psychotherapy.

In outpatient settings, clinicians have limited control over a patient's environment and must therefore rely on one-to-one interventions if the patient is willing to cooperate with treatment. With some patients, it may be necessary to convey a basic formulation of their behaviors, along with suggested approaches, to caregivers and affiliated health care professionals, such as internists, social workers, and visiting nurses. This communication is important when patients are vulnerable to self-harm or likely to cause significant disruptions in other settings when they are not understood and approached in a therapeutic manner. Table 35.2 suggests therapeutic approaches that clinicians can employ with various personality disorders.

Long-term-care settings allow more opportunities for intervention. A staff meeting or case conference

Table 35.2—Therapeutic Strategies for Personality Disorders in Late Life

Cluster A—Paranoid, Schizoid, Schizotypal Personality Disorders

- Always assess for and treat comorbid psychosis.

- Do not force social interactions, but offer support and problem-solving assistance in a professional and consistent manner.

- Do not challenge paranoid ideation; instead, solicit and empathize with emotional responses to the inner turmoil and fear of paranoid states.

Cluster B—Antisocial, Borderline, Histrionic, and Narcissistic Personality Disorders

- Assess for and treat underlying mood lability, depression, anxiety, and substance abuse.

- Adopt a consistent, structured, and predictable approach with strict boundaries to contain disruptive behaviors.

- Adopt a team approach with all involved clinicians to devise a common plan; avoid staff splits between "supporters" and "detractors" of the patient.

- Use behavioral contracts and authority figures when necessary to address recurrent disruptive behaviors.

- Do not personalize belligerent behaviors directed toward clinicians; instead, provide opportunities to ventilate frustration and negative thoughts and emotions with colleagues.

Cluster C—Avoidant, Dependent, and Obsessive-Compulsive Personality Disorders

- Assess for and treat underlying anxiety, panic, and depression.

- Provide regularly scheduled clinical contacts rather than on an as-needed basis.

- When possible, provide case managers to solicit the needs of avoidant patients, and to provide extra reassurance and attention to the needs of dependent and obsessive-compulsive patients.

Depressive and Passive-Aggressive Personality Disorders

- Differentiate between the depressive and negative attitudes and the actual symptoms of major depression. Provide appropriate and adequate antidepressant treatment.

- Avoid becoming too pessimistic or burnt-out with attempts at providing care; shift focus to a supportive and nonjudgmental therapeutic relationship, with minimal expectations on outcome.

- Encourage individual psychotherapy to identify underlying emotions and to redirect negative attitudes toward more constructive activities.

often provides the best forum to discuss disruptive persons and to coordinate a consistent treatment plan. Disruptive behaviors can sometimes be traced to particular activities or staff interactions, which can be adapted as part of an overall treatment strategy. Sometimes, disengagement from patients will reduce the intensity of disruptive interactions. In other situations, the continuity of staffing and of daily schedules is critical. In all situations, a treatment plan should be well documented and conveyed to the patient, as well as all involved staff and caregivers. All plans must provide appropriate limits to ensure the safety of patients and staff. A written contract, signed by all parties, may be needed with nonadherent persons in order to eliminate ambiguity. Although it is important to involve family members in the treatment plan, clinicians must recognize that patients with personality disorders often have conflictual relationships with them. Attention should also be given to individual staff members who must work with difficult patients. They need opportunities to vent feelings of anxiety and frustration, and to feel acknowledged and supported by administrative and clinical staff.

There have been no studies looking specifically at pharmacologic strategies for personality disorders in late life, and so clinicians must instead extrapolate from guidelines used for younger persons. Psychotropic medications can be targeted at a particular personality disorder, specific symptoms or symptom clusters, or comorbid depression, anxiety, or psychosis. The goal is not to cure the disorder, but to reduce the frequency and intensity of targeted symptoms. Antidepressants target symptoms of depression and anxiety found in most personality disorders. Mood stabilizers (eg, lithium carbonate and divalproex sodium) have been found to reduce mood lability and impulsivity in borderline patients, and they may be useful with similar symptoms in antisocial personality disorder. Antianxiety agents are commonly used for transient agitation seen in borderline, antisocial, narcissistic, and paranoid disorders, and they can target social anxiety and panic in avoidant and dependent patients. Antidepressants are used commonly to treat obsessive-compulsive persons, although without the efficacy established for the treatment of obsessive-compulsive disorder. Antipsychotic agents can treat the transient psychosis, agitation, and impulsivity seen in dramatic cluster and paranoid disorders, as well as the borderline psychosis and paranoia seen in odd cluster disorders.

In general, psychotropic medications are best used as adjuncts to psychotherapy. In older persons, multiple medications should be avoided when there is a history of nonadherence, confusion, or impulsivity. Attention must be given to potential interactions with multiple other medications used to treat medical disorders. It is important to obtain and document informed consent (or consent of family members or guardians) for the use of psychotropics when there is a history of dementia, recent delirium, paranoia, or conflictual doctor-patient relationships.

Finally, clinicians must recognize that in some cases it is best not to prescribe a psychotropic medication. Such cases include older persons with personality disorders and comorbid substance abuse, chronic nonadherence, or a history of or potential for abusive or self-injurious use of medications. Antisocial and borderline persons often demonstrate such behaviors. Dependent patients may insist upon medications as a means of fostering dependency on the clinician, while obsessive-compulsive patients may perpetuate a maladaptive relationship with the clinician through detailed and controlling discussions of medication management. In each example, medication management is corrupted by dysfunctional interpersonal behaviors that lie at the heart of personality disorders.

SOMATOFORM DISORDERS

Somatoform disorders encompass a heterogeneous group of seven diagnoses that have in common the presence of physical symptoms or complaints without objective organic causes, and that are strongly associated with psychologic factors. Clinical characteristics of each diagnosis are summarized in Table 35.3. These disorders are especially relevant to geriatric care because affected older persons are seen in all health care settings, and they commonly overutilize medical services. Somatoform disorders in late life have not been well studied, and existing research has usually focused on select diagnoses, such as hypochondriasis, in limited or biased samples. Research also has looked at somatic symptom reporting rather than at specific diagnoses. Prevalence rates in middle and late life have been found to be less than 1%, except for one study, which found a prevalence rate of more than 36% for somatization disorder in women over 55 years old seen in health care clinics. The presence of these disorders has not been found to be strongly associated with age, although there is weak evidence for a slight increase in hypochondriasis with age. Increased somatic preoccupation and symptoms are, however, associated with depression in late life, and older age of onset for depression may be most predictive. In addition to depression, increased somatic preoccupation is associated with the presence of the personality trait of neuroticism, in which a person displays a tendency to experience more negative emotions. Somatoform disorders are found more commonly in women and in lower socioeconomic groups. Late onset of a somatoform disorder may be suggestive of associated neurologic illness.

Table 35.3—Clinical Characteristics of Somatoform Disorders

Somatization Disorder

Multiple physical complaints in excess of what would be expected, given history and examination, prior to the age of 30 and lasting several years; complaints not fully explained by medical work-up; must include four different sites of pain, two gastrointestinal symptoms, one sexual symptom, one pseudoneurologic symptom (not pain).

Undifferentiated Somatoform Disorder

One or more physical complaints, lasting at least 6 months, that cannot be fully explained by appropriate medical work-up and that result in considerable social, occupational, or functional impairment.

Conversion Disorder

One or more motor or sensory deficits that cannot be fully explained by appropriate medical work-up and that appear to be causally related to psychologic factors.

Pain Disorder

Pain is the major focus of clinical presentation, and psychologic factors are believed to be playing a critical role in the onset, severity, exacerbation, and maintenance of the pain.

Hypochondriasis

A preoccupation with fears of having a serious illness, based on misinterpretation of bodily symptoms and resistant to appropriate medical evaluation and reassurance.

Body Dysmorphic Disorder

Preoccupation with an imagined defect in appearance. If there is an actual physical defect, this preoccupation greatly exceeds what would be expected.

Somatoform Disorder, Not Otherwise Specified

The presence of somatoform symptoms that do not meet the criteria for other categories.

Clinical Characteristics and Causes

It is important to recognize that somatoform disorders do not represent intentional, conscious attempts by older patients to present factitious physical symptoms. Somatoform symptoms are experienced by the affected person as real physical pain and discomfort, usually without insight into associated psychologic factors. Somatoform disorders do not represent delusional thinking as found in psychotic states (although body dysmorphic disorder can be associated with beliefs of delusional quality), and they are different from psychosomatic disorders, which are characterized by actual disease states with presumed psychologic triggers. Rather, somatoform disorders represent a complex interaction between mind and brain in which an affected person is unknowingly expressing psychologic stress or conflict through the body. It is not surprising, then, that depression and anxiety are associated with increased somatic expressions. In late life, somatoform disorders, in particular hypochondriasis, may be a way for a person to express anxiety and attempt to cope with accumulating fears and losses. These may include fears of abandonment by family and caregivers, loss of beauty and strength, financial setbacks, loss of independence, and loss of social role (eg, through retirement, loss of spouse, occupational disability). The psychologic distress and anxiety over such losses may be less threatening and more controllable when shifted to somatic complaints or symptoms. In turn, the adoption of a sick role might be reinforced by increased social contacts and support.

The causes of somatoform disorders are usually multifactorial, and often they are rooted in early developmental experiences and personality traits. Psychodynamic approaches suggest that these disorders result from unconscious conflict in which intolerable impulses or affects are expressed through more tolerable somatic symptoms or complaints. One reason for this may be the presence of alexithymia, in which a person is unable to identify and express emotional states, so that the body becomes the available mode of expression. The classic example of this would be a conversion disorder, in which intolerable, unconscious impulses are converted into motor or sensory dysfunction. Sigmund Freud first wrote about such a mechanism; his work was based upon his studies of women with what was then termed *hysteria*. Excessive and intolerable guilt or hostility are other psychologic sources for somatization, in particular for hypochondriasis. In such cases, physical symptoms serve as a means of self-punishment for unacceptable unconscious impulses.

Although psychodynamic explanations can apply across the life span, these conflicts often begin early in life, perhaps accounting for the relatively young age of onset for most somatoform disorders. In late life, psychologic conflict that results in significant depression and anxiety are for the most part the same conflicts that can lead to somatization. In addition, the presence of so many comorbid medical problems and the use of multiple medications may provide readily available somatic symptoms around which psychologic conflict can center. In long-term care, older persons are faced with many overwhelming losses, and their own bodies often serve as the last bastion of control. Somatic preoccupation thus serves as a means of coping with stress, even though it is maladaptive and can result in excessive and unnecessary disability.

Treatment

Somatoform disorders do not usually present as such; by their definition they present to clinicians with what appear to be legitimate somatic complaints with an unknown physical cause. It is only after repeated but fruitless work-ups, multiple and persistent complaints and requests, and sometimes angry and inappropriate reactions to treatment that clinicians begin to suspect a somatoform disorder. In some cases the manner of presentation and symptom complex is more immediately suggestive of a particular somatoform disorder. In any event, it is important for the clinician to remember that from the perspective of the patient, the symptoms and complaints are quite real and disturbing. It is never wise to challenge the patient or to suggest that the symptoms are "all in your mind," even after work-up has made it obvious that there are psychologic factors involved. The typical response to such advice is for the patient to seek additional opinions and medical tests, which in turn can perpetuate a cycle of somatization that never addresses the underlying issues.

Instead, the clinician should attempt to foster an ongoing, supportive, consistent, and professional relationship with the affected person. Such a relationship will serve to provide reassurance as well as to protect the patient from excessive and unnecessary medical visits and procedures. The clinician should focus on responding to individual complaints, perhaps with periodic but regularly scheduled appointments, and to set limits on work-up and treatment in a firm but empathic manner. This can be difficult to do when patients become demanding and attempt to consume excessive clinic time, but the clinician must endeavor to remain professional and not to personalize the situation or to feel that he or she is failing the patient. Overall, the role of the clinician is to focus on symptom reduction and rehabilitation, and not to attempt to force the patient to have insight into the potential psychologic nature of his or her symptoms. It would be hazardous to prematurely diagnose a somatoform disorder when there might actually be underlying organic pathology that has eluded diagnosis. For example, disorders such as multiple sclerosis, systemic lupus erythematosus, and acute intermittent porphyria commonly have complex presentations that elude initial diagnostic work-up. Moreover, many somatoform disorders coexist with actual disease states; for example, many persons with pseudoseizures also have an actual seizure disorder. At the same time, it is important for the clinician to set limits on what he or she can offer, and to make appropriate referrals to specialists and mental health clinicians.

The mental health clinician will play a more active role in addressing the somatoform disorder. Unfortunately, no particular treatment for any somatoform disorder has been found to have good efficacy, and most disorders tend to be lifelong. As a result, the goal of treatment is not to cure, but to control symptoms. The clinician first forms a therapeutic alliance based on empathic listening and acknowledging of physical discomfort, without trivializing the somatic complaints. Sometimes an offer to review all available medical records can be a tangible way of conveying one's seriousness to the patient. Underlying anxiety and depression must be identified and treated with psychotherapy and, when necessary, antidepressant or antianxiety medications, or both. Individual therapy that takes a psychodynamic approach focuses on helping the patient identify psychologic conflict and associated emotions, and then to discuss it within a safe environment. Cognitive-behavioral therapy focuses on identifying distorted thought patterns and anxious triggers, and replacing them with more realistic and adaptive strategies. For conversion disorder, hypnosis is sometimes used as both a diagnostic and a therapeutic tool. Body dysmorphic disorder can be approached much the same way as obsessive-compulsive disorder and treated with both cognitive-behavioral conditioning and anti-obsessive medications. Antidepressant medications are typically used for somatization and pain disorders, as well as for undifferentiated somatoform disorder.

REFERENCES

- Agronin ME, Maletta G. Personality disorders in late life: understanding and overcoming the gap in research. *Am J Geriatric Psychiatry*. 2000;8(1):4–18.

- Martin RL, Yutzy SH. Somatoform disorders. In: Hales RE, Yudofsky SC, Talbott JA, eds. *Textbook of Psychiatry*, 2nd ed. Washington, DC: American Psychiatric Press; 1994:591–622.

- Rosowsky E, Abrams RC, Zweig RA, eds. *Personality Disorders in Older Adults: Emerging Issues in Diagnosis and Treatment*. Mahwah, NJ: Lawrence Erlbaum Associates, Inc.; 1999.

- Sheehan B, Banerjee S. Somatization in the elderly. *Int J Geriatric Psychiatry*. 1999;14:1044–1049.

CHAPTER 36—SUBSTANCE ABUSE

The abuse and misuse of alcohol, psychoactive medications, illicit drugs, and nicotine have become significant public health concerns for the growing population of elderly people. This concern is highlighted by the growth in the literature demonstrating that the abuse of or dependence on these substances among older people is common. Moreover, older adults are particularly vulnerable to the effects of these substances, and clinicians and researchers need to change their thinking about the risks of use in this segment of the population. Typically, substance-use problems are thought to occur only in those persons who use substances in high quantities and at regular intervals. Among older adults, however, negative health consequences have been demonstrated at consumption levels previously thought of as light to moderate, and certainly not in the amounts usually associated with a diagnosis of substance dependence. A growing number of effective treatments for these problems lead not only to reductions in substance use but also to improvement in general health. Taken together, both the risks and the emergence of new treatments underscore the need to identify problems and provide appropriate treatment for those older adults suffering from the effects of misuse of these substances.

DEFINITIONS OF SUBSTANCE ABUSE

Establishing valid criteria for determining which older adults would benefit from reducing or eliminating their substance use is the first step in successful intervention. *Substance dependence* has been defined by the medical community as any use that imparts significant disability and warrants treatment. Many older adults are not recognized as having problems that are related to their substance use, partly because the diagnostic criteria are difficult to interpret and to apply consistently to older adults. For instance, many older people drink at home by themselves; thus, they are less likely than younger drinkers to be arrested, to get into arguments, or to have difficulties in employment. Moreover, because many of the diseases caused or affected by substance misuse (eg, hypertension, stroke, and pulmonary disease) are common disorders in late life, the clinician may overlook the effects of substance use on the older patient who presents with these disorders. The literature indicates that older problem drinkers are identified less often by clinicians and are less often referred for treatment than are their younger counterparts.

Because of the difficulties in assessing older adults for substance dependence, many of the experts have advocated screening to identify persons who are at risk for problem behaviors or who have problem use. *At-risk* use is defined as any use of a substance at a quantity or frequency greater than a recommended level. The level of use is often determined empirically on the basis of association with significant disability. For instance, the recommended upper limit of alcohol consumption for older adults has been established as no more than seven standard drinks per week with no more than two episodes of binge drinking (four or more drinks in a day) during a period of 3 months. *Problem substance* use is defined as the consumption of any amount of an abusable substance that results in at least one problem related to this use. For example, the use of benzodiazepines by a patient who has an unsteady gait would be considered problem use.

The most practical method for identifying persons who could benefit from intervention is to determine the quantity and frequency of their use of abusable substances. This method has advantages over formal diagnostic interviews because of its brevity, easily interpretable results, and absence of stigmatizing language, such as "addiction," "alcoholism," "alcoholic" or "alcohol dependence." For more on screening, see the section below on identifying substance-use disorders (p 237).

MAGNITUDE OF THE PROBLEM

Drug Use

Little is known about the epidemiology of substance-use disorders among older persons other than alcoholism. The general belief is that older drug addicts represent only younger addicts grown old and that few older adults initiate drug use in their later years. The Epidemiologic Catchment Area (ECA) study provides perhaps the only community study of the prevalence of drug abuse and dependence among older adults. Using the Diagnostic Interview Schedule to determine prevalence rates for psychiatric diagnoses as defined by the third edition of the *Diagnostic and Statistical Manual of Mental Disorders* (*DSM-III*), the study found the lifetime prevalence rates of drug abuse and dependence to be 0.12% for older men and 0.06% for older women. The lifetime history of illicit drug use was found to be 2.88% for men and 0.66% for women. No active cases were reported in either gender. In contrast, a more recent study of an elder-specific drug program in a veteran population found that one quarter had either a primary drug problem or concurrent drug and alcohol problems. This study may be a reflection of the growing number of older persons raised during a time of expanded drug experimentation. Other studies to determine the prevalence and incidence among older adults of substances use disorders involving nicotine, caffeine, benzodiazepines, marijuana, and opiates are needed.

Medication Use

Perhaps a unique problem with the older adults is the misuse or inappropriate use of prescription and over-the-counter medications. This problem includes the misuse of substances such as sedatives, hypnotics, opioids and non-opioids, diet aids, decongestants, and a wide variety of other over-the-counter medications. Community surveys have found that 60% of older persons are taking an analgesic, 22% are taking a central nervous system medication, and 11% are taking a benzodiazepine. Many medications used by older persons have the potential for inducing tolerance, withdrawal syndromes, and harmful medical consequences, such as cognitive changes, renal disease, hepatic disease and falls. There is a growing body of literature demonstrating an increase in morbidity and mortality associated with the misuse of prescription and nonprescription medications, even though this is not considered as a disorder by *DSM-IV*.

Health care professionals should carefully monitor older patients' medication use, avoiding the prescription of dangerous combinations of drugs, medications with a high potential for side effects, and ineffective or unnecessary medications. (See "Pharmacotherapy," p 35.) A careful, closely monitored balance between appropriate pharmacotherapy for symptom management (eg, pain relief) and inadequate prescribing with resultant debilitating symptoms must be struck. Intra- and inter-individual variation in responses to analgesic medications, particularly, requires considerable tailoring of drug therapies weighing therapeutic responses against adverse effects. Titration and individualization are key. A practical approach to monitoring psychoactive medication use is to reevaluate use every 3 to 6 months after dosing regimens and the patient are stabilized. Only patients with a documented response to the treatment should continue on to maintenance treatment. Patients without a response or partial response should be reevaluated to consider the appropriate diagnosis and further care. In such cases, consultation with a geriatric mental health professional could be advantageous. (See also "Depression and Other Mood Disorders," p 211; "Anxiety Disorders," p 220; "Psychotic Disorders," p 224; and "Personality and Somatoform Disorders," p 228.)

Alcohol Use

Community-based epidemiologic studies help to define the extent and nature of alcohol use in the older population. Typically, these studies report patterns of alcohol use by determining percentages of abstainers, heavy drinkers, and daily drinkers. Abstention from alcohol ranges from 31% to 58%, and daily drinking ranges from 10% to 22% in samples of older patients. "Heavy" drinking, defined as a minimum of 12 to 21 drinks per week, is present in 3% to 9% of the older population; alcohol abuse, as defined clinically, is present in approximately 2% to 4%.

Longitudinally designed community studies give valuable insight regarding the natural course of drinking patterns in older age groups. Studies that examined longitudinal alcohol use indicate an incidence of heavy drinking of 0.2% to 4% of older persons per year. It is also important to keep in mind that most of the literature on drinking indicates that although older persons are likely to decrease the quantity of alcohol consumed on a given day, the frequency of use or pattern of use changes very little over time.

Cultural and Demographic Factors

Numerous studies have shown that the prevalence of alcohol use and alcohol-related problems among older persons is much higher for men than for women. Among younger adults, however, the ratio of men to women drinkers has changed over the past several decades, with the result that more women present for treatment. These changes are likely to be reflected in the next generation of older women. Similar patterns by gender are seen with illicit drug use, except that benzodiazepines are much more commonly used by older women than by older men.

Conclusions are less clear from the few studies addressing differences among various ethnic groups. Depending on the study, older black Americans and older Hispanic Americans have been found to consume amounts of alcohol similar to or lower than the amounts consumed by older white Americans. The ECA data demonstrated nonsignificant differences in the 1-year diagnosis of alcohol abuse and dependence among black Americans (2.93% among men, 0.60% among women), white Americans (2.85% among men and 0.47% among women), and Hispanic Americans (6.57% among men and 0.0% among women). More relevant risk factors than race or ethnicity for alcohol consumption among older adults are increased leisure time and increased disposable income.

Clinical Settings

Adults aged 65 and older constitute the majority of admissions to acute-care facilities and are frequent users of outpatient medical services, including primary care. The prevalence rates for alcohol problems among hospital populations range from 20% to 50%. High prevalence rates for problems related to drinking are also becoming more common in retirement communities. Data from a survey of a Veterans Affairs nursing home has demonstrated that 35% of the patients interviewed had a lifetime diagnosis of alcohol abuse. A significant number of patients seen in outpatient clinics also have been found to have an active alcohol use disorder. The high prevalence of alcohol-related problems in hospital and outpatient populations underscores the need for thorough screening and treatment of older patients in health care settings.

RISKS AND BENEFITS OF SUBSTANCE USE

Benefits of Alcohol Consumption

Moderate alcohol consumption among otherwise healthy older adults has been promoted as having significant beneficial effects, especially with regard to cardiovascular disease and mortality. The findings from the cardiovascular literature have led to a host of articles in the popular press espousing the benefits of alcohol use; they have also led some people to recommend that persons who formerly did not drink start consuming alcohol. Epidemiologic studies have also suggested that moderate alcohol use helps reduce the risk of developing a dementing illness and cancer.

Alcohol in moderate amounts may improve self-esteem, promote relaxation, and thus enhance social pleasure. However, even though there are benefits of moderate drinking, the practice of recommending drinking to people who currently do not drink is not advocated. Many older adults do not drink because of past problems with drinking, family problems with drinking, the expense related to drinking, and the unpleasant taste or effects of intoxication. There is no evidence to support a therapeutic effect of alcohol for heart disease or any other condition in persons who previously did not drink.

Excess Physical Disability

Substance abuse has clear and profound effects on the health and well-being of people in all spheres of life. Older persons are prone to the toxic effects of substances on many different organ systems. The social and economic impact is also tremendous. Substance abuse has adverse effects on self-esteem, coping skills, and interpersonal relationships, which may be compounded by losses that are common in the late stages of life. Older adults are particularly prone to these toxic effects because of both the physiologic changes associated with aging and the changes associated with other illnesses common in late life. Toxins such as alcohol may have greater clinical impact on the older person, as the body is not able to adjust to even modest amounts of alcohol or other substances.

Levels of alcohol consumption above seven drinks per week, so called at-risk drinking, have been associated with a number of health problems, including an increased risk of stroke caused by bleeding, impaired driving skills, and an increased rate of injuries, such as falls and fractures. The risk of breast cancer in women who consume three to nine drinks per week has been shown to be increased by approximately 50% over that of women who drink fewer than three drinks per week. Of particular importance to older persons are the potential harmful interactions between alcohol and both prescribed and over-the-counter medications, especially psychoactive medications such as benzodiazepines, barbiturates, and antidepressants. Alcohol is also known to interfere with the metabolism of many medications, including digoxin and warfarin.

Older adults who consume more than an average of four drinks per day or whose drinking has led to a diagnosis of alcohol dependence are at greatest risk for excess physical disability and physical illness that are related to the drinking. The most common problems associated with alcohol dependence are alcoholic liver disease, chronic obstructive pulmonary disease, peptic ulcer disease, and psoriasis. Moreover, unexplained multisystem disease should alert the clinician to probe more closely for alcohol use. With smoking, the risks are much clearer, including increased rates of pulmonary disease, especially cancer. Medications such as benzodiazepines are also associated with excess physical disability, with increased rates of falls, and driving-related impairment. Research is beginning to demonstrate that the disability associated with these problems is also reversible with reductions in substance use.

Mental Health Problems

Substance use can be a significant factor in the course and prognosis of nearly all mental health problems of late life. Alcohol, benzodiazepine, opioid, and cigarette use have all been demonstrated to be related etiologically to mood disturbances, but they also complicate the treatment of concurrent mood disorders. Overall, older persons with alcohol abuse or dependence are nearly three times more likely to have a lifetime diagnosis of another mental disorder. Alcoholism has been implicated in mood disorders, suicide, dementia, anxiety disorders, and sleep disturbances. Moderate alcohol use has also been demonstrated to have negative effects on the treatment of late-life depression, further underscoring the need for reducing moderate use in the context of chronic health problems in older adults.

IDENTIFYING SUBSTANCE USE DISORDERS

Although examination remains the clinician's most valuable tool for identifying substance-use problems, screening instruments help increase the sensitivity and efficiency of diagnosing various disorders. Several instruments have been developed for identifying alcohol use disorders, including self-administered questionnaires and laboratory studies. Self-administered questionnaires provide the busy clinician with a rapid,

sensitive, and inexpensive method of screening for alcohol problems. Two questionnaires—the MAST and the CAGE (see Table 36.1)—have been developed with these principles in mind. Both of these instruments have high sensitivity and specificity for identifying alcohol use disorders in young and middle-aged persons. The geriatric version of the MAST (MAST–G, see the Appendix, p 386; see Table 36.2 for a short version), which asks questions relevant to an aging cohort, has been found to be 95% sensitive and 78% specific for identifying older persons with alcohol problems. Other widely used questionnaires include the Alcohol Use Disorders Identification Test (AUDIT) and the Drinking Problems Index. (For information about a number of screens for alcohol problems, see http://www.niaaa.nih.gov/publications/instable.htm.)

Biologic markers of substance use can be useful in managing patients with known substance-use disorders, but they have proved less valuable in detecting illness. These markers include γ-glutamyl transferase, which has a low sensitivity and a moderate specificity for diagnosing an alcohol use disorder; mean corpuscular volume, which has a low sensitivity but a high specificity; high-density lipoprotein, which shows a linear increase with alcohol use; and carbohydrate-deficient transferrin, which has a low sensitivity and low specificity. Urine drug screens are an effective method for screening for or identifying illicit drug use as well as prescription drug use.

TREATMENT

Older persons with a substance-use problem often present with a variety of treatment needs. It is therefore important to have an array of services available for older adults that can be tailored to these individual needs and to have the flexibility to adapt to changing needs over time. The spectrum of interventions for alcohol abuse in older adults range from prevention and education for persons who are abstinent or low-risk drinkers, to minimal advice or brief structured interventions for at-risk or problem drinkers, and formalized alcoholism treatment for drinkers who meet

Table 36.1—The CAGE Questionnaire

C	Have you ever tried to Cut down on your drinking?
A	Have you ever gotten Annoyed at someone for criticizing your drinking?
G	Do you ever feel Guilty about your drinking?
E	Have you ever had an Eye-opener to steady your nerves or get rid of a hangover?

A positive answer to one or more questions suggests problem drinking

Table 36.2—Short Michigan Alcoholism Screening Test—Geriatric Version (S-MAST-G) © The Regents of the University of Michigan, 1991

	YES (1)	NO (0)
1. When talking with others, do you ever underestimate how much you actually drank?		
2. After a few drinks, have you sometimes not eaten or been able to skip a meal because you didn't feel hungry?		
3. Does having a few drinks help decrease your shakiness or tremors?		
4. Does alcohol sometimes make it hard for you to remember parts of the day or night?		
5. Do you usually take a drink to relax or calm your nerves?		
6. Do you drink to take your mind off your problems?		
7. Have you ever increased your drinking after experiencing a loss in your life?		
8. Has a doctor or nurse ever said they were worried or concerned about your drinking?		
9. Have you ever made rules to manage your drinking?		
10. When you feel lonely, does having a drink help?		

Scoring: Two or more "yes" responses indicate an alcohol problem.

Reprinted with permission. For further information, contact Frederic C. Blow, PhD, at the University of Michigan Alcohol Research Center, 400 E. Eisenhower Parkway, Suite A, Ann Arbor, MI 48108. 734-930-5139.

criteria for abuse or dependence. The array of formal treatment options available includes psychotherapy, education, rehabilitative and residential care, and psychopharmacologic agents. An example of the necessity to tailor care is the contrast between the at-risk drinker or benzodiazepine user and the severely dependent patient. It is unlikely that the at-risk user will need the intensity of services required for the severely dependent patient. Indeed, requiring the at-risk drinker to accept a set of rigorous services may be more detrimental than helpful.

Dependency is managed by placing the patient on a 24-hour equivalent of the dosage of the drug on which the patient is dependent, tapering the dosage by 10% every three half lives, and by providing supportive counseling via groups, psychosocial support, and 12-step programs. Withdrawal symptoms from narcotics can be controlled when necessary with oral clonidine. Assuring that the patient enters a long-term treatment program increases the likelihood of long-term success.

Detoxification and Stabilization

The assessment of any substance abuser starts with a thorough history, physical, and laboratory examination. Included in the initial assessment is an assessment of the patient's potential to suffer acute withdrawal. Severe withdrawal such as that from alcohol use can be life threatening and warrants careful attention. Patients with severe symptoms of dependency or withdrawal potential and patients with significant medical or psychiatric comorbidity may require inpatient hospitalization for acute stabilization prior to implementing an outpatient management strategy. Detoxification is achieved by placing the patient on the minimum amount of drug that suppresses withdrawal symptoms and then decreasing the dosage by 10% every three half-lives. In general, longer acting formulations of the drug being abused are preferred to shorter acting formulations, but many clinicians find that prescribing the specific drug that a patient was abusing makes the process more acceptable to the patient and minimizes the time needed to determine the initial dose.

Outpatient Management

Traditionally, outpatient substance-abuse treatment has been reserved for specialized clinics focused on substance abuse. It is becoming increasingly apparent that this model is inadequate in addressing the broader public health demand, and there is a need to involve a variety of clinicians and clinical settings to deliver substance-abuse treatment. This is particularly important for older adults, who frequently seek medical services but rarely seek specialized addiction services. The traditional addiction clinic is focused on supportive group psychotherapy and encouragement to attend regular self-help group meetings such as Alcoholics Anonymous, Alcoholics Victorious, Rational Recovery, or Narcotics Anonymous. For older adults, peer-specific group activities are considered superior to mixed-age group activities. Outpatient rehabilitation, in addition to focusing on active addiction issues, usually needs to address issues of time management. Abstinence reduces the time spent in maintaining the substance-use disorder. The management of this time, which is often the greater part of a patient's day, is critical to the prognosis of treatment. Use of resources such as day programs and senior centers can be beneficial, especially for cognitively impaired patients. Social services such as financial support are often needed to stabilize the patient in early recovery. Supervised living arrangements, such as halfway houses, group homes, nursing homes, and residing with relatives, should also be considered.

Brief Interventions

Low-intensity, brief interventions have been suggested as cost-effective and practical techniques that can be used as an initial approach to at-risk and problem drinkers in primary care settings. Studies of brief intervention have been conducted in a wide range of health care settings, from hospitals and primary health care locations to mental health clinics. Two trials of brief alcohol intervention with older adults have been reported. Both studies were randomized trials of brief intervention to reduce hazardous drinking by older adults, and both used advice protocols in primary care settings. These studies have shown that older adults can be engaged in brief intervention protocols, that the protocols are acceptable in this population, and that there is a substantial reduction in drinking among the at-risk drinkers receiving the interventions in comparison with a control group.

Pharmacotherapy

The use of medications to support abstinence may be of benefit, but it is not well studied. Small-scale studies have demonstrated that naltrexone is well tolerated and efficacious in older patients. Studies are currently under way using various antidepressants, including the selective serotonin-reuptake inhibitors. Some of the general principles used in treating younger patients should be applied to older drinkers as well. For example, benzodiazepines are important in the treatment of alcohol detoxification, but they have no clinical place in maintaining long-term abstinence because of their abuse potential and the potential for fostering further alcohol or benzodiazepine abuse. Disulfiram may benefit some well-motivated patients, but cardiac and hepatic disease limits the use of this agent by the older alcoholic. The efficacy of other agents, such as lithium, antidepressants (eg, the selective serotonin-reuptake inhibitors and tricyclics), and naltrexone, is as yet

unproven, and at this time their use should be limited to research trials. The use of methadone maintenance has proven efficacy in opioid dependence. Older patients can be initiated and maintained on methadone, following the same principles of use as in younger patients. Comorbid medical and psychiatric disorders must be identified and properly treated, and they may necessitate the need for referral to, or consultation with, a psychiatrist with expertise in these areas.

Establishing abstinence from nicotine follows the same principles as that from other addicting substances. Initially, pharmacologic substitution with either nicotine gum or patch is followed by a gradual decrease in dosage. Several trials demonstrated that antidepressant medications improve rates of continued abstinence, but only bupropion has been approved for this purpose by the Food and Drug Administration. As with other abstinence regimens, psychotherapy plus pharmacotherapy is better than pharmacotherapy alone. See also "Respiratory Diseases and Disorders" (p 302).

REFERENCES

■ Blow F, Consensus Panel Chair. Substance abuse among older adults. In: *Treatment Improvement Protocol*, SAMHSA Center for Substance Abuse Treatment, 1998. Washington, DC: US Government Printing Office; 1998.

■ Fleming MF, Manwell LB, Barry KL, et al. Brief physician advice for alcohol problems in older adults: a randomized community-based trial. *J Fam Pract*. 1999;48(5):378–384.

■ Helzer JE, Burnam A, McEvoy LT. Alcohol abuse and dependence. In: Robins LN, Reiger DA, eds. *Psychiatric Disorders in America: The Epidemiologic Catchment Area Study*. New York: The Free Press; 1991.

■ Oslin D, Liberto JG, O'Brien J, et al. Naltrexone as an adjunctive treatment for older patients with alcohol dependence. *Am J Geriatr Psychiatry*, 1997; 5(4):324–332.

■ Ostbye T, Taylor DH, Jung SH. A longitudinal study of the effects of tobacco smoking and other modifiable risk factors on ill health in middle-aged and old Americans: results from the Health and Retirement Study and Asset and Health Dynamics among the Oldest Old survey. *Preventive Medicine*. 2002; 34(3):334–345.

CHAPTER 37—MENTAL RETARDATION

Mental retardation continues to be a widely used term to describe the condition of subaverage intellectual function in the presence of deficits in adaptive behavior. Critics have attacked this definition because of difficulties with its clinical usefulness: reliance on a person's performance on intelligence tests to demonstrate intellectual difficulties has been criticized because of difficulties in determining cut-off values for normality, the questionable cultural fairness of the tests, and the questionable relevance of the tests for performance in real-life situations. Similar controversies regarding the imprecision of definition and measurement of adaptive behavior remain unresolved. However, the key concept of a central, biologically based deficit in intellectual function appears to be valid; persons with mental retardation have a condition in which nearly every cognitive process that has been studied is deficient. This has a major biologic basis: for mild mental retardation, the same genetic and environmental influences appear to operate that determine individual differences throughout the normal range of variation in general cognitive ability. Importantly, the heritability of general cognitive ability is substantial, probably around 50%; the effects of shared environmental influences in families become negligible after adolescence, and genetic influence increases from infancy to adulthood. Persons with severe degrees of mental retardation are more likely to have structural defects of the brain or metabolic or chromosomal derangements.

PREVALENCE

The number of aging persons with mental retardation is increasing, probably because of increased longevity in persons with mental retardation (with life expectancy increasing from 20 years in the 1930s to 60 years in 1980; life expectancy has increased by about 30 years in those with Down syndrome). American and European societies are showing a demographic shift, with an increasing percentage of persons aged 60 and over (9% in 1960, 17% in 1990, and an estimated 20% in 2010). The prevalence of mental retardation and developmental disability (cerebral palsy, autism, epilepsy) is generally assumed to be around 1%; thus, estimates are that in the United States there are 525,000 persons aged 60 and over with these conditions; and the numbers are expected to double by 2030.

PSYCHIATRIC AND MENTAL DISORDERS IN AGING ADULTS WITH MENTAL RETARDATION

The prevalence of psychiatric disorders among adults with mental retardation is about five times that of age-matched control groups. Depending on the exact population studied and the type of diagnoses included, rates range from 10% to 40%.

Dementia

Adults with Down syndrome have an increased risk for the early onset of Alzheimer's disease: 100% develop the neuropathology by age 40. Although not all develop symptoms in their 40s, approximately 40% aged 50 and over have symptoms, with 50% developing the associated new onset of seizures. Approximately 75% in their 60s have symptoms of dementia (compared with a prevalence in the general population of 5% at age 65). Symptoms also include loss of adaptive skills and increased maladaptive behavior; the dementia is often associated with depression, indifference, and social inappropriateness. Average age at death for persons with Down syndrome and Alzheimer's disease is approximately 50. The incidence of dementia in mentally retarded persons without Down syndrome is the same as in the general population; however, these persons also have an increased prevalence of the neuropathology of Alzheimer's disease: 54% for ages 50 to 65, 76% for ages 66 to 75, 87% for ages > 75.

Other Major Mental Disorders

For persons with mental retardation, the lifetime prevalence of other major mental illnesses appears to be similar to or higher than that of the general population, as follows: schizophrenia 2% to 5% (1% in general population); bipolar illness 1% to 2% (1%); affective disorder 3% to 10% (6%). In those aged 65 and over, approximately 70% may reach criteria for a psychiatric diagnosis, often with higher rates than for a younger age group. For example: schizophrenia 3% (versus 1% in the younger group); depression 6% (4%); anxiety disorders 9% (5%). Autistic traits are common, occurring in up to approximately half of adults with learning disability or mental retardation. These traits are more common in those with severe or profound degrees of mental retardation and in younger individuals; they are typically associated with behavioral difficulties.

Adaptive Behavioral Difficulties

Difficulties with adaptive behavior are commonly severe. For example, surveys of adults with mental retardation have revealed that 25% have no useful speech and 10%, no receptive comprehension. Half do not have basic self-care skills, half have a physical disability, and half have a mobility impairment; 10% are totally dependent. Support services for these people are usually deficient.

Behavioral Disorders

As many as 50% to 60% of adults with mental retardation have a maladaptive behavior (such as withdrawal, self-injury, stereotypy) that is severe or that occurs frequently. The proportion decreases with age, except in Down syndrome, in which the proportion is higher and the incidence of behavioral problems increases with the degree of mental retardation. Aggression occurs with similar frequency in all age groups. About half of the persons with behavioral disorders have had an experience in the preceding 12 months that may have precipitated the disorder.

DIAGNOSIS AND TREATMENT

The diagnosis of a mental disorder is based on the same principles of history and examination as those applying in the general population. However, presentations of mental illness may be different in persons with mental retardation: typically, verbal skills are poor, and reports of mood or mental experiences are difficult to obtain. Often, mental disorders present as behavioral changes, for example, social withdrawal, apathy, and vegetative changes occurring in depressed persons, or agitation, sleeplessness, or aggression in those experiencing delusions or hallucinations. It is more difficult for persons with limited coping skills to adjust to changes in living or work situations, and inquiries should be made about whether such changes have occurred.

It is important to identify the cause of the person's mental retardation. Careful physical, laboratory, and neurologic investigation (electroencephalography and neuroimaging) may establish a cause in 40%. Different conditions are associated with different problems: for example, Down syndrome with hypothyroidism and Alzheimer's disease; Prader-Willi syndrome with hyperphagia, obesity, ritualistic behaviors, and aggression; fragile-X syndrome with autistic behaviors, gaze avoidance, and attentional difficulty; frontal lobe damage with apathy, irritability, distractibility, perseveration, and dysexecutive problems; temporal lobe lesions with Klüver-Bucy syndrome (hypersexuality, hyperorality, hypermetamorphosis, visual agnosia, diminished aggression, and anxiety) or Gastaut-Geschwind syndrome (an interictal syndrome with hypergraphia, irritability, elation, and paranoia). Older adults with mental retardation who have not been previously evaluated should be referred to a specialist for assessment if asymmetric neurologic signs are present, if there is a history of cognitive or neurologic deterioration, or if behavioral symptoms cannot be reversed.

Medical disorders commonly present as psychiatric or behavioral disorders, and they occur in persons with mental retardation twice as commonly as in the average psychiatric population: 20% to 40% of the illnesses may cause or exacerbate the psychiatric symptoms.

Maladaptive behaviors, such as aggression, are common in persons with mental retardation and may not indicate a mental disorder. An impulsive response to a stressor may reflect only suboptimal judgment in a particular situation. An appropriate treatment in such cases would be instructional or behavioral; the preferred behavior programs are ones that reward good behavior. A disorder of impulse control, however, may also produce aggressive responses; diagnosis of such a disorder requires a pattern of impulsivity that is disproportionate to the degree of intellectual impairment. With an impulse-control disorder, aggression may be preceded by a period of increasing tension and arousal, occur explosively and out of proportion to the stressor, and seem to have a driven, sustained nature. Appropriate treatment would consist of instructional and behavioral methods, but also with pharmacologic interventions to reduce impulsivity (eg, selective serotonin-reuptake inhibitors) or arousal (eg, β-blockers). Pharmacologic treatment of aggression is similar to that in the general population and includes the use of mood stabilizers, selective serotonin-reuptake inhibitors, β-blockers, and antipsychotic medications.

The diagnosis of dementia in mentally retarded persons is made according to the same principles as in the general population: a history showing cognitive and adaptive deterioration; demonstration of deficits on examination (preferably with longitudinal follow-up showing progression of deficits, or with tests that the person has had previously, to enable comparison of performance); exclusion of other possible causes of deterioration, such as medical or environmental factors, or other mental disorders, such as depression or delirium. Standardized scales are available that help structure the interview and history and produce a score that indicates the likelihood that dementia is present and its severity. Neuroimaging studies are important in helping to establish the diagnosis and in differentiating Alzheimer's disease from vascular dementia; longitudinal and volumetric studies may help differentiate normal aging from dementia. There are insufficient studies to demonstrate the efficacy of standard treatments (such as donepezil) in persons with mental retardation, although anecdotal data supports their use.

MEDICAL DISORDERS

Adults with mental retardation have more medical problems than do age-matched persons (approximately five per person; those with more severe mental retardation have more problems). Approximately two thirds of those in a community setting have chronic conditions or major physical disability. It is estimated that 50% of these medical conditions go undetected. Prompt detection and treatment is associated with better survival. Visual or hearing impairments are more common in persons with mental retardation; they increase with age and affect approximately 25%.

Persons with Down syndrome and others with mental retardation have similar age-specific mortality until ages 30 to 34, after which there is an exponential increase in mortality with age for those with Down syndrome, probably because of the onset of dementia. Life expectancy decreases with increasing severity of mental retardation, and with other morbidity such as inability to ambulate, lack of feeding skills, and incontinence. Life expectancy is lower than for the general population and is about 65 years. The commonest causes of death are cardiovascular and respiratory disorders, cancer, and dementia (particularly in Down syndrome).

SOCIAL CONDITIONS

At least 80% of adults with mental retardation live at home and are cared for by aging family members; 20% live in residential programs. Elderly nursing-home residents with mental retardation may have no one to act as an advocate, which can affect treatment decisions for acute illnesses. It is estimated that about 40% of eligible persons may not be served by the formal service system. This situation often leads to a crisis when the parent is no longer able to provide adequate care or is unable to manage a behavioral problem. It is estimated that about half of developmentally disabled adults with a behavior problem need a different living arrangement. Typically, more than half of the families have not made future care plans for the person with mental retardation; those in day programs or workshops do not typically have pensions or Social Security benefits to allow retirement.

REFERENCES

- Cooper SA. The relationship between psychiatric and physical health in elderly people with intellectual disability. *J Intellect Disabil Res.* 1999;43(Pt 1):54–60.

- Gedye A. *The Dementia Scale for Down Syndrome.* Vancouver, BC, Canada: Gedye Research and Consulting;1995. (To order, contact A. Gedye, Gedye Research and Consulting, PO Box 39081, Point Grey, Vancouver, BC, Canada V6R 4P1. Phone/Fax: 604-733-1950.)

- Plomin R. Genetic research on general cognitive ability as a model for mild mental retardation. *Int Rev Psychiatry.* 1999;11:34–46.

- Ryan R, Sunada K. Medical evaluation of persons with mental retardation referred for psychiatric assessment. *Gen Hosp Psychiatry.* 1997;19(4):274–280.

- Schaefer GB, Bodensteiner JB. Developmental anomalies of the brain in mental retardation. *Int Rev Psychiatry.* 1999;11:47–55.

COMMON GERIATRIC DISEASES, DISORDERS, AND HEALTH CONCERNS

CHAPTER 38—CARDIOVASCULAR DISEASES AND DISORDERS

AGE-RELATED CARDIOVASCULAR CHANGES

See Table 38.1.

ISCHEMIC HEART DISEASE

Epidemiology

Coronary artery disease (CAD) is the most common cause of death in persons aged 65 years and older. Autopsy studies show that 70% of persons older than 70 years have CAD with ≥ 50% atherosclerotic obstruction of one or more coronary arteries. More than 30% of persons aged 65 years and older have clinical manifestations of CAD. In one study the prevalence of CAD among 1802 community-dwelling persons (mean age = 80 years) was 33% among the white Americans, 35% among the black Americans, 35% among the Hispanic Americans, and 38% among the Asian Americans. Eighty percent of deaths from CAD occur in persons aged 65 years and older; 60% of persons hospitalized with acute myocardial infarction (MI) are aged 65 years and older. The prevalence of CAD and the incidence of new coronary events are similar among men and women aged 75 years and older, but they are higher among the men in those younger than 75. Eighty-three percent of MIs in women occur after menopause. Women are less likely than men to survive the initial MI.

CAD may be diagnosed in older persons if there is coronary angiographic evidence of significant CAD, a documented MI, a typical history of angina pectoris, or clinical findings of myocardial ischemia. The incidence of sudden cardiac death as the initial manifestation of CAD increases with age.

Risk Factors

Modifiable risk factors for CAD should be controlled in older persons. Cessation of cigarette smoking, treatment of hyperlipidemia, treatment of hypertension, ingestion of a diet low in saturated fat and cholesterol, maintenance of ideal body weight, and regular physical activity will lead to a reduction of CAD and new coronary events. Whether decreasing elevated plasma homocysteine levels by increasing folate supplements will reduce the incidence of new coronary events needs investigation.

If hypertension is present, the blood pressure should be lowered to < 140/90 mm Hg. If CAD or other vascular disease is present and the serum low-density lipoprotein (LDL) cholesterol is > 125 mg/dL despite use of the American Heart Association Step II diet, lipid-lowering drug therapy, preferably statin drug therapy, should be administered to lower the serum LDL cholesterol to < 100 mg/dL. If a second lipid-lowering drug is needed in addition to a statin drug to achieve this, a bile acid resin such as cholestyramine should be used.

The serum LDL cholesterol should also be lowered to < 100 mg/dL if the older person has diabetes mellitus or two or more risk factors that confer a 1-year risk for CAD of > 20%. The serum LDL cholesterol should be lowered to < 130 mg/dL in older persons with two or more risk factors and a 10-year risk for CAD of ≤ 20%. The serum LDL cholesterol should be lowered to < 160 mg/dL for persons with one or no risk factors.

Hypertriglyceridemia should be treated with gemfibrozil or nicotinic acid. Persons with CAD and a

Table 38.1—Age-Related Changes That Affect Heart Action and Circulation

Structure and Function	Change With Age
Myocytes	Progressive loss of cells; hypertrophy
Skeletal muscles	Deconditioning
Left-ventricular stiffness	Increased
Left-ventricular compliance	Decreased
Left-ventricular wall thickness	Increased
Left-ventricular diastolic filling	Decreased, with increased contribution to filling resulting from left atrial systole
Left-ventricular relaxation	Decreased
Maximal heart rate	Progressive decrease
Maximal cardiac output	Progressive decrease
Maximal Vo$_2$	Progressive decrease
Systemic vascular resistance	Increased
Vasodilator response to exercise	Decreased
Ability to secrete sodium	Decreased

low serum high-density lipoprotein (HDL) cholesterol in the presence of a normal serum LDL cholesterol should be treated with gemfibrozil. These recommendations may need to be modified in the presence of comorbid conditions.

Presentation

Dyspnea on exertion is a more common manifestation of myocardial ischemia caused by CAD in older persons than is the chest pain typical of angina pectoris. The dyspnea is caused by a transient increase in left ventricular (LV) end-diastolic pressure caused by ischemia superimposed on reduced ventricular compliance. A substernal location of anginal pain is less commonly observed in older persons. Angina pectoris in older persons may cause pain in the back and shoulders or a burning epigastric pain. The pain of angina pectoris in older persons may be described as less severe and of shorter duration. Myocardial ischemia may cause clinical heart failure. Acute pulmonary edema in older persons unassociated with acute MI may be a clinical manifestation of unstable angina pectoris resulting from extensive CAD.

Attacks of angina pectoris may vary in frequency from several a day to occasional episodes. They may increase in frequency (crescendo angina) to a fatal outcome or may gradually decrease or disappear if an adequate collateral circulation develops, if the ischemic area becomes infarcted, or if heart failure supervenes and limits activity.

The prevalence of clinically unrecognized Q-wave MI in older persons with MI documented by an electrocardiogram (ECG) is approximately 40%. The incidence of new coronary events is similar in older men and women with clinically recognized or unrecognized Q-wave MI. Non-Q-wave MI is commoner in older persons than in younger persons. Because body muscle mass is reduced in older persons, the increased plasma level of the MB isoenzyme of creatine kinase ($\geq$ 5%) resulting from acute MI may occur with a normal total creatine kinase level.

In studies of older patients with clinically recognized acute MI, the prevalence of presenting symptoms ranged from 19% to 66% for chest pain, 20% to 59% for dyspnea, 15% to 33% for neurologic symptoms, and 0% to 19% for gastrointestinal symptoms. Other symptoms associated with acute MI in older persons include sudden death, peripheral gangrene or increased claudication, palpitations, renal failure, weakness, pulmonary embolism, restlessness, and sweating. Older persons with acute MI are more likely than younger persons to die from the MI and to have pulmonary edema, congestive heart failure (CHF), LV systolic dysfunction, cardiogenic shock, conduction disturbances requiring insertion of a pacemaker, atrial fibril-lation (AF) or atrial flutter, and rupture of the LV free wall, septum, or papillary muscle.

Diagnostic Testing

Coronary angiography is the gold standard for detecting CAD and determining its severity. The resting ECG may be used to diagnose MI or ischemia, whether silent or symptomatic, in older persons. Diagnosis of CAD by treadmill exercise–induced ischemic ST-segment depression $\geq$ 1.0 mm in older persons has a sensitivity of 84% and a specificity of 70%. Diagnosis of CAD by upright bicycle exercise–induced ischemic ST-segment depression $\geq$ 1.0 mm in older persons has a sensitivity of 62% and a specificity of 93%. Older persons with exercise-induced hypotension, an inadequate blood-pressure response to exercise, marked ischemic ST-segment depression ($\geq$ 2.0 mm), ischemic ST-segment depression in both anterior and inferior leads, poor exercise duration ($<$ 6 minutes using a standard Bruce treadmill protocol), ischemic ST-segment depression occurring within 6 minutes of exercise, and persistence of ST-segment depression past 8 minutes in the recovery period are more likely to have multivessel CAD and a higher incidence of new coronary events. Older persons with CAD and complex ventricular arrhythmias or silent myocardial ischemia detected by 24-hour ambulatory ECG monitoring have a higher incidence of new coronary events.

Exercise stress testing using thallium perfusion scintigraphy or radionuclide ventriculography may be useful in the diagnosis and prognosis of CAD in older persons, especially for those in whom ST-segment changes cannot be reliably interpreted because of left bundle branch block, LV hypertrophy, or treatment with digitalis. In older persons unable to perform exercise stress testing because of musculoskeletal disorders or pulmonary disease, intravenous dipyridamole-thallium imaging may be used for the diagnosis and prognosis of CAD. The diagnosis of CAD by intravenous dipyridamole-thallium imaging in persons aged 70 years or older has a sensitivity of 86% and a specificity of 75%.

Echocardiography may be useful for detecting regional LV wall motion abnormalities, acute myocardial ischemia, and complications due to acute MI, LV aneurysm, cardiac thrombi, left main CAD, LV hypertrophy, and associated valvular heart disease; it is also useful for evaluating LV systolic and diastolic function and cardiac chamber size in older persons with CAD. Echocardiographic LV hypertrophy and abnormal LV ejection fraction are also associated with an increased incidence of new coronary events in older persons with CAD.

Stress echocardiography using exercise or dobutamine or adenosine to cause new or worsening wall-motion abnormalities and transient dyskinesia is useful in diagnosing CAD and determining the prognosis in older persons. Exercise echocardiography has a sensitivity of 85% and a specificity of 77% in diagnosing CAD in older persons. In persons aged ≥ 70 years, dobutamine stress echocardiography has a sensitivity of 87%, a specificity of 84%, and an accuracy of 86%. In persons aged ≥ 70 years, adenosine stress echocardiography has a sensitivity of 66%, a specificity of 90%, and an accuracy of 73%.

Management

The management decisions described below are based on data from randomized, controlled trials that included highly variable percentages of older persons. Few trials include older persons with serious comorbidities.

Stable Angina Pectoris

The clinician should identify and correct reversible factors that can aggravate angina pectoris and myocardial ischemia, for example, anemia, infection, obesity, hyperthyroidism, uncontrolled hypertension, arrhythmias such as AF with a rapid ventricular rate, and severe valvular aortic stenosis. Smoking should be stopped. Hypertension and hyperlipidemia should be treated. An exercise program will improve exercise tolerance. Aspirin 160 to 325 mg daily decreases the incidence of MI, stroke, and vascular death.

Nitrates relieve and prevent angina pectoris. Nitroglycerin administered as a sublingual tablet 0.3 to 0.6 mg or as a sublingual spray 0.4 mg is the drug most commonly used to relieve an acute anginal attack. Long-acting nitrates help prevent recurrent episodes of angina. A 12- to 14-hour nitrate-free interval every 24 hours is necessary to avoid nitrate tolerance.

β-Blockers are effective antianginal agents and are the drug of choice to prevent myocardial ischemia. They reduce MI, sudden coronary death, and mortality, and they should be given to all persons with CAD without contraindications to β-blockers. If anginal symptoms persist despite treatment with nitrates and β-blockers, a nondihydropyridine calcium channel blocker such as verapamil or diltiazem should be used in persons with normal LV ejection fraction and amlodipine or felodipine in persons with CHF or abnormal LV ejection fraction.

If persons with stable angina have persistent angina interfering with their quality of life despite therapy with nitrates, β-blockers, and calcium channel blockers, coronary revascularization by coronary artery bypass graft (CABG) surgery or by percutaneous transluminal coronary angioplasty (PTCA) should be considered.

Unstable Angina Pectoris and Non-Q-Wave Myocardial Infarction

Persons with unstable angina or non-Q-wave MI should be admitted to a coronary care unit, after treatment has been initiated in the emergency department. Reversible factors should be identified and corrected. Continuous nasal oxygen should be administered at 1 to 2 liters per minute to persons with cyanosis, respiratory distress, CHF, or high risk factors. Aspirin 160 to 325 mg should be given at admission and daily indefinitely. The first dose of aspirin should be chewed. Clopidogrel 75 mg daily may be used by persons unable to tolerate aspirin. Subcutaneous enoxaparin (a low-molecular-weight heparin) should replace unfractionated heparin as the antithrombin for the acute phase of management of persons with non-Q-wave MI or unstable angina pectoris. Platelet glycoprotein IIb/IIIa receptor blockade with administration of tirofiban or eptifibatide has been used as an adjunct to aspirin and enoxaparin in the treatment of persons with non-Q-wave MI or unstable angina.

Persons whose anginal symptoms are not fully relieved with three sublingual nitroglycerin tablets should be treated with continuous intravenous nitroglycerin for at least 24 hours. When the person is angina free for 24 hours, he or she can be switched to an oral or transdermal preparation of long-acting nitrates. β-Blockers, unless contraindicated, should be given in the emergency department. They should be given intravenously initially and then orally and continued indefinitely.

Approximately 90% of older persons with unstable angina can be stabilized with medical management. Persons who continue to have unstable angina 30 minutes after initiation of therapy or who have recurrence of unstable angina during hospitalization should have coronary angiography. Coronary revascularization is indicated in persons with

- significant left main CAD;
- significant three-vessel CAD plus abnormal LV ejection fraction;
- significant two-vessel CAD with proximal subtotal stenosis of the left anterior descending coronary artery plus abnormal LV ejection fraction;
- significant CAD and who
  —fail to stabilize with medical therapy,
  —have recurrent angina pectoris or myocardial ischemia at rest or with low-level activity,
  —have myocardial ischemia accompanied by CHF, an S_3 gallop, or new or worsening mitral regurgitation.

Cardiovascular Diseases and Disorders **245**

Acute Myocardial Infarction

Aspirin in a dosage of 160 mg to 325 mg daily should be administered as soon as acute MI is suspected, and it should be continued indefinitely. The first dose of aspirin should be chewed. Ticlopidine 250 mg twice a day or clopidogrel 75 mg daily may be used in persons unable to tolerate aspirin. Intravenous metoprolol or atenolol (the two β-blockers approved by the Food and Drug Administration for intravenous use in acute MI) should be administered at admission to older persons with acute MI without contraindications to β-blockers. Early intravenous blockade should be followed by oral β-blocker therapy continued indefinitely to reduce the incidence of recurrent MI and mortality.

In the absence of contraindications, older persons with ischemic symptoms of at least 30 minutes' duration occurring within 6 to 12 hours of clinical presentation and with at least 1 to 2 mm of ST-segment elevation in two or more ECG leads or the presence of left bundle branch block should be considered for reperfusion therapy with either thrombolytic therapy or PTCA. Intravenous heparin is recommended in persons with acute MI undergoing PTCA or CABG surgery and in persons with acute MI at high risk for systemic embolization, for example, persons with a large or anterior MI, atrial fibrillation, history of pulmonary or systemic embolus, or known LV thrombus. If intravenous heparin is not given, subcutaneous heparin should be administered to reduce the incidence of deep-vein thrombosis.

Nitrates may be used for the treatment of chest pain and CHF in older persons with acute MI. To reduce mortality, severe CHF, or severe LV systolic dysfunction, use angiotensin-converting enzyme (ACE) inhibitors to treat persons with acute MI who are hemodynamically stable (systolic blood pressure ≥ 100 mm Hg) with CHF, a large anterior MI, or an LV ejection fraction ≥ 40%. Calcium channel blockers are not recommended in the treatment of acute MI. Older persons taking calcium channel blockers before the onset of their acute MI should be switched to β-blockers at the time of their acute MI.

Prophylactic use of antiarrhythmic drugs other than β-blockers does not improve clinical outcome in persons with acute MI. The use of lidocaine during MI should be limited to the treatment of life-threatening ventricular arrhythmias. Supraventricular tachyarrhythmias may be treated with β-blockers or direct-current cardioversion.

Treatment After Myocardial Infarction

Coronary risk factors should be controlled after MI. Aspirin 160 to 325 mg daily should be administered indefinitely. Long-term oral anticoagulant therapy should be used as secondary prevention of MI in persons unable to tolerate daily aspirin, in persons with persistent AF, and in persons with LV thrombus.

Persons without contraindications to β-blockers should receive them indefinitely after MI. β-Blockers with intrinsic sympathomimetic activity should be avoided. High-risk subgroups of persons with a history of MI, for example, all older persons and persons with CHF, asymptomatic abnormal LV ejection fraction, complex ventricular arrhythmias, peripheral arterial disease, or diabetes mellitus, are most likely to benefit from the use of β-blockers.

ACE inhibitors are recommended for use indefinitely in older persons after MI if they have CHF, an anterior MI, or an LV ejection fraction ≥ 40% unless there are specific contraindications to their use. Calcium channel blockers should not be used after MI unless there is persistent angina pectoris despite the use of β-blockers and nitrates. On the basis of data from the Heart Estrogen/progestin Replacement Study, hormonal therapy should not be used in the treatment of postmenopausal women after MI.

β-Blockers are the only antiarrhythmic drugs that reduce mortality after MI. To reduce mortality in older persons with life-threatening ventricular tachycardia or ventricular fibrillation after MI, an automatic implantable cardioverter-defibrillator is indicated. Benefits of revascularization in older persons after MI are prolongation of life and relief of unacceptable symptoms that persist despite optimal medical management.

Risk Stratification After Myocardial Infarction

Clinical factors, including age and coronary risk factors, can be used to classify persons as high or low risk after MI (see Table 38.2). Exercise stress tests using thallium perfusion scintigraphy or radionuclide ventriculography and stress echocardiography using exercise or dobutamine or adenosine are useful for classifying persons as high or low risk after MI.

After MI, older persons with spontaneous episodes of myocardial ischemia or episodes of myocardial ischemia provoked by minimal exertion, before treatment of a mechanical complication of MI (eg, acute mitral valve regurgitation, postinfarction septal deficit, left ventricular free wall rupture, or ventricular aneurysm), or with persistent hemodynamic instability should be referred for coronary angiography and consideration of coronary revascularization.

HEART FAILURE
Epidemiology and Etiology

CHF is the most common cause of hospitalization and rehospitalization in persons aged 65 years and

Table 38.2—Factors Indicating a High Risk of New Coronary Events in Older Persons With a History of Myocardial Infarction

Abnormal LV ejection fraction detected by echocardiography or radionuclide ventriculography

Abnormal signal-averaged ECG

Complex ventricular arrhythmias or silent myocardial ischemia detected by a 24-hour ambulatory ECG

Echocardiographic LV hypertrophy

Exercise-induced hypotension

Exercise-induced ischemic ST-segment depression in both anterior and inferior leads

Exercise-induced marked ischemic ST-segment depression (≥ 2.0 mm)

Inadequate blood-pressure response to exercise

Ischemic ST-segment depression occurring within 6 minutes of exercise

Ischemic ST-segment depression on a resting ECG

Persistence of exercise-induced ST-segment depression past 8 minutes in the recovery period

Poor exercise duration ($<$ 6 minutes using a standard Bruce treadmill protocol)

NOTE: ECG = electrocardiogram (-graphy); LV = left ventricular.

---

older. The prevalence and incidence of CHF increase with age. One study determined that at 43-month follow-up of 922 men and 1971 women (mean age = 81 years), CHF developed in 27%. The study found male gender, hypertension, CAD, diabetes mellitus, and age to be significant independent risk factors for the development of CHF. CAD, hypertension, valvular heart disease, and cardiomyopathies are the commonest causes of CHF in older persons.

Not only do older persons experience an age-related decrease in LV diastolic relaxation and early LV diastolic filling (see Table 38.1), they are more likely to have LV diastolic dysfunction because they have an increased prevalence of hypertension, myocardial ischemia due to CAD, LV hypertrophy due to hypertension, valvular aortic stenosis, hypertrophic cardiomyopathy, and other cardiac disorders. In older persons, the increased stiffness of the LV and prolonged LV relaxation time impair LV early diastolic filling and cause higher LV end-diastolic pressures at rest and during exericse.

In CHF associated with LV systolic dysfunction, the LV ejection fraction is < 50%. The amount of myocardial fiber shortening is reduced, the stroke volume is decreased, the LV is dilated, and the patient is symptomatic.

In CHF associated with LV diastolic dysfunction with normal LV systolic function, the LV ejection fraction is normal ($\geq$ 50%). During exercise, persons with normal LV systolic function but abnormal LV diastolic function are unable to normally increase stroke volume, even in the presence of increased LV filling pressure. Myocardial hypertrophy, ischemia, or fibrosis causes slow or incomplete LV filling at normal left atrial pressures. Left atrial pressure rises to increase LV filling, resulting in pulmonary and systemic venous congestion.

The development of AF (the prevalence of which increases with age) may also cause a decrease in cardiac output and the development of pulmonary and systemic venous congestion, because of the loss of left atrial contribution to LV late diastolic filling and reduced diastolic filling time due to a rapid ventricular rate.

The prevalence of a normal LV ejection fraction associated with CHF increases with age and is higher in older women than in older men. In one study, for example, the prevalence of a normal LV ejection fraction associated with CHF in older persons (mean age = 81 years) was found to be 44% in 55 black American men, 58% in 110 black American women, 46% in 24 Hispanic American men, 56% in 34 Hispanic American women, 35% in 148 white American men, and 57% in 303 white American women. The clinician must measure LV ejection fraction in all persons with CHF, preferably by echocardiography (because of the additional information provided, eg, the presence and severity of valvular heart disease, LV thrombus), in order to determine appropriate therapy for CHF.

In a prospective study of 198 men and 418 women (mean age = 81 years) with CHF associated with prior MI, the 1-year mortality was 20% for men and 19% for women with normal LV ejection fraction and 41% for men and women with abnormal LV ejection fraction. The 5-year mortality was 75% for men and 74% for women with normal LV ejection fraction and 92% for men and women with abnormal LV ejection fraction. Significant independent risk factors for mortality in this study were age, hypertension, diabetes mellitus, and abnormal LV ejection fraction.

Presentation

Increased pulmonary capillary wedge pressure causes pulmonary congestion, resulting in dyspnea. Dyspnea may progress from exertional dyspnea to orthopnea, to paroxysmal nocturnal dyspnea, to dyspnea at rest, and to the development of acute pulmonary edema. Pulmonary congestion may cause coughing and wheezing. Decreased cardiac output may cause weakness, a feeling of heaviness in the limbs, nocturia, oliguria, confusion, insomnia, headache, anxiety, memory impairment, bad dreams or nightmares, and, rarely, psychotic manifestations. Congestive hepatomegaly may cause epigastric or right upper quadrant heaviness or a dull ache, a sense of fullness after eating, anorexia, nausea, and vomiting.

Systemic venous hypertension causes distention of the jugular veins. LV failure with transudation of fluid into the alveoli causes moist rales, which are heard over the lung bases posteriorly. Congestion of bronchial mucosa causes rhonchi and wheezes. During acute pulmonary edema, coarse, bubbling rales and wheezes are heard over the lung fields. Signs of pleural effusion may occur with left or right ventricular failure.

Right ventricular failure may cause an enlarged, tender liver and ascites. Compression causes the hepatojugular reflux sign. Pressure applied to the middle of the abdomen can cause abdominal jugular reflux sign. A pulsating liver indicates tricuspid regurgitation. Right ventricular failure causes edema that first occurs in the dependent parts of the body. Severe right ventricular failure will cause anasarca.

An LV third heart sound (best heard at the apex) and jugular venous distention are the most sensitive and specific physical findings in CHF. Most persons with CHF have cardiomegaly. However, CHF may develop in persons with acute MI or other conditions before the heart has had a chance to enlarge. In a study of 50 patients with chronic CHF, 96% were found to have an LV third heart sound; 50%, jugular venous distention; 20%, peripheral edema; and 19%; pulmonary rales. Heart murmurs due to valvular heart disease may become faint or absent because of a low cardiac output. Physical examination cannot distinguish between CHF associated with abnormal and CHF associated with normal LV ejection fraction.

Chest radiographs should be obtained for all persons with suspected CHF and will show pulmonary vascular congestion in those with LV failure. When the pulmonary capillary pressure exceeds 20 to 25 mm Hg, interstitial pulmonary edema is present. When the pulmonary capillary pressure exceeds 25 mm Hg, alveolar edema and pleural effusion occur.

Management

Underlying causes of CHF should be treated when possible, and precipitating causes should be identified and treated. Sodium intake should be decreased to 1.6 g (4 g of sodium chloride) daily. Hypertension should be treated with diuretics and ACE inhibitors. Myocardial ischemia should be treated with anti-ischemic drugs. Persons with CHF who are dyspneic at rest or at a low work level may benefit from a formal cardiac rehabilitation program. Disease management strategies, either self-or nurse-directed, have been shown to be effective at reducing rehospitalization rates among older persons with CHF. Frequent weighing, careful attention to symptoms, and adjustment of diuretic dosing are components of CHF disease management strategies.

Persons with myocardial ischemia due to severely stenotic coronary arteries without contraindications to coronary revascularization who have exercise-limiting angina, frequent episodes of angina occurring at rest, or recurrent episodes of acute pulmonary edema despite optimal medical management should have coronary angiography with CABG surgery or PTCA. Persons with CHF should have surgical correction of valvular lesions and surgical excision of a dyskinetic LV aneurysm.

Infection, anemia, fever, hypoxia, tachyarrhythmias, bradyarrhythmias, hyperthyroidism, hypothyroidism, and obesity should be treated. Anticoagulants should be given if there is prior systemic or pulmonary embolism, AF, or cardiac thrombi detected by echocardiography. A transvenous pacemaker should be implanted into the right ventricle of persons with CHF who have complete atrioventricular block or severe bradycardia.

Diuretics

Diuretics are the first-line choice of drug in the treatment of CHF associated with abnormal or normal LV ejection fraction (see Table 38.3). Mild CHF may be treated with a thiazide diuretic. However, the thiazide diuretic is ineffective if the glomerular filtration rate is < 30 mL per minute. Older persons with moderate or severe CHF should be treated with a loop diuretic such as furosemide. Persons with severe CHF or concomitant renal insufficiency may need metolazone in addition to the loop diuretic. Severe volume overload should be treated with intravenous diuretics and hospitalization. The minimum effective dose of diuretic should be given. Older persons with

Table 38.3—Drug Treatment of Congestive Heart Failure With Abnormal and Normal Left Ventricular Ejection Fraction

Abnormal left ventricular ejection fraction	Normal left ventricular ejection fraction
Use diuretics plus ACE inhibitors** plus β-blockers	Use diuretics plus β-blockers*
Consider spironolactone if severe CHF present	Use ACE inhibitors if CHF persists**
Use digoxin if CHF persists	Use isosorbide dinitrate plus hydralazine if CHF persists
Use isosorbide dinitrate plus hydralazine if CHF persists	Use a calcium channel blocker if CHF persists despite diuretics and the person is unable to tolerate β-blockers, ACE inhibitors, and isosorbide dinitrate plus hydralazine
Avoid calcium channel blockers	Avoid digoxin if sinus rhythm is present

NOTE: ACE = angiotensin-converting enzyme; CHF = congestive heart failure; MI = myocardial infarction.

* Use diuretics cautiously to avoid intravascular depletion.

**Use an angiotensin II type 1 receptor antagonist if the person cannot tolerate ACE inhibitors because of cough, rash, or altered taste sensation.

CHF associated with abnormal LV ejection fraction tolerate higher doses of diuretics than do older persons with CHF and normal LV ejection fraction. Older persons with CHF and normal LV ejection fraction need high LV filling pressures to maintain an adequate stroke volume and cardiac output, and they cannot tolerate intravascular depletion.

Angiotensin-Converting Enzyme Inhibitors

ACE inhibitors improve symptoms, quality of life, and exercise tolerance, and they decrease mortality and hospitalization for CHF in persons with CHF associated with abnormal LV ejection fraction. A review of 32 randomized trials of ACE inhibitors in persons with CHF and abnormal LV ejection fraction revealed that ACE inhibitors have been found to significantly reduce total mortality by 23% and mortality or hospitalization for CHF by 32%. ACE inhibitors should be administered to all persons with CHF and abnormal LV ejection fraction unless there are specific contraindications to their use (Table 38.3).

ACE inhibitors also improve symptoms, exercise tolerance, and LV systolic and diastolic function in persons with CHF and normal LV ejection fraction. One study reported that persons with CHF and normal LV ejection fraction treated with ACE inhibitors for 6 months had a 54% significant reduction in mortality and a 19% insignificant decrease in mortality or hospital readmission. ACE inhibitors should be given to persons with CHF and normal LV ejection fraction if CHF persists despite diuretic and β-blocker therapy (see Table 38.3).

Asymptomatic hypotension with a systolic blood pressure between 80 and 90 mm Hg and a serum creatinine level that increases but is < 2.5 mg/dL are side effects of ACE inhibitors that should not necessarily cause cessation of this drug, but should cause the physician to decrease the dose of diuretic if the jugular venous pressure is normal and to consider reducing the dose of ACE inhibitor. Contraindications to the use of ACE inhibitors are symptomatic hypotension, progressive azotemia, angioneurotic edema, hyperkalemia, intolerable cough, and rash.

Angiotensin II Type 1 Receptor Antagonists

Studies have found that older patients with CHF and abnormal LV ejection fraction treated with losartan have fewer adverse effects, such as cough, rash, or altered taste sensation, than do patients treated with captopril. In the second Evaluation of Losartan in the Elderly study, patients with CHF and abnormal LV ejection fraction treated with losartan were found to have a similar mortality and hospitalization for CHF as patients treated with captopril. This study found a significant reduction in mortality in persons receiving captopril who were also receiving β-blockers. Older persons with CHF should be treated with an angiotensin II type 1 receptor antagonist if they are unable to tolerate ACE inhibitors because of cough, rash, or altered taste sensation (Table 38.3).

Spironolactone

One study showed that among persons with severe CHF and abnormal LV ejection fraction treated with diuretics, ACE inhibitors, and digoxin, those randomized to spironolactone 25 mg daily had a 30% significant decrease in mortality and a 35% significant reduction in hospitalization for CHF at 2-year follow-up. These preliminary data warrant the use of spironolactone 25 mg daily in persons with severe CHF and abnormal LV ejection fraction that persist despite the use of diuretics and ACE inhibitors (Table 38.3).

β-Blockers

Chronic administration of β-blockers after MI reduces mortality, sudden cardiac death, and recurrent MI, especially in older persons. These benefits are more marked in persons with a history of CHF. One study showed that after 6 to 12 months of therapy, carvedilol caused a 65% significant reduction in mortality in patients with CHF and abnormal LV ejection fraction treated with diuretics, ACE inhibitors, and digoxin. At 1.3-year follow-up in a study of patients with New York Heart Association class III or IV CHF and abnormal LV ejection fraction who were treated with diuretics plus ACE inhibitors and optional digoxin, bisoprolol was shown to cause a 34% significant decrease in mortality. At 1-year follow-up of those with New York Heart Association class II, III, or IV CHF and abnormal LV ejection fraction who were treated with diuretics, ACE inhibitors, and optional digoxin, metoprolol was shown to cause a 34% significant reduction in mortality. Older persons with CHF and abnormal LV ejection fraction should be treated with diuretics, ACE inhibitors, and β-blockers (see Table 38.3).

β-Blockers are beneficial in the treatment of CHF associated with normal LV ejection fraction by:

- reducing the ventricular rate to < 90 beats per minute, thereby increasing LV diastolic filling time and causing an increase in LV end-diastolic volume;
- decreasing myocardial ischemia;
- reducing elevated blood pressure;

- decreasing LV mass; and
- improving LV relaxation.

The increase in ventricular rate that occurs with exercise can also be prevented with modest doses of β-blockers, especially in older persons. In one study, at 32-month follow-up of 158 older persons (mean age = 81 years) with prior MI and New York Heart Association class II or III CHF with an LV ejection fraction ≥ 40% treated with diuretics plus ACE inhibitors, those randomized to treatment with propranolol were found to have a 35% significant reduction in mortality and a 37% significant decrease in mortality plus nonfatal MI.

β-Blockers along with loop diuretics should be used to treat older persons with CHF and normal LV ejection fraction (Table 38.3). The initial dosage of β-blockers should be small (eg, carvedilol 3.125 mg twice daily or metoprolol CR 12.5 daily). This should be gradually increased at 3-week intervals, with the maintenance dosage (eg, carvedilol 25 mg twice daily or metoprolol 200 mg daily) reached over 3 months.

Digoxin

Digoxin should be used in the treatment of older persons with CHF and supraventricular tachyarrhythmias such as AF. At 37-month follow-up in the Digitalis Investigator Group trial, patients (mean age = 63 years) with CHF treated with diuretics plus ACE inhibitors were found to have a similar mortality rate if they were treated with digoxin or placebo. Patients with an LV ejection fraction ≤ 45% treated with digoxin were significantly less likely to be hospitalized for worsening CHF or for any cause. Digoxin was more beneficial in patients with an LV ejection fraction < 25%, nonischemic CHF, a cardiothoracic ratio > 0.55, or New York Heart Association class III or IV CHF. The effects of digoxin were consistent across all age groups, except that toxicity was increased at older ages. On the basis of the available data, digoxin should be given to older persons with CHF in sinus rhythm with abnormal LV ejection fraction who have persistent CHF despite diuretics, ACE inhibitors, and β-blockers (Table 38.3).

Digoxin should not be used for treating persons with CHF in sinus rhythm associated with a normal LV ejection fraction (Table 38.3). By increasing contractility through an increased intracellular calcium concentration, digoxin may increase LV stiffness in these persons, increasing LV filling pressure and aggravating CHF with normal LV ejection fraction.

Isosorbide Dinitrate Plus Hydralazine

The combination of oral isosorbide dinitrate and hydralazine may be beneficial in the treatment of CHF and abnormal or normal LV ejection fraction (Table 38.3). Isosorbide dinitrate plus hydralazine should be added

- if CHF with abnormal ejection fraction persists despite treatment with diuretics, ACE inhibitors, β-blockers, and digoxin, or
- if CHF with normal LV ejection fraction persists despite treatment with diuretics, β-blockers, and ACE inhibitors.

Calcium Channel Blockers

Calcium channel blockers such as nifedipine, diltiazem, and verapamil exacerbate CHF in patients with CHF and abnormal LV ejection fraction. Studies show that diltiazem significantly increases mortality in patients with pulmonary congestion and abnormal LV ejection fraction after MI and that the vasoselective calcium channel blockers amlodipine and felodipine do not significantly affect survival in patients with CHF and abnormal LV ejection fraction. In these studies, a significantly higher incidence of pulmonary edema and peripheral edema was observed in patients treated with amlodipine than in those treated with placebo, and a significantly higher incidence of peripheral edema was observed in patients treated with felodipine than in those treated with placebo. Therefore, calcium channel blockers should not be administered to older persons with CHF and abnormal LV ejection fraction. However, calcium channel blockers may be given to persons with CHF and normal LV ejection fraction if they have persistent CHF despite the use of diuretics and are unable to tolerate β-blockers, ACE inhibitors, and isosorbide dinitrate plus hydralazine (Table 38.3).

Self-Management

The number-one cause of recidivism in heart failure patients is volume and sodium retention. Patients need to be taught and encouraged to eat better. They need to weigh themselves daily and call the primary care clinician immediately if they gain more than 2 pounds in 1 day. Over-the-counter drugs to avoid that can exacerbate sodium and fluid retention include sodium-based antacids, high-dose aspirin, nonsteroidal anti-inflammatory drugs, ginseng (germanium), ginkgo, echinacea, and decongestants. Black licorice has the same effect and should also be avoided.

VALVULAR HEART DISEASE

Valvular Aortic Stenosis

Valvular aortic stenosis (AS) in older persons is usually due to stiffening, scarring, and calcification of the valve leaflets. Aortic cuspal calcium was found in one study to be present in 39% of 752 older men (mean age = 80 years) and in 40% of 1663 older women (mean age = 82 years). The prevalence of AS is similar in older men and women. In 1797 older persons (mean age = 81 years) the prevalence of severe AS (peak gradient across the aortic valve $\geq$ 50 mm Hg) was 2%, of moderate AS (peak gradient across the aortic valve 26 to 49 mm Hg) was 5%, and of mild AS (peak gradient across the aortic valve 10 to 25 mm Hg) was 9%.

Angina pectoris, syncope or near syncope, and CHF are the three classic manifestations of severe AS. Researchers found CHF, syncope, or angina to be present in 90% of 40 older persons with severe AS, in 69% of 96 older persons with moderate AS, and in 27% of 165 older persons with mild AS. Prolonged duration and late peaking of the aortic systolic ejection murmur occurred in 84% of older persons with severe AS, in 63% of older persons with moderate AS, and in 3% of older persons with mild AS. The same study found that a prolonged carotid upstroke time occurred in 53% of older persons with severe AS, in 33% of older persons with moderate AS, and in 3% of older persons with mild AS. Absent or decreased aortic second sound occurred in 74% of older persons with severe AS, in 49% of older persons with moderate AS, and in 5% of older persons with mild AS. Doppler echocardiography is used to diagnose the prevalence and severity of AS.

Older persons with AS have an increased incidence of new coronary events; those with symptomatic severe AS have a poor prognosis. However, those with asymptomatic severe AS are at low risk for death and can be followed until symptoms develop.

Antibiotics should be used to prevent bacterial endocarditis, according to American Heart Association guidelines (available at http://www.americanheart.org). Older persons with CHF, exertional syncope, or angina associated with moderate or severe AS should undergo aortic valve replacement promptly. Persons with asymptomatic AS should report the development of symptoms possibly related to AS immediately to their physician. Nitrates should be used with caution in persons with AS and angina to prevent orthostatic hypotension and syncope. Vasodilators should be avoided. Diuretics should be used with caution in persons with AS and CHF to prevent a decrease in cardiac output and hypotension.

If LV systolic dysfunction in persons with severe AS is associated with critical narrowing of the aortic valve rather than with myocardial fibrosis, it often improves after successful aortic valve replacement. Balloon aortic valvuloplasty should be considered for older persons with symptomatic severe AS who are not candidates for aortic valve surgery and possibly for persons with severe LV dysfunction, as a bridge to subsequent aortic valve surgery.

Aortic Regurgitation

Acute aortic regurgitation (AR) in older persons may be due to infective endocarditis, rheumatic fever, aortic dissection, trauma following prosthetic valve surgery, or rupture of the sinus of Valsalva. It causes sudden severe CHF. Chronic AR in older persons may be caused by aortic valve leaflet disease (secondary to any cause of AS, infective endocarditis, rheumatic fever, congenital heart disease, rheumatoid arthritis, ankylosing spondylitis, following prosthetic valve surgery, or myxomatous degeneration of the valve) or by aortic root disease.

The prevalence of AR increases with age; in one study it was found to be 31% among 554 older men and 28% among 1243 older women. Severe or moderate AR was present in 16% of these 1797 older persons. The AR murmur is typically a high-pitched blowing diastolic murmur that begins immediately after the aortic second sound. The diastolic murmur is best heard along the left sternal border in the third and fourth intercostal spaces when AR is due to valvular disease and is best heard along the right sternal border when AR is due to dilatation of the ascending aorta. The severity of AR correlates with the duration of the diastolic murmur, not with the intensity of the murmur. Doppler echocardiography is used to diagnose the presence and severity of AR.

Persons with acute AR develop symptoms as a consequence of the sudden onset of CHF. Persons with acute AR should have immediate aortic valve replacement because death may occur within hours to days. Persons with chronic AR may be asymptomatic for many years. The prognosis of older persons with CHF and unoperated severe AR is poor.

Prophylactic antibiotics should be used to prevent bacterial endocarditis in older persons with chronic AR, according to American Heart Association guidelines (available at http://www.americanheart.org). Older persons with asymptomatic chronic severe AR should be treated with ACE inhibitors to reduce the LV volume overload. Echocardiographic evaluation of LV end-systolic dimension should be performed yearly if the measurement is < 50 mm, but every 3 to 6 months if the measurement is 50 to 54 mm. Aortic valve replacement should be considered if the LV end-systolic dimension exceeds 55 mm, even in the absence of cardiac symptoms. Aortic valve replacement should also be considered when the LV ejection fraction approaches 50% before the decompensated state.

Mitral Regurgitation

One study found mitral regurgitation (MR) to be present in 32% of 554 older men and in 33% of 1243 older women. The most common cause of MR in older persons is mitral annular calcium. Other disorders causing MR in older persons include CAD, mitral valve prolapse, and rheumatic heart disease. Symptoms associated with severe MR are primarily those of CHF, especially dyspnea. The heart murmur associated with MR is heard as an apical holosystolic murmur, late systolic murmur, or early systolic murmur beginning with the first heart sound but ending in mid-systole. The presence of an LV third heart sound suggests that the MR is severe. Doppler echocardiography is used to diagnose the presence and monitor the severity of MR.

In MR, the LV ejection fraction should be > 55% to 60% and the LV end-systolic dimension < 45 mm. Mitral valve surgery should be considered in older persons with New York Heart Association class III or IV symptoms caused by MR or in older persons with severe MR and an LV ejection fraction < 50% or an LV end-systolic dimension above 45 to 50 mm.

Mitral Stenosis

The most common cause of mitral stenosis (MS) in older persons is mitral annular calcium. One study found the prevalence of MS among 1028 older persons with mitral annular calcium to be 8%. Rheumatic MS was found in one study to be present in 0.4% of 554 older men and in 2% of 1243 older women. In another study the prevalence of rheumatic MS among 1699 older persons was 6% in older persons with AF and 0.4% in older persons with sinus rhythm. Older persons with MS have a low-pitched mid-diastolic murmur heard at the point of maximum apical impulse with or without presystolic accentuation. Doppler echocardiography is used to diagnose the presence and severity of MS.

All older persons with MS, especially those with AF, should be treated with long-term oral warfarin therapy to reduce thromboembolic events. Mitral valvular surgery or valvuloplasty should be performed if the person has recurrent embolization on anticoagulants. A β-blocker will slow the ventricular rate if AF is present. Diuretics will control congestive symptoms.

In the absence of clot, MR, and severe subvalvular involvement, the therapy of choice for symptomatic MS is balloon valvuloplasty. However, many older persons with symptomatic MS have poor valve morphology for valvuloplasty (heavy calcification) and require mitral valve replacement. Older persons with MS and a critical valve area of 1.0 cm^2 need interventional therapy. Mitral valve replacement is usually necessary since most stenotic mitral valves in older persons are commonly calcified and severely deformed, with associated significant MR, and successful open mitral commissurotomy is not possible.

ARRHYTHMIAS

Ventricular Arrhythmias

The presence of three or more consecutive ventricular premature complexes on an ECG is diagnosed as ventricular tachycardia (VT). VT is considered sustained if it lasts ≥ 30 seconds and nonsustained if its lasts < 30 seconds. Complex ventricular arrhythmias (VAs) include VT or paired, multiform, or frequent (≥ 30 per hour on a 24-hour ambulatory ECG or ≥ 6 per minute on a 1-minute rhythm strip of an ECG) ventricular premature complexes. Researchers using a 24-hour ambulatory ECG to detect VAs in older persons found a prevalence of 10% for nonsustained VT (N = 554) and a rate of 55% for complex VAs (N = 843).

Nonsustained VT and complex VA are not associated with an increased incidence of new coronary events in older persons with no clinical evidence of heart disease, and asymptomatic persons should not be treated with antiarrhythmic drugs. Simple VA (ie, VAs that are not paired, multiform, or frequent) in older persons with heart disease should also not be treated with antiarrhythmic drugs. Nonsustained VT and complex VA are associated with an increased incidence of new coronary events in older persons with heart disease, especially in those with abnormal LV ejection fraction, LV hypertrophy, or silent myocardial ischemia.

Available data show that older persons with nonsustained VT or complex VA and heart disease should not be treated with any of the Class I antiarrhythmic drugs (ie, encainide, flecainide, lorcainide, moricizine, propafenone, quinidine, procainamide, disopyramide, mexiletine, phenytoin, and tocainide), calcium channel blockers, d-sotalol, or d,l-sotalol and should be treated with β-blockers if there are no contraindications to β-blockers. Amiodarone was found to not reduce mortality in persons with VT or complex VA associated with prior MI or CHF, and it had a high incidence of toxicity.

In a study of 245 persons (mean age = 81 years) with heart disease (64% with prior MI and 36% with hypertensive heart disease) and complex VA (32% with nonsustained VT and 33% with silent ischemia), those randomized to propranolol had at 29-month follow-up a 47% significant reduction in sudden cardiac death, a 37% significant decrease in total cardiac death, and a 20% borderline significant reduction ($P = 0.057$) in total mortality. Analysis of data from the Cardiac Arrhythmia Suppression Trial showed that β-blockers were an independent factor for decreasing arrhythmic death or cardiac arrest by 40%, for reducing all-cause mortality by 33%, and for decreasing occurrence of new or worsened CHF by 32%. However, the automatic implantable cardioverter-defibrillator is the most effective treatment for reducing mortality in older persons with life-threatening VT or ventricular fibrillation.

Atrial Fibrillation

The prevalence of AF increases with age. In a study of 2101 persons (mean age = 81 years), the prevalence of AF was found to be 16% in older men and 13% in older women. AF may be paroxysmal (lasting a few seconds to several weeks) or chronic. Older persons with AF may be symptomatic or asymptomatic, their arrhythmia detected by physical examination or by an ECG. In older men and women AF is associated with the increased incidence of mortality, death from cardiovascular causes, thromboembolic stroke, and CHF. In a study of 2101 older persons (mean age = 81 years) the 3-year incidence of thromboembolic stroke was found to be 38% in persons with AF and 11% in persons with sinus rhythm; the 5-year incidence of thromboembolic stroke was 72% in persons with AF and 24% in persons with sinus rhythm.

Management of AF includes treatment of the underlying disease (such as pneumonia, hyperthyroidism, or pulmonary embolus) when possible and treatment of precipitating factors. Immediate direct-current cardioversion should be performed in persons with paroxysmal AF with a very rapid ventricular rate associated with acute MI, chest pain caused by myocardial ischemia, hypotension, severe CHF, or syncope. Intravenous β-blockers, verapamil, or diltiazem may be used to slow immediately a very rapid ventricular rate associated with AF.

Digoxin is ineffective in slowing a rapid ventricular rate in AF if there is fever, hypoxia, hyperthyroidism, acute blood loss, or any condition with increased sympathetic tone, and digoxin is contraindicated in the Wolff-Parkinson-White syndrome or hypertrophic cardiomyopathy. It should be avoided in persons with sinus rhythm and a history of paroxysmal AF. An oral β-blocker, verapamil, or diltiazem should be added to digoxin if a rapid ventricular rate in AF occurs at rest or during exercise despite digoxin. Amiodarone may be used in persons with symptomatic life-threatening AF refractory to other drug therapy. Radiofrequency catheter modification of atrioventricular conduction or complete atrioventricular block produced by radiofrequency catheter ablation followed by permanent pacemaker implantation should be performed in persons with symptomatic AF in whom a rapid ventricular rate cannot be slowed by drug therapy.

Paroxysmal AF associated with the tachycardia-bradycardia syndrome should be treated with a permanent pacemaker, in combination with drugs used to slow a rapid ventricular rate in AF. A permanent pacemaker should also be implanted in persons with AF who develop cerebral symptoms such as dizziness or syncope associated with ventricular pauses > 3 seconds that are not drug-induced, as documented by a 24-hour ambulatory ECG.

At 1.1-year follow-up in the Stroke Prevention in Atrial Fibrillation III study, persons with AF at high risk for thromboembolic stroke randomized to adjusted-dose warfarin to achieve an international normalized ratio (INR) between 2.0 and 3.0 had a 1.9% incidence of ischemic stroke or systemic embolism. Persons randomized to aspirin 325 mg daily plus low-dose warfarin to achieve an INR between 1.2 and 1.5 had a 7.9% incidence of ischemic stroke or systemic embolism (76% relative reduction and 6% absolute reduction in risk by adjusted-dose warfarin).

Because maintenance of sinus rhythm with antiarrhythmic drugs may require serial cardioversions, exposes persons to the risks of proarrhythmia, sudden cardiac death, and other adverse effects, and requires the use of anticoagulants in persons with sinus rhythm who have a high risk of recurrence of AF, many cardiologists prefer the treatment strategy of ventricular rate control (preferably by β-blockers) plus anticoagulant therapy in older persons with AF. Older persons with chronic or paroxysmal AF at high risk for thromboembolic stroke or who have a history of hypertension and who have no contraindications to anticoagulants should receive long-term oral warfarin to achieve an INR between 2.0 and 3.0. Older persons with AF at low risk for thromboembolic stroke or who have contraindications to warfarin should receive 325 mg of oral aspirin daily.

PERIPHERAL ARTERIAL DISEASE

Aneurysms and Dissections

Aneurysms and dissections are primarily diseases of older persons. Aneurysms most commonly occur in the abdominal aorta, thoracic aorta, popliteal arteries, and iliac arteries, and they are usually atherosclerotic. Symptomatic aneurysms are medical emergencies that require immediate surgery. Asymptomatic aneurysms should be followed for rate of growth. Older persons with an abdominal aortic aneurysm > 5 cm should be considered for surgical repair. Elective surgical repair of a descending thoracic aortic aneurysm or a thoracoabdominal aortic aneurysm in older persons should be considered if the aneurysm is ≥ 5 cm in maximal diameter. All older persons considered for elective surgical repair should be evaluated for coexistent CAD.

The pain associated with thoracic aortic dissection is severe and often tearing. Stroke, paraplegia, syncope, pulse loss with or without ischemic pain, and CHF resulting from severe AR secondary to the dissection may occur. Diagnosis is best made by transesophageal echocardiography, magnetic resonance imaging, or computed tomography. Surgical intervention is the treatment of choice for acute proximal dissection and for complicated acute distal dissection (ie, complicated by rupture, expansion, saccular aneurysm formation, vital organ or limb ischemia, or continued pain). Endostenting, a new procedure for treating aneurysm, is under investigation. Medical treatment with afterload reduction and β-blockers is the treatment of choice for uncomplicated distal dissection, for stable, isolated arch dissection, and for uncomplicated dissection presenting 2 weeks or later after onset.

Occlusive Peripheral Vascular Disease

One study found the prevalence of symptomatic occlusive peripheral vascular disease (PVD) to be 20% in 467 men (mean age = 80 years) and 13% in 1444 women (mean age = 81 years). Significant independent risk factors for symptomatic PVD in older men and women in this study were age, cigarette smoking, hypertension, diabetes mellitus, serum LDL cholesterol, and serum HDL cholesterol (inverse association). Persons with diabetes mellitus commonly have more distal and diffuse atherosclerosis.

Atherosclerotic vascular disease affecting the lower extremities may cause asymptomatic arterial insufficiency or symptomatic disease presenting as intermittent claudication or pain at rest, ulceration, and gangrene. Since the superficial femoral and popliteal vessels are most commonly affected by the atherosclerotic process, the pain of intermittent claudication is most often localized to the calf. Atherosclerotic narrowing of the distal aorta and its bifurcation to the two iliac arteries may cause pain in the buttocks or thighs, as well as the legs. Persons with rest pain are at increased risk for developing ulcers and infection.

The diagnosis of PVD is usually made by a thorough history and physical examination. Persons with asymptomatic arterial insufficiency are identified by a low ankle-brachial index (ABI), which is determined by dividing the systolic blood pressure measured at the ankle by that obtained in the brachial artery. Lower-extremity arterial disease is defined as an ABI < 0.95 and usually ≤ 0.9. An ABI < 0.4 is indicative of severe disease that would require intervention to promote wound healing. Doppler flow velocity measurements may be useful in grading severity of vascular obstructions, predicting healing of ischemic ulcers, and studying diabetic patients with noncompressible arteries. Ultrasonic duplex scanning with color provides detailed information about the arterial system and should be performed when the person is scheduled for balloon angioplasty or direct arterial surgery; it is also useful in follow-up studies of these persons.

Medical therapy of PVD includes cessation of cigarette smoking and treatment of other risk factors. In the Scandinavian Simvastatin Survival Study, simvastatin, in comparison with placebo, was found to reduce the risk of new or worsening intermittent claudication by 38%. Exercise therapy is the most effective medical treatment for intermittent claudication. Aspirin therapy will delay the progression of PVD and will reduce the incidence of stroke, MI, or vascular death. The Clopidogrel versus Aspirin in Patients at Risk for Ischaemic Events trial compared aspirin 325 mg daily with clopidogrel 75 mg daily; clopidogrel was found to significantly reduce the annual incidence rate of stroke, MI, or vascular death by 24% in patients with significant PVD. Clopidogrel 75 mg daily should be considered in the treatment of persons with symptomatic PVD who have failed aspirin therapy. Vasodilators should be avoided. The use of pentoxifylline has generally been disappointing. However, this drug may be tried in persons with markedly reduced walking distances who cannot participate in exercise therapy.

Indications for percutaneous transluminal angioplasty with intravascular stenting or lower-extremity bypass surgery include:

- incapacitating claudication interfering with work or quality of life;
- limb salvage in persons with life-threatening ischemia, as indicated by one or more of the following: pain at rest, nonhealing ulcer, infection or gangrene;
- vasculogenic impotence.

Amputation is recommended for chronic institutionalized, neurologically impaired persons who are permanently nonambulatory.

VENOUS DISORDERS

Deep Venous Insufficiency

Chronic deep venous insufficiency usually results from prior deep-vein thrombosis (DVT). Symptoms of chronic deep venous insufficiency include edema of the lower extremities, with resolution following nighttime recumbency. Chronic edema with pigmentation of the leg and stasis ulcers may develop. Venous ulcers occur in the lower aspect of the tibial region, typically above the medial malleolus. Venous ulcers are best treated with pressure stocking and limb elevation.

Persons with chronic deep venous insufficiency are at increased risk for developing DVT, a potentially life-threatening disorder. The gold standard diagnostic test for DVT of the lower extremity is ascending phlebography. Other diagnostic tests include impedance plethysmography and venous doppler duplex ultrasonography. Low-molecular-weight heparin is considered the drug of choice for DVT prophylaxis for many surgical procedures because laboratory monitoring is not required.

Superficial Venous Insufficiency

Superficial venous insufficiency with development of varicose veins may be caused by primary valvular degeneration of veins or by chronic deep venous insufficiency. The most common symptom is aching leg pain, most often exacerbated by standing. Ulcers rarely occur unless deep venous insufficiency is present. Stasis dermatitis may also occur. Superficial phlebitis develops in severe cases as a result of localized clotting of the vessels. Treatment consists of limb elevation, elastic supportive stockings, and exercise to increase muscle tone. Anticoagulation is not indicated in the absence of deep venous disease.

REFERENCES

■ Antman EM, Cohen M, Radley D, et al. Assessment of the treatment effect of enoxaparin for unstable angina/non-Q-wave myocardial infarction: TIMI 11B-ESSENCE meta-analysis. *Circulation*. 1999;100(15):1602–1608.

■ Aronow WS, Ahn C, Kronzon I. Comparison of incidences of congestive heart failure in older African-Americans, Hispanics, and whites. *Am J Cardiol*. 1999;84(5):611–612.

■ Aronow WS, Ahn C, Kronzon I. Prognosis of congestive heart failure after prior myocardial infarction in older men and women with abnormal versus normal left ventricular ejection fraction. *Am J Cardiol*. 2000;85(11):1382–1384.

■ Berger AK, Schulman KA, Gersh BJ, et al. Primary coronary angioplasty vs thrombolysis for the management of acute myocardial infarction in elderly patients. *JAMA*. 1999;282(4):341–348.

■ Hamm CW, Heeschen C, Goldmann B, et al. Benefit of abciximab in patients with refractory unstable angina in relation to serum troponin T levels. *N Engl J Med*. 1999;340(21):1623–1629.

■ Lewis SJ, Moye LA, Sacks FM, et al. Effect of pravastatin on cardiovascular events in older patients with myocardial infarction and cholesterol levels in the average range: results of the Cholesterol and Recurrent Events (CARE) Trial. *Ann Intern Med*. 1998;129(9):681–689.

■ MERIT-HF Study Group. Effect of metoprolol CR/XL in chronic heart failure: Metoprolol CR/XL Randomised Intervention Trial in Congestive Heart Failure. *Lancet*. 1999;353(9169):2001–2007.

■ Ness J, Aronow WS, Ahn C. Risk factors for symptomatic peripheral arterial disease in older persons in an academic hospital-based geriatrics practice. *J Am Geriatr Soc*. 2000;48(3):312–314.

■ Packer M, Poole-Wilson PA, Armstrong PW, et al. Comparative effects of low and high doses of the angiotensin-converting enzyme inhibitor, lisinopril, on morbidity and mortality in chronic heart failure. *Circulation*. 1999;100(23):2312–2318.

■ Pitt B, Zannad F, Remme WJ, et al. The effect of spironolactone on morbidity and mortality in patients with severe heart failure. *N Engl J Med*. 1999;341(10):709–717.

CHAPTER 39—HYPERTENSION

EPIDEMIOLOGY AND PHYSIOLOGY

Blood pressure, particularly systolic pressure, increases with increasing age. The risk associated with hypertension does not decline with age, and the criteria that define hypertension, outlined in the Sixth Report of the Joint National Committee on Prevention, Detection, Evaluation, and Treatment of High Blood Pressure (JNC-VI; see Table 39.1), are not age adjusted. Epidemiologic studies, including the National Health and Nutrition Examination surveys, suggest that the prevalence of hypertension in persons aged 65 years and older is between 50% and 70%; the prevalence is highest among older black Americans. In contrast to younger hypertensive populations, among whom males predominate, older hypertensive populations show no apparent difference in the prevalence rates of men and women. Over the past 50 years the use of antihypertensive medications has increased, and the prevalence rates of elevated blood pressure, left ventricular hypertrophy, and cardiovascular and stroke mortality have all declined. However, these trends have been delayed among the older population, and blood pressure remains poorly controlled in many older patients despite treatment for hypertension.

Many of the physiologic changes that occur with aging contribute to the increase in blood pressure, but life-style factors such as obesity and physical inactivity and the presence of comorbid diseases are also important contributors. Several physiologic changes combine to increase peripheral vascular resistance, the physiologic hallmark of hypertension in older persons. Several mechanisms contribute to the age-associated increase in arterial vascular stiffness. Arterial stiffness, or reduced vascular compliance, provides the best explanation for the relatively greater increase in systolic pressure and the increase in pulse pressure (the difference between systolic and diastolic pressure) observed with aging. Decreased sensitivity of the baroreflex is also related to decreased arterial distensibility, increasing blood-pressure variability and sympathetic nervous system activity. The dynamic regulation of vascular tone is affected by impairments in vasodilator systems (eg, vascular endothelial cell production of nitric oxide and β-adrenergic receptor mediated vasodilatation) and heightened α-adrenergic receptor mediated vasoconstriction. Alterations in renal function as well as in neurohumoral systems that are involved in sodium balance combine to increase the proportion of older hypertensive persons whose blood pressure increases with increased sodium intake. Approximately two thirds of older hypertensive persons have sodium-sensitive hypertension.

The regulation of blood-pressure homeostasis may be impaired in older hypertensive persons, making older people with elevated systolic blood pressure more likely to develop both orthostatic and postprandial hypotension. Maintaining normal blood pressure and cerebrovascular and coronary perfusion in the face of hypotensive stimuli related to postural challenge, meals, or medications requires the integrated coordination of multiple compensatory mechanisms. The age-associated decline in baroreflex sensitivity and alterations in sympathetic nervous system function impair the dynamic regulation of blood pressure. Because of the blunted sensitivity of the baroreflex, a greater reduction in blood pressure occurs before the increase in heart rate and other compensatory mechanisms are activated. Other pathophysiologic changes that impair blood-pressure regulation include arterial and cardiac stiffness and a decrease in early diastolic filling.

CLINICAL EVALUATION

Accurate measurement of blood pressure is the most critical aspect of diagnosis of hypertension in the older patient. Because variability in blood pressure increases with age, the diagnosis of hypertension should be made by using the average of several blood-pressure readings taken on each of three visits. Ambulatory blood-pressure monitoring may be necessary for patients with extreme blood-pressure variability or possible "white-coat" hypertension. Clinicians should be aware of an auscultatory gap, which can lead to underestimation of the true systolic blood pressure and can indicate arterial stiffness. Determining the systolic blood pressure by palpation avoids this problem.

Once a diagnosis of hypertension has been made, the remainder of the clinical evaluation centers on excluding secondary forms of hypertension (using an approach similar to that used in younger patient

Table 39.1—Classification of Blood Pressure

Category	Systolic (mm Hg)		Diastolic (mm Hg)
Normal	< 130	and	< 85
High normal	130–139	and	85–89
Hypertension			
Stage 1	140–159	or	90–99
Stage 2	160–179	or	100–109
Stage 3	≥180	or	≥110–119

NOTE: Diagnoses should be based on the average of two or more readings taken at each of two or more visits after an initial screening.

SOURCE: Adapted from The sixth report of the Joint National Committee on Prevention, Detection, Evaluation, and Treatment of High Blood Pressure. *Arch Intern Med.* 1997; 157(21):2417.

populations), identifying target organ damage, and determining cardiovascular risk factors and the presence of comorbid conditions. Although most older patients have essential hypertension, secondary forms of hypertension should be suspected in the presence of malignant hypertension, a sudden increase in diastolic blood pressure, worsening level of control, or poorly controlled blood pressure on a regimen of three antihypertensive medications. Among the causes of secondary hypertension, renovascular disease is the most common among older hypertensive patients. Treatment decisions should take into account cardiovascular disease, target organ damage (eg, left ventricular hypertrophy), and diabetes mellitus. Finally, the patient's smoking history, dietary intake of sodium and fat, alcohol intake, and the level of usual physical activity should be determined to permit advice about life-style modifications to help control blood pressure as well as reduce overall cardiovascular disease risk factors.

TREATMENT

The overwhelming consensus derived from the results of several randomized, placebo-controlled clinical trials is that treatment of hypertension in older persons is safe and effective. Several randomized clinical trials of antihypertensive therapy in older patients have provided compelling evidence that treatment is effective in reducing cardiovascular (eg, chronic congestive heart failure) and cerebrovascular (eg, stroke) morbidity and mortality. A meta-analysis of outcome trials in systolic hypertension demonstrated that treatment was associated with significant reductions in overall mortality, cardiovascular events, and stroke. The treatment effect was largest in men, in those aged 70 years and over, and in those who had greater pulse pressures. Of note, few participants in randomized, controlled trials of hypertension treatment were over 80 years old and almost none were over 85 years. As the treatment effect is delayed about 5 years, consideration needs to be given to initiating or continuing antihypertensive medication in very old adults.

As with other chronic conditions in older patients, it is important to balance the recognized beneficial effects of antihypertensive therapy with the potential impact on the patient's functional status and quality of life (eg, the development of orthostatic hypotension). A treatment approach using modalities least likely to produce adverse effects and targeting a reduction in systolic blood pressure to 135 to 140 mm Hg and diastolic blood pressure to 85 to 90 mm Hg should be developed. For persons with markedly elevated systolic blood pressure, an intermediate target, such as 160 mm Hg, may be an appropriate initial goal in the absence of target organ damage. The major focus of

treatment should be on the systolic blood pressure and pulse pressure, since among older hypertensive persons, they are stronger predictors of adverse outcomes than is the diastolic blood pressure. The systolic blood pressure alone correctly classifies the JNC-VI blood-pressure stage of more than 99% of older hypertensive patients. In addition, analysis of data from the Systolic Hypertension in the Elderly Program study demonstrates a significant relationship between pulse pressure and the risk for stroke and overall mortality that was independent of the level of mean arterial pressure.

Life-Style Modification

Nonpharmacologic therapy may be effective for older persons with stage 1 hypertension (140 to 159 mm Hg systolic and 90 to 99 mm Hg diastolic blood pressure) and is an important adjunct to drug treatment because of synergistic effects with antihypertensive drugs and the benefits realized through the reduction in other cardiovascular risk factors (see Table 39.2). Life-style modifications that target the typical characteristics of the older hypertensive person—overweight, sedentary, and salt-sensitive—are likely to be effective. A randomized trial of nonpharmacologic interventions in older patients (the TONE study) that evaluated the effects of dietary sodium restriction and weight loss demonstrated that relatively modest reductions in dietary sodium intake (40 mmol per day) and in body weight (4 kg) were accompanied by a 30% decrease in the need to reinitiate pharmacologic treatment. A meta-analysis of randomized trials assessing the effects of dietary sodium restriction demonstrated a significant reduction in systolic (a mean decrease of 3.7 mm Hg for each decrease of 100 mmol per day in sodium intake) but not in diastolic blood pressure. This differential reduction in systolic pressure is particularly well suited for the older hypertensive patient. Persons with stage 1 hypertension (systolic blood pressure less than 160 mm Hg) who do not have diabetes mellitus should complete a 6-month trial of nonpharmacologic

---

Table 39.2—Nonpharmacologic Therapy for Stage 1 Hypertension

- Weight reduction

- Aerobic and strength-training exercise programs

- Smoking cessation

- Moderation of alcohol intake

- Dietary changes to decrease sodium, saturated fat, and cholesterol while maintaining adequate intake of potassium, magnesium, and calcium

therapy before adding an antihypertensive medication if the target blood pressure is not achieved.

Pharmacologic Treatment

The general approach to pharmacologic management of the older hypertensive patient is presented in the JNC-VI. Several points regarding drug selection are reviewed here and summarized in Table 39.3. Drug selection may be affected by whether the patient has simple hypertension or has hypertension complicated by one of several comorbid conditions (eg, diabetes mellitus, coronary artery disease or history of myocardial infarction, heart failure, prostatism) that may influence the choice for a person's drug treatment. For those with simple, uncomplicated hypertension, the initial antihypertensive drug choice given the available evidence to date is a thiazide diuretic. Beyond this general recommendation for initial therapy, there is no universally accepted approach to choosing alternative agents or combination therapies; these decisions should be made on an individualized basis that considers the advantages and disadvantages of the drug together with the patient's comorbidities. Finally, centrally acting agents (eg, clonidine, methyldopa) and those more likely to produce orthostatic hypotension should be avoided in most older patients.

Diuretics

Therapy with low-dose thiazide diuretics (eg, hydrochlorothiazide ≤ 25 mg daily, or the equivalent) has demonstrated significant benefits in mortality, stroke, and coronary events in randomized clinical trials in older hypertensive patients. These beneficial effects, combined with their relative safety, favorable adverse effect profile (their adverse metabolic effects—hypokalemia, hyperuricemia, and glucose intolerance—

Table 39.3—General Treatment Recommendations for Stage 1, Simple Hypertension

■ Begin with a nonpharmacologic approach (see Table 39.2).

■ Use a low-dose diuretic as the first choice for initial pharmacologic therapy.

■ Base alternative drug selection or combination therapies on individual patient characteristics.

■ When initiating drug therapy, begin at half of the usual dose, increase dose slowly, and continue nonpharmacologic therapies.

■ Focus treatment goal on systolic blood pressure reduction to 135 to 140 mm Hg.

■ Avoid excessive reduction in diastolic blood pressure (below 70 mm Hg).

■ Do not use aggressive therapy where adverse effects (eg, postural hypotension) cannot be avoided.

are attenuated at lower doses), once-daily dosing, and low cost have led to the recommendation that diuretics are preferred for initial therapy. Another advantage is that diuretic therapy leads to a disproportionate reduction in systolic relative to diastolic blood pressure, and it is better than other agents at achieving a reduction in systolic blood pressure. Thiazide diuretics are also well suited for use in combination therapies because of synergistic effects with other antihypertensive drug classes. It is worth noting that, despite these recommendations, only 23% of those who were on monotherapy at the time of their entry into the TONE study were treated with diuretics.

Calcium Channel Antagonists

Therapy with calcium channel antagonists (CCAs), in particular, long-acting agents in the dihydropyridine (nifedipine-like) class, has been shown in the Systolic Hypertension in Europe and China Trials to lead to significant reduction in stroke risk in older hypertensive patients. A Japanese Intervention Cooperative Study followed older hypertensive patients randomized to the dihydropyridine CCA nicardipine or a thiazide diuretic and reported no difference in the risk of cardiovascular events between groups. The pathophysiologic (reduction in peripheral vascular resistance) and adverse effect (absence of central or metabolic effects) profiles of the CCA class are other factors that support their use as an initial antihypertensive agent. Because of age-related changes in their pharmacokinetics, lower doses of CCAs should be used. Short-acting CCAs should not be used to treat hypertension.

β-Receptor Antagonists

β-Receptor antagonists are recommended in the JNC-VI report as another option for initial drug therapy for uncomplicated hypertension. However, analysis of evidence from randomized, controlled trials has questioned this recommendation for older hypertensive persons. Results from these studies suggest that therapy with a β-receptor antagonist is less effective than therapy with low-dose thiazide diuretics with respect to blood-pressure reduction and in the prevention of cardiovascular events and death. In addition, β-blockers were more likely to be discontinued because of adverse effects. Therefore, β-receptor antagonists should not be considered as first-line monotherapy for simple hypertension in older patients. Because of their effectiveness in the management of symptomatic coronary artery disease, in secondary prevention following myocardial infarction, and in certain congestive heart failure settings, β-receptor antagonists should be considered for older patients whose hypertension is complicated by these comorbid conditions. Glucose and lipid profiles may be slightly affected by treatment with β-receptor antagonists. In addition, lethargy may develop during β-receptor antagonist therapy.

Angiotensin-Converting Enzyme Inhibitors and Angiotensin-Receptor Antagonists

The effectiveness of angiotensin-converting enzyme (ACE) inhibitors and angiotensin-receptor antagonists in lowering blood pressure in older hypertensive patients has been documented. Drugs in these classes are generally well tolerated (with the exception of cough during ACE inhibitor therapy), and they do not adversely effect the central nervous system or metabolic profile. In the absence of data from randomized, controlled trials to support their benefit with respect to cardiovascular events and mortality, therapies from these classes generally should not be considered as initial monotherapy for simple hypertension. There are compelling benefits from using ACE inhibitors in those patients with coexisting diabetes mellitus (particularly when there is microalbuminuria), as well as in those with systolic dysfunction.

α-Receptor Antagonists

Although the reduction in peripheral vascular resistance that occurs with therapy using an α-receptor antagonist is particularly appropriate for the pathophysiologic profile of geriatric hypertension, and although these agents are effective in blood-pressure reduction, the development of postural hypotension has limited the widespread use of this class of antihypertensive for treating older patients. In the currently ongoing Antihypertensive and Lipid Lowering Treatment to Prevent Heart Attack Trial (ALLHAT), the treatment arm that included persons randomized to therapy with the α-receptor antagonist doxazosin was stopped early because of a higher rate of cardiovascular end points, including a twofold greater likelihood of being hospitalized for congestive heart failure. Consequently, this arm of the ALLHAT study was closed. α-Receptor antagonist therapy might be considered for treating older hypertensive men with prostatism since these drugs have been shown to be efficacious in improving obstructive urinary symptoms.

The J-Curve Hypothesis

Although it is clear that an increase in blood pressure above normal (> 130/85 mm Hg) is positively and linearly associated with morbidity and mortality, concerns have been expressed that reduction of blood pressure below a given threshold level may be linked to adverse outcomes. Some studies have shown an increase in mortality with blood-pressure reduction below a certain threshold, creating a J-shaped curve of mortality. The significance of these concerns remains controversial. Many of the studies that have suggested a J-curve relationship have been confounded by comorbid illnesses among those with the lowest blood pressures. However, the results from several longitudinal studies have identified an increased risk for stroke and overall mortality in persons in the lowest systolic and, particularly, diastolic blood-pressure levels. Until additional prospective data are available to provide guidance in this therapeutic dilemma, it is prudent to use caution in lowering blood pressure in older persons with hypertension much below 140/90 mm Hg. Excessive reductions in blood pressure (eg, diastolic levels below 70 mm Hg) and treatment-induced postural hypotension should be avoided.

Follow-Up Visits

The frequency of follow-up visits should reflect the patient's degree of blood-pressure elevation at presentation, with closer follow-up indicated for those with stage 3 hypertension (ie, a systolic blood pressure greater than 180 mm Hg). With the exception of hypertensive emergencies (discussed below), attempts to reduce the patient's blood pressure to target levels too rapidly are unnecessary and likely deleterious. For most patients, an interval of 1 to 2 months is appropriate between visits to determine the need for dose titration.

Given the age-related changes in systems that regulate blood pressure and impaired blood-pressure homeostasis, overtreatment of hypertension may result in situational (postural or postprandial) hypotension. At all follow-up visits, it is imperative to determine the supine and standing blood pressure (Table 39.4). It is good practice to titrate antihypertensive drug doses to achieve the target (seated) blood pressure only after determining whether postural hypotension is present.

The patient's adherence to his or her antihypertensive medication regimen should be assessed before an increased dosage is recommended or switching to an alternative medication is considered.

Table 39.4—Hypertension Management: Follow-Up Visits

- Assess adherence to therapy.
- Monitor for adverse effects, especially postural hypotension.
- Measure supine and upright blood pressure.
- Encourage self-monitoring of blood pressure.
- Reinforce life-style modifications (eg, diet, exercise).
- Titrate dose cautiously.
- Evaluate for refractory hypertension.

For some patients, additional information derived from blood-pressure measurements taken at home or another nonclinical setting may be important; home blood-pressure monitoring may also aid in promoting a patient's adherence to therapy. Patient education regarding the significant benefits to be gained from adequate blood-pressure control is of particular importance, since hypertension is usually asymptomatic. The interdisciplinary geriatric team is well suited to promote this approach (eg, nurses to provide feedback on the degree of blood-pressure control, dietitians to review dietary information and adherence, pharmacists to promote adherence to the medical regimen, and social workers to review and, where possible, alleviate the financial burden associated with the cost of medical therapy). This evaluation should include a careful review of the patient's other medications to identify those (eg, nonsteroidal anti-inflammatory drugs and corticosteroids) that may worsen blood-pressure control.

When a patient's blood pressure has not been successfully reduced to the target level, cautiously increasing the dose, adding another agent (particularly a thiazide diuretic, if the patient is not already receiving this drug), or switching to another class of medication should be considered. Patients also should be counseled to continue their life-style modifications. It may take many months to achieve the target blood-pressure goal. When this goal is not attained despite adherence to a three-drug regimen, an evaluation for refractory hypertension (especially renovascular disease) should be considered. Once a patient has achieved appropriate stable blood-pressure control for more than a year, step-down treatment may be considered; a cautious downward dosage titration may be attempted, with close blood-pressure monitoring. Patients who have been successful at achieving weight loss or other nonpharmacologic interventions are most likely to be successfully weaned from antihypertensive medications.

SPECIAL CONSIDERATIONS

Hypertensive Emergencies and Urgencies

Elevated blood pressure per se in the absence of signs or symptoms of target organ damage does not constitute a hypertensive emergency or urgency. Rapidly and overly aggressively reducing blood pressure in a patient with incidentally discovered elevated blood pressure is potentially harmful and may produce complications, such as coronary or cerebral hypoperfusion syndromes. Examples of true hypertensive emergencies in older patients include hypertensive encephalopathy, acute heart failure with pulmonary edema, dissecting aortic

aneurysm, and unstable angina. These situations will present with symptoms and signs of vascular compromise of the affected organs. The management of these emergencies requires an acute hospital setting, with the parenteral administration of an antihypertensive agent and continuous blood-pressure monitoring to achieve an immediate reduction in blood pressure, although not initially to a normal target level. Blood pressure should not be lowered emergently more than 25% within the first 2 hours, with a goal of achieving 160/100 mm Hg gradually over the first 6 hours of therapy. Hypertensive urgencies, situations in which blood pressure should be lowered within 24 hours to prevent the risk of target organ damage, are more common than true emergencies. The majority may be managed with oral administration of antihypertensive medications to achieve a gradual blood-pressure reduction.

Hypertension in the Long-Term-Care Setting

Approximately one third to two thirds of residents in long-term-care facilities have hypertension. Special considerations are warranted in the care of residents with respect to making the correct diagnosis and defining the goals of therapy and its effects on quality of life. Blood-pressure measurements in long-term-care settings may not be accurate. Inaccuracies result from measurement errors and from the temporal variability in blood pressure, particularly in relation to meals. Blood pressure appears to be highest in the morning before breakfast. Postprandial hypotension is common among long-term-care residents, affecting about one third of this population. The presence of postprandial hypotension has been associated with otherwise unexplained syncope, and it has been found to be a significant independent risk factor for falls, syncope, stroke, and overall mortality.

There are several factors to consider in the management of hypertension in this setting. First, the advanced average age of persons in long-term care raises controversy surrounding the question whether the benefits of antihypertensive therapy extend to the very old (ie, those aged 80 years and older). If the beneficial effects of treatment are less evident, the potential adverse effects and risks of therapy should be weighed more heavily in defining the goals of therapy. Even an intervention as seemingly innocuous as a sodium-restricted diet needs to be evaluated in the context of the high prevalence of protein-energy malnutrition among nursing-home residents. Second, the average resident in long-term care takes seven medications, and most have three or more comorbid conditions. The addition of an antihypertensive medication increases the possibility of an adverse drug event in this frail, at-risk group. Third, several studies have identified the use antihypertensive medications, particularly vasodilators, as a risk factor for falls in this high-risk population, who experience an average of two falls each year. It is therefore important to assess both postural and postprandial blood pressure in this population. Randomized, controlled trials that could provide clear risk-benefit evidence to support an approach to antihypertensive management in the long-term-care population have not yet been conducted. The available data suggest that diuretic therapy is effective in controlling systolic blood-pressure elevations and that blood-pressure reduction with diuretics lowered the prevalence of postural hypotension.

REFERENCES

- Jones RA, Stephens R. Issues and trends in care of the hypertensive client. *Holist Nurs Pract.* 2001;15(4):vi–xi.

- Staessen JA, Gasowski JG, Thijs L, et al. Risks of untreated and treated isolated systolic hypertension in the elderly: meta-analysis of outcome trials. *Lancet.* 2000;355:865–872.

- The sixth report of The Joint National Committee on Prevention, Detection, Evaluation, and Treatment of High Blood Pressure. *Arch Int Med.* 1997;157(21):2413–2445.

- Whelton PK, Appel LJ, Espeland MA, et al. Sodium reduction and weight loss in the treatment of hypertension in older persons: a randomized controlled trial of nonpharmacologic interventions in the elderly (TONE). TONE Collaborative Research Group. *JAMA.* 1998;279(11):839–846.

- Wright JM, Lee CH, Chambers GK. Systematic review of antihypertensive therapies: does the evidence assist in choosing a first-line drug? *CMAJ.* 1999;161:25–32.

CHAPTER 40—MUSCULOSKELETAL DISEASES AND DISORDERS

The prevalence of arthritis is 15% in adults and is projected to increase to 18% by 2020. Musculoskeletal complaints are among the commonest reasons adults seek medical attention. Studies of referral patterns from primary care physicians to rheumatologists suggest that in older adults conditions found most frequently by the rheumatologist are chronic soft tissue pain (soft tissue rheumatism) involving muscle and periarticular tissues, rather than true joint disease. Soft tissue rheumatism includes conditions such as chronic postural strain, acute muscle and ligamentous strain, bursitis, and fibromyalgia. Most of these conditions do not have a clear inflammatory basis, are sometimes very poorly localized, and can be confused with serious systemic rheumatologic diseases, such as systemic lupus erythematosus (SLE), vasculitis, polymyositis (PM), or polymyalgia rheumatica (PMR). Evaluation can be further confounded by the likely presence in older adults of nonrheumatologic diseases that may affect multiple organ systems.

CLASSIFICATION AND OVERVIEW OF RHEUMATOLOGIC DISORDERS

The rheumatologic disorders can be broadly classified into those presenting with musculoskeletal complaints and those presenting as systemic illness. True joint disease (arthritis) is revealed by symptoms and findings that refer specifically to joints. A history of joint swelling is strong evidence of true joint involvement. A history of pain in a joint with motion or weight bearing is also suggestive of arthritis. Patterns of joint involvement, the presence of morning stiffness or stiffness after periods of inactivity, the effect of activity, and the effect on sleep can greatly narrow diagnostic possibilities.

When symptoms of pain and fatigue are generalized and not specifically referable to joints or classic bursal areas, differentiation between inflammatory and noninflammatory conditions is paramount. In the inflammatory disorders that may present with generalized aching and pain, historical and physical findings usually lead to the correct diagnosis. The presence of rash, fever, stomatitis, dysphagia, Raynaud's phenomenon, true muscle weakness, or seizures suggests one of the autoimmune rheumatologic disorders. The absence of such symptoms makes generalized noninflammatory conditions, such as fibromyalgia, or regional conditions, such as chronic postural strain or myofascial pain, more likely.

Laboratory Testing in Rheumatologic Diseases

Laboratory testing plays a minor role in the diagnosis of rheumatologic diseases in older adults. Factors that make laboratory testing in older adults less useful are the lack of tests that are specific, the high incidence of osteoarthritis (OA) in this age group, and increased seroreactivity in later life, especially in women. Tests such as erythrocyte sedimentation rate (ESR) and rheumatoid factor are neither sensitive nor specific. The antinuclear antibody test has such a high sensitivity in SLE that a negative test essentially excludes the disease; however, a positive antinuclear antibody is of very low specificity. A few blood tests are specific. For example, either high titers of anti–double-stranded DNA antibodies or the presence of the anti-Sm antibody is specific for SLE, but unfortunately neither is sensitive. Most blood testing in rheumatologic conditions can, at best, only help confirm the clinical impression or provide prognostic data. Studies suggest that laboratory testing tends to be overutilized by older adults and by primary care clinicians.

Physical Activity

Physical activity reverses many physiologic consequences of aging; specifically, exercise preserves muscle and bone mass, reverses the increased fat-to-muscle ratio associated with aging, and preserves physical function. As recently as the mid-1980s typical instruction in the treatment of rheumatoid arthritis (RA) was that exercise should be avoided and even that total bed rest was a mainstay treatment for severe flares in disease activity. Conventional wisdom also held that weight bearing in OA would accelerate joint degeneration and exercise in PM would aggravate muscle inflammation. Increasingly, well-designed studies have disproved these old beliefs and have now shown the value of exercise in RA, OA, PM, and SLE. Rather than worsening these disorders, exercise preserves function, reduces symptoms, and reduces the number of sick days in the inflammatory rheumatologic disorders and OA. Prescribed exercise must now be considered an essential part of the treatment of all the rheumatologic disorders. (See also "Physical Activity," p 65.)

OSTEOARTHRITIS

Radiologic evidence of OA can be found in nearly 100% of adults aged 65 and over, and OA is the major cause of knee, hip, and back pain in older adults. Knee pain alone, according to data from NHANES III (National Health and Nutrition Examination Survey), affects more that 20% of adults aged 60 and over, with incidence rates approaching 30% in those aged 80 and over. NHANES data suggest that the rising incidence of knee pain can be attributed to the trends of worsening obesity and decreased physical activity in American society in recent decades.

OA is a degenerative disease of cartilage that correlates strongly with aging, yet pathologic changes in osteoarthritic cartilage are quite distinct from changes seen in normal aging cartilage. OA is also a heterogenous group of related joint disorders that have a variety of causes; they can be inborn, associated with metabolic disease, or due to joint malformation, joint trauma, or damage from other joint diseases. Distinct patterns of joint involvement are seen and are used to classify OA, ranging from isolated finger interphalangeal joint boney enlargement, to severe deterioration of weight-bearing joints, to isolated spinal involvement, and to generalized axial and peripheral joint degeneration. Primary OA appears to be genetically determined, with dominant expression in woman and recessive expression in men. It tends to avoid wrists, elbows, shoulders, and ankles. Involvement of these joints with OA suggests the presence of another disease or factor contributing to joint degeneration.

Underlying pathology in OA does not feature inflammation, though hypertrophy of synovium and accumulation of joint effusions are typical. Progressive changes in cartilage include poor chondrocyte function and death, altered cartilage composition with poor mechanical properties, cartilage surface fibrillation, and eventual gross cartilage destruction. Associated boney proliferation at the cartilage–bone interface leads to palpable and radiographically distinct osteophytes around affected joints.

Pain and reduced joint motion are the hallmarks of OA, with attendant ligamental instability and muscle atrophy. OA in weight-bearing joints is associated with gait abnormalities and increases the risk for falls and injury, which contribute substantially to OA morbidity, especially in the oldest and most frail persons.

The management of OA often begins with efforts to control pain. Rarely do analgesics alone accomplish pain control; by the time the clinician is asked to evaluate for symptomatic OA, function has likely worsened, with related muscle atrophy and limitation of joint motion. These collateral changes put an affected joint at a biomechanical disadvantage that both increases pain and predisposes to more rapid deterioration. It is critical to institute not only analgesic therapy but also early efforts to strengthen atrophied muscles related to the diseased joint and to improve joint motion. Analgesics play a role in allowing physical therapy to be used effectively, as in the long-term management of OA. Early referral to a physical therapist for evaluation and to define a set of exercises the patient can do daily at home is usually indicated. With OA of the weight-bearing joints, especially the knees, early mobilization and an ongoing walking exercise program may result in progressive functional improvement and reduction in pain rather than deterioration of the affected joints. Weight reduction can help reduce pain and improve function, especially if the lumbar spine or weight-bearing joints are involved. Joint injections with corticosteroids and joint injections with hyaluronic acid derivatives can be of temporary benefit with low risk for toxicity. Cartilage-preserving arthrotomy is effective for some patients. If nonsurgical management proves inadequate with knee or hip disease, total arthroplasty is an excellent solution. Hip and knee arthroplasties can have a significant impact on a patient's life style and function. The primary indication for this surgery is pain. Surgery is usually considered if the patient has pain at rest, if the pain interrupts sleep, or if walking is significantly limited (eg, < 300 meters) or requires an assistive device. In the final analysis, the patient must decide whether joint pain is affecting his or her function, life style, or independence enough to consider major surgery.

Recommendations for the choice of analgesics has changed in recent years, as research has shown that acetaminophen is as effective as any of the nonsteroidal anti-inflammatory drugs (NSAIDs) for mild to moderate pain. Considerable gastrointestinal and renal toxicity are both associated with NSAID use by older adults; therefore, acetaminophen is the first drug of choice in OA pain management. If acetaminophen is ineffective, nonacetylated salicylates, which have low gastrointestinal toxicity, can be given. The selective COX-2 inhibitors show promise as safer and highly effective analgesics with reduced gastrointestinal toxicity. In severe cases of debilitating OA, poorly responsive to non-pharmacological and other pharmacological therapies, or where adverse effects prevail, titrated use of continuous release (for continuous pain) and/or short-acting opioid formulations (for episodic pains), may be required. (See the Appendix, pp 411–412 for pain medications tables from the AGS guidelines on managing persistent pain.)

Hyaluronic acid is a major constituent of synovial fluid and is a major contributor to synovial fluid viscosity and a contributor to cartilage elasticity. Hyaluronic acid and hyaluronan polymers were approved by the Food and Drug Administration in 1997 for intra-articular injection for OA of the knee. This viscosupplementation therapy is given in a series of weekly knee joint injections, five for hyaluronic acid and three for hyaluronan polymers. Typical benefit for 6 months is reported; for some patients, this is longer than the relief obtained from a corticosteroid injection.

Glucosamine and chondroitin sulfate are components of glucosaminoglycan molecules that are important in maintaining the mechanical properties of connective tissue and cartilage. Both have been studied separately as treatments for OA, with evidence of benefit in the reduction of pain. In a 3-year randomized, controlled trial, glucosamine, in comparison with placebo, was found to be associated with less joint space narrowing and improved symptoms. The therapeutic benefit of chondroitin sulfate does not become apparent for several weeks after it is started, and improvement lasts for several weeks after it is stopped. Long-term studies are needed before chondroitin sulfate can be considered a disease-modifying drug in the treatment of OA. Glucosamine and chondroitin sulfate are available in combination as "nutriceuticals." Though glucosamine and chondroitin sulfate have few side effects, the dosage and bioavailability of available preparations of nutriceuticals are not established; therefore, the benefit seen in therapeutic trials cannot be predicted with the available over-the-counter preparations.

BACK PAIN AND SPINAL STENOSIS

See "Back Pain" (p 270).

GOUT

Gout is perhaps the oldest recognized form of arthritis. It was unmistakably described by Hippocrates, and Sydenham's clinical description of his own experience of gout in the late 17th century can hardly be improved upon today. Well into the 19th century, rheumatic fever was classified as a distinct form of arthritis, and other forms of joint disease were considered to be subtypes of gout, which is why terms like *rheumatoid gout* were used for the disease now called *rheumatoid arthritis*. These views prevailed until recognition about 150 years ago of the relationship of classic gout with high levels of uric acid in blood. Proof of intra-articular monosodium urate crystals as the specific cause of acute gout was not established until the early 1960s.

Gout often presents as acute monoarthritis, usually of the first metatarsal phalangeal joint, mid-foot, or ankle. With subsequent attacks, the knee, elbow, or wrist can be involved. Later in the course of untreated disease, attacks tend to be less intense but to last longer and may feature simultaneous involvement of more than one joint. Late in untreated disease, chronic low-grade inflammation in multiple joints occurs, and tophi (gross subcutaneous urate deposits on extensor surfaces) develop. In this late phase of untreated gout, the condition can be mistaken for nodular rheumatoid arthritis, with tophi being mistaken for rheumatoid nodules. Because gout and rheumatoid arthritis do not occur together and the two conditions are treated so differently, a strong case is made for microscopic evaluation of a joint fluid samples in the initial evaluation of chronic polyarticular, as well as acute monarticular, arthritis.

With rare exceptions, the clinical emergence of gout is preceded by a period of asymptomatic hyperuricemia. However, hyperuricemia is not uniformly present at the time of an acute gout attack, nor does the presence of hyperuricemia confirm a diagnosis of gout. Acute attacks can be precipitated by trauma, acute nonarticular illness requiring hospitalization, dehydration (acute gout is particularly common postoperatively), or medications that can perturb serum uric acid levels.

Diagnosis of gout is most directly and unequivocally established by observing the presence of strongly negatively birefringent needle-shaped crystals in a sample of joint fluid. Needle-shaped urate crystals can often be seen by ordinary or dark field microscopy of joint fluid samples, but confirmation of negative birefringence requires use of a polarizing microscope equipped with a compensator plate. Many laboratories and most rheumatologists have access to such a microscope. This type of microscope is essential in the diagnosis of pseudogout, described in the next section.

The treatment of gout is biphasic. The acute episode is best managed with a short course of an NSAID. The choice of the NSAID is not critical, as gastrointestinal toxicity is less likely to emerge during the 10 to 21 days needed for an acute attack to respond. Drugs, such as allopurinol or probenecid, that can acutely lower uric acid level should not be used in the management of acute gout, as premature lowering of uric acid level will paradoxically intensify and prolong an acute gout attack. Colchicine and corticosteroids are also effective treatments for acute gouty attacks.

Once the acute attack is resolved, attention can be turned to correcting the underlying problem of urate deposition. Urate accumulation in body tissues can be due to uric acid overproduction in the body, reduced renal elimination, or a combination of both. Ninety percent of chronic hyperuricemia is due to reduced renal excretion resulting from renal disease or the use of drugs, especially diuretics. Uric acid overproduction in older adults is seen in disorders with increased tissue turnover, such as lymphoproliferative disease, chronic hemolytic anemia, and psoriasis, and in rare genetic enzymatic defects.

Drugs, for example probenecid, that promote renal uric acid excretion can correct hyperuricemia in young adults who have normal renal function. In older adults, reduced renal function renders uricosuric drugs less effective. The most effective treatment for uric acid reduction is allopurinol, which acts by blocking formation of uric acid. Allopurinol dosage can be adjusted upward, starting with 100 mg daily and increasing stepwise by 100 mg increments in the daily dosage at 2- to 4-week intervals until serum uric acid levels are 5 or less.

During treatment to lower uric acid levels, the risk of recurrent acute gout attacks is raised. Prophylaxis against acute attacks is advisable for 3 to 6 months while treatment to lower uric acid is introduced and optimized. Although NSAIDs could be used for prophylaxis, the risk of gastrointestinal toxicity with chronic use must be considered. Colchicine can be effective for prophylaxis in older adults at a reduced dosage of 0.6 mg daily. This low dose is well tolerated and does not have associated risk of gastrointestinal ulceration. Colchicine should be avoided in persons with hepatic disease or advanced renal insufficiency and is contraindicated if both hepatic and renal disease are present.

CHONDROCALCINOSIS

Radiographically evident deposition of calcium pyrophosphate dihydrate (CPPD) crystals in articular tissue is markedly related to aging and can be seen in up to 50% of adults aged 90 and over. CPPD crystals can be found in synovial fluid and are associated with several clinical syndromes. CPPD crystals can cause attacks of acute monarthritis, most commonly the knee, wrist, and shoulder, a condition termed *pseudogout* because of the resemblance to acute (urate) gout. CPPD deposition can occur simultaneously in multiple joints and be responsible for chronic polyarticular synovitis reminiscent of RA. Radiographic chondrocalcinosis with or without CPPD crystals in the synovial fluid can also be present in joints with OA without any evidence of inflammation. The coexistence of CPPD crystals and OA is not surprising, as both conditions are common in older adults; however, controversy persists regarding the relationship of the two disorders. Differentiation of CPPD deposition arthropathy from urate gout and RA is important, as long-term treatment approaches are different.

Acute pseudogout attacks can be treated with an NSAID in a manner similar to that used to treat acute gout arthritis. Similarly, intra-articular corticosteroids will halt an attack in patients for whom an NSAID is contraindicated. Parenteral corticosteroids have been shown to be effective for acute pseudogout when NSAIDs and intra-articular corticosteroid injections are both contraindicated. Given once, with a possible repeat in 1 to 2 days, triamcinolone acetonide 60 mg intramuscularly (IM), betamethasone 7 mg IM, and methylprednisolone 125 mg intravenously (IV) have all proven safe and effective. Recurrent attacks of pseudogout can be prevented by the use of prophylactic oral colchicine 0.6 mg once or twice per day.

POLYMYALGIA RHEUMATICA

PMR is a distinct syndrome that occurs in older adults, as early as age 50 but predominantly after age 60.

Onset tends to be insidious, which commonly delays diagnosis. The classic symptom of PMR is remarkable stiffness of the proximal limb girdle and aching pain upon arising in the morning. ESR is so often markedly elevated that a high ESR is one of the essential diagnostic criteria. The syndrome may be accompanied by fatigue, low-grade fever, weight loss, and variable expression of synovitis of proximal joints of the upper, more than the lower, extremities. Studies of PMR have confirmed the presence of synovitis identical to that seen in RA, with synovial thickening, effusions, and lymphocytic synovial infiltration. PMR can progress to chronic polyarthritis that fulfills criteria for RA. Of more immediate clinical importance is the frequent coexistence of PMR with giant cell arteritis (GCA), a more serious, potentially life-threatening disease. This relationship is discussed below. Even with uncomplicated PMR, treatment with corticosteroids is associated with significant iatrogenic long-term morbidity, including diabetes mellitus, osteoporotic fracture, muscle atrophy, hypertension, glaucoma, and acceleration of cataracts and skin atrophy.

The cause of PMR is unknown. Studies to identify infectious agents responsible for triggering the syndrome have been inconclusive. Type II human leukocyte antigen (HLA) gene associations have been found, but associations differ from those seen with RA.

The standard treatment for PMR is oral prednisone, starting with 15 mg daily. Dramatic improvement is so expected that some have proposed that low-dose corticosteroid responsiveness confirms the diagnosis of PMR. Normalization of ESR corresponds to initial symptomatic improvement. The prednisone dose can be tapered over succeeding months on the basis of control of symptoms. PMR often runs a course of 2 to 3 years, and many patients are able to discontinue prednisone by then. Unfortunately, mean time to the first adverse event on corticosteroid therapy for PMR is about 1.6 years. Occasional patients with PMR respond to NSAIDs. Though long-term prednisone has significant toxicity, prednisone may be safer than NSAIDs for use by older adults, provided that the prednisone dose can be minimized and ongoing efforts are made to protect bone mass. A randomized trial of methylprednisolone acetate 120 mg IM every 3 to 4 weeks found that this regimen controlled PMR with fewer fractures, less weight gain, and lower cumulative dose than did daily oral prednisone.

GIANT CELL ARTERITIS

GCA is the commonest form of vasculitis that affects older adults. This form of vasculitis predominantly affects proximal branches of the aorta; inflammatory and ischemic manifestations, therefore, are mostly seen in the head and upper extremities. Occasionally, gross inflammation with tender, nodular swelling and erythema of the temporal arteries can be seen. In the absence of gross findings, symptoms of temporal headache, jaw and tongue claudication, and sudden vision loss are also seen. Diagnosis can be confirmed by biopsy of a temporal artery, thus the often-used synonym *temporal arteritis*. Recognition of GCA is often preceded by several months of a nonspecific systemic illness that includes weight loss, fever, and muscle aching that is indistinguishable from or identical to PMR. GCA can also present with sudden blindness with no prior systemic illness or with upper-extremity limb claudication. Other manifestations can include stroke, ischemic necrosis of tongue or scalp, or, rarely, myocardial infarction. Aortic aneurysm, predominantly thoracic, is a late manifestation of GCA even when previously appropriately treated. The incidence of aneurysm in GCA is about 10%, with discovery of thoracic and abdominal aneurysm 5.9 and 2.5 years, respectively, after GCA diagnosis.

The cause of GCA is unknown. Infectious agents have long been suspected, but none has yet been confirmed as causative. Studies of biopsy material revealed the presence of parvovirus B19 DNA. In another study, serum immunoglobulin M antibodies (implying recent infection or reinfection) against type I parainfluenza virus correlated extremely well with biopsy-positive GCA.

Diagnosis of GCA may require a high index of suspicion combined with a finding of an otherwise unexplained elevated ESR above 40 mm per hour. Combined elevation of ESR and C-reactive protein is more specific (97%) than elevated ESR alone for biopsy-positive GCA. Because of the risk of sudden blindness, most clinicians would start high-dose oral prednisone as soon as the possibility of GCA is seriously considered, and then proceed to biopsy. The administration of prednisone does not change arterial histology for weeks. Diagnosis can sometimes even be established or reestablished after a few years of prednisone treatment. Arterial involvement is patchy, and diagnostic histologic changes can be missed by biopsy. This oversight can be minimized by biopsy of the symptomatic side and by obtaining a several centimeters' length of artery. Multiple longitudinal sections as well as cross-sections of artery should be examined by the pathologist. Still, biopsies are occasionally negative in cases where suspicion remains high. Biopsy of the opposite side is recommended by some; however, in a study of bilateral temporal artery biopsy in 150 patients suspected of GCA, results from the two sides were found to agree in 97% of the cases.

Since 25% of cases of GCA are associated with PMR, there is a longstanding dilemma about deciding which patients with PMR should undergo temporal artery biopsy. There are no clear data to guide decision making in this situation. One reasonable criterion would be to obtain temporal artery biopsies in cases of PMR in which symptoms or physical findings are suggestive of arteritis, that is, temporal headache; visual changes; tongue, jaw, or limb claudication; neck or chest pain; or neurologic changes suggestive of central nervous system ischemia. The temporal artery can also be involved with other forms of systemic vasculitis. Vasculitides other than GCA should be considered whenever the temporal artery biopsy shows necrotizing vasculitis but absence of giant cells.

Treatment of GCA requires high-dose prednisone initially. No other treatment has been shown to be as effective. Clinicians differ on the definition of high dose, with some recommending starting doses as high as 120 mg daily. There are no data that show doses above 40 mg daily are more effective. Older adults are highly susceptible to corticosteroid toxicity, and toxicity increases markedly with total dose. The use of higher doses should be individualized and considered when there is resistance to initial treatment or unusually severe disease is present. Response is confirmed when the ESR falls rapidly over the first month of therapy. Tapering of corticosteroid should begin at the rate of 10% to 20% of the total dose per month as soon as the ESR is normalized. Published studies of methotrexate as a steroid-sparing agent have not consistently shown methotrexate to be effective.

RHEUMATOID ARTHRITIS

RA with late-life onset appears to be clinically different from the same disease with onset earlier in life. The condition in the older adult is more likely to have rapid onset, involve fewer and more proximal joints, and to be rheumatoid-factor negative. Nodules are less likely, and joint destruction may be less severe. Overall prognosis may be better than with earlier onset, seropositive, nodular, erosive disease. Nevertheless, RA is a chronic disease that persists indefinitely, with a high risk for progressive joint damage and functional impairment, and reviews confirm that late-onset RA is still a serious disease. Treatment is almost always indicated, and therapeutic options have increased since 1998, with the introduction of a variety of entirely new drugs. In more severe cases, consultation with a rheumatologist is indicated.

NSAIDs are often recommended as first-line medications for symptom control in RA. Because of the increased risk of gastrointestinal ulcer and bleeding in the older adult using NSAIDs, therapy with a low-dose corticosteroid such as prednisone may be preferable, provided that doses can be limited to 5 mg daily and precautions are taken to preserve bone density. The nonacetylated salicylate, salsalate, has minimal gastric mucosal toxicity yet has preserved anti-inflammatory activity. Celecoxib was approved in late 1998 as the first of a new class of NSAIDs, the selective COX-2 inhibitors. Rofecoxib was approved in mid-1999 for OA and pain; it is not yet approved for use in patients with RA. COX-2 inhibitors are thought to be as effective as such older drugs as naproxen in treating RA, and they show promise as oral anti-inflammatory and analgesic agents, with possibly a lower risk for gastrointestinal ulceration and bleeding. Available COX-2 inhibitors do not interfere with platelet aggregation. Celecoxib has a sulfonamide side chain and is contraindicated in patients with a sulfa allergy. Though the higher cost of COX-2 inhibitors is an important factor to consider in choosing medications for RA patient, their cost of may be offset by the fact that they may help reduce the multisystem toxicities of corticosteroids. COX-2 inhibitors should still be considered potentially toxic to gastric mucosa. They have effects on intrarenal prostaglandin production that resemble those of other NSAIDs and must be used with caution in patients with diabetes mellitus or renal insufficiency, or who are also using diuretics or angiotensin-converting enzyme inhibitors.

RA is a lifelong systemic disease associated with progressive joint and extra-articular organ involvement leading to functional decline and shortened longevity. Disease-modifying drugs should be considered in all cases of RA. Longitudinal studies have confirmed the preservation of function when disease-modifying drugs are instituted early and maintained over the long term.

The use of parenteral gold, penicillamine, azathioprine, and cyclophosphamide has markedly declined in the past decade because of the availability of safer drugs. Methotrexate has been approved for more than a decade for treating RA and has become established as the disease-modifying agent of choice. When given daily, methotrexate can cause hepatic injury, with cirrhosis and end-stage hepatic failure. Low-dose, weekly, oral pulse therapy dramatically reduces the risk of hepatic toxicity, provided ethanol intake is completely avoided. Methotrexate can be used in combination with other immunosuppressive agents to yield proven additive or synergistic benefit. Since 1991, more than 100 cases of lymphoproliferative disease have been reported in patients with RA who are under treatment with methotrexate. Usually, the lesion is extranodal non-Hodgkin's lymphoma, and remission is often seen when methotrexate is stopped. At least one population-defined study did not find excess cancer in RA patients treated with methotrexate who were compared with RA cases who never received methotrexate.

Randomized, controlled studies have now confirmed that minocycline 100 mg twice daily is effective in treating RA with minimal toxicity. Minocycline would be a good choice for mild disease or when there is need to start therapy even when the initial phase of diagnostic uncertainty has not passed. Similarly, hydroxychloroquine is well tolerated and does not require blood-test monitoring for toxicity. When doses are limited to 5 mg per kg per day, the risk of retinal toxicity is very low. Weekly oral methotrexate can be added if hydroxychloroquine alone is ineffective. Sulfasalazine is more effective than hydroxychloroquine but requires divided daily dosing, has high incidence of gastrointestinal intolerance, and cannot be given in the presence of sulfa allergy.

Cyclosporine is approved for use in treating severe RA, either alone or in combination with methotrexate. Toxicity remains a concern, and the role of cyclosporine in treating RA is still evolving.

Leflunomide, approved in 1998, is the first disease-modifying antirheumatic drug introduced for more than a decade and is the first such drug approved both for symptomatic improvement of RA and to prevent radiographic progression in joint damage. Leflunomide exerts its action through inhibition of mitochondrial dihydroorotate dehydrogenase, thus blocking an important step in de novo pyrimidine synthesis. In T and B lymphocytes, the effect is cytostatic rather than cytocidal, resulting in reduced immunoglobulin production. It has relatively fast onset of action (about 4 weeks) in comparison with older disease-modifying drugs.

Etanercept was approved in late 1998 for use in treating RA that has failed at least one other disease-modifying agent. Etanercept is a tumor necrosis factor inhibitor produced by recombinant DNA techniques consisting of the ligand-binding portion of human tumor necrosis factor receptor fused with the Fc portion of human immunoglobulin G. Etanercept is given in twice-weekly subcutaneous injections, and it is expensive. Clinical benefit is seen within 1 to 12 weeks of the start of therapy, and the drug must be given indefinitely to maintain benefit. The major risk of etanercept is the development of serious infections. Headache is a common side effect. Clinically insignificant autoantibody production can be detected in about 10% of patients receiving etanercept.

Infliximab was approved in late 1999 in combination with methotrexate for the treatment of RA. Infliximab is a mouse-human chimeric monoclonal antibody that prevents interaction of tumor necrosis factor α with its receptor. Tumor necrosis factor α is a potent trigger of multiple aspects of the inflammatory process. Infliximab must be given by intravenous infusion. Clinical trials show marked initial response to a single infusion of infliximab, but continued response to bimonthly infusions requires concomitant administration of oral methotrexate. Adverse effects include postinfusion reactions of fever, chills, headache,

chest pain, and dyspnea. Antibody formation is common, but it is reduced by the concurrent use of methotrexate.

SYSTEMIC LUPUS ERYTHEMATOSUS

Although it is thought of as a disease in younger women, predominantly of black women, SLE can present in later life. SLE is a multisystem disorder that can have a wide variety of presentations and predominant organ system involvement at any age. SLE is diagnosed with high specificity when any four of eleven criteria are documented singly or together at any time during the patient's life. Defining diagnostic criteria in this way implies that cases will represent a heterogenous group. It is not surprising that patterns of organ involvement are different in older adults. Criteria include malar rash, discoid rash, photosensitivity, stomatitis, nonerosive arthritis, serositis (pleurisy or pericarditis), seizure, nephropathy (urinary casts or heavy proteinuria), cytopenias (leukopenia, hemolytic anemia, or thrombocytopenia), positive antinuclear antibody, and any one of other immunologic abnormalities (anti–double-stranded DNA, anti-Sm, false-positive test for syphilis, or hypocomplementemia). Fever, Raynaud's phenomenon, migraine, antiphospholipid syndrome, and Sjögren's syndrome are also often seen in SLE. Numerous studies suggest that late-onset SLE affects women and men more equally (3:1 in older adults versus 10:1 in young adults), with relatively more white older adults affected than black. Late-onset SLE is less likely to involve rash, arthritis, Raynaud's phenomenon, nephropathy, and the central nervous system and more likely to involve serositis, Sjögren's syndrome, and positive rheumatoid factor. In older adults, SLE onset may be more insidious, with fewer organ systems involved per case and fewer relapses. As nephropathy and central nervous system involvement are related to mortality in younger women, late-onset lupus has been sometimes thought of as a milder disease. Despite the impression of milder disease in older adults, immunosuppressive and cytotoxic medications are required as often among older persons as among younger persons with SLE.

Hormonal factors may be partly responsible for the differences between early- and late-onset SLE. Estrogens are suspected of being an aggravating factor in young women. Studies of administration of postmenopausal estrogen for 2 years or more in women is associated with a fivefold increase in SLE risk. Increased risk is somewhat less if estrogen is combined with a progestational agent. SLE remains an uncommon disease. SLE in women has been associated with doubled overall incidence of cancer in a population-based study.

The treatment of SLE in older adults follows principles similar to those for treating early-onset disease. Corticosteroids are less well tolerated by the older adult and should be reserved as much as possible for organ- or life-threatening SLE flares. Hydroxychloroquine has been shown to be of benefit in SLE skin involvement and to reduce the overall number of disease relapses in younger adults. Hydroxychloroquine is well tolerated and has few serious side effects in doses of 5 mg per kg per day or less. Dapsone, azathioprine, and weekly oral methotrexate are used by some clinicians as alternatives to corticosteroids or as corticosteroid-sparing agents. Monthly intravenous pulse cyclophosphamide is reserved for severe or life-threatening disease.

SJÖGREN'S SYNDROME AND SJÖGREN'S DISEASE

Sjögren's syndrome, as xerostomia and keratoconjunctivitis sicca, has been long recognized as occasionally complicating RA. The incidence of Sjögren's syndrome in other connective tissue diseases is also higher. The involvement of salivary and lacrimal glands is responsible for the sicca symptoms seen in the Sjögren's that is associated with other connective tissue diseases. Dry eye and dry mouth symptoms without confirmation of Sjögren's syndrome occur in up to 40% of older adults who do not have a connective tissue disease. Many of the medications often prescribed to older adults undoubtedly contribute to this finding. (See "Oral Diseases and Disorders," p 307.) Treatment of sicca symptoms and uncomplicated Sjögren's syndrome is symptomatic and includes the use of artificial tears and artificial saliva and ophthalmological and dental preventive care. Pilocarpine 5 mg three times a day can help stimulate saliva flow.

Sjögren's disease is a systemic, multiorgan chronic disease that features lymphocytic infiltration of exocrine glands throughout the body, including the lacrimal and salivary, as well as the respiratory tree, intestinal tract, pancreas, liver, kidney, and vagina. In addition, cutaneous vasculitis and central nervous system involvement are often seen. The peak onset for Sjögren's disease is in mid-life to early late life.

There is no single diagnostic test for Sjögren's disease. Unexplained interstitial lung disease, renal impairment, hepatic dysfunction, esophageal dysfunction, malabsorption, or central nervous system disease resembling multiple sclerosis or multi-infarct state should raise suspicion of Sjögren's disease. Antinuclear, anti–Sjögren's syndrome antigen A (SS-A), and anti–Sjögren's syndrome antigen B (SS-B) antibodies are usually present. Rheumatoid factor and a variety of autoantibodies against gastric parietal cells, mitochondria, smooth muscle, and thyroid are often seen. Examination by an ophthalmologist can confirm the presence of keratoconjunctivitis, and biopsy of a lip or lacrimal gland can confirm the presence of characteristic lymphocytic infiltration. Biopsy of a rash can verify the presence of cutaneous vasculitis.

Symptomatic and preventive treatments are indicated for sicca symptoms, as described above. Trial therapy with hydroxychloroquine may help stabilize disease activity, as in SLE. Dapsone may be effective for cutaneous vasculitis. Corticosteroids and other cytotoxic drug should be reserved for organ- or life-threatening disease.

POLYMYOSITIS AND DERMATOMYOSITIS

PM is a heterogeneous group of inflammatory diseases of striated muscle that are not unique to older adults; however, late-onset PM is evaluated and treated somewhat differently in older adults. The onset of PM is often insidious. The cardinal symptom is muscle weakness, most marked in proximal muscle groups. Muscle tenderness is usually not prominent. Exercise tolerance is reduced, and the inability to perform simple tasks, such as reaching above the head or ascending stairs, may be present. Other organ system involvement is common in PM and reminiscent of other connective tissue diseases, including rash, arthritis, esophageal dysmotility, and Raynaud's phenomenon. Cardiac involvement is not rare and usually presents with dysrhythmias. Rash may involve the eyelids (heliotrope), the nose and malar areas, or be more generalized. Rash with dorsal thickening over the interphalangeal joints (Gottron's papules) are distinctly different from the dorsal phalangeal rash of systemic lupus that spares the interphalangeal joints. When rash is present, PM is referred to as *dermatomyositis* (DM).

In contrast to childhood PM, adult-onset PM affects women more often than men and blacks more often than whites. In older adults esophageal involvement and respiratory failure complicated by bacterial pneumonia are more likely. Up to 50% of cases of late-onset PM, and especially DM, are associated with underlying malignancy. No one cancer type seems most strongly associated. Colon, lung, breast, prostate, uterus, and ovary cancers are all well represented with PM and DM. Ovarian cancer is the most commonly associated gynecologic tumor underlying PM and DM. Mortality in adult PM and DM is usually associated with esophageal disease, respiratory failure with bacterial pneumonia, and malignancy.

Serum levels of muscle enzymes are usually markedly elevated in PM. Electromyography reveals changes consistent with myositis, provided affected muscle is tested. Paraspinal muscle involvement is constant and should be included in muscles tested. Diagnosis is confirmed with muscle biopsy that reveals inflammatory cellular infiltrates. Diagnosis of PM or DM in older adults should prompt further investigation for underlying malignancy.

An important histologic and clinical subtype of PM is inclusion-body myositis. Rimmed vacuoles and the accumulation of amyloid in muscle fibers are seen on muscle biopsy. Inclusion-body myositis predominantly affects men and is more likely to involve distal muscle groups including the volar forearm flexor and ankle dorsiflexor muscles. Onset and progression are slower than in PM. Inclusion-body myositis is thought to be relatively resistant to anti-inflammatory therapy.

Remission of PM and DM after treatment of an underlying malignancy may be seen. Therapy should also generally be directed at the inflammatory process itself. Corticosteroids are almost always the first drug of choice. Prednisone at 1 mg per kg per day is a typical starting dosage. Some clinicians advocate pulse parenteral steroid therapy to begin treatment of severe PM or DM, which consists of 1000 mg methylprednisolone IV daily for 3 consecutive days. Pulse therapy would then be followed with the usual oral dosage of prednisone, 1 mg per kg per day thereafter. In the absence of prospective data, this high-dose regimen should be individualized. Prednisone can be tapered after an initial phase of improvement of muscle strength and normalization of muscle enzyme levels. Rates of tapering of 10% to 20% of the total dose per month are typical. Methotrexate, given parenterally, in a weekly pulse regimen can be combined with corticosteroids. Somewhat higher methotrexate doses than those used for RA are given by some clinicians, up to 50 mg weekly. Methotrexate may also have a steroid-sparing effect in long-term therapy. Weekly oral methotrexate is effective in managing refractory skin manifestations of DM. Azathioprine may also have a steroid-sparing effect, but it is not as well accepted in the treatment of PM. Supervised exercise over 6-week and 6-month study periods has proven beneficial in PM, with improved function and without aggravation of the underlying disease.

REFERENCES

- Agudelo CA, Wise CM. Crystal-associated arthritis. *Clin Geriatr Med.* 1998;14(3):495–513.

- Boyev LR, Miller NR, Green WR. Efficacy of unilateral versus bilateral temporal artery biopsies for the diagnosis of giant cell arteritis. *Am J Ophthalmol.* 1999;128(2):211–215.

- Clarke J. Patient education: dealing with joint and muscle pain. *The Nurse Practitioner.* 2001;26(7):23–25.

- Creamer P, Flores R, Hochberg MC. Management of osteoarthritis in older adults. *Clin Geriatr Med.* 1998;14(3):435–454.

- Evans JM, Hunder GG. Polymyalgia rheumatica and giant cell arteritis. *Clin Geriatr Med.* 1998;14(3):455–473.

- Holland NW, Gonzalez EB. Soft tissue problems in older adults. *Clin Geriatr Med.* 1998;14(3):601–611.

- Lawrence RC, Helmick CG, Arnett FC, et al. Estimates of the prevalence of arthritis and selected musculoskeletal disorders in the United States. *Arthritis Rheum.* 1998;41(5):778–799.

- Lee AG, Brazis PW. Temporal arteritis: a clinical approach. *J Am Geriatr Soc.* 1999; 47(11):1364–1370.

- Marie I, Hatron PY, Levesque H, et al. Influence of age on characteristics of polymyositis and dermatomyositis in adults. *Medicine.* 1999;78(3):139–147.

- Matteson EL. Current treatment strategies for rheumatoid arthritis. *Mayo Clin Proc.* 2000;75(1):69–74.

- Reginster JY, Deroisy R, Rovati LC, et al. Long-term effects of glucosamine sulphate on osteoarthritis progression: a randomized, placebo-controlled clinical trial. *Lancet.* 2001;357(9252):251–256.

- Sewell KL. Rheumatoid arthritis in older adults. *Clin Geriatr Med.* 1998;14(3):475–494.

- Turner E, Stein M. Management of osteoarthritis in the nursing home patient. *Annals of Long Term Care.* 2002;10(9):39–44.

CHAPTER 41—BACK PAIN

Back problems are still the third most common cause for physician visits by older persons, and degenerative conditions of the spine are the most common cause. Less common systemic conditions that can cause back pain, such as tumors, infections, and visceral lesions, occur more commonly in older than in younger patients and may require emergent treatment. Anatomic abnormalities are commonly found in diagnostic imaging tests of an older person's lumbar spine. These abnormalities, often unrelated to the patient's pain, add to the diagnostic challenge. Finally, even though the natural history of low-back pain in younger persons has been well described, the patterns and natural history of back problems in older persons are less clear.

A systematic approach to low-back pain in older patients requires knowledge of the typical presentation of common back conditions of persons aged 65 and over, an understanding of the anatomy of the lumbar spine, the identification of physical findings associated with common abnormalities, and the judicious use of diagnostic imaging studies.

CAUSES OF BACK PAIN

The causes of back pain in the older adult can be classified as systemic, nonsystemic, or osteoporotic (see Table 41.1).

Systemic causes of back pain in the older adult include tumors, infection of the vertebrae or intervertebral area, and referred pain from such visceral problems as abdominal aortic aneurysms.

Nonsystemic back pain can be usefully divided into two categories—neurogenic and mechanical, each with acute and chronic characteristics. Neurogenic back pain results from direct neural compression. It is often

described as sharp, stabbing, or electrical, and it usually has a radicular component. It is more likely to be constant and less likely to be associated with position or activity. It is often accompanied by combinations of numbness, tingling, and weakness. Herniation of the nucleus pulposus leads to acute neurogenic pain, and spinal stenosis is a cause of chronic neurogenic pain.

Mechanical back pain results from abnormal, excessive movement within the *motor segment*, which is defined as two adjacent vertebrae and the interfacing disc. With excessive motion, there is the possibility of intermittent neural irritation or irritation of adjacent structures such as muscle, ligament, and facet joint capsule. Mechanical pain is usually localized to the back and is often described as a dull, boring, toothache-like pain. It is more likely to be intermittent; its intensity is often directly related to activity or position.

Specific examples of conditions causing back pain in older adults are listed in Table 41.2.

Systemic Causes

Back pain due to systemic cause merits immediate attention and intervention. The pattern of pain with these conditions can be distinctive. Tumors or infections of the spine usually have an insidious onset of pain that becomes more and more persistent with time. This pain is usually nonpositional and associated with systemic systems and signs; it often persists through the night. The likelihood of cancer as a cause of back pain increases in patients aged 50 and older, those with a previous history of cancer, and those with pain that persists for longer than 1 month. Patients with cancer are more apt to be anemic and have an elevated erythrocyte sedimentation rate.

Fever, discrete local vertebral tenderness, upper lumbar or thoracic pain, and nonpositional pain may indicate vertebral infection. Approximately 10% of patients with endocarditis have back pain. Infection may produce back pain in patients at risk for endovascular infections, such as those on hemodialysis, with chronic indwelling venous access catheters, a history of recent or chronic urinary tract infections, or a history of intravenous drug abuse.

A number of visceral problems, from abdominal aortic aneurysms to intra-abdominal infections or tumor, can present with back pain. Referred pain from these conditions should be suggested by the historical pattern of the pain, the absence of positional changes, and a normal physical examination of the lumbosacral spine.

Table 41.1—Classification of Causes of Back Pain

Systemic
  Infection
  Neoplasm
  Osteoarthritis
  Referred visceral condition (eg, abdominal aortic aneurysm)

Nonsystemic
  Mechanical
    Acute (eg, lumbar spinal strain)
    Chronic (eg, unstable lumbar spine)
  Neurogenic
    Acute (eg, herniated nucleus pulposus)
    Chronic (eg, lumbar spinal stenosis)

Osteoporotic
  Vertebral compression fracture
  Osteoporotic sacral fracture

Table 41.2—Conditions Causing Back Pain in Older Persons

Condition	History	Examination	Laboratory Tests, Imaging
Tumor	Persistent, progressive pain at rest; systemic symptoms	No focal abnormalities on examination	Anemia, elevated ESR, abnormal bone scan or MRI
Infection	Persistent pain, fever; at-risk patient (indwelling catheter)	Tender spine	Elevated ESR, WBC; positive bone scan or MRI
Unstable lumbar spine	Recurring episodes of pain on change of position	Pain going from flexed to extended position	One disc space narrowed and sclerotic spondylolisthesis
Lumbar spinal stenosis	Pain on standing and walking relieved by sitting and lying	Immobile spine; L4, L5, S1 weakness	MRI or CT scan showing stenosis
Sciatica	Pain in the posterior aspect of leg; may be incomplete	Often positive straight leg raise; L4, L5, S1 weakness	Variable diagnostic imaging findings
Vertebral compression fracture	Sudden onset of severe pain resolves in 4–6 weeks	Pain on any movement of spine; no neurologic deficits	Vertebral end-plate collapse; compression fracture seen on plain film
Osteoporotic sacral fracture	Sudden low-back, buttock, or hip pain	Sacral tenderness	H-shaped uptake on bone scan

NOTE: CT = computed tomography; ESR = erythrocyte sedimentation rate; MRI = magnetic resonance imaging; WBC = white blood cell count.

Nonsystemic Causes

Neurogenic Causes

Lumbar spinal stenosis results from a narrowing of either the central or lateral aspect of the lumbar spine. This narrowing may be due to facet joint osteophytes, encroachment of the annulus fibrosus of the lumbar disc, or hypertrophy of the ligamentum flavum. Diagnostic imaging tests often demonstrate spinal stenosis in patients without back pain, or with other causes of pain; the clinician must recognize the characteristic historical and physical features of this condition.

Flexion of the lumbar spine causes an increase in spinal canal volume and decrease in nerve root bulk. Extension of the lumbar spine produces a decreased volume of the spinal canal with an increased nerve root bulk. As a result of these anatomical changes, positions that flex the spine, such as sitting, bending forward, walking uphill, and lying in a flexed position, all relieve symptoms. Extension of the lumbar canal, which occurs with prolonged standing, walking, and walking downhill, exacerbates symptoms.

Lumbar spinal stenosis produces pain either in the back or in the legs, made worse by standing or walking. Pain in the calf when walking can often mimic the claudication of arterial insufficiency and is referred to as *pseudoclaudication*. Continued walking after this point may produce combinations of paresthesia, numbness, and weakness in one or both legs. Walking uphill is easier than walking downhill, and walking with an assistive device, such as a shopping cart, which allows some flexion of the lumbar spine, is usually better tolerated. These symptoms are usually progressive and consistent, not intermittent. There is often subtle weakness in the muscles innervated by L4–L5, L5, and L5–S1. (See Table 41.3 and the assessment section, p 272.)

Sciatica is a pain that can be felt from the buttock down to the foot, or in just isolated regions of the distribution of the nerve. In older persons there are two common patterns of sciatica. Sciatic pain that comes on only with standing and walking and that limits the person's ability to walk at a relatively constant distance is usually a result of lumbar spinal stenosis. Other older patients may develop the relatively sudden onset of sciatic pain, present at rest and exacerbated by sudden maneuvers, such as getting out of a bed or chair. This abrupt and persistent pain, not necessarily related to the erect position, usually resolves spontaneously in several weeks. This condition is most likely due to displacement of soft tissue, such as the annulus fibrosus of the intervertebral disc adjacent to the nerve root. The diagnosis of sciatica can be confirmed by the demonstration of muscle weakness of the L4, L5, and L5–S1 innervated muscles of the foot, ankle, and hip. (See Table 41.3 and the assessment section, below.)

Mechanical Causes

Acute mechanical pain occurs when a motion or activity stresses the soft tissue supporting structures of the spine (muscle, ligament, facet joint capsule) to their failure, resulting in a lumbar sprain syndrome, caused by partial or complete tear of these structures. This pain is usually abrupt at onset, localized to the lumbar region, and self-limited. The time required to heal this injury varies, and treatment is symptomatic.

Herniation of the nucleus pulposus of the intervertebral disc is uncommon after the age of 60. As

Table 41.3—Innervation of Lower Extremities

Function	Muscle	Peripheral Nerve	Nerve Root
Great toe dorsiflexion	Extensor hallucis longus	Deep peroneal	L5
Ankle dorsiflexion	Tibialis anterior	Deep peroneal	L4, L5
Ankle eversion	Peroneus longus, brevis	Superficial peroneal	L5, S1
Ankle plantar flexion	Gastrocnemius, soleus	Tibial	S1, S2
Knee extension	Quadriceps	Femoral	L3, L4
Hip flexion	Iliopsoas	Femoral	L2, L3
Hip adduction	Adductor magnus, brevis, longus	Obturator	L3, L4
Hip abduction	Gluteus medius	Superior gluteal	L4, L5
Hip extension	Gluteus maximus	Inferior gluteal	L5, S1

the nucleus pulposus becomes less gel-like, it is less apt to herniate. The evaluation of disc disease in older patients can be obscured by changes commonly seen in radiographic imaging of the older lumbar spine. Population studies have found no correlation between diffuse disc space narrowing and vertebral osteophytosis and back pain.

Lumbar degenerative disc disease may produce an unstable lumbar spine. Patients with this condition often have episodes of severe pain in the back or in the distribution of the sciatic nerve. This pain usually comes on suddenly, often following abrupt movements. It usually lasts only minutes to hours, but recurs frequently. This pain also comes on with significant flexion or extension of the lumbar spine. On physical examination, the patient often has guarded movements of the lumbar spine and pain when moving from the flexed to extended position. The presence in radiographs of significant changes at one disc and facet joint level, out of proportion to the other disc spaces, may point to instability of the lumbar spine as the cause of back pain.

Osteoporotic Vertebral Compression Fracture

Vertebral compression fractures are a common cause of back pain in older persons. Many of these fractures, however, are found incidentally and are asymptomatic. The pain from an acute vertebral fracture usually lasts from 2 weeks to 2 months. The onset of pain is abrupt and pain is intense; it is felt deep at the site of the fracture. There is often marked tenderness over the involved vertebra. The pain is usually worse on standing and walking, and relieved with lying down. Although the pain commonly radiates to the flank, abdomen, and legs, neurologic sequelae should not occur in patients with spontaneous osteopenic fractures. Symptomatic fractures most often affect the lower thoracic and lumbar vertebrae.

The acute pain resolves slowly. One study found that analgesic use decreased by 16% by day 5 and 33%

by day 14. Patients often have trouble walking for 2 weeks and have approximately 1 month of restricted activity.

The impact of these fractures, and osteoporosis in general, on chronic back pain and the function of older persons is unclear. Some studies have found that multiple fractures are associated with more disability, frailty, and back pain; others have not demonstrated a correlation between osteoporosis and chronic back pain.

Osteoporotic Sacral Fractures

Low-back pain in older women may be due to osteoporotic sacral fractures. This pain often occurs spontaneously, usually involving the lower back. Pain can also be felt in the buttock or hip area. Sacral tenderness on physical examination is found in a majority of patients. There is a high incidence of associated additional osteoporotic fractures.

Plain radiographs are usually negative. Technetium bone scans show a characteristic H-shaped uptake over the sacrum. A computed tomography (CT) scan shows displacement of the anterior border of the sacrum. These fractures have an excellent prognosis for recovery, with no neurologic deficits. The pain usually resolves in 4 to 6 weeks.

ASSESSMENT

History

Pain that is insidious in onset, progressive in its course, nonpositional, associated with night pain and systemic symptoms or signs, and persists for more than 1 month should raise concerns about tumor or infection. Nonsystemic causes of pain are characterized by intermittent, often positional, pain that is worse at onset and usually improves with time.

Diseases of the hip often produce pain in the back and leg in a distribution that resembles that of back disease. Back disease is more apt to cause pain when a patient goes from the supine to the sitting position or when bending or stooping. Hip disease can cause pain after prolonged sitting and when moving from a sitting to a standing position

Physical Examination

The physical examination of the back, hips, and legs is essential in the assessment of an older patient with back pain. The finding of subtle but asymmetric weakness of the hip, ankle, and feet muscles innervated by the lumbar and sacral nerves can help elucidate the cause of back and lower-extremity pain.

The back can be thoroughly examined only in the upright position. The back should be moved through all four planes of movement of the lumbar spine, side flexion to the right, side flexion to the left, forward flexion, and extension. Asymmetric limitation of the range of motion of the lumbar spine, or reproduction of the patient's pain with these maneuvers, often indicates mechanical disease of the lumbar spine. The pain of lumbar spinal stenosis is often produced by spinal extension.

The remainder of the examination should be performed with the patient in the supine position. A straight leg raise test can be informative if positive, but a negative test does not exclude any condition. Each patient with a back complaint should have a complete examination of the hips, as hip disease often mimics back disease. The passive range of motion of the hip should be assessed. The examiner should be able to abduct the hip to 40 degrees before the pelvic starts to tilt. The hip should flex beyond 110 degrees, externally rotate 50 to 60 degrees, and internally rotate 15 to 20 degrees.

The manual examination of the muscles of the lower extremities can be helpful. This examination should distinguish between weakness due to a nerve root problem and weakness due to a peripheral neuropathy. The third and fourth lumbar roots innervate the hip adductors and knee extensors (quadriceps); the fourth and fifth lumbar roots innervate the ankle dorsiflexors and the hip abductors; the fifth lumbar root innervates the great toe extensors; and the fifth lumbar and first sacral roots innervate the ankle evertors and the hip extensors. Great toe extension, ankle dorsiflexion, and ankle eversion weakness, with no involvement of the hip abductors and hip extensors, suggests a peripheral neuropathy rather than lumbar spine disease. A patient with lumbar spine disease is more likely to have weakness of lumbar and sacral innervated hip, as well as ankle and feet, muscles. A patient should be observed closely both rising from a chair and walking. Unless the patient has significant sciatica, back disease should not cause a limp. A significant limp suggests hip disease as a cause of the patient's pain.

Laboratory Tests and Imaging

Plain radiographs remain the most useful starting point in a back pain work-up of an older patient. Although these films are not recommended in the initial evaluation of back pain in younger patients, they are appropriate for patients aged 70 and over. This single test can demonstrate degenerative disc and joint disease, vertebral compression fractures, deformities such as spondylolisthesis and scoliosis, systemic disorders such as osteoporosis and Paget's disease, and, in some cases, infectious processes and neoplasms. A complete blood cell count with erythrocyte sedimentation rate is perhaps the most useful laboratory test among patients for whom there is a concern about an underlying systemic disease.

A technetium bone scan is useful in evaluating a suspected infection or neoplasm. CT and magnetic resonance imaging (MRI) have largely replaced myelography in assessing the neural canal. CT imaging is, in many cases, slightly superior in demonstrating the bony architecture of the spine, whereas the MRI is more sensitive to morphology of soft tissue, including disc, ligamentum flavum, neoplasm, and infection. Either CT or MRI studies are necessary to document spinal stenosis should surgical treatment be contemplated.

The utility of diagnostic imaging studies is tempered by the high false-positive rates of these studies in older persons. A diagnostic imaging study simply identifies an anatomic abnormality; it does not demonstrate that this abnormality is the cause of the patient's pain. One study found that 57% of persons aged 60 and older, with no history of low-back pain or sciatica, had abnormal lumbar spine MRIs. Of these persons, 36% had a herniated nucleus pulposus and 21% had lumbar spinal stenosis. Another study found that only 36% of asymptomatic persons had normal discs at all levels; the prevalence of disc abnormalities did increase in older persons. Other studies have shown similarly high rates of abnormal findings in asymptomatic persons. These studies reinforce the need to correlate carefully the patient's history and physical examination with the findings on diagnostic imaging studies.

MANAGEMENT

Management of back pain is hampered by the common difficulty of making a definitive diagnosis. Patients can do well, however, with a therapeutic approach that addresses the structural problems most likely to be causing their pain. Table 41.4 summarizes the therapies discussed below.

Table 41.4—Management of Back Pain in Older Persons

Condition	Treatment
Acute lumbar sacral strain	Analgesia
	Progressive exercise program
Unstable lumbar spine	Abdominal stabilizing exercises
	Lumbar sacral corset
	Spinal fusion if necessary
Lumbar spinal stenosis	Analgesics
	Progressive exercise program
	Laminectomy with or without fusion
Vertebral compression fracture	Spinal extension exercises
	Calcitonin may be helpful

NOTE: Also see the pain guidelines in the Appendix, pp 429–431.

Acute neurogenic pain is caused by nerve compression or rotation. This category is often self-limited, but symptoms may persist for several weeks. Initial treatment is symptomatic, including limitation of activities and analgesia. Once acute symptoms have resolved, progressive back-strengthening exercises should be undertaken in an attempt to prevent future recurrences.

Chronic neurogenic pain is the result of chronic nerve compression, almost always as a result of structural changes in the lumbar spine. Lumbar spinal stenosis is a classic example of this type of pain. The options for management are limited because of the structural changes of the vertebral column. The initial therapy of spinal stenosis could be conservative, with the combined use of analgesics, physical therapy, and possibly epidural spinal steroid injections. Spinal stenosis is the most common indication for spinal surgery in older adults. Long-term benefit from laminectomy, or laminectomy combined with fusion, is about 50% to 70%, regardless of whether the stenosis is central or lateral. In a prospective study of surgery for spinal stenosis, the ideal candidates for surgery were found to be those patients with severe narrowing of the spinal canal, minimal associated back pain, no coexisting conditions that affect walking, and symptom duration of less than 4 years.

Treatment of acute mechanical pain is symptomatic. Nonopioid analgesics are often helpful in the early stages. As soon as the acute symptoms subside, a gentle, progressive exercise program should be initiated that is designed to strengthen and improve the efficiency of the spinal and abdominal musculature. An aquatic program offers the dual benefits of rapid rehabilitation with a low incidence of reinjury. Walking in chest-high water against resistance and performing the flutter kick are two simple aquatic exercises.

Chronic mechanical pain is based on excessive vertebral motion that is more pronounced and repetitive. The pain is usually associated with advanced degenerative disc and facet joint disease. Management is aimed at eliminating or reducing motion. This can be done internally by strengthening the paraspinous and abdominal muscles, thus providing an internal "brace" for the lumbar spine. It must be stressed that this exercise should be a lifetime commitment. Lumbar sacral corsets and braces provide an external method of immobilizing the lumbar spine. The third option, a structural alteration to limit motion, is accomplished by surgical fusion. Despite the potential complications, surgical fusion can offer significant relief to an older patient with spinal instability who has failed conservative management.

Analgesia is the most important goal of treatment of vertebral compression fractures, while trying to avoid the complications of the bed rest required by the patient's pain. Braces and corsets are rarely required, as the natural history of the acute pain is relatively brief. Corsets may offer symptomatic relief if the pain is persistent. Spinal extension exercises also may be helpful. Calcitonin has an analgesic as well as antiresorptive effect on bone and may shorten the period of acute pain.

REFERENCES

- Bigos SJ, Bowyer OR, Braen GR, et al. *Acute Low Back Problems in Adults. Clinical Practice Guideline No. 14.* Rockville, MD: US Department of Health and Human Services, Public Health Service, Agency for Health Care Policy and Research; December 1994. AHCPR Pub. No. 95-0642.

- Boden SD, Davis DO, Dina TS, et al. Abnormal magnetic-resonance scans of the lumbar spine in asymptomatic subjects. *J Bone Joint Surg Am.* 1990;72(3):403–408.

- Borenstein DG, Burton JR. Lumbar spine disease in the elderly. *J Am Geriatr Soc.* 1993;41(2):167–175.

- Deyo RA, Kiehl AK. Cancer as a cause of back pain: frequency, clinical presentation, and diagnostic strategies. *J Gen Intern Med.*1988;3(3):230–238.

- Feldt K. Improving assessment and treatment of pain in cognitively impaired nursing home residents. *Annals of Long-Term Care.* 2000;8(9):36–41.

- Lavsky-Shulan M, Wallace RB, Kohout FJ, et al. Prevalence and functional correlates of low back pain in the elderly: the Iowa 65+ Rural Health Study. *J Am Geriatr Soc.* 1985;33(1):23–28.

- Silverman SL. The clinical consequences of vertebral compression fracture. *Bone.* 1992;13(suppl 2):S27–S31.

- Svara CJ, Hadler NM. Back pain. *Clin Geriatr Med.* 1988;4(2):395–410.

CHAPTER 42—DISEASES AND DISORDERS OF THE FOOT

Foot problems lead to some of the most distressing and disabling symptoms and conditions affecting older patients. The ability to remain pain free and ambulatory is a key element in successful aging. Foot and related problems and their sequelae may be local, or they may be associated with systemic conditions caused by disease. The medical conditions that place older patients most at risk for serious foot problems are vascular, neurologic, and endocrinologic diseases, as well as arthritis.

Feet are fairly rigid structures that carry heavy physical workloads, both static and dynamic. The foot itself is in the shape of a modified rectangle and bears static forces in a triangular pattern. Flat and hard surfaces force the foot to absorb shock, creating prolonged and repetitive micro- and macrotrauma. Any inability of the foot to adapt to stress produces inflammatory changes in bone and soft tissue, which may manifest in many mechanical disorders, including but not limited to synovitis, fasciitis, and arthritis.

There may be progressive loss of muscle mass and atrophy of tissue as a consequence of disease, decreased function, or lack of activity, all of which increase the risk of osteopenia in older adults. Because even minor trauma can result in a fracture, a stress fracture should be suspected when foot pain is severe, prolonged, and not otherwise explained. Manifestations of degenerative processes affecting older persons that are specific to the foot include plantar fasciitis, atrophy of the plantar fat pad, and hammertoe formation (see Table 42.1 for definitions and descriptions of several foot disorders and deformities). These conditions can cause pain, limit mobility, and thus threaten ambulatory status. As the ambulatory status of a older person changes, the foot problems change.

AGE-RELATED CHANGES AND THE IMPACT OF CHRONIC STRESS

With aging, the skin, ligaments, muscles, neurovascular structures, and bones undergo changes. The skin is one of the first structures to demonstrate change with aging. Trophic changes, such as a loss of hair below the knee and on the dorsum of the foot and toes, are common. The skin may become atrophic and resemble parchment. It also loses the normal oils and becomes xerotic. Brownish pigmentations are often related to the deposition of hemosiderin. A combination of physiologic changes in the skin coupled with continuing repetitive pressure and atrophy of soft tissue prompts hyperkeratosis to form as a normal protective function. When the hyperkeratosis becomes excessive, it tends to act as a foreign body, increasing pressure and creating local ischemia, which can lead to tissue breakdown. Localized pressure can create subkeratotic hemorrhage, and the resultant hematoma becomes the predisposing factor for the development of ulcerations.

The toenails undergo degeneration and trophic changes (onychopathy) with thickening or longitudinal ridging (onychorrhexis) that is the consequence of repeated microtrauma, disease, and nutritional impairment. Onychodystrophy (nail malformation), subungual hematoma, discoloration, onycholysis, onychauxis (thickening) (see Figure 42.1), subungual keratosis, and deformity are also prevalent among older adults. Deformities of the toenails may become more pronounced and may be complicated by xerotic changes in the periungual nail folds as onychophosis (hyperkeratosis) and tinea unguium (onychomycosis) with periungual infection.

Degenerative diseases commonly impact the older person's foot as a consequence of severe or repetitive trauma, inflammation, metabolic change, repeated and chronic microtrauma, strain, obesity, and osteoporosis. Manifestations of these processes that may involve the foot include stress fractures, tendonitis, residual deformities (including rotational digital deformities), joint swelling, anterior imbalance, bursitis, neuritis, and neuromas. Manifestations of degenerative processes that are specific to the foot include plantar fasciitis, spur formation, periostitis, tenosynovitis, pes planus, pes valgo planus, pes cavus, hallux valgus, hallux limitus, hallux rigidus, atrophy of the plantar fat pad, metatarsal prolapse, metatarsalgia, digiti flexus, Morton's syndrome, Haglund's deformity, tailor's bunion, and entrapment syndrome. (See Table 42.1 for definitions and descriptions.) These conditions can increase pain, limit mobility, and threaten the older person's ambulatory status.

ASSESSMENT AND TREATMENT OF SPECIFIC DISORDERS

Older patients should be asked about foot pain and paresthesias. Findings in the foot examination may include pain, stiffness, swelling, limitation of movement, and deformity. An important part of the foot examination is the neurologic assessment, including vibratory sensation, sharp and dull perception, joint position sense, and monofilament sensation. The examination also includes vascular, dermatologic,

Table 42.1—A Glossary of Foot Disorders

Disorder	Definition or Description
Calcaneal spur	A calcification of the attachment of the plantar fascia, usually at the medial plantar tuberosity of the calcaneus. The spur projects anteriorly and is the consequence of chronic repetitive trauma or stress resulting from biomechanical and pathomechanical change. When ligamentous calcification occurs, inflammation and associated pain at the attachment is the result. This may be referred to as *heel pain syndrome* and may be related to plantar fascitis.
Cystic erosion	Areas of radiolucency usually noted with arthritic changes, such as rheumatoid arthritis, and usually occurring in the metatarsal heads with associated joint changes.
Digiti flexus	May be fixed or flexible flexion at the metatarsal phalangeal joints; ie, hammertoe.
Digiti quinti varus	Refers to a valgus displacement or splaying of the fifth metatarsal, with a resulting varus or inward deviation of the fifth toe.
Entrapment syndrome	Occurs when a nerve is compressed by ligamentous or other soft tissue inflammation, resulting in pain and possible numbness and neuropathic symptoms. The most common sites are the posterior tibial nerve and the intermetatarsal nerves, plantarly.
Hallux abducto valgus	An alternative clinical diagnosis for hallux valgus, or bunion. There is a varus splaying of the first metatarsal with a valgus and rotational deformity of the phalanges of the great toe.
Hallux limitus and rigidus	A degenerative joint change involving the first metatarsal phalangeal joint, resulting from dorsal spurs, with a marked limitation or absence of any range of motion. The difference between hallux limitus and rigidus is based on the radiographic interpretation and difference in function
Hallux valgus	Deviation of the tip of the great toe, or main axis of the toe, toward the outer or lateral side of the foot; also, *bunion*
Haglund's deformity	A hyperostosis of the posterior and superior portion of the calcaneus, which expands the shape of the calcaneus, which can in turn place pressure on the attachment of the Achilles tendon. The presence of the deformity also can produce a pressure area for the counter of the shoe. It is easily demonstrated on a lateral radiograph of the foot and is clinically significant, with pain associated with tendonitis or bursitis, usually resulting from a foot to shoe last incompatibility.
Metatarsal prolapse	Marked prominence of the metatarsal head, usually associated with atrophy or plantar displacement of the anterior plantar fat pad, pes cavus, or digital contractures, which force the metatarsal heads in a plantar projection.
Metatarsalgia	Pain in the forefoot near the heads of the metatarsals.
Morton's syndrome	A congenital shortening of the first metatarsal shaft, which creates an abnormal metatarsal arc. Excessive weight is placed on the second metatarsal head during gait and stance. The dynamics and pathomechanics of the foot are modified and provide one of the causes of hallux valgus, abducto valgus, and rotational deformity of the hallux.
Periostitis	Inflammation of the periosteum.
Disorder	Definition or Description
Pes cavus	Represents a higher than normal arch and is commonly associated with neurologic change. In the older patient, excessive pressure is usually placed on the metatarsal heads. With atrophy of the plantar fat pad and displacement, pressure is increased, which can serve as a predisposing cause for pain and ulceration.
Pes planus	A flattening of the medial longitudinal arch, where the calcaneal pitch on a radiograph is usually below 15 degrees.
Pes valgo planus	Represents the same clinical picture as pes cavus, with an addition of pronation, demonstrated by a lateral deviation of the Achilles tendon and an outward and rotational deformity of the foot, which presents a compensatory deformity due to complex biomechanical imbalance.
Plantar fasciitis	An inflammation and pain involving repetitive microtrauma to the plantar fascia, particularly at its posterior calcaneal attachment; associated with biomechanical and pathomechanical changes in the function of the foot. It is related to calcaneal spurs, ligamentous calcification, and tissue atrophy.
Tailor's bunion	An enlargement of the fifth metatarsal phalangeal joint, usually with a lateral deviation of the fifth metatarsal shaft and head and a medial and rotational deformity of the fifth toe. It is usually associated with a splaying of the fifth metatarsal and can present with bursitis, capsulitis, and degenerative joint change.
Tenosynovitis	Inflammation of a tendon and enveloping sheath.

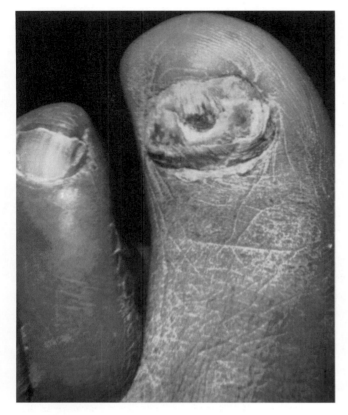

Figure 42.1—Onychauxis, subungual diabetic ulcer, with arterial insufficiency and onychomycosis.

and biomechanical evaluation, which includes foot type, angulations, muscle power, contractions, and other deformities that affect both weight-bearing and non-weight-bearing ability (eg, hip contraction increases pressure on ipsilateral heel). Assessment may also include radiography (weight- and non-weight-bearing).

Xerosis

Excessive dryness, or xerosis, is associated with a lack of hydration and lubrication and is a related keratin dysfunction. Fissures develop as a result of dryness and associated stress on the heel. Management aims to prevent infection and further complications. A 20% or 40% urea solution or 12% ammonium lactate may be helpful as a mild and safe keratolytic. A heel sleeve made of mineral oil or heel cup can help to minimize trauma to the heel, thus reducing the potential for complications.

Primary Nail Problems

Disorders of the toenails are common in older patients. Toenails undergo changes much more than do fingernails, as a consequence of trauma, the environment of the shoe or sock, and the forces associated with ambulation. The toenails may undergo degeneration and become thickened (onychorrhexis) in response to repeated microtrauma. When the nail is thickened without mycosis present, it is termed *onychauxis*. Untreated or neglected onychauxis is termed *onychogryphosis* or ram's horn nails (Figure 42.2). The nails can become so long that they encircle the entire toe.

Onychomycosis, fungal infection of the nail plate, is a common disorder of older adults. (See also "Dermatologic Diseases and Disorders," p 372.) It is a chronic and communicable disease that may spread from one nail to the next and may also infect the skin (tinea pedis). Bathing in the same tub or shower can seed the fungus from another individual. Onychomycosis is common in toenails because of the wearing of shoes. It is caused by repeated microtrauma in the internal environment of most footwear, which is dark, warm, and moist, thus serving as a medium for infection. Fungal nail infection may lead to deformity and pain that results from the nail's rubbing on the nail bed or encircling the nailbed. Ulcerations or abscesses are not uncommon. The mainstay of treatment is debridement of the nails. Topical antifungal agents are of little help. Ciclopirox, an antifungal nail lacquer approved by the Food and Drug Administration, may help. Oral antifungal agents are effective but carry the risk of possible drug interactions and adverse effects.

Ingrown toe nails are relatively common in older adults and are usually the consequence of deformity and improper self-care. When the nail penetrates the

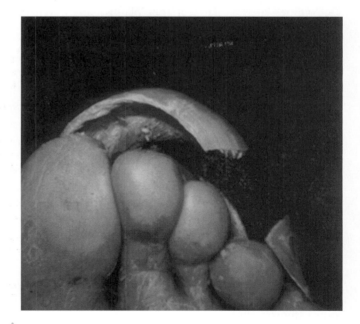

Figure 42.2—Onychogryphosis, onychomycosis, tinea pedis.

skin, an abscess and infection may result. If an ingrown nail is not managed early, periungual granulation tissue may form and complicate treatment. Onychia, inflammation of the soft tissue adjacent to the nail plate, is usually precipitated by local trauma or pressure, but may be a complication of systemic disease or an early sign of infection. Mild erythema, swelling, and pain are the most prevalent findings. Management includes removing all pressure, applying tepid saline compresses, and using antibiotics if needed. Lamb's wool, tube foam, or shoe modification may reduce pressure. Paronychia, inflammation of the nail matrix plus the deeper and surrounding structures, may develop with infection and abscess of the posterior nail wall. It is a serious problem because of the potential for bone involvement as a result of the close association of the nail with the distal phalanx. Management includes surgical debridement and antibiotic treatment, if needed.

Older adults may also develop subungual hemorrhage from trauma of the shoes or trauma from the bed covers. Bleeding under the nail may result in an ulcer or loss of the toenail (onycholysis) if it is substantial.

Subungual heloma (also known as a corn or clavus) is usually associated with a subungual exostosis, spur, or hypertrophy of the tufted end of the distal phalanx. Initial management includes debridement and protection of the toe involved, as well as the use of a shoe with a high toe box. Surgical excision of the osseous deformity may be required if the condition cannot be successfully treated in a conservative manner.

Pathomechanics

Deformities such as flat feet (pes planus), high arched feet (pes cavus), bunions, and hammertoes create pain and a reduction in the ability of the older patient to ambulate. Management should be directed toward relief of pain and improved ability to ambulate. *Hammertoe* is a general term applied to several types of contracture deformities of the toes. It is usually seen in the lesser toes, but a hallux (great toe) hammertoe may develop in the presence of coexistent neurologic abnormalities. The classic hammertoe is dorsiflexion at the metatarsophalangeal joint and plantar contraction of the proximal interphalangeal joint. Mallet toes and claw toes are different variations. A cock-up toe occurs when the contracture provides no contact between the toe and plane of support. Rotational deformities and overlapping toes (see Figure 42.3) due to hallux valgus and arthritis are also referred to clinically as hammertoes. These deformities are related to atrophy of interossei muscles of the foot and contractures of the long extensor tendons. The deformities can be classed as flexible, semi-rigid, or rigid, depending on the

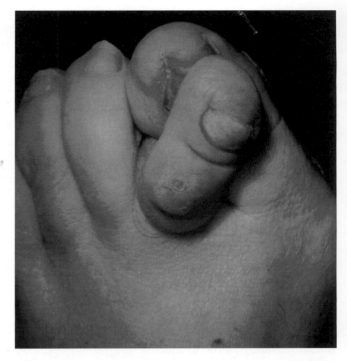

Figure 42.3—Hallux abducto valgus, hammertoe, subluxated second toe, onychodystrophy, onychodysplasia.

motion demonstrated and the ability to reduce the deformity. The toes may also become rotated, and with arthritic changes, they may become dislocated and subluxed (as in rheumatoid arthritis). These deformities increase the formation of corns, especially in the presence of ill-fitting foot wear. In older patients the heads and bases of the phalanges are commonly enlarged, and degenerative changes can often be demonstrated at the tufted end of the distal phalanx.

Management strategies depend on the causes and symptoms. When deformity is noted, shoe modification is important and should include a high toe box. Silicone molds can be used to maintain a more normal position of the toes, acting as a digital brace. Where hyperkeratosis is noted, debridement should be completed to reduce the possibility of ulceration. Padding with materials such as lamb's wool, silicone, or foam can help reduce pressure. For most older patients conservative treatment strategies are effective in controlling the pain associated with the deformity. Surgical revision remains an option when conservative measures are not successful.

Heel and Arch Pain

Plantar fasciitis is a common syndrome that causes pain in the sole of the foot. This heel pain is usually due to a strain of the plantar fascial attachment, which inserts on the medial plantar tuberosity of the calcaneus. A calcaneal spur may develop as a result of chronic stress on the attachment. The injury represents a prototypical wear-and-tear pattern that usually results in an absence of overt residual pain. Conservative management is usually effective for the older patient. Oral analgesics and physical medicine are the mainstays of therapy. Orthotics can reduce pressure on the heel by changing biomechanics during the gait cycle and transferring weight elsewhere.

Heel pain may also be caused by the rubbing of the shoe on the back of the heel. This may result in inflammation known as Haglund's disease. Constant pressure can result in bursal formation. Conservative management is usually effective.

Metatarsalgia refers to pain in the anterior metatarsal area. It can be functional in nature or associated with metatarsophalangeal abnormalities. It can be associated with anterior fat pad atrophy or displacement, retrograde pressure from hammertoe deformities on the metatarsal heads, and other pathomechanical changes. It may also be due to obesity, ill-fitting foot wear, and foot deformities that increase the angle at which the foot hits the ground.

Management depends on the cause and includes padding, orthotics such as a metatarsal pad, shoe modifications, physical therapy, local corticosteroid injection, digital molds to help transfer an anteriorly displaced fat pad, and analgesics if the problem is related to degenerative joint changes. A metatarsal bar is a transverse bar used to transfer weight over the metatarsal heads and is usually placed on the plantar surface or sole of the shoe. It may be placed between the insole and outsole.

SYSTEMIC DISEASES AND THE FOOT

Diabetes Mellitus

Diabetes is the most important disease affecting foot health in older persons. (See also "Endocrine and Metabolic Disorders," p 319.) It has been estimated that 50% to 75% of all amputations in diabetic patients could be prevented by periodic assessment, early intervention, and foot health education. The ocular complications impact on the ability of the older person to see ingrown toenails, corns, and ulcers. Delayed wound healing is another important factor.

The foot problems commonly seen in older diabetic patients include vascular impairment, neuropathy, dermopathy, atrophy of the muscles and soft tissues, and deformity. Neuropathy is the precursor to ulcers and is of utmost importance. Insensitivity, paresthesias, diminished or lost Achilles and patellar reflexes, decreased vibratory sense, and motor weakness may be noted.

Vascular impairment causes pallor, a loss or decrease in the posterior tibial and dorsalis pedis pulse, dependent rubor, decreased capillary filling time in the toes, and venous swelling. Severe vascular disease may result in rest pain that typically occurs at night. There is usually a loss of the plantar metatarsal fat pad, which predisposes the patient to ulceration in relation to bony deformities of the foot.

Foot ulcers are important problems for older diabetic patients. The most common causes are pressure, venous insufficiency, arterial insufficiency, and neuropathy. Other causes include tumors, polycythemia vera, and self-inflicted improper care. There may be overlap in the cause of ulceration. Other systemic conditions that can impact on the foot include hypothyroidism, congestive heart failure, renal failure, and lymphedema.

Clinicians should examine the feet of diabetic patients at each visit, as patients may be unaware of problems because of poor vision and neuropathy. Daily foot inspection by the patient or caregiver is ideal. Preventive strategies include management of the underlying disease process as well as treatment of peripheral neuropathy, arterial disease, limited joint mobility, elevated plantar pressures, bony deformities, hyperkeratosis, and onychodystrophy. Reducing excessive plantar pressure, shock, and shear by accommodating, stabilizing, and supporting deformities by weight diffusion and dispersion is important to ulcer prevention.

The key elements in the management of diabetic ulcers in the older patient include education, assessment, and prevention. Education is directed toward the professional, the patient, and the caregiver. Programs that have been professionally developed for patients and their families are available through national and regional diabetes associations. Also available are programs for professional education and assessment protocols that help identify and stratify risk. The key component in prevention is assessment of foot problems and stratification of risk. The risk of ulcer development is related to the effectiveness of management and the presence of vascular or renal complications. Components that interact to affect risk include daily activity, footwear, chemical exposure, hyperkeratosis, deformities, prior surgery and ulceration, neuropathy, and ischemia. When an ulcer is present, assessment should address location, duration, inciting event or trauma, prior ulcerations, infection, ischemia, neuropathy, hospitalization, wound care, off-loading procedures, edema, and Charcot joints.

The general foot examination includes an evaluation of the vascular, neurologic, and dermatologic systems along with structural deformity identification. Imaging is essential and may include plain radiography, computed tomography, technetium bone scans, indium scans, and magnetic resonance imaging. Vascular studies may be noninvasive and include doppler and transcutaneous oxygen tension as well as vascular consultation where the results are abnormal and with nonhealing lesions. The Semmes-Weinstein monofilament, vibratory perception, and Bio-Thesiometer as well as reflex changes all help assess the diabetic foot and ulceration, which may be present.

Appropriate footwear alone is not the total answer to prevention. A team approach to management of the ulcer, including proper medical management of the patient's diabetes, is useful. The general principles of management include debridement, pressure relief, off-loading, no or limited weight bearing, proper wound management, managing infection with antibiotics early, managing ischemia, medical management of comorbidities, and hospitalization and surgical management if needed. Weight bearing can be modified by the use of crutches, wheelchairs, and bed rest, as well as contact casts, walkers, boots, braces, total contact orthosis, and surgical shoes and boots as modified and appropriate dressings. A wide variety of dressings and topical agents are available; selection must be guided by nature of the ulcer and its complications. Topical agents include saline, antiseptics, topical antibiotics, enzymes, growth factors, and dermal skin substitutes. Physical medicine modalities and procedures should also be used early in management.

Empiric antibiotic therapy should be instituted early, especially if infection may become limb threatening; for limb-threatening infection, hospitalization may also be indicated. The choice of antibiotic is based on the clinical symptoms, culture and sensitivity, and the presence of deep infection, bone exposure, and sepsis, as well as whether soft tissue or bone is infected.

Peripheral Vascular Disease

Older adults with peripheral vascular disease demonstrate many of the same signs and symptoms as those with diabetes mellitus. (See "Cardiovascular Diseases and Disorders," p 243.) In contrast to neuropathic ulcers, vascular ulcers are extremely painful.

Arthritis

Osteoarthritis is common in older adults as a consequence of normal aging with chronic trauma, strain, obesity, and deformity. It occurs in weight-bearing joints and causes pain, swelling, stiffness, limitation of movement, and deformity. Gouty arthritis results early in intense pain and erythema and later in joint damage.

Rheumatoid arthritis affects the hands and feet equally and results in muscle wasting and marked deformity. The metatarsophalangeal joints become dis-located or subluxed; there is increased protrusion of the metatarsal heads, and walking becomes painful. If conservative treatment with orthotics and special shoes do not relieve the pain, surgery is helpful to allow less painful ambulation. (See "Musculoskeletal Diseases and Disorders," p 261.)

SPECIAL SHOES AND ORTHOTICS

Foot pain and stress can be relieved through weight diffusion and weight dispersion. Weight diffusion is accomplished with an increase in the thickness of an orthosis or sole of a shoe that is placed between the foot and the plane of support, such as the floor. Weight dispersion is accomplished by diverting pressure away from painful areas of the foot by making specific adjustments to an orthosis or insole or by some form of internal or external shoe modification. Examples include balance padding, metatarsal padding, and external shoe wedges or bars. The primary treatment goals of both approaches are to relieve pain, restore maximum function, and maintain restored function once it is achieved.

Special footwear and orthotics aim to reduce shock and shear, transfer weight from painful areas, correct or support flexible deformities, accommodate fixed deformities, and control or limit joint motion. Shoes with depth or extra-depth lasts are usually suggested to accomplish these objectives. (The *last* is the model over which shoes are made.) A *depth shoe* is a shoe that usually has a filler or insole that extends from heel to toe and that provides at least 3/16" of additional depth in the shoe so that an orthotic or customized insole can be placed in the shoe and prevent the top of the foot from being compressed against the underside of the toe box. An *extra-depth shoe* provides a 1/4" additional depth, and a *super-depth shoe* provides an additional 1/2" of depth for total-contact orthoses or inserts. Custom shoes are recommended for patients with severe deformity, amputation, or other foot problems for which special lasts are required.

Shoe modifications that are often useful for older patients include mild calcaneal wedges to limit motion and alter gait, metatarsal bars to transfer weight, Thomas heels to increase calcaneal support, long shoe counters to increase mid-foot support and control foot direction, heel flares to add stability, shank fillers or wedges to produce a total weight-bearing surface, steel plates to restrict motion, and rocker bars to prevent flexion and extension. Additional internal modifications include longitudinal arch pads, wedges, bars, lifts, and tongue or bite pads. Orthoses are available in rigid, semi-rigid, and flexible varieties, made from an array of materials, of which plastic, leather, and laminates are the most useful.

Medicare provides for what are termed *therapeutic shoes* (depth, super-depth, or custom) and multidensity inserts. To be eligible, patients must have a history of diabetes mellitus or other disease affecting foot health, evidence of a comprehensive management plan for the disease process that specifies that therapeutic shoes are needed, and documentation that he or she has one or more of the following conditions: peripheral neuropathy with evidence of callus formation, a history of pre-ulcerative calluses, a history of a previous ulceration, a foot deformity, previous amputation of all or part of the foot, or poor circulation. Appropriate footwear is effective in the prevention of serious foot complications.

REFERENCES

- Alexander I. *The Foot, Examination and Diagnosis.* 2nd ed. New York: Churchill Livingstone; 1997.

- Birrer RB, Dellacorte MP, Grisafi PJ. *Common Foot Problems in Primary Care.* 2nd ed. Philadelphia: Henley & Belfus, Inc.; 1998.

- Gray JA. Onychomycosis: new treatments are effective. *Clinician Reviews.* 2002;12(9):7–88.

- Helfand AE, ed. The geriatric patient and considerations of aging. *Clinics in Podiatric Medicine and Surgery.* Philadelphia: W.B. Saunders Co.; Vol I, January 1993; Vol II, April 1993.

- Helfand AE. Public health strategies to develop a comprehensive chronic disease and podogeriatric protocol. *National Academies of Practice Forum.* 1999;1(1):49–57.

- Helfand AE, Jessett DF. Foot problems. In: MSJ Pathy, ed. *Principles and Practice of Geriatric Medicine.* 3rd ed. Edinburgh: John Wiley & Sons; 1998:1165–1176.

CHAPTER 43—NEUROLOGIC DISEASES AND DISORDERS

A number of neurologic signs increase in frequency with age. One study of nearly 500 older adults noted that, among those over the age of 84 years, the following signs could not be attributed to a medical or a neurologic disease: diminished arm swing (present in 29% of those examined), diminished toe vibration sense (21%), hyperreflexia in arms (10%), unequal nasolabial folds (9%), absent pupillary response (9%), Babinski's sign (7%), diminished toe position sense (7%), and reduction in arm strength (5%). One implication of these findings is that the diagnosis of neurologic disease may be more difficult in the setting of these "normal" signs.

CEREBROVASCULAR DISEASES

Stroke is a leading cause of disability and death. The incidence of stroke increases with advancing age, approximately doubling with each decade. The incidence of stroke for men is 2.1 per 1000 at ages 55 to 64 years, 4.5 per 1000 at ages 65 to 74 years, and 9.3 per 1000 at ages 75 to 84 years. The incidence of stroke in women is 25% to 30% lower than that of men in comparable age groups, but it surpasses that of men in the group who are ≥ 85 years old.

Throughout the latter half of the century the incidence of stroke has decreased. This decline may be attributable to better control of modifiable risk factors. These risk factors include hypertension, heart disease, diabetes mellitus, cigarette smoking, elevated blood lipids, and alcohol use. Hypertension is the most prevalent risk factor for stroke, and its treatment results in a substantial reduction in the risk of stroke. Treatment of isolated systolic hypertension in older persons reduces the risk of stroke by nearly 40%. (See "Hypertension," p 256.) Heart disease is also an important risk factor for stroke, including atherosclerotic coronary heart disease, left ventricular hypertrophy, valvular heart disease, valve replacement, and valvular and nonvalvular atrial fibrillation. (See "Cardiovascular Diseases and Disorders," p 243.) Several studies have confirmed a two- to fourfold increased risk of stroke in patients with diabetes mellitus. Studies have suggested that tight control of blood sugar levels reduces the risk of stroke in patients with diabetes mellitus, although the evidence is less compelling than that for reduction of other vascular complications (eg, retinopathy, nephropathy) with tight glucose control. (See "Endocrine and Metabolic Disorders," p 319.) Cigarette smoking independently increases the risk of stroke as much as threefold, according to the Framingham Study. The incidence of stroke declines significantly even after 2 years of cessation of smoking, and after 5 years the level of risk returns to that of nonsmokers. Elevated blood lipids and alcohol use are other important risk factors for stroke. (See "Substance Abuse," p 234.)

The fatality rate within 1 month of an acute stroke is 20% to 30% across all age groups. Survival in part depends on the location and severity of the stroke. Common causes of death are myocardial infarction, arrhythmia, congestive heart failure, all due to comorbid coronary artery disease, and aspiration pneumonia. Age in itself does not influence the gross neurologic aspects of stroke, but older age is associated with lesser recovery in activities of daily living. Older stroke patients can benefit from formal rehabilitation.

Internal Carotid Artery Disease

A lesion in the internal carotid artery may present as transient monocular blindness (amaurosis fugax) or a cerebral hemispheric deficit (eg, focal motor, sensory, or cognitive symptoms or signs) because both the retina and cerebral hemispheres derive their blood supply from the internal carotid artery. Cerebral hemispheric deficits may include hemiparesis, hemisensory loss, aphasia, or apraxia. The initial evaluation of patients with these symptoms or signs usually includes a neuroimaging study (computed tomography or magnetic resonance imaging) and noninvasive imaging of the carotid arteries (B-mode ultrasonography and Doppler ultrasonography or magnetic resonance angiography). Data from the North American Symptomatic Carotid Endarterectomy Trial (NASCET) indicate that the optimal treatment for symptomatic carotid stenosis of greater than 70% is carotid endarterectomy, provided the patient has few comorbidities and the institution performs a high number of endarterectomies. The optimal treatment for symptomatic carotid stenosis of less than 70% or of asymptomatic carotid stenosis is still not clear; treatment options include carotid endarterectomy or medical management with antiplatelet agents (aspirin, clopidogrel) or anticoagulation (warfarin).

Aspirin is the mainstay of stroke prevention in cases of carotid artery disease where surgery is not indicated or is declined. Many studies on the use of aspirin in stroke prevention suggest that higher dosages than 325 mg of aspirin per day do not add therapeutic benefit, but the minimum necessary dosage has not been fully investigated. Many physicians routinely prescribe 81 to 650 mg per day; as little as 75 mg per day may be as effective, although even the lower dosage may also cause gastrointestinal irritative symptoms and blood loss. Clopidogrel 75 mg once daily is an alternative for patients who cannot tolerate aspirin. Warfarin is used for stroke prevention in older patients with atrial fibrillation.

Vertebrobasilar Arterial Diseases

Syndromes associated with vascular lesions in the posterior circulation (vertebral and basilar arteries) result in cranial nerve involvement or involvement of the descending motor or ascending sensory tracks within the brain stem. Because of the large number of pathways passing through the brain stem, vertebrobasilar occlusion may result in a myriad of syndromes, including drop attacks; abnormal eye movements; Horner's syndrome; motor and sensory abnormalities in the face, arm, or leg; and even stupor or coma. Treatment of posterior circulation cerebrovascular disease is medical, as no surgical approach to improving the posterior circulation has been shown to improve outcomes. Many clinicians prefer warfarin anticoagulation over antiplatelet agents for patients with vertebrobasilar disease. However, no formal studies have confirmed better clinical outcomes with warfarin.

Lacunar Disease

Lacunar disease, the occlusion of small penetrating vessels, is presumably the consequence of lipohyalinosis (lipid deposition and hyalinization). Lacunar strokes may result in several well-defined syndromes, including pure motor hemiplegia, pure hemisensory stroke, ataxic hemiparesis, and dysarthria–clumsy hand syndrome. Risk factors include hypertension and diabetes mellitus, and the most effective means of managing lacunar disease is aggressive treatment of these risk factors. Many clinicians prescribe aspirin for stroke prevention in patients who have suffered lacunar strokes, although it has not been shown to prevent lacunar strokes specifically. Lacunar strokes may occur independently or concurrently with large-vessel cerebrovascular disease.

Intracerebral Hemorrhage

Intracerebral hemorrhage accounts for 15% to 20% of all strokes. Approximately 80% occur during the 40s, 50s, and 60s. A racial distribution suggests that black Americans and Chinese Americans may be at slightly higher risk than white Americans.

The most common cause of intracerebral hemorrhage is hypertension, which accounts for 75% to 80% of the cases. Excessive use of alcohol is also associated with a higher incidence. Common locations for hypertensive bleeds are the putamen, thalamus, cerebellar hemisphere, pons, and cerebrum. Treatment is primarily control of hypertension and supportive care. In older patients a common cause of cerebral lobar hemorrhage is cerebral amyloid angiopathy, which usually occurs without systemic amyloidosis. In these cases intracranial bleeds tend to be recurrent. Acute treatment is supportive; prevention is limited to controlling hypertension.

Treatment

The current protocol for acute care of the older stroke patient includes optimizing hydration status; controlling blood pressure while avoiding acute hypotension; preventing deep-vein thrombosis; detecting and treating coronary ischemia, congestive heart failure, and cardiac arrhythmias; and initiating full anticoagulation in patients with nonhemorrhagic embolic strokes. For large embolic strokes (eg, involving most of the middle cerebral artery territory or involving both middle and anterior cerebral artery territories), one generally waits 48 hours before beginning anticoagulation. Dehydration on presentation is common, but rehydration must be gradual because of the risk of fluid overload. In patients with clinically evident cerebrovascular disease immediately after the occurrence of an ischemic cerebral infarction, it is appropriate to withhold treatment of hypertension (unless blood pressure is very high, eg, > 200/100 mm Hg) until the situation has been stabilized. Even when treatment has been withheld temporarily, the eventual goal is to reduce blood pressure gradually while avoiding orthostatic hypotension. The target systolic blood pressure should be 10 to 20 points higher than the patient's baseline pressure; if the baseline is unknown, systolic pressure should not be lowered beyond 160 mm Hg. Patients with acute ischemic stroke who are treated with fibrinolytic agents require careful blood-pressure monitoring, especially over the first 24 hours after treatment is started. Elevated blood pressure should gradually be brought down to the upper end of the normal range. Patients with a history of ischemic heart disease or arrhythmia and patients with large strokes should be monitored by electrocardiography for several days.

Many medical centers and clinicians are now using recombinant tissue–plasminogen (rt-PA) in the treatment of acute ischemic stroke. The benefits of this treatment, however, must be weighed against the increased the risk of intracranial hemorrhage, which can be fatal or can result in neurologic disability. If the patient presents within 3 hours of onset of stroke symptoms, has been assessed by a physician with expertise in stroke, and has CT evidence of less than major vessel infarction, thrombolysis with rt-PA should be considered.

EPILEPSY

A seizure is a paroxysmal excessive or hypersynchronous cerebral neuronal discharge, or both, that results in a transient change in sensation, motor function, and mental state. Recurrent seizures are the defining feature of epilepsy. Seizures may be broadly classified as partial (eg, simple focal seizures, partial complex seizures) or generalized (eg, absence attacks, generalized tonic-clonic seizures).

New-onset seizures occur in a bimodal pattern with respect to age, with an initial peak in incidence within the first year of life and a second peak after the age of 60 years. Disease-specific causes of epilepsy are more common in older adults, and one-half or more of older adult patients with new-onset epilepsy have an underlying cause. Common causes include vascular disease, neurodegenerative diseases, and brain tumors. Related to this is the observation that the incidence of partial seizures increases in older adults, whereas the incidence of generalized tonic-clonic seizures remains constant with respect to age. Beyond the age of 65, approximately one half of new-onset cases of epilepsy have a complex partial pattern. This pattern may be explained by the greater incidence of underlying focal lesions in older age groups.

Because of this propensity for new-onset cases of epilepsy to be harbingers of focal lesions, the work-up of older adults to exclude an underlying treatable cause is particularly important. The neurologic history and examination should aim to clinically characterize the seizure and localize its source, as well as elicit other signs of a focal lesion or a metabolic disturbance (eg, uremia, hepatic failure). Blood studies (blood urea nitrogen; serum levels of sodium, glucose, creatinine, magnesium, and calcium; and liver function tests), neuroimaging studies, and electroencephalogram (either a standard study with drowsiness or sleep, if possible, or a longer term 24- to 48-hour ambulatory monitoring) play important roles.

The treatment of epilepsy in older adults is particularly challenging, for a variety of reasons. First, the prevalence of adverse drug-disease and drug-drug interactions increases with age. For example, because of the tendency of lamotrigine to prolong the PR interval on the electrocardiogram, caution should be used when using it in patients with concomitant cardiac disease. Cimetidine and propranolol increase the serum concentrations of phenytoin and carbamazepine, respectively. Second, age-related changes in renal and hepatic function may alter drug metabolism significantly, so that older adults must often be placed on lower doses of antiepileptic drugs (AEDs). A sizable fraction of many AEDs is bound to plasma-binding proteins (eg, albumin). Since aging causes a reduced synthesis of albumin, it may be important to monitor free (unbound) levels of AEDs (eg, phenytoin). Third, older adults may be particularly sensitive to medication side effects. For example, AEDs may intensify an underlying dementia or exacerbate mild cognitive decline. Finally, there are a variety of reasons why older adults may have difficulty with adherence. It is particularly important in treating older adults to involve caregivers so that the goals of the treatment, side effects, and monitoring of progress may be understood.

There are a variety of AEDs, and most must be started slowly and the dose increased gradually (see Table 43.1). Reduction in seizure frequency and severity and the onset of side effects are the parameters that should be followed, not the blood level. If monotherapy has not adequately controlled the seizures and the dose has been maximized, then add-on therapy may be tried. Epilepsy surgery has become an increasingly common choice of patients whose seizures have proven refractory to pharmacologic management. Discontinuing AEDs should be considered if the patient has not had a seizure for several years, particularly if the original seizure activity was a single or poorly characterized event.

HEADACHES

There is evidence to suggest that the prevalence of headaches diminishes with age. One study demonstrated that although 74% of men and 92% of women between the ages of 21 and 34 years had headaches, these proportions dropped to 22% and 55% after the age of 75 years. Headache is one of the most common medical complaints in young persons, and yet one study suggests that it is the 10th most common symptom in older women and the 14th most common symptom in older men. Headache incidence also declines with age; only 2% of all sufferers of an initial migraine are over the age of 50 years.

Persistent headaches are more likely to represent systemic or intracranial lesions (ie, nonbenign conditions) in older adults than in younger adults. One study demonstrated that among younger patients, 10% of headaches represented systemic or intracranial lesions; in older adults, this proportion was 34%. These nonbenign conditions include intracranial masses (eg, primary or secondary tumors, subdural hematomas), cervical spondylosis, chronic obstructive pulmonary disease, carbon monoxide poisoning, and giant cell arteritis. In addition, many commonly used medications can cause headaches that are dull, diffuse, and nondescript, including vasodilators (eg, nitrates), hypotensives (eg, reserpine, atenolol, methyldopa), anti-Parkinsonian agents, and stimulants.

As in younger persons, the common primary headache disorders may be classified into migraines (with or without aura) and tension-type headaches. Migraines are often unilateral, pulsating headaches of moderate or severe intensity associated with nausea, vomiting, or photophobia. Auras, when they occur, usually precede the headache and are manifested by transient neurologic symptoms that are localizable to the cerebral cortex or brain stem. Visual phenomena

Table 43.1—Antiepileptic Therapy in Older Patients

Drug	Dosage (*mg*)	Target Blood Level (*µg/mL*)	Comments (Metabolism, Excretion)
Carbamazepine	200–600 bid	4–12	Many drug interactions; mood stabilizer; sustained-release form also available (L, K)
Gabapentin	300–600 tid	n.a.	Used as adjunct to other agents; adjust dose on basis of creatinine clearance (K)
Lamotrigine	100–300 bid	2–4	Prolongs PR interval; when used with valproic acid, begin at 25 mg qd, titrate to 25–100 mg bid (L, K)
Phenobarbital	30–60 bid–tid	20–40	Many drug interactions; not recommended for use in older patients (L)
Phenytoin	200–300 qd	5–20*	Many drug interactions; exhibits nonlinear pharmacokinetics (L)
Tiagabine	2–12 bid–tid	n.a.	Side-effect profile in older persons less well described (L)
Topiramate	25–100 qd–bid	n.a.	May affect cognitive functioning at high doses (L, K)
Valproic acid	250–750 bid–tid	50–100	Can cause weight gain; several drug interactions; mood stabilizer (L)

NOTE: K = metabolized via kidneys; L = metabolized via liver; n.a. = not available.

*Phenytoin is extensively bound to plasma albumin. In cases of hypoalbuminemia or marked renal insufficiency, calculate adjusted phenytoin concentration (C):

$$C_{adjusted} = \frac{C_{observed} \ (\mu g/mL)}{0.2 \times albumin \ (g/dL) + 0.1}$$

If creatinine clearance < 10 mL/min, use:

$$C_{adjusted} = \frac{C_{observed} \ (\mu g/mL)}{0.1 \times albumin \ (g/dL) + 0.1}$$

Obtaining a free phenytoin level is an alternate method for monitoring phenytoin in cases of hypoalbuminemia or marked renal insufficiency.

SOURCE: Adapted from Reuben DB, Herr K, Pacala JT, et al., eds. *Geriatrics At Your Fingertips*. 2003 ed. Malden, MA: Blackwell Science, Inc., for the American Geriatrics Society; 2003:102. Adapted with permission.

are among the most common types of auras. In contrast to migraines, tension-type headaches are often more diffuse, have a pressing or a tight quality, and are not associated with nausea or vomiting.

Headaches in older adults, however, may present in atypical ways. With migraines in particular, auras tend to disappear with age, and in some individuals, the reverse occurs (headaches disappear while auras remain). The occurrence of an isolated visual or sensory aura in the absence of a headache can be diagnostically challenging in the sense that these symptoms may be signs of transient ischemic attacks as well.

The treatment of headaches may be categorized as either abortive (ie, treating an attack that has already begun) or preventive. Apart from various over-the-counter preparations, abortive therapies include ergotamines or triptans (eg, sumatriptan, zolmitriptan), which act by central serotonergic mechanisms. These medications are available as injections, tablets, or nasal sprays. Though injections have the most rapid onset and carry the highest efficacy rates, oral and nasal preparations are more convenient. Preventive therapies include β-blockers (propranolol, timolol), valproic acid, methysergide, tricyclic antidepressants, calcium channel blockers, and selective serotonin-reuptake inhibitors. The choice of an agent should be guided by an effort to avoid side effects and drug interactions.

Older adults may not be tolerate headache medications as well as younger patients do; moreover, in some older patients a medication may be contraindicated by comorbidities or existing drug regimens. For example, β-blockers and tricyclic antidepressants, which are often used as preventive therapy, may be associated with lethargy or sedation, and the use of ergotamines and sumatriptan are contraindicated for patients with coronary artery disease.

MOVEMENT DISORDERS

A movement disorder may be defined simply as abnormal involuntary movements. These movements are not the result of weakness or sensory deficits; they are the result of dysfunction of the basal ganglia or the extrapyramidal motor system. Movement disorders may be classified as hyperkinesias (excessive movement) or hypokinesias (paucity of movement). A particular movement disorder (eg, Parkinson's disease) may be characterized by several types of involuntary movements (eg, tremor, bradykinesia, dystonia). Several movement disorders are especially common among older persons.

Essential Tremor

Essential tremor is the most common form of abnormal tremor. The tremor is an action tremor, which is present when the limbs are in active use (eg, while writing or while holding a cup). The tremor most commonly involves the arms, although the head and voice are also commonly involved. Other areas of the body may include the chin, tongue, and legs. The tremor is often slightly worse in one arm than in the other. One of the striking features of the tremor is that is has a varying amplitude so that during some moments the tremor is mild or even absent and during others it can be severe. The tremor disappears when the arms are relaxed, that is, when the person is sitting with hands in his or her lap or when standing or walking with arms held at the sides. Functionally, the tremor may interfere with many daily activities, such as eating, writing, or fastening buttons, and stress or anxiety can exacerbate the tremor. The frequency of the tremor is in the 4- to 12-Hz range; because age is inversely related to the frequency of the tremor, older persons have slower tremor, which is often in the 4- to 8-Hz range.

The prevalence of the disorder increases with advancing age, with as many as 1% to 5% of persons aged 60 years and older affected. The age of onset seems to have a bimodal distribution, with peaks in the teens and 20s and in the 50s through the 70s. The prevalence rates among men and women are similar, although head tremor may be more common among women.

Between 17% and 100% of affected persons report having an affected relative, which suggests that there is a familial form of the tremor. In some families, many individuals are affected over several generations. Familial forms of the tremor have been linked to regions on chromosomes 2p and 3q. There are no apparent clinical differences between the familial and sporadic forms of essential tremor. The cause of the sporadic form of the illness is not known; age is the only known risk factor for essential tremor.

It may be difficult to distinguish essential tremor from several other conditions. Physiologic tremor, which is present in all people, varies in amplitude, and it may be more noticeable in some individuals. It may also be enhanced by anxiety, stimulants, hypoglycemia, medications, or certain illnesses (eg, hyperthyroidism). The tremor is often faster than that of essential tremor (8 to 12 Hz) and the amplitude lower. Inertial loading during a tremor analysis recording may also reveal differences between the two conditions. Although patients with Parkinson's disease most typically have a tremor at rest, they may also have an action tremor, and in some instances have only an action tremor. In addition, if essential tremor is severe enough, it may even be present at rest. However, other features of Parkinson's disease (bradykinesia and rigidity) should not be present in persons with essential tremor.

The main indications for treatment of essential tremor are embarrassment and disability. The latter may manifest itself either as difficulty performing certain tasks such as eating and writing, the use of two hands to perform these tasks, modification in the way the task is performed (eg, only drinking with a straw out of closed cups), and even avoidance of certain tasks. Initial therapy includes β-blocking agents (eg, propranolol, atenolol), primidone, phenobarbital, diazepam, and newer agents, including gabapentin and clozapine. The response to these agents is patchy (ie, some patients experience moderate to marked improvement, whereas others experience none), and the tremor is rarely reduced to asymptomatic levels. Depression and male impotence are side effects of propranolol (less so with atenolol), and β-blockers are contraindicated for those with asthma. Primidone, phenobarbital, and diazepam are associated with unwanted sedation. Clozapine has been shown to be effective in one placebo-controlled trial, but there is a need to monitor the white blood cell count weekly because of the risk of agranulocytosis. Gabapentin has shown mixed results in placebo-controlled trials but is an attractive option, given the paucity of drug interactions or side effects. Some patients with severe, medically refractory tremor may undergo deep brain (thalamic) stimulator surgery in which the VIM nucleus of the thalamus is stimulated at high frequency with an implanted electrode. The treatment has been shown to be highly effective in controlling tremor.

Parkinson's Disease

Parkinson's disease is a progressive neurodegenerative disease in which cell death in the substantia nigra and consequent reduction in brain dopamine levels results in a constellation of signs, including tremor at rest, bradykinesia, rigidity, and postural instability. The pathologic hallmark of the disease is the Lewy body, an intracellular inclusion body found in the substantia nigra.

The incidence increases dramatically with age, and the incidence rate among people in their 70s and 80s in the United States is approximately 200 cases per 100,000 (0.2%). The incidence among those in their 70s and 80s in other countries (Iceland, India, Scotland, Australia) has been estimated to be even higher, approaching 1000 to 2000 per 100,000 (1% to 2%). The disease most commonly appears between the ages of 50 and 79 years. In a small proportion of cases, the disease clusters within families and has a genetic basis. In a small number of these families, the disease has been linked to a region on the long arm of chromosome 4 that encodes the neuronal protein α-synuclein.

In addition, environmental toxins (eg, manganese and pesticides) have been associated with some forms of the disease.

The disease begins insidiously and asymmetrically. The clinical manifestations include tremor, usually in one hand or sometimes in both, classically involving the fingers in a pill-rolling motion. The tremor (usually 3 to 5 Hz) is present at rest and usually decreases with active, purposeful movement. Muscular rigidity is usually readily evident on passive movement of a limb. Passive movement may demonstrate a smooth resistance or superimposed ratchet-like jerks (cogwheel phenomenon). The term *bradykinesia* is often used to describe either a slowness in initiating movement (ie, a paucity of spontaneous movements) or movements themselves that are slow, and the term *freezing* is used to describe sudden interruption of movement. Tachykinesia, which is the tendency for movements to become smaller and faster, may accompany speech (tachyphemia is the tendency during a sentence to speak more and more rapidly until all of the words run together into a mumble), handwriting (as the person attempts to draw loops across a page, the loops become smaller and tighter), gait (festination is the process by which the steps may inadvertently quicken and become smaller, and the patient may break into a run), and rapid finger taps in which the amplitude of the movements lessen and the movements become more rapid until the fingers seem stuck together. Postural abnormalities are evident in the erect and sitting positions; an erect posture is not readily assumed or maintained. The head tends to fall forward on the trunk. The tendency to fall forward (propulsion) or backward (retropulsion) results from the loss of postural reflexes. Bradykinesia prevents the patient from stopping the fall, either by taking a step or moving the arms. The face can become mask-like, with lack of expression and diminished eye blinking. Micrographia and difficulty with activities of daily living (eg, tying shoes) often develop.

Mood abnormalities, usually depression or anxiety, are common, as is cognitive impairment and dementia. These may place severe restrictions on the medications that might be used to relieve the tremor, bradykinesia, and rigidity.

One of the diagnostic challenges may be distinguishing mild early parkinsonism from the changes that often accompany normal aging (slowing down, loss of balance, stiffness, difficulty walking, stooped posture). However, the bradykinesia and rigidity of Parkinson's disease are usually asymmetric at onset, with one side slightly affected and the other remaining normal. In addition, tremor at rest is not a feature of normal aging, and although older persons may complain of stiffness, true extrapyramidal rigidity is uncommon.

The diagnosis is made clinically, although deoxyglucose positron emission tomography (FDG-PET) scan of the brain often reveals an abnormal pattern of increased glucose metabolism in the globus pallidum, which is characteristic of Parkinson's disease.

Treatment programs should be individualized. This caution applies especially to older adults, who have reduced tolerance for dopaminergic and anticholinergic agents, the mainstays of parkinsonism therapy. Nonpharmacologic therapy includes a regular exercise program. An older patient who is limber and active will have more reserve when facing a disease associated with progressively increasing stiffness and slowness. Many older patients benefit from a course of physical therapy aimed at restoring their confidence in walking and maintaining balance, as well as teaching them simple tricks to help them manage unpredictable and disabling freezing episodes, and, when needed, selecting a cane or walker of the appropriate size and weight. A home visit by an occupational therapist may help to plan the appropriate placement of wall rails, grab bars, and other such assistive devices that reduce the possibility of falling.

Treatment of the motor manifestations of parkinsonism is important, but many older patients also complain of difficulty with constipation and insomnia. Constipation is particularly bothersome to older patients taking levodopa, which tends to exacerbate the constipation associated with reduced levels of physical activity. Treatment includes a diet rich in fruit and fiber, prune and other juices, frequent consumption of liquids, and use of medications. It is important to emphasize to patients that they should take medications for constipation on a daily basis as part of a regular routine and not wait to take the medications as a response to severe constipation. One medication that is particularly effective is senna concentrate, one to six tablets per day. Older Parkinson's disease patients with insomnia should also be given individualized treatment. Some patients wake up at night because of a low dopamine state, which results in feelings of stiffness, malaise, low energy, and doom that are severe enough to awaken the patient from a light sleep. Higher bedtime doses of levodopa or even sustained-release forms of levodopa are appropriate. Patients may also experience insomnia because they are sleeping too much during the day, which may be a side effect of levodopa therapy. In these cases, it may be important to reduce the dosage of levodopa and correct the reversed sleep-wake cycle. Because urinary urgency may be a feature of Parkinson's disease, many patients must wake up at night to micturate, and this may be the cause of their frequent night-time awakenings.

Depression is also a common feature of parkinsonism. However, the side effects of many antidepressant medications limit their use, particularly the anticholinergic side effects of tricyclic antidepressants. The selective serotonin-reuptake inhibitors (including fluoxetine, sertraline, paroxetine) are preferred because of their favorable side-effect profiles.

The major factor impacting the treatment of older patients with Parkinson's disease is their propensity to develop confusion and toxic psychosis on antiparkinsonian medications. In general, the therapeutic regimen should be kept simple. Rather than prescribing small doses of multiple medications, prescribe higher doses of one or two medications; toxic side effects are less likely to occur. Levodopa provides the most improvement in the motor manifestations of Parkinson's disease relative to its toxic side effects on the central nervous system, whereas those with stronger anticholinergic properties (anticholinergic agents such as trihexyphenidyl and amantadine) provide the least benefit. The dopamine agonists (bromocriptine, pergolide, ropinirole, pramipexole) fall in between. Although low levels of toxic psychosis may be treated effectively with clozapine, olanzapine, or quetiapine, which have fewer extrapyramidal side effects than other antipsychotic agents, confusion and disorientation may be treated only by lowering the doses of antiparkinsonian medications. In this setting, anticholinergic medications should be the first to be discontinued, followed by selegiline, dopamine agonists, and, finally, levodopa.

The first step in treating the older patient with Parkinson's disease is to accomplish dopamine replacement by using levodopa combined with carbidopa. Levodopa is converted to dopamine in both the central nervous system and the periphery. To reduce peripheral conversion, use levodopa combined with carbidopa (a peripheral decarboxylate inhibitor), which does not cross the blood-brain barrier. Treatment usually begins with a half tablet of the 25:100 combination (ie, 25 mg carbidopa to 100 mg levodopa) once or twice a day. Every 1 to 2 weeks, the dose can be increased by one half to one tablet, to reach a dose of one full tablet three times a day, if needed and if side effects are tolerable. If disabling bradykinesia, rigidity, postural instability, or tremor are still present, the dose can be gradually increased further, with cautious observation of side effects. Older adults, particularly if cognitively impaired, rarely tolerate more than 1000 mg per day of levodopa. Common side effects include nausea, abdominal cramping, orthostatic hypotension, and confusion. A controlled-release form (25:100 and 50:200) generally requires a slightly higher total daily dose. Although levodopa is generally very effective in treating idiopathic Parkinson's disease, it is less effective in treating symptoms of secondary parkinsonism, which usually requires higher doses to achieve a mild benefit.

Levodopa-carbidopa is often given in combination with dopamine agonists (eg, bromocriptine, pergolide, ropinirole, pramipexole), although these other drugs may also be used as single therapies. A cautious induction period with each is required, as nausea, orthostatic hypotension, and confusion are common side effects. Bromocriptine is begun with 1.25 mg per day and gradually increased by 1.25-mg increments every 2 to 5 days, to a total daily dose of 10 to 30 mg. Pergolide is begun at 0.05 mg per day, with increments of 0.05 mg every 2 or 3 days until a daily dose of 1 to 3 mg is reached. Other newer dopamine agonists include ropinirole (given in starting dosages of 0.25 mg per day and increased as needed to dosages of 3 mg per day) and pramipexole (given in starting dosages of 0.125 mg per day and increased as needed to dosages of 4.5 mg per day). The latter two have been associated with sudden sleep attacks in which patients fall asleep at the steering wheel while driving. COMT (catechol O-methyltransferase) inhibitors such as tolcapone extend the benefit of levodopa-carbidopa by inhibiting the metabolic breakdown of dopamine.

Amantadine, a drug particularly useful for treating tremor, is generally prescribed at 100 mg two to three times daily. Amantadine's mild anticholinergic effects appear to play a role in its antiparkinsonian effects. It also promotes dopamine release in the corpus striatum.

Selegiline (a monoamine oxidase-B inhibitor) in dosages of 5 mg twice a day may be used in an early stage to prevent or slow disease progression. The drug inhibits oxidative metabolism of dopamine. Trials indicate that selegiline can delay the need for additional antiparkinsonian agents. However, whether selegiline slows the disease progression or just suppresses symptoms is controversial. The drug is generally well tolerated, although some patients may experience side effects, including nausea, insomnia, confusion, anxiety, and feeling "revved up." Although chemically related to other monoamine oxidase inhibitors, selegiline does not require dietary restrictions.

A new approach to replenishing the dopamine deficit by transplantation or grafting of fetal nigral cells to the corpus striatum shows promise, although data from a double-blinded, placebo-controlled trial are still being collected. Nigral cells harvested from aborted fetuses are stereotactically inserted in the striatum of patients with Parkinson's disease. These cells appear to remain viable, to form neural connections, and to be capable of producing dopamine. Other surgical therapies include stereotactic pallidotomy (primarily to reduce severe dyskinesias as well as improve bradykinesia and rigidity) and either thalamotomy or implantation of deep brain (thalamic) stimulator electrodes to treat disabling, pharmacologically refractory tremors.

Shy-Drager Syndrome

Shy-Drager syndrome is a multisystem degenerative disease with involvement of central (preganglionic) autonomic, cerebellar, basal ganglia, pyramidal, and spinal motor neurons. The major feature differentiating Shy-Drager syndrome from Parkinson's disease is the prominence and severity of the autonomic failure. The mean age of onset is 55 years, and more men than women are affected. No genetic predisposition has been shown. The disease is progressive, and death occurs 7 to 10 years after the onset of neurologic symptoms. Cardiac arrhythmias, aspiration, sleep apnea, and pulmonary emboli are common causes of death.

The major manifestation is autonomic insufficiency, with wide swings in blood pressure with little or no change in pulse rate. Patients complain of dizziness, lightheadedness, or syncope on standing, and of postexertional weakness, gait unsteadiness, and dimming of vision. Impaired temperature control, reduced sweating, sphincter disturbance with urinary or fecal incontinence, diarrhea, constipation, nocturnal diuresis, impotence, iridic atrophy, impaired eye movements, Horner's syndrome, and anisocoria may also occur. Central neuron degeneration is manifested by parkinsonian features, intention tremor, ataxia, dysarthria, and, in some cases, corticobulbar and corticospinal tract signs. Anterior horn cell degeneration leads to wasting and fasciculation of distal muscles. Intellectual and emotional function is preserved until late in the disease course. Laboratory studies are usually normal. The electromyogram may show anterior horn cell involvement.

Orthostatic hypotension is often the most disabling symptom. Nonpharmacologic treatment of the autonomic dysfunction includes avoiding large meals, getting up rapidly, and excessive straining at stool. Compressive clothing and elastic stockings, increased salt and fluid intake, and sleeping in a reverse Trendelenburg position may ameliorate some of the orthostatic symptoms. Drugs that are sometimes useful in treating the orthostatic hypotension include midodrine and fludrocortisone. Use of these medications sometimes results in supine hypertension so that blood pressure needs to be monitored closely. Treatment of the parkinsonism with dopamine agonists or with levodopa usually worsens the orthostatic hypotension.

Progressive Supranuclear Palsy

Progressive supranuclear palsy is a rare disorder characterized by parkinsonian symptoms, a supranuclear gaze palsy, square wave jerks (defined next page), and cognitive impairment. Approximately 4% of patients with parkinsonism have progressive supranuclear palsy. Onset usually occurs during or after the 50s. The pathogenesis is unknown. Evidence of a transmissible cause is lacking, and familial cases are rare. The disease usually progresses rapidly, with marked incapacity occurring within 3 to 5 years and death within 10 years, generally as a result of intercurrent infection or other complications of immobility.

Pathologic examination shows degenerative changes in the brain stem, diencephalon, basal ganglia, and cerebral cortex. Microscopic findings include nerve cell loss and neurofibrillary tangles, which are different from those seen in Alzheimer's disease.

The clinical manifestations include progressive impairment of voluntary gaze of supranuclear origin, with vertical-gaze palsy (downward more than upward) being most prominent. The progressive supranuclear palsy patient is unable to fully direct his or her gaze on command, but eye movements are less impaired when the patient's gaze is fixed on a point while the head is moved by the examiner. Square wave jerks (fixation instability) are also prominent. Other findings are gait unsteadiness with falling (often backward), dysarthria, dysphagia, rigidity, bradykinesia, deep nasolabial folds, and dystonic neck extension. Tremor at rest is often not prominent.

No fully effective treatment is available. Treatment with levodopa, amitriptyline, or anticholinergic medications may be partially effective, although the dramatic response to levodopa that is experienced by patients with Parkinson's disease is usually lacking. Idazoxan, an α_2 presynaptic inhibitor that increases norepinephrine transmission, may improve the motor manifestations of this disorder. Electroconvulsive therapy has been of limited benefit as well for improving bradykinesia, rigidity, and gait difficulties, although transient confusion is a common side effect.

Chorea

Chorea is a flowing, continuous, random movement that flits from one part of the body to another. A variety of conditions are associated with chorea in the older patient (Table 43.2). The pathologic basis for chorea is dysfunction of the striatum.

Choreiform movements that sometimes occur as an isolated symptom in persons 60 years and older are then called *senile chorea*. Involuntary complex movements of the face, mouth, and tongue may occur alone or with unilateral or bilateral limb movements. Neither mental disturbance nor family history of Huntington's chorea is associated with senile chorea. Pathologic findings often include degeneration of the putamen or caudate nucleus, or both.

Chorea may be treated with dopamine-receptor blocking medications (eg, haloperidol), but a potential side effect is tardive dyskinesia. Agents that block the release of dopamine presynaptically (eg, reserpine) are

Table 43.2—Conditions Associated With Chorea in Older Persons

Condition	Comments
Huntington's disease	Autosomal dominant condition, often with an age of onset in the 40s and 50s
Hyperthyroidism	Usually associated with other signs of hyperthyroidism
Medications	Dopamine replacement therapy, estrogen replacement therapy
Post-pump chorea	Following cardiopulmonary bypass surgery
Senile chorea	Movements of the face, mouth, and tongue
Vascular chorea	Usually unilateral in the setting of a stroke

another option, as they are not associated with tardive dyskinesias; however, reserpine can be associated with depression and orthostatic hypotension. Metyrosine is an agent that inhibits the enzyme tyrosine hydroxylase, which catalyzes the conversion of tyrosine to dihydroxyphenylalanine (DOPA). Therefore, metyrosine blocks the formation of dopamine and can be effective in treating chorea. Though not associated with tardive phenomena, the medication may cause some somnolence. All of these medications can produce parkinsonism as a side effect, which is usually dose-dependent and reversible when the medication is discontinued.

Drug-Induced Movement Disorders

A variety of different types of involuntary movements may arise as a result of the use of medications (Table 43.3). It is important to distinguish acute drug effects, chronic but reversible drug effects, and chronic and irreversible drug effects. The most common acute drug effect is an acute dystonic reaction that occurs with exposure to antipsychotic medications and often results in oral, lingual, or nuchal dystonia. If it is severe enough, treatment with intravenous diphenhydramine is required, although this approach in older adults should be exercised with caution, given the propensity for this agent to produce somnolence or confusion. Chronic reversible drug effects (effects that resolve upon discontinuation of the causative medication) include action tremor (eg, lithium, theophylline, valproic acid), parkinsonism (antipsychotic medications), chorea (estrogen, antiepileptic medications), or dystonia (dopamine replacement therapy in Parkinson's disease). Chronic irreversible drug effects or tardive phenomena often begin after the medication (usually an antipsychotic medication) has been in use for weeks to months. Movements may include orobuccal dyskinesias, dystonia, akathisia (sensation of needing to move), myoclonus, and tics. Advanced age and duration of treatment with antipsychotic medications are

Table 43.3—Movement Disorders Associated With Medications

Movement Disorder	Drug or Chemical
Action tremor	Bronchodilator inhalers
	Corticosteroids
	Lithium
	Methylxanthines (coffee, tea)
	Theophylline
	Thyroid hormones
	Valproic acid
Parkinsonism	Antipsychotic medications
	Calcium channel blockers
	Lithium
	Methyldopa
	Metoclopramide
	Reserpine
Chorea	Amphetamines
	Anticholinergic drugs
	Antiepileptic drugs
	Antiparkinsonian drugs
	Estrogen replacement therapy
Dystonia	Antipsychotic medications
	Dopamine agonists
	Levodopa replacement therapy

the only well-established risk factors for developing tardive movement disorders. Once the diagnosis of a tardive phenomenon is established, the clinician should attempt to reduce the dosage of medication or discontinue it. Treatment for tardive dyskinesia or tardive dystonia includes anticholinergic agents (trihexyphenidyl), baclofen, reserpine, or clozapine, each of which must be used with caution in older adults. In cases of severe tardive dystonia in which there is neck jerking or sustained eye closure, intramuscular injections of botulinum toxin may reduce the frequency and severity of movements. The Abnormal Involuntary Movement Scale (see the Appendix, p 424) can be helpful in assessing and monitoring drug-induced movement disorders.

MYELOPATHY

Myelopathy or spinal cord dysfunction is most often a result of either intrinsic or extrinsic compression of the spinal cord. The region most commonly involved in older patients is the cervical spinal cord. Intrinsic compression is often the result of spinal cord tumors or vascular events (infarcts or hemorrhages). Extrinsic compression is more prevalent; common causes among older patients are cervical spondylosis (with resultant osteophyte formation and degenerative disc disease), disc prolapse or herniation, rheumatoid arthritis resulting in vertebral body subluxation, or spinal metastases. Nearly 80% of patients aged 70 years or older have radiographic evidence of osteophyte formation with significant narrowing of the cord; the majority of these

cases are asymptomatic. Spinal stenosis is a congenitally abnormally narrow spinal canal. When disc protrusion occurs in a patient with spinal stenosis, it further compromises the capacity of a spinal canal that is already limited. Narrowing of the cervical canal may lead to neck stiffness and pain; radicular pain, sensory loss, or weakness in the arm; and weakness and upper motor neuron signs (hyperreflexia, spasticity, Babinski's sign) in the lower extremities. Narrowing of the lumbar canal may lead to lower back pain, to radicular pain, sensory loss, or weakness in the leg(s), and to upper motor neuron signs in the legs.

Other symptoms of spinal cord compression include gait disturbance, falls, or complaints of "numb, clumsy hands." On examination, the patient may exhibit spastic paraparesis (symmetric or asymmetric), sensory loss at a particular cord level, or problems with micturition.

Evaluation is most commonly in the form of magnetic resonance imaging of the spine. If the patient cannot tolerate this because of the presence of metallic objects, a pacemaker, or claustrophobia, then spinal computed tomogram with intrathecal contrast should be performed.

Conservative management, particularly if neck pain is an associated feature, includes activity modification, neck immobilization with a cervical collar, massage, heat treatment, physical therapy, and medications (muscle relaxants and pain medications including nonsteroidal anti-inflammatory agents). Decompressive surgery is recommended for persistent pain or a progressive neurologic deficit. Older patients are more prone to have multiple levels of involvement, and some studies have suggested that their prognosis after surgery is poorer than that of younger patients.

MOTOR NEURON DISEASE

Motor neuron disease (MND) is a neurodegenerative condition involving both upper and lower motor neuron cell bodies; it is characterized clinically by a progressive weakness and wasting of skeletal muscles, often in combination with bulbar palsy and respiratory failure. The incidence increases with age but reaches a plateau in the 60s. To date, age remains the single most clearly identifiable risk factor for this progressive and fatal disorder.

Patients frequently present with gait disturbance, falls, foot drop, weakness in grip, dysphagia, or dysarthria. On neurologic examination, patients may have a combination of weakness with upper motor neuron signs (hypertonia, hyperreflexia, clonus, extensor plantar responses) and lower motor neuron signs (atrophy, hyporeflexia). In addition, there are signs of involvement of the lower motor neuron cell bodies (fasciculations). Although cranial nerves may be involved, with resulting facial weakness, palatal weakness, and tongue weakness, the extraocular movements are usually spared. The electromyogram demonstrates findings consistent with diffuse denervation (diffuse fibrillation potentials, positive sharp waves) and poor recruitment of motor units. The differential diagnosis includes lesions at the level of the foramen magnum or the high cervical cord and vitamin B_{12} deficiency. The prognosis is poor, with the average survival on the order of 2 to 3 years. The presence of bulbar signs carries a poorer prognosis.

Although most new cases of MND occur in older adults, the incidence and prevalence of this disorder relative to other more common neurologic disorders is low. Therefore, gait disturbance and focal motor weakness may be attributed to the more common cerebrovascular diseases or to cervical radiculomyelopathy rather than to MND. Older adults are also more likely to have coexisting neuropathology, adding to the challenge of and delay in diagnosing MND. One study showed that those over the age of 65 years were diagnosed after 19 months, in comparison with those who were less than 65 years of age, who were diagnosed after 3 months.

The treatment is mostly supportive. Riluzole, which has demonstrated modest effects upon survival or time to tracheostomy, is now in widespread use. The action of riluzole is thought to protect against glutamate toxicity, which may be involved in the pathogenesis of MND.

Amyotrophic lateral sclerosis (ALS) is the most common neuron disorder and affects upper and lower motor neurons. The most common symptom onset with ALS patients is in the limbs. Approximately 25% present with bulbar symptoms. Bulbar symptoms frequently occur in older individuals and are the presenting sign in 50% of all patients. Rapid progression of ALS is associated with age of onset and the presence of bulbar symptoms. The diagnosis of ALS is made by history, examination, with blood and imaging studies to exclude other causes. Muscle denervation with preserved nerve conduction velocities are seen in an electromyogram. The treatment for ALS is consistent with other motor neuron diseases and focuses on supportive care.

RADICULOPATHY

Radiculopathy is a disruption of the peripheral nervous system at the level of the spinal roots after they exit the spinal cord. Among older adults, this may be the result of herniated discs or osteophyte formation. Symptomatic nerve root compression may result in complaints of pain radiating down the neck, back, arm, or leg, and on neurologic examination, this may be accompanied by motor and sensory deficits as well as diminution of reflexes in the distribution of a particular spinal root or roots.

PERIPHERAL NEUROPATHY

The prevalence of peripheral neuropathy in older adults has been estimated to be as high as 20%, and some degree of subclinical decrement in peripheral nerve function on electromyography is probably universal in healthy older adults. Peripheral neuropathy may be particularly devastating in older adults because of gait impairment due to sensory and motor deficits and thus a propensity to fall. In developed countries, diabetic neuropathy is the most common form of neuropathy, with up to 60% of patients who have diabetes mellitus and who are over the age of 60 years having a peripheral neuropathy. Several types of neuropathy are associated with diabetes mellitus, including a distal symmetric neuropathy, asymmetric neuropathies that may involve cranial nerves, roots, or plexus, and mononeuropathy multiplex. Other common causes of peripheral neuropathy in older adults are medications (eg, amiodarone, colchicine, phenytoin, lithium, vincristine, isoniazid), alcohol abuse, and nutritional deficiencies (eg, vitamins B_6 and B_{12} deficiency, as well as deficiencies of thiamine, folate, and niacin), renal disease (ie, uremia), monoclonal gammopathy (eg, multiple myeloma), and neoplasm (eg, infiltration of peripheral nerves by malignant cells, paraneoplastic syndromes associated with oat cell carcinoma of the lung, breast cancer, ovarian cancer, renal cell carcinoma, and prostate cancer).

The treatment of the neuropathy depends on the cause, ranging from withdrawal of the causative agent (alcohol, medications) to nutritional supplementation (nutritional deficiency), or treatment of the primary cancer (neoplastic neuropathy). There is some evidence that optimizing glucose control may lessen the severity of diabetic neuropathy. Treatment of neuropathic pain includes the use of tricyclic antidepressants, AEDs (eg, carbamazepine, phenytoin, clonazepam, gabapentin), selective serotonin-reuptake inhibitors, and topical agents. Topical agents include capsaicin analgesic cream and local anesthetic agents.

MYOPATHY

Myopathies are characterized by proximal muscle weakness, wasting, and diminished or absent reflexes, and they may be accompanied by elevations in serum enzymes (creatinine kinase) and a myopathic pattern on electromyogram and on muscle biopsy (ie, fiber degeneration follows a random pattern). Older adults may attribute mild or moderate muscle weakness to aging and therefore may not immediately consult a physician. Proximal muscle weakness, which results in difficulty rising from a chair, difficulty in climbing stairs, or difficulty washing the hair, is particularly likely to be attributed to aging or arthritis.

The most common myopathies in older adults are polymyositis, endocrine myopathies, toxic myopathies, and myopathies associated with carcinoma. Polymyositis is a disorder of skeletal muscle of diverse causes characterized by an infiltration of the muscles with lymphocytes. Muscle biopsy usually shows signs of degeneration, regeneration, and infiltration by lymphocytes. Treatment with prednisone should be used with caution in older adults because of its propensity to produce psychosis. In thyrotoxic myopathy, weakness and wasting are greatest in the pelvic girdle muscles and to some extent in the muscles of the shoulder region. Reflexes may be normal, and the diagnosis is made by the distribution of muscle weakness in a patient with thyrotoxicosis. Improvement of the myopathy follows treatment of the underlying endocrine disorder. Hypothyroidism may also cause a myopathy that improves with thyroid replacement therapy. Myopathy may occasionally be the result of a remote effect of a cancer (ie, a paraneoplastic disorder), with complaints of weakness often preceding the establishment of a diagnosis of cancer. Several drugs are known to cause myopathy, including corticosteroids, lipid-lowering agents, procainamide, and diuretics that produce hypokalemia.

SUBDURAL HEMATOMA

A collection of blood between the dura and the arachnoid is referred to as a *subdural hematoma*. It is usually due to head trauma, although the trauma may be mild, particularly in older adults. In approximately 15% of cases, the hematomas are bilateral.

Perhaps most relevant in the older patient is the chronic subdural hematoma. The incidence of chronic subdural hematoma increases with age, from 0.13 per 100,000 for those in their 20s to 7.4 per 100,000 for those in their 70s. In 50% of chronic subdural hematomas, there is no history of head injury, although other risk factors include clotting disorders, shunting procedures (eg, ventriculo-peritoneal shunting for normal-pressure hydrocephalus may separate the blood vessels from the dura, resulting in tears), and seizures.

The symptoms of chronic subdural hematoma are headache, slight or severe impairment in cognition, and hemiparesis. Some patients may have seizures. Focal neurologic signs (weakness, sensory loss, change in sensation) may be present. Neuroimaging studies reveal an extra-axial collection of blood.

The treatment of the hematoma varies, depending on whether it is symptomatic or an incidental finding on a neuroimaging study. If symptomatic and the patient's condition is worsening, then removal of the clot may be attempted. If asymptomatic or if the patient's condition is improving, then clinical monitoring is appropriate, as the hematoma may shrink and disappear without surgery.

RESTLESS LEGS SYNDROME

See "Sleep Problems" (p 201).

REFERENCES

- Cancellor AM, Hendry A, Caird FI, et al. Motor neuron disease: a disease of old age. *Scot Med J.* 1993;38:178–182.

- Caplan L. Cerebrovascular disease and stroke. In: Cassel CK, Cohen HJ, Larson EB, et al, eds. *Geriatric Medicine, 3rd ed.* New York: Springer-Verlag: 1997:923–938.

- Charles PD, Esper GJ, Davis TL, et al. Classification of tremor and update on treatment. *Am Fam Physician.* 1999;59(6):1565–1572.

- Edmeads J. Headaches in older people. *Postgraduate Medicine.* 1997;101:91–100.

- Odenheimer G, Funkenstein HH, Beckett L, et al. Comparison of neurologic changes in "successfully aging" persons vs the total aging population. *Arch Neurol.* 1994;51:573–580.

- Pancioli AM, Broderick J, Kothari R, et al. Public perception of stroke warning signs and knowledge of potential risk factors. *JAMA.* 2000;279:1288–1292.

- Wilmore JL. Management of epilepsy in the elderly. *Epilepsia.* 1996;37 (suppl 6):S23–S33.

CHAPTER 44—INFECTIOUS DISEASES

Infection is the major cause of mortality in 40% of those aged 65 years and older, and it contributes to death in many others. Infection is also a significant cause of morbidity in older adults, often exacerbating underlying illness or leading to hospitalization. Biologic, cultural, and societal factors all influence susceptibility to infection, the presentation of disease, and the management of infections in older adults.

PREDISPOSITION TO INFECTION

Fundamental alterations in the immune response occur with aging in large measure because of comorbidities, but also because of a phenomenon known as *immune senescence* (Table 44.1). The major features of immune senescence are depressed T-cell responses and T-cell–macrophage interactions (clinically reflected as delayed-type hypersensitivity responses). The cause(s) of immune dysfunction in older adults have yet to be elucidated fully.

Comorbidities have the greatest impact on those arms of the immune response that are not specific to a given organism or antigen: eg, skin integrity and cough or gag reflexes are local defense mechanisms that are often impaired. Perhaps the best example is chronic obstructive pulmonary disease, in which impaired mucociliary clearance and alveolar macrophage dysfunction are likely to be factors that increase the risk of lower respiratory tract infection. Comorbid diseases also indirectly complicate infections in older persons. For example, community-acquired pneumonia in otherwise healthy patients under age 50 is typically treated on an outpatient basis and rarely causes mortality; however, in older patients with community-acquired pneumonia and multiple comorbid conditions, the greatly increased risk of morbidity and mortality often necessitates hospitalization. Furthermore, cognitive impairment and other barriers to adherence may increase the difficulty of treating older patients, increasing complications and costs.

A major influence on immune function in the older person is nutritional status. Global (protein and calorie) undernutrition is present in 30% to 60% of persons aged 65 years or older on admission to the hospital. In the outpatient arena, 11% of older adults suffer from undernutrition, 90% of which is due to reversible underlying conditions (depression, poorly controlled diabetes mellitus, medication side effects). Delayed wound healing, increased risk of nosocomial infection, extended lengths of hospital stay, and increased mortality are all associated with malnutrition. Even mildly undernourished older adults (those with a

Table 44.1—Changes in Immune Function Associated With Aging

	Change With Age*		
	Direction	Degree	Comment
Innate immunity			
Skin, mucous membranes	decrease	+++	Skin thins and dries with aging
Complement		—	Most changes are due to comorbidity
Polymorphonuclear neutrophils			Most changes are due to comorbidity
Adherence, chemotaxis		—	
Ingestion		—	
Intracellular killing	decrease	+	Most changes are due to comorbidity
Adaptive immunity			
Thymic hormones	decrease	+++	
Lymphocyte subsets			
T cells		+++	Shift from naive to memory subtypes
Natural killer cells	decrease	++	Number increases, but function declines
Lymphocyte functions			
Proliferative responses	decrease	++	
Cytokine production, secretion			
IL-2, IL-2 receptor	decrease	+++	
IL-4	increase	++	
IL-6	increase	++	
IL-10	increase	++	
IFN-γ	increase	+	
PGE$_2$	increase	++	
Delayed-type hypersensitivity	decrease	++	
Autoimmunity	increase	++	Autoantibodies common, but of unclear significance

NOTE: — = no age-related changes; + = mild; ++ = moderate; +++ = marked; IL = interleukin; IFN = interferon; PGE$_2$ = prostaglandin E$_2$.

serum albumin of 3.0 to 3.5 g/dL) have evidence of immune compromise, poor vaccine responses, and diminished cytokine responses to specific challenges. Nutritional interventions may boost immune function in some older adults. One study demonstrated that vitamin E supplementation in older adults can augment delayed-type hypersensitivity and antibody responses. A second study using a multivitamin and mineral supplement showed a reduction in the median number of days of illness due to infection. Importantly, these two studies were performed in older adults who were not obviously vitamin deficient at the start of the trial, but additional studies are needed to define the role of multivitamin or specific nutritional supplements for augmenting immune response of older adults. (See "Malnutrition," p 182.)

Institutionalization places older persons at risk for epidemic disease. High levels of antibiotic use is a major risk factor for acquiring disease that is due to more resistant organisms. Methicillin-resistant *Staphylococcus aureus,* vancomycin-resistant enterococci, and multiply resistant gram-negative rods are more common causes of infection in institutionalized older persons. Resistance is fostered in the nursing home by debilitated hosts, close proximity of residents, and high levels of antibiotic use.

DIAGNOSIS AND MANAGEMENT OF INFECTIONS

Presentation

It has long been recognized that older adults commonly present with significant infection in the absence of classic signs or symptoms. Fever, the most readily recognized feature of infection, may be absent in 30% to 50% of frail, older adults with serious infections, even pneumonia or endocarditis. The cause of impaired febrile responses in older adults is incompletely understood, but diverse mechanisms of thermoregulation are involved, including blunted thermogenesis by brown adipose tissue.

Because of the altered febrile response to infection, many authors have suggested a redefinition of *fever* in older adults. Given the sensitivity, specificity, and positive and negative predictive values, fever in older nursing-home residents aged 65 and over can be redefined appropriately as a temperature > 2°F (1.1°C) over baseline (if a baseline is available) or, perhaps more practically, an oral temperature > 99°F (37.2°C) or a rectal temperature > 99.5°F (37.5°C) on repeated measures. This definition of fever has a sensitivity of 82.5% in nursing-home residents, and the specificity remains high at 89.9% (Table 44.2). Although these data were generated in a trial with frail, older, veteran men in a nursing home, it would seem reasonable to apply the same definitions to frail, older adults of either gender in the community. However, well older adults may be more appropriately managed by the use of conventional definitions of fever.

The absence of fever is only one way that infectious diseases may present atypically in the older person. For example, infective endocarditis may be heralded by a nonspecific decline in baseline functional status, such as confusion or falling. Subsequent anorexia and decreased oral intake may follow, and exacerbation of an underlying illness (eg, atrial fibrillation) may become the predominant feature. Cognitive impairment further contributes to the atypical presentation of infections in older adults. Many cognitively impaired older patients are unable to communicate symptoms accurately, and clinicians must be ready to pursue objective assessments such as laboratory and radiologic evaluations at a lower threshold, unless advance directives indicate otherwise.

Antibiotic Management

Drug distribution, metabolism, excretion, and interactions may be altered with age. Aging in the absence of any comorbid disease is associated with a reduction in renal function by about age 70, and antibiotic dose reductions may be required in the older patient. (See "Renal Diseases and Disorders," p 357.) Furthermore, antibiotic interactions occur with many medications commonly prescribed for older persons. Digoxin, warfarin, oral hypoglycemic agents, theophylline, antacids, lipid-lowering agents, antihypertensive medications,

Table 44.2—Defining Fever in Frail, Older Residents of Long-Term-Care Facilities

Definition	Sensitivity	Specificity	(+) Likelihood Ratio	(−) Likelihood Ratio
T > 101°F (38.3°C)	40.0%	99.7%	133	0.6
T > 100°F (37.7°C)	70.0%	98.3%	41	0.3
T > 99°F (37.2°C)	82.5%	89.9%	8	0.2

NOTE: (+) Likelihood ratio = sensitivity / (1−specificity); (−) Likelihood ratio = (1−sensitivity) / specificity; T = temperature.

SOURCE: Data from Castle SC, Yeh M, Toledo S, et al. Lowering the temperature criterion improves detection of infections in nursing home residents. *Aging Immunol Infect Dis.* 1993;4(2):67–76.

and H_2-receptor antagonists all have significant interactions with commonly prescribed antibiotics. Drug concentrations can increase (eg, enhanced digoxin toxicity associated with macrolides, tetracyclines, and trimethoprim) or decrease (eg, reduced absorption of fluoroquinolones [FQs] with antacids) with concomitant drug administration. Atrophic gastritis, a common problem in older adults, and H_2 blockers or proton pump inhibitors can reduce the absorption of some antibiotics, such as ketoconazole or itraconazole. Drug interactions, such as that between FQs and antacids, may also reduce absorption. Finally, adherence to prescribed regimens may be limited as a consequence of poor cognitive function, impaired hearing or vision, and multiple medications.

The choice and timing of antibiotics may also be important in the treatment of older infected adults. In sepsis, a preponderance of data suggests that initially broad coverage is warranted, since outcomes (mortality, length of stay in intensive care) are improved when the offending organism is covered by the initial antibiotic regimen. In older adults with pneumonia, data suggest that delaying initiation of therapy 8 or more hours after admission to the hospital is associated with an increased risk of mortality.

INFECTIOUS SYNDROMES

Bacteremia and Sepsis

Bacteremia is a common cause of hospitalization for older patients. Older patients with bacteremia are less likely than their younger counterparts to have chills or sweating, and fever is commonly absent. Gastrointestinal and genitourinary sources of bacteremia are more common; thus, the causative bacteria are more likely to be gram-negative rods.

Bacteremia carries a poor prognosis in older adults. For example, nosocomial gram-negative bacteremia carries a mortality rate of 5% to 35% for young adults, but in older adults the mortality rate is 37% to 50%. Major contributing factors include the more common use of invasive devices (eg, intravenous or urinary catheters) that make eradication of organisms difficult and coexisting diseases that reduce physiologic reserve.

The management of bacteremia and sepsis in older and younger patients is similar. Rapid administration of appropriate antibiotics aimed at the most likely sources is essential. Despite many randomized trials, there is still no proven immune modulatory therapy for sepsis.

Pneumonia

Patients aged 65 years and older account for more than 50% of all pneumonia cases, and annual hospital-ization rates for pneumonia range from 12 per 1000 among community-dwelling adults aged 75 and older to 32 per 1000 among nursing-home residents. Pneumonia mortality in older adults is approximately three to five times that of young adults, but the rate is profoundly influenced by comorbidity. Comorbidity is the strongest independent predictor of mortality in community-acquired pneumonia in older adults, with a relative risk of 4.1 (in the article that determined this relative risk, comorbidity was defined as cancer, collagen vascular disease, or advanced liver disease). Other independent risk factors include age of 85 years and older, debility (decreased motor function), serum creatinine > 1.5 mg/dL, and the presence of hypothermia (< 36.1°F), hypotension (< 90 mm Hg systolic), or tachycardia (> 110 beats per minute) on admission. Long-term follow-up data also suggest that community-acquired pneumonia in older adults indicates a higher risk of subsequent all-cause mortality over the next 12 years as a consequence of both recurrent pneumonia (relative risk 2.1 [1.3 to 3.4]) and cardiovascular disease (relative risk 1.4 [1.0 to 1.9]).

The causes of pneumonia in older adults differ from those of their younger counterparts. *Streptococcus pneumoniae* is still the predominant organism, but gram-negative bacilli (eg, *Haemophilus influenzae*, *Moraxella catarrhalis*, *Klebsiella* spp.) are much more common, particularly in patients with chronic obstructive pulmonary disease or who reside in long-term-care facilities. *S. aureus* and respiratory viruses are also common causes of community-acquired pneumonia in nursing-home residents (Figure 44.1).

Pneumonia therapy has changed significantly in the past few years because of the emergence of resistant bacteria, particularly drug-resistant *S. pneumoniae*, leading many practitioners to rely heavily on FQs, even for routine community-acquired pneumonia. This practice, however, has led to increased rates of FQ resistance in several areas of the world, and some FQs can have significant side effects, including dizziness and cardiac conduction abnormalities (QT prolongation), that may limit their use in certain older adults. The current Infectious Diseases Society of America treatment guidelines for community-acquired pneumonia suggest the following as first-line therapy in adults over the age of 60 with or without comorbidity: a β-lactam and β-lactamase combination or advanced-generation cephalosporin (ceftriaxone or cefotaxime) with or without a macrolide. Alternatively, one of the newer FQs with enhanced activity against *S. pneumoniae* (levofloxacin, sparfloxacin, moxifloxacin, gatifloxacin) may be used. Given the resistance already emerging to FQs, it is prudent to use these drugs only in situations with highest risk for drug-resistant *S. pneumoniae* or other resistant organisms. In the outpatient setting,

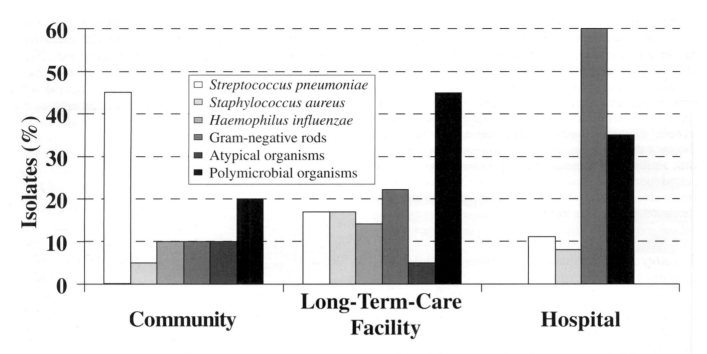

Figure 44.1—A specific cause for pneumonia is isolated only 30% to 50% of the time. Isolates here were pooled from several studies and were microbiologically confirmed. When a specific causative agent is identified, the predominant organisms vary by domiciliary setting, as indicated. Atypical organisms include *Mycoplasma pneumoniae*, *Chlamydia pneumoniae*, viruses, and rarely *Legionella* spp.

this is limited to residents of long-term-care facilities or patients with marked chronic obstructive pulmonary disease (FEV$_1$ < 30% predicted). In the inpatient setting, the sicker the patient (ie, the closer they are to needing intensive care), the stronger the justification for use of an FQ. This is true because the margin for error is small, FQs are currently the most effective therapy for drug-resistant *S. pneumoniae*, they are effective against most gram-negative bacilli, and they can be used to treat atypical organisms such as such as *Legionella* spp. that are more likely in the intensive-care setting.

The prevention of pneumonia in older adults is a complex issue, and a multipronged approach is most likely to be effective. Immunization of at-risk persons is far and away the most well-studied measure (see "Prevention," p 59). In addition to vaccines, smoking cessation and aggressive treatment of comorbidities (eg, minimizing aspiration risk in post-stroke patients, limited use of sedative-hypnotics) may reduce the risk of infection. Finally, system changes with attention to infection control (isolation, cohorting, skin testing for tuberculosis with purified protein derivative [PPD], and immunization policies) may be particularly effective in the nursing home.

Urinary Tract Infection

Urinary tract infection (UTI) is among the most common of clinical illnesses in older adults, with an incidence of 10.9 per 100 person years in men and 14 per 100 person years in women aged 65 and older. As in young adults, gram-negative bacilli (eg, *Escherichia coli*, *Enterobacter* spp., *Klebsiella* spp., *Proteus* spp.) are most common, but there is an increase in more resistant isolates, such as *Pseudomonas aeruginosa*, and gram-positive organisms, including enterococci, coagulase-negative staphylococci, and *Streptococcus agalactiae* (group B strep).

Asymptomatic Bacteruria

Up to 15% of women in the community and 40% of women in nursing homes will have asymptomatic bacteruria, whereas the incidence in men is approximately half that for women. Rates are even higher with the use of condom catheters (87%) or Foley catheters (nearly 100%). Numerous studies have suggested that there is no clinical benefit from the treatment of asymptomatic bacteruria, and that treatment is associated with significant side effects, expense, and the potential for selection of resistant organisms. Thus, no treatment is recommended. The clinical difficulty faced almost daily by clinicians is deciding what is symptomatic. The presentation of infection can be quite subtle in older adults, and a change in functional status often prompts the collection of a urine specimen even in the absence of fever, dysuria, or other typical clinical feature. However, since no controlled trial has ever shown a decreased incidence of urosepsis or mortality with antibiotic treatment of asymptomatic bacteruria, a period of observation rather than a therapeutic trial would seem most prudent when symptoms are not clearly related to bacteruria.

Urinary Tract Infection in Women

In contrast to asymptomatic bacteruria, symptomatic UTI does require therapy. Therapy is based on the location of infection (upper versus lower tract disease) and likely causative agent. Lower tract UTI (cystitis), characterized by dysuria, frequency, and urgency (note: not fever, which generally indicates upper tract disease) are often treated in young women for 1 to 3 days, but the efficacy of this practice for older women is not established. Most experts recommend 3 to 7 days of therapy for cystitis in older women, and culture is not required unless first-line therapy fails. Trimethoprim-sulfamethoxazole (TMP-SMX) is the drug of choice for patients who are not allergic to sulfa. Other reasonable choices include amoxicillin, first-generation cephalosporins, or FQs.

Upper UTI (pyelonephritis), characterized by fever, chills, nausea, and flank pain and commonly accompanied by lower tract symptoms, requires more prolonged therapy, 7 to 21 days. Because of the excellent bioavailability of many antibiotics, particularly the FQs, intravenous therapy is not essential if the patient can tolerate oral medications. A study comparing FQs to TMP-SMX for upper tract UTI in younger women (aged 18 to 58) suggests that FQs are more effective (microbiologic cure rate 99% versus 89% for TMP-SMX; clinical cure rates 96% versus 83%, respectively) because of the presence of TMP-SMX–resistant organisms. This is likely to be true in older adults as well, but, as noted above, FQs may have significant side effects in older adults and should be used with caution in this age group. Intravenous administration of antibiotics remains the standard of care for patients with suspected urosepsis, those with upper tract disease due to relatively resistant bacteria such as enterococci, or those unable to tolerate oral medications. Culture and sensitivity data are more useful in guiding antimicrobial therapy in upper tract UTIs than in lower tract disease and should be obtained in most cases.

Prophylactic antibiotics intended to prevent frequently recurrent UTIs in older women are not recommended because of the high incidence of the development of resistant organisms. Several measures may decrease the frequency of recurrence, including intravaginal or systemic estrogen replacement that changes the vaginal flora, thus reducing the risk of UTI, or ingestion of at least 300 mL of cranberry juice each day.

Urinary Tract Infection in Men

Prostatic disease (primarily hyperplasia) or functional disability, such as autonomic neuropathy from diabetes mellitus with incomplete bladder emptying, account for the majority of both lower and upper UTIs in older men. Thus, short-course therapy for UTIs in older men is inappropriate and should be avoided. A minimum of 14 days of therapy should be provided, and if prostatic involvement is suspected (ie, acute or chronic prostatitis), at least 6 weeks of therapy is usually required. The causative organisms and treatment choices are similar to those outlined above for older women. FQs and TMP-SMX are most widely used when prostatic involvement is suspected and culture data confirms the organism's susceptibility because, of the available agents, these two penetrate the prostate most adequately. Because treatment for all UTIs in men is generally longer than in women and the prostate is a common reservoir for recurrent UTIs, culture and sensitivity data should guide therapy for virtually all UTIs in men.

Tuberculosis

Worldwide, approximately 1.7 billion persons are infected with *Mycobacterium tuberculosis* (MTB), 16 million in the United States. Adults aged 65 and older account for one quarter of all active tuberculosis cases in the United States. The vast majority of active MTB in older adults occurs in community-dwelling persons aged 65 and over, but long-term-care residents represent a focus of particularly high risk: skin test studies show prevalence rates of skin test reactivity in the range of 30% to 50%. This high prevalence is due to MTB exposure in the early 1900s, when it was estimated that 80% of all persons were infected with MTB by the age of 30. Most active cases of tuberculosis in older adults are, therefore, due to reactivation disease, but primary infection may account for 10% to 20% of cases and is of particular concern in nursing-home outbreaks.

As with most other infections, tuberculosis may not present in classic fashion (cough, sputum, fever, night sweats, weight loss) in the older patient. Often fatigue, anorexia, decreased functional status, or low-grade fever are the presenting manifestation. Most tuberculous disease in older persons occurs with lung involvement (75%), and pneumonic processes in older adults, particularly those that occur in a postacute manner, should raise a high index of suspicion for MTB. Older adults are more likely than their younger counterparts to have extrapulmonary disease. Other sites include miliary (disseminated) disease, tuberculous meningitis or osteomyelitis, and urogenital disease, but virtually any body structure can be involved, and that organ system can account for the major presenting symptom.

A diagnosis of active disease usually requires isolation of the organism from sputum, urine, or other clinical specimen. Current techniques have improved the speed of diagnosis, particularly for identifying the species of *Mycobacterium* after isolation. This is now typically accomplished within 24 hours of obtaining a positive culture by use of DNA probes. Direct polymerase chain reaction of clinical specimens or other rapid diagnostic techniques are not available or reliable in most local laboratories, but such tests can be obtained in research settings. They are most likely to be helpful for establishing a diagnosis from cerebrospinal or pleural fluid, which yields positive cultures in only 10% to 15% of cases.

The most confusing area of MTB diagnostics for most practitioners is the interpretation of the results of PPD skin tests. In all populations, induration of ≥ 15 mm 48 to 72 hours after placement of a 5-tuberculin-unit PPD indicates a positive test. Induration ≥ 10 mm is considered a positive test in nursing-home residents, recent converters (previous PPD < 5 mm) under the age of 35, immigrants from countries with high endemicity of MTB, underserved populations in the United States (homeless persons, black Americans, Hispanic Americans, and Native Americans), and persons with specific risk factors (gastrectomy, > 10% below ideal body weight, chronic renal failure, diabetes mellitus, or immune suppression, including that caused by corticosteroids or malignancy). In patients infected with human immunodeficiency virus (HIV), those with a history of close contact with persons with active MTB, and those with chest radiographs consistent with MTB, ≥ 5 mm induration is considered a positive PPD test. Anergy panel testing in conjunction with PPD testing is of little value and is not recommended.

Long-term-care facilities should employ a two-step procedure for PPD testing during the initial evaluation of residents. Two-step testing requires retesting of patients with < 10 mm induration within 2 weeks. If the second skin test results in ≥ 10 mm of induration or the increase in the size of the induration from the first to the second skin test is ≥ 6mm, the patient is considered PPD positive.

The treatment of active MTB in the older person is similar to that in young adults. Four-drug therapy (usually isoniazid [INH], rifampin, pyrazinamide, and ethambutol or streptomycin) is recommended as initial therapy, with tapering to one of several two- or three-drug regimens once susceptibility testing is available. The most common regimen is INH, rifampin, and pyrazinamide for 2 months, followed by INH and rifampin for an additional 4 months.

Prophylaxis with 6 to 12 months of INH for asymptomatic persons with a positive PPD should be provided *regardless of age* in adults who are recent converters (defined in persons > 35 years of age with a PPD that has gone from < 10 mm to ≥ 15 mm within 2 years), or regardless of duration of PPD positivity if one is afflicted with any of the specific risk factors highlighted above. A patient with a positive PPD of unknown duration does not require INH prophylaxis in the absence of one of the indicated conditions. Close monitoring of patients on antituberculous therapy for symptoms and signs of peripheral neuropathy (due to INH and preventable by coadministration of pyridoxine) and hepatitis (due to INH, rifampin, or pyrazinamide) is recommended.

Infective Endocarditis

Since the early part of the 20th century, infective endocarditis (IE) has undergone a transformation, from a disease of young adults primarily due to rheumatic or congenital valve anomalies to one of older adults associated with degenerative valvular disorders and prosthetic valves. Native-valve endocarditis is typically caused by viridans streptococci, *S. aureus,* and occasional infections due to HACEK organisms (a group of typically nonfermenting gram-negative rods that primarily inhabit the oral cavity and include the genuses *Haemophilus, Actinobacillus, Cardiobacterium, Eikenella, Kingella*). Gastrointestinal and genitourinary organisms, such as enterococci and gram-negative rods, are more common in native-valve IE in older adults, and coagulase-negative staphylococci are a frequent cause of prosthetic-valve endocarditis, particularly in the first 60 days following placement of a prosthetic valve.

The diagnosis of endocarditis is often difficult in the older patient. Fever and leukocytosis are less common in older than in younger patients, occurring in only 55% and 25%, respectively, versus 80% and 60%, respectively. Blood culture positivity rates do not vary by age; however, degenerative, calcific valvular lesions and prosthetic valves lower the sensitivity of transthoracic echocardiography (TTE) to 45% in older patients sensitivity is 75% in younger patients. Transesophageal echocardiography (TEE) improves the diagnostic yield for IE, but the absence of positive findings on TEE never excludes IE. TEE is of particular value in resolving the clinical problem of *S. aureus* bacteremia. Positive findings on TEE support prolonged antibiotic administration (4 to 6 weeks) versus short-course (2-week) therapy. On the other hand, TEE is invasive and expensive. Interestingly, age does not appear to play a major role in mortality risk, with a 2-year survival of 75% for IE in all age groups unless major comorbidities are also present.

Antibiotic treatment of IE is directed at the identified pathogen or the most likely causes, if blood cultures are negative. Therapy is administered intravenously for 2 to 6 weeks. Surgical therapy should be considered for severe valvular dysfunction, recurrent emboli, marked heart failure, myocardial abscess formation, fungal endocarditis, or the failure of appropriate antibiotics to sterilize blood cultures.

Effective prophylaxis is available for bacterial endocarditis in at-risk patients undergoing dental, upper respiratory tract, gastrointestinal, or genitourinary procedures. Recommendations for endocarditis prophylaxis have been published and are widely available (eg, the American Heart Association, see http://www.americanheart.org).

Prosthetic Device Infections

Permanent implantable prosthetic devices are common in the ≥65 age group. Prosthetic joints, cardiac pacemakers, artificial heart valves, intraocular lens implants, vascular grafts, penile prostheses, and a variety of other devices are more often placed in older than in younger adults. A discussion of all prosthetic device infections is beyond the scope of this chapter, but several general concepts can be summarized.

Prosthetic device infections are usually separated into early versus late infection because the causative agents differ significantly. Early prosthetic device infection (PDI), most commonly defined as occurring less than 60 days after device implantation, is primarily due to contamination at the time of implantation or events associated with the acute hospitalization (such as occult bacteremias due to intravenous catheters).

In general, hardware removal is required to clear PDIs. However, early antibiotic intervention, in some instances combined with aggressive surgical drainage, may be successful. Patients should be referred to an infectious disease specialist for consultation. Infected prosthetic devices are usually surrounded by microbial biofilms, such as microbe-derived glycocalyx. Biofilms reduce antibiotic penetration and greatly increase the bactericidal concentrations of antibiotic without changing the inhibitory concentrations (ie, the amount of drug necessary to inhibit the organism does not change, but it takes tremendously increased concentrations to kill the organism). Furthermore, many conditions associated with infected prostheses are also accompanied by poor blood flow to the area. Thus, it is preferable to use bactericidal antibiotics, often in combination with a second agent that penetrates biofilms and poorly perfused areas (eg, rifampin for staphylococci).

The use of prophylactic antibiotics in situations other than prosthetic heart valves remains a point of contention. Antimicrobial prophylaxis is indicated for dental, gastrointestinal, and genitourinary procedures for patients with prosthetic valves and is probably reasonable for vascular grafts, particularly within the first few months after placement, but no randomized, controlled trial has ever clearly shown benefit. The need for prophylaxis for patients with prosthetic joints, intraocular lens implants, cerebrospinal fluid shunts, breast implants, or less common prostheses is even less clear.

Bone and Joint Infections

Native bone and joint infections in the absence of prostheses occur in older adults. Septic arthritis is more likely to occur in joints with underlying pathology (rheumatoid changes, gout, osteoarthritis), and early arthrocentesis is indicated in any mono- or oligo-articular syndrome to exclude infection. *S. aureus* is the most likely pathogen, with rare infections due to gram-negative bacilli and streptococci. Aggressive antibiotic therapy combined with serial arthrocentesis may be as effective as open surgical drainage in uncomplicated septic arthritis, and it preserves better functionality in the joint. Surgical drainage is required for patients failing this more conservative strategy.

Osteomyelitis in older adults can be due to hematogenous seeding from a bacteremia or contiguous spread from an adjacent focus. *S. aureus* is the predominant organism, but gastrointestinal and genitourinary flora are again more common in older adults and emphasize the advantage of a specific microbiologic diagnosis to guide therapy. Infections of pressure ulcers and diabetic foot infections are very common, particularly in institutionalized older adults, and they frequently require surgical consultation combined with aggressive antimicrobial therapy aimed at mixed aerobic and anaerobic bacteria.

HIV Infection and AIDS

HIV infection in older adults was initially limited to those who had received blood transfusions for surgical procedures. However, older Americans with HIV have increasingly acquired their infection via sexual activity. Adults aged 65 and over constitute approximately 10% of all new diagnoses of acquired immunodeficiency syndrome (AIDS) in the United States, but this group suffers from a lack of HIV awareness among their medical providers. Nonspecific symptoms such as forgetfulness, anorexia, weight loss, and recurrent pneumonia are often dismissed as age-related, and HIV testing can be delayed. HIV infection in the older person tends to pursue a more rapid downhill course, perhaps because of impaired T-cell replacement mechanisms with advanced age and the impact of additional comorbidities. Antiretroviral therapy with combination treatment regimens and opportunistic infection prophylaxis is similar to that used in younger persons. Indications that HIV therapies may accelerate atherosclerosis and glucose intolerance suggest that an aggressive approach to cardiovascular prevention in older HIV-infected adults is warranted.

HIV prevention is rarely discussed in the geriatric community but is important if the trend of sexual acquisition of HIV in older adults is to be reversed. Most older women do not feel they are at risk for HIV infection, yet heterosexual activity is the primary mode of infection in this group. The concept of HIV-risky behavior is not pervasive in the geriatric community because HIV was not a problem during their adolescence or young adulthood. Older persons must be included in educational programs aimed at ensuring safe sexual practices and increasing awareness of the benefits of testing and effective HIV therapy.

Miscellaneous Infectious Syndromes

Bacterial meningitis is most common at the extremes of life, and older adults account for the majority of meningitis-associated fatalities. *S. pneumoniae* remains the most common cause in older adults, but gram-negative bacilli (20% to 25%), *Listeria* spp. (up to 10%), and tuberculosis are more common than in young adults. Because many *S. pneumoniae* are now resistant to β-lactam antibiotics (up to 30% penicillin resistance and 10% ceftriaxone resistance nationwide), ceftriaxone or cefotaxime *plus* vancomycin are recommended as empiric therapy for bacterial meningitis in older adults until a specific isolate can be tested for antimicrobial susceptibility. Ampicillin is the drug of choice for *Listeria* spp., and more resistant gram-negative rods (eg, *Pseudomonas* spp.) require ceftazidime or an extended-spectrum penicillin with or without intrathecal aminoglycoside therapy.

Neurosyphilis remains one of the most perplexing diagnoses in medicine. It is often raised as a possible underlying process in stroke or dementia in older adults. Syphilis should also be considered in unilateral deafness, gait disturbances, uveitis, and optic neuritis. A positive cerebrospinal fluid VDRL is diagnostic of neurosyphilis, but the sensitivity of this test is approximately 75% in most series. Other diagnostic tests are controversial. The ratio of intrathecal to serum-specific treponemal antibody (standardized to the total immunoglobulin G in cerebrospinal fluid and serum) may also be helpful, with ratios of 3.0 or greater indicating likely infection. Optimal treatment of neurosyphilis remains penicillin G, but a study in HIV-infected patients suggests that ceftriaxone may be an acceptable alternative.

Advancing age is the major risk factor for reactivated varicella-zoster virus, herpes zoster or "shingles"; the most disabling complication, post-herpetic neuralgia, is common in older persons. (See "Dermatologic Diseases and Disorders," p 372, for diagnosis and treatment.)

Facial nerve palsy (Bell's palsy) is common in older adults and associated with at least three infectious causes: herpes simplex virus, varicella zoster virus, and *Borrelia burgdorferi* (which causes Lyme disease). There are no strong data, at present, to suggest benefit of antiviral therapy for facial nerve palsies due to herpes simplex virus, but trials are under way. If facial nerve palsy occurs as part of an episode of varicella zoster virus, treatment is indicated as outlined above. If Lyme disease is suspected on a clinical basis, the patient should receive 14 days of oral amoxicillin, 500 mg four times a day; or doxycycline, 100 mg twice a day; or intravenous ceftriaxone, 2 g per day.

Gastrointestinal infections are common among older persons. Diverticulitis, appendicitis, cholecystitis, intra-abdominal abscess, and ischemic bowel can present particular diagnostic dilemmas in the absence of fever or elevated white blood cell counts. A high index of suspicion is necessary in older adults. Computed tomography or labeled white cell studies are most likely to be of value in establishing the diagnosis of intra-abdominal infection, and ultrasound is an easy, readily available tool to assist in diagnosing cholecystitis, appendicitis, or abscess. Ischemic bowel often requires angiography.

Infectious diarrhea is also common in older persons. Older patients with achlorhydria are at particular risk because a lower bacterial inoculum is necessary to cause disease. Decreased intestinal motility associated with specific medications and advanced age may further increase susceptibility to infection. Epidemics occurring in the long-term-care setting are commonly due to *E. coli*, viruses, salmonellae, or *Shigella* spp. Frequent use of antimicrobials in older adults also increases the risk for *Clostridium difficile* colitis. Standard therapies for infectious diarrhea should be used in older patients.

FEVER OF UNKNOWN ORIGIN

Fever of unknown origin (FUO) is currently defined as temperature greater than 38.3°C (101°F) that lasts for at least 3 weeks and is undiagnosed after 1 week of medical evaluation. Several studies have examined this syndrome in older patients and demonstrated interesting differences between older and younger adults. The cause of FUO can be determined in more than 90% of cases in older persons, and one third have treatable infections, such as intra-abdominal abscess, bacterial endocarditis, tuberculosis, perinephric abscess, or occult osteomyelitis, with an incidence of infection similar to that in younger patients. In contrast, collagen vascular diseases are more common causes of FUO in older than in younger patients. These are primarily due to giant cell arteritis, polymyalgia rheumatica, and polyarteritis nodosa, but rarely due to Wegener's granulomatosis. In several published series, more than 25% of all FUOs in older persons were due to collagen vascular diseases (Table 44.3). Neoplastic disease accounts for another 20%, but, with rare exception, fever due to cancer is primarily confined to hematologic malignancies (eg, lymphoma and leukemia), and not solid tumors. Drugs are another cause of FUO in older persons. Rare causes in this age group include deep-vein thrombosis with or without recurrent pulmonary emboli and hyperthyroidism.

A diagnostic approach to FUO in older adults is presented in Table 44.4.

Table 44.3—Fever of Unknown Origin in Older Adults

Causes	Approximate % of Cases
Infections	35
Intra-abdominal abscess	12
Infective endocarditis	10
Other	7
Tuberculosis	6
Collagen vascular disorders	28
Giant cell arteritis, polymyalgia rheumatica	19
Polyarteritis nodosa	6
Other	3
Malignancy	19
Lymphoma	10
Carcinoma	9
Others (pulmonary emboli, drug fever)	9
No diagnosis	5–10

SOURCE: Data pooled from multiple studies: Esposito AL, Gleckman RA. Fever of unknown origin in the elderly. *J Am Geriatr Soc.* 1978;26(11):498; Knockaert DC, Vanneste LJ, Bobbaers HJ. Fever of unknown origin in elderly patients. *J Am Geriatr Soc.* 1993;41(11):1187–1192.

Table 44.4—Evaluation of Fever of Unknown Origin in Older Adults

1. Confirm fever; conduct thorough history (include travel, MTB exposure, drugs, constitutional symptoms, symptoms of giant cell arteritis) and physical examination. Discontinue nonessential medications.
2. Initial laboratory evaluation: CBC with differential, liver enzymes, ESR, blood cultures × 3, PPD skin testing, TSH, antinuclear antibody, consider antineutrophilic cytoplasmic-antibody or HIV-antibody testing in specific cases.
3. a) Chest/abdomen/pelvic CT scan—if no obvious source; *or*
   b) Temporal artery biopsy—if symptoms or signs consistent with giant cell arteritis or polymyalgia rheumatica and increased ESR; *or*
   c) Site-directed work-up on basis of symptoms or laboratory abnormalities, or both.
4. If 3a is performed and no source is found, then 3b, and vice versa.
5. a) BM biopsy—yield best if hemogram abnormal—send for H&E, special stains, cultures, *or*
   b) Liver biopsy—very poor yield unless abnormal liver enzymes or hepatomegaly.
6. Indium-111 labeled white blood cell or gallium-67 scan—nuclear scans can effectively exclude infectious cause of FUO if negative.
7. Laparoscopy or exploratory laparotomy.
8. Empiric trial—typically reserved for anti-tuberculosis therapy in rapidly declining host or high suspicion for tuberculosis (ie, prior [+] PPD).

NOTE: BM = bone marrow; CBC = complete blood cell count; CT = computed tomography; ESR = erythrocyte sedimentation rate; FUO = fever of unknown origin; HIV = human immunodeficiency virus; H&E = hematoxylin and eosin stain; MTB = *Mycobacterium tuberculosis*; PPD = (tuberculin) purified protein derivative; TSH = thyroid stimulating hormone.

REFERENCES

■ AIDS among persons aged > 50 years—United States, 1991–1996. *MMWR Morb Mortal Wkly Rep.* 1998;47(2):21–27.

■ Bentley DW, Bradley S, High K, et al. Practice guideline for evaluation of fever and infection in long-term care facilities. *J Am Geriatr Soc.* 2001;49(2):210–222.

■ Brown S. Systematic review of nursing management of urinary tract infections in the cognitively impaired elderly client in residential care: is there a hole in holistic care? *Int J Nurs Pract.* 2002;8(1):2–7.

■ Conte HA, Chen Y, Mehal W, et al. A prognostic rule for elderly patients admitted with community-acquired pneumonia. *Am J Med.* 1999;106(1):20–28.

■ Talan DA, Stamm WE, Hooton TM, et al. Comparison of ciprofloxacin (7 days) and trimethoprim-sulfamethoxazole (14 days) for acute uncomplicated pyelonephritis in women: a randomized trial. *JAMA.* 2000;283(12):1583–1590.

■ Zimmerli W, Widmer AF, Blatter M, et al. Role of rifampin for treatment of orthopedic implant-related staphylococcal infections: a randomized controlled trial. *JAMA.* 1998;279(19):1537–1541.

CHAPTER 45—RESPIRATORY DISEASES AND DISORDERS

AGE-RELATED ALTERATIONS IN PULMONARY PHYSIOLOGY

Older persons often present clinicians with special challenges because of age-related differences in the presentation of common respiratory illnesses, as well as notable differences in their management. As a consequence of age-associated alterations in connective tissue and the development of emphysema or bronchiolar injury, the older person's airway size decreases and the alveolar sacs become shallow. Chest wall compliance is reduced because of kyphoscoliosis, calcification of the costal cartilage, and arthritic changes in the costovertebral joints. Diaphragmatic strength is reduced by 25%, and intercostal muscle atrophy also develops after the 40s. The sum effect of these processes results in a decline of forced vital capacity and FEV_1 of 25 to 30 mL per year in nonsmokers and approximately double that (60 to 70 mL per year) in smokers. The normal A-a gradient increases with age and can be approximated by the following formula: (age / 4) + 4. The Pao_2 also decreases with age and can be approximated by the following equation: $Pao_2 = 110 - (0.4 \times age)$. Age-specific alterations in pulmonary function are complicated by important comorbidities commonly experienced by older persons, including smoking-related diseases, occupational and industrially related exposures, and other significant organ dysfunction, such as congestive heart failure or deconditioning.

COMMON RESPIRATORY SYMPTOMS AND COMPLAINTS

There is a common misperception that older persons tend to exaggerate pulmonary symptoms. In reality, however, older persons often adjust their activity level to compensate for insidiously shrinking lung function and disabling dyspnea. Such changes in life style often go unnoticed by family members, the patient's physician, and even the patient. Many clinicians consequently tend to underestimate the magnitude of dyspnea in older adults, and too often these patients present with advanced disease. The clinician should maintain a high level of suspicion for pulmonary or cardiac disorders, or both, whenever modifications in an older person's life style become apparent. Another complicating feature of symptom recognition in older persons is that they commonly have more than one explanation for their problems. Overlapping symptoms of dyspnea, cough, wheezing, and choking may occur because an older patient has a combination of diseases, such as asthma or emphysema, obstructive sleep apnea, congestive heart failure, and a hiatal hernia.

Although dyspnea may be overlooked even with significant disease, it becomes the overriding symptom of patients with end-stage lung diseases, such as chronic obstructive pulmonary disease (COPD) and idiopathic pulmonary fibrosis. The level of dyspnea is the best predictor of quality of life, yet it does not correlate with either oxygenation or pulmonary function tests. Rather than subject the patient to a myriad of potentially harmful and expensive diagnostic tests to determine the cause of dyspnea, the clinician should rely instead on a thorough history and physical examination to tailor both testing and empirical treatment choices. For example, in an older person presenting with dyspnea and associated nocturnal cough, one would first consider common diseases such as asthma, emphysema, allergic rhinitis with postnasal drip, and gastroesophageal reflux disease. Minimal testing (eg, pulmonary function tests only) followed by an empiric trial directed toward the most likely cause would be a reasonable approach. In the same patient, significant weight loss or constitutional symptoms (fever, night sweats) would make one consider other diseases, such as malignancy or tuberculosis. Less common yet important differential diagnostic considerations of wheezing and cough in older persons would include drug effects (eg, angiotensin-converting enzyme inhibitors), "cardiac asthma," laryngeal dysfunction, *Bordetella pertussis* infection, postviral cough or secondary bacterial infections, recurrent aspiration, bronchiectasis, airway tumors, and pulmonary embolism.

MAJOR PULMONARY DISEASES IN OLDER PERSONS

Asthma

After childhood, there is a second peak in the prevalence of asthma beyond the age of 65, with 5% to 10% of older persons meeting criteria for obstruction and bronchial hyperreactivity. The rate of death from asthma has increased most significantly in those aged 65 or over, accounting for up to 45% of all asthma deaths. This is likely due to the patient's reduced awareness of bronchial constriction (with delays in seeking medical attention), as well as under-recognition and undertreatment on the part of clinicians. Therapy of asthma in older persons differs in several ways from that in younger patients. Inhaled corticosteroids (see next section) or other controller drugs such as leukotriene receptor antagonists represent the mainstay of therapy. Cromolyn and nedocromil are adjunctive therapies for the prevention of asthma and exercise-induced bronchospasm. They are not bronchodilators and should not be used to treat acute asthma attacks. Theophylline is fraught with side effects and drug interactions, and it should be considered a third-line drug used only as a daily medication in the evening for severe asthmatics or emphysema patients, targeting a level of 10 to 12 mg per dL. It is controversial whether the response to β-agonists varies with age, but these drugs remain a mainstay as an as-needed reliever medication. The adverse effects of β-agonists, such as hypokalemia or possible QT prolongation in cardiac patients on digoxin or other medications, warrant care in their use for asthmatic patients to minimize excessive reliance on β-agonists. The importance of adequate instruction in the proper use of peak expiratory flow monitoring (because of a decreased perception of bronchoconstriction by older patients) and activation of the metered-dose inhaler cannot be overemphasized. It is well documented that neurologic, muscular, and arthritic diseases can lead to suboptimal timing and discoordination in the older person's actuation of the inhaler device. A clinician should check the patient's ability by observing him or her actually using the inhaler.

Emphysema or COPD

COPD affects approximately 15 million people in the United States and is the fourth most common cause of death after heart disease, cancer, and stroke. Its prevalence and mortality rate are increasing, especially in older persons. Episodes of acute respiratory failure that require mechanical ventilation have hospital mortality rates ranging from 11% to 46%. The costs of care for COPD are astounding, and the National Lung Health Education Program Executive Committee has noted that the morbidity and mortality of COPD account for more than $15 billion per year in U.S. medical care expenditures. Hospitalization continues to represent the largest component of cost for COPD patients. Efforts to keep COPD patients out of the hospital by improved outpatient management would potentially reduce costs and improve quality of life for older persons with this disease. The salient issues concerning the presentation of dyspnea, wheezing, cough associated with emphysema, and other overlapping comorbid illnesses are discussed above. Regarding the use of the clinical examination to diagnose air-flow limitation, the following points are worth noting:

- No single item or combination of items from the clinical examination excludes air-flow limitation.

- Wheezing noted on physical examination is the most potent predictor of air-flow limitation, and patients with obstructive air-flow limitation are 36 times more likely to have wheezing than are patients without this problem.

- Other findings associated with an increased likelihood of air-flow limitation include a barrel-shaped chest, hyperresonance on percussion, and a forced expiratory time of greater than 9 seconds measured during the clinical bedside examination.

- The best finding associated with decreased likelihood of air-flow limitation is a history of never having smoked cigarettes (especially in patients without a history of wheezing and without wheezing on examination).

Smoking cessation at any age has been shown to slow the decline in lung function, and aggressive cessation efforts are appropriate even in the oldest-old persons. The basic elements of the approach are the "Four *A*'s" (see Table 45.1).

The chief components of daily drug therapy for emphysema consist of a β-agonist, ipratropium bromide, or both drugs in combination. For more severe disease, the use of long-acting β-agonists, such as salmeterol, along with a combined albuterol and ipratropium bromide metered-dose inhaler can achieve long-term control and improved adherence. Inhaled corticosteroids have now been tested in several multicenter randomized, controlled trials for COPD with negative results overall; however, there does appear to be a benefit in subgroup analyses of patients with "asthmatic COPD," as defined by pulmonary function tests with documented bronchodilator responsiveness (see the asthma section, above, for issues related to β-agonist and theophylline use by elderly persons). One investigation documented that the use of systemic corticosteroids (intravenous followed by oral) reduced the duration and recurrence of acute exacerbations of COPD for up to 6 months. There was no benefit to a course of systemic corticosteroids

Table 45.1—The "Four *A*'s" of Smoking Cessation

Ask the patient about smoking cessation.

Advise the patient to quit.

Assist the patient in the quit attempt with aids, such as a local cessation program, and pharmacologic agents, such as bupropion, buspirone, or nicotine replacement.

Arrange both a quit date and a follow-up visit or contact to discuss the quit attempt.

SOURCE: The Agency for Health Care Policy and Research Smoking Cessation Clinical Practice Guideline. *JAMA.* 1996;275(16):1270–1280. Reprinted with permission. ©1996, American Medical Association.

longer than 14 days. For the few (5% to 10%) patients who do benefit from chronic use or who require prolonged use of corticosteroids, the risks should be considered, discussed, and documented. This risk list should include (but not be limited to) peptic ulcer disease, hypertension, cataracts, diabetes mellitus, osteoporosis, psychosis, seizures, poor wound healing, infections, and aseptic necrosis of the hip. Appropriate preventive measures should also be taken in these circumstances of prolonged use. For example, osteoporosis prevention would consist of the use of the lowest possible dose of corticosteroids and supplemental vitamin D, calcium, weight-bearing exercise, and bisphosphonates; peptic ulcer disease prevention, the avoidance of nonsteroidal anti-inflammatory drugs.

Other possible therapies for older emphysema patients include pulmonary rehabilitation via exercise training and respiratory therapy and education. Major depression and anxiety have each been shown to occur in up to 40% of COPD patients, and treatment of these problems must be addressed. In fact, unprovoked, episodic, and transient anxiety attacks that resemble posttraumatic stress disorder often result in patients' unnecessarily seeking help in emergency departments, being admitted to the hospital, and being treated with potentially avoidable courses of oral corticosteroids.

Obstructive Sleep Apnea

Sleep-related breathing disorders are very common in persons 65 years and older (up to 40%), and obstructive sleep apnea may be present in as many as one in five older patients. Obstructive sleep apnea has been associated with cerebrovascular accidents, myocardial infarctions, and a threefold increase in mortality, which may be greater in the older age group because of its frequent occurrence as a comorbid condition in this patient population. Most patients with obstructive sleep apnea remain undiagnosed and therefore without treatment of this life-threatening, yet potentially correctable disease. A helpful mnemonic to screen for obstructive sleep apnea in the midst of a busy clinical practice is the "I SNORED" (see Table 45.2). In a recent investigation of 251 patients evaluated for sleep disturbed breathing, 6 of 7 positive answers to this "I SNORED" mnemonic were found to have a 100% positive predictive value. In this study, the highest prevalence of disease (75%) occurred in the 60 patients older than 60 years. Treatment options include addressing upper airway obstruction, losing weight, avoiding alcohol and sedatives, sleeping on one's side or upright, correcting metabolic disorders such as hypothyroidism, and using continuous positive airway pressure (CPAP) with a nasal mask. Treatment issues

Table 45.2—The "I SNORED" Screen for Obstructive Sleep Apnea

Insomnia
Snoring
Nocturnal awakenings or Not breathing at night
Obesity
Restorative sleep or do you feel Refreshed in the morning?
Excessive daytime somnolence (eg, falling asleep on the phone)
Driving difficulties due to sleepiness, as well as Drugs that might affect sleepiness or keep you awake

SOURCE: Data from Namen AM, Haponik EF, McCall Z, et al. I SNORED: An acronym of sleep disordered breathing symptoms. *Am J Respir Crit Care Med.* 2001; 163:A387.

are generally the same for young and old patients, and the major consideration for the clinician is to remain alert for signs and symptoms of this underdiagnosed disease.

Idiopathic Pulmonary Fibrosis

There are more than 100 causes of restrictive lung diseases. The history, examination, serologic testing, and biopsy often leave the patient with the diagnosis of idiopathic pulmonary fibrosis. This disease is increasing in prevalence with the aging population, and in rare situations it can be an inherited disorder. Pulmonary fibrosis exhibits relentless progression and a median survival of 3 to 5 years. The presentation is normally one of insidious dyspnea (often unrecognized because of a decrease in the patient's activity level) and cough. Clubbing is commonly a prominent finding on physical examination in idiopathic pulmonary fibrosis, as opposed to emphysema, which rarely causes clubbing (prompting a search for another disease such as occult lung cancer). Three to 6 months of oral corticosteroids (0.5 mg per kg per day) is the initial therapeutic maneuver most commonly taken, yet only 10% to 20% of patients respond. Early referral to a subspecialist is warranted if the patient wishes to consider further therapeutic attempts, so that steroid-sparing agents such as azathioprine or enrollment into a randomized, controlled trial of newer pharmacologic agents (eg, interleukin-10 or interferon gamma) can be considered.

Pulmonary Thromboembolism

The incidence of pulmonary thromboembolism triples between the ages of 65 and 90 years and has a reported 10% recurrence rate within 1 year. Age greater than 70 years has been independently associated with missed antemortem diagnosis. It is important to realize that 10% to 20% of patients with documented pulmonary embolism have an entirely normal blood gas. Realization of this fact may help avoid a missed diagnosis. General risk factors are well recognized, but age-specific risk factors are often present as well, such as hypercoagulability due to increases in fibrinogen, malignancy, stasis (decreased mobility due to stroke, heart failure, or arthritis), or vessel injury (due to trauma or varicosities). The diagnostic work-up, which is beyond the scope of this chapter, does not differ for young and the old patients. Anticoagulant therapy is imperative and generally is guided by the same principles in young and old patients; however, with less cardiopulmonary reserve, the older patient must achieve therapeutic levels of heparinization quickly to avoid major adverse hemodynamic or oxygenation defects. The trend toward increased utilization of outpatient low-molecular-weight heparin preparations, while achieving anticoagulation with warfarin, is supported by large and appropriately designed randomized, controlled trials. There should be an overlap of approximately 1 to 3 days between heparinization and adequate warfarin therapy, with an international normalized ratio target of 2 to 3. Duration of therapy for 6 months has been shown to be superior to a duration of 3 months, and the shorter duration should be used only for those with either a specific risk factor that is now removed or those in whom the risk of prolonged anticoagulant therapy clearly outweighs that of completing 6 months of therapy. Indeed, patients with multiple ongoing risk factors for pulmonary thromboembolic disease are to be considered for anticoagulation therapy indefinitely. (For oral anticoagulation guidelines, see the Appendix, pp 406–407.)

Pneumonia

See "Infectious Diseases" (p 293) and "Eating and Feeding Problems" (p 191).

Lung Cancer

See "Oncology" (p 349).

MECHANICAL VENTILATION IN CRITICAL ILLNESS

Data from the Study to Understand Prognoses and Preferences for Outcomes and Risks of Treatments (SUPPORT) showed that physician error rates in approximating patient's preferences for mechanical ventilation increased from 36% at age less than 50 up to 79% at age greater than 80. Furthermore, SUPPORT data also showed that age was a predictor of less aggressive care in the intensive care unit (ICU) even after adjusting for severity of illness, gender, race, and diagnosis. A report from a cohort of mechanically ventilated patients in a medical ICU, on the other hand, showed that persons older than 75 years spent the same amount of time on the ventilator as did younger patients, but had a lower cost of ICU and in-hospital care. These outcomes were not explained by differences in mortality, since both groups had similar survival rates. Accordingly, the decision to use mechanical ventilation should not be based on age alone, and the appropriate use of ventilatory support in the older patient requires further prospective evaluation.

When the potential benefits of ICU care and mechanical ventilation are chosen to treat an older person with respiratory failure, special issues concerning weaning from the ventilator appear to be important. In contrast to the general medical ICU population mentioned above, patients with acute lung injury and acute respiratory distress syndrome do appear to have a steadily higher mortality with each decade of life. Research suggests that older adults recover from other pulmonary physiologic abnormalities, such as hypoxemia and ventilatory disturbances, as often as their younger counterparts, but they require more time to be weaned from mechanical ventilation. Despite similar rates of recovery for many pulmonary problems requiring mechanical ventilation, older adults in the ICU often succumb to other nonpulmonary conditions. Therefore, clinicians should pay particular attention to other nonpulmonary conditions commonly seen in older ICU patients. Specific examples of precautions include the judicious use of sedative and analgesic medications and monitoring for persistent delirium, occult systolic or diastolic heart failure, hypothyroidism, electrolyte disturbances, oropharyngeal dysfunction and aspiration due to support devices or cerebrovascular accidents, and malnutrition, each of which can develop rapidly in the hospital setting.

PREOPERATIVE PULMONARY EVALUATION

There are many tools to determine the perioperative risk factors for cardiac complications; however, the development of pulmonary complications has been less extensively studied. In reality, the development of pulmonary complications is at least as common (if not more so) than cardiac complications.

The independent importance of age in the development of postoperative pulmonary complications has not been studied in a manner that would control for coexisting conditions. The presence of COPD has been determined to carry a threefold higher risk of postoperative pulmonary complications. There are no data to support the notion that age-related changes in lung function increase postoperative pulmonary complications. Even among those with severe COPD, age has not been shown to be an independent risk factor for pulmonary complications. Much like the situation with mechanical ventilation (discussed above), chronologic age is less predictive of pulmonary postoperative complications than are coexisting conditions. Therefore, advanced age alone should not be a reason to withhold the benefits of contemporary surgical procedures from an older person. Routine perioperative pulmonary function tests have not been shown to result in better outcomes in the general older adult population. Rather, these tests should be performed selectively in patients who demonstrate significant risk for adverse outcomes.

Postoperative pulmonary complications have been reported to prolong the hospital stay of older patients by an average of 1 to 2 weeks. The in-hospital mortality rate for those with postoperative respiratory failure is around 40%, versus 5% for those without respiratory failure. Potential patient-related factors for the development of postoperative pulmonary complications include smoking, comorbidity, age, obesity, COPD, neurologic status, cardiovascular status, and intravascular volume shifts. Procedure-related risk factors include the site of the incision, length of the surgery, and type of anesthesia. The risk of pulmonary complications increases as the incision approaches the diaphragm, with upper abdominal and thoracic procedures carrying the greatest risk (10% to 40%).

REFERENCES

■ Chan ED, Welsh CH. Geriatric respiratory medicine. *Chest.* 1998;114(6):1704–1733.

■ Ely EW, Evans GW, Haponik EF. Mechanical ventilation in a cohort of elderly patients admitted to an intensive care unit. *Ann Intern Med.* 1999;131(2):96–104.

■ Ely EW, Wheeler AP, Thompson BT, et al. Recovery rate and prognosis in older persons who develop acute lung injury and the acute respiratory distress syndrome. *Ann Intern Med.* 2002;136(1):25–36.

■ Johnson AP. The elderly and COPD. *J Gerontol Nurs.* 1988;14(12):20–24.

■ Lynn J, Ely EW, Zhong Z, et al. Living and dying with chronic obstructive pulmonary disease. *J Am Geriatr Soc.* 2000;48(5 suppl):S91–S100.

■ Niewoehner DE, Erbland ML, Deupree RH, et al. Effect of systemic glucocorticoids on exacerbations of chronic obstructive pulmonary disease: Department of Veterans Affairs cooperative study group. *N Engl J Med.* 1999;340(25):1941–1947.

■ Smetana GW. Preoperative pulmonary evaluation. *N Engl J Med.* 1999;340(12):937–944.

The oral cavity is responsible for initiating food intake, producing speech, and protecting the alimentary tract and upper airway. Dysfunction and disease in the mouth can profoundly affect overall health and social functioning, and may be particularly important for older patients who are frail or nutritionally at risk. Findings prevalent in older patients (eg, decay, missing teeth, periodontal disease, and salivary hypofunction) do not represent normal aging, and patients with such findings should be urged to seek preventive and therapeutic care.

THE AGING OF THE TEETH

Most age-related changes in teeth are subtle (see Table 46.1) but become significant in the presence of environmental factors or disease. For a combination of reasons, the teeth of an older person are typically less sensitive or wholly insensitive to temperature changes and, importantly, to the sensations that commonly herald dental disease in younger adults. It is not uncommon to observe profound yet asymptomatic untreated dental disease in an older person's mouth.

DENTAL DECAY

Dental *caries*, or decay, is a bacterially derived demineralization and cavitation that can attack teeth throughout the life span. *Recurrent caries* refers to decay at the interface between a dental restoration (such as a filling or crown) and the tooth. (See Figure 46.1 for the anatomy of the tooth.) Older persons have more restored teeth (and usually the restorations are older and more extensive) and thus are more likely to have recurrent caries. The teeth of older persons may feature more caries of the root surfaces than are typically observed in younger persons because prior periodontal disease exposes the root surface, thereby predisposing it to demineralization and increased risk for caries. Both recurrent and root caries are generally asymptomatic and may become advanced before discovery, often resulting in destruction of much or all of the tooth.

Advanced caries commonly results in necrosis of the remaining pulp, which usually leads to acute or chronic dental abscess. Even if such infections do not cause pain, they should not be ignored, since severe metastatic infections of dental and oral origin have been reported in virtually every organ system. In particular, α-hemolytic (viridans) streptococci of the oral cavity have long been implicated in close to one third of the cases of bacterial endocarditis reported annually in the United States, and bacteria associated with dental abscesses (eg, *Staphylococcus aureus*) have been cultured from the aspirates of infected hip arthroplasties.

The risk factors for dental caries are the same at any age, but many of the risk factors increase in prevalence as people age. A primary risk factor is poor oral hygiene, which often occurs in an older person when visual acuity, manual dexterity, or upper-extremity flexibility is impaired, or when salivary flow is diminished. Another risk factor is frequent ingestion of sticky foods with a high content of sucrose, such as cake, candy, and cookies. Other risk factors include infrequent dental visits because of financial, access, or educational barriers; the presence of permanent or removable artificial teeth (more common with increasing age); and limited lifetime exposure to fluoride, widely used in the United States only in the past four decades. White older Americans display a higher incidence of root caries than either older black Americans or older Hispanic Americans, but they are more likely to have received dental treatment for the lesions.

Table 46.1—The Clinical Significance of Selected Age-Related Changes in Oral Tissues

Tissue Affected	Nature of Change	Clinical Significance
Tooth dentin	Increased thickness	Diminished pulp space
	Diminished permeability due to sclerosis of dentinal tubules	Diminished sensitivity of dentin; diminished susceptibility to effects of bacterial metabolites; increased tooth brittleness
Dental pulp	Diminished volume	Diminished reparative capacity; diminished sensitivity and alteration in nature of sensitivity
	Shift in proportion of nervous, vascular, and connective tissues	Diminished reparative capacity; diminished sensitivity and alteration in nature of sensitivity
Salivary glands	Fatty replacement of acini	Possibly less physiologic reserve

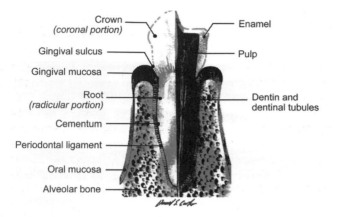

Figure 46.1—Dental and periodontal anatomy.

The prevention of caries involves daily oral hygiene with fluoride toothpaste, limitation of sugar intake, and regular dental examinations. Treatment of dental caries includes high-potency fluoride for remineralization, removal of demineralized tooth structure ("drilling"), and replacement with fillings or crowns. When caries involves the dental pulp, root canal treatment becomes necessary. This in turn usually requires reinforcement of the remaining tooth structure with a crown ("cap").

DISEASES OF THE PERIODONTIUM

The investing tissues of the teeth, termed the *periodontium*, consist of the gingiva, the alveolar bone, and a collagenous sleeve (termed the *periodontal ligament*) located between the tooth root and the surrounding bone. Periodontal disease occurs when microorganic colonies (*plaque*) form on the teeth near the gingiva and between the gingiva and the root surface within the gingival sulcus. The most common form of periodontal disease is gingivitis, in which the inflammatory reaction to plaque is limited to the gingiva. Gingivitis develops more rapidly in healthy older adults than in younger ones, but in both groups the changes—including gingival edema and light bleeding on brushing—are rapidly reversible following removal of plaque. If the inflammatory process extends to the periodontal ligament and alveolar bone, the process is termed *periodontitis*. In periodontitis there is destruction of the hard and soft tissues of the periodontium. In most adults periodontitis is a process marked by long periods of disease quiescence punctuated by bursts of localized destructive inflammation. Surveys demonstrate that 20% to 40% of dentate adults have active periodontitis at any point in time. By their 50s, more than 90% of Americans with teeth show 2 mm or more of lost alveolar bone height, the primary marker of prior periodontal disease activity. In advanced cases of periodontitis, the decreased support around a tooth leads to its malposition, loosening, and eventual loss.

Epidemiologic data support the concept that those who reach advanced age without significant periodontal bone loss will not likely experience a worsening of the disease in senescence. In contrast, other adults who have experienced a more rapid rate of bone loss commonly will have lost teeth in their 40s and 50s. In addition to age, risk factors for periodontitis include smoking and poor oral hygiene. Black and Hispanic Americans have a significantly higher prevalence of advanced periodontitis than do white Americans. Preventing gingivitis and periodontitis is largely a matter of oral hygiene and regular dental examinations and cleanings. Managing periodontal disease involves debriding the roots below the gingiva, which may require surgical access. Topical antibiotics (chlorhexidine, tetracycline) and systemic antibiotics (minocycline, metronidazole) are increasingly used as an adjunct to other periodontal therapy.

Periodontitis has been long reported to be worse in patients with poorly controlled diabetes mellitus. Investigations also support the contention that periodontitis, as an active infection, impairs diabetic control. Periodontal disease may be rapidly destructive in a patient whose immune system is impaired by disease or immunosuppression therapy. Epidemiologic data also correlate osteoporosis and tooth loss due to periodontitis. Periodontal disease and the pathogens responsible for it have been linked epidemiologically and immunologically with peripheral vascular disease, cerebrovascular disease, and pneumonia. Similar correlations have been reported for coronary heart disease, although one report disputes this. There is also epidemiologic association between gram-negative pneumonia, gram-negative periodontal pathogens, salivary hypofunction, and impaired swallowing function.

Prevention and control of periodontal disease revolve around daily oral care: tooth brushing and flossing to remove bacterial plaque on the teeth, particularly within the gingival sulcus. Regular dental evaluation, every 6 to 12 months, is important to ensure that the periodontium is healthy or to provide early intervention if it is not.

TOOTHLESSNESS

Advanced age was once considered synonymous with the need for false teeth, but that stereotype has passed. In the early 1960s more than 70% of adult Americans aged 75 or over were edentulous. By the 1990s fewer than 40% of this group were edentulous, most likely because of exposure to some level of preventive and restorative dental care in childhood or early adulthood.

Nevertheless, removal of one or more teeth in an older adult may be necessitated by various combinations of physiologic and behavioral factors. The leading cause is inability or unwillingness to access and pay for restorative dental treatment in the face of a symptomatic dental disease, usually stemming from dental caries. A second common cause is loosening of teeth due to periodontal disease to the point that mastication becomes painful or ineffective, or both. The third common cause is removal of otherwise healthy teeth that, because of the absence or loss of other teeth for the preceding or other reasons, would hinder the fabrication or function of a dental prosthesis.

Nearly 50% of Americans aged 85 and over have no natural teeth, and there are unique problems associated with the edentulous state. Functionally, the teeth aid in mastication and enunciation. Aesthetically, the teeth support the lips and cheeks and keep the nose and chin at a fixed distance apart. When a person has lost all teeth and there are no prosthetic replacements, the facial appearance is dramatically changed because of the lack of tissue support and diminished vertical height in the lower half of the face. Chewing ability is severely compromised, yet the impact on nutritional intake is difficult to characterize. One longitudinal study employing diet diaries demonstrated a correlation between loss of teeth and increased carbohydrate intake, decreased protein intake, and diminished intake of selected micronutrients.

As a modality of compensation for loss of all of the teeth, removable dentures can aid in speech and restore diminished facial contours, but they are less predictably successful in restoring the ability to masticate. Edentulous persons with dentures are generally capable of eating a wider range of foods than edentulous persons without dentures. Yet dentures restore, on average, only about 15% of the chewing ability of the natural dentition. The range of foods regularly eaten by denture wearers is significantly restricted in comparison with the dietary range of persons with natural teeth. Denture wearers also have to chew more times before they swallow food, and they swallow their food in larger particles. Older patients and their physicians who hope that dentures will restore oral intake in cases of malnutrition or unexplained weight loss are usually disappointed, whereas those who hope for a more socially acceptable appearance, clearer speech, and modest improvement in chewing comfort and range of dietary choices are more likely to be satisfied.

Dentures often are a considerable source of discomfort, dysfunction, and embarrassment for older people. This is because the alveolar processes that originally held the natural teeth continually remodel and diminish in volume once the natural teeth are gone. For most patients, dentures require frequent professional adjustment and periodic replacement. Alveolar ridge resorption is most severe in the oldest patients who have had the longest time without natural teeth; this effect is more pronounced in those with osteoporosis.

For health of the oral mucosa, dentures should be kept clean by removing them and cleaning them after meals, and soaking them in a commercial disinfectant several times each week. Dentures should remain out of the mouth for several hours each day; most people choose to leave their dentures out during sleep. Fractured or broken dentures, as well as denture looseness or soreness, should be brought to a dentist's attention without delay. However, since neither dental services nor dentures are currently covered by Medicare and fewer than 10% of older Americans have private dental insurance, many older people continue to use inadequate or even damaging dentures.

SALIVARY FUNCTION IN AGING

Saliva is critical for protecting the tissues of the oral cavity and maintaining their function in speech, mastication, swallowing, and taste perception. Saliva buffers the intraoral pH, contains a wide spectrum of antimicrobial factors, remineralizes and lubricates the oral surfaces, and keeps the taste pores patent. In the absence of disease, the major salivary glands undergo regressive histologic changes with age. Yet data from the Baltimore Longitudinal Study on Aging and the Veterans Affairs Dental Longitudinal Study have demonstrated that with healthy aging, flow from the parotid glands under both resting and stimulated conditions is essentially unchanged with aging. Both groups of investigators have reported that flow from the submandibular glands undergoes no change with age; other centers have reported a measurable but clinically minor decrease. It has been suggested that the major salivary glands show "organ reserve" in which the capacity of youthful glands exceeds ordinary demands, but that with age-related changes, functional reserves dwindle. By extreme old age, healthy glands function adequately under normal conditions but are more susceptible to factors that impede function, such as dehydration or drug-induced hypofunction.

Complaints of dry mouth are very common among older people. The leading causes are the commonly prescribed drugs that have this adverse effect. Commonly implicated are drugs with anticholinergic effects, including tricyclic antidepressants, opioids, antihistamines, and anti-arrhythmic agents. Separate studies have found that 72% of institutionalized older patients received at least one (and some as many as five) potentially xerostomic medications daily and that 55% of more than 4000 rural community-dwelling older persons took at least one potentially xerostomic medication daily. Dry mouth may also be due to local disease, such as salivary gland tumors and blocked ducts, or to systemic disease. Sjögren's syndrome affects approximately 3 million Americans—predominantly women—aged 50 or over. Depression has been reported to diminish saliva flow, as have poorly controlled diabetes mellitus and hypothyroidism.

Dry mouth is also an adverse effect of therapeutic irradiation of the head and neck. In the total dose range administered for oral and oropharyngeal squamous cell carcinoma, salivary flow is commonly obliterated as a consequence of short-term direct effects on the glands and long-term fibrosis of their vascular supply. Patients who have undergone radiation of the head may experience rapidly destructive dental caries and painful oral mucositis, which may affect nutritional status. (See "Malnutrition," p 182.)

Treatment of the older person with dry mouth requires attention to both diagnosis and prevention. Diminished oral secretions increase the risk for serious oral disease. A history of irradiation of the head and neck as well as systemic causes should be excluded. Medications that reduce salivary flow should be decreased, discontinued, or substituted for, if possible. Patients who have had irradiation should be considered for a 3-month course of oral pilocarpine (5 to 10 mg three times a day), which may restore some salivary function. Saliva substitutes and oral lubricants, available without prescription and used as needed, can provide transient relief but have none of the protective properties of saliva. Patients should be counseled on the greatly elevated risk for oral disease and educated on the need to limit sugar in their diet and optimize their daily oral hygiene practices.

ORAL MUCOSAL PROBLEMS

Squamous cell carcinoma accounts for 96% of oral and oropharyngeal malignancies. Of the 28,000 new cases of oral cancer reported in the United States annually, more than 95% occur in people aged 40 or over; age is the primary risk factor identified in epidemiologic analyses. The 5-year survival rate for white Americans is approximately 55% and for black Americans, 34%. Carcinoma of the lip, tongue, and floor of mouth represents more than 65% of all oropharyngeal cases. Lip cancer affects men eight times more frequently than women; most other sites affect men at a ratio slightly below 2:1. Oral cancer is strongly linked with the use of tobacco, particularly cigarettes. Lip cancer has a strong correlation with pipe and cigar smoking. Ethanol is a potent cofactor that enhances the effects of tobacco. Other potential risk factors—dentures, poor oral care, oral viral disease, oral lichen planus, candidosis—have been suggested, but none has shown the unambiguous associations of age, smoking, and alcohol use.

Oral malignancy appears clinically as painless red, white, or mixed red and white areas of the oral mucosa that may be ulcerated or indurated. Red and mixed lesions (termed *erythroplakia*) display cellular atypia in as many as 93% of cases and should be biopsied immediately. White lesions (*leukoplakia*) are malignant or premalignant less than 10% of the time and merit close monitoring; biopsy is indicated if a lesion does not disappear in 14 days or is increasing in size. Clinicians also have less invasive diagnostic tools available for determining whether a white or red lesion in the mouth merits biopsy, such as scraping (exfoliative cytology) and in situ staining. Early identification markedly improves outcome: 5-year survival without nodal involvement in white Americans is 80% and in black Americans 69%, but survival rates decline with nodal involvement (41% and 30%, respectively) and with distant metastases (18% and 12%). A thorough oral cancer screening, which can be completed in less than 2 minutes, consists of a head and neck nodal assessment followed by inspection of the oral cavity using gauze to retract the tongue and tongue blades to enhance visualization of the cheeks, lips, and vestibules. Although oral cancer screening is easy to learn, straightforward to perform, requires minimal instrumentation, and causes no discomfort to the patient, few older smokers receive oral evaluations as part of the routine physical examination.

The treatment of localized oral squamous cell carcinoma is generally surgical, although large but localized tumors can be managed with radioactive implants. More extensive disease necessitates surgery followed by beam irradiation. Concern over the deleterious adverse effects of irradiation described above has led to development of techniques that seek to limit destruction of healthy tissues surrounding a tumor. Radiation alone has been used to shrink inoperable tumors. Newer protocols combine surgery and chemotherapy with the goal of a cure.

Candidiasis presents as diffuse erythema, cracking at the corners of the mouth, curd-like white patches, or erythema in denture areas; it can result in taste dysfunction, burning, itching, and pain. Older patients are particularly susceptible to candidiasis because of denture use, salivary hypofunction, prevalence of diabetes mellitus, and use of antibiotics for pulmonary and urologic diseases. Patients who use inhaled corticosteroids also are at higher risk and should be instructed to rinse out their mouth after using the inhaler. Management of candidiasis involves, first, ruling out any immunopathic cause for the disease, followed by administration of topical or systemic antifungal agents and optimal oral and denture hygiene.

Burning mouth syndrome is a chronic oral-facial pain disorder usually without other clinical signs. It usually affects women aged 50 or over, with a particularly high attack rate in Asian Americans and Native Americans. The pain most commonly affects the lips, tongue, and palate. Multiple causes have been suggested, including xerostomia, denture use, candidiasis, nutritional deficiencies, and psychiatric disorders. Treatment is empirical.

CHEMOSENSORY PERCEPTION

Olfactory function declines with age. A decreased ability to identify odors and to rank their intensities affects both older men (to the greater extent) and women. Several drugs have been implicated in smell dysfunction, as has Alzheimer's disease, among other disorders common among older persons. Impaired olfaction in older persons has been anecdotally implicated as a risk factor for eating spoiled food or failing to notice gas leaks or domestic fires.

Taste perception changes with aging. Changes in subjectively perceived saltiness and sweetness show blunting with advancing age, which potentially have clinical significance, possibly playing a role in a person's tendency to oversalt foods or crave sweets.

Complaints of taste and smell dysfunction are common among older persons. Often the complaint derives from medication use, but other causes are possible (see Table 46.2 and Table 46.3). Some drugs

Table 46.2—Nonpharmacologic Causes of Taste and Smell Dysfunction in Older Persons

Gustatory dysfunction
　Oral causes
　　Burning mouth syndrome
　　Candidiasis
　　Laceration
　　Malignancy
　　Salivary hypofunction
　　Therapeutic irradiation of head
　　Thermal or chemical burn
　Nonoral causes
　　Alzheimer's disease, other neurodegenerative disorders
　　Central nervous system tumor
　　Endocrinopathies (eg, diabetes mellitus, Cushing's syndrome, adrenocortical insufficiency, hypothyroidism)
　　Head trauma
　　Nutritional deficiencies (vitamin B$_{12}$, zinc)
　　Psychiatric disorder
　　Stroke
Olfactory dysfunction
　Upper aerodigestive and respiratory causes
　　Dental infection
　　Periodontal disease
　　Poor oral hygiene, including poor denture hygiene
　　Sinusitis
　　Tobacco smoking or use of nasal snuff
　　Tumor of airway or sinus
　　Upper respiratory infection (bacterial or viral)
　Other causes
　　Alzheimer's disease, other neurodegenerative disorders
　　Central nervous system tumor
　　Exposure to volatile or particulate toxins
　　Head trauma
　　Nutritional deficiencies (niacin, zinc)
　　Psychiatric disorder
　　Stroke

Table 46.3—Drugs That Interfere With Gustation (Taste) and Olfaction (Smell)

Gustation		
Acetazolamide	Dexamethasone	Methimazole
Allopurinol	Diazoxide	Methotrexate
Amiloride	Diltiazem	Methylthiouracil
Amphetamine	Dipyridamole	Metronidazole
Amphotericin B	Doxorubicin	Nifedipine
Ampicillin	Enalapril	Nitroglycerin patch
Azathioprine	Ethacrynic acid	Phenylbutazone
Baclofen	Ethambutol	Phenytoin
Bleomycin	hydrochloride	Propyl uracil
Captopril	Etidronate	Sulfasalazine
Carbamazepine	Glipizide	Tetracyclines
Chlorpheniramine	Gold	Thiouracil
maleate	Griseofulvin	Trifluoperazine
Colchicine	Hydrocortisone	Vincristine sulfate
D-Penicillamine	Idoxuridine	Vitamin D
	Iron sorbitex	
	Levodopa	
	Lithium carbonate	
Olfaction		
Amitriptyline	Hydromorphone	Nifedipine
Amphetamine	hydrochloride	Propylthiouracil
Codeine	Methimazole	Streptomycin
Diltiazem	Methyl uracil	
	Morphine	

SOURCE: Data from Schiffman SS. Drugs influencing taste and smell perception. In: Getchell TV, Bartoshuk LM, Doty RL, et al., eds. *Smell and Taste in Health and Disease.* New York: Raven Press;1991:846–847.

may have no primary effect on taste but cause diminished saliva flow and lead to impaired taste perception. One's sense of "taste" may actually be more accurately termed "flavor"—that is, the full range of sensations that accompany eating, including temperature, texture, sound, and smell in addition to the perception of sweet, salt, sour, and bitter. Flavor perception is prone to impairment in the older person because of changes in olfaction and oral stereognosis, salivary hypofunction, and the presence of dentures, which present physical and thermal barriers.

REFERENCES

- Beck JD, Pankow J, Tyroler HA, et al. Dental infections and atherosclerosis. *Am Heart J.* 1999;138(5 part 2): S528–S533.

- Hujoel PP, Drangsholt M, Spiekerman C, et al. Periodontal disease and coronary heart disease risk. *JAMA.* 2000;284(11):1406–1410.

- Kaugars GE, Silverman S Jr, Ray AK, et al. The use of exfoliative cytology for the early diagnosis of oral cancers: is there a role for it in education and private practice? *J Cancer Educ.* 1998;13(2):85–89.

- Ship JA. The influence of aging on oral health and consequences for taste and smell. *Physiol & Behav.* 1999;66(2):209–215.

- Walton JC, Miller T, Tordecilla L. Elderly oral assessment and care. *Head and Neck Nursing.* 2002;20(2):12–19.

CHAPTER 47—GASTROINTESTINAL DISEASES AND DISORDERS

The structure and function of the gastrointestinal tract are affected both by physiologic changes of aging and by the effects of accumulating disorders involving many body systems. In association with advancing age, there can be changes in connective tissue that limit the elasticity of the gut and alterations in the nerves and muscles that impair motility. Accumulating disorders and diseases are often associated with increased use of medications by older persons, many of which have direct effects on intestinal mucosa and motility. Some disease states, like atherosclerosis and diabetes mellitus, can adversely influence gastrointestinal function and lead to symptoms and complications. Gastrointestinal problems may quickly compromise the older person's ability to maintain adequate nutrition and lead to fatigue and weight loss.

ESOPHAGUS

Dysphagia

Dysphagia implies either the inability to initiate a swallow or a sensation that solids or liquids do not pass easily from the mouth into the stomach; it is a common problem among older adults. Dysphagia among patients with dyspepsia requires immediate evaluation and therapy. Patients with *oropharyngeal* dysphagia complain of food's getting stuck shortly after they swallow, nasal regurgitation, and coughing. In contrast, patients with *esophageal* dysphagia usually point to the sternum when asked to localize the site. Dysphagia for both solids and liquids from the onset usually implies a motility disorder of the esophagus. In contrast, dysphagia for solids that progresses later to involve liquids suggests mechanical obstruction. Progressive dysphagia results from either cancer or peptic stricture, whereas intermittent dysphagia is most often related to a lower esophageal ring or esophageal dysmotility, such as achalasia or diffuse esophageal spasm. It is particularly important to obtain a detailed review of medications, because anticholinergics, antihistamines, and certain antihypertensive agents can reduce salivary flow. Slurred speech may indicate weakness or incoordination of muscles involved in articulation and swallowing. Dysarthria and nasal regurgitation of food suggest weakness of the soft palate or pharyngeal constrictors. Food regurgitation, halitosis, a sensation of fullness in the neck, or a history of pneumonia accompanying dysphagia may be the result of a pharyngoesophageal (or Zenker's) diverticulum, which may be associated with a poorly relaxing or hypertensive upper esophageal sphincter. Painful swallowing (odynophagia) typically results from infection or malignancy.

Endoscopy is the best first test to evaluate dysphagia; it allows biopsies and therapeutic interventions, such as dilation. However, lower esophageal rings or extrinsic esophageal compression can be overlooked during endoscopy. In such cases, radiologic evaluation with a 13-mm barium tablet or a solid bolus with barium, such as a marshmallow or bread, may identify the level and nature of obstruction. If results of these tests are normal, an esophageal motility study should be performed. For patients with oropharyngeal dysphagia, videofluoroscopy allows detailed analysis of swallowing mechanics, identifies whether aspiration is present, and evaluates the effects of different barium consistencies. Nasopharyngolaryngoscopy is a bedside procedure that evaluates the oropharynx, vallecula, and piriform sinuses, as well as the larynx and perilaryngeal regions, for pooled secretions or retained food; its utility is uncertain.

The treatment of dysphagia depends on its underlying cause. Esophageal cancer requires resection, chemotherapy, or radiation therapy. Following stroke, head or neck surgery, or in degenerative neurologic diseases, swallowing rehabilitation and dietary modifications to facilitate oral intake are required. In some cases, feeding with a cup, straw, or spoon may improve swallowing. Endoscopic dilation is performed in patients with esophageal webs or strictures. Cricopharyngeal myotomy may benefit patients who have inadequate pharyngeal contraction, pharyngoesophageal diverticulum, or lack coordination between the pharynx and the upper esophageal sphincter. Botulinum toxin injection to the cricopharyngeus muscle is an alternative to surgery for patients with cricopharyngeal achalasia.

Gastroesophageal Reflux Disease

Gastroesophageal reflux disease (GERD) is defined as chronic symptoms or mucosal damage produced by the abnormal reflux of gastric contents into the esophagus. Highly specific symptoms for GERD include heartburn, regurgitation, or both, which occur often after meals and are aggravated by recumbency and relieved by antacids. Among persons aged 65 and over, symptoms of heartburn or acid regurgitation occur at least weekly in 20% of the population and at least monthly in 59% of the population, rates similar to those observed in younger adults.

In more than 80% of patients, GERD is caused by transient inappropriate lower esophageal sphincter relaxations that lead to acid reflux into the esophagus. Some patients may have reduced lower esophageal sphincter tone, which permits reflux when intra-abdominal pressure rises. Sliding hiatal hernia occurs in about 30% of patients aged 50 years or over and may contribute to acid reflux and regurgitation. Poor esophageal peristalsis leads to delayed clearance of the refluxate and increased acid exposure time. In patients receiving anticholinergic drugs, reduced salivary secretion decreases the buffering capacity of the esophagus against refluxed acid and may aggravate mucosal injury.

Patients with uncomplicated heartburn or regurgitation should be treated empirically with acid-suppressing drugs. If such therapy is unsuccessful, or if there are symptoms suggesting complicated disease, an upper endoscopy should be performed. Individuals, particularly white men, who have longstanding symptoms or who require continuous therapy need endoscopic screening for Barrett's esophagus. The frequency and severity of reflux symptoms are poorly predictive of the presence of Barrett's esophagus, particularly in patients aged 65 or over.

The presence of anemia, dysphagia, gastrointestinal bleeding, recurrent vomiting, and weight loss suggests complicated GERD. Patients with these signs and symptoms should be considered for endoscopy. This is the procedure of choice to evaluate mucosal integrity and confirm the diagnosis of dysplasia or cancer in cases of Barrett's esophagus. However, many patients with reflux symptoms do not have esophagitis. In such cases, 24-hour ambulatory esophageal pH testing helps to confirm the diagnosis. This noninvasive test is also useful for patients with noncardiac chest pain or reflux-associated pulmonary and upper respiratory symptoms or to monitor the esophageal acid exposure in patients with refractory symptoms. Esophageal manometry is used to document the presence of effective esophageal peristalsis in patients in whom antireflux surgery is being considered.

Proton pump inhibitors are the treatment of choice for patients with GERD, but they are expensive. Use of these drugs heals esophagitis in 85% of cases and eradicates heartburn and regurgitation in 80%. In comparison, H_2 antagonists ameliorate symptoms and heal esophagitis in only 60% of cases. Regardless, therapy should be maintained for at least 8 weeks. After acute medical therapy alleviates symptoms, the patient should be given a trial off medication. Endoscopy, esophageal motility, and ambulatory 24-hour pH monitoring should be performed if the most potent medical therapy still results in a poor response.

Recurrence of symptoms is common after therapy is stopped, and lifelong therapy is commonly needed. Intermittent therapy with an H_2 antagonist or proton pump inhibitor may be successful in some patients with mild to moderate symptoms without severe esophagitis. Depending upon the initial therapy rendered, the medical regimen is adjusted in a step-up or step-down fashion to the most cost-effective regimen. The need for maintenance medical therapy is determined by the rapidity of recurrence. Recurrent symptoms in less than 3 months suggest that the disease will be best managed with continuous therapy, whereas remissions in excess of 3 months can be adequately managed with intermittent therapy. Induction of hypergastrinemia and gastric carcinoid tumors in rats treated with omeprazole has raised safety concerns about the long-term safety of proton pump inhibitors. However, although patients treated with omeprazole for up to 5 years have shown gastritis and gastric atrophy, no neoplastic changes have been seen. Since gastric acidity normally protects against ingested pathogens, another concern with gastric acid inhibition is an increased risk of enteric infections.

Older patients with large hiatal hernia, with persistent regurgitation despite proton pump inhibitor therapy, or who do not wish to take proton pump inhibitors over the long term, should be considered for antireflux surgery. This can be performed laparoscopically, with success rates of more than 90%.

Drug-Induced Esophageal Injury

Old age and decreased esophageal peristaltic clearance may be associated with pill retention. Esophageal injury may then occur as a result of prolonged contact of the caustic contents of the medication with the esophageal mucosa. The site of injury is commonly at the level of the aortic arch, the level of an enlarged left atrium, or the level of the esophagogastric junction. Because salivation and swallowing are markedly reduced during sleep, pill intake immediately prior to recumbency and without adequate fluid bolus favors pill retention and injury. Patients with medication-induced esophageal injury present with sudden odynophagia to a degree that even swallowing saliva is difficult. A classic example is the older patient in a nursing home given a number of medications with a small amount of water while recumbent prior to sleep.

Tetracyclines, particularly doxycycline, are the most common antibiotics that induce esophagitis. Aspirin and all of the nonsteroidal anti-inflammatory drugs (NSAIDs) can also damage the esophagus. Other offenders include potassium chloride, quinidine, iron, and alendronate, which is increasingly used for the treatment of osteoporosis in older adults. Because of this, alendronate should be cautiously used in patients with esophageal dysfunction and taken with at least 8 ounces of water to minimize the risk of the tablet's getting stuck in the esophagus and causing damage. Patients should stand or sit upright for at least 30 minutes and should not eat during this interval.

Etidronate, another bisphosphonate used to treat postmenopausal osteoporosis and Paget's disease, does not cause esophageal injury.

Upper endoscopy, the most sensitive diagnostic tool, may reveal a discrete ulcer of variable size with normal surrounding mucosa. These lesions typically heal spontaneously within a few days, and it is unclear whether therapy is needed. Suspension of sucralfate provides a protective coat on the esophageal mucosa and promotes healing. Strictures may be noted in users of NSAIDs. Endoscopic dilation may be needed if a stricture is found. If possible, potentially caustic oral medications should be discontinued or substituted with a liquid preparation.

Endoscopic Palliation of Esophageal Cancer

Esophageal cancer is commonly diagnosed at an advanced, incurable stage in older patients who are not candidates for tumor resection. These patients are plagued by symptoms of esophageal obstruction or fistula formation, dysphagia, aspiration, and weight loss. In such instances, endoscopic palliation can be achieved with either laser therapy or a single stent placement. Laser therapy with neodymium-yttrium-aluminum-garnet (Nd:YAG) laser fulgurates the malignant obstructing tissue and restores luminal patency in more than 90% of cases, with a 5% risk of perforation. Relief may last for up to several months, but treatments may be repeated. Photodynamic therapy uses a photosensitizing agent in combination with endoscopic laser exposure. It is more effective than Nd:YAG laser for palliation and has fewer complications, but it may cause skin photosensitivity.

Stenting with self-expanding metal stents is preferable therapy for patients with a malignant stricture or an esophago-bronchial fistula, as it relieves dysphagia and aspiration in up to 95% of patients with a low complication rate. Disadvantages of stents include their high cost, tumor ingrowth, and stent migration.

STOMACH

Dyspepsia

Dyspepsia implies chronic or recurrent pain or discomfort in the upper abdomen. The major causes of dyspepsia are gastric or duodenal ulcer, gastroesophageal reflux, and gastric cancer. Because symptom pattern is inadequate for accurate diagnosis, endoscopy is the test of choice. Endoscopy is normal in up to 60% of patients, who are then classified as having functional dyspepsia. It is unclear whether *Helicobacter pylori* gastritis causes symptoms of dyspepsia.

Because the incidence of gastric cancer increases with age, upper endoscopy should be considered in older patients presenting with new onset of dyspepsia. Treatment is then targeted at the underlying diagnosis. For patients with ulcer and documented *H. pylori* infection, a trial of anti–*H. pylori* therapy should heal the ulcer and abolish the ulcer diathesis. For the majority of patients with functional (or nonulcer) dyspepsia, reassurance and a course of antisecretory therapy using either H_2-receptor antagonists or proton-pump inhibitors is recommended.

Treatment of *H. pylori* may lead to or possibly exacerbate reflux esophagitis. One possibility is that ammonia production by *H. pylori* buffers acid. Alternatively, reversal of *H. pylori*–induced gastritis (and associated hypochlorhydria) may increase gastric acid secretion and precipitate previously asymptomatic reflux. Despite this association, eradication of *H. pylori* should not be avoided solely to prevent the development or exacerbation of reflux esophagitis.

NSAID-Induced Gastric Complications

The risk of ulcers and their complications is three times greater in NSAID users than in nonusers. For those aged 60 or over, the relative risk increases even more, to fivefold. Older patients, particularly women, are two to four times more likely than younger patients to be hospitalized with peptic ulcer disease. The presence of *H. pylori* infection does not increase the risk for NSAID-induced ulcer disease. Older patients with NSAID-induced ulcers tend to present with anemia, bleeding, or perforation without the warning symptoms of dyspepsia or abdominal pain. In addition, older NSAID users frequently require emergency surgery for serious complications, have higher rebleeding rates, greater transfusion requirements, longer hospital stays, and higher mortality rates than do younger patients. Risk factors for upper gastrointestinal complications of NSAIDs use, besides advanced age, are shown in Table 47.1.

The COX-2 inhibitors, a new class of drugs for arthritis, have equal analgesic and anti-inflammatory efficacy but a better safety and tolerability profile than standard NSAIDs, and they are preferred for patients who are at high risk for gastrointestinal complications, such as perforation or bleeding.

Peptic Ulcer Disease

In the United States, *H. pylori* infection is responsible for about 80% of duodenal ulcers and approximately 60% of gastric ulcers. Most older patients with ulcers complain of dyspepsia, although bleeding, anemia, and acute abdominal pain may occur. Typically, the diagnosis of peptic ulcer is made by upper gastrointestinal

Table 47.1—Risk Factors for Upper Gastrointestinal Adverse Events in Patients Treated With Nonsteroidal Anti-Inflammatory Drugs

Age 65 years and older
Comorbid medical conditions
Use of oral glucocorticoids
History of peptic ulcer disease
History of upper gastrointestinal bleeding
Use of anticoagulants

SOURCE: Data from American College of Rheumatology Subcommittee on Osteoarthritis Guidelines: recommendations for the medical management of osteoarthritis of the hip and knee, 2000 update. *Arthritis Rheum.* 2000;(43):1905–1915.

radiography or endoscopy. Endoscopy is more sensitive and specific than double-contrast barium study (92% versus 54% and 100% versus 91%, respectively). It is important to differentiate benign gastric ulcers from gastric cancer by obtaining multiple endoscopic biopsies.

The goal in evaluating an older patient with upper gastrointestinal symptoms is to quickly establish a definitive diagnosis, avoiding costly and risky diagnostic procedures. Drugs that may cause dyspepsia, especially NSAIDs, should be eliminated when possible. If early satiety, weight loss, occult gastrointestinal bleeding, or otherwise unexplained anemia is present, an endoscopy should be performed to exclude malignancy.

Among patients with dyspepsia who test positive for *H. pylori*, antibiotic therapy may be beneficial for up to 30% of those with underlying peptic ulcer, but those with nonulcer (functional) dyspepsia will have a variable response. *H. pylori* testing should not be performed in asymptomatic people.

BILIARY DISEASE

Gallstones primarily form in the gallbladder and may obstruct the cystic or common bile duct, causing biliary pain, cholecystitis, and cholangitis. When stones obstruct the ampulla, pancreatitis may occur. Biliary pain is acute, severe upper abdominal pain, usually in the epigastrium or right upper quadrant, that lasts for more than 1 hour. The pain may radiate to the back or scapula, and is often associated with restlessness, nausea, or vomiting. Episodes are typically separated by several weeks. Postprandial epigastric fullness, fatty food intolerance, and regurgitation are nonspecific symptoms and are not related to gallstones. If biliary disease is suspected in older patients, ultrasonography should be the initial imaging modality. Computed abdominal tomography scanning may be used if common bile duct stones or ductal obstruction are suspected. Magnetic resonance cholangiography (MRC) and endoscopic ultrasonography are two new, very accurate imaging modalities to detect common bile duct pathology, including gallstones. However, for patients with obstructive jaundice, cholangitis, or sus-

pected biliary pancreatitis where the probability of common bile duct stones is high, therapeutic endoscopic retrograde cholangiopancreatography (ERCP) is preferred.

Isolated alkaline phosphatase elevation without jaundice may be a presenting manifestation of biliary obstruction in older patients and should always be evaluated. If cholelithiasis is detected in patients with biliary pain, laparoscopic cholecystectomy is the procedure of choice. However, this procedure is not indicated in patients with gallstones without biliary pain or complications. The incidental finding of gallstones in a patient with dyspepsia may lead to an unnecessary cholecystectomy and a poor long-term outcome. In the rare older patient who is unable to undergo surgery, treatment with ursodeoxycholic acid or lithotripsy, or both, may be attempted. In patients with common bile duct obstruction due to gallstones, endoscopic sphincterotomy and bile ductal drainage is adequate in preventing recurrent cholangitis, and the gallbladder may be left in situ. In any older patient with gallstones, the possibility of gallbladder cancer should be entertained. In older patients presenting with biliary pain who have had a cholecystectomy, a retained common bile duct stone should be suspected and evaluated by ERCP, MRC, or endoscopic ultrasonography. In patients with abnormal liver function tests, right upper quadrant pain, and an increased common bile duct diameter, biliary manometry should also be considered. If sphincter of Oddi dysfunction is confirmed, endoscopic sphincterotomy should be performed. For patients with malignant jaundice, treatments are mostly palliative, with either surgery, or percutaneous or endoscopic stenting. Such drainage improves quality of life, decreases pruritus, and improves the nutritional state of the patient but does not improve survival.

COLON

Constipation

Chronic constipation affects about 30% of adults aged 65 years or older, more commonly women. Although it frequently occurs as a side effect of drugs, it may be a manifestation of metabolic or neurologic disease. Regardless, colonic obstruction must always be excluded. Constipation has been defined as a stool frequency of less than three per week. However, some individuals may complain of straining at defecation or a sense of incomplete defecation despite a daily bowel evacuation. A more objective diagnosis of constipation is based upon colonic transit times.

Patients with irritable bowel syndrome often complain of constipation, which alternates with periods of diarrhea or normal bowel evacuation. Such patients have normal colonic transit times. Lumbosacral spinal disease may lead to colonic hypomotility and dilatation, decreased rectal tone and sensation, and impaired defecation. Older patients with Parkinson's disease may have constipation worsened by physical inactivity or medication use. Acquired laxity of the pelvic floor muscles that contribute to the external sphincter of the rectum can occur in middle-aged and older women, contributing to problems with fecal incontinence.

Most patients with prolonged colonic transit have colonic inertia, defined as the delayed passage of radiopaque markers through the proximal colon. Outlet delay is a form of idiopathic constipation in which markers move normally through the colon but stagnate in the rectum. This is typically seen in older patients with fecal impaction and megarectum, and in women with pelvic floor dyssynergia who demonstrate abnormal responses of the pelvic floor muscles during defecation. Older patients with megacolon or megarectum have chronic fecal retention, increased rectal compliance and elasticity, and blunted rectal sensation, all leading to fecal impaction and soiling.

For most patients with constipation and normal colonic transit time, fluids, dietary fiber, and bulk laxatives, such as psyllium seed or and calcium polycarbophil, are effective in increasing the frequency and softening the consistency of stool with a minimum of adverse effects. Patients who respond poorly or who do not tolerate fiber may require laxatives. Chronic use of stimulant laxatives such as bisacodyl and senna may lead to hypokalemia, protein-losing enteropathy, and impairment of bowel motility. Stool softeners such as docusate sodium have few side effects but are less effective than laxatives. Constipation among patients with dementia is common, especially if psychotropic medications are being used. Because the patient cannot be relied upon to describe symptoms, a proactive approach is needed.

Management of slow-transit constipation requires daily osmotic laxatives, such as sorbitol, lactulose, or a polyethylene glycol solution. Severe intractable colonic inertia with megacolon may require subtotal colectomy and ileorectostomy. Pelvic floor dysfunction requires biofeedback, relaxation exercises, and the use of suppositories.

Patients with fecal impaction should first have their colon evacuated with enemas or polyethylene glycol electrolyte solution until cleansing is complete. Recurrence of fecal impaction is then prevented with a fiber-restricted diet together with cleansing enemas twice weekly or daily oral intake of 12 to 16 fluid ounces of polyethylene glycol solution.

Fecal Incontinence

Fecal incontinence, defined as the recurrent uncontrolled passage of fecal material for at least 1 month, is a disturbing disability because it affects quality of life and may lead to social isolation. Fecal incontinence may be minor, with inadvertent passage of flatus or soiling of underwear with liquid stool, or it may be major, with involuntary leakage of feces. Fecal incontinence affects 2% to 7% of adults, mostly older persons in poor general health.

Fecal continence depends on many factors, such as mental function, stool consistency, colonic transit, rectal compliance, internal and external anal sphincter function, as well as anorectal sensation and reflexes. Normal defecation is a complex sequential process that starts with the entry of stool into the rectum that leads to reflex relaxation of the internal anal sphincter. If defecation is desired, the anorectal angle is voluntarily straightened, and abdominal pressure is increased by straining. This results in descent of the pelvic floor, contraction of the rectum, and inhibition of the external anal sphincter, which causes evacuation of the rectal contents.

Decreased anal sphincter tone can result from trauma (eg, anal surgery) or neurologic disorders (eg, spinal cord injury or a secondary effect of diabetes mellitus). Vaginal delivery associated with anal sphincter tears or trauma to the pudendal nerve may result in fecal incontinence immediately or after many years. Decreased rectal compliance resulting from ulcerative or radiation proctitis leads to increased fecal frequency and urgency. Impaction is a common cause of fecal incontinence in older persons because it inhibits the internal anal sphincter tone, permitting leakage of liquid stool. Idiopathic fecal incontinence caused by denervation of the pelvic floor musculature occurs most commonly in middle-aged and older women.

The history and physical examination often provide clues on the cause of fecal incontinence. A flexible sigmoidoscopy may be considered in order to exclude inflammation or tumor. The next step is anorectal manometry, which measures resting anal sphincter tone, the squeeze pressure, the rectoanal inhibitory reflex, rectal sensation, and rectal compliance. Abnormalities of the anal sphincters, the rectal wall, and the puborectalis muscle can be further evaluated by the use of endorectal ultrasound. Typically, a defect in the internal anal sphincter is associated with low resting sphincter pressure, whereas defects in the external sphincter are associated with lower anal squeeze pressure.

Medical therapy is aimed at reducing stool frequency and improving stool consistency. The former is achieved with antidiarrheal drugs, such as loperamide; the latter, by supplementing the diet with a bulking agent, such as methylcellulose. Older patients with incontinence related to cognitive impairment or physical debility may benefit from a regular defecation program. Biofeedback therapy is a painless noninvasive method of retraining the pelvic floor and the abdominal wall musculature and is recommended for patients with fecal incontinence associated with structurally intact sphincter. Surgery may involve sphincter repair or implantation of an artificial sphincter. Colostomy may be needed for patients with intractable symptoms in whom other treatments have failed. A synthetic sphincter device, consisting of an inflatable cuff that maintains continence, is a valve that allows the cuff to deflate for defecation.

Diverticular Disease

The prevalence of diverticular disease is age-dependent, increasing to 30% by age 60 and to 65% by age 85. Although most patients remain asymptomatic, 20% develop diverticulitis, and 10% may develop diverticular bleeding. Therefore, the mere presence of diverticulosis does not require specific therapy. A diet high in fiber appears to be associated with a reduced risk of the development of diverticular disease and may reduce the risk of subsequent complications.

Uncomplicated diverticulosis is often an incidental finding on screening sigmoidoscopy, colonoscopy, or barium enema. Some patients may complain of nonspecific abdominal cramping, bloating, flatulence, and irregular bowel habits. Diverticular bleeding is usually painless and self-limited, and it rarely coexists with acute diverticulitis. Diverticulitis usually presents with left lower quadrant pain, although nausea, vomiting, constipation, diarrhea, and dysuria or frequency may occur. The physical examination usually reveals left lower quadrant tenderness, a tender mass, and abdominal distention. Generalized tenderness suggests free perforation and peritonitis. Low-grade fever and leukocytosis are common, but their absence in older patients does not exclude the diagnosis. Urinalysis may reveal sterile pyuria induced by adjacent colonic inflammation; the presence of mixed colonic flora on urine culture suggests a colovesical fistula. Other complications that can occur include perforation, obstruction, and abscess formation.

Computed tomographic (CT) scanning is the optimal imaging method in acute diverticulitis. CT features of acute diverticulitis include increased density of soft tissue within pericolic fat and colonic diverticula, bowel wall thickening, soft-tissue masses (phlegmon), and pericolic fluid collections (abscess formation). CT can also identify peritonitis, obstruction, and fistula to the bladder, vagina, and abdominal wall. However, in approximately 10% of patients, diverticulitis cannot be distinguished from colon cancer, since both may show focal thickening of the bowel wall. In such cases, upon resolution of the acute inflammation, a colonoscopy is indicated. In older persons, CT-guided percutaneous drainage of localized abscesses may obviate emergent surgery and permit single-stage elective surgical resection.

The majority of patients (85%) with simple diverticulitis respond to medical therapy. In contrast, all patients with complicated diverticulitis require surgery. Indications for emergency surgery are free perforation with peritonitis, obstruction, clinical deterioration or failure to improve with conservative management, and an abscess that cannot be drained percutaneously. Indications for elective surgical intervention are recurrent or intractable symptoms, persistent mass, obstruction, and fistula or abscess formation.

Mild diverticulitis with left lower quadrant pain, low-grade fever, and minimal physical findings is often treated on an outpatient basis, with clear liquids and oral antibiotics, such as ciprofloxacin 500 mg twice a day, or metronidazole 500 mg three times a day, or both. Hospitalization is needed only if the patient fails to improve. Once the episode resolves, diet is reintroduced and the colon is evaluated, preferably by colonoscopy. For patients with moderate to severe symptoms, treatment with bowel rest, fluids, and intravenous antibiotics is initiated, with the aim to avoid urgent surgery. Antibiotics should be active against gram-negative rods and anaerobes. A single antibiotic active against both aerobes and anaerobes, such as cefoxitin or piperacillin-tazobactam, is as effective as combination therapy, like gentamicin and clindamycin. If there is no improvement, the diagnosis is incorrect or an abscess, peritonitis, fistula, or obstruction is present. Older, immunosuppressed patients with multiple underlying medical conditions may present with minimal symptoms or signs even with frank peritonitis, and the diagnosis is commonly delayed. In such cases, early surgical intervention should be considered. Diffuse peritonitis requires fluid resuscitation, broad-spectrum antibiotics, and emergency laparotomy. Colonic resective surgery removes the septic focus, corrects the obstruction or fistula formation, and restores bowel continuity. In most elective cases, resection and primary anastomosis are possible, since the disease is well localized or has significantly resolved.

After successful medical therapy of the first episode of diverticulitis, one third of patients will remain asymptomatic, another third will have episodic abdominal cramps (painful diverticulosis), and the remaining will proceed to a second attack of diverticulitis. Therefore, elective surgery is not necessary for all patients with diverticulitis who respond to medical therapy. If surgery is performed, progression of diverticulosis in the remaining colon occurs in only 15%, and the need for further surgery in reduced to less than 10%.

Occult Gastrointestinal Bleeding

Older patients are commonly noted to have a positive stool test for occult blood or are diagnosed with unexplained iron-deficiency anemia. Although colorectal cancer is a leading concern in such patients, many other causes, such as esophagitis, peptic ulcers, esophageal and gastric malignancies, intestinal or colonic angiodysplasia, benign colon polyps, inflammatory bowel disease, or hemorrhoids may be the cause. A positive fecal occult blood test should not be attributed to esophageal varices or colonic diverticula, because it is rare for such lesions to bleed in an occult fashion. The presence of fecal occult blood should not be attributed to aspirin or warfarin use or alcohol ingestion.

Detection of occult blood in the stool has a low sensitivity and a high rate of false-positive results, leading to more invasive and expensive tests. Despite these limitations, annual screening is currently recommended and has been associated with up to a 33% reduction in mortality from colorectal cancer. Because of the high prevalence of colorectal cancer and adenomatous polyps in older adults with a positive fecal occult blood test, colonoscopy is performed and, if negative, is followed by an upper endoscopy. If symptoms of upper gastrointestinal disease are present, there is a high likelihood for a positive endoscopy. However, in older patients at risk for colon cancer, the presence of a proximal lesion should not preclude evaluation of the colon. Patients with normal upper and lower tract may require evaluation for a small bowel source. The most common cause for bleeding from the small bowel is angiodysplasia, followed by tumors or ulcers that are commonly caused by NSAIDs. Unrecognized gluten-sensitive enteropathy can result in iron-deficiency anemia, since iron is absorbed in the proximal small bowel.

In one prospective study that evaluated patients with iron-deficiency anemia and presumed occult fecal blood loss with colonoscopy, endoscopy, and, if these tests were negative, radiographic examination of the small intestine, a source of bleeding was identified in 62%. A lesion was seen on colonoscopy in 25%, on upper endoscopy in 36%, and on both in 1% of patients. Peptic ulcer disease was the primary abnormality in the upper gastrointestinal tract, but cancer was detected in 11% of patients on colonoscopy.

Colonic Angiodysplasia

The terms *angiodysplasia*, *arteriovenous malformation*, and *vascular ectasia* have been used interchangeably. Angiodysplasias occur most often in the cecum and ascending colon, where they may cause bleeding, particularly in patients aged 60 or over. However, angiodysplasias occur throughout the gastrointestinal tract and may be multiple or coexist in several different regions of the gastrointestinal tract. They may be asymptomatic or cause occult or clinically overt gastrointestinal bleeding.

Angiodysplasias are dilated, thin-walled vessels in the mucosa and submucosa that are lined by endothelium or by smooth muscle. Although they are mostly tortuous veins, arteriovenous communications or enlarged arteries may be present, leading to brisk bleeding. The pathogenesis of angiodysplasias is not well understood. They may result from local ischemia associated with cardiac, vascular, or pulmonary disease. More recently, increased expression of angiogenic factors, basic fibroblast growth factor and vascular endothelial growth factor, has been detected in segments of colon with angiodysplasia.

Angiodysplasias are usually diagnosed during colonoscopy, appearing as 5- to 10-mm cherry-red, ectatic blood vessels radiating from a central vascular core. Angiodysplasias can also be diagnosed by angiography. If they are serendipitously detected during routine endoscopy or colonoscopy, angiodysplasias should not be treated. In contrast, an actively bleeding angiodysplasia should be treated. Whether angiodysplasias were the cause of bleeding in patients who have stopped bleeding and, in particular, in patients who are found to have both angiodysplasias and diverticula is a more difficult problem. In such cases, bleeding from angiodysplasias is almost always from the cecum or ascending colon.

Many endoscopic ablation techniques have been used in the treatment of angiodysplasias. Although acute bleeding can be successfully controlled with these approaches, rebleeding is common. Angiography may localize the site of active bleeding and allows embolization or infusion of vasopressin. Surgical resection is definitive for lesions that have been clearly identified as the source of bleeding. However, recurrent bleeding may occur from other proximal or distal lesions in more than 30% of cases. Hormonal therapy with estrogen (with or without progesterone) has also been used in women, but its benefit should be weighed against the potential risks of thromboembolic disease, estrogen-dependent tumors, or uterine bleeding.

Colonic Polyps

Polyps are usually asymptomatic, but they may bleed or predispose the patient to cancer. Colonic polyps are usually classified as neoplastic (adenomas) and nonneoplastic (hyperplastic). Approximately 40% of the U.S. population aged 50 or over have one or more adenomas. Detection and removal of adenomas significantly decreases the morbidity and mortality associated with colorectal cancer. Old age and male gender are major risk factors. First-degree relatives of patients with adenomas are also at increased risk for colorectal cancer and should undergo screening.

Adenomas are most often detected by colon cancer screening tests, primarily sigmoidoscopy. Because adenomas do not typically bleed, the fecal occult blood testing is an insensitive screening method. Older age, villous histology, and size are independent risk factors for malignancy within an adenoma. The risk of colon cancer also increases with the number of high-risk adenomas that are present.

Colonoscopy with endoscopic polypectomy is the ideal examination for the detection and removal of adenomatous polyps. Large adenomas that cannot be safely or completely resected endoscopically should generally be removed by segmental colectomy. If a polyp is detected by barium enema, colonoscopy is recommended to establish the histology, remove the polyp, and search for other lesions. If a single polyp is detected by sigmoidoscopy, it should be biopsied. If the polyp is hyperplastic, colonoscopy is not required. If the polyp is adenomatous, full colonoscopy is warranted.

A 3-year interval for surveillance colonoscopy is safe and cost-effective for most patients with adenomas. If only a small tubular adenoma is found, the interval may be extended to 5 years; in contrast, after removal of a large villous adenoma, a 1-year follow-up is recommended. After a negative screening or surveillance colonoscopy, an examination interval of 5 years appears to be safe. Patients with colorectal cancer should also have regular colonoscopic surveillance for adenomas, since these patients have adenoma recurrence rates of 25% to 30% at 3 years.

REFERENCES

- American Gastroenterological Association medical position statement: evaluation of dyspepsia. *Gastroenterology.* 1998;114(3):579–581.

- De Lillo AR, Rose S. Functional bowel disorders in the geriatric patient: constipation, fecal impaction, and fecal incontinence. *Am J Gastroenterol.* 2000; 95(4):901–905.

- Gostout CJ. Gastrointestinal bleeding in the elderly patient. *Am J Gastroenterol.* 2000; 95(3):590–595.

- Richter JE. Gastroesophageal reflux disease in the older patient: presentation, treatment and complications. *Am J Gastroenterol.* 2000; 95(2):368–373.

- Williams SG, DiPalma JA. Medication-induced digestive system injury in the elderly. *Geriatr Nurs.* 1992;13(1):39–42.

CHAPTER 48—ENDOCRINE AND METABOLIC DISORDERS

Impaired homeostatic regulation, a hallmark of aging, occurs in many endocrine functions but may become manifest only during stress. For example, fasting blood glucose levels change little with normal aging, increasing 1 to 2 mg per dL per decade of life. In contrast, glucose levels after a glucose challenge increase much more in healthy older persons than in young adults. In some cases, a loss of function in one aspect of endocrine function may result in a compensatory change in endocrine regulation and associated alterations in catabolism that maintain homeostasis. For example, the reduction in testicular testosterone production that occurs in many older men may be partially compensated for by an increase in pituitary luteinizing hormone secretion and a decrease in testosterone metabolism. In other instances, compensatory changes or alterations in hormone catabolism do not fully offset age-related impairment in endocrine functions, as illustrated by the age-related decline in basal serum aldosterone levels. In this case, a decline in aldosterone clearance fails to offset the decrease in aldosterone secretion.

As with diseases in other organ systems, endocrine disorders in older adults often present with nonspecific, muted, or atypical symptoms and signs. Some of these presentations are well-defined syndromes that are seen almost exclusively in older adults, such as apathetic thyrotoxicosis or hyperosmolar nonketotic state in patients with diabetes mellitus. However, more commonly, endocrine disorders present with subtle, nonspecific symptoms, such as cognitive impairment, or an absence of any complaints. For example, "silent" presentation of myocardial infarction is more likely to occur in older than in younger patients with diabetes mellitus. Indeed, the diagnosis of endocrinopathies such as hyperparathyroidism, diabetes mellitus, hypothyroidism, and hyperthyroidism in older adults is commonly established as a result of abnormalities found on routine laboratory screening.

Laboratory evaluation of older adults for endocrine disorders may be complicated by coexisting medical illnesses and medications. For example, the presence of serious acute nonthyroidal illness may lead to the mistaken impression of a thyroid disorder, because of the reduction in free thyroxine (T_4) levels and sometimes increased or decreased thyrotropin (TSH) levels in sick but euthyroid older patients. Furthermore, ranges of normal laboratory values for endocrine testing are commonly established in younger adults, and even age-adjusted norms for laboratory tests may be confounded by the inclusion of older adults who are ill. Therefore, normal ranges for healthy older people are not available for most laboratory tests.

THYROID DISORDERS

With aging, a reduction in T_4 secretion is balanced by a decrease in T_4 clearance, resulting in unchanged circulating T_4 levels. Triiodothyronine (T_3) levels are unchanged until extreme old age, when they decrease slightly. However, T_3 levels are commonly reduced in the setting of nonthyroidal illness because of decreased T_4-to-T_3 conversion. TSH levels are unchanged or minimally changed in healthy older people.

Because nonspecific, atypical, or asymptomatic presentations of thyroid disease are common in older adults, laboratory testing is the most reliable way to identify cases of hypothyroidism or hyperthyroidism in this age group. Given a 1.4% prevalence of thyroid disease in ambulatory women aged 50 and over, some clinicians recommend routine screening with a highly sensitive TSH test, but treatment may not affect outcomes. In addition, the prevalence of hypothyroidism or hyperthyroidism is sufficiently high to warrant TSH testing in all older adults with a recent decline in clinical, cognitive, or functional status, or upon admission to the hospital or nursing home. However, the results of thyroid function testing may be confusing in euthyroid patients with significant concurrent illnesses, as discussed below.

Hypothyroidism

Most prevalence estimates of hypothyroidism in older adults range from 0.5% to 5% for overt disease, and from 5% to 10% for subclinical hypothyroidism, depending on the population studied. As in younger people, most cases of hypothyroidism in older adults are due to chronic autoimmune thyroiditis.

Symptoms of hypothyroidism are often muted, nonspecific, or atypical in older adults. Some clinical features of hypothyroidism (eg, dry skin, decreased skin turgor, slowed mentation, weakness, constipation, anemia, hyponatremia, arthritis, paresthesias, gait disturbances, alopecia, elevated myocardial band of creatine phosphokinase) may misleadingly suggest other diseases. Furthermore, these symptoms usually have an insidious onset and a slow rate of progression. As a result, the diagnosis of hypothyroidism is recognized on clinical examination in only 10% to 20% of cases in older adults, and laboratory screening is necessary to detect most cases of hypothyroidism in this population. In addition, older patients with mild

hypothyroidism who develop serious nonthyroidal illness may rapidly become severely hypothyroid, and older adults are more susceptible to myxedema coma in this setting. Demented older people with hypothyroidism rarely recover normal cognitive function with thyroid replacement, but cognition, functional status, and mood may improve with treatment of the hypothyroidism.

Subclinical hypothyroidism, with elevated serum TSH and normal free T_4 levels, occurs in up to 15% of people aged 65 and over, and is more common in women. Data indicate that subclinical hypothyroidism is an important risk factor for atherosclerosis and myocardial infarction in older women. The presence of elevated thyroid antimicrosomal antibody titers portends the eventual development of thyroid failure and overt hypothyroidism, and it is appropriate to initiate T_4 replacement therapy in these patients. Alternatively, if antibody titers are low or are not obtained, patients should be followed with serial (every 3 weeks) TSH levels and observed for the development of symptoms and signs of hypothyroidism. Hormone replacement is warranted in older adults with progressively increasing TSH levels or a TSH level persistently above 10 mIU/L.

By itself, an increased TSH level is usually due to primary hypothyroidism, but TSH levels may be transiently elevated during recovery from acute illnesses. Therefore, the diagnosis of hypothyroidism should be confirmed with the combination of an elevated TSH level and a decreased free T_4 or free T_4 index, or by the demonstration of a persistently increased TSH level, or both. Other potentially confusing scenarios in the diagnosis of hypothyroidism include the *low T4 syndrome*, seen in euthyroid patients with severe nonthyroidal illnesses and presenting with a decreased free T_4 index without an increase in TSH levels. Free T_4 levels are usually normal in the low T_4 syndrome, with elevated levels of reverse T_3. Thyroid hormone supplementation has not been shown to be beneficial in these patients. A normal (or low) TSH together with a low free T_4 level may also suggest *secondary hypothyroidism*, which is differentiated from the low T_4 syndrome by the presence of hypopituitarism (deficiencies in other pituitary hormones) and decreased reverse T_3 levels. Finally, older people with primary hypothyroidism may also present with inappropriately normal TSH levels resulting from suppression of TSH by fasting, acute illnesses, and medications such as dopamine, phenytoin, or glucocorticoids. However, it is uncommon for TSH levels to be suppressed into the normal range in these patients.

T_4 replacement is usually initiated at a low dosage (eg, 25 µg per day) in older adults, increasing the dose every few weeks until TSH levels normalize. However, in patients with cardiac disease, it is prudent to begin replacement therapy at even lower dosages (eg, 12.5 µg per day). In these patients, thyroid replacement should not be withheld for fear of exacerbating cardiac disease; instead, the goal is to reduce or eliminate symptoms of hypothyroidism without causing intolerable exacerbation of symptoms, such as angina. Older adults who are severely hypothyroid at presentation should receive larger initial T_4 replacement doses of 50 to 100 µg, or as high as 400 µg intravenously for those with myxedema stupor or coma, even if there is preexisting heart disease. Such patients should also receive testing to exclude concomitant adrenal insufficiency as well as stress doses of glucocorticoids prior to receiving T_4 to avoid precipitating an adrenal crisis with T_4 replacement.

Thyroid hormone requirements decrease with aging because of a reduction in clearance rate, and T_4 replacement doses are as much as a third lower in older than in younger adults. The average T_4 replacement dosage in older adults is approximately 110 µg per day. Overreplacement of thyroid hormone should be avoided, because osteopenia related to increased bone turnover and exacerbation of heart disease may occur. With correction of the hypothyroid state, the clearance rate of medications such as anticonvulsants, digoxin, and opiate analgesic agents may be affected, necessitating dosage adjustments. T_4 supplementation may have beneficial effects on some parameters of cognitive and cardiac function in some older adults with subclinical hypothyroidism, although randomized trials of such treatment have yielded mixed results. Finally, elevations in total and low-density lipoprotein cholesterol levels in hypothyroid patients may resolve with restoration of the euthyroid state, suggesting that T_4 replacement may reduce the risk of atherosclerotic vascular disease in older adults with good long-term survival prospects.

Hyperthyroidism

Hyperthyroidism develops in 0.5% to 2.3% of adults aged 65 and over, and 15% to 25% of all cases of thyrotoxicosis occur in adults aged 60 and over. In the United States, most cases in older adults are due to Graves' disease, but toxic multinodular goiter and autonomously functioning adenomas are more common in older than in young adults, especially in populations with low iodine intake.

Hyperthyroidism often presents with vague, atypical, or nonspecific symptoms in frail older patients. Many findings that are common in younger adults (eg, tremor, heat intolerance, tachycardia, ophthalmopathy, increased perspiration, goiter, brisk reflexes) are less common or absent in older persons, whereas other manifestations, such as atrial fibrillation, congestive heart failure signs and symptoms, constipation, anorexia, muscle atrophy, and weakness, are more

common in older adults. Older persons may present with *apathetic thyrotoxicosis*, a well-known clinical presentation of hyperthyroidism that is rarely seen in younger persons, in which the usual hyperkinetic presentation is replaced by depression, inactivity, lethargy, or withdrawn behavior, often in association with symptoms such as weight loss, muscle weakness, or cardiac symptoms. A low TSH level is associated with a threefold higher risk of developing atrial fibrillation within 10 years, and hyperthyroidism is present in 13% to 30% of older people with atrial fibrillation. Hyperthyroidism is a cause of secondary osteoporosis and should be considered in the evaluation of patients presenting with decreased bone mass.

A highly sensitive TSH test is adequate as an initial test for hyperthyroidism in relatively healthy older patients, but the diagnosis should be confirmed with a free T_4 test. Most asymptomatic older adults with low serum TSH levels are euthyroid and have normal T_4 and T_3 levels, with normal TSH on repeat testing 4 to 6 weeks later. In addition, serious illnesses, malnutrition, and medications such as glucocorticoids, dopamine agonists, and phenytoin may suppress TSH levels. *T_3 thyrotoxicosis*, with elevated T_3 but normal T_4 levels, occurs in a minority of hyperthyroid patients, but it is more common with aging, especially in patients with toxic adenomas or toxic multinodular goiter. However, in contrast to young adults, many older persons with hyperthyroidism do not have increased T_4 or T_3 levels, probably because of decreased conversion of T_4 to T_3 associated with aging and nonthyroidal illness. Diagnostic confusion may occasionally occur in euthyroid patients with conditions or medications causing elevated T_4 levels (*high T_4 syndrome*). The high T_4 syndrome may occur with drugs or illnesses that decrease T_4-to-T_3 conversion (high-dose glucocorticoids or β-blocking agents, acute fasting) or that increase circulating levels of thyroid-binding globulin (estrogens, clofibrate, hepatitis).

Subclinical hyperthyroidism is present in less than 2% of older people and is associated with adverse cardiovascular events such as atrial fibrillation, osteoporosis, and neuropsychiatric effects. Accordingly, treatment for this condition may be justifiable, but there is a lack of data from randomized, controlled trials to support this approach.

Thyroid scanning and measurements of radioactive iodine uptake may be useful in confirming hyperthyroidism and defining the cause. Radioactive iodine therapy is the treatment of choice for most older people with hyperthyroidism. Higher or repeated doses are often necessary for patients with toxic multinodular goiter. Antithyroid drugs such as propylthiouracil are given prior to radioactive iodine, to control symptoms and to avoid a worsening of thyrotoxicosis due to transient release of thyroid hormone after radioactive iodine. β-Blocking agents are helpful to manage symptoms such as tachycardia, tremor, and anxiety, but patients should be monitored for changes in cardiopulmonary function. Following radioactive iodine therapy, patients should be followed with serial TSH levels for the eventual development of hypothyroidism, or persistent or recurrent hyperthyroidism. With resolution of hyperthyroidism, the clearance rate of other drugs may decrease, necessitating dosage adjustments to avoid excessive drug levels.

Nodular Thyroid Disease and Thyroid Cancer

The incidence of multinodular goiter increases with aging, and approximately 90% of women aged 70 years and over, and 60% of men aged 80 years and over have thyroid nodules. Most of these are nonpalpable. Multinodular goiters often have autonomously functioning areas, but administration of exogenous thyroid hormone to suppress these goiters may cause iatrogenic hyperthyroidism. Older persons with multinodular goiter may develop iodine-induced thyrotoxicosis after receiving radiocontrast or amiodarone.

Solitary thyroid nodules are more likely to be malignant in people over 60 years of age, especially men. The incidence of differentiated thyroid cancers is similar in older and younger adults, whereas anaplastic thyroid carcinomas occur almost exclusively in older adults. However, even well-differentiated papillary and follicular carcinomas are more aggressive and are associated with increased mortality in older persons. Accordingly, a new solitary nodule or an enlargement of an existing nodule warrants a careful evaluation, including a fine-needle aspiration.

DISORDERS OF PARATHYROID AND CALCIUM METABOLISM

Important changes occur with aging in several systems that regulate calcium homeostasis, ultimately leading to a reduction in bone mass and in some cases osteoporosis in older people (Table 48.1). The net effect of these changes is to increase circulating levels of parathyroid hormone (PTH), which increases 30% between 30 and 80 years of age. Serum calcium levels remain normal as a result of the increase in PTH, but the balance between bone resorption and bone formation is altered in favor of resorption, resulting in a decrease in bone mass and an increased risk of osteoporosis with aging.

When dietary calcium intake is low, older people are less able than younger adults to compensate by

Table 48.1—Age-Related Alterations in Calcium Homeostasis

Factors leading to decreased 1,25(OH)$_2$D levels

  Decreased renal 1α-hydroxylase activity, leading to decreased renal PTH responsiveness

  Decreased vitamin D synthesis by the skin

  Decreased sunlight exposure (housebound and institutionalized elderly persons)

Factors leading to decreased intestinal absorption of dietary calcium

  Inadequate dietary calcium and vitamin D intake

  Decreased intestinal responsiveness to 1,25(OH)$_2$D

  Decreased gastric acid secretion

  Lactase deficiency (avoidance of dairy products)

Factors leading to age-related increase in serum PTH levels

  Slight decrease in serum calcium levels

  Decreased renal clearance of PTH

  Decreased 1,25(OH)$_2$D levels

NOTE: 1,25(OH)$_2$D = 1,25 dihydroxyvitamin D; PTH = parathyroid hormone.

increasing their intestinal absorption of ingested calcium. Older adults are therefore more dependent on an adequate dietary calcium intake, yet most take in far less calcium than they need. In addition, vitamin D deficiency is extremely common in older adults, occurring in a third to over half of medical inpatients, nursing-home residents, and older homebound community-dwelling adults. However, adequate dietary calcium and vitamin D supplementation may reverse age-related hyperparathyroidism, increase bone mineral density, and reduce osteoporotic fracture rates.

Hypercalcemia

Primary hyperparathyroidism and malignancy-associated hypercalcemia are the most common causes of hypercalcemia in older adults. The annual incidence of primary hyperparathyroidism is approximately 1 per 1000, and the disease is threefold more prevalent in women than in men. Most patients with primary hyperparathyroidism are asymptomatic, and the diagnosis is made after an incidental finding of hypercalcemia. When the disease is symptomatic, older persons are more likely than younger adults to present with neuropsychiatric symptoms such as depression and cognitive impairment, neuromuscular symptoms such as proximal muscle weakness, or osteoporosis. In addition to hypercalcemia, laboratory findings of primary hyperparathyroidism may include low to low-normal phosphate, elevated alkaline phosphatase levels, and hypercalciuria. The diagnosis is confirmed with an elevated or high normal PTH level by the use of an assay for intact PTH, in the presence of hypercalcemia. Surgery is the treatment of choice for primary hyperparathyroidism with serum calcium levels > 12 mg/dL, 24-hour urine calcium levels > 400 mg, and overt manifestations including markedly decreased cortical bone density or nephrolithiasis. Patients with serum calcium levels < 12 mg/dL who are asymptomatic and managed conservatively should avoid thiazide diuretics, dehydration, and immobilization; serum calcium, 24-hour urine calcium, creatinine clearance, and bone densitometry should be monitored. In addition, these patients should be followed clinically for the development of nephrolithiasis, minimal trauma fractures, and neuropsychiatric or neuromuscular symptoms. Medical management options for hyperparathyroidism also include β-blocking agents, estrogens in women, oral phosphate in patients with low serum phosphate levels and good renal function, and possibly bisphosphonates.

Patients with nonparathyroid causes of hypercalcemia have undetectable or markedly decreased PTH levels. In hospitalized patients, the most common cause of hypercalcemia is a malignancy that produces PTH-related peptide, with hypercalcemia resulting primarily from increased net bone resorption. The presence of an underlying cancer is usually evident on examination and routine diagnostic testing. Squamous cell cancers of the lung or head and neck are common causes of hypercalcemia due to PTH-related peptide production. Other common malignancies associated with hypercalcemia include breast cancer, lymphoma, and myeloma, although the mechanism of the hypercalcemia is different for many of these cancers. Acute treatment for hypercalcemia includes volume replacement with intravenous saline, followed by diuresis with a loop diuretic when rehydration is complete. A parenteral bisphosphonate such as pamidronate should be given, along with treatment of the underlying malignancy, if possible. In addition to their usefulness in the treatment of hypercalcemia, bisphosphonates may decrease bone pain and the risk of pathologic fractures in patients with osteolytic bone metastases from a variety of cancers.

Paget's Disease of Bone

Paget's disease is characterized by localized areas of increased bone remodeling, resulting in a change in bone architecture and an increased tendency to deformity and fracture. Its prevalence increases with aging, affecting 2% to 5% of people aged 50 years and over. Paget's disease is usually asymptomatic and is often diagnosed as an incidental finding on radiographs or during evaluation for an unexplained elevation in serum alkaline phosphatase. The most commonly affected sites are the pelvis, spine, femur, and skull. When Paget's disease is symptomatic, pain is the most common presenting symptom, either localized to the affected bones or resulting from secondary osteoarthritic changes, often in the hips, knees, and vertebrae. When bone deformities occur, the long bones of the lower extremities are usually affected, often with a bowing of the involved extremity. Skull involvement may result in compression of the eighth cranial nerve and sensorineural hearing loss. Treatment is not usually necessary for asymptomatic disease, unless there is concern for hearing loss from skull involvement, nerve root or spinal cord compression from vertebral involvement, or hip fracture from femoral neck involvement. Bisphosphonates suppress the accelerated bone turnover and bone remodeling that is characteristic of this disease, and they are the treatment of choice. During treatment, patients should be monitored clinically for changes in bone pain, joint function, and neurologic status, and with biochemical indices of bone formation (eg, serum osteocalcin or bone-specific alkaline phosphatase) or resorption (eg, urinary N-telopeptide), or both.

HORMONAL REGULATION OF WATER AND ELECTROLYTE BALANCE

Unlike young adults, older persons are predisposed to both volume depletion and free water excess. This impairment in regulation of volume status and osmolality is multifactorial, reflecting alterations in antidiuretic hormone (ADH) secretion, osmoreceptor and baroreceptor systems, urine-concentrating capability, renal hormone responsiveness, and thirst sensation. ADH secretion tends to be excessive in older people, with normal to elevated basal ADH levels, increased ADH responses to osmoreceptor stimuli such as hypertonic saline infusion, and decreased ethanol-induced inhibition of ADH secretion. This state of relative ADH excess with aging, together with the common occurrence of renal insufficiency, congestive heart failure, hypothyroidism, and diuretic use, predisposes older adults to hyponatremia by impairing free water clearance.

Under other circumstances, older people are at increased risk of volume depletion. With aging, basal aldosterone secretion declines disproportionately to the decrease in clearance, with a net reduction in circulating aldosterone levels of about 30% by the age of 80 years. At the same time, atrial natriuretic hormone secretion (and renal responsiveness to this hormone) increases with aging. Atrial natriuretic hormone inhibits aldosterone production and causes natriuresis and diuresis through its effects on the kidneys. Taken together, these changes predispose older people to volume depletion by decreasing the ability of the kidneys to conserve sodium under conditions of fluid deprivation. Baroreceptor ADH responses to hypotension and hypovolemia are decreased in older people, placing them at additional risk of dehydration. Moreover, renal responsiveness to ADH is decreased with aging, resulting in a decreased ability of the kidneys to maximally concentrate urine. Finally, even healthy older adults have decreased thirst sensation and may not be aware that they are becoming dehydrated. Demented and immobile older people are at the highest risk for severe dehydration.

In addition to predisposing to volume depletion, age-related hyporeninemic hypoaldosteronism also increases the risk of hyperkalemia, especially in patients with diabetes mellitus or renal insufficiency. The addition of angiotensin-converting enzyme inhibitors, nonsteroidal anti-inflammatory drugs, β-blocking agents, and diuretics with aldosterone-antagonist properties may lead to potentially lethal hyperkalemia in some of these patients.

DISORDERS OF THE ADRENAL CORTEX

Basal serum cortisol levels do not change with aging, because decreased cortisol secretion is balanced by a decrease in clearance. Adrenocorticotropic hormone (ACTH) stimulation of cortisol production is unchanged, and cortisol and ACTH responses to stress and secretagogues are unimpaired with aging. Clinically, acute cortisol responses to stress may be higher and more prolonged in older than in younger adults. Accordingly, unless it is emergent, adrenal function testing should be deferred at least 48 hours after major stressors, such as surgery or trauma. In older patients with a normal ACTH stimulation test in whom adrenal insufficiency is suspected, endocrinology consultation is recommended to assist with further testing.

Hypoadrenocorticoidism

Chronic glucocorticoid therapy is also the most common cause of adrenal failure in older adults, because of chronic suppression of adrenal function. Recovery of adrenal axis function is variable and may take several months to occur. Autoimmune-mediated adrenal failure is less common in older than in younger adults, but tuberculosis, adrenal metastases, and adrenal hemorrhage in anticoagulated patients are more common causes of adrenal insufficiency in older persons. Older patients with chronic adrenal insufficiency may present with nonspecific symptoms such as anorexia, weight loss, or impaired functional status, and hyperkalemia may not be present initially. Accordingly, a high index of suspicion is required to make the diagnosis. When adrenocortical insufficiency is suspected, the ACTH stimulation test should be performed and therapy initiated. In older people who are stopping chronic glucocorticoid therapy, the replacement regimen should be tapered gradually, and stress dose coverage should be given for major surgery and other acute physiologic stresses until adrenocortical function has normalized.

Hyperadrenocorticoidism

Exogenous glucocorticoids are the most common cause of Cushing's syndrome in older adults, often causing adverse effects, including psychiatric and cognitive symptoms, osteoporosis, myopathy, and glucose intolerance. For patients beginning long-term glucocorticoid therapy, baseline and follow-up bone densitometry measurements are indicated, and calcium, vitamin D, and antiresorptive treatments such as bisphosphonates should be initiated.

Adrenal Androgens

In contrast to cortisol, circulating levels of the principal adrenal androgen, dehydroepiandrosterone (DHEA), decline progressively with aging and are only 10% to 20% of young adult levels in octogenarians. Low DHEA levels are associated with poor health, whereas DHEA levels are positively correlated with some measures of longevity and functional status. Given these associations, there is considerable interest in the potential therapeutic effects of DHEA administration in older adults.

Some trials of up to 6 months of DHEA therapy in middle-aged and older adults reported subjective improvements in physical and psychologic well-being, increased serum insulin-like growth factor-I levels, and, at supraphysiologic doses, increased lean body mass and some measures of muscle strength. However, DHEA was found to decrease circulating high-density lipoprotein cholesterol levels, suggesting potential long-term atherogenic effects. Furthermore, DHEA is metabolized to estrogens and to androgens, including testosterone and dihydrotestosterone, and its effects on the risk of breast cancer in women and prostate cancer in men are unknown. Finally, higher doses of DHEA may cause androgenization in some women and gynecomastia in men. Thus, although these data are intriguing, the safety and efficacy of DHEA supplementation have not been established, and its use is inappropriate outside of clinical studies.

TESTOSTERONE

Despite former controversy, there is now general agreement that total and free testosterone levels and testosterone secretion are lower in healthy older men than in younger men. Many healthy older men exhibit moderate primary testicular failure, with decreased sperm production, testosterone levels, and testosterone secretory responses to gonadotropin administration. In addition, many of these men have inappropriately normal (ie, not increased) gonadotropin levels in the presence of low testosterone levels, suggesting secondary (hypothalamic or pituitary) testicular failure. Overt testicular failure is common in chronically ill and debilitated older men, manifested by total testosterone levels well below the normal range and symptoms suggesting androgen deficiency, including decreased libido and potency, gynecomastia, and hot flashes. Testosterone replacement therapy is generally warranted in these patients, as in hypogonadal young men. However, it is more common to encounter older men with low-normal or mildly decreased serum testosterone levels and nonspecific manifestations, such as decreased libido, weakness, decreased muscle mass, osteopenia, and memory loss. In most cases, these manifestations have multiple causes, but it has been hypothesized that declining testosterone levels with aging contribute to their development, and that testosterone supplementation may help to prevent or treat these disorders.

Men with suspected hypogonadism should be evaluated with a serum free or bioavailable (non–sex hormone–binding globulin-bound) testosterone level, either measured by equilibrium dialysis or calculated from measurements of total testosterone and sex hormone–binding globulin. Concentrations of sex hormone–binding globulin, the main circulating binding protein for testosterone, increase with age. Therefore, the age-related decline in serum free or bioavailable testosterone is greater than that of total testosterone, and total testosterone measurements do not accurately reflect the decrease in biologically active testosterone with aging. Direct radioimmunoassays using "analog" kits for free testosterone are widely used but are not recommended because they may underestimate androgen deficiency in older men and overestimate androgen deficiency in men with low sex hormone–binding globulin (eg, moderately obese men). Luteinizing hormone and follicle-stimulating hormone levels should be obtained. In addition, a review (and if possible, discontinuation) of medications that may suppress gonadotropins (eg, glucocorticoids and central nervous system–active drugs) and a prolactin level are indicated if gonadotropins are low-normal or low in the presence of low testosterone levels. High prolactin levels inhibit gonadotropin secretion and could be due to either a pituitary adenoma or hypothalamic disorder. Further studies may be warranted in such patients, including magnetic resonance imaging of the pituitary fossa and assessment of other pituitary functions (eg, cortisol response to ACTH and T_4). Baseline bone densitometry measurements should be obtained in men with decreased testosterone levels to exclude osteoporosis.

Small controlled studies of testosterone supplementation in older men of up to 3 years' duration have reported improvements in muscle strength, lean body mass, bone mass, cognitive functioning, and sense of well-being. However, it is unknown whether these benefits are clinically important, or whether the benefits outweigh the potential risks. Bearing these uncertainties in mind, a trial of androgen supplementation may be appropriate in older men with serum total testosterone levels < 3.0 ng/mL and clinical features suggesting hypogonadism (eg, osteoporosis, muscle wasting or weakness, mild anemia of unclear cause, loss of libido). However, androgen replacement therapy is inappropriate in asymptomatic older men with low-normal total testosterone levels. In the absence of decreased libido, erectile dysfunction in older men does not usually respond to testosterone therapy. Men should be monitored closely for adverse androgenic effects of treatment, including polycythemia and potential exacerbation of prostatic disease. However, there is no direct evidence that testosterone therapy increases the risk of prostate cancer or symptomatic benign prostatic hyperplasia. (See also "Disorders of Sexual Function," p 339.)

GROWTH HORMONE

Growth hormone secretion declines with aging, and by 70 to 80 years of age, about half of adults have no significant growth hormone secretion over 24 hours. A corresponding decline occurs in levels of insulin-like growth factor 1, which mediates most of the effects of growth hormone and falls to levels comparable to growth hormone–deficient children in 40% of adults 70 to 80 years of age.

Adults with growth hormone deficiency due to hypothalamic pituitary disease exhibit decreased muscle strength, lean body mass, and bone density; increased abdominal obesity; unfavorable lipid profiles; and an increased risk of cardiovascular disease; all are reversible with growth hormone replacement. Older adults without hypothalamic pituitary disease have many of the same conditions, leading to the hypothesis that growth hormone supplementation may have a beneficial effect on these clinically important age-related disorders.

Small randomized trials of growth hormone supplementation in older adults have reported increased lean body mass and bone density, and decreased fat mass, but no improvements in functional status were demonstrated. Furthermore, significant side effects were common, including carpal tunnel syndrome, arthralgias, edema, and gynecomastia,

Short-term growth hormone supplementation may improve nitrogen balance in older persons with severe illness and catabolic states. However, growth hormone is very expensive, and at present it is not recommended for clinical use in older people without established hypothalamic pituitary disease.

MELATONIN

Melatonin is a hormone secreted by the pineal gland that is thought to be involved in the regulation of circadian and seasonal biorhythms. Melatonin secretion is inhibited by exposure to light, resulting in a marked circadian variation in circulating melatonin levels, and its sedative effects suggest a role in sleep induction. Production of melatonin gradually decreases throughout life after early childhood, but the physiologic significance of this decline in melatonin secretion is unclear. Numerous claims have been made in the lay press regarding the "anti-aging" benefits of melatonin supplementation for various conditions, including insomnia, immune deficiency, cancer, and the aging process itself. Although melatonin may have sleep-inducing properties in older people with insomnia, the long-term risks and benefits of melatonin supplementation have not been established for insomnia or any other indication.

DIABETES MELLITUS

Diabetes mellitus is a group of metabolic diseases characterized by hyperglycemia due to abnormalities in insulin secretion, insulin action, or both. It is one of the most common chronic diseases affecting older persons. Estimates of the prevalence among persons aged 65 years and over range between 15% and 20%, with the higher rates associated with persons over age 75. Because the disease may be asymptomatic for many years, it is estimated that one third of older adults with diabetes mellitus are unaware of their condition. Despite the early asymptomatic period, diabetes mellitus is a serious condition associated with significant morbidity and a shortened survival. Older persons with diabetes can expect a 10-year reduction in life expectancy and a mortality rate nearly twice that of persons without this disease. When the diabetes is poorly controlled, hyperglycemia alone can be the cause of insidious decline in an older patient. Uncontrolled or undiagnosed diabetes mellitus can be characterized by fatigue, weight loss, muscle weakness, cognitive changes, infections, and functional impairments. Complications of this disease over the longer term include loss of vision, renal insufficiency, atherosclerosis, and neuropathies. The rates of myocardial infarction, stroke, and renal failure are increased approximately

twofold, and the risk of blindness is increased approximately 40% in older persons with diabetes.

Pathophysiology and Diagnosis

The American Diabetes Association classifies diabetes mellitus affecting older adults into three types. Type 1 is the result of an absolute deficiency in insulin secretion due to autoimmune destruction of the β cells of the pancreas. Type 2 is most commonly due to tissue resistance to insulin action and relative insulin deficiency. A third category is reserved for other specific types of diabetes, such as injuries to the exocrine pancreas; endocrinopathies characterized by excesses of hormones, such as growth hormone, cortisol, glucagon, and epinephrine, which antagonize insulin action; drug- or chemical-induced diabetes; infections leading to the destruction of the β cells of the pancreas. In about 90% of cases, older adults with diabetes have the type 2 form of the disease. This is the form in which hyperglycemia is characteristic, but ketosis is not a common part of the clinical syndrome. The reasons for the increased prevalence of type 2 diabetes among older persons are not fully known; there appears to be an interaction among several factors, including genetics, life style, and aging influences. There is a strong genetic predisposition to type 2 diabetes. Obesity and decreased physical activity, common among older persons, contribute to impairments in insulin action. Glucose intolerance has also been shown to be related to aged-associated decline in pancreatic β-cell function and to reductions with aging of the insulin-signaling mechanisms that limit the mobilization of glucose transporters needed for insulin-mediated glucose uptake and metabolism in muscle and fat. The heterogeneity in the severity of hyperglycemia among older patients with type 2 diabetes is related to the varying contributions of each of these factors in each individual.

The pathophysiology of the complications of diabetes is similar in younger and older persons. Prolonged hyperglycemia leads to glycosylation of proteins; the accumulation of these abnormal proteins can cause tissue damage. Also, metabolic products of the aldose-reductase system, such as sorbitol, accumulate in the presence of hyperglycemia. These products can impair cellular energy metabolism and contribute to cell injury and death.

The American Diabetes Association diagnostic criteria for diabetes mellitus published in 2001 do not include any adjustments based on age. Three ways to establish the diagnosis of diabetes mellitus are possible, and each must be confirmed, on a subsequent day, by any one of three methods:

- Symptoms of polyuria, polydipsia and unexplained weight loss plus a casual plasma glucose concentration of ≥ 200mg/dL (11.1 mmol/L). Casual is defined as any time of day without regard to time since last meal.

- A plasma glucose concentration after an 8-hour fast ≥ 126 mg/dL (7.0 mmol/L).

- A plasma glucose concentration of ≥ 200 mg/dL (11.1 mmol/L) measured 2 hours after ingestion of 75 g of glucose in 300 mL of water administered after an overnight fast.

During the comprehensive evaluation of a patient with suspected diabetes mellitus, several issues deserve special attention. A drug history is important because certain medications can contribute to hyperglycemia (eg, diuretics, adrenergic agonists, glucocorticoids, caffeine, nicotine, alcohol, and phenytoin). Because of the genetic determinants of diabetes, a family history of the disease can provide useful information. Diabetes is a well-established risk factor for atherosclerotic cardiovascular disease, so other risk factors such as smoking, family history, hypertension, and hyperlipidemia should also be explored.

Management

The principles of managing diabetes mellitus are similar to those of managing many other chronic illnesses. As the evidence of benefit among older, particularly frail persons is less compelling than among Type 1 and younger Type II diabetics, attention to tradeoffs between risk and benefit is particularly important. It is important that the patient understands the mechanisms of the metabolic derangements and their management, becomes fully involved in monitoring and treating the disease and its complications, and, in conjunction with the treating practitioner, sets realistic goals. These goals may vary, depending on the patient's preferences, level of commitment, and life expectancy, the number and severity of coexisting health problems, and the availability of supportive services. Some recommended goals suggested by the American Diabetes Association are shown in Table 48.2. Other health professionals such as diabetes educators, nurses, dietitians, pharmacists, and social workers may play an important role in formulating a comprehensive treatment plan and in providing education and support.

Diet and physical activity remain cornerstones of the initial and ongoing management of patients with diabetes. The specific dietary recommendations must be tailored for each individual, but there are guidelines that are widely applicable. Moderate caloric restriction of 250 to 500 kcal less than usual daily intake is a reasonable goal, unless the patient is significantly undernourished. A low-fat diet in which calories from fat are limited to 25% to 30% of total calories is advisable. It is often recommended that meals, especially carbohydrate intake, be spaced throughout the day to avoid large caloric loads. Physical activity programs should also be individualized; however, at a minimum, it is reasonable to follow the recommendations of the Surgeon General's Report on Physical Activity and Health that a person accumulate at least 30 minutes of moderate physical activity on most days.

There are many options for drug therapy in older persons with type 2 diabetes and no clearly preferred algorithm. Regimens can consist of any of the classes of drugs shown in Table 48.3, used alone or in combination. It is common to adjust the regimen over the course of the illness as goals change, the disease progresses, or complications develop. Sulfonylurea preparations have a long record of safety and effectiveness. Hypoglycemia is an important side effect, and these drugs must be used cautiously in patients with significant renal and hepatic insufficiency, since the liver is the primary site of metabolism and they are excreted by the kidneys. α-Glucosidase inhibitors impair the breakdown of carbohydrates in the gut and limit absorption. The residual carbohydrates in the intestinal lumen are responsible for diarrhea in about 25% of patients who use this drug. The biguanide preparations also have gastrointestinal side effects and can cause lactic acidosis in patients with renal insufficiency. It is recommended that metformin not be

Table 48.2—ADA Goals for Glucose Control Among Patients With Type II Diabetes Mellitus

Measurement	Normal Value	Goal Value	Additional Action Suggested
Whole blood values			
Average preprandial glucose (mg/dL)	< 100	80–120	< 80 or > 140
Average bedtime glucose (mg/dL)	< 110	100–140	< 100 or > 160
Plasma values			
Average preprandial glucose (mg/dL)	< 110	90–130	< 90 or > 150
Average bedtime glucose (mg/dL)	< 120	110–150	< 110 or >180
Hemoglobin A$_{1c}$ (%)	< 6	< 7	> 8

NOTE: ADA = American Diabetes Association.

Table 48.3—Oral Medications Used in the Management of Type 2 Diabetes Mellitus

Medication	Daily Dose Range	Comments
α-Glucosidase inhibitors		Delay glucose absorption
Acarbose	25–100 mg three times daily just before meals	GI side effects common; avoid if creatinine > 2; monitor liver function tests
Biguanides		Insulin sensitizers
Metformin	500–2550 mg divided	Avoid in patients with renal insufficiency, congestive heart failure, abnormal liver function test
Sulfonylureas		Stimulate insulin secretion
Glimepiride	1–8 mg once or divided	Numerous drug interactions, long-acting
Glipizide	2.5–20 mg once or divided	Short-acting
Glyburide	1.25–20 mg once or divided	Long-acting, risk of hypoglycemia
Micronized glyburide	1.5–12 mg once	
Thiazolidinediones		Insulin resistance reducers
Pioglitazone	15–45 mg once	Check liver function tests at start and every 2 months for first year; avoid in patients with liver disease
Rosiglitazone	2–8 mg once or divided	Check liver function tests at start and every 2 months for first year; avoid in patients with liver disease

SOURCE: Data from Reuben DB, Herr K, Pacala JT, et al. *Geriatrics at Your Fingertips: 2003 Edition.* Malden, MA: Blackwell Science, Inc., for the American Geriatrics Society; 2003:52–53.

prescribed to patients with a serum creatinine of 1.5 mg/dL or greater. The thiazolidinedimes are generally well tolerated, but there is a risk of idiosyncratic hepatic toxicity. Finally, insulin can be used effectively in patients with type 2 diabetes. It is often possible to achieve good glycemic control with one or two injections a day of an intermediate-acting insulin preparation. The greatest risk of insulin therapy is hypoglycemia, which can be managed with either oral glucose solutions or injectable glucagon.

One of the primary reasons for treating diabetes is to avoid the long-term complications of the metabolic abnormalities. Patients with diabetes can be asymptomatic for many years, making it difficult to date the onset of the condition. For this reason, as soon as the diagnosis of diabetes has been established, it is appropriate to examine the patient for early signs of complications. Hypertension should be aggressively controlled; the Sixth Report of the Joint National Committee on Prevention, Detection, Evaluation, and Treatment of High Blood Pressure recommends maintaining the blood pressure below 130/85. A referral to ophthalmology is recommended to monitor the patient for retinopathy due to diabetes, an important cause of blindness. Because diabetes is an important risk factor for atherosclerosis, a careful examination of the heart and peripheral blood vessels, with special attention to the feet, is very important. Symptoms and signs of neuropathy should be explored, again, with special attention to early sensory changes in the feet, such as loss of light touch sensation or proprioception. Genitourinary complaints, such as recurrent cystitis, urinary incontinence, and sexual dysfunction, can be related to diabetes. Since the kidney is an organ commonly affected by diabetes, it is important to screen for early glomerulopathy by measuring albumin secretion. Glomerular disease should be suspected if more than 30 mg of albumin are measured in a 24-hour collection of urine. It is also possible to calculate the albumin-to-creatinine ratio in a random urine specimen. A ratio exceeding 30 μg of albumin per mg of creatinine is considered consistent with nephropathy. If microalbuminuria is confirmed by a second measurement within 3 to 6 months, an angiotensin-converting enzyme inhibitor should be started in an effort to slow the progression of renal disease. Serum lipids should also be measured to complete the detailed evaluation of cardiovascular risk factors in patients with diabetes. According to the National Cholesterol Education Program, among patients with diabetes, the target low-density lipoprotein cholesterol concentration is less than 100 mg/dL.

In the United States, diabetes mellitus is a very common chronic disease among older adults. There may be a prolonged asymptomatic period before the illness is detected. Once it is recognized, careful attention to glycemic control and managing the related comorbid conditions will offer the best opportunity for minimizing the complications and extending the years of high-quality life for patients with this disease.

REFERENCES

- American College of Physicians. Clinical guideline, part 1: screening for thyroid disease. *Ann Intern Med.* 1998;129:141–143.

- American Medical Directors Association. *Managing Diabetes in the Long-Term Care Setting: Clinical Practice Guideline*; 2002.

- Helfand M, Redfern CC. Clinical guideline, part 2: screening for thyroid disease: an update. *Ann Intern Med.* 1998;129:144–158.

- American Diabetes Association: Clinical practice recommendations 2002. *Diabetes Care.* 2002;25(suppl 1):S1–S147.

- Chiovato L, Mariotti S, Pinchera A. Thyroid diseases in the elderly. *Baillieres Clin Endocrinol Metab.* 1997;11:251–270.

- DeFronzo RA: Pharmacologic therapy for type 2 diabetes mellitus. *Ann Intern Med.* 1999;131:281–303.

- Gruenewald DA, Matsumoto AM. Aging of the endocrine system. In: Hazzard WR, Blass JP, Ettinger WH Jr, et al., eds. *Principles of Geriatric Medicine and Gerontology.* 4th ed. New York: McGraw-Hill; 1999:949–965.

- Miller M. Fluid and electrolyte homeostasis in the elderly: physiological changes of aging and clinical consequences. *Baillieres Clin Endocrinol Metab.* 1997;11:367–387.

CHAPTER 49—HORMONE REPLACEMENT THERAPY

Many of the symptoms and signs of hormone deficiency mimic those classically associated with aging. The fact that many hormones also decline with aging has led to an enthusiasm for attempting to reverse unwanted changes associated with aging by the use of hormonal replacement. The evidence for this approach is limited, with the exception of that for estrogen replacement in women and, to a lesser extent, testosterone replacement in men.

TREATMENT OF MENOPAUSAL SYMPTOMS

Estrogen replacement therapy (ERT) is approved by the Food and Drug Administration for the treatment of menopausal symptoms and urogenital dryness and for the prevention and treatment of osteoporosis, but it is used by clinicians for other reasons as well, in both women and men. The common short- and long-term uses, common prescribing practices, and risks of ERT are reviewed herein.

Menopause on average occurs at age 51 in the United States; with a life expectancy of 78 years, the average woman is postmenopausal one third of her life. Despite some controversy about the need for ERT, many women and their clinicians choose to treat or prevent the sequelae of estrogen deficiency in menopause.

Vasomotor symptoms or hot flushes are the most common symptom of the climacteric, occurring in 40% to 60% of perimenopausal women. Symptoms persist beyond 5 years in 25% of women and are lifelong in a small minority. Although the cause of the vasomotor response remains unknown, vasomotor symptoms are usually relieved within the first cycle of estrogen treatment. Low-dose therapy can be initiated and estrogen doses titrated until symptoms improve. When estrogen is contraindicated or not acceptable, progestins are considered the second most effective therapy; clonidine, methyldopa, or sustained-release tablets of belladonna alkaloids, phenobarbital, and ergotamine tartrate may relieve some symptoms.

TREATMENT OF UROGENITAL SYMPTOMS

Estrogen deficiency causes atrophy of both the vagina and urethra. (See "Gynecologic Diseases and Disorders," p 334, and "Disorders of Sexual Function," p 339.) Both have a high density of estrogen receptors. Although randomized trials are lacking, clinical experience with oral and vaginal estrogen indicates that they may relieve dysuria, incontinence, and urethral pressure in some cases.

PREVENTION AND TREATMENT OF OSTEOPOROSIS

Estrogen therapy is approved by the Food and Drug Administration for the prevention of osteoporosis. Estrogen prevents bone loss and hip and spine fractures in early postmenopausal women, and studies suggest that it likely benefits older postmenopausal women. Estrogen decreases markers of bone turnover in both early and later postmenopausal women. A few studies also demonstrate increased distal radius and spinal bone mineral density. Moreover, withdrawal of estrogen after age 65 produces a decline in bone density resembling the loss at menopause. The Framingham Study showed that women taking estrogen for more than 7 years had greater bone density than did women not on estrogen.

Osteoporotic fractures are no longer considered an indication for ERT, with many treatment options other than estrogen available. Women with osteopenia or osteoporosis who have not sustained a fracture should be considered for preventive treatment, although caution should be used until more information about the risk of estrogen-progesterone therapy is available. (See "Osteoporosis and Osteomalacia," p 174.)

Estrogen therapy is effective in maintaining bone density in postmenopausal women; the addition of progestogens does not reduce the efficacy. The oral, transdermal, and implant routes are all effective. Available preparations and dosages are given in Table 49.1. Dosages of 0.3 to 0.625 mg per day of conjugated equine estrogen, 0.5 mg per day of micronized estrogen, or 2 mg per day of estradiol valerate are adequate to maintain bone. Several studies of lower dose estrogen, including a study of 822 postmenopausal women receiving ¾ and ½ the usual dose, have demonstrated preservation of bone similar to that seen with typical doses of estrogen. These studies include the use of adequate calcium and vitamin D with estrogen, a combination that may work synergistically, allowing lower doses of estrogen to be used. (See "Osteoporosis and Osteomalacia," p 174.)

PREVENTION OF CARDIOVASCULAR DISEASE

The net benefit or risk of ERT in cardiovascular disease remains unclear. Although cardiovascular death rates increase exponentially with age, the rate of increase begins in women aged 65 to 74 years rather than at menopause. Age at menopause is inversely correlated with risk of cardiovascular disease.

Three meta-analyses of observational studies have demonstrated an association of ERT use in women with a reduction in heart disease by half. Current use of estrogen is the factor most strongly associated with reducing risk, and prolonged use is the second most important factor. The association occurs whether or not cardiovascular disease risk factors are present. Preliminary studies suggest that the effects are similar when progesterone is added.

However, long-term prospective studies are needed to decide if the cardiovascular benefit of ERT is as great as that suggested by epidemiologic studies. Estrogen users are healthier, more health conscious, and seek more medical care than women not on estrogen, factors that confound interpretation of these results. The benefit of ERT on overall mortality comes from cardiovascular health, and that benefit had needed further clarification. There are now several randomized controlled trials to address the question of ERT effects on cardiovascular disease. A randomized, controlled trial of estrogen with progesterone replacement in women with established coronary disease did not find that estrogen improved cardiac outcome. The estrogen treatment group demonstrated increased mortality in the first year on therapy and improved outcomes in years 2 through 5. Further open-labeled follow-up of the trial failed to demonstrate continued benefit in years 6 and 7 of the trial. Overall, there was no difference in cardiovascular events or mortality in the ERT or placebo groups. Further confirmatory studies have shown that ERT for secondary prevention is not warranted; one study shows no benefit seen by angiography, and another indicates increased levels of unstable angina in women recently begun on ERT. Primary prevention of coronary disease has also been suggested from observational studies. An arm of the Women's Health Initiative estrogen-progesterone trial was discontinued early (at 5.2 years of follow-up) partly because of the increased risk of cardiovascular events. The study found a 29% increase in cardiovascu-

Table 49.1—Common Hormone Replacement Therapies for Prevention and Treatment of Osteoporosis

Preparation	Dose
Estrogens	
Conjugated equine estrogen	0.3–0.625 mg/day
Estradiol valerate	0.5–2.0 mg/day
Transdermal estrogen	0.025–0.1 mg patches twice weekly
Progesterones	
Medroxyprogesterone	2.5–10.0 mg/day
Micronized progesterone	100–200 mg/day
Estrogen-progesterone combinations	
Conjugated estrogen	0.625 mg
with	
Medroxyprogesterone	2.5 mg
Conjugated estrogen	0.625 mg
with	
Medroxyprogesterone	5.0 mg

NOTE: The selective estrogen receptive modulators are becoming available.

lar events, mostly in the nonfatal myocardial infarctions. The study demonstrated no difference in myocardial death or revascularization procedures. In addition, it indicated that there is an increased risk of thrombotic events, including stroke (41% increased risk). The arm of the study with unopposed estrogen (for women with prior hysterectomy) is ongoing and will further address the questions of estrogen role without progesterone.

TREATMENT AND PREVENTION OF COGNITIVE DISORDERS

Observational studies have suggested that estrogen may be neuroprotective. Proposed mechanisms include increased synthesis of neurotransmitters, suppression of apolipoprotein E, and increased cerebral blood flow. Case-control studies of women with and without dementia and epidemiologic studies have demonstrated mixed results. Studies of estrogen in women with mild dementia demonstrate improved memory, orientation, and calculation skills, but these studies are small and limited by selection bias. A placebo-controlled trial of estrogen replacement given to 120 women with early to moderate Alzheimer's dementia for 1 year found no improvement in affective or cognitive outcomes. A primary prevention trial is ongoing. (See "Dementia," p 113.)

BREAST CANCER AND ESTROGEN REPLACEMENT THERAPY

Evidence that estrogen causes or promotes breast cancer is strong. Breast cancer is associated with nulliparity, early menarche, and late menopause. Early oophorectomy protects against breast cancer. Whether ERT causes breast cancer is less clear. Two of the four meta-analyses found no increased risk of breast cancer with ERT; the remaining two found a relative risk of 1.3 and 1.06. These meta-analyses found that women using estrogen for 5 years or less had no increased risk of breast cancer but that treatment for 15 years or more was associated with a 30% increased risk.

Meta-analyses may underestimate the actual risk of breast cancer since women on estrogen are more likely to have had oophorectomy, more physician visits, and more preventive care and screening for breast cancer prior to estrogen use. The largest study evaluating estrogen use by postmenopausal women, the Nurses Health Survey, found that women currently using estrogen had an increased risk of breast cancer but that past users did not. The few studies that have evaluated the estrogen-progesterone combination show inconsistent results, with a suggestion of an increased risk, specifically in two of the larger cohort analyses by a

collaborative group at the National Cancer Institute and the Nurses Health Study. There is some suggestion that cyclic therapy may worsen the risk, but there is insufficient information on the use of continuous progesterone to compare. Similarly, there is not adequate information to discriminate the effects of micronized and synthetic progesterones. The Postmenopausal Estrogen/Progestin Interventions (PEPI) trial found increased breast density with medroxyprogesterone or micronized progesterone, cyclically or continuously. Finally the Women's Health Initiative trial, a randomized prospective trial of estrogen-progestin therapy, found an increased risk of invasive breast cancer at 5.2 years of follow-up in women treated with estrogen-progestin 638 versus 30 per 10,000 person-years).

Hormone therapy in women with a history of breast cancer is controversial and under study. Historically, opponents believed that it would activate micrometastasis; proponents believed that the presumed cardiovascular benefits and improved bone mineral density outweighed the risk in women successfully treated for breast cancer. Now, with alternate treatments for osteoporosis that also protect from breast cancer and with the lack of benefit with regard to cardiovascular health, estrogen is avoided in those with a history of breast cancer.

ENDOMETRIAL CANCER AND ESTROGEN REPLACEMENT THERAPY

Unopposed estrogen (either endogenous or exogenous) increases the risk for endometrial cancer by 2% to 8%. Progesterone was not usually used with estrogen until discovery of this association. The risk of endometrial cancer increases with increasing duration of use in the usually prescribed dosages; risk is also probably increased with lower dosages. Any mode of administration that results in significant systemic levels of estrogen has similar effects on the endometrium. Most cancers caused by exogenous estrogen use are detected as early, low-grade lesions in the course of investigation of bleeding. (See the section on postmenopausal bleeding in "Gynecologic Diseases and Disorders," p 334.) Aggressive, anaplastic endometrial cancers also can arise during estrogen therapy.

Progesterone reduces or negates the risk of endometrial cancer associated with estrogen. Endometrial hyperplasias without atypia usually can be treated with progestins. Those with atypia are treated surgically. The best proven therapy to prevent hyperplasia is to use a progestin at least 10 to 12 days per month. Daily low-dose combination therapy is also effective.

There is no evidence that estrogen increases the risk of ovarian cancer and little information on the effects of estrogen on vulvar or cervical cancer.

ESTROGEN REGIMENS

Who Should Be Treated

The potential risks and benefits of estrogen should be discussed with postmenopausal women. With the discontinuation of the Women's Health Initiative trial, caution should be used in prescribing estrogen for conditions other than those approved by the FDA until more information is available from trials of low-dose estrogen or the estrogen formulation. Women at high risk for osteoporosis or with established osteoporosis have alternate approved treatments available but may be considered for long-term low-dose therapy, since estrogen is beneficial for osteoporosis. The answer is less clear for cognitive benefits and information available at this time suggests that estrogen should not be used for cardioprotective reasons.

Contraindications

Women with breast or endometrial cancer should not be given ERT. Undiagnosed vaginal bleeding or active thromboembolic disease are also contraindications. Whether to treat those with a history of breast or endometrial cancer is being studied but most likely will not be recommended if no cardiovascular benefits exist. Other conditions, including a history of gallbladder disease and menstrual migraine headaches, are considered relative contraindications to ERT. Continuous estrogen dosing may prevent such headaches. It is unclear whether estrogen can be used safely in women with cardiovascular disease.

Regimens

Estrogen is delivered orally, topically to vaginal mucosa, or by the transdermal route (see Table 49.1). Intramuscular estrogen is not recommended. Nonvaginal preparations that ensure systemic treatment are preferred if systemic effects are desired. Estrogen may be given daily or cyclically, since efficacy does not differ. However, each regimen has characteristics that may affect adherence. The addition of medications mid-month or the resumption of withdrawal bleeding may dissuade some from using cyclic therapy; the uncertainty of vaginal bleeding may dissuade others from continuous therapy. The optimal dosage is also not clearly defined. It is prudent to use the lowest effective dose of estrogen to minimize side effects and ensure symptom relief or disease prevention. Conju-

gated equine estrogen 0.625 mg and 50 μg of 17β-estradiol stabilize bone, and both are associated with improved cardiovascular health, but little information is available on lower doses of estrogen.

Progestin Regimens

With an intact uterus, progestins—most commonly medroxyprogesterone acetate—must be given to avoid the increased risk of endometrial cancer. Progestins may be given cyclically (10 to 14 days per month) or continuously. With cyclic therapy, 80% of women experience withdrawal bleeding. Endometrial biopsies reveal hyperplasia rates to be ≤ 1%. Continuous therapy diminishes bleeding and protects against endometrial hyperplasia; amenorrhea is achieved in 50% to 90% of women at 12 months of therapy, and endometrial biopsies are atrophic or hypotrophic in 50% to 75%. (See "Gynecologic Diseases and Disorders," p 334.)

Adverse Effects

The most common adverse effect of estrogen is breast tenderness, which usually subsides after 2 to 3 months. If tenderness is troublesome for more than 4 months, the dose can be reduced but with less clear benefit. Headaches and rarely idiosyncratic elevation in blood pressure have been described. The adverse effects of progesterone include fluid retention, depression, and irritability. Estrogen therapy has consistently been found to increase the risk of venous thromboembolism two- to fourfold. One study found risk factors to be lower-extremity fracture, cancer, the first 90 days following inpatient surgery or nonsurgical hospitalization, and a history of myocardial infarction. Women using aspirin or statins were found to be at lower risk.

Continuing Estrogen Treatment

Only about 10% of American postmenopausal women receive ERT. Reasons women report for having started ERT are that it was recommended by a physician, they needed symptom relief, and they received reassurance that the cancer risk is low. Women most likely to begin ERT have higher socioeconomic status, lower body weight, and an active life style. Studies show that 20% to 30% of women never fill the prescription for ERT, 10% use it sporadically, and 20% stop treatment within 9 months. The reasons women give for stopping treatment include these: that the symptoms abated, the symptoms were not adequately alleviated, the regimen was too complex, and the adverse effects were unacceptable. This will most likely change dramatically in coming years following the information revealed in the Women's Health Initiative trial.

ANDROGEN DEFICIENCY

Testosterone Therapy in Aging Women

Testosterone levels decrease by 28% at menopause because of a decrease in adrenal androstenedione. Testosterone increases libido in women whose baseline testosterone levels are low. Low testosterone levels are correlated with higher fracture risk in women. There have been no studies of testosterone alone in women with osteoporosis, but in studies comparing estrogen-testosterone implants with estrogen alone, the combination demonstrated either greater or comparable bone mineral density. One study demonstrated that the combination produced higher markers of bone formation and similar suppression of resorption. Adverse effects of testosterone include mild hirsutism, acne, and decreased high-density lipoprotein cholesterol.

Androgen Deficiency in Aging Men

The decline in testosterone levels has been associated in some studies with symptoms of decreased libido, decreased energy, decreased muscle strength, increased fat mass, and low bone mass. Testosterone replacement in men with low levels of testosterone has resulted in reports of modest increase in bone mass, gains in strength, decrease in body fat, and increase in lean body mass. The long-term effects of testosterone replacement are not fully known. Prostate-specific antigen levels increase very little in studies of up to 3 years' duration, but the number of men included in clinical trials has been very small. To date, there, are no data to address whether androgens enhance the progression of preclinical to clinical prostate cancer. Nested case-control studies from two large population-based epidemiologic studies have revealed contradictory results regarding an association between baseline testosterone levels and subsequent risk of developing prostate cancer. Men receiving testosterone replacement should be monitored for changes in prostate examination or increases in prostate-specific antigen level. Additional adverse effects that should be monitored are increased hematocrit and precipitation of sleep apnea. Testosterone preparations that are aromatized to estrogen do not appear to affect lipid levels; the effects of testosterone on cardiovascular risk are not known. Testosterone may be given intramuscularly, via patch (scrotal or transdermal), or as a topical gel.

Growth Hormone

See "Endocrine and Metabolic Disorders" (p 319).

Testosterone Replacement in Men

See "Endocrine and Metabolic Disorders" (p 319).

Dehydroepiandrosterone

See "Endocrine and Metabolic Disorders" (p 319).

REFERENCES

■ Grady D, Herrington D, Bittner V, et al; HERS Research Group. Cardiovascular disease outcomes during 6.8 years of hormone therapy: Heart and Estrogen/progestin Replacement Study follow-up (HERS II). *JAMA.* 2002; 288(1):49–57.

■ Grady D, Wenger NK, Herrington D, et al. Postmenopausal hormone therapy increases risk for venous thromboembolic disease. *Ann Intern Med.* 2000;132(9):689–696.

■ Herrington DM, Reboussin DM, Brosnihan KB, et al. Effects of estrogen replacement on the progression of coronary artery atherosclerosis. *N Engl J Med.* 2000;343(8):522–529.

■ Hulley S, Furberg C, Barrett-Connor E, et al; HERS Research Group. Noncardiovascular disease outcomes during 6.8 years of hormone therapy: Heart and Estrogen/ progestin Replacement Study follow-up (HERS II). *JAMA.* 2002;288(1):58–66.

■ Hulley S, Grady D, Bush T, et al. Randomized trial of estrogen plus progestin for secondary prevention of coronary heart disease in postmenopausal women. *JAMA.* 1998; 280(7):605–613.

■ Mulnard RA, Cotman CW, Kawas C, et al. Estrogen replacement therapy for treatment of mild to moderate Alzheimer disease: a randomized controlled trial. *JAMA.* 2000; 283(8):1007–1015.

■ Rossouw JE, Anderson GL, Prentice RL, et al. Writing Group for the Women's Health Initiative Investigators. Risks and benefits of estrogen plus progestin in healthy postmenopausal women: principal results from the Women's Health Initiative randomized controlled trial. *JAMA.* 2002; 288(3):321–333.

■ Tenover JL. Testosterone and the aging male. *J Androl.* 1997;18(2):103–106.

CHAPTER 50—GYNECOLOGIC DISEASES AND DISORDERS

Most older women do not seek regular gynecologic care. This may be in part because they are reticent about discussing personal gynecologic problems. Important and treatable disorders consequently go undiagnosed until they become severely disabling. For example, although urinary incontinence affects 16 million adults in the United States, the average time between onset and reporting to a clinician is 8.5 years; gynecologic problems such as genital prolapse and atrophic vaginitis often exacerbate urinary incontinence. Full gynecologic examination should be a routine part of a complete history and physical examination for all older women.

HISTORY AND PHYSICAL EXAMINATION

The latest American College of Obstetrics and Gynecology recommendations for primary care of women aged 65 and older include inquiring about not only routine gynecologic issues but also about involuntary loss of urine or feces, sexual behavior patterns and potential exposure to sexually transmitted diseases, use of alternative medical treatments, and immunizations. Nongynecologic medical problems that can have significant gynecologic effects should be noted in the history. As such, breast cancer therapy typically leads to severe urogenital atrophy, obesity can result in hyperestrogenic states due to peripheral conversion of androgens to estrogen, and osteoporotic lordosis causes increased intra-abdominal pressure and resultant predisposition to genital prolapse. Previous obstetrical events may cause pelvic floor neuromuscular damage and eventual development of urinary incontinence and genital prolapse. If a woman is on hormonal replacement, the regimen should be reviewed annually to assure adherence and absence of abnormal side effects. If the uterus is present, estrogen must be combined with a progestin in order to prevent the development of endometrial hyperplasia (see "Hormone Replacement Therapy," p 329). The history should also include inquiry about abdominal distention (sign of ovarian cancer) and abnormal vaginal discharge or bleeding (signs of endometrial, cervical, or vaginal cancer).

The pelvic examination also presents an opportunity to discuss sexual function with the patient. Although the lack of available, sexually capable men may limit an older woman's sexual activities, many are interested in maintaining sexual relationships. Issues related to sexual activity such as atrophy-related dyspareunia, postcoital bleeding, and sexually transmitted diseases should be addressed. Many require reassurance that enjoyable sexual activity is possible and normal at their age. Also, women who maintain regular sexual activity are less likely to have significant vaginal atrophy.

Most ambulatory older patients can assume the lithotomy position. Because the vaginal introitus may be small and stenotic, smaller speculums may be needed. The dorsal position, in stirrups for a pelvic examination, requires flexion and external rotation of the hips. Patients with osteoarthritis who find the lithotomy position uncomfortable or impossible to assume will need to use an alternative position. The left lateral decubitus position is an alternative. The patient lies on her left side, with knees flexed. The upper hip (right) is flexed to a greater degree and the right leg is elevated, exposing the perineum. An adequate speculum and bimanual examination can usually be done in this position. To examine a bedbound patient, position an inverted bedpan under the sacrum to elevate the pelvis. Lubricants facilitate the examination but should be avoided if a Pap smear will be performed.

In performing the pelvic examination of an older woman, the examiner should:

- examine the vulva for abnormal pigmentation, erythema, or raised lesions;

- look for signs of urogenital atrophy, including urethral caruncle, vaginal dryness, pale vaginal mucosa, loss of rugae, and reduced vaginal caliber and depth;

- have the patient perform Valsalva's maneuver to evaluate for pelvic organ prolapse and urinary incontinence;

- carefully palpate for pelvic masses or ovarian enlargement on bimanual examination;

- perform a Pap smear if indicated (see the section on cervical cancer in "Prevention," p 60).

The presence of significant vaginal mucosal atrophic changes may lead to inadequate or abnormal Pap smear interpretation. In this situation, the Pap smear should be repeated after 2 to 3 months of local estrogen therapy. Bimanual examinations and perineal inspection performed annually remain critical for the detection of vulvar, vaginal, and ovarian pathology. A rectal examination should also be performed in order to identify masses, detect occult bleeding, and evaluate the anal sphincter.

Ovaries become smaller with aging, and any palpable adnexal tissue should be investigated to exclude malignancy. Although uterine fibroids are common, any increase in uterine size should be investigated. An ovarian or uterine mass should be evaluated by abdominal or pelvic ultrasound (using a vaginal probe) to determine location and character. Sonography, however, cannot definitively establish the nature (benign or malignant) of the mass.

UROGENITAL ATROPHY

The lower genital tract is exquisitely sensitive to estrogen. Proliferation and maturation of the vaginal epithelium depends on adequate estrogen stimulation. With reduction of estrogen production, genital blood flow decreases, leading to further decline in delivery of estrogen to those tissues. This reduction in microvascularity leads to vaginal dryness, mucosal pallor, decreased rugation, mucosal thinning, inflammation with discharge, and, ultimately, decreased vaginal caliber and depth. With progressive atrophy, the vaginal Pap smear–maturation index shows atrophic changes with a decrease in mucosal superficial cells and an increase in intermediate and basal cells. Many women experience dyspareunia, burning, and even vaginal bleeding in some cases (Figure 50.1).

These changes are readily reversed with the administration of local estrogen. The intravaginal use of estrogen cream, one half an applicator (2 g) as infrequently as two nights per week, allows topical estrogen therapy with minimal absorption, endometrial proliferation, or other systemic effects. The available prescription estrogen creams appear to be therapeutically equivalent. Intravaginal estradiol tablets are also available; they allow less messy insertion with preloaded applicator. The estrogen ring may be used for 3 months per ring. Estrogen cream is also an excellent lubricant for use during intercourse or for pessary insertion. All the currently available forms of low-dose local estrogen therapy appear to be equivalent in treating vaginal atrophy. Creams may lead to a more prompt response, but maintenance therapy may be accomplished with either formulation. (See also "Disorders of Sexual Function," p 339.)

VULVOVAGINAL INFECTION AND INFLAMMATION

Postmenopausal women are at least as susceptible as other women to the broad range of vulvovaginal infections. Candidal infection, common in diabetic and obese patients who are plagued with moisture and

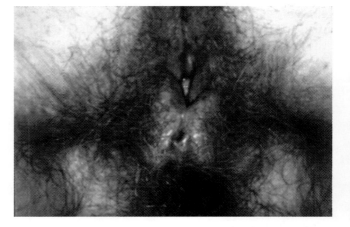

Figure 50.1—Severe vulvovaginal atrophy, including labial fusion secondary to lichen sclerosus.

irritation, is treated with intravaginal and topical antifungal agents. Patients should be questioned about their ability to insert a vaginal applicator before beginning therapy. Topical corticosteroids can be used to hasten relief of symptoms. Oral antifungal agents such as fluconazole are also effective. Combination therapy may be necessary, as older women commonly present with more chronic, untreated candidal infections that spread from the vulva to the inguinal areas. Other vaginal infections common in reproductive age women such as trichomonas and *Gardnerella* vaginosis are less common in elderly women, likely because of the higher vaginal pH. A wet preparation revealing sheets of inflammatory cells without bacterial forms may represent advanced atrophy rather than an infectious cause. Local estrogen cream should be prescribed.

DISORDERS OF THE VULVA

With aging, the skin of the vulva loses elasticity, and the underlying fat and connective tissues undergo degeneration, with loss of collagen and thinning of the epithelial layer. Consequently, postmenopausal women not on estrogen are predisposed to a variety of dermatologic disorders and symptoms. The assessment of vulvar complaints must include direct examination. Any pigmented lesion or lesions that do not respond to topical corticosteroid or estrogen treatment *must* be promptly biopsied.

Vulvar skin irritation occurs from a variety of agents and causes burning, itching, and edema. Hygienic products used for urinary or fecal incontinence may lead to chemical dermatitis, as does urine itself. Correction of incontinence is paramount to solving this problem. Vulvar burning is rarely due to estrogen deficiency, and this complaint should be investigated rather than treated with ever-increasing doses of estrogen. Vulvar excoriation can result from scratching of an inflamed vulva. Local corticosteroids such as hydrocortisone 1% ointment applied daily, sitz baths, or use of a bidet can help alleviate vulvar irritation. Any chronically irritated area should be biopsied to exclude a malignancy.

Vulvar dystrophy is a somewhat outdated term used to describe both benign and malignant vulvar squamous changes. The preferred terminology set out by the International Society for the Study of Vulvovaginal Disease outlines three classes of non-neoplastic vulvar lesions. These are lichen sclerosus, squamous cell hyperplasia, and other dermatoses. A separate classification is used for biopsy-proven dysplastic lesions. These vulvar intraepithelial neoplasias (VIN) are graded on the basis of the level of atypia (dysplasia).

Nonneoplastic Vulvar Lesions

Lichen sclerosus causes over one third of all vulvar dystrophies and may extend beyond the vulva to the perirectal areas. It is rarely precancerous. There is epithelial thinning with edema and fibrosis of the dermis. It can progress to shrinkage and agglutination of the labia minora and reduction in introital caliber. Lesions are typically shiny, white or pink, and parchment-like. Lesions may be asymptomatic or may cause itching, vaginal soreness, and dyspareunia. Diagnosis is confirmed on biopsy of the involved vulvar areas. Recommended treatment involves daily application of a rather potent topical corticosteroid, clobetasol propionate 0.05%. Treatment should be continued for at least 3 months. Testosterone had been the mainstay of therapy but has been shown to be significantly less effective than clobetasol. Further measures include wearing cotton underwear and avoiding irritant soaps. Topical emollient agents including lanolin can be helpful, but petroleum jelly should be avoided.

Squamous hyperplasia appears as thickened, hyperplastic, elevated white keratinized lesions that can be difficult to distinguish from VIN or condylomata on a clinical basis. However, it is benign. Biopsy should precede treatment. Topical mid-potency corticosteroids such as triamcinolone 0.1% twice daily for a few weeks (or longer with thick lesions) resolves the lesions; intermittent therapy may be necessary.

Other vulvar lesions include lichen simplex chronicus, which presents with vulvar pruritus, and lichen planus, which presents as erosive, ulcerative lesions that can result in significant vulvar scarring. Mid-potency corticosteroids topically or intravaginally applied are recommended. In lichen planus involving the vagina, local estrogen cream should also be used.

Vulvar Neoplasia

All suspicious, unusual, or symptomatic vulvar lesions should be biopsied. VIN lesions are not usually precancerous. VIN is most often seen in postmenopausal women, but the incidence of VIN does not increase with age. Over half of cases are asymptomatic. When symptoms are present, the most common is pruritus. The clinical appearance is the same as squamous hyperplasia or may be simply pigmentation. Lesions are often multifocal.

Invasive cancer of the vulva is an age-related malignancy; half of all cases occur after age 70. The vast majority are squamous cell carcinomas. Malignant melanoma, sarcoma, basal cell, and adenocarcinoma account for under 20% of cases. Treatment involves surgery (radical vulvectomy), occasionally accompanied by radiation.

DISORDERS OF PELVIC FLOOR SUPPORT

Child bearing and activities that increase intra-abdominal pressure cause progressive weakening of the connective tissue and muscular supports of the genital organs and can lead to genital prolapse. Conditions such as constipation, chronic coughing, and heavy lifting commonly increase intra-abdominal pressure. Common symptoms of prolapse include pelvic pressure, low-back pain, urinary or fecal incontinence, difficulty with rectal emptying, or a palpable mass. Traditional classification of vaginal prolapse differentiated protrusion of the posterior vaginal wall (enterocele or rectocele), descent of the anterior vaginal wall (cystocele), or prolapse of the vaginal apex. These conditions are demonstrated by having the patient bear down or cough while in the dorsal lithotomy position, but the full extent of prolapse is better appreciated with a standing Valsalva's maneuver. Vaginal prolapse represents a pelvic organ hernia through the vaginal hiatus.

The 1995 American College of Obstetrics and Gynecology classification of pelvic organ prolapse is outlined in Table 50.1. The International Continence Society and the American Urogynecologic Association adopted a new, rather complex prolapse classification system based on measurement of the distance between vaginal anatomic sites and the hymeneal ring. The purpose of this classification, which is used by specialty societies, is to more objectively and reproducibly describe a patient's degree of prolapse.

Mild prolapse (1st or 2nd degree; see Table 50.1) can be retarded with adequate estrogenization and Kegel's exercises to strengthen the pelvic floor musculature. Genital prolapse does not always mean bladder

Table 50.1—Classification of Pelvic Organ Prolapse

Class	Description
1st degree	Extension to the mid-vagina
2nd degree	Approaching the hymenal ring
3rd degree	At the hymenal ring
4th degree	Beyond the hymenal ring

SOURCE: Data from The American College of Obstetricians and Gynecologists. *Pelvic Organ Prolapse*. Washington, DC: American College of Obstetricians and Gynecologists. Technical Bulletin No. 214; 1995.

dysfunction and should not be assumed to be the cause of incontinence (see "Urinary Incontinence," p 134). Correcting the prolapse will in some cases cause or exacerbate incontinence. On the other hand, large cystoceles or rectoceles may produce urinary retention, and reduction of the cystocele may restore bladder function.

Pessaries

Pessaries are commonly employed in an effort to delay or avoid surgery. Their use in older women may be indicated to provide comfort and restore bladder function when comorbid illness makes surgery undesirable. Such women may elect long-term pessary use under medical supervision. Available pessaries are made from rubber, plastic, or silicone. A variety of shapes and sizes are available: doughnuts, rings, cubes, inflatable balls, and foldable models (Figure 50.2). Pessary care requirements (Table 50.2) often influence the selection of a device and the amount of follow-up required.

The choice of pessary is influenced by the degree of prolapse, presence of incontinence, type of accompanying tissue relaxation, and ease of care. Patients with prolapse and no incontinence require only space-occupying (eg, doughnut, inflatable) types. Those with stress incontinence benefit from a foldable (eg, Smith, Hodge) type (Figure 50.2C, D, E, H), which restores bladder neck support. Ring pessaries are easier to insert and remove and may be preferred by older women. Gellhorn pessaries (Figure 50.2L, M, N) may be difficult to insert, but are the best choice for large anterior vaginal wall prolapse. Doughnut pessaries (Figure 50.2X) provide excellent support but are more difficult to insert. Cube pessaries (Figure 50.2F, G) may be easier to insert, but care must be taken on removal to avoid vaginal mucosal trauma, as the sides of the cube may adhere strongly to the vaginal walls. Inflatable pessaries (Figure 50.2W) may cause vulvar irritation because of the presence of a stalk that rubs on the perineum.

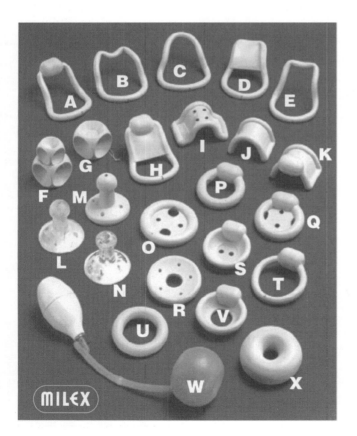

Figure 50.2—Currently available types of vaginal pessaries:
- A. Hodge with Knob (Silicone)
- B. Risser (Silicone)
- C. Smith (Silicone)
- D. Hodge with Support (Silicone)
- E. Hodge (Silicone)
- F. Tandem Cube (Silicone)
- G. Cube (Silicone)
- H. Hodge with Support + Knob (Silicone)
- I. Regula (Silicone)
- J. Gehrung (Silicone)
- K. Gehrung with Knob (Silicone)
- L. Gellhorn 95% Rigid (Silicone)
- M. Gellhorn Flexible (Silicone)
- N. Gellhorn Rigid (Acrylic)
- O. Ring with Support (Silicone)
- P. Ring with Knob (Silicone)
- Q. Ring with Support + Knob (Silicone)
- R. Shaatz (Silicone)
- S. Incontinence Dish with Support (Silicone)
- T. Ring Incontinence (Silicone)
- U. Ring (Silicone)
- V. Incontinence Dish (Silicone)
- W. Inflatoball (Latex)
- X. Doughnut (Silicone)

SOURCE: Courtesy, Milex Products, Inc. Chicago, Illinois 60634.

Table 50.2—Recommendations for Pessary Care

- If mobility and manual dexterity are adequate, remove 2 nights per week; if not, receive assistance at office visit or from visiting home nurse
- Wash with soap and water
- Reinsert using water-soluble lubricant
- Use vaginal estrogen cream (1 g) two nights per week
- Report any unusual discharge, bleeding, or discomfort
- Report any changes in bladder or bowel function
- Have pelvic examination every 6 to 12 months

SOURCE: Reproduced with permission from Davila GW. Vaginal prolapse: management with nonsurgical techniques. *Postgrad Med.* 1996;99(4):181. ©The McGraw-Hill Companies.

Pessary selection often proceeds by trial and error; the optimal pessary fits snugly but comfortably and allows voiding and defecating without difficulty. After pessary selection and insertion, clinical follow-up within a few days is essential. After initial fitting and recheck, silicone pessaries should be removed, cleaned, and the vaginal vault inspected. Ideally, patients should be instructed to remove nightly for cleaning. In those who are incapable of pessary self-care, the pessary should be reinserted for 4 to 6 weeks. If discomfort is present or the device becomes uncomfortable, a different size or type should be tried. Pessaries do not work as well with marked vaginal outlet relaxation. If a pessary is left in place for long periods without monitoring, fibrous tissue may form around the pessary, and surgical removal may be necessary.

Surgery for Prolapse

Surgical treatment of vaginal prolapse can be classified as either reconstructive or obliterative. Reconstructive procedures are designed to restore normal anatomy, whereas obliterative procedures result in closure of the vaginal canal. Vaginal reconstructive procedures include sacrospinous fixation (for vault prolapse), anterior repairs (for a cystocele), and posterior repairs (for a rectocele). These can safely be done under regional anesthesia, minimizing anesthetic risks. Abdominal reconstructive procedures include sacrocolpopexy (for vault prolapse) and paravaginal repairs (for a cystocele). They typically require general anesthesia. Urinary incontinence procedures can be done either vaginally or abdominally at the time of the prolapse surgery. (See "Urinary Incontinence," p 134.)

Obliterative procedures are restricted to older women who are not, and will not be, sexually active. In a LaForte colpocleisis, the anterior and posterior vaginal walls are sutured together, obliterating the vaginal canal. The simplicity and safety are very attractive for the oldest-old women, as the procedure can be done under local anesthesia in the outpatient setting. Anti-incontinence procedures can be done at the same time, as well.

Surgical success rates are high, exceeding 90% in most cases. Limitation of physical activities and intra-abdominal pressure increase for 6 to 12 weeks postoperatively; performance of pelvic floor exercises and use of vaginal estrogen cream are key in optimizing the success rate of surgical therapy. The impact on quality of life of prolapse surgery for the patient can be quite remarkable, as a large, exteriorized prolapse can markedly limit a woman's ability to perform physical and social activities.

POSTMENOPAUSAL VAGINAL BLEEDING

Postmenopausal bleeding (defined as bleeding after 1 year of amenorrhea) occurs in a significant number of patients. The challenge is not only to exclude gynecologic malignancies but also to alleviate the symptoms and eliminate the cause of benign conditions. Causes of bleeding can be grouped according to anatomic areas and endocrine dysfunction (Table 50.3). Not all complaints of postmenopausal bleeding are related to the reproductive organs but may be confused by the patients as originating from these areas. Proper evaluation involves complete physical examination and directed diagnostic studies. Endometrial hyperplasia and

Table 50.3—Causes of Postmenopausal Vaginal Bleeding

Cervical
  Carcinoma
  Cervicitis
  Polyp

Endocrinologic
  Exogenous hormones
  Perimenopausal ovarian function

Ovarian
  Functioning ovarian tumor

Uterine
  Endometrial atrophy
  Hyperplasia
  Neoplasia
  Polyp
  Submucosal leiomyoma

Vaginal
  Atrophy
  Inflammation
  Tumor
  Ulceration

Vulvar
  Carcinoma
  Laceration or ulceration
  Urethral caruncle

Other
  Coagulation disorder
  Rectal lesion
  Urinary tract infection

cancer can be evaluated with endometrial biopsy or by measuring the endometrial thickness on vaginal probe ultrasound. An endometrial thickness of less than 5 mm essentially excludes hyperplasia and malignancy; however, neither ultrasound nor biopsy can completely exclude the possibility of malignancy. Dilation and curettage is reserved for cases where tissue cannot otherwise be adequately sampled or when bleeding persists. The use of direct visualization (hysteroscopy) during the procedure is the most accurate method for tissue sampling.

Exogenous hormone replacement is an increasingly common cause of postmenopausal bleeding. Women on continuous combined estrogen-progesterone replacement who continue to have bleeding after 1 year must be evaluated. Some specialists recommend biopsy if bleeding persists beyond 6 months. Women on cyclic hormone therapy who bleed at an unexpected time during the cycle should also be evaluated. (See also "Hormone Replacement Therapy," p 329.)

CLIMACTERIC SYNDROMES

See "Hormone Replacement Therapy" (p 329).

REFERENCES

- American College of Obstetricians and Gynecologists. *Vulvar Non-neoplastic Epithelial Disorders*. ACOG Educational Bulletin No. 241. Washington, DC: American College of Obstetricians and Gynecologists; 1997.

- Bash KL. Review of vaginal pessaries. *Obstet Gynecol Surv.* 2000;55(7):455–460.

- Bump RC, Mattiason A, Bo K, et al. The standardization of terminology of female pelvic organ prolapse and pelvic floor dysfunction. *Am J Obstet Gynecol.* 1996;175(1):10–17.

- Davila GW. Vaginal prolapse: management with nonsurgical techniques. *Postgrad Med.* 1996;99(4):171–176, 181, 184–185.

- Handa VL, Bachus KE, Johnston WW, et al. Vaginal administration of low-dose conjugated estrogens: systemic absorption and effects on the endometrium. *Obstet Gynecol.* 1994;84(2):215–218.

- Holley RL, Varner RE, Gleason BP, et al. Sexual function after sacrospinous fixation for vaginal vault prolapse. *J Reprod Med.* 1996;41(5):355–358.

CHAPTER 51—DISORDERS OF SEXUAL FUNCTION

During the past there has been a significant increase in our understanding of sexual function and dysfunction in older men. However, there is less scientific information on the sexuality of older women. The latter may be in part due to the difficulty of measuring the female sexual response and the exclusion of older adults from research. For example, a study of adult sexual behavior, the National Health and Social Life Survey, sampled adults only up to age 59.

MALE SEXUALITY

Age-Associated Changes

As men age, their sexuality changes. The frequency of sexual intercourse and the prevalence of engaging in any sexual activity decreases. Young men report having intercourse three to four times per week, whereas only 7% of men aged 60 to 69 years and 2% of those aged 70 years and older report the same frequency. Fifty percent to 80% of men 60 to 70 years old engage in any sexual activity, a prevalence rate that declines to 15% to 25% among those aged 80 years and older. However, sexual interest often persists despite decreased activity. The man's level of sexual activity,

interest, and enjoyment in younger years often determines his sexual behavior with aging. Factors contributing to a man's decreased sexual activity include poor health, social issues, partner availability, decreased libido, and erectile dysfunction.

Aging is associated not only with changes in sexual behavior but also with changes in the stages of sexual response. During the excitement phase, there is a delay in erection, decreased tensing of the scrotal sac, and loss of testicular elevation. The duration of the plateau stage is prolonged, and pre-ejaculatory secretion is decreased. Orgasm is diminished in duration and intensity, with decreased quantity and force of seminal emission. During the resolution phase, there is rapid detumescence and testicular descent. The refractory period between erections is also prolonged. However, erectile dysfunction is not a part of healthy aging.

Erectile Dysfunction

Erectile dysfunction is the inability to achieve or maintain an erection adequate for sexual intercourse. The prevalence of erectile dysfunction increases with age; by age 70, 67% of men have erectile dysfunction. This high prevalence is important; in a study comparing affected and unaffected men, men with sexual dysfunction reported impaired quality of life.

The most common cause of erectile dysfunction in older men is vascular disease. Risk for vascular erectile dysfunction increases with traditional vascular risk factors such as diabetes mellitus, hypertension, hyperlipidemia, and smoking. In fact, erectile dysfunction is a predictor of future major atherosclerotic vascular disease (ie, myocardial infarction and stroke).

Obstruction from atherosclerotic arterial occlusive disease likely impedes the intracavernosal blood flow and pressure needed to achieve a rigid erection. In addition, atherosclerotic disease may cause ischemia of trabecular smooth muscle and result in fibrotic changes leading to failure of venous closure mechanisms. Venous leakage leading to vascular erectile dysfunction may also result from Peyronie's disease, arteriovenous fistula, or trauma-induced communication between the glans and the corpora. In anxious men who have excessive adrenergic-constrictor tone and in men with injured parasympathetic dilator nerves, erectile dysfunction can occur from insufficient relaxation of trabecular smooth muscle.

The second most common cause of erectile dysfunction in older men is neurologic disease. Disorders that affect the parasympathetic sacral spinal cord or the peripheral efferent autonomic fibers to the penis impair penile smooth muscle relaxation and prevent the vasodilation necessary for erection. In spinal-cord injury patients the extent of erectile dysfunction largely depends on the completeness and the level of the spinal injury; those who have complete lesions or injury to the sacral spinal cord are more likely to have loss of erectile function. Common health problems such as diabetes mellitus, stroke, and Parkinson's disease can cause autonomic dysfunction that results in erectile failure. Finally, surgical procedures such as radical prostatectomy, cystoprostatectomy, and proctocolectomy commonly disrupt the autonomic nerve supply to the penis, resulting in postoperative erectile dysfunction.

Numerous commonly used medications have been associated with erectile dysfunction for which the mechanism, for the most part, is unknown. Those with anticholinergic effects, such as antidepressants, antipsychotics, and antihistamines, may cause erectile dysfunction by blocking parasympathetic-mediated penile artery vasodilatation and trabecular smooth muscle relaxation. Almost all antihypertensive agents have been associated with erectile dysfunction, but with higher incidence for β-blockers, clonidine, and thiazide diuretics. One mechanism may be the lowering of blood pressure below the critical threshold needed to maintain sufficient blood flow for penile erection, especially in those men who already have penile arterial

disease. Over-the-counter medications such as cimetidine and ranitidine may also cause erectile dysfunction. Cimetidine, a H_2-receptor antagonist, acts as an antiandrogen and increases prolactin secretion and thus has been associated with loss of libido and erectile failure. Ranitidine can also increase prolactin secretion, although less commonly than does cimetidine.

The prevalence of psychogenic erectile dysfunction correlates inversely with age. Psychogenic erectile dysfunction may occur via increased sympathetic stimuli to the sacral cord, inhibiting the parasympathetic dilator nerves and thus inhibiting erection. Common causes of psychogenic erectile dysfunction include relationship conflicts, performance anxiety, childhood sexual abuse, and fear of sexually transmitted diseases. Older men may have "widower's syndrome," in which the man involved in a new relationship feels guilt as a defense against subconscious unfaithfulness to his deceased spouse.

The role of androgens in erection is unclear. Hypogonadal men show smaller and slower developing erections in response to fantasy, which is improved with androgen replacement. However, even men with castrate levels of testosterone can attain erections in response to direct penile stimulation. It may be that erection to certain types of sexual stimuli (ie, direct penile stimulation) are androgen independent, whereas response to fantasy may be androgen sensitive. Overall, testosterone appears to play a minor role in erectile function and a larger role in libido.

Hyperthyroidism, hypothyroidism, and hyperprolactinemia have been associated with erectile dysfunction. However, less than 5% of erectile dysfunction is caused by endocrine abnormalities. Thus, endocrine evaluation of men with erectile dysfunction but intact libido is of limited value.

Evaluation of Erectile Dysfunction

The initial step in evaluation is a sexual, medical, and psychosocial history. Sexual history should clarify whether the problem consists of inadequate erections, decrease in libido, or orgasmic failure. The onset and duration of erectile dysfunction, the presence or absence of sleep-associated erections, and associated decline in libido may lead the clinician to the likely cause.

Sudden onset suggests psychogenic or drug-induced erectile dysfunction. A psychogenic cause is likely if there is sudden onset but sleep-associated erections or erections with masturbation or another partner are intact. However, if the sudden onset is accompanied by lack of sleep-associated erections and lack of erection with masturbation, temporal association with new medication should be sought. A gradual onset of erectile dysfunction associated with loss of libido suggests hypogonadism.

Medical history is directed at discerning those factors likely to be contributing to erectile dysfunction. Vascular risk factors include diabetes mellitus, hypertension, coronary artery disease, peripheral arterial disease, hyperlipidemia, and smoking. Neurogenic risk factors include diabetes mellitus, history of pelvic injury or surgery, spinal injury or surgery, Parkinson's disease, multiple sclerosis, and alcoholism. An extensive medication review, including over-the-counter medications, is also essential. Finally, the psychosocial history should assess the patient's relationship with the sexual partner, the partner's health and attitude toward sex, economic or social stresses, living situation, alcohol use, and affective disorders.

On physical examination, signs of vascular or neurologic diseases must be sought. Peripheral pulses should be palpated. Signs of autonomic neuropathy and loss of the bulbocavernosus reflex suggest neurologic dysfunction. The genital examination should include palpating the penis for Peyronie's plaques and assessing for testicular atrophy. A loss of secondary sexual characteristics, the presence of small testes, and gynecomastia suggest hypogonadism.

Laboratory evaluation would include urinalysis, cholesterol level, and serum testosterone concentration. If the serum testosterone is low, further hormonal evaluation may be done using free-testosterone, luteinizing hormone, and prolactin serum concentrations.

A diagnostic screening tool that can help direct treatment of erectile dysfunction is intracavernous injection of a vasoactive drug, such as papaverine or prostaglandin E_1 (PGE_1). An initial test dose of 15 to 30 mg papaverine is used if the history and examination suggests a neurogenic cause. A 30-gauge needle and 1-cc syringe are typically used for the injection. Hold the glans of the penis with one hand and clean the injection site with an alcohol swab. Then, holding the needle parallel to the floor, insert the needle into the side of the penis to avoid the urethra. Inject the vasoactive agent over 30 to 60 seconds. After withdrawing the needle, apply pressure to the injection site for 1 minute to prevent bruising. An erectile response will occur within 15 minutes and may last up to 40 minutes. A poor response suggests arteriogenic or venogenic cause, inadequate dose of vasoactive agent, or anxiety with excessive adrenergic tone. A second trial injection at the next office visit with a higher dose (30 to 60 mg papaverine) or PGE_1 (5 to 20 μg) may be used.

More extensive diagnostic tools are available but not commonly used. Nocturnal penile tumescence testing is of little value, except to confirm a psychogenic cause. The penile brachial pressure index may be helpful in assessing arteriogenic erectile dysfunction. This index measures the loss of systolic pressure between the arm and the penis. When measured before and after exercise, it can be used to assess for a pelvic steal syndrome, which is the loss of erection associated with initiation of active thrusting, presumably due to the transfer of blood flow from the penis to the pelvis musculature. More invasive and expensive tests such as Doppler ultrasound to assess penile arterial function, dynamic infusion cavernosometry to assess venous leakage syndrome, and penile arteriography are generally reserved for research or penile vascular surgery candidates.

Treatment of Erectile Dysfunction

Multiple effective therapeutic options are now available for the treatment of erectile dysfunction. Treatment should be individualized and based on cause, personal preference, partner issues, cost, and practicality of the therapeutic modality (Table 51.1).

Oral therapy for erectile dysfunction consists of sildenafil citrate. Sildenafil is a type-5 phosphodiesterase inhibitor that potentiates the penile response to sexual stimulation. It is effective in improving the rigidity and duration of erection. It is taken 1 hour prior to sexual activity and has no effect until sexual stimulation occurs. Potential side effects include headache, flushing, dyspepsia, and transient color blindness. It is contraindicated for concomitant use with nitrate drugs, since the combination can produce profound and fatal hypotension.

Vacuum tumescence devices are an effective and accepted treatment. The apparatus consists of a plastic cylinder with an open end into which the penis is inserted. A vacuum device attached to the cylinder creates negative pressure within the cylinder, and blood flows into the penis to produce penile rigidity. A penile constriction ring placed at the base of the penis then traps the blood in the corpora cavernosa to maintain an erection for about 30 minutes. The vacuum device is effective for psychogenic, neurogenic, and venogenic erectile dysfunction, but it requires manual dexterity. Local pain, swelling, bruising, coolness of penile tip, and painful ejaculation are potential side effects. It is important to remove the constriction ring after 30 minutes.

Intracavernous injection of vasoactive drugs such as papaverine, phentolamine, and PGE_1 are effective in producing erections adequate for sexual activity. PGE_1, which is the only agent approved by the Food and Drug Administration for intracavernous injection, produces erections that last 40 to 60 minutes. Phentolamine is mainly used in combination therapy with papaverine or PGE_1, or both. Potential side

Table 51.1—Treatment Options for Erectile Dysfunction

Treatment	Administration	Applicable Conditions	Onset	Duration of Action	Dosage	Side Effects
MUSE	Intraurethral	N, A?, V?	10 min	60–80 min	250–1000 μg	Penile pain or burning, hypotension
Papaverine*	Intracavernosal	N, A?, V?	10 min	30–60 min	15–60 mg	Prolonged erection, fibrosis, ecchymosis
Penile prosthesis	Surgical	N, A, V		replacement in 5–10 yrs		Infection, erosion, mechanical failure
PGE₁	Intracavernosal	N, A?, V?	10 min	40–60 min	5–20 μg	Prolonged erection, pain, fibrosis
Phentolamine*	Intracavernosal	N, A?, V?	10 min	30–60 min	0.5–1 mg	Prolonged erection, fibrosis, headache, facial flushing
Sex therapy	Counseling	psychogenic	weeks	years	weekly	Anxiety
Sildenafil	Oral	N, A?, V?	60 min	4 hrs	25–100 mg	Headache, flushing, rhinitis, dyspepsia, transient color blindness; contraindicated with nitrate use
Vacuum device	External	N, V, A?	< 5 min	30 min	—	Petechiae, bruising, painful ejaculation

NOTE: A = arteriogenic; MUSE = medicated urethral system for erection; N = neurogenic; P = psychogenic; PGE₁ = prostaglandin E₁; V = venogenic; ? = possibly.
* Not approved by the Food and Drug Administration for this use.

effects are bruising, ecchymoses or hematoma, local pain, fibrosis from repeated injections, and priapism. PGE₁ appears to cause less scarring and priapism than papaverine. If an erection lasts longer than 4 hours, detumescence is necessary by aspiration of blood from the corpora cavernosa or injection of phenylephrine, since there is the potential for intracavernous hypoxia and fibrosis of trabecular smooth muscle, which may prevent future erections.

PGE₁ can also be administered intraurethrally using MUSE (medicated urethral system for erection). This system contains a small pellet of PGE₁ that is placed within the urethra and is rapidly absorbed through the urethral mucosa to produce an erection within 10 to 15 minutes. Possible side effects are penile pain, urethral burning, and a throbbing sensation in the perineum.

Moxisylyte, a peripheral vasodilator, has also been shown to induce penile rigidity when injected intracavernously, but it is less efficacious than PGE₁ and has more systemic side effects. A combination of vasoactive intestinal polypeptide and phentolamine may be an alternative for those who have failed previous therapy with PGE₁ or papaverine.

Testosterone supplementation increases libido and may improve erectile dysfunction in men with true hypogonadism. It is available as an intramuscular injection (testosterone enanthate or cyprionate) or topical transdermal patch and gel. Possible side effects associated with testosterone include polycythemia, increase in prostate size, gynecomastia, and fluid retention. It is important to perform a digital rectal examination to assess the prostate and obtain a baseline prostate-specific antigen level prior to initiation of therapy. If there is a rise in prostate-specific antigen or hematocrit with testosterone therapy, it usually occurs within 6 months. Therefore, it is advisable to check these levels at 3-month intervals during the first year of therapy, then every 12 months thereafter.

Surgical implantation of a penile prostheses is another therapeutic option. Mechanical failure, infection, device erosion, and fibrosis are possible complications. Penile revascularization surgery has limited success.

FEMALE SEXUALITY

Age-Associated Changes

Many factors play an important role in the sexual response of older women, including changes that occur with menopause, cultural expectations, relationship problems, previous sexual experiences, chronic illnesses, and depression. American women live about 29 years after menopause and outlive their spouses an average of 8 years. Although the frequency of intercourse decreases with aging, sexuality remains important for older women. One study found that among Swedish women aged 61 years, 59% were sexually active, but 43% experienced vaginal dryness and 10% vaginal burning. In a study of British women aged 55 to 85, only 24% were found to be sexually active; 62% did not have a sexual partner. Lack of sexual activity among women with partners was found to be due to lack of the woman's interest in intercourse (43%), lack of the man's interest (24%), or the man's illness or erectile dysfunction (29%).

The female sexual response cycle changes with aging. During the excitement phase, the clitoris may require longer direct stimulation, and genital engorgement is decreased. Vaginal lubrication is reduced, although with increased foreplay and gentle stimulation lubrication is usually adequate for intercourse. During the plateau phase, there is less expansion and vasocongestion of the vagina. During orgasm, fewer and weaker contractions occur, although older women can still achieve multiple orgasms. Occasionally during orgasm, the older woman experiences spastic and painful contractions of the uterine musculature. During the resolution phase, vasocongestion is lost more rapidly. Most of these changes are thought to be due to a decline in serum estrogen concentration after menopause, but a vasculogenic component may contribute to postmenopausal sexual dysfunction.

Female Sexual Dysfunction

For the most part, menopause is accompanied by decreased sexual function, with decreased sexual interest, responsiveness, and coital frequency. In addition, there is an increase in urogenital symptoms, often not discussed with the clinician. For example, a study of older British women found that 16% reported urinary urgency, dysuria, or frequency, 9% urinary incontinence, 11% vaginal itching, 8% vaginal dryness, and 2% painful intercourse. Among the women affected by vaginal dryness or painful intercourse, 33% did not seek professional advice and 36% resorted to over-the-counter medication (ie, lubricating jelly).

Dyspareunia, defined as pain with intercourse, can be due to organic or psychologic factors, or a combination of the two. For example, a woman may experience an episode of dyspareunia because of postmenopausal vaginal atrophy. With each subsequent sexual encounter she anticipates pain, causing inadequate arousal with decreased lubrication. Because of this cycle, the woman continues to experience dyspareunia, even after the vaginal atrophy has been treated. The most common organic cause of dyspareunia is atrophic vaginitis due to estrogen deficiency. Other causes include localized vaginal infections, cystitis, Bartholin's cyst, retroverted uterus, pelvic tumors, excessive penile thrusting, or improper angle of penile entry.

Estrogen replacement can improve vaginal lubrication and sense of well-being, but it has little effect on libido. Libido is thought to be dependent on testosterone (even in women), rather than estrogen.

The ovaries and adrenals are the main sources of androgens in women. Many investigators believe that there is a female androgen deficiency syndrome. The effects of female androgen deficiency were originally identified in women treated for advanced breast cancer with oophorectomy and adrenalectomy. When deprived of androgens, these women reported loss of libido. Surgically menopausal women receiving estradiol and testosterone replacement reported higher sexual desire, arousal, and more frequent fantasies than women on estradiol alone or placebo. In naturally postmenopausal women, some, but not all, studies have shown that the addition of testosterone to estrogen replacement therapy improves sexual function. (See also "Hormone Replacement Therapy," p 329.)

Older women commonly have multiple medical ailments, some of which affect sexuality. However, there are limited scientific studies of the effect of chronic diseases and medications on the sexuality of older women. Nevertheless, women with diabetes mellitus report decreased libido and lubrication, and longer time to reach orgasm. Rheumatic diseases affect sexuality via functional disability. After mastectomy for breast cancer, 20% to 40% of women experience sexual dysfunction. This may be due to disruption of body image, marital and family problems, spousal reaction, adjuvant therapy, or the psychologic impact of a breast cancer diagnosis. Several drugs can adversely affect sexual function, including antihistamines, antihypertensives, antidepressants, antipsychotics, antiestrogens, central nervous system stimulants, narcotics, alcohol, and anticholinergic drugs.

Psychosocial factors have an important role in sexual dysfunction. Women often marry men older than themselves and live longer than men. Consequently, heterosexual older women are likely to spend the last years of their lives alone. Even when a partner is available, he might have erectile dysfunction. Finally, lack of privacy may be a problem when the older couple lives with their children or in a nursing home.

Evaluation and Treatment

The history is the most important part of the evaluation, and careful questioning can detect problems that the woman might not otherwise volunteer. First, it is important to attempt to provide a comfortable atmosphere. Clinicians should ask about dyspareunia, lack of vaginal lubrication, and previous negative experiences, like rape, child abuse, or domestic violence. Medications should be carefully reviewed. A woman with dyspareunia should undergo a pelvic examination to exclude organic causes.

Dyspareunia due to atrophic vaginitis and decreased lubrication responds well to topical or systemic estrogen therapy. However, it is important to explain to the patient that complete restoration of vaginal tissue function may take up to 2 years. A vaginal estradiol ring delivers low-dose estrogen locally with lower systemic absorption and risks of systemic side effect than do vaginal estrogen creams. The ring is inserted into the upper third of the vaginal vault and replaced every 3 months. If the patient is not a candidate for or does not want to use estrogen, water-soluble vaginal lubricants (eg, Replens, Astroglide, K-Y jelly) are beneficial. Importantly, local stimulation through regular intercourse helps maintain a healthy vaginal mucosa. Longer foreplay allows more time for vaginal lubrication, just as older men often need longer and more direct stimulation to achieve an adequate erection.

Decreased libido may respond to testosterone. Testosterone for women is available in combination with estrogens and is approved by the Food and Drug Administration for moderate to severe vasomotor symptoms not improved with estrogens alone. Therapy is usually initiated with oral esterified estrogen 0.625 mg and methyltestosterone 1.25 mg. If symptoms do not improve, the dose can be doubled to esterified estrogen 1.25 mg and methyltestosterone 2.5 mg. Pharmacokinetic studies identifying appropriate replacement doses are lacking. The masculinizing side effects of testosterone, such as increased facial hair, are infrequent, dose dependent, and, for the most part, reversible upon discontinuation. Hepatic toxicity has been noted only in female-to-male transsexuals receiving very high doses of oral methyltestosterone.

Estrogen-androgen replacement is contraindicated in women with liver disease, and testosterone may limit the beneficial cardiovascular effects of estrogen replacement therapy. In a 9-week study in postmenopausal women, esterified estrogens (1.25 mg a day) were found to decrease low-density lipoproteins and increase high-density lipoproteins, while the same dose of estrogens plus methyltestosterone (2.5 mg a day) decreased high-density lipoproteins with no change in low-density lipoproteins. Before starting estrogen-androgen replacement, the woman's lipid profile should be checked. If borderline, it should be repeated every 6 months. Further studies of the best dosage, delivery system, long-term efficacy, and safety of testosterone are needed. (See also "Hormone Replacement Therapy," p 329.)

Sildenafil was tested in a 12-week placebo-controlled trial of 583 women with sexual dysfunction that included female sexual arousal disorder. Although well tolerated, sildenafil did not produce different outcomes of self-reported sexual functioning when compared with placebo.

Finally, the older woman should receive education about male sexual aging in addition to female sexual aging. Otherwise, she might mistakenly attribute her partner's diminished erection and need for more genital stimulation to her own inability to arouse her partner. Other psychologic issues, including depression, history of sexual abuse, and relationship problems, should be addressed and treated with antidepressant, psychotherapy, and marital therapy, as necessary. Table 51.2 summarizes treatments for female sexual dysfunction.

Table 51.2—Treatment Options for Sexual Dysfunction in Older Women

Symptom	Possible Cause	Therapy
Decreased desire	Postmenopausal	Estrogen ± testosterone
	Chronic illness	Treat underlying illness
	Depression	Antidepressant
	Relationship problems	Marital therapy
	Drugs	Review drugs ingested
Decreased lubrication	Postmenopausal	Longer foreplay, regular intercourse, lubricants, estrogen
	Anticholinergic drugs	Review medications, including over-the-counter drugs
Delayed or absent orgasm	Postmenopausal	Estrogen ± testosterone
	Psychological	Sex therapy, antidepressant
Pain with intercourse	Organic cause	Treat underlying physical condition
	Vaginal dryness, atrophy	Longer foreplay, regular intercourse, lubricants, estrogen
	Vaginismus (involuntary vaginal contractions)	Sex therapy

REFERENCES

- Barlow DH, Cardozo LD, Francis RM, et al. Urogenital aging and its effect on sexual health in older British women. *Br J Obstet Gynaecol.* 1997; 104(1):87–91.

- Bhasin S, Bagatell CJ, Bremner WJ, et al. Issues in testosterone replacement in older men. *J Clin Endocrinol Metab.* 1998; 83(10): 3435–3448.

- Gingell JC. New development in self-injection therapy for erectile dysfunction. *Br J Urol.* 1998; 81(4): 599–603.

- Mathias RE, Lubben JE, Atchison KA, et al. Sexual activity and satisfaction among very old adults: results from a community-dwelling Medicare population survey. *Gerontologist.* 1997; 37(1): 6–14.

- Padero MC, Bhasin S, Friedman TC. Androgen supplementation in older women: too much hype, not enough data. *J Am Geriatr Soc.* 2002; 50(6):1131–1140.

- Rendell MS, Rajfer J, Wicker PA, et al. Sildenafil for treatment of erectile dysfunction in men with diabetes: a randomized controlled trial. *JAMA.* 1999; 281(5): 421–426.

- Rosenberg MJ, King TD, Timmons MC. Estrogen-androgen for hormone replacement: a review. *J Reprod Med.* 1997; 42(7):394–404.

CHAPTER 52—HEMATOLOGIC DISEASES AND DISORDERS

The hematologic system shows minimal declines in function with advancing age. The major effects are a decreased ability to respond to a maximum stimulation and, once all pathologic factors have been excluded, a modest increase in the prevalence of anemia. This is particularly noted in older men (> 75), who in cross-sectional studies have a significantly lower values than their younger counterparts (< 65). This large effect has not been noted in longitudinal studies. The mechanism for the difference probably reflects the presence of comorbid illness or reduced erythropoietin drive as a result of declines in androgen concentrations.

Numerous animal studies have shown a reduced ability of the aged hematopoietic system to respond to stimulation. Thus, the rate of return of the hemoglobin to normal following phlebotomy is blunted and the ability to mount a granulocyte response to infection is reduced. These reductions are similar to the age-related decline in the ability of the immune system to respond to a stimulatory challenge. Studies in humans have not been as conclusive. (See also "Biology," p 1.) There does not appear to be an impaired ability of older persons to increase their granulocyte count following the injection of granulocyte colony-stimulating factor or to increase their hematocrit in response to erythropoietin injection. There is little evidence to suggest that leukocyte counts are lower in older persons with bacterial infections or in response to a surgical insult. One study has suggested that the presence of comorbid conditions combined with aging do result in significant differences. Thus, the severity of neutropenia following chemotherapy for small cell cancer of the lung is greater in patients who are underweight and malnourished than in those who are not. Age appears to reduce the hematopoietic reserve capacity. This, however, is of no clinical relevance unless another abnormality that also adversely affects function (eg, protein energy malnutrition) is present. Thus, the evidence is that aging and illness combined lead to significant abnormalities.

Aging does not appear to affect the circulating concentrations of erythropoietin and colony-stimulating factors; the increase in response to anemia or infection in older people is equal to that noted in their younger counterparts. However, in response to stress, the blunted hematopoietic response seen with age has been attributed to an impaired ability to release growth factors. This might explain the age-related reduced neutrophil response to infection seen in animal studies and may contribute to increased infection-induced morbidity with aging. The production of certain growth factors, particularly interleukin-6, appears to increase with aging. (See Table 44.1, p 293.) This has led to the notion that aging is accompanied by dysregulation of growth factor production with overproduction of some and underproduction of other cytokines. An important question is whether aging affects the ability of the hematopoietic system to respond to injected growth factors such as erythropoietin and granulocyte colony-stimulating factor. Current information suggests that in the absence of comorbidity the response is unaffected.

ANEMIA

Clearly, the most common age-related hematologic abnormality, anemia, occurs in both older men and older women. The increase in incidence is significant for men as they age, and the incidence rate remains relatively constant in women with advancing age. It has been suggested that reduced sensitivity to erythropoietin occurs because of declines in testosterone concentrations. This contributes to the lower hemoglobin concentrations in men. In very mild anemia (hemoglobin > 11.5 gm/dL for women, and > 12.0 gm/dL for men), comprehensive work-up commonly fails to identify a cause. Studies of such cases have shown an associated reduction in neutrophil counts that suggests that the lower hemoglobin may be a marker of decreased hematopoietic reserve capacity. An evaluation of anemia when values are < 10.5 gm/dL invariably identifies a pathologic cause.

Because of heterogeneity of presentation, the evaluation of anemia on the basis of red cell size and shape has very limited utility. A more rational approach is one in which anemia is classified functionally as due to increased red cell destruction (hemolytic anemia), ineffective production (ineffective anemia), or reduced production (hypoproliferative anemia).

Hemolytic anemia is diagnosed by the presence of a significant reticulocytosis and an elevated indirect bilirubin. In the older adult the most common cause is immunologic (Coombs' serum test positive). In contrast to younger persons, in older persons an obvious cause for a Coombs'-positive hemolytic anemia can often be identified (lymphoma, chronic lymphatic leukemia, drug-related effects).

Ineffective erythropoiesis is characterized by increased red cell production, but, because of structural abnormalities, the red cells are destroyed in the bone marrow and never enter the peripheral blood. Laboratory features include anemia, reticulocytopenia, and an elevated indirect bilirubin. The most common causes of ineffective erythropoiesis in older adults is either vitamin B_{12} or folate deficiency. Macrocytosis is invariably present in the anemic patient, and the diagnosis is made by measuring levels of serum B_{12} and serum and red cell folate. The latter is almost always the result of alcohol ingestion or drug-related interference of folate metabolism. Sideroblastic anemia must be considered in an older person with evidence of ineffective erythropoiesis. Not infrequently, the anemia is severe, it is associated with microcytosis, and the serum iron and the transferrin saturation are increased. The diagnosis is made by bone marrow aspirate and biopsy. Usually no cause is identified. A fraction of these patients respond to treatment with pharmacologic doses of pyridoxine. This anemia may also be secondary to inflammation, cancer, or drug side effect (eg, isoniazid). The myelodysplastic syndrome is another cause of ineffective erythropoiesis in older adults. The syndrome consists of a group of stem cell disorders that present with refractory anemia with or without ringed sideroblasts. Cytogenetic abnormalities are common in this condition, the most frequent being 5q-deletion. This condition is found almost exclusively in older persons. These patients have a macrocytic anemia, mild leukopenia, and normal to increased platelet counts. Treatment is supportive, and the condition carries a relatively good prognosis. Di Guglielmo's syndrome is related to myelodysplastic syndrome and is primarily a disease of older persons. In addition to red cell abnormalities, myeloid and megakaryocytic dysplasia occur. This condition frequently evolves into an acute myelogenous leukemia characterized by pancytopenia and immature nucleated red cells and primitive myeloid and megakaryocytic precursors in the peripheral blood. Treatment is supportive. (See "Oncology," p 349.)

Hypoproliferative anemia remains the most common type of anemia in older persons. Inadequate iron supply for erythropoiesis is the main cause. Although still common in older persons, iron-deficiency (blood-loss) anemia is not the most common type in persons over the age of 70. Laboratory features include a low serum iron, elevated total iron-binding capacity (> 400 µg/dL), and transferrin saturation < 20%. Iron stores are absent, and as a consequence the serum ferritin level is invariably lower than 100 ng/mL. Once it is diagnosed, an aggressive evaluation to identify a source of blood loss is essential for both women and men. A gastrointestinal cause (acute gastritis, polyps, cancer) is common. In a relatively large number of cases, however, no obvious cause can be identified. This may be due to the high prevalence of angiodysplasia of the large bowel in older persons. In older persons with iron deficiency, a coagulopathy should be considered. Acquired factor-VIII deficiency and acquired von Willebrand's disease are generally diseases of older persons. In older persons with significant and continued bleeding in whom no obvious cause can be identified, an evaluation of coagulation should be considered.

A more common cause of anemia in older persons is the so-called *anemia of chronic disease*. Pathophysiologically, this condition is caused by an inability of macrophages to release iron from the breakdown of senescent red cells. As a consequence, the serum iron falls, and as with blood-loss anemia, there is inadequate iron supply for erythropoiesis. In contrast to blood-loss anemia, in which iron stores are absent, in the anemia of chronic disease, iron stores are normal or increased. Laboratory features include a mild anemia, a low serum iron, low transferrin saturation, and normal to increased iron stores (ferritin > 100 ng/mL, low total iron-binding capacity < 250 µg/dL). Classic causes include acute and chronic infections, pressure ulcers, inflammatory conditions such as polymyalgia rheumatica, and the anemia of cancer. It is critical that this condition be distinguished from iron-deficiency (blood-loss) anemia, to avoid unnecessary gastrointestinal tests to identify a cause for blood loss and to prevent the inappropriate prescription of oral iron therapy.

Because of the high prevalence of iron deficiency in menstruating women and in children, many of our foods are now fortified with iron. For this, and perhaps other reasons, reduced iron stores from blood-loss anemia are now much rarer in menstruating women than was noted in the 1970s. This has been accompanied by a gradual increase in tissue iron stores in both men and women. Of concern are reports linking increased tissue iron stores to a higher risk of both heart disease and an array of cancers. For this reason, iron fortification is clearly not recommended in iron-replete individuals and should be avoided in postmenopausal women and in men. Many older people take daily multivitamin supplements that contain the recommended daily allowance (18 mg) of iron or more. It is now recommended that if a supplement is used, that it not contain iron. Fortunately, a number of companies are now making inexpensive supplements that are iron free.

COAGULATION

The concentrations of a large number of coagulation enzymes have been shown to increase with age. These include factors VII and VIII and fibrinogen. In centenarians, highly significant increases in the concentrations of these factors are noted, as are levels of factors IX and X and thrombin-antithrombin complexes. Fibrin formation is also increased, as evidenced by higher concentrations of fibrinopeptide A. In addition, elevated levels of D-dimers suggest increased hyperfibrinolysis. These facts suggest that aging may be accompanied by increased hypercoagulability. This may well be a contributory factor to the increased prevalence and incidence of thrombotic episodes in older persons. This is further supported by the higher concentrations of D-dimer in frail, functionally dependent older persons, who are at even greater risk of thrombotic episodes. However, the very high level of clotting factors and evidence of hypercoagulability in remarkably healthy centenarians has led to the suggestion that elevated coagulation factors may not be markers of increased risks of thrombosis.

Bleeding diatheses are not uncommon in older persons. Unexplained bruises, repeated nosebleeds, gastrointestinal losses, or excessive blood loss during surgery or following dental extraction are common presentations. In these patients, screening platelet counts and coagulation studies should be obtained. Bleeding times can also be of value, provided they are meticulously standardized and done by a person with experience in the procedure. Thrombocytopenia is a common cause of bleeding problems in older persons. A level less than 150,000 mL is considered significant, but bleeding usually occurs at much lower levels. Common causes include decreased production of platelets in the bone marrow, sequestration in enlarged spleens, and increased peripheral destruction. Decreased production of platelets occurs in the leukemias, marrow aplasia, or most frequently in older persons in association with drugs that suppress platelet production. The major cause of increased peripheral destruction is immune thrombocytopenia. A lymphoma, collagen vascular disease, or a drug-induced cause is common in older persons with autoimmune thrombocytopenia. Treatment of thrombocytopenia depends upon the cause. For decreased production, platelet transfusion should be considered if there is significant blood loss, irrespective of the platelet count. Generally, bleeding occurs when the count drops to 20,000 per μL or less. Since the immune thrombocytopenia is usually secondary in older persons, the initial approach is to identify and treat the primary cause. If no cause is found, a trial of corticosteroids is warranted.

Bleeding may also occur because of a platelet function disorder (thrombopathy), although uncommon significant bleeding can occur with aspirin therapy in older persons. Aspirin irreversibly acetylates cyclooxygenase affecting arachidonic acid metabolism. The net effect is significant loss of platelet function. In the rare circumstance, spontaneous bleeding may occur or may be precipitated by injury or surgery. Platelet transfusions may be needed. Hereditary von Willebrand's disease may present initially in older persons. The disease is caused by a reduction in concentration of von Willebrand's factor (vWF) that is accompanied by reductions in factor-VIII concentrations. vWF is essential for normal platelet function, so bleeding occurs because of a platelet function defect. Acquired von Willebrand's disease, although rare, is a disease of older persons. It is commonly associated with monoclonal gammopathies, lymphomas, or myeloma. Monoclonal factor VIII does not contain the vWF factor, and viral contamination may occur with cryoprecipitates (which used to be the treatment of choice for von Willebrand's disease). When treatment is necessary, desmopressin acetate may be used. This synthetic analogue of arginine vasopressin stimulates endothelial cells to release stored vWF. Treatment is often successful, but adverse effects are common. In this circumstance, factor VIII concentrates that have high doses of vWF should be used. The concentrate should be processed to inactivate viruses.

Liver disease must always be considered in patients who present with excessive bleeding. The prothrombin time is prolonged even in mild to moderate liver disease. The partial thromboplastin time remains normal until liver disease becomes severe. With the exception of factor VIII (which is produced by endothelial cells), liver disease causes reductions in all clotting factors. Liver disease is also associated with disseminated intravascular coagulation, particularly in the liver. Fibrin degradation products are not cleared as well, and platelet function may be affected. The treatment of a bleeding diathesis in liver disease is fresh frozen plasma.

Bleeding can also occur because of clotting factor deficiencies, which in the older person are usually acquired and caused by the presence of circulating clotting factor inhibitors. The most common is an acquired inhibitor to factor VIII. The onset is often sudden, titers to anti-factor VIII antibodies can be very high, and presentation is with bleeding into joints and muscle, similar to that in hemophilia A. Treatment involves factor replacement; depending on the severity, immunosuppression with prednisone or cyclophosphamide may also be needed.

Deficiency of the vitamin K–dependent clotting factors tends to occur in older persons with major illnesses. Disorders of the hepatobiliary tree, antibiotics that neutralize bowel bacteria (a major source of the vitamin), malabsorption, and severe malnutrition are the causes. Even if the patient is not on coumadin, inappropriate use must be considered. The deficits are readily treated with parenteral vitamin K injections.

A bleeding disorder will be thought of only if it is appropriately included in a differential diagnosis. This particularly applies to chronic blood loss from the gastrointestinal system. In those in whom endoscopic evaluation does not identify a cause, careful evaluation of platelets, including platelet functions and coagulation, should always be considered.

VITAMIN B$_{12}$, FOLATE, AND HOMOCYSTEINE

Older persons are more likely than younger persons to have lower levels of vitamin B$_{12}$ and folate. In epidemiologic studies, approximately 10% of apparently healthy persons aged 70 and over were found to have vitamin B$_{12}$ levels that are deficient, and 5% to 10% have low folate values. These low values may well be clinically important. Methylmalonic acid levels are increased in the urine and serum, marrow deoxyuridine suppression is abnormal, and excretion of formiminoglutamic acid is increased. These tests tend to indicate functional abnormalities as a direct consequence of low vitamin B$_{12}$ or folate. Pernicious anemia is a rare cause of vitamin B$_{12}$ deficiency. Atrophic gastritis leading to vitamin B$_{12}$ malabsorption is the

likely cause in the majority of cases. This can also contribute to low folate levels in older persons. However, alcohol abuse, drug interactions with folate absorption, and inadequate dietary intake are the most common causes of low folate levels. Low vitamin B$_{12}$ and folate levels are not necessarily accompanied by macrocytosis or evidence of megaloblastic anemia. Studies have shown that the mean corpuscular volume does increase, as does the number of neutrophil lobes, as the vitamin B$_{12}$ and folate levels become progressively more deficient.

There is some evidence to suggest that low vitamin B$_{12}$ levels may contribute to cognitive decline in older persons. There is no question that severe vitamin B$_{12}$ deficiency can result in cognitive loss and significant neurologic deficits. In the older population with low vitamin B$_{12}$ levels, there is little evidence at the current time to indicate an important relationship between the vitamin and dementia. Nevertheless, aggressive replacement must always be undertaken when a demented patient presents with low levels of vitamin B$_{12}$ or folate.

Low levels of vitamin B$_{12}$ or folate are accompanied by increased levels of homocysteine. In recent years a great deal of attention has focused on the role of raised homocysteine levels in coronary artery disease risk. It has been suggested that this abnormality can account for a substantial fraction of myocardial infarctions in those who do not have hypercholesterolemia. A relationship may well exist between coronary artery disease and low vitamin B$_{12}$ and elevated homocysteine in older persons. Levels of homocysteine can be reduced by prescribing 400 μg of folate acid once or twice daily.

It is clear that deficiencies of vitamin B$_{12}$ and folate are common in older persons and that the reductions have clinical relevance. Should levels of the vitamins be routinely obtained in older persons? It is unlikely that this would be cost-effective. Nevertheless, measurements should be obtained in those who present with cognitive loss, in whom deficiencies are likely (eg, alcoholism), and who have a high risk of coronary artery disease. Empiric prescription of vitamin B$_{12}$ or folate for older persons with ischemic heart disease may be reasonable. Even in patients with atrophic gastritis, oral vitamin B$_{12}$ is generally adequate; 10% will be absorbed by mass action alone and not require the presence of intrinsic factor. Thus, a daily dose of 1 mg vitamin B$_{12}$ will replete a person with levels in the low-normal range. Parenteral replacement should be used in severe deficiencies with vitamin B$_{12}$, that is, levels below 100 pg/mL.

It has been suggested that in older patients with low normal (< 350 pg/ml) B$_{12}$ level, methylmalonic acid (MMA) levels be checked to exclude metabolically active B$_{12}$ deficiency. Renal failure can artificially raise the serum MMA level. A few authors have suggested that even for less than 500 pg/ml, replacement therapy be considered. Those patients with low-normal B_{12} levels and macrocytosis (with or without anemia) or neurologic changes should be considered for vitamin replacement, particularly if the MMA level is elevated.

REFERENCES

- Ajmani RS, Rifkind JM. Hemorheological changes during human aging. *Gerontology.* 1998;44(2):111–120.

- Carmel R. Cobalamin, the stomach and aging. *Am J Clin Nutr.* 1997;66(4):750–759.

- Ioannou GN, Spector J, Scott K, et al. Prospective evaluation of a clinical guideline for the diagnosis and management of iron deficiency anemia. *Am J Med.* 2002;113(4):281–287.

- Izaks GJ, Westendorp RG, Knook, DL. The definition of anemia in older persons. *JAMA.* 1999;281(18):1714–1717.

CHAPTER 53—ONCOLOGY

Prevalence studies indicate that cancer is primarily a burden for geriatric populations. In fact, the median age for cancer in the United States is 70 years. Though cancer has long been recognized as a disease of older people, emphasis on geriatric issues and cancer is a recent development.

Three questions have arisen that form the underpinnings of this new emphasis

- Why are tumors more common in older persons?
- Is there a difference in tumor aggressiveness with advancing age?
- Should treatment be different for the older patient?

Experimental data and clinical experience have indicated that tumors are not resistant to treatment by virtue of age alone. However, age is associated with slight reductions in certain organ functions, and these deficiencies in physiologic reserve might be magnified by comorbid conditions. Cancer treatments, especially chemotherapy, may therefore be associated with an increase in adverse events, and treatment should be tailored to the individual, taking into consideration potential increased toxicities and balancing this with expectations of survival in the context of comorbidities.

A review of the National Cancer Institute's Surveillance, Epidemiology and End Results (SEER) data revealed that more than 50% of all cancers are diagnosed in patients aged 65 years and older, and this older patient population incurs more than 60% of all cancer deaths. The data also reveal important trends. Whereas between 1968 and 1985 cancer mortality decreased 23% in patients younger than 55 years (primarily reflecting advances in the therapy of acute leukemias, Hodgkin's disease, non-Hodgkin's lymphomas, and testicular cancers), cancer mortality for those aged 55 years and older increased by 17%. Thus, in the older age groups we are faced with an increasingly prevalent disease for which modern therapies have not improved overall survival. We have much to learn about providing optimal management of cancer in older persons, but an emphasis on disease prevention and screening remains a logical priority.

CANCER BIOLOGY AND AGING

Explaining the Increased Prevalence of Cancer With Age

There are at least three reasons for the increased prevalence of cancer with age. First, cancers, particularly those that occur after menopause, are thought to develop over a long period, perhaps decades. This is best exemplified by the current understanding of colon cancer, which has been shown to develop because of an accumulation of several damaging genetic events occurring in a stochastic manner over time. Thus, if mutations are acquired at a constant rate, older people are more likely to have lived long enough to develop the 8 to 10 genetic lesions it takes to develop a malignancy. In contrast, lymphomas are just as likely to occur in young as old people. Lymphocytes normally undergo gene rearrangements and mutations to generate antigen receptors, and these processes appear to be particularly vulnerable to errors that may lead to lymphoma at any age.

A second reason for the greater prevalence of cancer with advancing age is that DNA repair mechanisms are thought to decline with age. As a consequence, cells may accumulate damage. Normally, a dividing cell pauses in G1 (the gap following mitosis

[M] and before DNA replication [S]) and in G2 (the gap following S and before M) to take inventory and repair any damage before proceeding to the next phase. These are the G1 or the G2 checkpoints. Older cells may fail to detect or repair damage and fail to control DNA replication accurately. This leads to aneuploidy and to uncontrolled proliferation. In younger people, these aberrations may trigger the death of the cell; in older people, the errors may be tolerated and fail to signal cell death. Cells without functioning checkpoints are vulnerable to loss of growth control.

A third contribution to increased cancer incidence in older people may be a decline in the function of the immune system, particularly in cellular immunity. A number of findings suggest that the immune system can recognize and control certain cancers. A decline in immune function may lead to the emergence of a cancer in an older person that was controlled when that person was younger.

The Different Characteristics of Cancer

There has been a long-held but incompletely documented clinical dogma that cancers in older people are less aggressive or slower growing. However, epidemiologic data from tumor registries or large clinical trials have not supported this notion. Such data may be confounded by geriatric problems that shorten survival independently of the cancer (eg, comorbidity, multiple medications, clinician or family bias regarding diagnosis and treatment in older persons, and age-associated life stresses). These factors may counter any primary influence that aging might have on tumor aggressiveness. However, there is experimental support for the contention that there is reduced tumor aggressiveness with age. Data obtained from laboratory animals with a wide range of tumors under highly controlled circumstances demonstrate slower tumor growth, fewer experimental metastases, and longer survival in old mice. Tumor growth involves several levels of interaction between the tumor and the host. It may be that tumor angiogenesis is impaired in older people, thereby controlling the rate of tumor growth. The clinical importance of this is limited, inasmuch as it is difficult to know in any given patient whether the course of the disease will be characterized by an indolent or aggressive pattern of growth.

Breast cancer is the most notable clinical example of age-associated decline in tumor aggressiveness. Older patients are more likely to have more favorable histologic types, higher levels of estrogen and progesterone receptor expression, lower growth fraction, and less frequent metastases. In a published series on breast cancer patients with primary tumors of 1 cm (diameter) or less, the single most important predictor of metastasis to axillary nodes has consistently been found to be patient age: patients under the age of 50 years have the highest likelihood of spread, whereas those over the age of 70 years have the lowest likelihood of spread. Stage for stage, older patients seem to have longer survival than younger patients.

By contrast, Hodgkin's disease seems to be a more aggressive disease in older patients. The most likely reason for the age-associated differences in prognosis is that Hodgkin's disease is a different disease in patients aged 45 years and over than in younger patients. Incidence data demonstrate two distinct peak incidence rates, one at age 32 years and one at age 84 years. The frequency of particular histologic subtypes of Hodgkin's disease is different in younger and older patients; nodular sclerosis is the most common subtype in younger patients, mixed cellularity is the most common in older patients. In all reported treatment series, older age is an independent prognostic factor. Additional study is necessary to document age-associated differences in tumor cell biology.

Acute leukemia, like Hodgkin's disease, appears to be a different disease in older people; the MDR1 drug resistance pump is more commonly expressed, patients respond less well to treatment, and survival is shorter than in younger patients. However, for most cancer types, the molecular biology and clinical behavior of the tumor is similar across the age span.

PRINCIPLES OF CANCER MANAGEMENT

Current forms of cancer treatment include surgery, radiation, cytotoxic chemotherapy, hormone manipulation, and biologic therapy. Age alone does not preclude any of these approaches, but because of normal changes with age in certain organs and also age-associated conditions (comorbidities), special considerations are warranted.

Randomized clinical trials are the most reliable instrument to study medical intervention, and treatment decisions are best founded on the results of such work. However, despite efforts from the cooperative oncology groups, patients entered onto trial are by and large younger and presumably healthier than the typical geriatric patient with the same disorder. Furthermore, common end points of these trials are length of survival (for therapeutic interventions) or disease-specific deaths (for prevention studies), and these end points are not always the most appropriate outcomes for older patients (because of their inherently limited life expectancies on the basis of age alone).

Clinical researchers are making a start at addressing issues of geriatric oncology. New, more geriatrics-oriented trials focus more on symptom reduction and quality of life than life expectancy. Surveys have indicated that older patients, when fully informed, most often choose life-extending treatments, even at the risk of toxicity. It is the clinician and the patient's family that are most focused on quality-of-life issues. Furthermore, for the most part, tumors are not more resistant to treatment in older patients. It is also commonly appreciated that acute toxicities (nausea, vomiting, hair loss) are less prominent in older patients. Thus, although quality of life remains a primary treatment consideration, efforts at extending life should not be denied older patients on the basis of their age alone.

Cancer Screening

Two issues are barriers to screening older persons for cancers. First, most of the large cancer clinical studies that have documented the efficacy of screening have systematically omitted the study of older people. Thus, it is not clear whether the benefits of a particular screening test initiated at age 50 extends to people at age 70 or 75. For prostate cancer, it is felt that screening is not indicated for someone with less than 10 years' life expectancy. For men without other comorbidities, this rule would suggest that men older than age 80 should not be screened. Data are not available in other cancers.

A second issue that complicates screening older persons is adherence with the screening schedule. Barriers to screening include a person's lack of infor-

mation about the nature and value of screening and limited availability of economic and social support. The primary care provider has a central role in promoting screening. Published investigations have revealed that physician recommendation is the most important factor influencing cancer-screening adherence.

Several methods of improving adherence have been investigated. These include personal invitation letters, a plastic pocket-sized card as a reminder of screening deadlines, and personal visits with members of volunteer organizations who escort the person through the screening process. Adherence may be improved by streamlining the process, avoiding redundancies, prolonging the time interval between screening sessions, and coupling screening sessions with other office visits. An increase in the percentage of women aged 65 and older undergoing mammography may indicate the success of these approaches. (See "Prevention," p 59.)

Chemotherapy

Aging may be associated with changes in key pharmacologic parameters of antineoplastic agents and in the susceptibility to end-organ toxicity.

The most consistent pharmacokinetic change of aging is a progressive delay in the elimination of renally excretable drugs because of a reduction in glomerular filtration rate (Table 53.1). The more prolonged

Table 53.1—Chemotherapy Issues in Geriatric Oncology

Issue	Description
General	Comorbidities and multiple medications add complexity.
Pharmacokinetic changes	A progressive delay with age in the elimination of renally excreted drugs, due to a reduction in glomerular filtration rate, may account, in part, for more severe toxicity.
Pharmacodynamic changes	Pharmacodynamic changes may include enhanced resistance to antitumor agents. An increased expression of the multidrug resistance gene has been reported in some older patients. Other proteins that result in drug efflux have also been shown to have prognostic importance, but age-associated changes have not been described. Another factor that would influence drug distribution and metabolism is the observation in a murine model of increased tumor hypoxia with age.
Toxicity	Mucositis, cardiotoxicity, and peripheral and central neurotoxicity become more common and more severe with aging. Cardiotoxicity is a complication of anthracyclines and anthraquinones, mitomycin C, and high-dose cyclophosphamide. The incidence of cardiotoxicity also increases with age. Vincristine peripheral neurotoxicity is more common and more severe in older patients. Similarly, the incidence of cerebellar toxicity from high-dose cytosine arabinoside increases with age.
Myelotoxicity	Whereas chemotherapy-related myelotoxicity may become more severe and more prolonged with aging, moderately toxic treatment regimens, such as CMF (cyclophosphamide, methotrexate, fluorouracil), cisplatin and fluorouracil, and cisplatin and etoposide are tolerated by many patients aged 70 and older without life-threatening neutropenia or thrombocytopenia. However, infections are markedly increased among older acute leukemia patients undergoing intensive induction treatment. In these cases it is possible that the disease itself, rather than an age-associated change in "marrow reserve," is responsible for the depletion of hemopoietic stem cells.
Recent advances	Granulocyte colony-stimulating factor and granulocyte-macrophage colony-stimulating factor have reduced the incidence of neutropenic infections in patients receiving intensive treatment, and their effectiveness does not appear to be diminished with advancing patient age. Also, certain new drugs or new formulations may be particularly suitable to the older patient. Included in these would be oral etoposide and fludarabine, gemcitabine, and vinorelbine.

half-life of these agents may account in part for more severe toxicity. In a study of women aged 65 and older with metastatic breast cancer, doses of methotrexate and cyclophosphamide were modified according to the creatinine clearance. As a consequence, the myelotoxicity was markedly reduced without compromise of the therapeutic effect.

Owing to differences in their pharmacokinetics and pharmacodynamics, certain drugs may be particularly suitable for treating older patients. Oral etoposide provides valuable palliation for small cell cancer of the lung and large cell lymphoma, with minimal risk of complications. Fludarabine, which is very active in lymphoproliferative neoplasms, induces apoptosis of cancer cells, a process that may be altered in malignancies occurring in older persons. Vinorelbine and gemcitabine are two newer agents that are active against lung and breast cancer and are well tolerated and effective in older patients.

Hormonal Therapy

Hormonal treatment is effective in cancers of the breast, the prostate, and the endometrium. Tamoxifen, a selective estrogen receptor modulator, has antagonistic and partial agonistic effects. It is a useful therapy in adjuvant treatment of breast cancer and also has estrogen-like positive effects on cardiovascular risk factors and bone disease. Other more selective drugs in this category, such as raloxifene, are in clinical testing. Although inactive as single agent, tamoxifen is synergistic with chemotherapy in the management of malignant melanoma. Currently used hormonal agents are listed in Table 53.2. Most of these are well tolerated by older persons and commonly are the treatment of choice in this age group. Diethylstilbestrol is an estrogenic compound with serious cardiovascular risks (stroke, heart attack, thromboembolism) when used to treat prostate cancer in older men.

Table 53.2—Hormonal Agents Commonly Used in Treating Cancer

Breast
    Antiestrogens: tamoxifen, toremifene
    Progestational: medroxyprogesterone acetate
    Aromatase inhibitors: aminoglutethimide, letrozole, anastrozole

Prostate
    LH-RH analogs: goserelin, leuprolide
    Estrogens: diethylstilbestrol
    Antiandrogens: flutamide, bicalutamide

Endometrium
    Progestational
    Antiestrogens

Biologic Therapy

Modulation of immune response is a particularly attractive option in treating the older person, whose natural defenses against cancer may be impaired by immune senescence. Only a limited number of options are clinically available, and these are clearly inadequate to restore a normal immune response in the aged person.

Recombinant α-interferon at moderate doses (eg, 3 million units, three times weekly) is reasonably well tolerated by patients of all ages. At higher doses α-interferon causes myelodepression, severe fatigue, flu-like illness, malaise, fever, neuropathy, and abnormalities of liver enzymes. There are reports of delirium, depression, and dementia following α-interferon use in persons aged 65 and older. More information on the safety of this compound in the older patient would be desirable. This is particularly important because interferon has been shown to be effective therapy for chronic myeloid leukemia, hairy cell leukemia, and multiple myeloma, hematologic malignancies that occur more commonly among older people. It may also prolong survival after chemotherapy for follicular lymphoma. It is being tested at higher, more toxic doses in patients with stage II melanoma after surgical resection of the primary lesion. About 15% of patients with metastatic melanoma may experience a partial response from α-interferon.

Interleukin-2 is used to treat metastatic melanoma and renal cancer. When administered daily at 3 million units per square meter, it may produce partial responses in about 15% of patients and complete remissions in about 5% of patients, many of which responses are long lasting. Interleukin-2 can produce severe dose-related toxicity, including capillary leak syndrome, hypotension, adult respiratory distress syndrome, cardiac arrhythmias, peripheral edema, renal failure (prerenal), cholestatic liver dysfunction, skin rashes, and thrombocytopenia. These complications tend to appear gradually in less severe form; generally, patients do not suddenly deteriorate. The toxicities reverse completely within a few days of stopping the drug. It is a strong clinical impression that interleukin-2 toxicities are less severe and develop later in older patients.

Monoclonal antibodies directed against CD20 (rituximab) expressed on B-cell lymphomas and against HER-2/*neu* (trastuzumab) expressed on breast cancer and other epithelial malignancies are effective treatments. In most patients the antibodies are given just before combination chemotherapy; the antibodies appear to augment the response to the drugs. These humanized antibodies generally have mild toxicities. Patients may develop hypotension or shortness of breath with the first infusion because of complement fixation. Symptoms clear when the infusion rate is slowed down, and such symptoms rarely recur. Other antibodies against cancers are in development.

Radiation Therapy

Radiation therapy provides palliation for virtually all cancers, and it may be part of a treatment plan for lymphomas and cancers of the prostate, bladder, cervix, esophagus, breast, and head and neck area. In combination with cytotoxic chemotherapy, radiation therapy has allowed organ preservation in cancers of the anus, bladder, and larynx, and in extremity sarcomas. A central issue for radiation therapy in the older patient is safety. There has been a trend for almost five decades to use radiation therapy as an alternative to surgery in poor surgical candidates, mainly patients aged 65 and older, with the implied expectation that such an approach was less toxic. In fact, published reports have indicated that radiation therapy is both safe and effective in older patients. However, there remains concern when treatment involves irradiation of the whole brain (fear of neurologic sequelae, including dementia) or pelvis (fear of marrow aplasia or myelodysplasia or radiation enteritis), but no systematic investigation has categorically substantiated these concerns.

Advances in radiation therapy include techniques that allow a more restricted radiation field, especially partial brain irradiation, new applications of brachytherapy (insertion of radiation sources into the tumor bed), the development of radiosurgery (gamma ray knife, a precisely focused external beam of radiation) that allows destruction of small lesions (diameter $\leq$ 4 cm) of the central nervous system without craniotomy, and the development of new radiosensitizers.

Surgery

Concerns related to cancer surgery in the older person are safety and rehabilitative potential. Several reports indicate that age itself is not a risk factor for elective cancer surgery, but the length of hospital stay and the time to full recovery become more prolonged with advancing age of the patient. Similar results have been reported both from referral centers and community hospitals.

In contrast, the complications and the mortality of emergency surgery increase significantly with age. The most common cause of death is septic shock following emergency abdominal surgery. These results are not unexpected. Because of a decline in the functional reserve of many organ systems, the ability to cope with stress becomes progressively more limited with aging.

Advances in anesthesia and surgery have benefited the older patient. Included among these are new endoscopic procedures that provide valuable palliation for the many tumors of the gastrointestinal tract, and the more widespread use of spinal anesthesia for major abdominal interventions, with a substantial decline in perioperative complications and mortality. More widespread use of laparoscopic surgical techniques and application of laser and photodynamic therapy is also broadening the surgical armamentarium and providing more older patients with potential palliation and cure.

The trend to manage cancer without deforming surgery may preclude the need for complex rehabilitation and may be of special value for older people. Organ preservation without compromise of treatment outcome is obtainable for cancer of the anus and of the larynx, and is being studied for cancers of the oropharynx, the esophagus, the bladder, and the vulva. Also, the use of initial (neoadjuvant) chemotherapy before primary surgery has been shown to be effective in patients with large primary breast and lung cancers. Such an approach results in less extensive and potentially more curative surgical procedures.

Quality-of-Life Issues

Several studies have determined that the perception of quality of life is highly subjective and is poorly reproduced by external observers, even when these are close relationships or health care providers are very familiar with a person's physical condition. Furthermore, there is considerable discrepancy between the physician's determination of the patient's quality of life and patient's own assessment; physicians tend to underestimate the patient's quality of life.

Early assessments of quality of life focused on functional status and freedom from pain, but these factors, though important, are inadequate to evaluate far-reaching consequences of serious diseases on all domains of life. In the past decade several instruments for the measurement of quality of life have been validated and have been successfully used to study specific problems, such as the effects on quality of life of intensive care, the consequences of limb amputation, of partial and total mastectomy, and of iatrogenic impotence. These instruments are questionnaires requesting a person to rate his or her own well-being in several dimensions with a categorical or a visual analog scale. Unfortunately, these instruments have not been adjusted to the special needs of the older person. It is reasonable to assume that the importance of some factors, such as professional or job satisfaction, may decline with age, while the importance of others, including social support and the perception of family burden, may become more prominent.

Other problems related to assessing quality of life include the complexity of some questionnaires, which may overburden some older persons. In addition, little progress has been made in the assessment of quality of life in the cognitively impaired. Studies of pain in demented persons have demonstrated the reliability of repetitive behavioral testing in the assessment of discomfort, even in patients with cognitive impairment. Perhaps the same principles may be applied to the assessment of quality of life in demented patients.

At present, the main application of quality-of-life assessment in clinical decision making concerns the choice between interventions yielding comparable survival. An area of potential use is in medical decisions involving limited survival benefits at the price of a decline in quality of life. At present, the value of this trade-off is evaluated with measures known as "quality of life adjusted survival" or "quality-adjusted time without symptoms or toxicity," both of which include complex interviews of limited application to persons aged 70 and older.

SPECIFIC CANCERS

Breast Cancer

Controversy surrounds several critical issues in the management of this most common malignancy in older women. These include the following.

Postoperative Irradiation Following Lumpectomy

Although irradiation following lumpectomy is safe in women aged 65 and older, it may be a source of significant inconvenience and cost to them. The value of postoperative irradiation has been questioned because the local recurrence rate of breast cancer may decrease with age, and the inconvenience of daily radiation treatment protocols may outweigh the limited benefits for some.

Need for Axillary Lymphadenectomy

Given the benefits regardless of nodal status of adjuvant tamoxifen in all postmenopausal women with estrogen-receptor positive breast cancer, axillary dissection when the axilla is clinically negative may add unnecessary morbidity. This is particularly true if the procedure requires general anesthesia. However, proponents of lymphadenectomy claim that the procedure not only has a staging function but may also improve the curability of breast cancer or reduce the duration of adjuvant tamoxifen treatment. In some centers, axillary dissection is being replaced by biopsy of the sentinel node, the first lymph node draining the area of the breast that harbors the cancer. This is determined

at operation by injecting a dye into the site of the resected lump and removing the first node that turns blue. Early data suggest that sentinel node sampling is just as accurate as axillary dissection but considerably less toxic.

Adjuvant Hormonal Treatment

A meta-analysis of randomized trials established that adjuvant treatment with tamoxifen for at least 2 years prolongs both the disease-free survival and the overall survival of postmenopausal women. The benefits and risks of more prolonged treatment, especially for women over 70, are still controversial. Aromatase inhibitors are currently licensed as second-line hormonal treatment for patients who have progressed on tamoxifen. Trials of aromatase inhibitors have established them as first-line treatment in women with estrogen-receptor positive tumors. They are both more effective and less toxic than tamoxifen.

Initial Management of Metastatic Breast Cancer

Women aged 65 and older with metastatic, hormone receptor-positive breast cancer are likely to have effective palliation with hormonal therapy, such as tamoxifen. Hormonal treatment has also been shown to benefit older patients with hormone receptor–poor tumors, but chemotherapy has been shown to be safe and effective in this group of patients, as well.

Lung Cancer

Lung cancer is becoming increasingly common in older women for reasons that are not completely understood. The increase may be due to the more widespread smoking among women. In addition, some data suggest that women are at greater risk of developing lung cancer per unit of tobacco exposure. Lung cancer currently is the leading cause of cancer death in men and is second behind breast cancer in women. Early recognition and surgical resection remain the best chance for cure. For patients with lesions in a location that precludes surgery, occasionally localized radiation produces long-term survival. Over the past decade chemotherapy has been shown to produce clinical responses and provide effective palliation for a portion of the patients with metastatic disease. Prolongation of survival has been demonstrated, but the added increment is measured in weeks to months. New chemotherapeutic agents, such as vinorelbine and gemcitabine, and more established agents such as paclitaxel or docetaxel used in lower-dose weekly schedules, have proven to be effective treatments for older patients with lung cancer.

Colon Cancer

Two thirds of colon cancer cases occur in persons aged 65 years and over. With advancing age, there is a greater likelihood of right-sided lesions and presentations with anemia rather than pain. Colonoscopy has become the mainstay of diagnosis, primarily because it enables the gastroenterologist direct visualization and biopsy of the entire colon. Surgical excision may be adequate for lesions confined to the colon, but if extension to regional nodes is observed, postoperative adjuvant chemotherapy (usually 5-fluorouracil plus leucovorin) has been found to reduce recurrence by 40% to 50%. Survival of patients with disease metastatic to liver or other organs remains disappointing, despite the appearance of new drugs, such as irinotecan, capable of inducing partial remissions in a subset of patients. New drugs that target tyrosine kinase (an integral enzyme for cellular proliferation) within tumor cells are currently in development, and these offer great promise for future patients. Surgical excision of solitary hepatic lesions has been shown to offer survival advantage for selected patients, primarily those with smaller lesions, five or fewer lesions confined to a single hepatic lobe, and a longer interval from original tumor resection until the diagnosis of hepatic metastasis.

Prostate Cancer

See "Prostate Disease" (p 366).

Hematologic Malignancies

Leukemias

Acute myeloid leukemia (AML) following myelodysplastic syndromes, as occurs more commonly among older patients, is more likely to be refractory to treatment and to have a smoldering course, requiring only supportive care. What is not clear is whether the prevalence of unfavorable cytogenetic abnormalities and of multilineage neoplastic involvement increases with age in de novo AML. The subset of myelodysplasia patients who do not have excess blasts or overt leukemia but are neutropenic and have recurrent infections may benefit from intermittent granulocyte colony-stimulating factor.

In a trial with older patients with AML, the effectiveness of delayed treatment was found to be much inferior to that of immediate treatment. Although this study established the value of timely chemotherapy, the choice of treatment (whether full-dose induction or low-dose cytarabine) remains controversial. In one study the survival of older patients with leukemia treated with low-dose cytarabine was found to be superior to the survival of those receiving standard induction, because of lower treatment-related mortality. Others have obtained different results and claimed the superiority of standard treatment.

Chronic Lymphocytic Leukemia

Chronic lymphocytic leukemia (CLL) is the most common form of leukemia in the Western world; about 12,500 cases are diagnosed each year in the United States. The incidence is declining for unknown reasons. The median age at diagnosis is 61 years. The diagnosis is most often made incidentally when a peripheral white blood cell count reveals leukocytosis with a small lymphocyte count above 4,000/μL. Treatment is generally withheld until it is required to control a life-threatening or symptomatic complication. The major complications of the disease are infection and marrow failure. Because about 25% of patients develop autoimmune anemia or thrombocytopenia some time in the course of the disease, it is important to investigate the mechanism of any decline in peripheral blood cell counts. Autoimmune mechanisms can be treated with glucocorticoids or splenectomy, whereas marrow infiltration by tumor cells requires antitumor therapy. Chlorambucil and fludarabine are the two most active agents. Median survival varies with the stage of disease. Once anemia or thrombocytopenia develop as a consequence of marrow failure, median survival is about 18 months.

Non-Hodgkin's Lymphoma

The prognosis of low- and intermediate-grade non-Hodgkin's lymphoma worsens with age, but the explanation remains unclear. It is possible that older patients have more aggressive variants or, equally likely, that older patients are increasingly susceptible to the complications of intensive treatment.

The treatment of older persons with intermediate-grade large cell lymphoma is controversial. As many as 30% of such patients obtain a durable complete remission with standard treatment (CHOP, ie, cyclophosphamide, doxorubicin, vincristine, prednisone). Administration of lower-than-normal doses results in a poorer outcome. Whether hematopoietic growth factors can lessen the hematopoietic toxicity of treatment in the older age groups has not been specifically addressed.

Hodgkin's Disease

Hodgkin's disease exhibits a curious bimodal age-incidence curve, with a second peak late in life. There have been earlier reports that older patients with advanced disease respond less well to therapy and that their survival is shorter. It is not clear whether this represents a shift to less a favorable histologic type, more extensive disease at presentation, or either greater toxicity with standard treatment regimens or the provision of less aggressive treatment. There are published reports that would indicate that each of these factors is involved. Most older patients tolerate full doses of ABVD (ie, doxorubicin, bleomycin, vinblastine, dacarbazine) without life-threatening bone-marrow toxicity.

Multiple Myeloma

Multiple myeloma is diagnosed in about 14,400 people each year in the United States. The median age at diagnosis is 68 years; it is rare in people younger than 40 years. Black Americans have twice the incidence of white Americans. The classic triad of myeloma is marrow plasmacytosis (> 10%), lytic bone lesions, and a serum or urine, or both, monoclonal gammopathy. Monoclonal gammopathy is common in older people, estimated at 6% of persons aged 70 or older. Distinguishing myeloma from monoclonal gammopathy of uncertain significance is important. When an abnormal paraprotein is discovered on serum immuno-electrophoresis, the best diagnostic test to identify myeloma is a skeletal survey. Patients with monoclonal gammopathy of uncertain significance do not have lytic bone lesions and usually do not have the other features of myeloma, including hypercalcemia, renal failure, anemia, or susceptibility to infection, and marrow plasma cells are less than 10% of the total cell number. Patients with myeloma require treatment when the lytic bone lesions become symptomatic or progressive, recurrent infections occur, or the serum paraprotein increases. Standard treatment consists of intermittent pulses of an oral alkylating agent and prednisone given for 4 to 7 days every 4 to 6 weeks. Supportive care includes bisphosphonates to decrease bone turnover, erythropoietin and other hematinics for the anemia, intravenous immunoglobulin for recurrent infections, radiation to specific symptomatic bone lesions, maintenance of hydration to preserve renal function, and adequate analgesia.

PRINCIPLES OF MANAGEMENT

The principles of managing older patients with cancer are summarized in Table 53.3. Older patients get cancer more commonly, and they more often present

Table 53.3—General Considerations in Cancer Among Older Persons

- Older patients are more likely to develop cancer.
- Older patients are likely to present with more advanced disease.
- Cancer in older patients may demonstrate more indolent patterns of growth and spread.
- There has been no demonstrated inherent resistance to chemotherapy on the basis of age.
- Surgery, radiation, chemotherapy, and biologic therapy all are demonstrated to be safe and effective for older patients, but for each modality, certain precautions are exercised on the basis of the patient's existing comorbidities, vital organ functions, and other medications.

with advanced-stage disease. Efforts to screen the older population for common cancers (such as colon, breast, and prostate) before they experience symptoms are likely to discover earlier and more curable lesions. Older patients may have less physiologic reserve than younger patients, but unless a specific comorbid illness is influencing baseline organ function, cancer treatments with curative or palliative potential should be offered to most patients in most settings, regardless of age. Curative surgical procedures may require more prolonged convalescence, but recovery from most procedures is expected. Radiation therapy is safe and effective in the same settings it is used in younger patients. Chemotherapy may need to be adjusted to the individual patient's level of tolerance of the side effects, but usually the changes should be made in the face of toxicities actually encountered rather than toxicities anticipated. Biologic therapies are usually safe; some produce less toxicity in older than in younger patients.

See also "Dermatologic Diseases and Disorders" (p 372) for the diagnosis and treatment of skin cancers, and "Palliative Care" (p 103) for the management of pain and end-of-life care.

REFERENCES

- Balducci L, Beghe C. Prevention of cancer in the older person. *Clin Geriatr Med.* 2002;18(3):505–528.

- Balducci L, Extermann M, eds. Cancer in the elderly: current concepts and future directions. *Hematol Oncol Clin North Am.* 2000;14(1):1–291.

- Balducci L, Lyman GH, Ershler WB, eds. *Geriatric Oncology.* 2nd ed. Philadelphia: JB Lippincott Company; 1997.

- Cleary JF, Carbone PP. Palliative medicine in the elderly. *Cancer.* 1997; 80(7):1335–1347.

- Edwards BK, Howe HL, Ries LA, et al. Annual report to the nation on the status of cancer, 1973–1999, featuring implications of age and aging on U.S. cancer burden. *Cancer.* 2002;94(10):2766–2792.

- Ershler WB, Longo DL. Aging and cancer: issues of basic and clinical science. *J Natl Cancer Inst.* 1997;89(20):1489–1497.

- Monfardini S, Audisio R, Zagonel V, et al., eds. Guidelines for the management of cancer in the elderly. *Crit Rev Oncol Hematol.* 1998;27(2):85–168.

- Sundararajan V, Grann VR, Jacobson JS, et al. Variations in the use of adjuvant chemotherapy for node-positive colon cancer in the elderly: a population-based study. *Cancer J.* 2001;7:213–219.

CHAPTER 54—RENAL DISEASES AND DISORDERS

NORMAL AGING CHANGES IN RENAL FUNCTION

Renal function declines after age 40 years at a mean rate of approximately 1% per year, accelerating some in the later years. This observation was first reported in cross-sectional studies and confirmed in a population of normal aging persons followed over time. However, although two thirds of individuals followed for up to 20 years in the Baltimore Longitudinal Study developed a decline in glomerular filtration rate (GFR) with aging, one third had no decline, indicating that a decline in renal function with age is not inevitable.

Although there is loss of glomerular mass with aging, the loss of tubular mass is proportional, so that glomerular-tubular balance is usually maintained. Despite significant anatomic and functional changes, the older kidney is capable of maintaining homeostasis of body fluids and electrolytes under most circumstances. However, under environmental and disease-related stresses, such as volume changes or alterations in acid-base status, the older kidney is slower to respond to correct the abnormality.

CLINICAL PRESENTATIONS OF RENAL DISEASE

In general, the presentation of renal disease in older and younger adults is not significantly different. It is important to recognize a decline in renal function to permit early diagnosis of treatable causes of renal insufficiency. If no treatment is available, then interventions to retard disease progression should be started whenever possible. Equally important, the impact of renal function on other aspects of a person's health care, such as nutrition and medication dosing, needs to be considered.

The medical history and physical examination may be very helpful in determining the cause of renal insufficiency. The clinical symptoms and signs are variable but often are related to the underlying disease.

Nephrotic syndrome may present with edema and hypertension. Renal stones may present with flank pain, hematuria, nausea, and vomiting. These same symptoms are also seen with acute renal artery embolization. Amyloidosis may be suggested by increased serum globulin and peripheral nephropathy with proteinuria. Renal artery stenosis may be silent or present with multiple episodes of pulmonary edema. The symptoms commonly reported as a direct result of renal failure (eg, fatigue, nausea, cognitive difficulties) are generally not seen until the creatinine clearance (CrCl) is less than 20 mL/min.

The first hint of renal disease may be seen on a screening urinalysis with asymptomatic abnormalities (hematuria, proteinuria, pyuria, casts). It may also present with an asymptomatic elevated serum urea nitrogen or serum creatinine concentration. It is important to remember that muscle mass decreases with age. Therefore, a normal serum creatinine may represent a decline in renal function. For example, a serum creatinine of 1.0 mg/dL in an 80-year-old person weighing 65 kg corresponds to an estimated CrCl of 54 mL per minute. It also is helpful to look for changes in serum creatinine over time. A change in serum creatinine from a steady-state level of 0.7 mg/dL to 1.4 mg/dL indicates that the renal function has decreased by 50% and should alert the clinician to the need for further evaluation.

In summary, the finding in an older adult of hematuria, proteinuria, abnormal urinary sediment, or a decreased CrCl should alert the clinician to more fully evaluate renal function. Although it is not clear that age alone is a risk factor for renal insufficiency, the comorbidity associated with the aging process, including vascular disease, diabetes mellitus, and cardiac disease, place older adults at increased risk for a renal insult.

Hematuria

Whether macroscopic or microscopic (> 3 to 5 red blood cells per high-power field), hematuria in older adults deserves evaluation. A microscopic examination of the urine may suggest the source of the hematuria. Dysmorphic red blood cells that have lost their biconcave shape or red cell casts in a freshly voided urine suggest a glomerular source. Associated proteinuria or an elevated serum creatinine concentration also suggest renal parenchymal disease. Biconcave red blood cells suggest a disease of the collecting system. It is also important to consider systemic coagulation defects. In addition to a microscopic urine evaluation, the work-up of isolated hematuria should include a urine culture, imaging (renal ultrasound or intravenous pyelography) to exclude a renal parenchymal mass, and, if these are nondiagnostic, a urologic consultation for cystoscopy. In addition, a platelet count, prothrombin time, and partial thromboplastin time should be obtained to exclude a coagulopathy. In approximately 80% of older adults, the source of hematuria is the bladder, prostate, or urethra. Malignancies, most often bladder but also hypernephroma and prostate, account for one third of the cases of hematuria. Less than 10% of the hematuria is glomerular in origin (in the absence of proteinuria). It is important to remember that hematuria in patients on coumadin is not normal and suggests underlying pathology. Where hematuria is noted on dipstick examination of the urine and no red blood cells are seen on the microscopic examination, the clinician needs to look for the presence of myoglobulin.

Proteinuria

Normal protein excretion in older and younger adults does not differ significantly. Significant proteinuria is defined as greater than 150 mg per 24 hours. The urine dipstick is a good screening method for the detection of proteinuria, but it detects only albumin; light chains, which would be present in a patient with multiple myeloma, and low-molecular-weight protein (tubular protein) need to be detected by the use of a sulfa salicylic acid test. This test may be easily performed in the outpatient clinical setting.

When urinary proteins are primarily albumin and higher-molecular-weight proteins, the pathology is likely glomerular. Three grams of protein in a 24-hour urine sample is used to distinguish nephrotic from non-nephrotic proteinuria. The evaluation of proteinuria should begin with a careful examination of fresh urinary sediment (cells, casts), as this can provide helpful clues as to the mechanism of the proteinuria.

The urine dipstick method for detection of proteinuria is relatively insensitive, requiring urinary albumin concentrations of nearly 30 mg/dL. This means that a person with a urine output of 1 liter per day must be excreting nearly 300 mg of albumin per day before proteinuria can be detected. Microalbuminuria, defined as a urinary albumin excretion of more than 30 mg per day (less than that detectable with the dipstick method), can be quantified with Chemstrip Micral (Boehringer Mannheim Corporation, Indianapolis, Indiana 46256). Microalbuminuria is an early indicator of progressing renal injury. This has become important because antihypertensive therapy, specifically, angiotensin-converting enzyme (ACE) inhibitors, are being used to lower glomerular capillary pressures. This therapy reduces the proteinuria, which itself may be nephrotoxic, and retards the further development of renal damage, not only in diabetic but in nondiabetic renal disease. Quantification of the severity of microalbuminuria does not require a 24-hour urine sample, as accurate enough estimates can be obtained with a timed early morning sample or simultaneous measurement of urinary creatinine concentration, or both.

Renal Insufficiency

The most useful measure of renal function is an estimate of the GFR, as decreases in all other functions (eg, tubular functions, concentrating ability, acid excretion) tend to parallel decreases in GFR. The CrCl is the most reproducible measure of GFR available for clinical decision making. In older persons creatinine production falls at nearly the same rate as the renal clearance of creatinine and, as noted previously, a normal serum creatinine may actually reflect a decline in renal function. This pattern of change is important to recognize when the older patient is using drugs cleared primarily by the kidney. The relationship between serum creatinine and GFR has prompted a number of investigators to suggest that one could properly correct for the confounding variables, so they have developed formulas to estimate CrCl as a measure of GFR. The most widely used formula is that of Cockroft and Gault (see box below).

This formula was developed and validated on highly selected samples of older adults that did not include many very old individuals. Only moderate correlations have subsequently been found between

$$\text{Estimated CrCl (mL/min)} = \frac{(\text{weight in kg})\,(140 - \text{age in years})}{(72)\,(\text{serum creatinine in mg/dL})} \times (0.85 \text{ if female})$$

calculated and actual CrCls, especially in older populations. Currently, no available method of estimating GFR from easily obtainable variables, such as age, sex, weight, and serum creatinine, is very accurate, and no method will be available until we have an easy method for estimating muscle mass. A timed CrCl should be obtained when a precise estimate of GFR is needed, for example, when prescribing drugs cleared by the kidney with narrow therapeutic or toxic margins. Nevertheless, in clinical practice, the use of an estimated GFR from the Cockroft and Gault formula will provide a prompt and reasonable guide for clinical decision making in most situations. Finally, it is important to recognize that certain commonly prescribed drugs (trimethoprim-sulfamethoxazole, cimetidine, and cefoxitin) compete with creatinine for tubular secretion, causing an increase in serum creatinine concentration without changing GFR.

IMAGING TECHNIQUES AND RENAL BIOPSY

A variety of imaging techniques are available to evaluate the genitourinary system. Ultrasonography is noninvasive and safe, and it can provide many diagnostic clues, showing kidney size, hydronephrosis of the collecting system, and solid and cystic parenchymal renal masses. An intravenous pyelogram shows more detail of the collecting system, including sites of obstruction and other pathology, such as papillary necrosis. However, it is best to avoid intravenous contrast in older adults with diabetes mellitus, renal insufficiency, hypertension, and, most notably, multiple myeloma, given the increased risk for contrast media–induced acute renal failure (ARF), especially if the person is dehydrated. If intravenous contrast absolutely must be used, the patient should be well hydrated before the procedure and for at least 24 hours after the procedure. Computed tomography scans, magnetic resonance imaging, isotopic renography, and angiography are additional techniques available to further evaluate selected renal disorders.

For patients with suspected primary glomerular disease or unexplained renal failure, a renal biopsy may be indicated after all other available means for establishing a diagnosis have been exhausted. Renal biopsy should not be withheld because of age alone. At least half of all primary glomerular lesions responsible for the nephrotic syndrome are potentially treatable (eg, membranous glomerulopathy, minimal-change disease, vasculitis), and trials of immunosuppressive or corticosteroid therapies, or both, are warranted. On the other hand, when a lesion unresponsive to these agents is diagnosed, such as primary amyloidosis, it is important not to subject older adults to the potentially serious side effects of these medications. One study has

looked at more than 200 renal biopsy samples in adults aged 60 and over with ARF to evaluate whether the renal biopsy was useful in predicting renal and patient survival. The authors found that in over 90% of the biopsies, a diagnosis was made for ARF; in many of these cases, a treatment was available; and in 30% of the cases, the diagnosis on biopsy did not match the clinical diagnosis. In summary, when a cause for ARF is unclear on the basis of clinical and laboratory evaluation, a renal biopsy is warranted. The exception would be the older adult who is unable to tolerate any treatment because of comorbidity. It is important for the clinician to work with the nephrologist and make certain that the patient is clinically optimized for the procedure. This includes optimum blood-pressure control and holding medications that might increase the risk of bleeding, for example, aspirin.

DISEASES OF THE KIDNEY AND VASCULAR SYSTEM

A retrospective analysis examining the reason for renal biopsy in 1368 older adults showed the three most common reasons for referral were nephrotic syndrome (31%), acute renal insufficiency (26%), and chronic renal insufficiency (25%).

The incidence of nephrotic syndrome is at least as common in older adults as it is in younger persons. The most common cause in older adults is membranous nephropathy (35%), followed by minimal-change disease (16%) and primary amyloidosis (12%). The incidence rates for membranous nephropathy, crescentic glomerulonephritis (GN), and amyloidosis are higher in older adults, those for proliferative GN and immunoglobulin A nephropathy are lower, and the incidence rate for minimal-change disease is comparable to that for young adults but much lower than the rate seen in children. Diabetic nephropathy is probably the most common cause of nephrotic syndrome in older adults. The diagnosis is usually made on the basis of a long (15- to 20-year) history of diabetes mellitus and the finding of diabetic retinopathy, and a biopsy is not necessary. Glomerulopathies resulting from systemic disease are more common in older adults because of the increased incidence of underlying diseases, such as amyloidosis (dysproteinemias), collagen vascular diseases (vasculitis), and neoplastic disease.

Membranous nephropathy (MN) is the most common form of primary renal disease in older adults and is twice as common in older than in younger persons. Possible causes of MN include medications (eg, nonsteroidal anti-inflammatory drugs or NSAIDs, penicillamine), malignancies, and hepatitis B infection. One review reported that 11% of patients with MN had an underlying malignancy. In most patients the malignancy is clinically evident when the diagnosis of

MN is made, and probably only 1% to 2% of patients have an occult malignancy. Screening older adults with MN for malignancy should probably include a complete history and physical examination, chest radiograph, fecal occult blood tests, and colonoscopy. It does appear that older patients are more susceptible to the extra-renal complications of the nephrotic syndrome and its treatment, most notably, cardiovascular, thrombotic, and infectious events. It is important for the primary clinician to be aware of this. As the primary care clinician is likely the first person called when acute symptoms develop, it is essential they are aware of these potential complications.

Minimal-change nephropathy presents similarly in young and old patients, but older persons are more likely to have nonselective proteinuria, microscopic hematuria, hypertension, and renal insufficiency.

As few type 1 (insulin-dependent) diabetics survive to become older adults, most older adults with diabetic nephropathy have type 2 (non-insulin-dependent) diabetes. Control of blood pressure is important in slowing the rate of deterioration of renal function. The use of ACE inhibitors or angiotensin-II receptor blockade agents, even in normotensive diabetic patients, promotes efferent arteriolar vasodilatation and decreases glomerular capillary pressure, which also slows the rate of deterioration of renal function. Although tight control of blood glucose has been shown to slow the course of renal deterioration in type 1 diabetes, little evidence exists that it affects the course in type 2 diabetes. Nevertheless, it seems reasonable to assume that it does.

After diabetes, the next most common group of systemic diseases associated with renal disease in older adults is the dysglobulinemias. These include amyloidosis, multiple myeloma, fibrillary GN, essential mixed cryoglobulinemia, and macroglobulinemia.

Acute Renal Insufficiency or Failure

ARF is at least as common in older as in younger adults. Controversy remains as to whether the prognosis is poorer in older adults, but there are no technical reasons to deny treatment for ARF, using any of the available techniques, on the basis of age. In older adults, azotemia and other consequences of ARF may induce acute behavioral changes that are usually reversible, and treatment should not be stopped on the assumption that the patient's mental status is irreversible. The primary clinician is in a unique position to impact acute renal insufficiency, both in terms of prevention and early detection. With a comprehensive medical history, physical examination, laboratory values, and urinalysis, it is usually possible to determine whether the cause of acute renal insufficiency is pre-renal, intra-renal, or post-renal. In general, a nor-

mal urinalysis suggests the cause is either pre-renal or post-renal.

There are two clinical situations to consider. The first is the development of acute renal insufficiency in the hospitalized or institutionalized patient being treated for a non-nephrologic illness. In this setting, intravascular volume depletion and acute tubular necrosis (ATN) are the major contributors—both of which may often be avoided with appropriate measures. The diagnosis is usually made on the basis of the history, physical examination, and laboratory data, so that a renal biopsy is not necessary. ARF has been reported in up to 8% of acutely hospitalized older adults aged 60 years and older. Although the studies vary, in general, ATN accounts for approximately 40% to 50% of the cases of ARF, and intravascular volume depletion for most of the remaining cases.

The second clinical situation to consider is whether acute renal insufficiency results from a primary renal disease or is secondary to a systemic disease, such as diabetes mellitus, hypertensive or atherosclerotic vascular disease, or collagen vascular disease. Post-renal obstruction should always be excluded, as it is usually amenable to treatment.

Pre-renal Acute Renal Insufficiency

Pre-renal ARF occurs when poor perfusion is causing the failure of renal function. This type of ARF is of special importance in older adults. With acute hypotension, the decrease in renal perfusion stimulates sympathetic activity and release of vasoconstrictor substances that further reduce GFR, contributing to ARF. Once the hemodynamic disturbances are corrected, the patient usually, but not always, recovers from the ARF. Loss of fluids (intravascular volume depletion), internal redistribution, decreased cardiac output, sepsis, and certain drugs (diuretics, ACE inhibitors) are responsible for the vast majority of cases of pre-renal ARF. In several series, intravascular volume depletion alone was found to account for more than half of the cases of pre-renal ARF in older adults. The slow response to sodium retention, the decreased urinary concentrating ability, and, most importantly, the impairment of thirst regulation, all characteristics of the older patient, contribute to this high incidence.

The use of drugs that alter intrarenal hemodynamics is a growing cause of pre-renal ARF in older adults. The rapid development of pre-renal ARF in a patient recently started on an ACE inhibitor should make the clinician think about bilateral renal arterial stenosis. However, in one series, two thirds of the ACE inhibitor–related cases of ARF were found to have occurred in persons without renal arterial stenosis. Other factors that alter intrarenal hemodynamics include cardiac failure, concomitant use of NSAIDs (which inhibit prostaglandin production, an important regulator of renal blood flow and GFR), diabetes mellitus, and volume depletion from any cause. (See the section on renal disease associated with NSAID use, p 380.)

It is important to distinguish between pre-renal ARF and ATN, which can develop in the more severe cases. In patients who are oliguric, a urinary osmolality > 500 mOsm/kg, a urinary sodium concentration of < 20 mEq/L, a urine-to-plasma creatinine ratio > 40, or a fractional excretion of sodium < 1% suggests pre-renal ARF. Generally, with pre-renal ARF the ratio of blood urea nitrogen to serum creatinine is > 20. These urinary indices are not always reliable in differentiating pre-renal ARF from other forms of ARF. Probably the most reliable indicator of the pre-renal state is the response to treatment with volume (salt and water) repletion, but, again, older patients may have a delayed response to volume expansion.

Acute Tubular Necrosis

ATN can be either ischemic or nephrotoxic in origin. The causes of ischemic ATN are basically the same as those described in the preceding section as causes of pre-renal ARF, only more severe. In addition, surgical interventions, most notably cardiac surgery and repair of aortic aneurysms, as well as sepsis, account for most of the remaining cases in older adults. Hypotension during and after surgery, postoperative fluid loss, and arrhythmias may be important contributors. Measures to decrease the risk of ATN in the postoperative patient include careful attention to nutritional issues, avoidance of hypotension, prevention and treatment of postoperative infection, and appropriate medication dosing and hydration.

Most of the antibiotics effective in treating serious infections have been associated with nephrotoxic ATN. Age is a well-known risk factor for the development of aminoglycoside nephrotoxicity. Preexisting renal dysfunction and volume depletion may contribute to medication accumulation, leading to ATN. When it is necessary to use an aminoglycoside antibiotic in an older person, monitoring blood levels is essential.

Older adults also are at increased risk of developing radiocontrast-induced ARF. Although the non-ionic contrast dye has been reported in the literature to be less toxic to the kidneys, in practice, the risk of an acute renal insult is likely not significantly reduced. As mentioned earlier, it is best to avoid the use of intravenous contrast dye in any person with preexisting impairment of renal function, multiple myeloma, vascular disease, intravascular volume depletion, or diabetes. Hydration before and after procedures employing use of contrast agents has been reported to be effective in reducing the incidence and severity of ARF in high-risk patients.

Clearly, when ARF develops, it needs to be dealt with promptly—but perhaps one of the most important roles of the clinician is preventing hospital-acquired ARF. With daily attention to changes in fluid intake, urine production, weight, and orthostatic blood-pressure measurements, the development of intravascular volume contraction in many older adults may be identified before significant symptoms develop. Another common cause of intravascular volume depletion is the order for "nothing by mouth" written in anticipation of a procedure, or the order for enemas written as a bowel preparation. When a procedure is delayed and maintenance intravenous fluids are not given, symptomatic intravascular volume depletion may develop in the frail older adult, with all the associated risks, including falls. Although the older kidney is able to defend against changes in volume, the response to correction is delayed. Avoiding the simultaneous use of multiple medications that may interact also is of benefit. For example, in the treatment of congestive heart failure, the combination of a diuretic and an ACE inhibitor together with an NSAID is a recipe for the potential development of renal insufficiency unless the patient is carefully monitored. When an older hospitalized patient is being treated by several physicians, it may be prudent to write orders for "no NSAIDs" when appropriate.

Other Intrarenal Causes of Acute Renal Failure

In one review of 259 renal biopsies done for ARF on adults aged 60 and older (remembering that when the cause of ARF has been established by the history, physical examination, and laboratory data, a renal biopsy is not done), the following diagnoses were made: pauci-immune crescentic GN (with or without arteritis) in 31% of the biopsy samples, acute interstitial nephritis (AIN) 19%, ATN with nephrotic syndrome 8%, atheroemboli 7%, ATN alone 7%, light chain cast nephropathy 6%, postinfectious GN 5.5%, anti-glomerular membrane antibody nephritis 4.0%, and immunoglobulin A nephropathy or Henoch-Schönlein syndrome 4%.

Acute GN in older adults often presents with circulatory congestion that suggests heart failure, in contrast to the hypertension and edema seen in younger patients. This observation, together with low urinary sodium concentrations and high ratios of blood urea nitrogen to serum creatinine that suggests pre-renal ARF, results in the misdiagnosis of acute GN as heart failure.

Acute or subacute GN may be an immunologic consequence of a systemic disease, for example, lupus erythematosus, vasculitis, Wegener's granulomatosis, mixed cryoglobulinemia, or a primary renal disease of unknown cause, for example, crescentic GN with or without glomerular immune deposits. Other forms of proliferative GN include mesangioproliferative GN (including immunoglobulin A nephropathy), focal proliferative GN, crescentic GN (including antiglomerular basement membrane disease), and vasculitis. It is important to remember that acute postinfectious GN remains a common entity.

AIN is caused by a variety of agents and probably has no special implications for older adults except for the higher prevalence of NSAID-induced AIN, discussed below, and the fact that older adults tend to be on multiple medications.

Renal vascular causes of ARF are discussed below. Rhabdomyolysis with ARF is seen in the setting of acute immobilization, infectious diseases, stroke, hyperosmolar states, hyponatremia and hypernatremia, and after falls associated with muscle trauma.

Obstructive Nephropathy

Urinary obstruction is one of the most common causes of ARF in older adults. It is an important diagnosis to make because it is usually reversible. Prostatic hypertrophy or carcinoma is the most common cause, but one should also consider retroperitoneal or pelvic neoplasia, such as lymphoma and carcinoma of the bladder, cervix, uterus, ovaries, or rectum. Another cause of post-renal obstruction may be a blocked indwelling Foley catheter.

Laboratory findings with obstructive ARF tend to be nonspecific, with high urinary sodiums and decreased osmolalities and a nondiagnostic urinalysis. The ratio of blood urea nitrogen to serum creatinine is usually increased. Ultrasonography is safe and readily available, and it has become the initial evaluation of choice in most settings. In most cases, but not all, the diagnosis of obstruction can be made on the basis of a dilated collecting system or large distended bladder.

Renal Vascular Disease

Nearly half of both normotensive and hypertensive person aged 60 and over with evidence of atherosclerotic aortoiliac or peripheral vascular disease, or both, show some obstruction (> 50% narrowing) of the renal artery. In most of these patients, the obstruction goes unrecognized and is not clinically important. However, in some individuals, severe hypertension or progressive renal insufficiency, or both, may develop. Correction of stenosis may reverse these consequences. Therefore, any patient with suspected severe renal artery stenosis should have a diagnostic work-up. If a significant stenosis is found, the patient should be referred for evaluation for either percutaneous transluminal renal angioplasty or surgical revascularization of the renal artery. Clues suggesting hemodynami-

cally significant renal artery stenosis include the new onset of severe hypertension, significant worsening of preexistent hypertension, failure to control hypertension on previously effective medications, repeated episodes of pulmonary edema, and renal insufficiency in the absence of urinary abnormalities or other known cause. The last may be most dramatic in patients started on ACE inhibitors. A vascular bruit may be heard in the mid-abdomen or flank.

Occlusive arterial disease can cause either acute or chronic renal failure with or without changes in the urinalysis and urinary sediment. Renal arterial embolization or thrombosis may occur in patients with acute myocardial infarction, chronic atrial fibrillation, and subacute bacterial endocarditis. Symptoms vary from a slowly progressive, clinically silent event to severe acute flank pain and tenderness, hematuria, hypertension, fever, nausea, and vomiting. Serum lactic dehydrogenase concentrations increase dramatically after 1 to 2 days and remain elevated for a week or more.

Renal cholesterol embolization may occur after either aortic surgery or angiography in patients with diffuse atherosclerosis (dislodging atheromatous material), or spontaneously. The usual course is a progressive renal insufficiency and worsening hypertension, but it can be acute with oliguria or anuria, fever, eosinophilia, and with embolization to other organs and the extremities (digital infarctions). Hints to this diagnosis include livedo reticularis and cholesterol emboli on a dilated funduscopic examination (which should be performed on every patient when this diagnosis is suspected). If the diagnosis remains unclear or other diagnoses exist as valid possibilities, a definitive diagnosis may be made on visualization of cholesterol crystals on a biopsy of the skin or kidney.

Renal Diseases Associated With NSAID Use

NSAIDs are widely consumed by older adults because of their effectiveness in relieving pain in a variety of common chronic musculoskeletal disorders. Older persons are more predisposed than younger adults to the adverse renal effects of NSAIDs because of the age-associated decline in renal function, the increased prevalence of such comorbid conditions as heart failure, hypertension, cirrhosis, and renal insufficiency, and the high use of concomitant drugs that affect kidney function (eg, diuretics, antihypertensives). It should be possible to use these drugs safely in older adults and maintain a low risk-to-benefit ratio, as those who are at risk for NSAID-induced renal disease can be identified and monitored.

As mentioned above, NSAIDs may alter intrarenal hemodynamics and decrease GFR. NSAIDs may induce a variety of acute and chronic renal lesions. AIN can follow the use of nearly all NSAIDs. The typical clinical picture includes the nephrotic syndrome with acute renal insufficiency in a patient who has been on NSAIDs for months. An increase in eosinophils in blood or urine, or both, with NSAID-induced AIN is not nearly as common as in AIN due to penicillin and other agents. The renal abnormalities usually improve after discontinuation of the medication, with or without corticosteroid therapy, but chronic renal insufficiency, and even end-stage renal disease (ESRD), may occur. The AIN results primarily from a delayed hypersensitivity response to NSAID, and the nephrotic syndrome results from changes in glomerular permeability mediated by prostaglandins and other hormones. Less commonly, nephrotic syndrome may occur without AIN; rarely, an immune complex glomerulopathy is observed. Patients taking NSAIDs for months or years may develop papillary necrosis, chronic interstitial nephritis, and even ESRD. Case-control studies show that patients at increased risk are older men with chronic heart disease and renal hypoperfusion. Impaired medullary circulation and direct toxicity due to a drug metabolite appear to play a critical role in inducing interstitial fibrosis, which can be facilitated by a sustained production of some growth factors and cytokines. The newer COX-2 inhibitors may also cause renal dysfunction.

Chronic Renal Failure

An examination of renal biopsy results in older adults with chronic renal failure showed that the most common histologic findings were hypertensive nephrosclerosis, focal segmental glomerulosclerosis, interstitial nephritis, and amyloidosis. Again, in persons with chronic renal failure where a cause is clear from the history and physical examination (eg, diabetes mellitus), no biopsy would be necessary. There are several points to be made with regard to chronic renal insufficiency in the older adult.

First, although chronic elevation of serum creatinine represents a loss of renal function that likely will not be recovered, defining the underlying pathology may help to prevent further decline in function. Second, the degree of renal failure may be much greater than indicated by the serum creatinine, so that cognitive difficulties may develop at lower than expected serum creatinine levels. Third, although this area needs considerable research, some data suggest that erythropoietin serum levels do not change with age. Data also suggest that anemia secondary to erythropoietin deficiency may occur with more mild cases of renal insufficiency than previously thought. Fourth, some data suggest that renal insufficiency is an independent risk factor for all-cause mortality in older

adults with congestive heart failure, likely because of decreased ability to compensate volume, which supports the argument for maximizing renal function whenever possible. Preventing a further decline in renal function or the development of "acute or chronic" renal failure is critical. This requires careful attention to medication dosing, measurement of serum blood levels of medications when available, and avoidance of medications known to accumulate in renal insufficiency, including magnesium-containing compounds and meperidine. In addition, the older adult with renal insufficiency is even less able than the healthy older adult to defend against physiologic stress, including a free water load, salt challenge, or acidosis; this should be taken into consideration during acute illness.

Nutrition

It is important for older adults with chronic renal insufficiency or ESRD to have a consultation with an expert in renal nutrition. The U.S. Multicenter Modification of Diet in Renal Disease Study has shown a benefit of a low-protein diet (0.7 gm/kg of body weight) to those with a CrCl < 55 mL/min/L in slowing the progression of chronic renal failure. However, the benefits must be weighed against the nutritional consequences, as this study showed there were also small declines in various indices of nutritional status (protein-calorie malnutrition). It is important for the clinical team, including a nephrologist and *renal dietitian*, to determine what is best given each patient's individual nutritional needs.

Early Referral to a Nephrologist

Early referral of older adults with evidence of renal insufficiency to a nephrologist is important. A plan should be instituted to maximize renal function and prevent complications associated with comorbidity and multiple medications. Data suggest that beginning dialysis early in older adults may improve clinical outcomes and patient survival; early referral contributes to this positive outcome.

Dialysis and Transplantation

A 1999 report from the U.S. Renal Data System indicates that in 1997 more than half of all patients on chronic dialysis were aged 65 years or older. Diabetes mellitus, hypertension, GN, and obstructive nephropathy were the most common causes of ESRD in this group. The increased number of older adults started on dialysis has occurred for two reasons. First, there is increased referral and acceptance of older adults, especially those with serious comorbid conditions. Second, the increased survival rates of other competing diseases, such as coronary artery disease or diabetes, increase the chances that a person will survive to develop ESRD.

The results of studies looking at life satisfaction and functional status in older adults on dialysis have varied. One prospective cohort study found that life satisfaction of older adults on dialysis and those in the control group did not differ significantly at 3 years. For some older adults living alone or in isolation, time spent on dialysis was a time to interact both with their "neighbors" on dialysis and with nursing staff; in a sense, this becomes their social life. It is also clear that rehabilitation (occupational and physical therapy) is important in slowing the loss of function in the dialysis patient. The choice of hemodialysis or peritoneal dialysis (generally, chronic ambulatory peritoneal dialysis) depends on the patient's wishes and overall condition, the clinician's expertise, and available resources. Neither method offers any advantage in survival rates when patients with similar risk factors are compared.

An alternative therapy for ESRD in older adults is renal transplantation. The results have improved because of better patient selection, improved perioperative care, and the use of safer, more effective immunosuppression. Despite improved survival, renal transplantation in persons aged 65 years and over remains uncommon and controversial, largely because of a reluctance to allocate a scarce resource (the donor kidney) to an older adult with a limited life expectancy. As older adults have a senescent immune system, they may require less aggressive immunotherapy.

One report comparing older adults with a renal transplant to those on dialysis (matched by age, underlying diagnosis leading to ESRD, and number of comorbid conditions) showed that after adjusting for known prognostic factors, the transplant patients had a much better (twofold) survival probability than did the patients on dialysis. The 5-year survival rates were 81% and 51% for transplant and dialysis patients, respectively. In addition, a study comparing graft survival in patients aged 18 to 59 with that in patients 60 years and older found that in the absence of risk factors (pretransplant history of nonskin cancer, vascular disease, or being an active smoker), the survival rates were similar. These findings will have important implications in the future for the management of ESRD patients aged 60 years and older.

FLUID AND ELECTROLYTE DISTURBANCES

Hyponatremia and Hypernatremia

Surveys of older adults in both acute and long-term-care facilities show a high prevalence of hyponatremia (serum sodium concentration < 132 mmol/L). By definition, these persons have an excess of water relative to solute. Clinically, older adults with hyponatremia can be separated into those with decreased extracellular fluid (ECF) volume (eg, gastrointestinal losses, adrenal and renal salt-losing conditions), increased ECF volume (eg, congestive heart failure), or normal ECF volume (eg, syndrome of inappropriate antidiuretic hormone, or SIADH). The last is the most common. Regardless of cause, nonosmotic (baroreceptor) stimulation of arginine vasopressin (AVP) release is a major factor in the development of hyponatremia. Older persons appear to have an increased osmoreceptor sensitivity, as evidenced by the greater increase in serum AVP in response to any given increase in serum osmolality. Postoperative and diuretic-induced hyponatremia are much more common in older than in younger persons.

Hyponatremia does not usually produce symptoms until the serum sodium concentration falls below 125 mmol/L. At about this level, central nervous symptoms begin to appear, including somnolence, cognitive impairment, seizures, and ultimately coma, secondary to brain edema. Although therapy is not different for older adults, it is important to proceed slowly and to monitor regularly the older patient's response to avoid the development of cardiovascular or neurologic symptoms, or both.

Hypertonic dehydration (serum sodium > 148 mmol/L) is common in older adults, especially among acutely hospitalized and nursing-home patients. It also is largely avoidable. A number of factors may contribute to this condition. Body water is decreased as a proportion of total body weight because of the relative increase in fat content of normal older adults. Although AVP release from the posterior pituitary is normal (or even supernormal) in response to hypertonicity in older adults, the ability to concentrate the urine in response to AVP is decreased. Probably most important is the blunted or even absent thirst response to hypertonicity seen in normal older adults. This thirst response is even more impaired in patients with cerebral disease, such as stroke. In hot weather and in the absence of air conditioning, it is therefore important to make certain that older adults know to increase their consumption of fluids. An inability to obtain water because of functional or cognitive barriers may further limit the older person's ability to adequately replenish lost body fluids. It is helpful to instruct older adults to drink a specific amount of water each day. For institutionalized older adults, particularly those with decreased mobility or impaired cognition, placing a specific amount of fluid within easy reach and assuring that it is gone by the end of the day is helpful. In addition, on very hot days, it may be wise to hold or decrease the dose of diuretics in some patients. Symptoms of hypernatremia (obtundation, lethargy, coma) are predominantly neurologic, presumably because of shrinkage of the brain cells. As intravascular volume is preserved at the expense of cell water, changes in blood pressure, pulse rate, and skin turgor may not be evident early on.

Hypokalemia and Hyperkalemia

There is a long list of potential causes of hypokalemia in older adults. A low serum potassium measurement usually represents total body potassium depletion. This may be secondary to gastrointestinal losses, as occurs with vomiting, diarrhea, nasogastric suction, or fistula drainage. Vomiting produces a metabolic alkalosis that shifts potassium into cells and increases urinary potassium losses. Another commonly overlooked cause of hypokalemia is excessive use of purgatives and enemas.

Total body depletion of potassium may also occur secondary to renal losses. In older adults this is commonly secondary to diuretic usage and may be completely avoided with supplemental potassium. Although the liquid form of potassium supplement has an unpleasant taste, it is generally absorbed better than potassium tablets and is not associated with the same risk of gastric ulceration. Renal potassium wasting may also result from excessive adrenal hormone production or a primary underlying renal disease. Primary and secondary aldosteronism (the latter from renal artery stenosis or volume contraction resulting from diuretic usage in patients with cardiac, hepatic, or renal disease) may be a contributing factor. Hypomagnesemia-induced hypokalemia with ongoing renal potassium wasting is also seen with diuretic usage.

Potassium deficiency affects the cardiovascular system, neurologic system, muscles, and kidneys. The major side effects affecting the cardiovascular system are hypokalemia-induced ventricular arrhythmias. Muscle symptoms include weakness, easy fatigability, cramping, myalgias, and muscle tenderness secondary to rhabdomyolysis. Renal effects include polyuria and development of a metabolic alkalosis with paradoxical aciduria (low urine pH).

Since an alkalosis (chloride depletion) usually accompanies hypokalemia and is responsible for a shift of potassium intracellularly, replacement therapy should be with potassium chloride. The exception is the patient with renal tubular acidosis, in which case the alkaline salts of potassium should be given. Azotemia and age are the two significant risk factors for life-threatening hyperkalemia in potassium-supplemented patients. The latter may be related to the lower levels of aldosterone seen in the older patient under any given set of conditions (low-salt versus high-salt diet, supine versus upright posture).

Most episodes of hyperkalemia are seen in patients with impaired renal function. However, patients with chronic renal failure do not develop significant hyperkalemia until the azotemia becomes life threatening or another factor contributes, such as an increased endogenous or ingested potassium load, severe acidosis, administration of a diuretic to block sodium potassium exchange (triamterene, spironolactone), a deficiency of endogenous aldosterone or mineralocorticoid, or, importantly, administration of drugs, such as NSAIDs or ACE inhibitors. Older persons with an interstitial nephritis, especially diabetic patients, develop a failure of the renin-aldosterone system with a hyperkalemia and mild metabolic acidosis, often referred to as *type IV renal tubular acidosis.*

REFERENCES

■ Brown W, ed. Aging and the kidney. *Adv Renal Replacement Ther.* 2000;7(1):1–92.

■ Cameron JS. Nephrotic syndrome in the elderly. *Semin Nephrol.* 1996;16(4):319–329.

■ Doyle SE, Matas AJ, Gillingham K, et al. Predicting clinical outcome in the elderly transplant recipient. *Kidney Int.* 2000;57(5):2144–2150.

■ Faubert PF, Porush JG. *Renal Disease in the Elderly.* New York: Marcel Dekker, Inc; 1998.

■ Giatras I, Lau J, Levey AS. Effect of angiotensin-converting enzyme inhibitors on the progression of non-diabetic renal disease: a meta-analysis of randomized trials. *Ann Intern Med.* 1997;127(5):337–345.

■ Haas M, Spargo BH, Wit EC, et al. Etiologies and outcome of acute renal insufficiency in older adults: a renal biopsy study of 259 cases. *Am J Kidney Dis.* 2000;35(3): 433–447.

■ Johnson DW, Herzig K, Purdie D, et al. A comparison of the effects of dialysis and renal transplantation on the survival of older uremic patients. *Transplantation.* 2000;69(5):794–799.

■ Kleinknecht D. Interstitial nephritis, the nephrotic syndrome, and chronic renal failure secondary to non-steroidal antiinflammatory drugs. *Semin Nephrol.* 1995;15(3):228–235.

■ Levey AS, Greene T, Beck GJ, et al. for the Modification of Diet in Renal Disease (MDRD) study group. Dietary protein restriction and the progression of chronic renal disease: what have all the results of the MDRD study shown. *J Am Soc Nephrol.* 1999; 10(11):2426–2439.

CHAPTER 55—PROSTATE DISEASE

BENIGN PROSTATIC HYPERPLASIA

Epidemiology

Benign prostatic hyperplasia (BPH) is a noncancerous enlargement of the epithelial and fibromuscular components of the prostate gland. The epithelial component normally makes up 20% to 30% of prostate volume and contributes to the seminal fluid. The fibromuscular component comprises 70% to 80% of the prostate and is responsible for expressing prostatic fluid during ejaculation. Age and long-term androgen stimulation induce BPH development. Microscopic appearance of BPH may occur as early as age 30, is present in 50% of men by age 60, and in 90% of men by age 85. In half of these cases, microscopic BPH develops into palpable macroscopic BPH. Of those with macroscopic BPH, only half develop into clinically significant disease brought to medical attention. BPH is one of the most common conditions in aging men; in the United States annually it accounts for more than 1.7 million office visits and 250,000 surgical procedures.

Prostatism, or Lower Urinary Tract Symptoms

The symptoms of BPH are nonspecific; other diseases can result in identical symptoms. The pathophysiology of BPH symptoms is not completely understood, but presumably involves the periurethral zone of the prostate gland, which results in obstructed urine flow and compensatory responses of the urinary bladder, such as hypertrophy and decreased capacity. The urethral obstruction has both mechanical (obstructing mass) and dynamic (smooth muscle contractions) components. The resulting lower urinary tract symptoms (LUTS) are divided into irritative (frequency, urgency, nocturia) and obstructive (hesitancy, intermittency, weak stream, incomplete emptying) manifestations. The American Urological Association developed a quantitative symptom index for severity assessment and treatment response monitoring, which was adopted by the World Health Organization and is known as the International Prostate Symptom Score (IPSS; see Appendix, p 389). Symptom severity has not been found to correlate with prostate size, urine flow rates, or postvoid residual volume. BPH primarily affects quality of life, although complications such as recurrent urinary tract infection, bladder stones, urinary retention, chronic renal insufficiency, and hematuria can develop.

Diagnosis

BPH in men with LUTS is a diagnosis of exclusion. Differential diagnoses include endocrine disorders (especially diabetes mellitus), neurologic disorders, urinary tract infections, sexually transmitted diseases, kidney or bladder stones, and medication effects (especially anticholinergics, antihistamines, or diuretics). Digital rectal examination (DRE) may be unremarkable or reveal an enlarged, smooth, rubbery, symmetrical gland. Urinalysis is routinely performed to evaluate for urinary tract infection, hematuria, and glycosuria. A baseline serum creatinine assesses renal function and the possibility of obstructive uropathy or intrinsic renal disease, or both. Additional optional tests include postvoid residual urine volume, urine flow rates, and pressure flow studies. These tests may be considered when the diagnosis is uncertain or an invasive treatment is being planned.

Treatment Approaches

BPH therapy is patient dependent and driven by the impact of symptoms on the patient's quality of life. All patients should be educated regarding life-style modification: fluid adjustments (avoid caffeine) and avoidance of medications (especially anticholinergics) that aggravate symptoms. Patients with mild to moderate symptoms may be satisfied with life-style modification only. Both medical and surgical treatments are also available, with medication the usual first approach. Indications for surgical treatment include patient preference, dissatisfaction with medication, and refractory urinary retention, as well as renal dysfunction, bladder stones, recurrent urinary tract infections, or hematuria if these are clearly due to prostatic obstruction.

Medical Treatment

The two main pharmacologic approaches are α-adrenergic antagonists and 5α-reductase inhibitors.

α-Adrenergic antagonists, or α-blockers, are directed at the dynamic component of urethral obstruction. Smooth muscle of the prostate and bladder neck has a resting tone mediated by α-adrenergic innervation. α-Blockers relax the smooth muscle in the hyperplastic prostate tissue, prostate capsule, and bladder neck, thus decreasing resistance to urinary flow. Of the two major α-adrenergic receptors, α_1 receptors predominate in the prostate, and the α_{1a} subtype comprises 70% of these receptors. α-Blockade development for BPH therapy has progressed from selective α_1 agents (prazosin, alfuzosin) to long-acting selective α_1 agents (terazosin, doxazosin) and now to long-acting

α_{1a} subtype selective agents (tamsulosin). The most common adverse effects of α_1 agents are dizziness, mild asthenia (fatigue or weakness), and headaches. Postural hypotension occurs infrequently and can be minimized by careful dose titration. Tamsulosin (α_{1a} subtype) does not affect blood pressure or heart rate and therefore does not cause postural hypotension or require dose titration. Tamsulosin does increase abnormal ejaculation and rhinitis.

The enzyme 5α-reductase is required for the conversion of testosterone to the more active dihydrotestosterone. Finasteride is an inhibitor of this enzyme and reduces tissue levels of dihydrotestosterone, thus reducing prostate gland size. Improvements in symptom scores and urine flow rates may not be evident for up to 6 months. Finasteride is most effective in men with larger prostates (> 40 g, about the size of a plum). Because finasteride reduces serum prostate-specific antigen (PSA) levels an average 50%, baseline serum PSA determination is advocated for men in whom prostate cancer surveillance is planned. Subsequently, after a 6-month trial if continued finasteride therapy is desired, a PSA level on treatment is obtained and PSA velocity is measured annually for cancer surveillance.

Surgical Treatment

Surgical management includes transurethral resection of the prostate, transurethral incision of the prostate, open prostatectomy, transurethral vaporization of the prostate, and device insertion such as stent placement. Surgical approaches offer the best chance for symptom improvement but also have the highest rates of complications. The benefits of surgical treatments are generally considered equivalent, but complication rates differ. Transurethral resection of the prostate is the standard of care to which other BPH treatments are compared and has an 80% likelihood of successful outcome in properly selected patients. Usually performed under spinal anesthesia, a transurethral resection of the prostate involves the passage of an endoscope through the urethra to remove surgically the inner portion of the prostate. Long-term complications may include retrograde ejaculation, urethral stricture, bladder neck contracture, incontinence, and impotence. Transurethral incision of the prostate is an endoscopic procedure via the urethra to make one to two cuts in the prostate and prostate capsule, relieving urethral constriction. Limited to small prostate glands (< 30 g), transurethral incision of the prostate offers lower rates of retrograde ejaculation, bleeding, and contractures. Open prostatectomy involves removal of the inner portion of the prostate through a retropubic or suprapubic incision. It is best used for patients with larger prostates or with complicating conditions such as

bladder stones or urethral strictures. Open prostatectomy is associated with incisional morbidity, longer hospitalization, and greater risk of impotence. Transurethral vaporization of the prostate uses a high-energy electrode inserted via the urethra to vaporize the prostate. This approach has little bleeding but creates more prolonged irritative voiding. Prostatic stents are used to maintain expansion of the prostatic urethra and are employed for temporary and permanent uses.

PROSTATE CANCER

Incidence and Epidemiology

Cancer of the prostate (CaP) is the most common noncutaneous cancer and the second leading cause of cancer deaths among men in the United States. In the United States it was estimated that in 2002, 189,000 new cases of prostate cancer would be diagnosed and 30,200 men would die from CaP. CaP incidence increases with age and is rare in men younger than 40 years. In autopsy studies where the entire prostate is examined, incidental histologic evidence of CaP is found in 30% of men over 50 and 80% of men over 80. The incidence of disease varies according to race, with American blacks having the highest risk in the world. Among black men CaP occurs at an earlier age, has a higher mortality rate, and tends to be at a more advanced stage of disease at diagnosis. Family history is a contributing factor. Men with one first-degree relative affected have more than a twofold increased risk, and with two first-degree relatives affected, more than an eightfold increased risk. Androgens are necessary for CaP pathogenesis; the disease does not occur in men castrated before puberty. Diets high in total fat consumption are associated with increased CaP risk. The association between CaP and early onset of sexual activity, sexually transmitted disease, or vasectomy is inconclusive.

Symptoms

CaP usually arises in the peripheral zone of the prostate. The majority of patients, especially those with early-stage, potentially curable disease, are asymptomatic. CaP spreads by three routes: direct extension, the lymphatics, and the blood stream. Direct invasion of the urethra and bladder can lead to irritative voiding symptoms, urinary incontinence, and hematuria. Extension of disease to adjacent nerves may cause impotence and pelvic pain. Nodal metastasis may cause extrinsic ureteral obstruction. Leg edema may develop from lymphatic obstruction. Hematogenous metastasis to bone may cause severe local pain, normochromic normocytic anemia, pathologic fractures, and spinal cord compression. Less commonly, hematogenous metastasis involves viscera—namely, the lung, liver, and adrenal glands.

Screening Controversy

Early detection and treatment of CaP are controversial. At the heart of the CaP screening debate is the fact that no direct evidence exists to show that early detection decreases CaP mortality rates. There is a large reservoir of CaP that does not need to be diagnosed because the majority of men with CaP die with the disease, not from it. The well-recognized burden of progressive CaP is the impetus for early detection and management. The American Urological Association and the American Cancer Society advocate annual screening, recommending the PSA test and DRE beginning at age 50 for men with at least a 10-year life expectancy and earlier (age 40) for men at high risk (black men, first-degree relative affected). Groups that use explicit criteria to develop evidence-based practice guidelines (eg, U.S. Preventive Services Task Force) have concluded that there is insufficient evidence to recommend for or against routine screening for CaP using PSA testing or digital rectal examination. The Canadian Task Force on the Periodic Health Examination is in the process of updating their recommendations. Guidelines are in agreement that the controversy surrounding CaP screening should be discussed with patients in order to achieve individualized, informed courses of action. The effectiveness of PSA screening is particularly questionable in older men.

Screening and Diagnostic Tests

DRE of the prostate allows palpation of the posterior surfaces of the lateral lobes, where cancer most often begins. Cancer characteristically is hard, nodular, and irregular. DRE enhances screening efforts by detecting some cancers with a normal PSA level. DRE is inherently inaccurate because parts of the prostate gland cannot be reached. About half of the cancers thought to be "confined" to the prostate on the basis of DRE are found during surgery to have already spread. DRE produces many false-positive results; about one third of positive DRE tests are shown to be cancer by biopsy. Local extension of CaP into the seminal vesicles can often be detected by DRE. Despite its limitations, DRE remains important for screening and staging.

The serum PSA test is not specific for CaP. PSA elevations occur in benign conditions of the prostate, namely, hypertrophy and prostatitis, and in transient response to conditions such as ejaculation and prostatic massage. The sensitivity of the PSA test is also imperfect. Declines in PSA values have been associated with acute hospitalization and use of medications such as finasteride and saw palmetto. Normal PSA levels are found in 30% to 40% of men with cancer confined to the prostate (false-negative tests). The reported positive predictive value of PSA in screening studies is 28% to 35%: about one third of men with elevated PSA levels have CaP demonstrated by fine-needle biopsy.

Several approaches to improve the accuracy of PSA testing have been developed. PSA density is derived from the PSA concentration divided by the volume of the gland (measured by ultrasound). CaP produces higher PSA levels per unit volume than BPH and should therefore yield a higher PSA density. The PSA rate of change or velocity is more specific for CaP than a single PSA measurement. Using a PSA velocity value of $\geq$ 0.75 ng/mL/year achieves 90% specificity, whereas using a single PSA level > 4 ng/mL achieves 60% specificity. This high specificity for PSA velocity is realized even in normal-range serum PSA levels (< 4 ng/mL). Another approach involves age-adjusted PSA reference ranges because PSA values increase with age. Finally, one can measure the ratio of free-to-complexed PSA, recognizing that PSA bound to α_1-antichymotrypsin accounts for a larger proportion of total PSA with CaP than with BPH.

Abnormal DRE or PSA tests lead to transrectal ultrasound–guided biopsy of the prostate for pathologic diagnosis. Cancer may appear as a hypoechoic density, but ultrasound is not specific enough to be used as a screening tool. Spring-loaded core needle biopsies are routinely taken from the base, middle, and apex of each lobe (six samples total). Biopsies may also be taken from specific palpable nodules.

Grading

The Gleason grading system is the most commonly used system that is based on the histologic appearance of the CaP. The Gleason grade ranges from 1, or well differentiated, to 5, or poorly differentiated. The Gleason score is the sum of the most common Gleason grade observed plus the next most common Gleason grade seen. The Gleason score ranges from 2 to 10. Gleason scores are sometimes grouped as 2–4, well differentiated; 5–7, moderately differentiated; 8–10, poorly differentiated. Well-differentiated tumors have a favorable prognosis; poorly differentiated tumors, an unfavorable prognosis. Most clinically detected tumors are moderately differentiated.

Staging

Staging of CaP is necessary for planning disease management. Two systems are used to classify CaP: the tumor, regional node, metastasis (TNM) system and the Whitmore-Jewett (ABCD) system (Table 55.1). Usually detected by transurethral resection of the prostate, incidentally discovered cancers are staged according to the amount of tissue involved (T1 or A). Stage T1c reflects the growing number of tumors detected because of an elevated PSA level. Tumors detectable by DRE and confined to the prostate (T2 or B) are subdivided on the basis of the amount of tumor palpable. The degree of extension and invasion of surrounding structures stage tumors that extend beyond the prostatic capsule (T3 to T4 or C). Advanced disease (M1 or D) has metastasized.

The initial staging evaluation includes PSA level, DRE findings, and transrectal ultrasonography results. Bone scans may be performed on patients with PSA values greater than 10 ng/mL or complaints of bone pain. For patients electing active treatment, surgical assessment of lymph node involvement (pelvic lymphadenectomy) is performed by itself or in conjunction with prostate surgery or implantation of radioactive seeds. Computed tomography (CT) scans are often employed for active treatment planning.

In the past, CT scans, magnetic resonance imaging scans, pedal lymphangiography, and pelvic lymph node dissection were routinely employed in variable combinations to evaluate the extent of CaP. These tests should be eliminated in the initial staging evaluation of CaP patients because they have been associated with unacceptably high false-negative and false-positive results. A subset of patients appears to benefit from CT scans combined with fine-needle aspiration. Patients who have a PSA > 25 ng/mL, a Gleason score > 6, and a palpable abnormality on DRE are currently recommended to undergo a CT scan with fine-needle aspiration if a lymph node larger than 6 mm is present. Many of these patients will be diagnosed with nodal metastasis and thus spared the need for bilateral pelvic lymph-node dissection and its associated morbidity.

The serum PSA level should be used to eliminate the staging radionuclide bone scan. In the asymptomatic, newly diagnosed, previously untreated CaP patient, a PSA concentration ≤ 10 ng/mL has been associated with rare (0% to 0.8%) findings of skeletal metastases. Adopting recommendations to eliminate the staging radionuclide bone scan in this population

Table 55.1—TNM and Jewett-Whitmore Staging Systems for Prostate Cancer

TNM Stage	Jewett-Whitmore Stage	Description
TX		Tumor cannot be assessed
T0		No evidence of tumor
T1a	A1	Tumor an incidental finding at TURP involving 5% or less of tissue resected
T1b	A2	Tumor an incidental finding at TURP involving more than 5% of tissue resected
T1c	B0	Nonpalpable tumor identified because of elevated PSA
T2a	B1	Tumor involves one half of a lobe or less
T2b	B1	Tumor involves more than one half of a lobe, but not both lobes
T2c	B2	Tumor involves both lobes
T3a	C1	Unilateral extracapsular extension
T3b	C1	Bilateral extracapsular extension
T3c	C2	Tumor invades one or both seminal vesicles
T4a	C2	Tumor invades bladder neck and/or external sphincter and/or rectum
T4b	C2	Tumor invades levator muscles and/or is fixed to the pelvic sidewall
NX		Regional lymph nodes cannot be assessed
N0		No regional lymph node metastasis
N1	D1	Metastasis in a single lymph node, 2 cm or less at greatest dimension
N2	D1	Metastasis in a single lymph node more than 2 cm, but not more than 5 cm, at greatest dimension, or in multiple lymph nodes none more than 5 cm at greatest dimension
N3	D1	Metastasis in a lymph node more than 5 cm at greatest dimension
MX		Presence of distant metastasis cannot be assessed
M0		No distant metastasis
M1	D2	Distant metastasis

NOTE: TNM = tumor, regional node, metastasis; TURP = transurethral prostatectomy.

SOURCE: AUA Prostate Cancer Clinical Guidelines Panel. *Report on the Management of Clinically Localized Prostate Cancer.* Baltimore, MD: American Urological Association; 1995. Reprinted with permission.

will substantially reduce testing, because 50% to 60% of men with newly diagnosed CaP have a serum PSA concentration in this range.

Management of Localized Disease

Localized cancer lends itself to cure, but the prevalence of men dying with CaP (often asymptomatic) but not from CaP questions the necessity of treatment (see also "Oncology," p 349). Recent evidence, however, suggests that radical prostatectomy reduces cancer-specific mortality by almost 50% when compared with treatment with watchful waiting. Three approaches to localized CaP are routinely advocated: watchful waiting, radical prostatectomy, and radiation therapy.

Watchful waiting (also called *expectant* or *conservative management; surveillance*) is the approach offered most commonly to men with less than a 10-year life expectancy, who have significant medical comorbidities, or whose tumor is small and well to moderately differentiated. Conservative management studies have shown that 10-year disease-specific survival is 89% to 96% for Gleason score 2–5 tumors, 70% to 82% for Gleason score 6 tumors, 30% to 58% for Gleason score 7 tumors, and 13% to 40% for Gleason score 8–10 tumors. Because most men with CaP are asymptomatic, watchful waiting attempts to spare men the burden of unnecessary treatment. However, awaiting symptoms in men with CaP before initiating treatment means sacrificing the opportunity for cure. Patients are offered palliation if and when symptoms develop.

Radical prostatectomy involves the surgical removal of the entire prostate gland and the seminal vesicles. It can be performed through a perineal (incision near the rectum) or retropubic (lower abdominal incision) approach. The perineal approach allows an easier vesicourethral anastomosis and less bleeding, whereas the retropubic approach allows access to the pelvic lymph nodes and spares the neurovascular supply to the corpora cavernosa (with improved potency). The major morbidities of this treatment are urinary incontinence and erectile dysfunction. A population-based study of men undergoing radical prostatectomy for clinically localized prostate cancer found that 18 months later, 60% were impotent and 8% were incontinent. The goal of surgery is cure. Biochemical progression (PSA $\geq$ 0.4 ng/mL) has been reported in 40% of men 10 years after radical prostatectomy for localized disease. Actuarial metastasis-free survival at 15 years is 82%. Thus this treatment can be offered to men with locally confined disease, with greater than a 10-year life expectancy, and with absence of surgical contraindications.

Radiation therapy is provided through external beam radiation or through implantation of radioactive sources (known as *brachytherapy*). The standard regimen of external beam radiation delivers a total of 6000 to 7000 rads over a 7-week period. Pelvic lymph nodes can be radiated as well. Acute proctitis and urethritis are common side effects. Chronic complications include erectile dysfunction, urinary incontinence, and chronic proctitis. Local control and cancer survival rates are comparable to those of radical prostatectomy. Conformal radiation therapy is a mode of high-precision external-beam radiation that uses high-resolution CT scan data and advanced computer technology to conform the radiation dose to the three-dimensional configuration of the tumor. This new technology shows promise in reducing complications and side effects.

Brachytherapy involves retropubic or perineal implantation of radioactive seeds, usually iridium or palladium. Improvements in three-dimensional imaging of the prostate through CT scan or ultrasound guidance have allowed more uniform distribution of seeds throughout the prostate and overcome many of the past limitations of brachytherapy. Potency is better preserved with seed implants. Currently no evidence suggests that brachytherapy is more effective than external beam radiation or prostatectomy.

Management of Locally Advanced CaP

Locally advanced CaP extends beyond the capsule or invades the seminal vesicle, without evidence of distant or nodal metastasis. Radiation therapy is the recommended treatment, and adjuvant androgen deprivation provides additional benefit toward increased survival and freedom from metastases. However, controversy exists as to when androgen deprivation should be initiated. Patients may have a prolonged asymptomatic cancer period, while significant negative quality-of-life changes from long-term androgen deprivation occur, including loss of stamina, increased fatigue, hot flashes, diminished muscle mass, and premature osteoporosis. Patients should therefore be given the choice of early versus delayed androgen deprivation.

Management of Advanced Disease

Advanced disease is treated with androgen ablation and symptom-specific approaches, such as focal radiation therapy to painful bone metastasis. Androgen ablation aims to eliminate CaP growth stimulation and includes orchiectomy or luteinizing hormone-releasing hormone (LHRH) agonists with antiandrogens. Orchiectomy and LHRH agonists are equally effective at reducing androgens to castration levels. Orchiectomy is the oldest, safest, least expensive approach but is rejected by nearly half of U.S. men. LHRH agonists such as leuprolide and goserelin produce castration levels about a month after an initial increase in serum testosterone levels. Antiandrogens (eg, flutamide) are often given before initiation of LHRH agonists to blunt the effects of the initial testosterone increase. Antiandrogens inhibit the binding of androgen to its receptor. After castration a small amount of adrenal androgen exists and may allow continued stimulation of CaP growth. Antiandrogens may be combined with chemical or surgical castration, a practice called *complete androgen ablation.* Survival rates for antiandrogens alone are inferior to those for chemical or surgical castration alone; complete androgen ablation offers slight improvement in survival over that offered by castration only.

Radiation therapy is useful for relieving the pain of isolated bone metastasis and reducing the risk of fracture of bones with significant destruction. Diffuse bone metastases require alternative approaches. Bone-seeking radiopharmaceuticals such as strontium can be beneficial for pain control. Androgen deprivation decreases bone pain in two thirds of symptomatic patients.

PROSTATITIS

Etiology

Prostatitis is an inflammatory condition of the prostate that may represent acute bacterial, chronic bacterial, or nonbacterial causes. The most common sources of acute or chronic infection are ascending urethral infection or reflux of infected urine into the prostatic ducts, or both. Direct extension or lymphatic spread from the rectum or hematogenous spread also occurs. Acute prostatitis is an infectious process that is more common in young men. Pathogens in men 35 years and younger often include *Neisseria gonorrhea* and *Chlamydia trachomatis.* In older men acute prostatitis is associated with indwelling urethral catheter use, and coliforms are the suspected bacterial cause. More than 80% of patients with prostatitis have no identifiable infectious agent.

Diagnosis

Acute bacterial prostatitis is characterized by fever, chills, dysuria, and a tense or boggy, extremely tender prostate. Because bacteremia may result from manipulation of the inflamed gland, minimal rectal examination is indicated. Gram's stain and culture of the urine can identify the causative agent.

Chronic bacterial prostatitis presents classically as recurrent bacteriuria caused by the same organism, although most patients will not have this presentation. Patients have varying degrees of obstructive or irritative voiding symptoms and perineal pain. The prostate often feels normal. First-void or midstream urine is compared with expressed prostatic secretion or postmassage urine collection. The expressed sample should reveal leukocytosis and the causative agent. Sterile expressant with leukocytosis suggests nonbacterial prostatitis.

Treatment

Acute bacterial prostatitis is treated with antibiotics and may require hospitalization. The severe inflammation allows antibiotics to penetrate the prostate, and prompt response to empiric therapy is expected. CT or magnetic resonance imaging should be considered to evaluate for an abscess if recovery is delayed. Antibiotic selection should be based initially on urine Gram's stain results, with subsequent consideration of sensitivity profiles. Fluoroquinolones are highly effective in most cases.

Antibiotics are less effective for chronic bacterial prostatitis because of the poor penetration of the prostate by most of these drugs. Prolonged therapy of 6 to 16 weeks offers a cure rate of 30% to 40%. Continuous low-dose antibiotic suppression therapy can be offered for those with frequent symptomatic relapse. Total prostatectomy offers cure but at a high risk-to-benefit ratio. Transurethral resection of the prostate is safer but cures only one third of patients.

Nonbacterial prostatitis is treated symptomatically. A small percentage of cases may involve occult infections, and empiric antibiotic therapy is often used. Efforts to reduce pain and discomfort include anti-inflammatory agents, sitz baths, fluid adjustments (avoid caffeine), anticholinergic agents, and α-adrenergic antagonists.

REFERENCES

- Letran JL, Brawer MK. Disorders of the prostate. In: Hazzard WR, Blass JP, Ettinger WH Jr, et al., eds. *Principles & Practice of Geriatric Medicine and Gerontology.* 4th ed. New York: McGraw Hill; 1999:809–821.

- Medina JJ, Parra RO, Moore RG. Benign prostatic hyperplasia (the aging prostate). *Med Clin North Am.* 1999;83(5):1213–1229.

- Nickel JC. Prostatitis: evolving management strategies. *Urol Clin North Am.* 1999;26(4):737–751.

- Moorhouse DL, Robinson JP, Bradway C, et al. Behavioral treatments for post-prostatectomy incontinence. *Ostomy Wound Manage.* 2001;47(12):30–42.

- Stanford JL, Feng Z, Hamilton AS, et al. Urinary and sexual function after radical prostatectomy for clinically localized prostate cancer: The Prostate Cancer Outcomes Study. *JAMA.* 2000;283(3):354–360.

CHAPTER 56—DERMATOLOGIC DISEASES AND DISORDERS

Skin disease increases with aging and sun exposure. Dermatologic care in the older patient requires an awareness of cutaneous changes of aging and cumulative ultraviolet (UV) radiation exposure as well as specific knowledge of common tumors, inflammatory diseases, and infections seen in older persons.

AGING AND PHOTOAGING

Skin is composed of the epidermis, dermis, basement membrane zone (the area between the epidermis and dermis that serves to hold the two together), and the subcutaneous fat. In normal young skin the epidermis interdigitates with the dermis. Over time these interdigitations are flattened, with decreased contact between the epidermis and dermis. This results in less nutrient transfer and increased skin fragility. There is also a change with age in the barrier function because fewer lipids are present in the top layer of the skin, leading to dryness and roughness. The turnover of epidermal cells is slower and may account for decrease in the rate of wound healing. In aging skin, there is a decrease in the number of immune antigen-presenting cells, such as Langerhans cells, which may have consequences for cutaneous immune surveillance. Changes in the dermis, such as decreased ground substance, correlate with wrinkling and atrophy of the skin in the older person. A decrease in the amount of collagen and elastin is associated with striking changes in fiber orientation, notably a fragmented, less ordered, and more haphazard architecture.

Changes in hair in the older person include graying of hairs, due to changes in follicular melanocytes, and a decrease in scalp hair density secondary to shortening of anagen (the growth phase of the hair cycle) duration and an increase in the proportion of hairs in telogen (the resting phase).

Photoaging refers to the effects of UV exposure on skin. The depth of penetration of UV light depends on the wavelength, and shorter wavelengths are more biologically active. UVB (290 to 320 nm) radiation causes most of the acute and chronic damage. UVA (320 to 400 nm) also plays an important role because it makes up more of the sunlight that reaches the earth's surface and has greater depth of penetration. Mechanisms by which UV light causes changes in the skin probably include DNA injury or decreased DNA repair or both, oxidative damage, lysosomal damage, and altered collagen structure.

Photodamaged skin appears wrinkled, coarse, or rough, and it has mottled pigmentation (due to solar lentigos, seborrheic keratoses, and ephelides or freckles), hypopigmentation, and telangiectasias. Cutaneous malignancies are also more common in photodamaged skin. Skin phototypes are characterized by response to sun exposure. Prevention of photodamage includes the use of broad-spectrum sunscreens—sunscreens that protect against both UVB and UVA radiation—as well as the avoidance of direct sunlight and use of protective clothing along with hats and sunglasses. Although there are claims that various topical agents decrease photodamage, only topical tretinoin has been shown to increase thickness of the superficial skin layers, reduce pigmentary changes and roughness, and increase collagen synthesis. However, to induce these changes, it must be used at high concentrations for a long period of time.

Surgical therapies are used to treat photodamage through controlled partial injury to the skin. These include chemical peeling agents, dermabrasion, and laser resurfacing. All rely on the destruction of surface populations of keratinocytes, followed by repopulation of the surface with keratinocytes deep from within the sun-protected follicular structures. Controlled trials to evaluate the effectiveness of these expensive modalities are rare and inconclusive.

SEBORRHEIC DERMATITIS

Seborrheic dermatitis is a common chronic dermatitis that is characterized by erythema and greasy-looking scales in areas rich in sebaceous glands, such as the hairline (scalp), nasolabial fold, and midline chest areas. Dandruff may be an early precursor of this condition. The prevalence of dandruff is higher in persons infected with human immunodeficiency virus (HIV) and those with Parkinson's disease. At all ages, seborrheic dermatitis is more common in males than females.

Although the cause of seborrheic dermatitis is unclear, it is thought that the normal yeast flora (*Pityrosporum orbiculare* or *Malassezia furfur*) play some role in inducing inflammation of the skin, which leads to increased epidermal proliferation and desquamation. The name is misleading, and patients affected with seborrheic dermatitis do not have more seborrhea than the normal population. On the face, it can involve only the eyebrows, glabella, and nasolabial folds, or it can cause a mild blepharitis with red eyelid margins. It should be stressed to patients that seborrheic dermatitis can be suppressed but not cured. It is often treated with medicated shampoos that act against yeast, including selenium sulfide, ketoconazole, and various tar shampoos. Acute forms can also be treated with mild topical corticosteroids such as hydrocortisone 1% to 2%. Once the dermatitis is under control, patients can use the medicated shampoos for maintenance.

ROSACEA

Rosacea (Figure 56.1) is a common condition in fair-skinned persons and affects young to middle-aged as well as older persons. The cause of rosacea remains elusive; recurrent facial flushing resulting from a variety of stimuli is a common symptom. The flushing is often induced by sunlight exposure, alcohol, hot beverages, and drugs that cause vasodilatation. Rosacea has several variants, each of which requires a different approach to treatment. Usually the central convex areas of the face are affected (nose, forehead, cheeks, and chin) with erythema and telangiectasias. More advanced cases show follicular and nonfollicular papules and pustules. Recurrent flushing and edema cause thickening of the skin; in the most severe cases a rhinophyma may

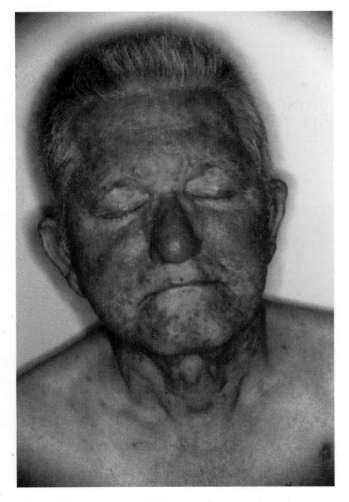

Figure 56.1—Rosacea. Diffuse erythema and erythematous papules and papulopustules are seen on the cheeks, forehead, and chin. The nose shows thickening of the skin and changes consistent with an early rhinophyma.

develop. Rosacea can also involve the eye, causing irritation and burning that may present as conjunctival injection, blepharitis, episcleritis, chalazion, or hordeolum.

Treatment of rosacea is based on the clinical picture. It is important for patients to understand that it is a chronic condition with frequent flares. They should be educated on avoiding skin irritants or strong soaps and cleansers, and instructed to reduce sun exposure and regularly apply sunscreens. Oral antibiotics such as tetracylines (doxycycline, minocycline) and erythromycin are used to treat the moderate to severe papular-pustular rosacea. Topical anti-infective agents such as erythromycin, clindamycin, and metronidazole can be used for mild rosacea or as maintenance once the oral antibiotics have been tapered. Severe or refractory rosacea can be treated with oral isotretinoin. The erythema and telangiectasias are difficult to treat. The availability of lasers, such as the potassium-titanyl-phosphate (KTP) laser, has provided an option for patients to reduce the redness and improve cosmetic appearance. Rhinophyma occurs less commonly and can be treated with surgical excision or CO_2 laser ablation.

XEROSIS

Dryness of the skin, often a concern for the older patient, is due to the reduction in water content and barrier function of the aging epidermis. It is exacerbated by environmental factors, such as decreased humidity from cold weather or central heating, irritation by hot water, and too frequent washing with harsh soaps and cleansers. Skin findings are often more pronounced on the legs. Depending on the severity of the dryness, xerosis can present as rough, itchy skin or as scales that give the skin a dry, cracked appearance known as *eczema craquelé* (Figure 56.2).

The patient's awareness of exacerbating factors and regular use of tepid showers and emollients immediately after bathing can be quite helpful. Moisturizing agents containing lactic acid or α-hydroxy acids can reduce the roughness and scaliness. When irritation or inflammation is a prominent finding, episodic use of mild topical corticosteroids for a short time provides relief.

NEURODERMATITIS

Neurodermatitis is a nonspecific term that is used to refer to chronic, pruritic conditions of unclear cause. Another term commonly used is *lichen simplex chronicus*. The lesions show signs of chronic scratching, such as hyperpigmentation and lichenification (leathery thickness), along with redness and scaling. Scratching

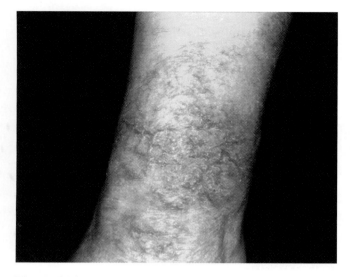

Figure 56.2—Eczema craquelé. Dry, erythematous, fissured, and cracked skin is seen on the lower legs of this patient.

these lesions often leads to pleasure and a vicious cycle of skin changes that then induce more pruritus. Treatment consists of potent topical corticosteroids, often under occlusion, emollients, as well as behavior modification. Other causes of pruritus such as irritant or allergic contact dermatitis must be excluded.

INTERTRIGO

Intertrigo (Figure 56.3) is more common in older persons because of the increased skin folds secondary to decreased dermal elasticity; environmental factors such as decreased mobility, moisture, friction, and poor hygiene also contribute. Diabetic and obese patients are more prone to develop intertrigo.

Commonly involved areas, such as the inframammary abdominal folds, groin, and axillae, will appear erythematous, macerated, moist, and mildly malodorous. Often there is secondary candidal or mixed bacterial colonization. Frequent airing, keeping involved areas dry, and using topical antifungal powders and creams, such as 2% miconazole powder or nystatin cream, constitute the treatment. Occasionally, a very mild topical corticosteroid such as 1% to 2% hydrocortisone is needed for a short period to reduce inflammation and irritation. (See also the section, p 396; on candidiasis.)

BULLOUS PEMPHIGOID

Most cases of bullous pemphigoid (Figure 56.4) occur in patients in their 60s and 70s. This is an autoimmune blistering disorder characterized by large tense blisters on normal or erythematous skin. The blisters heal

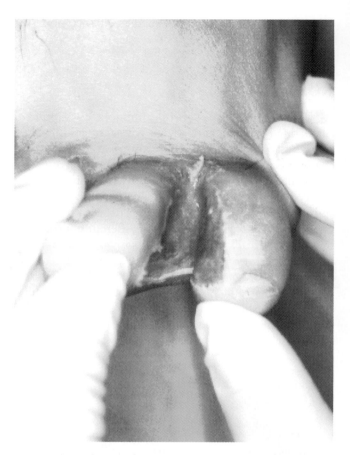

Figure 56.3—Intertrigo and candidiasis are commonly found in the web space between the 4th and 5th toes. Moist erythema, maceration, and superficial erosion is apparent.

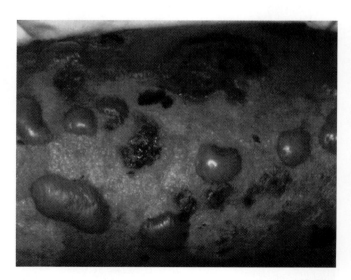

Figure 56.4—Bullous pemphigoid. Tense, fluid-filled, and hemorrhagic bullae on an erythematous base were seen on the trunk and extremities. Some of the bullae have ruptured and left a scab with crusting.

without scar formation. They are usually filled with clear fluid but on occasion may be hemorrhagic and can be found anywhere on the body. Mucous membranes are involved in up to a third of patients and show erosions or blisters on the mucosa. In some cases there is intense pruritus, and instead of blisters, one may find urticarial lesions.

The antibodies directed against bullous pemphigoid are antigens in the hemidesmosomes (proteinaceous plaques that help the epidermis adhere to the basement membrane). One of the antigens, called *desmoplakin* (also known as BP antigen I), anchors the keratin intermediate filaments to the desmosome and is inside the cell. Patients also have an antibody to type XVII collagen (also known as BP antigen II), which is a transmembrane protein. The cause of antibody formation is still unclear. It is thought that the antibodies bind to the bullous pemphigoid antigen, which then activates the complement cascade. The activated complement components then attract leukocytes and cause degranulation of mast cells, and proteases from these cells cause separation of the epidermis from the basement membrane.

Diagnosis is made by biopsy and immunofluorescence studies. On histopathology, one sees that the blister occurs below the epidermis. Direct immunofluorescence reveals immunoreactants in a linear pattern at the basement membrane between the epidermis and dermis. C3 is detected in all almost all patients, and immunoglobulin G is found in most patients. One can also measure antibodies to the basement membrane antigens in sera through indirect immunofluorescence; however, the antibody titer does not correlate with disease activity.

Though it may last for months to years, bullous pemphigoid is often a self-limited disease. Treatment depends on severity. When the lesions are localized, they may be treated with topical corticosteroids. More extensive disease can be treated with oral corticosteroids, especially for control of acute flares. Because of the adverse effects of corticosteroids, particularly in older persons, other immunosuppressive, steroid-sparing agents, such as azathioprine or cyclophosphamide, are usually added as steroids are tapered. Combination therapy with tetracylines and niacinamide has been shown to be effective.

PRURITUS

Pruritus, a very common skin complaint, is associated with many cutaneous and systemic conditions. In older persons pruritus at times can be very severe, compromising quality of life. Although xerosis is the most common cause of pruritus in the older patient, it is important to perform a complete history and examination to exclude skin conditions such as scabies, allergic, irritant or atopic dermatitis, or bullous pemphigoid. Systemic diseases such as renal disease, cholestasis or chronic liver disease, thyroid disease, anemia, occult malignancies, or drug side effects must also be considered.

Treatment depends on the underlying cause; symptomatic relief can often be achieved with topical corticosteroids, emollients, or menthol in calamine preparations. Oral antihistamines should be used with caution in older persons. For severe, refractory cases, UVB phototherapy has been used.

PSORIASIS

Psoriasis (Figure 56.5) affects 2% of the population and has bimodal incidences: one in the mid-20s and the other at about 50 to 60 years of age. There is a genetic predisposition, with multigene mode of inheritance, and environmental factors also play a role in triggering the disease.

The skin findings in psoriasis are rather characteristic: well-demarcated erythematous papules and plaques with overlying silvery scale. Extensor surfaces, areas prone to trauma, scalp, and nails are commonly involved. Various forms of psoriasis exist:

- inverse pattern, where lesions occur in skin folds, such as the neck, axillae, and genital area;
- guttate, where small 1-cm papules appear over the upper trunk and proximal extremities, usually after an infection;
- pustular, which is acute with generalized eruption of 2- to 3-mm sterile pustules and fever;
- palmoplantar; and
- erythrodermic psoriasis, in which the patient has generalized erythema.

Various factors may trigger psoriasis. Physical trauma (known as Koebner's phenomenon), infections, stress, medications (oral corticosteroids, lithium, β-blockers, angiotensin-converting enzyme inhibitors, as well as nonsteroidal anti-inflammatory drugs) have been shown to initiate or exacerbate psoriasis. Five percent to 8% of patients with psoriasis also suffer from psoriatic arthritis, which is characterized by pain, swelling, and stiffness in the small joints. Some patients may also suffer from spondylitis or sacroiliitis. Radiologic findings are often indistinguishable from rheumatoid arthritis.

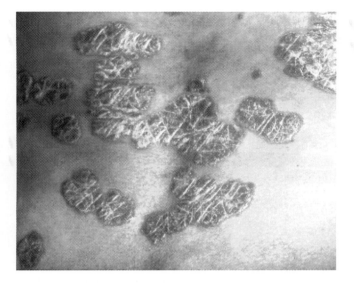

Figure 56.5—Psoriasis. Characteristic well-demarcated beefy red plaques with overlying silvery-white scales are evident on the back of this patient.

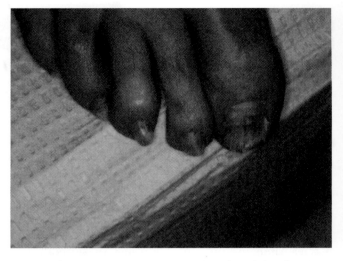

Figure 56.6—Onychomycosis. Nails infected by fungi are often yellow, thickened, and friable, with yellow-brown debris under the nail plate.

Several treatment options are available for patients with psoriasis, but each method must be evaluated in terms of risks and benefits for the older patient. Topical treatments such as corticosteroids, vitamin D derivatives (calcipotriene), topical retinoids (tazarotene), salicylic acid, or tar compounds may be sufficient to treat and control mild plaque psoriasis. Some of these treatments may be irritating or messy to apply. Long-term use of topical corticosteroids is limited by the cutaneous atrophy and decreased potency (tachyphylaxis) that occur over time. Patients who do not improve with topical treatments may be candidates for systemic treatment, such as phototherapy or immunosuppressive agents. UV therapy, including PUVA (psoralen with UVA light) and UVB therapies, can be adjunctive treatment along with topical agents; several treatments per week may be required. Patients with longstanding psoriasis who receive phototherapy must be carefully examined for skin cancer. Agents such as cyclosporine and methotrexate are quite effective in treating psoriasis. However, each of these medications has significant side effects that require careful monitoring through laboratory tests and physical examinations. In addition to drug interactions, systemic illnesses such as poor renal function, hypertension, and lung disease may limit the use of these medications.

ONYCHOMYCOSIS

Fungal infections account for 20% of all nail disease and are almost exclusively found in adults. Onychomycosis (Figure 56.6) can be caused not only by dermatophytes (fungi that infect keratinized tissues), but also by certain yeasts and nondermatophytic molds. The most common dermatophytes causing onychomycosis are *Trichophyton rubrum*, *Trichophyton mentagrophytes* var. *interdigitale*, and *Epidermophyton floccosum*. *Candida albicans* can infect the nails in chronic mucocutaneous candidiasis; however, other candida species (such as *C. parapsilosis*) can infect the nails of otherwise healthy persons. Nondermatophytic onychomycosis usually occurs in previously diseased nails or aged nails. It can often be difficult to determine whether a positive nondermatophytic nail culture is truly infection or contamination. In most cases of onychomycosis, there is preceding and or concomitant tinea pedis.

Onychomycosis can be divided into four clinical subtypes: distal subungual onychomycosis, proximal subungual onychomycosis, white superficial onychomycosis, and candidal onychomycosis. Distal subungual onychomycosis is most common, and proximal subungual onychomycosis is least common. On clinical examination, infected nails have whitish or brownish-yellow discoloration. In response to the infection, hyperproliferation of the nail bed occurs, leading to subungual hyperkeratosis (yellow-brown debris under the nail bed). Diagnosis can be confirmed by potassium hydroxide (KOH) preparation or fungal culture of the nail plate or subungual debris.

A decision to treat is usually made because of the cosmetic concern of a yellow friable nail, other comorbidities (particularly diabetes mellitus, where the break in the epidermal barrier due to the fungal infection can serve as a route for bacterial infections), and occasionally because of pain. Topical agents have not been effective in the past. A topical nail lacquer, ciclopirox (which is applied daily for 1 year) has been made available to treat onychomycosis, but in clinical studies it was found that less than 12% of patients achieved clear or almost clear toenails with its use. Griseofulvin was the standard of treatment, but poor absorption, side effects, and drug interactions have limited adherence and efficacy. Regimens with newer agents, such as oral terbinafine, fluconazole, and itraconazole, have fewer side effects and drug interactions. Fluconazole can be used to treat candidal infections. It is well tolerated and has an excellent safety profile. When prescribing itraconazole, it is imperative to review all other medications the patient is taking; itraconazole interacts with warfarin, digoxin, and many other drugs through the cytochrome P-450 liver enzyme system. Terbinafine is the only orally active fungicidal agent. It has fewer drug interactions but may interact with tricyclic antidepressants. Regardless, the rate of relapse of onychomycosis is high, and treatment can take 3 to 4 months.

For other conditions involving the feet, see "Diseases and Disorders of the Foot" (p 275).

HERPES ZOSTER

More than two thirds of reported cases of herpes zoster (Figure 56.7) occur in persons aged 50 years and older. The incidence of herpes zoster is 20 to 100 times higher in immunosuppressed patients than in other groups, and the severity and likelihood of recurrence is also higher. Patients with herpes zoster are contagious to those who lack immunity, but less so than patients with varicella. Patients with uncomplicated dermatomal zoster spread infection by means of direct contact with their lesions, whereas patients with disseminated zoster may also transmit infection in aerosol and thus need respiratory isolation.

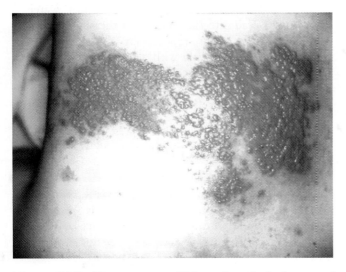

Figure 56.7—Herpes zoster. This patient had clusters of vesicles and pustules on an erythematous base involving a thoracic dermatome.

The pathogenesis of zoster is due to the passage of the varicella zoster virus (VZV) from skin and mucosal surfaces into sensory nerves and then into sensory ganglia, where latent infection is established. Although reactivation is associated with several immunosuppressive conditions, such as such as HIV infection, malignancy, or the use of immunosuppressive drugs or corticosteroids, the most important is the senescence of the cellular immune response to VZV with increasing age. (See Table 44.1, p 293.) These settings lead to reactivation of the virus, with the neuronal necrosis and inflammation that account for the severe neuralgia. The infection spreads down the sensory nerve and is released around the sensory nerve endings in the skin, producing the characteristic lesions: a cluster of vesicles on an erythematous base in a dermatomal pattern that is unilateral and does not cross the midline. Patients often complain of symptoms of pain, burning, paresthesias, tenderness, pruritus, or hyperesthesia several days before the rash appears. The vesicles turn into pustules and eventually crust over in 7 to 10 days.

Ten percent to 15% of cases of herpes zoster involve the ophthalmic branch of the trigeminal nerve. Involvement of the nasociliary branch, which presents as vesicles on the tip of the nose (known as Hutchinson's sign), requires careful ophthalmic examination to monitor for complications, such as neurotrophic keratitis and ulceration, scleritis, or uveitis. Involvement of the facial or auditory nerves that presents as herpes zoster of the external ear or tympanic membrane leads to facial palsy with or without tinnitus, vertigo, and deafness. This is known as Ramsay-Hunt syndrome. Another complication is secondary bacterial infection. Pain is a chief complaint of patients with zoster; it can precede, be concomitant with, or persist after the rash. Pain that persists or appears after the rash has healed or at 30 days after onset of rash is called *post-herpetic neuralgia*. Age is the most significant risk factor, and post-herpetic neuralgia occurs in 70% of zoster patients aged 70 and older. It is often difficult to treat.

Although the symptoms of herpes zoster can be confused with a variety of conditions causing localized pain (eg, pleurisy, myocardial infarction, renal colic, cholecystitis, glaucoma), the lesions and their distribution make the diagnosis rather easy. However, it is very difficult, if not impossible in some situations, to differentiate herpes simplex from zoster. In both infections, a Tzanck smear from the base of vesicle (stained with either hematoxylin-eosin, Giemsa, or Papanicolaou) shows multinucleated giant cells and epithelial cells containing intranuclear inclusion bodies. A smear from the base of the vesicle can be sent for direct fluorescent antibody staining. This test can differentiate between herpes simplex virus and the

VZV. Definitive diagnosis is made by viral culture; however, isolation of the virus can be difficult.

If the patient's immunity is intact, herpes zoster is usually self-limited. Treatment in all patients should be initiated early, within 72 hours of the onset of rash. Acyclovir is effective, and in patients aged 50 years and older is dosed at 800 mg five times a day for 7 to 10 days. Valacyclovir or famciclovir are prodrugs of acyclovir that provide greater oral bioavailability and allow less frequent dosing. Early treatment halts progression of disease, increases the rate of clearance of virus from vesicles, decreases the incidence of visceral and cutaneous dissemination, decreases the ocular complications when the eye is involved, and in some cases may decrease pain and the incidence of post-herpetic neuralgia. Wet compresses and topical antibiotics such as bacitracin or mupirocin can treat secondary bacterial infection.

There is no definitive treatment for post-herpetic neuralgia. Narcotics, nonsteroidal anti-inflammatory drugs, epidural injection of local anesthetics, glucocorticoids, antidepressants, capsaicin, and acupuncture are some of the therapies that are mentioned in literature. Debate over the efficacy of corticosteroids given with antiviral therapy has been fueled by two large randomized, controlled trials that reached opposite conclusions. However, risks do not appear to be significantly increased with the use of corticosteroids for zoster, especially when used with antiviral therapy, and the steroids may decrease the acute neuropathic pain and reduce pain medication requirements. Capsaicin, an extract of hot chili peppers that depletes substance P, is the only compound licensed for use in post-herpetic neuralgia. Unfortunately, many patients cannot tolerate the burning associated with this topical medication.

CANDIDIASIS

Factors that contribute to intertrigo also predispose a person to candidiasis. (See the section, p 392, on intertrigo.) Involved areas appear clinically similar to intertrigo, but there may be peripheral satellite pustules. Candida pustules can also occur on the backs of bedridden patients and on other areas prone to moisture and occlusion. Oral thrush may also develop in patients on corticosteroid inhalers, antibiotics, or immunosuppressive medications or with concomitant systemic illnesses, such as diabetes mellitus. To confirm the diagnosis, a KOH preparation of scrapings of the involved site is performed. The presence of spores and pseudohyphae is consistent with candidiasis.

Treatment resembles that of intertrigo: keeping the moist areas dry, improving hygiene, and treating with topical or oral treatment with anticandidal agents such as nystatin or ketoconazole.

SCABIES

Scabies refers to infestation with the human mite *Sarcoptes scabiei*. It is spread by person-to-person contact and is common in institutionalized older persons. Epidemics are described in long-term-care facilities, and eradication can be difficult. The adult female mite becomes fertilized on skin and burrows into the top superficial layer, where she lays eggs. The clinical manifestations occur days to weeks later when the patient develops hypersensitivity reaction to the mite saliva and excretions. Therefore, it is often difficult to pinpoint the initial infested patient, and spreading of mites may have occurred before diagnosis.

Infested patients complain of severe pruritus, especially of the hands, axillae, genitalia, and peri-umbilical region. Clinically one finds erythematous papules and occasionally nodules along with linear burrows (crooked, raised lines). The patient may have scratched to the point of causing bleeding or weeping eczematous lesions. Scabies should be suspected in anyone who complains of pruritus or displays signs of excoriation. Diagnosis is confirmed by performing a scraping on a suspected lesion and finding mite excreta, eggs, or, rarely, the mite itself, under the microscope.

Treatment of scabies is often initiated when there is strong clinical suspicion of infestation. Treatment involves eradicating the mite, decreasing the pruritus, and treating any contacts. Topical permethrin 5% is most commonly used. It is applied from the neck to the toes and rinsed off after 8 to 12 hours. This treatment should be repeated in 1 week in patients still having severe pruritus or skin lesions. Persons who may have been exposed should be treated once. Topical corticosteroids may help to reduce pruritus, but it is important to reassure patients that the itching may persist for weeks or months. Cleaning the bedding, clothes, and towels (bath, linen) with hot water is sufficient to eradicate the mite from the surroundings.

There have been reports in the literature of treating scabies effectively with a one-time oral dose of an antihelminthic agent called ivermectin (200 µg per kg). However, there are no long-term studies, and it is not yet approved for this use by the Food and Drug Administration.

LOUSE INFESTATIONS

Lice can infest the body (pediculosis corporis), scalp (pediculosis capitis), or pubic hair (pediculosis pubis). With pediculosis corporis or capitis, lice is spread from person to person through physical contact or fomites. Pediculosis pubis is usually spread by sexual contact. In all cases, patients complain of pruritus of the involved areas, and there can be secondary infection. In cases of pediculosis corporis, the lice feed on the body but live on clothing, where they lay eggs, often near the seams.

In cases of pediculosis capitis, the lice lay eggs on the proximal part of the hair shaft. The eggs (or nits) are visible as white specks cemented to the hair at an oblique angle. Patients with pediculosis pubis also have nits on the pubic hair and commonly have more organisms.

Treatment involves eradicating the lice and larvae, treating close contacts, and treating the secondary infection. Pyrethrins or its derivatives (permethrin) are ovicidal and can be used as single 10-minute topical treatment for patients and those who have been exposed. Combs, brushes, hats, clothing, bedding, and towels (bath, linen) must be washed with hot water.

ACTINIC KERATOSES

Actinic keratoses (also known as *solar keratoses*) are lesions caused by chronic UV radiation (Figure 56.8). Although they are usually considered premalignant growths, the majority resolve without treatment. It is unclear how many progress to squamous cell carcinoma; reports vary from 0.24% to 20%. They appear as poorly circumscribed, occasionally scaly, erythematous macules and papules on sun-exposed areas, such as the face, ears, and dorsum of hands and arms. Some may have an overlying thick, hard growth known as a *cutaneous horn*. Lesions on the lips are called *actinic cheilitis*.

Actinic keratoses are most often treated to prevent progression to squamous cell carcinoma but also to decrease discomfort. They respond to a variety of treatments, such as cryotherapy with liquid nitrogen, topical acids, topical 5-fluorouracil, or excision. Although treating the lesions with liquid nitrogen for 10 to 15 seconds is very effective, it can be somewhat uncomfortable and can cause pigmentary changes. When there are several lesions in an area, treatment that the patient can perform at home, such as topical 5-fluorouracil twice a day to the entire affected area, is helpful because it can also treat subclinical lesions. However, patients must be monitored and warned about the bright erythema and discomfort that occurs with 5-fluorouracil treatment.

SQUAMOUS CELL CARCINOMA

Squamous cell carcinoma (SCC) is the second most common form of skin cancer. It affects patients in mid- to late life and occurs most commonly on chronically sun-exposed areas. Squamous cell carcinomas cause local tissue destruction if not treated and have a low risk (but greater risk than basal cell carcinomas) to metastasize. The larger the tumor, the greater the risk of recurrence. SCC presents as chronic erythematous papules, plaques, or nodules with scaling, crusting, or ulceration. They also have a propensity to occur in

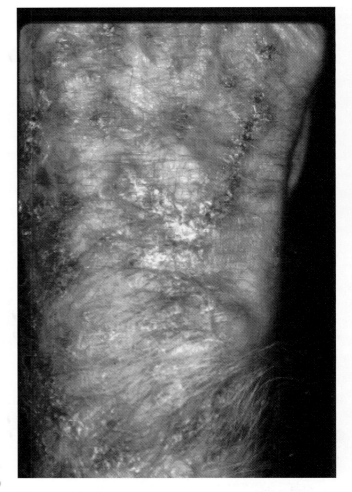

Figure 56.8—Actinic keratoses are rough, scaly, red-brown macules on sun-exposed skin and are premalignant.

longstanding nonhealing wounds and in burn and radiation scars.

Treatment consists of surgical excision. In cosmetically important areas, Mohs micrographic surgery is performed. In patients who are poor surgical candidates or who have multiple comorbidities, destruction with cryotherapy or local radiation has been used.

BASAL CELL CARCINOMA

Basal cell carcinoma is the most common cancer in the United States. As with other cutaneous malignancies, fair-skinned persons with chronic sun exposure are at risk. It presents in three major clinical patterns:

- nodular—this is the most common variant and appears as a waxy, translucent papule with overlying telangiectasias;
- morpheaform—this has a scar-like appearance and can look atrophic;
- superficial—this appears as an erythematous macule or papule with fine scale or superficial erosion.

Some basal cell carcinomas appear as superficial ulcers with characteristic rolled borders (Figure 56.9). Others may be pigmented and confused for melanoma.

Treatment of basal cell carcinoma is also surgical excision. Some basal cell carcinomas, particularly those located in cosmetically important areas, those that are nodular or morpheaform, and those that are recurrent should be excised by use of Mohs micrographic surgery to ensure adequate excision and tissue sparing. Like squamous cell carcinomas, basal cell carcinomas occurring in poor surgical candidates can also be treated with ablative methods, such as cryosurgery, radiation, and curettage with electrodessication.

MELANOMA

The incidence of melanoma continues to increase, and it affects all adult age groups. The risk factors for melanoma include very fair skin type, family history, dysplastic or numerous nevi, and sunlight exposure, particularly intermittent blistering sunburns in childhood. Melanomas are usually asymptomatic; thus, regular skin examinations and early recognition are key for favorable prognosis.

A new pigmented skin lesion or a change in the color, size, surface, or borders of a preexisting mole should be suspected for melanoma and biopsied. There are four clinical types:

- lentigo maligna—the type seen most commonly on atrophic, sun-damaged skin of an older patient; this appears as an irregularly shaped tan or brown macule that has been enlarging slowly;

- superficial spreading—this type can occur anywhere and presents often as an irregularly shaped macule, papule, or plaque with great variation in color (Figure 56.10);

- nodular—a papule or nodule, often black or gray in color, that has been growing rapidly;

- acral lentiginous—this type is found on the palms, soles, or nail beds (Figure 56.11); it is found in all skin types and presents as a dark brown or black patch; its incidence is highest in persons aged 65 or older.

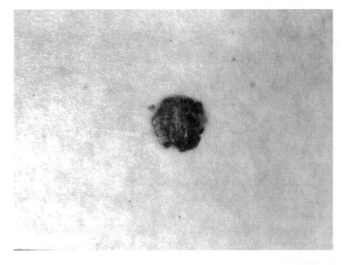

Figure 56.10—Melanoma. This lesion has irregular variegation in pigment (shades of brown and blue-black) as well as irregular borders, suggesting melanoma.

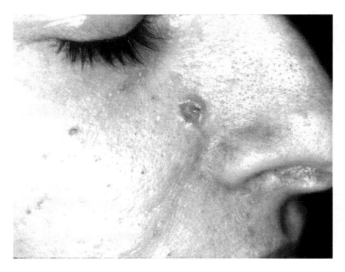

Figure 56.9—Basal cell carcinoma, ulcerated. This is also a pearly, fleshy papule but is ulcerated in the center and has a characteristic rolled border.

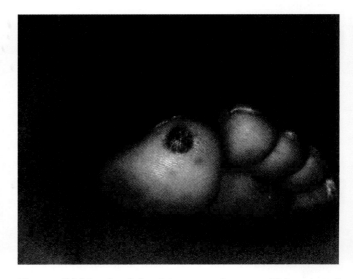

Figure 56.11—Acral lentiginous melanoma. This type of melanoma presents as a dark macular growth with irregular borders on volar surfaces of palms and soles (as in this case), and nails.

The treatment of melanoma consists of surgical excision and, depending on depth, may also involve lymph node dissection or adjuvant therapy.

REFERENCES

- Chosidow O. Scabies and pediculosis. *Lancet.* 2000;355(9206):819–826.

- Fleischer AB. Pruritus in the elderly. *Advances in Dermatology.* 1995;10:41–59.

- Hedderwick S, Kauffman CA. Opportunistic fungal infections: superficial and systemic candidiasis. *Geriatrics.* 1997;52(10):50–54.

- Lawrence N. New and emerging treatments for photoaging. *Dermatologic Clinics.* 2000;18(1):99–112.

- Lebwohl M. Advances in psoriasis therapy. *Dermatologic Clinics.* 2000;18(1):13–19.

- Palmissano C, Norman RA. Geriatric dermatology in chronic care and rehabilitation. *Dermatol Nurs.* 2000; 12(2):116–123.

- Thiboutot DM. Acne and rosacea. New and emerging therapies. *Dermatologic Clinics.* 2000;18(1):63–71.

- Schmader K. Herpes zoster in the elderly: issues related to geriatrics. *Clinical Infectious Diseases.* 1999;28(4):736–739.

APPENDIX CONTENTS

Activities of Daily Living
  Physical Self-Maintenance Scale (ADLs) 384
  Instrumental Activities of Daily Living Scale (IADLs)... 385
Alcoholism: The Michigan Alcoholism Screening Test—Geriatric Version (MAST-G) 386
Anticoagulation
  Oral Anticoagulation for Older Adults.. 387
  Reversal of Anticoagulants 388
  Initiation and Monitoring of Anticoagulants.. 388
  Anticoagulation When Surgical Procedure Is Planned... 388
Benign Prostatic Hyperplasia (BPH): The International Prostate Symptom Score 389
Depression: The Geriatric Depression Scale (short form, GDS)..................................... 390
Falls: Recommendations from the American Geriatrics Society Guidelines for the Prevention of Falls 391
Health Survey: The SF-36 Health Survey 393
Hearing: Hearing Handicap Inventory for the Elderly—Screening Version (HHIE-S)................... 399
Home Safety: Checklist 400
Functional Abilities: Functional Activities Questionnaire (FAQ)................................... 401
Geriatric Screening: Screening in Primary Care... 402
Incontinence: Prevention and Management—Behavioral Treatment 403
Mobility and Movement
  Abnormal Involuntary Movement Scale (AIMS) 405
  Performance-Oriented Mobility Assessment (POMA).. 407
NICHE Ready Sheet 409
Nutrition Screening: DETERMINE Your Nutritional Health Checklist 410
Pain Management
  Systemic Pharmacotherapy for Persistent Pain Management 411
Pressure Ulcers
  Braden Scale for Predicting Pressure Sore Risk 413
  The Pressure Ulcer Scale for Healing (PUSH)... 415
Resources
  What Can You Find on the AGS Web Site? 417
  Directory of Agencies and Organizations for Geriatric Clinicians 418

ACTIVITIES OF DAILY LIVING

Physical Self-Maintenance Scale (ADLs)

In each category, circle the item that most closely describes the person's highest level of functioning and record the score assigned to that level (either 1 or 0) in the blank at the beginning of the category.

A. Toilet _____
1. Care for self at toilet completely; no incontinence. 1
2. Needs to be reminded, or needs help in cleaning self, or has rare (weekly at most) accidents. 0
3. Soiling or wetting while asleep more than once a week. 0
4. Soiling or wetting while awake more than once a week. 0
5. No control of bowels or bladder. 0

B. Feeding _____
1. Eats without assistance. 1
2. Eats with minor assistance at meal times and/or with special preparation of food, or help in cleaning up after meals. 0
3. Feeds self with moderate assistance and is untidy. 0
4. Requires extensive assistance for all meals. 0
5. Does not feed self at all and resists efforts of others to feed him or her. 0

C. Dressing _____
1. Dresses, undresses, and selects clothes from own wardrobe. 1
2. Dresses and undresses self, with minor assistance. 0
3. Needs moderate assistance in dressing and selection of clothes. 0
4. Needs major assistance in dressing, but cooperates with efforts of others to help. 0
5. Completely unable to dress self and resists efforts of others to help. 0

D. Grooming (neatness, hair, nails, hands, face, clothing) _____
1. Always neatly dressed, well-groomed, without assistance. 1
2. Grooms self adequately with occasional minor assistance, eg, with shaving. 0
3. Needs moderate and regular assistance or supervision with grooming. 0
4. Needs total grooming care, but can remain well-groomed after help from others. 0
5. Actively negates all efforts of others to maintain grooming. 0

E. Physical Ambulation _____
1. Goes about grounds or city. 1
2. Ambulates within residence or about one block distant. 0
3. Ambulates with assistance of (*check one of a–e*) a. ( ) another person, b. ( ) railing, 0
   c. ( ) cane, d. ( ) walker, e. ( ) wheelchair (*check 1 or 2*) 1. ____ Gets in and out without help. 2. ____ Needs help getting in and out.
4. Sits unsupported in chair or wheelchair, but cannot propel self without help. 0
5. Bedridden more than half the time. 0

F. Bathing _____
1. Bathes self (tub, shower, sponge bath) without help. 1
2. Bathes self with help getting in and out of tub. 0
3. Washes face and hands only, but cannot bathe rest of body. 0
4. Does not wash self, but is cooperative with those who bathe him or her. 0
5. Does not try to wash self and resists efforts to keep him or her clean. 0

NOTE: For scoring interpretation and source, see note following the next instrument.

Instrumental Activities of Daily Living Scale (IADLs)

In each category, circle the item that most closely describes the person's highest level of functioning and record the score assigned to that level (either 1 or 0) in the blank at the beginning of the category.

A. Ability to Use Telephone _____
1. Operates telephone on own initiative; looks up and dials numbers. 1
2. Dials a few well-known numbers. 1
3. Answers telephone, but does not dial. 1
4. Does not use telephone at all. 0

B. Shopping _____
1. Takes care of all shopping needs independently. 1
2. Shops independently for small purchases. 0
3. Needs to be accompanied on any shopping trip. 0
4. Completely unable to shop. 0

C. Food Preparation _____
1. Plans, prepares, and serves adequate meals independently. 1
2. Prepares adequate meals if supplied with ingredients. 0
3. Heats and serves prepared meals or prepares meals, but does not maintain adequate diet. 0
4. Needs to have meals prepared and served. 0

D. Housekeeping _____
1. Maintains house alone or with occasional assistance (eg, heavy-work domestic help). 1
2. Performs light daily tasks such as dishwashing, bedmaking. 1
3. Performs light daily tasks, but cannot maintain acceptable level of cleanliness. 1
4. Needs help with all home maintenance tasks. 1
5. Does not participate in any housekeeping tasks. 0

E. Laundry _____
1. Does personal laundry completely. 1
2. Launders small items; rinses socks, stockings, etc. 1
3. All laundry must be done by others. 0

F. Mode of Transportation _____
1. Travels independently on public transportation or drives own car. 1
2. Arranges own travel via taxi, but does not otherwise use public transportation. 1
3. Travels on public transportation when assisted or accompanied by another. 1
4. Travel limited to taxi or automobile with assistance of another. 0
5. Does not travel at all. 0

G. Responsibility for Own Medications _____
1. Is responsible for taking medication in correct dosages at correct time. 1
2. Takes responsibility if medication is prepared in advance in separate dosages. 0
3. Is not capable of dispensing own medication. 0

H. Ability to Handle Finances _____
1. Manages financial matters independently (budgets, writes checks, pays rent and bills, goes to bank); collects and keeps track of income. 1
2. Manages day-to-day purchases, but needs help with banking, major purchases, etc. 1
3. Incapable of handling money. 0

NOTE: Scoring interpretation: For ADLs, the total score ranges from 0 to 6, and for IADLs, from 0 to 8. In some categories, only the highest level of function receives a 1; in others, two or more levels have scores of 1 because each describes competence that represents some minimal level of function. These screens are useful for indicating specifically how a person is performing at the present time. When they are also used over time, they serve as documentation of a person's functional improvement or deterioration.

SOURCE: Lawton MP, Brody EM. Assessment of older people: self-maintaining and instrumental activities of daily living. *Gerontologist.* 1969; 9:179–186. Reprinted with permission.

ALCOHOLISM

The Michigan Alcoholism Screening Test—Geriatric Version (MAST-G)

© The Regents of the University of Michigan, 1991

	Yes (1)	No (0)
1. After drinking have you ever noticed an increase in your heart rate or beating in your chest?	1. ____	____
2. When talking with others, do you ever underestimate how much you actually drink?	2. ____	____
3. Does alcohol make you sleepy so that you often fall asleep in your chair?	3. ____	____
4. After a few drinks, have you sometimes not eaten or been able to skip a meal because you don't feel hungry?	4. ____	____
5. Does having a few drinks help decrease your shakiness or tremors?	5. ____	____
6. Does alcohol sometimes make it hard for you to remember parts of the day or night?	6. ____	____
7. Do you have rules for yourself that you won't drink before a certain time of day or night?	7. ____	____
8. Have you lost interest in hobbies or activities you used to enjoy?	8. ____	____
9. When you wake up in the morning, do you ever have trouble remembering part of the night before?	9. ____	____
10. Does having a drink help you sleep?	10. ____	____
11. Do you hide your alcohol bottles from family members?	11. ____	____
12. After a social gathering, have you ever felt embarrassed because you drank too much?	12. ____	____
13. Have you ever been concerned that drinking might be harmful to your health?	13. ____	____
14. Do you like to end an evening with a nightcap?	14. ____	____
15. Did you find your drinking increased after someone close to you died?	15. ____	____
16. In general, would you prefer to have a few drinks at home rather than go out to social events?	16. ____	____
17. Are you drinking more now than in the past?	17. ____	____
18. Do you usually take a drink to relax or calm your nerves?	18. ____	____
19. Do you drink to take your mind off your problems?	19. ____	____
20. Have you ever increased your drinking after experiencing a loss in your life?	20. ____	____
21. Do you sometimes drive when you have had too much to drink?	21. ____	____
22. Has a doctor or nurse ever said they were worried or concerned about your drinking?	22. ____	____
23. Have you ever made rules to manage your drinking?	23. ____	____
24. When you feel lonely does having a drink help?	24. ____	____

NOTE: A score of: 5 or more "yes" responses is indicative of an alcohol problem.

SOURCE: Reprinted with permission. For further information, contact Frederic Blow, PhD, at University of Michigan Alcohol Research Center, 400 E. Eisenhower Parkway, Suite A, Ann Arbor, MI 48104, (734) 930-5139. See "Substance Abuse" (p 234) for a shorter version of this instrument.

ANTICOAGULATION

Oral Anticoagulation for Older Adults

Thromboembolic Disorder	INR	Duration	Clinical Comments
Venous thromboembolism			
Prophylaxis (eg, high-risk surgery)		Perioperative	Perioperative use of LMW heparin or adjusted-dose unfractionated heparin is appropriate in most patients
	Target 2.5; range 2.0–3.0	≤ 3 months or until ambulatory	Warfarin may be considered for use until patients become ambulatory
Treatment: single episode (DVT or PE)	Target 2.5; range 2.0–3.0	Reversible or time-limited risk factor: 3–6 months	At or above the knee
		Idiopathic DVT or PE: ≥ 6 months	Initial treatment with LMW heparin or adjusted dose unfractionated IV heparin for at least 5 days and to overlap warfarin at a therapeutic level for 2–4 days
Treatment: recurrent DVT or PE or continuing risk factor (cancer, congenital thrombophilic states, antiphospholipid antibody, etc.)	Target 2.5; range 2.0–3.0	Indefinite	At or above the knee
			Initial treatment with LMW heparin or adjusted dose unfractionated IV heparin for at least 5 days and to overlap warfarin at a therapeutic level for 2–4 days
Prevention of Systemic Embolism			
AF	Target 2.5; range 2.0–3.0	Indefinite	Age < 65, no risk factors (ie, no prior TIA, systemic embolus or stroke, hypertension, poor LV function, rheumatic mitral valve disease): ASA recommended
			Age 65–75, no risk factors: aspirin or warfarin recommended
			Age 65–75 with risk factors or > age 75: warfarin recommended
AF: cardioversion	Target 2.5; range 2.0–3.0	3 weeks prior for patients in AF > 48 hours; continue until NSR stable for 4 weeks	Indefinite anticoagulation as above for those who do not return to NSR
Acute MI	Target 2.5; range 2.0–3.0	≤ 3 months	ASA (160–325 mg enteric) daily indefinitely
			When no thrombolytics given, give heparin followed by warfarin to patients at increased embolic risk (anterior Q-wave MI, severe LV dysfunction, CHF, prior emboli, 2D echo evidence of mural thrombus, AF)
Cardiomyopathy	Target 2.5; range 2.0–3.0	Indefinite	Consider for patient with ejection fraction = 25%
Recurrent systemic embolism	Target 2.5; range 2.0–3.0	Indefinite	Criteria for recurrence: events, temporal and etiologic relationships
Valvular heart disease	Target 2.5; range 2.0–3.0	Indefinite	Consider patients with a history of SE, AF, or LA diameter ≥ 5.5 cm
			If recurrent SE occurs on warfarin, add ASA (80–100 mg/day) or increase target INR to 3.0 (range 2.5–3.5)
Tissue prosthetic heart valve	Target 2.5; range 2.0–3.0	3 months (absent AF)	Prosthetic mitral or aortic valve or positions without AF; then ASA (162 mg/day)
			If history of SE or LA thrombus at surgery, consider treating indefinitely
Mechanical heart valve	Target 3.0; range 2.5–3.5	Indefinite	If high embolic risk, add ASA (81mg/day)

NOTE: AF = atrial fibrillation ; ASA = aspirin; CHF = congestive heart failure; DVT = deep-vein thrombosis; INR = international normalized ratio; IV = intravenous; LA = left atrial; LMW = low molecular weight; LV = left ventricular; MI = myocardial infarction; NSR = normal sinus rhythm; PE = pulmonary embolus; SE = systemic embolism; TIA = transient ischemic attack.

Reversal of Anticoagulants

INR 2.0–5.0	No bleeding or minor bleeding	Withhold warfarin or lower dosage if above the therapeutic range and monitor INR Resume at same or lower dosage as INR approaches the desired range
INR 5.0–9.0	No bleeding	Withhold warfarin for one to two doses Monitor INR frequently Restart warfarin at lower dosage when INR falls into therapeutic range
	No bleeding but increased risk	Withhold one dose of warfarin Vitamin K (1.0–2.5 mg) po
	Minor bleeding	Withhold warfarin, monitor INR Vitamin K (1.0–2.5 mg) po or SC
INR > 9.0	No bleeding or minor bleeding	Withhold warfarin, monitor INR Vitamin K (3–5/mg) po or SC
	Severe bleeding	Discontinue warfarin Vitamin K (5–10 mg, slow IV infusion as increased risk of anaphylaxis) Administer fresh frozen plasma May repeat vitamin K every 12 hours
	Life-threatening bleeding	Discontinue warfarin Vitamin K (10 mg, slow IV infusion as increased risk of anaphylaxis) Administer fresh frozen plasma (prothrombin complex concentrate can be considered if insufficient time to thaw fresh frozen plasma)

NOTE: INR = international normalized ratio; IV = intravenous; po = by mouth; SC = subcutaneously.

Initiation and Monitoring of Anticoagulants

1. A baseline INR (and APTT if on heparin) should be obtained.

   ▪ In acute thrombotic episodes, warfarin treatment should be initiated during therapy with unfractionated or low-molecular-weight heparin. Dosing can begin with an estimated average maintenance dose, often 2.5 to 5.0 mg in the elderly patient. The two treatments should overlap for 2 to 4 days following a therapeutic INR.

   ▪ In non-urgent situations, such as chronic stable AF, warfarin treatment can begin in the absence of heparin treatment, following the above regimen.

2. The INR should be monitored daily until a stable and therapeutic level is achieved (usually 5 to 7 days).

3. The INR can be monitored 2 to 3 times weekly for 1 to 2 weeks, then weekly for 1 month, and monthly thereafter. More frequent monitoring may be required in some patients and is indicated during antibiotic therapy, during diet changes, or during changes affecting medications that interact with warfarin binding or metabolism.

NOTE: AF = atrial fibrillation; APTT = activated partial thromboplastin time; INR = international normalized ratio.

Anticoagulation When Surgical Procedure Is Planned

Hold warfarin for 3 days prior to planned procedure

INR < 2.0	Consider heparin until 4 hours prior to procedure Procedure at INR < 1.5 Post-procedure, consider heparin until INR is theraputic
INR 5.0–9.0	Withhold warfarin, monitor INR until < 2.0 Consider vitamin K (1.0 mg) po if rapid correction of INR required Consider heparin when INR < 2.0 until 4 hours prior to procedure Procedure at INR < 1.5 Post-procedure, administer heparin until INR is therapeutic
INR > 9.0	Withhold warfarin, monitor INR until < 2.0 Vitamin K (2.0–4.0 mg) po; may repeat in 24 hours if INR still high Consider heparin when INR < 2.0 until 4 hours prior to procedure Procedure at INR < 1.5 Post-procedure, administer heparin until INR is therapeutic

Post-procedure—Restart warfarin at regular maintenance dosage

NOTE: INR = international normalized ratio; po = by mouth.

SOURCE: Geriatric Recommendations adapted by Laurie G. Jacobs, MD, with assistance from Milayna Subar, MD, and the Clinical Practice Committee of the American Geriatrics Society (AGS). Supported by an educational grant from DuPont Pharmaceuticals Company. Last updated January 1, 2000. Modified with permission from *Chest*. 1998;114:439S–769S.

BENIGN PROSTATIC HYPERPLASIA (BPH)

The International Prostate Symptom Score

The following questionnaire was developed by the American Urological Association (AUA) to help men evaluate the severity of their symptoms from BPH. This self-administered test can help determine which treatment is needed, if any. Symptoms are classified as mild (1 to 7); moderate (8 to 19); or severe (20 to 35). Generally, no treatment is needed if symptoms are mild; moderate symptoms usually call for some form of treatment; and severe symptoms most often indicate that surgery is necessary.

Circle one number on each line.	Not At all	Less than 1 time in 5	Less than half the time	About half the time	More than half the time	Almost always
1. Over the past month, how often have you had a sensation of not emptying your bladder completely after you finished urinating?	0	1	2	3	4	5
2. Over the past month, how often have you had to urinate again less than two hours after you finished urinating?	0	1	2	3	4	5
3. Over the past month, how often have you found you stopped and started again several times when you urinated?	0	1	2	3	4	5
4. Over the past month, how often have you found it difficult to postpone urination?	0	1	2	3	4	5
5. Over the past month, how often have you had a weak urinary stream?	0	1	2	3	4	5
6. Over the past month, how often have you had to push or strain to begin urination?	0	1	2	3	4	5
	None	1 time	2 times	3 times	4 times	5 times
7. Over the past month, how many times did you most typically get up to urinate from the time you went to bed at night until the time you got up in the morning?	0	1	2	3	4	5

Total Score: _____

NOTE: According to the Clinical Practice Guidelines on BPH from the Agency for Health Care Policy and Research (AHCPR), no further diagnostic tests are needed when the AUA symptom index is 0 to 7 and no abnormalities are found in the evaluation.

SOURCE: Barry MJ, Fowler FJ Jr, O'Leary MP, et al. The American Urological Association symptom index for benign prostatic hyperplasia. *J Urol.* 1992;148(5):1549–1557. Reprinted with permission.

DEPRESSION

The Geriatric Depression Scale (short form, GDS)

Choose the best answer for how you felt over the past week.

1. Are you basically satisfied with your life?	yes/**no**
2. Have you dropped many of your activities and interests?	**yes**/no
3. Do you feel that your life is empty?	**yes**/no
4. Do you often get bored?	**yes**/no
5. Are you in good spirits most of the time?	yes/**no**
6. Are you afraid that something bad is going to happen to you?	**yes**/no
7. Do you feel happy most of the time?	yes/**no**
8. Do you often feel helpless?	**yes**/no
9. Do you prefer to stay at home, rather than going out and doing new things?	**yes**/no
10. Do you feel you have more problems with memory than most?	**yes**/no
11. Do you think it is wonderful to be alive now?	yes/**no**
12. Do you feel pretty worthless the way you are now?	**yes**/no
13. Do you feel full of energy?	yes/**no**
14. Do you feel that your situation is hopeless?	**yes**/no
15. Do you think that most people are better off than you are?	**yes**/no

NOTE: Score bolded answers. One point for each of these answers. Cut-off: normal = 0–5; above 5 suggests depression. For additional information on administration and scoring, refer to the following references:

1. Sheikh JI, Yesavage JA. Geriatric Depression Scale: recent evidence and development of a shorter version. *Clin Gerontol.* 1986;5:165–172.
2. Yesavage JA, Brink TL, Rose TL, et al. Development and validation of a geriatric depression rating scale: a preliminary report. *J Psych Res.* 1983;17:27.

SOURCE: Courtesy of Jerome A. Yesavage, MD. Reprinted with permission.

FALLS

Recommendations from the American Geriatrics Society Guidelines for the Prevention of Falls

The aim of this guideline is to assist health care professionals in their assessment of fall risk and in their management of older patients who are at risk of falling and those who have fallen. The Panel on Falls Prevention assumes that health care professionals will use their general clinical knowledge and judgment in applying the general principles and specific recommendations of this document to the assessment and management of individual patients. Decisions to adopt any particular recommendation must be made by the practitioner in light of available evidence and resources. (The key to strength of recommendations, indicated by letters A–D, is located in the note on next page.)

Assessment

Approach to older persons as part of routine care (not presenting after a fall):

- All older persons who are under the care of a health professional or their caregivers should be asked at least once a year about falls.

- All older persons who report a single fall should be observed as they stand up from a chair without using their arms, walk several paces, and return (ie, the "Get Up and Go Test"). Those demonstrating no difficulty or unsteadiness need no further assessment.

- Persons who have difficulty or demonstrate unsteadiness performing this test require further assessment.

Approach to older persons presenting with one or more falls or who have abnormalities of gait or balance, or both, or who report recurrent falls:

- Older persons who present for medical attention because of a fall, report recurrent falls in the past year, or demonstrate abnormalities of gait or balance, or both, should have a fall evaluation performed. This evaluation should be performed by a clinician with appropriate skills and experience, which may necessitate referral to a specialist (eg, geriatrician).

- A fall evaluation is defined as an assessment that includes the following: a history of fall circumstances, medications, acute or chronic medical problems, and mobility levels; an examination of vision, gait and balance, and lower-extremity joint function; an examination of basic neurologic function, including mental status, muscle strength, lower-extremity peripheral nerves, proprioception, reflexes, tests of cortical, extrapyramidal, and cerebellar function; and assessment of basic cardiovascular status, including heart rate and rhythm, postural pulse and blood pressure, and, if appropriate, heart rate and blood-pressure responses to carotid sinus stimulation.

Multifactorial Interventions

- Among *community-dwelling* older persons (ie, those living in their own homes), multifactorial interventions should include: gait training and advice on the appropriate use of assistive devices (B); review and modification of medication, especially psychotropic medication (B); exercise programs, with balance training as one of the components (B); treatment of postural hypotension (B); modification of environmental hazards (C); and treatment of cardiovascular disorders, including cardiac arrhythmias (D).

- In *long-term care and assisted-living settings*, multifactorial interventions should include: staff education programs (B); gait training and advice on the appropriate use of assistive devices (B); and review and modification of medications, especially psychotropic medications (B).

- The evidence is insufficient to make recommendations for or against multifactorial interventions in *acute hospital* settings.

Single Intervention: Exercise

- Although exercise has many proven benefits, the optimal type, duration, and intensity of exercise for falls prevention remain unclear (B).
- Older people who have had recurrent falls should be offered long-term exercise and balance training (B).
- Tai Chi C'uan is a promising type of balance exercise, although it requires further evaluation before it can be recommended as the preferred balance training (C).

Single Intervention: Environmental Modification

- When older patients at increased risk of falls are discharged from the hospital, a facilitated environmental home assessment should be considered (B).

Single Intervention: Medications

- Patients who have fallen should have their medications reviewed and altered or stopped, as appropriate, in light of their risk of future falls. Particular attention to medication reduction should be given to older persons taking four or more medications and to those taking psychotropic medications (C).

Single Intervention: Assistive Devices

- Studies of multifactorial interventions that have included assistive devices have demonstrated benefit. However, there is no direct evidence that the use of assistive devices alone will prevent falls. Therefore, while assistive devices may be effective elements of a multifactorial intervention program, their isolated use without attention to other risk factors cannot be recommended (C).

Single Intervention: Behavioral and Educational Programs

- Although studies of multifactorial interventions that have included behavioral and educational programs have demonstrated benefit, when used as an isolated intervention, health or behavioral education does not reduce falls and should not be done in isolation (B).

NOTE:

Key to Strength of Recommendation: A: Directly based on Class I evidence; B: Directly based on Class II evidence or extrapolated recommendation from Class I evidence; C: Directly based on Class III evidence or extrapolated recommendation from Class I or II evidence; D: Directly based on Class IV evidence or extrapolated recommendation from Class I, II, or III evidence.

Key to Categories of Evidence: Class I: Evidence from at least one randomized, controlled trial or a meta-analysis of randomized, controlled trials; Class II: Evidence from at least one controlled study without randomization or evidence from at least one other type of quasi-experimental study; Class III: Evidence from nonexperimental studies, such as comparative studies, correlation studies, and case-control studies; Class IV: Evidence from expert committee reports or opinions and/or clinical experience of respected authorities.

SOURCE: Adapted from American Geriatrics Society, British Geriatrics Society, and American Academy of Orthopaedic Surgeons Panel on Falls Prevention. Guidelines for the prevention of falls in older persons. *J Am Geriatr Soc* 2001;49(5):664–672. Reprinted by permission of Blackwell Science, Inc.

The SF-36™ Health Survey

Your Health and Well-Being

This survey asks for your views about your health. This information will help keep track of how you feel and how well you are able to do your usual activities. *Thank you for completing this survey!*

For each of the following questions, please mark an ⊠ in the one box that best describes your answer.

1. In general, would you say your health is:

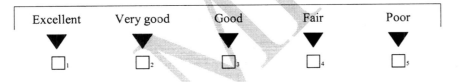

2. **Compared to one year ago**, how would you rate your health in general now?

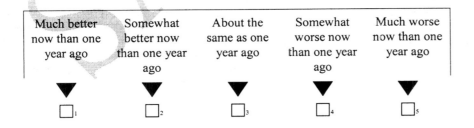

3. The following questions are about activities you might do during a typical day. Does <u>your health now limit you</u> in these activities? If so, how much?

	Yes, limited a lot ▼	Yes, limited a little ▼	No, not limited at all ▼
a <u>Vigorous activities</u>, such as running, lifting heavy objects, participating in strenuous sports	☐₁	☐₂	☐₃
b <u>Moderate activities</u>, such as moving a table, pushing a vacuum cleaner, bowling, or playing golf	☐₁	☐₂	☐₃
c Lifting or carrying groceries	☐₁	☐₂	☐₃
d Climbing <u>several</u> flights of stairs	☐₁	☐₂	☐₃
e Climbing <u>one</u> flight of stairs	☐₁	☐₂	☐₃
f Bending, kneeling, or stooping	☐₁	☐₂	☐₃
g Walking <u>more than a mile</u>	☐₁	☐₂	☐₃
h Walking <u>several hundred yards</u>	☐₁	☐₂	☐₃
i Walking <u>one hundred yards</u>	☐₁	☐₂	☐₃
j Bathing or dressing yourself	☐₁	☐₂	☐₃

4. During the <u>past 4 weeks</u>, how much of the time have you had any of the following problems with your work or other regular daily activities <u>as a result of your physical health</u>?

	All of the time	Most of the time	Some of the time	A little of the time	None of the time
	▼	▼	▼	▼	▼
a Cut down on the <u>amount of time</u> you spent on work or other activities	☐1	☐2	☐3	☐4	☐5
b <u>Accomplished less</u> than you would like	☐1	☐2	☐3	☐4	☐5
c Were limited in the <u>kind</u> of work or other activities	☐1	☐2	☐3	☐4	☐5
d Had <u>difficulty</u> performing the work or other activities (for example, it took extra effort)	☐1	☐2	☐3	☐4	☐5

5. During the <u>past 4 weeks</u>, how much of the time have you had any of the following problems with your work or other regular daily activities <u>as a result of any emotional problems</u> (such as feeling depressed or anxious)?

	All of the time	Most of the time	Some of the time	A little of the time	None of the time
	▼	▼	▼	▼	▼
a Cut down on the <u>amount of time</u> you spent on work or other activities	☐1	☐2	☐3	☐4	☐5
b <u>Accomplished less</u> than you would like	☐1	☐2	☐3	☐4	☐5
c Did work or other activities <u>less carefully</u> than usual	☐1	☐2	☐3	☐4	☐5

6. During the <u>past 4 weeks</u>, to what extent has your physical health or emotional problems interfered with your normal social activities with family, friends, neighbors, or groups?

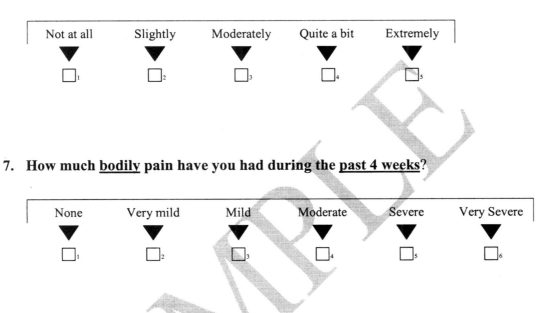

Not at all	Slightly	Moderately	Quite a bit	Extremely
□₁	□₂	□₃	□₄	□₅

7. How much <u>bodily</u> pain have you had during the <u>past 4 weeks</u>?

None	Very mild	Mild	Moderate	Severe	Very Severe
□₁	□₂	□₃	□₄	□₅	□₆

8. During the <u>past 4 weeks</u>, how much did <u>pain</u> interfere with your normal work (including both work outside the home and housework)?

Not at all	A little bit	Moderately	Quite a bit	Extremely
□₁	□₂	□₃	□₄	□₅

9. **These questions are about how you feel and how things have been with you during the past 4 weeks.** For each question, please give the one answer that comes closest to the way you have been feeling. How much of the time during the past 4 weeks...

	All of the time	Most of the time	Some of the time	A little of the time	None of the time
a Did you feel full of life?	☐₁	☐₂	☐₃	☐₄	☐₅
b Have you been very nervous?	☐₁	☐₂	☐₃	☐₄	☐₅
c Have you felt so down in the dumps that nothing could cheer you up?	☐₁	☐₂	☐₃	☐₄	☐₅
d Have you felt calm and peaceful?	☐₁	☐₂	☐₃	☐₄	☐₅
e Did you have a lot of energy?	☐₁	☐₂	☐₃	☐₄	☐₅
f Have you felt downhearted and depressed?	☐₁	☐₂	☐₃	☐₄	☐₅
g Did you feel worn out?	☐₁	☐₂	☐₃	☐₄	☐₅
h Have you been happy?	☐₁	☐₂	☐₃	☐₄	☐₅
i Did you feel tired?	☐₁	☐₂	☐₃	☐₄	☐₅

10. **During the past 4 weeks, how much of the time has your physical health or emotional problems interfered with your social activities (like visiting friends, relatives, etc.)?**

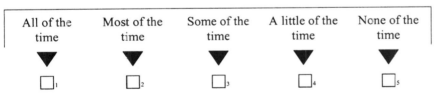

All of the time	Most of the time	Some of the time	A little of the time	None of the time
☐₁	☐₂	☐₃	☐₄	☐₅

11. How TRUE or FALSE is <u>each</u> of the following statements for you?

	Definitely true ▼	Mostly true ▼	Don't know ▼	Mostly false ▼	Definitely false ▼
a I seem to get sick a little easier than other people	☐1	☐2	☐3	☐4	☐5
b I am as healthy as anybody I know	☐1	☐2	☐3	☐4	☐5
c I expect my health to get worse	☐1	☐2	☐3	☐4	☐5
d My health is excellent	☐1	☐2	☐3	☐4	☐5

THANK YOU FOR COMPLETING THESE QUESTIONS!

HEARING

Hearing Handicap Inventory for the Elderly—Screening Version (HHIE-S)

	Yes (4)	Sometimes (2)	No (0)
Does a hearing problem cause you to feel embarrassed when meeting new people?	___	___	___
Does a hearing problem cause you to feel frustrated when talking to members of your family?	___	___	___
Do you have difficulty hearing when someone speaks in a whisper?	___	___	___
Do you feel handicapped by a hearing problem?	___	___	___
Does a hearing problem cause you difficulty when visiting friends, relatives, or neighbors?	___	___	___
Does a hearing problem cause you to attend religious services less often than you would like?	___	___	___
Does a hearing problem cause you to have arguments with family members?	___	___	___
Does a hearing problem cause you difficulty when listening to TV or radio?	___	___	___
Do you feel that any difficulty with your hearing limits or hampers your personal or social life?	___	___	___
Does a hearing problem cause you difficulty when in a restaurant with relatives or friends?	___	___	___

NOTE: Range of total points, 0–40; 0–8, no self-perceived handicap; 10–22, mild to moderate handicap; 24–40, significant handicap.

SOURCE: Ventry IM, Weinstein BE. Identification of elderly people with hearing problems. *Asha.* July 1983;25(7):37. Reprinted with permission from the American Speech-Language-Hearing Association.

HOME SAFETY

Checklist

Safety Item	Yes	No	Comment
1. Are emergency numbers kept by the phone and regularly updated?			
2. Do family members and other caregivers know how to report an emergency?			
3. Are patient, family, and caregivers aware of the dangers of smoking, especially in bed?			
4. If oxygen is used, do patient and caregivers know correct use of equipment, how to operate and clean it correctly?			
5. Are firearms stored unloaded and locked up?			
6. Are all poisons (medications, detergents, insecticides, cleaning fluids, polishes, etc.) kept out of reach of children and discarded when no longer needed?			
7. Is there a fire alarm and extinguisher? Do patient and caregivers know how to use it?			
8. Do the family and caregivers have an escape plan in case of fire or other disaster?			
9. Are throw rugs eliminated or fastened down?			
10. Are all electrical cords in working order, in the open, and not run under rugs or carpets or wrapped around nails?			
11. Are non-slip mats placed in bathtubs and showers?			
12. Are banisters or railings placed along stairways?			
13. Are stairs, halls, and doorways free of clutter?			
14. Are all steps and sidewalks clear of tools, toys, and other articles?			
15. Does adaptive or medical support equipment function adequately?			
16. Do patient and caregivers know safe and effective use of equipment?			
17. Do patient and caregivers know procedures to follow if equipment malfunctions?			

SOURCE: Ferrell BA. Home care. In: Cassel CK, Cohen HJ, Larson EB, et al., eds. *Geriatric Medicine*. 3rd ed. New York: Springer Verlag; 1997:115. ©Springer-Verlag. Reprinted with permission.

FUNCTIONAL ABILITIES

Functional Activities Questionnaire (FAQ)

The FAQ is an informant-based measure of functional abilities. Informants provide performance ratings of the target person on 10 complex, higher-order activities. For use, see "Dementia" (p 113).

Individual Items

1. Writing checks, paying bills, balancing checkbook.
2. Assembling tax records, business affairs, or papers.
3. Shopping alone for clothes, household necessities, or groceries.
4. Playing a game of skill, working on a hobby.
5. Heating water, making a cup of coffee, turning off stove.
6. Preparing a balanced meal.
7. Keeping track of current events.
8. Paying attention to, understanding, discussing TV, books, magazines.
9. Remembering appointments, family occasions, holidays, medications.
10. Traveling out of neighborhood, driving, arranging to take buses.

The levels of performance assigned ranged from dependent to independent and are rated as follows:

Dependent = 3
Requires assistance = 2
Has difficulty but does by self = 1
Normal = 0

Two other response options can also be scored:
Never did [the activity] but could do now = 0
Never did and would have difficulty now = 1

A total score for the FAQ is computed by simply summing the scores across the 10 items. Scores range from 0 to 30. A cutpoint of 9 (dependent in three or more activities) is recommended.

SOURCE: Pfeffer RI, Kurosaki TT, Harrah CH, et al. Measurement of functional activities of older adults in the community. *J Gerontol.* 1982;37(3):323–329. Copyright 1982, Gerontological Society of America. Reprinted with permission.

GERIATRIC SCREENING

Screening in Primary Care

Problem	Screening Measure	Positive Screen	Supporting Data
Vision	Two parts: Ask: "Do you have difficulty driving or watching television or reading or doing any of your daily activities because of your eyesight?" If yes, then: Test each eye with Snellen chart while patient wears corrective lenses (if applicable).	Yes to the question and inability to read greater than 20/40 on Snellen chart.	Question: derived from some of the most reliable items on the Boston Activities of Daily Vision Scale; test-retest reliability is 0.8; Snellen chart: gold standard.
Hearing	Use audioscope set at 40 dB. Test hearing using 1000 and 2000 Hz.	Inability to hear 1000 or 2000 Hz in both ears; or inability to hear frequencies in either ear.	In physicians' offices: sensitivity = 0.94; specificity = 0.72.
Leg mobility	Time the patient after asking: "Rise from the chair. Walk 10 feet (3 meters) briskly, turn, walk back to the chair and sit down."	Unable to complete task in 10 seconds.	Timed "Get Up & Go": inter-rater and test-retest reliability = 0.99; good correlations with other measures of gait and balance (0.6 to 0.8).
Urinary incontinence	Two parts: Ask: "In the past year, have you ever lost your urine and gotten wet?" If yes, then ask: "Have you lost urine on at least 6 separate days?"	Yes to both questions.	83% agreement between patient response and urologic assessment.
Nutrition, weight loss	Two parts Ask: "Have you lost 10 lbs. over the past 6 months without trying to do so?" Weigh the patient.	Yes to the question or weight < 100 lb.	Question: relative risk of death = 2.0* (NHEFS); weight: PPV of malnutrition = 0.99.
Memory	Three-item recall.	Unable to remember all three items after 1 minute.	Likelihood ratios for dementia: recalls all 3 = 0.06; recalls 2 = 0.5; recalls < 2 = 3.1.
Depression	Ask: "Do you often feel sad or depressed?"	Yes to the question.	Sensitivity = 0.78; specificity = 0.87.
Physical disability	Six questions: "Are you able to . . . "Do strenuous activities like fast walking or bicycling?" "Do heavy work around the house like washing windows, walls, or floors?" "Go shopping for groceries or clothes?" "Get to places out of walking distance?" "Bathe, either a sponge bath, tub bath, or shower?" "Dress, like putting on a shirt, buttoning and zipping, or putting on shoes?"	No to any of the questions.	Coefficient of reproducibility 0.96; test-retest reliability 0.88; good correlation with other measures of physical function = 0.63–0.89.

NOTE: NHEFS = National Health Epidemiologic Follow-up Study; PPV = positive predictive value.

SOURCE: Adapted with permission from Moore AA, Siu AL. Screening for common problems in ambulatory elderly: clinical confirmation of a screen instrument. *Am J Med.* 1996;100(4):440 (with personal communication from Tamara B. Harris, MD). Copyright 1996. Reprinted with permission from Excerpta Medica, Inc.

INCONTINENCE

Prevention and Management—Behavioral Treatment

Behavioral treatment for urinary incontinence depends on careful instruction of the patient. The following tools are examples of patient education materials for bladder training, bladder urge control, and pelvic muscle (Kegel's) exercises that have been found to be clinically useful. See "Urinary Incontinence" (p 134) for discussion of the use of behavioral approaches.

BLADDER TRAINING

Bladder training involves following a strict schedule for bathroom visits during the day. The schedule starts with bathroom visits every 2 hours or so, but the time between visits is gradually increased. The longer stretch of time between bathroom visits gives you increased bladder control and independence.

If you have a habit of using the bathroom more than once every 2 hours due to urgency—with or without urge incontinence—you may benefit from bladder training. Bladder training has been shown to be effective for both stress and urge incontinence.

Goals

Bladder training has several goals. It helps you

- Lengthen the amount of time between bathroom visits.
- Increase the amount of urine that the bladder can comfortably hold.
- Improve self-control over bladder urges by voiding on a schedule, not when the urge strikes.
- Reduce or eliminate incontinence.
- Increase independence in bladder management.

How To Do Bladder Training

Bladder training requires motivation for starting and maintaining a schedule for voids. Each week, as incontinence decreases, the schedule is changed slightly so that your bathroom visits occur less often. Bladder training will take between 6 and 8 weeks for success, but noticeable improvements will occur early in the program.

- Start with a Bladder Diary. Record your bathroom visits and urine leaks on the Bladder Diary for 48 hours. Measure the urine you produce during bathroom visits with a calibrated cup. This will help determine the amount of urine your bladder is able to hold.
- Review the Bladder Diary with your clinician, who will set a bladder training schedule according to the amount of time between your usual bathroom visits. For many people, the bathroom visits are scheduled for every 1-2 hours.
- For the first week, use the bathroom strictly according to the schedule. If a strong bladder urge strikes, use the Bladder Urge Control Procedure (below) to regain control and wait until the next scheduled time to void. If the urge is too strong and it cannot be entirely suppressed, use the bathroom, but then resume the bladder schedule
- Each week, increase the time between bathroom visits by 30 minutes, as tolerated. As incontinence decreases week by week, the schedule can be further increased. For many individuals, bathroom visits every 3 to 6 hours is desirable. For most older persons, every 3 to 4 hours is optimal.
- Monitor the number of urine leaks each day and for the entire week. Also monitor the amount of each leak. For example, a person may have 2 leaks a day, but instead of large leaks that saturate a pad, they are small dribbles that slightly dampen the pad. This is considered good improvement.
- If the number of urine leaks does not lessen in 1 week, then maintain the same bladder training schedule for another week. Adjust the schedule in the next week when urine leaks decrease.

BLADDER URGE CONTROL PROCEDURE

When a bladder urge strikes, you may be tempted to rush to the bathroom to prevent incontinence. This response can cause more harm than good, since the already overactive bladder becomes more stimulated and irritated with the rushed movement to the toilet. To get control over the bladder, practice the Bladder Control Procedure when the urge strikes. In this procedure, you

- Stand quietly or sit still. This prevents overstimulation of the bladder.
- Take slow, relaxed breaths.
- Contract the pelvic floor muscles repeatedly (see pelvic muscle exercises below). This helps keep the urethra closed to prevent urine from leaking. This also calms the bladder through special signals that are carried to the brain.
- Concentrate on making the urge go away. Use mental imagery and self-talk to help suppress the urge. Think to yourself, "I am in control of my bladder and this bladder has one job only and that is to hold urine until I am ready to go to the toilet." Imagine the urge as a wave that has peaked and now is fading away.
- Use mental distraction to reduce the awareness of the discomfort of the urge. Hum a tune or do mathematical calculations (subtract 7 from 100, then continue subtracting 7).
- When the urge subsides, do not use the toilet until the next scheduled void.
- If the urge does not completely subside, you may use the toilet.

When used with every urge, this procedure becomes more effective and gives you greater control over your bladder. Be encouraged by even small improvements in your symptoms. Although progress may seem slow, you are developing entirely new habits for bladder control. These healthy bladder habits will remain an important part of your life style. This takes both time and patience, but the rewards are worth the effort.

PELVIC MUSCLE (KEGEL'S) EXERCISES

Pelvic muscles, like other muscles, can become weak or damaged. Pelvic muscle exercises strengthen weak muscles around the bladder.

- Start by doing your pelvic muscle exercises 3 to 4 times each week. Usually it takes about 10 minutes to do the exercises. Your clinician will give you exact instructions about how many times you should perform the exercises and the number of times a day.
- Practice anywhere and any time. It is usually best to begin practicing them when lying on your bed. Once you have mastered the exercises lying down, practice them sitting in a chair. Then advance to practicing them standing. Soon you will be able to do them anywhere.
- Never use your stomach, thigh, or buttock muscles. To find out whether you are also contracting your stomach muscles, place your hand on your abdomen while you squeeze your pelvic muscle. If you feel your abdomen move, then you are also using these muscles.
- Avoid holding your breath. Inhale and exhale slowly while counting. In time, you will learn to practice effortlessly.
- If you forget to do your exercises for several days, do not be discouraged. When you have realized you have forgotten, begin your program again as instructed. Do not try to make up for lost days by doing more exercises or you will have sore muscles.

After 4 to 6 weeks of following your prescribed exercise routine, you will begin to notice that you are having fewer urinary accidents. After 3 months, you will see an even bigger difference. It may help to keep a diary of the times you practice your exercises and the times that you leak urine. This will give you a picture of the progress you are making. If you are having problems, your clinician may suggest biofeedback, weighted vaginal cones, or electrostimulation to help you with pelvic muscle exercises.

SOURCE: Adapted from Busby-Whitehead J, Kinkade J, Granville L. *Urinary Incontinence: Management in Primary Practice.* Tool Kit 2, Practicing Physician Education Project, Robinson BE, ed. New York: The John A. Hartford Foundation and The American Geriatrics Society; 2000. Reprinted with permission.

MOBILITY AND MOVEMENT

Abnormal Involuntary Movement Scale (AIMS)

Examination Procedure

Either before or after completing the Examination Procedure, observe the patient unobtrusively, at rest (eg, in waiting room).

The chair to be used in this examination should be a hard, firm one without arms.

1. Ask patient to remove shoes and socks.
2. Ask patient whether there is anything in his/her mouth (ie, gum, candy, etc.) and if there is, to remove it.
3. Ask patient about the **current** condition of his/her teeth. Ask patient if he/she wears dentures. Do teeth or dentures bother patient **now**?
4. Ask patient whether he/she notices any movements in mouth, face, hands, or feet. If yes, ask to describe and to what extent they **currently** bother patient or interfere with his/her activities.
5. Have patient sit in chair with hands on knees, legs slightly apart, and feet flat on floor. (Look at entire body for movements while in this position.)
6. Ask patient to sit with hands hanging unsupported. If male, between legs, if female and wearing a dress, hanging over knees. (Observe hands and other body areas.)
7. Ask patient to open mouth. (Observe tongue at rest within mouth.) Do this twice.
8. Ask patient to protrude tongue. (Observe abnormalities of tongue movement.) Do this twice.
9. Ask patient to tap thumb with each finger as rapidly as possible for 10–15 seconds; separately with right hand, then with left hand. (Observe facial and leg movements.)
10. Flex and extend patient's left and right arms (one at a time). (Note any rigidity.)
11. Ask patient to stand up. (Observe in profile. Observe all body areas again, hips included.)
12. Ask patient to extend both arms outstretched in front with palms down. (Observe trunk, legs, and mouth.)
13. Have patient walk a few paces, turn, and walk back to chair. (Observe hands and gait.) Do this twice.

Instructions: Complete examination procedure before making ratings. Rate highest severity observed.

Code:
1 = None
2 = Minimal, may be extreme normal
3 = Mild
4 = Moderate
5 = Severe

Facial and Oral Movements

1. Muscles of facial expression (eg, movements of forehead, eyebrows, periorbital area, cheeks; including frowning, blinking, smiling, grimacing)

   1 2 3 4 5

2. Lips and perioral area (eg, puckering, pouting, smacking)

   1 2 3 4 5

3. Jaw (eg, biting, clenching, chewing, mouth opening, lateral movement)

4. Tongue (rate only increase in movement both in and out of mouth, NOT inability to sustain movement)

   1 2 3 4 5

Extremity Movements

5. Upper (arms, wrists, hands, fingers). Include choreic movements (ie, rapid, objectively purposeless, irregular, spontaneous), athetoid movements (ie, slow, irregular, complex, serpentine). Do NOT include tremor (ie, repetitive, regular, rhythmic).

   1 2 3 4 5

6. Lower (legs, knees, ankles, toes). (Eg, lateral knee movement, foot tapping, heel dropping, foot squirming, inversion and eversion of foot.)

   1 2 3 4 5

Trunk Movements

7. Neck, shoulders, hips (eg, rocking, twisting, squirming, pelvic gyrations)

    1 2 3 4 5

Global Judgments

8. Severity of abnormal movements:
    1   None, normal
    2   Minimal
    3   Mild
    4   Moderate
    5   Severe

9. Incapacitation due to abnormal movements
    1   None, normal
    2   Minimal
    3   Mild
    4   Moderate
    5   Severe

10. Patient's awareness of abnormal movements (rate only patient's report)
    1   No awareness
    2   Aware, no distress
    3   Aware, mild distress
    4   Aware, moderate distress
    5   Aware, severe distress

Dental Status

11. Current problems with teeth and/or dentures
    1   No
    2   Yes

12. Does patient usually wear dentures?
    1   No
    2   Yes

SOURCE: Adapted from Department of Health and Human Services, Public Health Service, Alcohol, Drug Abuse and Mental Health Administration, National Institute of Mental Health. *Treatment Strategies in Schizophrenia Study.* ADM-117. Revised 1985.

Performance-Oriented Mobility Assessment (POMA)

BALANCE

Chair

Instructions: Place a hard, armless chair against a wall. The following maneuvers are tested.

1. Sitting down
    0 = unable without help *or* collapses (plops) into chair *or* lands off center of chair
    1 = able and does not meet criteria for 0 or 2
    2 = sits in a smooth, safe motion *and* ends with buttocks against back of chair and thighs centered on chair

2. Sitting balance
    0 = unable to maintain position (marked slide forward or leans forward or to side)
    1 = leans in chair slightly or slight increased distance from buttocks to back of chair
    2 = steady, safe, upright

3. Arising
    0 = unable without help or loses balance or requires > three attempts
    1 = able but requires three attempts
    2 = able in ≤ two attempts

4. Immediate standing balance (first 5 seconds)
    0 = unsteady, marked staggering, moves feet, marked trunk sway or grabs object for support
    1 = steady but uses walker or cane *or* mild staggering but catches self without grabbing object
    2 = steady without walker or cane or other support

Stand

5a. Side-by-side standing balance
    0 = unable *or* unsteady *or* holds ≤ 3 seconds
    1 = able *but* uses cane, walker, or other support *or* holds for 4–9 seconds
    2 = narrow stance without support for 10 seconds
5b. Timing ____ ____ . ____ seconds
6. Pull test (subject at maximum position attained in 5, examiner stands behind and exerts mild pull-back at waist)
    0 = begins to fall
    1 = takes more than two steps back
    2 = fewer than two steps backward and steady
7a. Able to stand on right leg unsupported
    0 = unable *or* holds onto any objects *or* able for < 3 seconds
    1 = able for 3 or 4 seconds
    2 = able for 5 seconds
7b. Timing ____ ____ . ____ seconds
8a. Able to stand on left leg unsupported
    0 = unable *or* holds onto any object *or* able for < 3 seconds
    1 = able for 3 or 4 seconds
    2 = able for 5 seconds
8b. Timing ____ ____ . ____ seconds
9a. Semi-tandem stand
    0 = unable to stand with one foot half in front of other with feet touching *or* begins to fall *or* holds for ≤ 3 seconds
    1 = able for 4 to 9 seconds
    2 = able to semi-tandem stand for 10 seconds
9b. Timing ____ ____ . ____ seconds
10a. Tandem stand
    0 = unable to stand with one foot in front of other *or* begins to fall *or* holds for ≤ 3 seconds
    1 = able for 4 to 9 seconds
    2 = able to tandem stand for 10 seconds
10b. Timing ____ ____ . ____ seconds

11. Bending over (to pick up a pen off floor)
    0 = unable *or* is unsteady
    1 = able, but requires more than one attempt to get up
    2 = able and is steady
12. Toe stand
    0 = unable
    1 = able but < 3 seconds
    2 = able for 3 seconds
13. Heel stand
    0 = unable
    1 = able but < 3 seconds
    2 = able for 3 seconds

GAIT

Instructions: Person stands with examiner and then walks down 10-foot walkway (measured). Ask the person to walk down walkway, turn, and walk back. The person should use customary walking aid.

Bare Floor (flat, even surface)

1. Type of surface: 1 = linoleum or tile; 2 = wood; 3 = cement or concrete; 4 = other [not included in scoring]
2. Initiation of gait (immediately after told to "go")
    0 = any hesitancy or multiple attempts to start
    1 = no hesitancy
3. Path (estimated in relation to tape measure). Observe excursion of foot closest to tape measure over middle 8 feet of course.
    0 = marked deviation
    1 = mild or moderate deviation *or* uses walking aid
    2 = straight without walking aid
4. Missed step (trip or loss of balance)
    0 = yes, and would have fallen *or* more than two missed steps
    1 = yes, but appropriate attempt to recover *and* no more than two missed steps
    2 = none
5. Turning (while walking)
    0 = almost falls
    1 = mild staggering, but catches self, uses walker or cane
    2 = steady, without walking aid
6. Step over obstacles (to be assessed in a separate walk with two shoes placed on course 4 feet apart)
    0 = begins to fall at any obstacle *or* unable *or* walks around any obstacle *or* > two missed steps
    1 = able to step over all obstacles, but some staggering and catches self *or* one to two missed steps
    2 = able and steady at stepping over all four obstacles with no missed steps

SOURCE: Courtesy of Mary E. Tinetti, MD. Adapted with permission.

NICHE READY SHEET

When you begin to think about doing NICHE, please consider the following questions:

1. Does your hospital have a vision or goal for the kind of care it wants to provide to its older patients?

2. Is your hospital receptive to collaborating with experts in geriatric care and other hospitals to improve care for older adults?

3. Is your hospital willing to undertake a period of self-assessment that will lead to quality improvements in geriatric care?

4. Is hospital management committed to improving geriatric care?

5. Is hospital management willing to dedicate the resources to carry out the changes necessary to improve geriatric care?

6. Are staff at the hospital willing to dedicate the time necessary to adapt innovations in geriatric care to make them their own?

7. Do you have a geriatric nurse specialist on staff who could help develop and deliver continuing education programs?

8. Is there a staff person willing to take on day-to-day management of a new program in geriatric care?

9. Do you have a quality improvement program that involves the individuals who provide clinical care?

10. Has your hospital begun a program that examines care for a specific population? If so, was it successful?

SOURCE: Reprinted with permission. The John A. Hartford Foundation Institute for Geriatric Nursing; 2002.

NUTRITION SCREENING

DETERMINE Your Nutritional Health Checklist

The nutrition screen is based on these warning signs of poor nutrition:

Disease
Eating poorly
Tooth loss, mouth pain
Economic hardship
Reduced social contact
Multiple medicines
Involuntary weight loss or gain
Need for assistance in self-care
Elderly (age > 80)

The mnemonic DETERMINE represents the warning signs and the questions in the screen.

Read the statements below. Circle the number in the "YES" column for those that apply to you or someone under your care. For each "YES" answer, score the number in the box. Total your nutrition score.

	YES
1. I have an illness or condition that made me change the kind and/or amount of food I eat.	2
2. I eat fewer than 2 meals per day.	3
3. I eat few fruits or vegetables, or milk products.	2
4. I have 3 or more drinks of beer, liquor, or wine almost every day.	2
5. I have tooth or mouth problems that make it hard for me to eat.	2
6. I don't always have enough money to buy the food I need.	4
7. I eat alone most of the time.	1
8. I take 3 or more different prescribed or over-the-counter drugs a day.	1
9. Without wanting to, I have lost or gained 10 pounds in the last 6 months.	2
10. I am not always physically able to shop, cook, and/or feed myself.	2
TOTAL: _____	

NOTE: Scoring: 0–2 = good; 3–5 = moderate nutritional risk; 6 or more = high nutritional risk.

SOURCE: Reprinted with permission of the Nutrition Screening Initiative, a project of the American Academy of Family Physicians and The American Dietetic Association, funded in part by a grant from Ross Products Division, Abbott Laboratories Inc.

PAIN MANAGEMENT

Systemic Pharmacotherapy for Persistent Pain Management (oral dosing unless otherwise specified)

Drug	Starting Dose	Usual Effective Dose (Maximum Dose)	Titration	Comments
NON-OPIOIDS				
Acetaminophen (Tylenol)	325 mg q 4h–500 mg q 6 h	2–4 g/24 h (4 g/24 h)	after 4–6 doses	Reduce maximum dose 50%–75% in patients with hepatic insufficiency; hx of alcohol abuse
Choline magnesium trisalicylate (Tricosal, Trilisate)	500–750 mg q 8 h	2,000–3,000 mg/24 h (same)	after 4–6 doses	Long half-life may allow qd or bid dosing after steady state is reached
Salsalate (e.g., Disalcid, Mono-Gesic, Salflex)	500–750 mg q 12 h	1,500–3,000 mg/24 h (3000 mg/24 h)	after 4–6 doses	In frail patients or those with diminished hepatic or renal function, it may be important to check salicylate levels during dose titration and after reaching steady state
Celecoxib (Celebrex)	100 mg bid or 200 qd	200 mg/24 h (400 mg/24 h)	after 2–3 days	Higher doses may be associated with a higher incidence of GI side effects; patients with indications for cardio-protective ASA require aspirin supplement
Rofecoxib (Vioxx)	12.5 mg qd	25 mg/24 h (50 mg/24 h)	after 2–3 days	Higher doses may be associated with a higher incidence of GI side effects; patients with indications for cardio-protective ASA require aspirin supplement
Valdecoxib (Bextra)	10 mg bid	20 mg/24 h (40 mg/24 h)		Higher doses may be associated with a higher incidence of GI side effects; patients with indications for cardio-protective ASA require aspirin supplement
Corticosteroids (prednisone) (e.g., Deltasone, Liquid Pred, Orasone)	5.0 mg qd	variable (NA)	after 2–3 doses	Use lowest possible dose to prevent chronic steroid effects; anticipate fluid retention and glycemic effects
Tricyclic antidepressants*; desipramine (Norpramin), nortriptyline (Aventyl, Pamelor)	10 mg hs	25–100 mg hs (variable)	after 3–5 days	Significant risk of adverse effects in older patients, anticholinergic effects
Anticonvulsants —carbamazepine (Tegretol)	100 mg qd	800–1,200 mg/24 h (2,400 mg/day)	after 3–5 days	Monitor LFTs, CBC, BUN/Creat., electrolytes
—chlonazepam (Klonopin)	0.25–0.5 mg hs	0.05–0.2 mg/kg/day (20 mg)	after 3–5 days	Monitor sedation, memory, CBC
—gabapentin (Neurontin)	100 mg hs	300–900 mg tid (3,600)	after 1–2 days	Monitor sedation, ataxia, edema
Mexiletine (Mexitil)	150 mg	150 mg tid–qid (variable)	after 3–5 days	Avoid use in patients with conduction block, bradyarrhythmia; monitor ECG
Baclofen (Lioresal)	5 mg	5–20mg bid–tid 200 mg	after 3–5 days	Monitor muscle weakness, urinary function; avoid abrupt discontinuation because of CNS irritability

Systemic Pharmacotherapy for Persistent Pain Management (oral dosing unless otherwise specified) (continued)

Drug	Starting Dose	Usual Effective Dose (Maximum Dose)	Titration	Comments
OPIOIDS				
Tramadol (Ultram)	25 mg q 4–6 h	50~100 mg (300 mg/24 h)	after 4–6 doses	Mixed opioid and central neurotransmitter mechanism of action; monitor for opioid side effects, including drowsiness and nausea
Hydrocodone (e.g., Lorcet, Lortab, Vicodin, Vicoprofen)	5 mg q 4–6 h	5–10 mg (see comments)	after 3–4 doses	Useful for acute recurrent, episodic, or breakthrough pain; daily dose limited by fixed-dose combinations with acetaminophen or NSAIDs
Oxycodone, immediate release (OxyIR)	5 mg q 4–6 h	5–10 mg (see comments)	after 3–4 doses	Useful for acute recurrent, episodic, or breakthrough pain; daily dose limited by fixed-dose combinations with acetaminophen or NSAIDs
Oxycodone, sustained release (OxyContin)	10 mg q 12 h	variable (variable)	after 3–5 days	Usually started after initial dose determined by effects of immediate-release opioid
Morphine, immediate release (e.g., MSIR, Roxanol)	2.5–10 mg q 4 h	variable (variable)	after 1–2 doses	Oral liquid concentrate recommended for breakthrough pain
Morphine, sustained release[†] (e.g., MSContin, Kadian, Avinza)	15 mg q 12 h 20 mg q 24 h	variable (variable)	after 3–5 days	Usually started after initial dose determined by effects of immediate-release opioid; toxic metabolites of morphine may limit usefulness in patients with renal insufficiency or when high-dose therapy is required; continuous-release formulations may require more frequent dosing if end-of-dose failure occurs regularly
Hydromorphone (Dilaudid, Hydrostat)	2 mg q 3–4 h	variable (variable)	after 3–4 doses	For breakthrough pain or for around-the-clock dosing; a sustained-release formulation is currently under FDA review
Transdermal fentanyl (Duragesic)	25 µg/h patch q 72 h	variable (variable)	after 2–3 patch changes	Usually started after initial dose determined by effects of immediate-release opioid; currently available lowest dose patch (25 µg/h) recommended for patients who require 60 mg per 24-h oral morphine equivalents; peak effects of first dose takes 18–24 h. Duration of effect is usually 3 days, but may range from 48 h to 96 h

NOTE: ASA = acetylsalicylic acid; BUN = blood urea nitrogen; CBC = complete blood cell count; CNS = central nervous system; Creat. = serum creatinine; CV = cardiovascular; ECG = electrocardiogram; FDA = U.S. Food and Drug Administration; GI = gastrointestinal; hx = history; LFT = liver function test; NA = not applicable; NSAIDs = nonsteroidal antiinflammatory drugs; hs = bedtime; qd = daily; bid = twice daily; tid = three times daily.

* Amitriptyline is not recommended.

† Different formulations have different dosages and durations of action.

SOURCE: AGS Panel on Persistent Pain in Older Persons. The management of persistent pain in older persons. *J Am Geriatr Soc.* 2002;50:S205–S224. Adapted with permission.

PRESSURE ULCERS
Braden Scale for Predicting Pressure Sore Risk

Patient's Name _____ Evaluator's Name _____ Date of Assessment

Sensory Perception Ability to respond meaningfully to pressure-related discomfort	**1. Completely limited:** Unresponsive (does not moan, flinch, or grasp) to painful stimuli because of diminished level of consciousness or sedation OR limited ability to feel pain over most of body surface.	**2. Very limited:** Responds only to painful stimuli; cannot communicate discomfort except by moaning or restlessness OR has a sensory impairment that limits the ability to feel pain or discomfort over ½ of body.	**3. Slightly limited:** Responds to verbal commands, but cannot always communicate discomfort or need to be turned OR has some sensory impairment that limits ability to feel pain or discomfort in 1 or 2 extremities.	**4. No impairment:** Responds to verbal commands. Has no sensory deficit that would limit ability to feel or voice pain or discomfort.
Moisture Degree to which skin is exposed to moisture	**1. Constantly moist:** Skin is kept moist almost constantly by perspiration, urine, etc. Dampness is detected every time patient is moved or turned.	**2. Very moist:** Skin is often, but not always moist. Linen must be changed at least once a shift.	**3. Occasionally moist:** Skin is occasionally moist, requiring an extra linen change approximately once a day.	**4. Rarely moist:** Skin is usually dry; linen only requires changing at routine intervals.
Activity Degree of physical activity	**1. Bedfast:** Confined to bed	**2. Chairfast:** Ability to walk severely limited or nonexistent. Cannot bear own weight and/or must be assisted into chair or wheelchair.	**3. Walks occasionally:** Walks occasionally during day, but for very short distances, with or without assistance. Spends majority of each shift in bed or chair.	**4. Walks frequently:** Walks outside the room at least twice a day and inside room at least once every 2 hours during waking hours.
Mobility Ability to change and control body position	**1. Completely immobile:** Does not make even slight changes in body or extremity position without assistance.	**2. Very limited:** Makes occasional slight changes in body or extremity position but unable to make frequent or significant changes independently.	**3. Slightly limited:** Makes frequent though slight changes in body or extremity position independently.	**4. No limitation:** Makes major and frequent changes in position without assistance.
Nutrition *Usual* food intake pattern	**1. Very poor:** Never eats a complete meal. Rarely eats more than ⅓ of any food offered. Eats 2 servings or less protein (meat or dairy products) per day. Takes fluids poorly. Does not take a liquid dietary supplement OR is NPO and/or maintained on clear liquids or IVs for more than 5 days.	**2. Probably inadequate:** Rarely eats a complete meal and generally eats only about ½ of any food offered. Protein intake includes only 3 servings of meat or dairy products per day. Occasionally will take a dietary supplement OR receives less than optimum amount of liquid diet or tube feeding.	**3. Adequate:** Eats over half of most meals. Eats a total of 4 servings of protein (meat, dairy products) each day. Occasionally will refuse a meal, but will usually take a supplement if offered OR is on a tube feeding or TPN regimen that probably meets most of nutritional needs.	**4. Excellent:** Eats most of every meal. Never refuses a meal. Usually eats a total of 4 or more servings of meat and dairy products. Occasionally eats between meals. Does not require supplementation.

Friction and Shear	1. Problem:	2. Potential problem:	3. No apparent problem
Requires moderate to maximum assistance in moving. Complete lifting without sliding against sheets is impossible. Frequently slides down in bed or chair, requiring frequent repositioning with maximum assistance. Spasticity, contractures, or agitation leads to almost constant friction.	Moves feebly or requires minimum assistance. During a move skin probably slides to some extent against sheets, chair, restraints, or other devices. Maintains relatively good position in chair or bed most of the time but occasionally slides down.	Moves in bed and in chair independently and has sufficient muscle strength to lift up completely during move. Maintains good position in bed or chair at all times.	

Total Score

NOTE: IVs = intravenous fluids; NPO = nothing by mouth; TPN = total parenteral nutrition.

SOURCE: © Copyright Barbara Braden and Nancy Bergstrom, 1988. Reproduced by permission. For additional information on administration and scoring, refer to the following: Braden BJ, Bergstrom N. Clinical utility of the Braden Scale for Predicting Pressure Sore Risk. *Decubitus.* 1989;2(3):44–51.

The Pressure Ulcer Scale for Healing (PUSH)

Patient Name, ID#: _____

Ulcer Location: _____

Date: _____

Directions: Observe and measure the pressure ulcer. Categorize the ulcer with respect to surface area, exudate, and appearance, and record in the column labeled "Ulcer Category." Multiply the Ulcer Category times the appropriate Weight Factor for each subscale and record in the column labeled "Weighted Sub-Score." Add the Weighted Sub-Scores to obtain the Total Score. A comparison of Total Scores measured over time provides an indication of the improvement or deterioration in pressure ulcer healing.

Surface Area	1 < 0.3 cm^2	2 0.3–0.9 cm^2	3 1.0–1.9 cm^2	4 2.0–5.0 cm^2	5 > 5.0 cm^2	Ulcer Category (1–5) _____	Weight Factor $\times 2$	Weighted Sub-Score _____
Exudate	1 $\leq \frac{1}{4}$	2 $\frac{1}{4}$ to $\frac{1}{2}$	3 $\frac{1}{2}$ to $\frac{3}{4}$	4 $> \frac{3}{4}$		Ulcer Category (1–4) _____	Weight Factor $\times 3$	Weighted Sub-Score _____
Appearance (predominant tissue)	1 epithelial	2 granulation	3 slough	4 necrotic eschar		Ulcer Category (1–4) _____	Weight Factor $\times 3$	Weighted Sub-Score _____
							Total Score	

Surface Area: Measure the greatest length (head to toe) and the greatest width (side to side) using a centimeter ruler. Multiply these two measurements (length × width) to obtain the surface area in square centimeters (cm^2). **Caveat:** Do not guess! Always use a centimeter ruler and the same method each time the ulcer is measured.

Exudate: Estimate the portion of the pressure-ulcer bed covered by drainage following removal of all dressings, but prior to any cleansing. Divide the ulcer into four imaginary quadrants, each representing about ¼ of the ulcer surface. Estimate the portion of the ulcer covered by exudate.

Appearance: Divide the pressure ulcer into four imaginary quadrants, each representing about ¼ of the original ulcer surface. Estimate the portion or amount of each tissue type on the ulcer. Identify the predominant tissue type on the ulcer and record the predominant tissue type in the space provided.

    Epithelial tissue: New pink or red skin that covers the original ulcer surface, growing in at the edges or in spots on the ulcer surface.

    Granulation tissue: Pink or beefy red tissue with a shiny, moist, granular appearance.

    Slough: Yellow or white tissue that adheres to the ulcer bed in strings or thick clumps.

    Necrotic eschar: Black or brown tissue that adheres firmly to the wound bed or ulcer edges and may be either firmer or softer than surrounding skin.

Pressure Ulcer Healing Chart

(use a separate page for each pressure ulcer)

Patient Name, ID#: _____

Ulcer Location: _____

Date: _____

Directions: Observe and measure pressure ulcer wounds at regular intervals using the PUSH scale. Date and record PUSH Weighted Sub-scale and Total Scores on the Pressure Ulcer Healing Record below.

PRESSURE ULCER HEALING RECORD															
DATE															
Surface Area															
Exudate															
Appearance															
Total Score															

Graph the PUSH Total Score on the Pressure Ulcer Healing Graph below.

PUSH Total Score	PRESSURE ULCER HEALING GRAPH														
34															
31															
29															
26															
23															
20															
17															
14															
11															
Healed 8															
DATE															

SOURCE: © 1997 National Pressure Ulcer Advisory Board. www.npuap.org. Reprinted with permission.

RESOURCES

What Can You Find on the AGS Website?
http://www.americangeriatrics.org
e-mail: info.amger@americangeriatrics.org

- **What is the American Geriatrics Society?** AGS mission and goals, current activities, history, AGS staff/contact information, list of Board of Directors and Committee Chairs and their affiliations.

- **Membership Opportunities and Benefits**. Includes a membership application, change-of-address form, order form for the Membership Directory, and a **Members Only** section that offers special resources and opportunities exclusively to AGS members.

- Complete list of AGS publications, including the *Geriatrics Review Syllabus: A Core Curriculum in Geriatric Medicine (GRS)*, and *Geriatrics At Your Fingertips*, a comprehensive clinical guide to the diseases and disorders that most commonly affect older adults. Other publications include the *Journal of the American Geriatrics Society*, the *Annals of Long-Term Care: Clinical Care and Aging*, the *AGS Newsletter*, and full-text versions of **AGS Position Papers, Statements, and Guidelines.**

- **Geriatrics Training Initiatives**–an overview of three AGS/John A. Hartford Foundation special initiatives that promote geriatrics to a much larger audience.

- **Professional Education** opportunities, including information on the **Geriatrics Recognition Award (GRA)**, and listings of continuing education courses and AGS co-sponsored events.

- **Consumer Education**–includes a series of **Patient Education Forums (PEFs)** that address common health problems facing older adults, and information on *The American Geriatrics Society's Complete Guide to Aging & Health*, the Society's comprehensive "public book."

- **Public Policy**–an overview of AGS public policy and legislative activities.

- **Council of State Affiliates Representatives (COSAR)**–AGS state affiliates promote geriatrics at the local level.

- **Links** to dozens of aging/health/education-related web sites.

- **AGS/AFAR Annual Meeting**–program and hotel information.

- **Junior Faculty Development Opportunities**–the Pfizer/FHA Postdoctoral Fellowships for Research on Health Outcomes in Geriatrics, additional junior faculty award opportunities, and links to other valuable resources.

- **Directory of Geriatrics Health Care Services Managed Care Directory**–a resource of AGS members currently responsible for geriatrics programs in managed care organizations.

- **AGS/Pfizer Managed Care Report** order form for expert panel's report on ways managed care organizations (MCOs) could improve the delivery of quality healthcare to older adults

- **AGS Website Assessment Survey** for health care professionals and the general public.

Directory of Agencies and Organizations for Geriatric Clinicians

While this list represents a comprehensive guide to organizations that address the clinical care needs of older people, it is not a resource of all social service agencies and organizations assisting older citizens. If you have questions that do not specifically relate to one of the following organizations, please contact your state and/or area agency on aging as listed by the Administration on Aging (AOA). These agencies provide information on, and refer callers to, local services for senior citizens. To locate state and area agencies on aging, visit the AOA website at http://www.aoa.dhhs.gov/agingsites/state.html or call the Eldercare Locator service (1-800-677-1116) operated by the National Association of Area Agencies on Aging.

Note: The organizations on this list are arranged in categories in the following order:

- *GENERAL AGING*
- *END-OF-LIFE ISSUES*
- *EDUCATION*
- *LEGAL ISSUES AND ELDER ABUSE*
- *RESOURCES ON SPECIFIC HEALTH PROBLEMS:*

Cancer	Neurologic Problems
Diabetes Mellitus	Nutritional Concerns
Digestive Problems	Pain
Head and Neck Problems	Psychological Problems
Hearing Problems	Sexuality and Sexual Concerns
Heart and Circulation Problems	Sight Problems
Joint, Muscle, and Bone Problems	Skin Problems
Lung and Breathing Problems	Urinary Problems
Memory and Thinking Problems	

GENERAL AGING

Administration on Aging
330 Independence Avenue, SW
Washington, DC 20201
Tel: (202) 619-0724
Fax: (202) 401-7620
Website: http://www.aoa.gov
E-Mail: aoainfo@aoa.gov

National Aging Information Center (NAIC)
(A Service of the Administration on Aging)
330 Independence Avenue, SW, Room 4656
Washington, DC 20201
Telephone: (202) 619-7501
TTY: (202) 401-7575
Fax: (202) 401-7620
Website: http://www.aoa.gov/naic
E-Mail: naic@aoa.gov

Agency for Health Care Research and Quality (AHRQ), formerly the Agency for Health Care Policy and Research
Clinical Practice Guidelines
Government Printing Office
Superintendent of Documents
Washington, DC 20402
Tel: (202) 512-1800
On-line retrieval:
http://www.ahrq.gov

Aging Network Services
4400 East-West Hwy.
Bethesda, MD 20814
Tel: (301) 657-4329
Fax: (301) 657-3250
Website: http://www.agingnets.com
E-Mail: ans@agingnets.com

Alliance for Aging Research
2021 K Street, NW, Suite 305
Washington, DC 20006
Tel: (202) 293-2856
Fax: (202) 785-8574
Website: www.agingresearch.org

American Academy of Home Care Physicians
PO Box 1037
Edgewood, MD 21040
Tel: (410) 676-7966
Fax: (410) 676-7980
Website: www.aahcp.org
E-Mail: aahcp@mindspring.com

American Association of Homes & Services for the Aging
901 E Street, NW, Suite 500
Washington, DC 20004-2011
Tel: (202) 783-2242
Fax: (202) 783-2255
Website: www.aahsa.org
E-Mail: info@aahsa.org

American Association of Retired Persons
601 E Street, NW
Washington, DC 20049
Tel: (800)424-3410
Website: www.aarp.org
E-Mail: member@aarp.org

American College of Health Care
  Administrators
1800 Diagonal Road
Suite 355
Alexandria, VA 22314
Tel: (703) 549-5822
Fax: (703) 739-7901
Toll Free: (888) 888-ACHCA
  (22422)
Website: www.achca.org
E-Mail: info@achca.org

American Federation for Aging
  Research
1414 Avenue of the Americas
New York, NY 10019
Tel: (212) 752-2327
Fax: (212) 832-2298
Website: www.afar.org
E-Mail: amfedaging@aol.com

American Geriatrics Society
The Empire State Building
350 Fifth Avenue, Suite 801
New York, NY 10118
Tel: (212) 308-1414
Fax: (212) 832-8646
Website: www.americangeriatrics.org
E-Mail:
info.amger@americangeriatrics.org

American Health Care Association
1201 L Street, NW
Washington, DC 20005
Tel: (202) 842-4444
Fax: (202) 842-3860
Toll Free for Publications Only
  (800) 321-0343
Website: www.ahca.org

American Hospital Association
1 North Franklin
Chicago, IL 60606
Tel: (312) 422-3000
Fax: (312) 422-4796
Website: www.aha.org

American Medical Directors
  Association
10480 Patuxent Parkway, Suite 760
Columbia, MD 21044
Tel: (410) 740-9743
Toll Free: (800) 876-2632
Fax: (410) 740-4572
Website: www.amda.com

American Occupational Therapy
  Association
PO Box 31220
Bethesda, MD 20824-1220
Tel: (301) 652-2682
Fax: (301) 652-7711
Website: www.aota.org

American Red Cross
Attn: Public Inquiry Office
431 18th Street NW
Washington, DC 20006
Tel: (202) 639-3520
Website: www.redcross.org

American Senior Fitness Association
PO Box 2575
New Smyrna Beach, FL 32170
Tel: (904) 423-6634
Fax: (904) 427-0613
Website: www.seniorfitness.net
E-Mail: sfa@ucnsb.net

American Seniors Housing
  Association
1850 M Street, NW, Suite 540
Washington, DC 20036
Tel: (202) 974-2300
Fax: (202) 775-0112
Website: www.nmhc.org
E-Mail: info@nmhc.org

American Social Health Association

Hotlines under the auspices of
  the ASHA
CDC National AIDS Hotline
  (English)-Toll Free (800)
  342-AIDS
CDC National AIDS Hotline
  (Spanish)-Toll Free: (800)
  344-7432
CDC National AIDS Hotline- TTY
  Toll Free: (800) 243-7889
CDC National STD Hotline- Toll
  Free: (800) 227-8922
CDC National Immunization
  Information Hotline-Toll Free
  (800) 232-2522
Website: www.ashastd.org

American Society on Aging
833 Market Street, Suite 511
San Francisco, CA 94103-1824
Tel: (415) 974-9600
Fax: (415) 974-0300
Website: www.asaging.org
E-Mail: info@asaging.org

American Society of Consultant
  Pharmacists
1321 Duke Street
Alexandria, VA 22314-3516
Tel: (703) 739-1300
Fax: (703) 739-1321
Toll Free Tel: (800) 355-2727
Toll Free Fax: (800) 707-ASCP
Fast Fax: (800) 220-1321
Website: www.ascp.com
E-Mail: info@ascp.com

Assisted Living Federation of
  America
10300 Eaton Place, Suite 400
Fairfax, VA 22030
Tel: (703) 691-8100
Fax: (703) 691-8106
Website: www.alfa.org
E-Mail: info@alfa.org

B'nai B'rith
1640 Rhode Island Avenue, NW
Washington, DC 20036-3278
Tel: (202) 857-6600
Fax: (202) 857-1099
Toll Free: (888) 388-4224
Senior Housing
Tel: (202) 857-6581
Fax: (202) 857-0980
E-Mail: senior@bnaibrith.org

Catholic Charities
1731 King Street, Suite 200
Alexandria, VA 22314
Tel: (703) 549-1390
Fax: (703) 549-1656
Website:
www.catholiccharitiesusa.org

Children of Aging Parents
1609 Woodbourne Road
Suite 302-A
Levittown, PA 19057
Tel: (215) 945-6900
Fax: (215) 945-8720
Toll Free Information/Referral:
  (800) 227-7294
Website: www.careguide.net

CDC National Prevention
  Information Network
For information on HIV, AIDS,
  STD, TB
PO Box 6003
Rockville, MD 20849-6003
Tel: (301) 562-1098
Toll Free Tel: (800) 458-5231
Toll Free Fax: (888) 282-7681
Toll Free TTY: (800) 243-7012
Website: www.cdcnpin.org
E-Mail: info@cdcnpin.org

Commission on Accreditation for
  Rehabilitation Facilities (CARF)
4891 East Grant Road
Tucson, AZ 85712
Tel: (520) 325-1044
Fax: (520) 318-1129
Website: www.carf.org

Department of Veteran Affairs
Office of Public Affairs
810 Vermont Avenue, NW
Washington, DC 20420
Tel: (202) 273-5700
Fax: (202) 273-6705
Website: www.va.gov

Disabled American Veterans
807 Maine Avenue, SW
Washington, DC 20024
Tel: (202) 554-3501
Fax: (202) 554-3581
Website: www.dav.org

Family Caregivers Alliance
690 Market Street
Suite 600
San Francisco, CA 94104
Tel: (415) 434-3388
Fax: (415) 434-3508
Toll Free: (800) 445-8106
Website: www.caregiver.org.
E-Mail: info@caregiver.org

Gerontological Society of America
1030 15th Street, NW, Suite 250
Washington, DC 20005
Tel: (202) 842-1275
Fax: (202) 842-1150
Website: www.geron.org

Healthcare Information and
  Management Systems Society
230 East Ohio Street, Suite 500
Chicago, IL 60611-3269
Tel: (312) 664-4467
Fax: (312) 664-6143
Website: www.himss.org

Interfaith Caregivers Alliance
One West Armour Blvd.
Suite 202
Kansas City, MO 64111
Tel: (816) 931-5442
Fax: (816) 931-5202
Website:
  www.interfaithcaregivers.org
E-Mail: info@interfaithcaregivers.org

Joint Commission on Accreditation
  of Healthcare Organizations
  (JCAHO)
One Renaissance Boulevard
Oakbrook Terrace, IL 60181
Tel: (630) 792-5000
Fax: (630) 792-5005
Website: www.jcaho.org

Medicare Hotline
Toll Free English & Spanish:
(800) MEDICARE (633-4227)
Website: www.medicare.gov

National Adult Day Services
  Association
409 Third Street, SW
Washington, DC 20024
Tel: (202) 479-6682
Fax: (202) 479-0735
Website: www.ncoa.org/nadsa
E-Mail: nadsa@ncoa.org

National Asian Pacific Center on
  Aging
Melbourne Tower, Suite 914
1511 Third Avenue
Seattle, WA 98101
Tel: (206) 624-1221
Fax: (206) 624-1023
Website: www.napca.org

National Association of Area
  Agencies on Aging
927 15th Street NW
6th Floor
Washington, DC 20005
Tel: (202) 296-8130
Fax: (202) 296-8134
Website: www.n4a.org
E-Mail: rseay@n4a.org
Toll Free Eldercare Locator:
  (800) 677-1116, operated as a
  cooperative partnership of the
  Administration on Aging, the
  National Association of Area
  Agencies on Aging, and the
  National Association of State
  Units on Aging.

National Association of Directors of
  Nursing Administration
10999 Reed Hartman Highway,
  Suite 233
Cincinnati, OH 45242
Tel: (513) 791-3679
Fax: (513) 791-3699
Toll Free: (800) 222-0539
Website: www.nadona.org
Email: info@nadona.org

National Association for Home Care
228 7th Street, SE
Washington, DC 20003
Tel: (202) 547-7424
Fax: (202) 547-3540
Website: http://www.nahc.org

National Association of Professional
  Geriatric Care Managers
1604 North Country Club Road
Tucson, AZ 85716
Tel: (520) 881-8008
Fax: (520) 325-7925
Website: www.caremanager.org

National Association for the Support
  of Long Term Care
1321 Duke Street, Suite 304
Alexandria, VA 22314
Tel: (703) 549-8500
Fax: (703) 549-8342
Website: www.NASL.org

National Caucus and Center on
  Black Aged, Inc.
1424 K Street, NW
Washington, DC 20005
Tel: (202) 637-8400
Fax: (202) 347-0895
Website: www.ncba-blackaged.org
E-Mail: ncba@aol.com

National Citizens' Coalition for
  Nursing Home Reform
1424 16th Street, NW, Suite 202
Washington, DC 20036-2211
Tel: (202) 332-2275
Fax: (202) 332-2949
Website: www.nccnhr.org
E-Mail: nccnhr1@nccnhr.org

National Council on the Aging
409 3rd Street, SW
Washington, DC 20024
Tel: (202) 479-1200
Fax: (202) 479-0735
Website: www.ncoa.org
E-Mail: info@ncoa.org

National Council on Patient
  Information and Education
4915 Saint Elmo Avenue
Suite 505
Bethesda, MD 20814-6053
Tel: (301) 656-8565
Fax: (301) 656-4464
Website: www.talkaboutrx.org
Email: ncpie@erols.com

National Family Caregivers
  Association
10400 Connecticut Avenue
500
Kensington, MD 20895-3944
Tel: (301) 942-6430
Fax: (301) 942-2302
Toll Free: (800) 896-3650
Website: www.nfcares.org
E-mail: info@nfcares.org

National Health Information Center
PO Box 1133
Washington, DC 20013-1133
Tel: (301) 565-4167
Toll Free: (800) 336-4797
Fax: (301) 884-4256
Website: www.health.gov/nhic
E-Mail: info@nhic.org

National Indian Council on Aging
10501 Montgomery Boulevard NE
Suite 210
Albuquerque, NM 87111-3846
Tel: (505) 292-2001
Fax: (505) 292-1922
Website: www.nicoa.org
E-Mail: dave@nicoa.org

National Institute on Aging
Information Clearinghouse
P.O. Box 8057
Gaithersburg, MD 20898-8057
Toll Free Tel: (800) 222-2225

National Institute on Aging
Building 31, Room 5C27
31 Center Drive
MSC 2292
Bethesda, MD 20892-2292
Tel: (301) 496-1752
Fax: (301) 496-1072
Website: www.nih.gov/nia

National Institute on Disability and
  Rehabilitation Research
ABLEDATA
8630 Fenton Street
Suite 930
Silver Spring, MD 20910
Tel: (301) 608-8998
Fax: (301) 608-8958
Toll Free: (800) 227-0216
Website: www.abledata.com
E-Mail: adaigle@macroint.com

National Rehabilitation Information
  Center
1010 Wayne Avenue
Suite 800
Silver Spring, MD 20910
Toll Free: (800) 346-2742
Fax: (301) 562-2401
Website: www.naric.com/naric

National Subacute Care Association
7315 Wisconsin Avenue,
  Suite 424E
Bethesda, MD 20814
Tel: (301) 961-8680
Fax: (301) 961-8681
Website: www.nsca.net
E-Mail: nsca@tiac.net

Projecto Ayuda
1452 West Temple Street, Suite 100
Los Angeles, CA 90026
Tel: (213) 487-1922
Fax: (213) 202-5905

United Seniors Health Cooperative
409 Third Street SW
Washington, DC 20024
Tel: (202) 479-6973
Fax: (202) 479-6660
Website: unitedseniorshealth.org

Visiting Nurse Associations of
  America
11 Beacon Street, Suite 910
Boston, MA 02108
Tel: (617) 523-4042
Fax: (617) 227-4843
Website: www.vnaa.org

Well Spouse Foundation
610 Lexington Avenue, Suite 208
New York City, NY 10022
Tel: (212) 644-1241
Fax: (212) 644-1338
Toll Free: (800) 838-0879
Website: www.wellspouse.org
E-Mail: wellspouse@aol.com

END-OF-LIFE ISSUES

Americans for Better Care of the
  Dying
2175 K Street, NW, Suite 820
Washington, DC 20037
Tel: (202) 530-9864
Fax: (202) 467-2271
Website: www.abcd-caring.com
E-Mail: caring@erols.com

Center to Improve Care of the
  Dying
Rand Corporation
1200 South Hayes Street
Arlington, VA 22202
Tel: (703) 413-1100
Website: www.medicaring.org

Choice in Dying, Inc.
1035 30th Street, NW
Washington, DC 20007
Tel: (202) 338-9790
Fax: (202) 338-0242
Toll Free: (800) 989-WILL (9455)
Website: partnershipforcaring.org

Compassion in Dying
6312 SW Capital Hwy, PMB 415
Portland, OR 97201
Tel: (503) 221-9556
Fax: (503) 228-9160
Website:
   www.compassionindying.org
E-Mail: info@compassionindying.org

GriefNet
Internet Address: www.rivendell.org

Hospice Association of America
228 Seventh Street, SE
Washington, DC 20003
Tel: (202) 546-4759
Fax: (202) 547-9559
Website: www.hospice-america.org

Hospice Education Institute
190 Westbrook Road
Essex, CT 06426-1510
Tel: (860) 767-1620
Fax: (860) 767-2746
Toll Free for Publications: (800)
   331-1620
Hospice Link Referral Service—
   Toll Free: (800) 331-1620
Website: www.hospiceworld.org
E-Mail: hospiceall@aol.com

Hospice Foundation of America
2001 S Street NW, Suite 300
Washington, DC 20009
Tel: (202) 638-5419
Toll Free: (800) 854-3402
Fax: (202) 638-5312
Website: www.hospicefoundation.org
E-Mail: hfa@hospicefoundation.org

The Last Acts Campaign
Barksdale Ballard & Co.
1951 Kidwell Drive, Suite 205
Vienna, VA 22182
Tel: (703) 827-8771
Fax: (703) 827-0783
Website: www.lastacts.org

Life With Dignity
1744 Riggs Place NW
Suite 300
Washington, DC 20009
Tel: (202) 986-0118
Website:
   http://members.aol.com/lwdfdn
E-Mail: lwdfdn@aol.com

National Hospice and Palliative
   Care Organization
1700 Diagonal Road
Suite 300
Alexandria, VA 22314
Tel: (703) 837-1500
Website: www.nhpco.org
E-Mail: info@nhpca.org

EDUCATION

Association for Gerontology in
   Higher Education
1030 15th Street, NW, Suite 240
Washington, DC 20005-1503
Tel: (202) 289-9806
Fax: (202) 289-9824
Website: www.aghe.org

Association of American Medical
   Colleges
2450 N Street, NW
Washington, DC 20037-1126
Tel: (202) 828-0400
Fax: (202) 828-1125
Website: www.aamc.org

LEGAL ISSUES AND ELDER ABUSE

Legal Services for the Elderly
130 West 42nd Street, 17th Floor
New York, NY 10036
Tel: (212) 391-0120
Fax: (212) 719-1939
E-Mail: hn4923@handsnet.org

National Academy of Elder Law
   Attorneys
1604 North Country Club Road
Tucson, AZ 85716
Tel: (520) 881-4005
Fax: (520) 325-7925
Website: www.naela.org
E-Mail: info@naela.com

National Center on Elder Abuse
A consortium of the following
   six partners with NASUA the
   lead agency:
National Association of State Units
   on Aging (NASUA)
Commission on Legal Problems of
   the Elderly of the American Bar
   Association (ABA)
The Clearinghouse on Abuse and
   Neglect of the Elderly of the
   University of Delaware CANE)
The San Francisco Consortium for
   Elder Abuse Prevention of the
   Goldman Institute on Aging
   (GIOA)
The National Association of Adult
   Protective Services
   Administrators (NAAPSA)
The National Committee to Prevent
   Elder Abuse (NCPEA)

National Association of State Units
   on Aging
1225 I Street
Suite 725
Washington, DC 20005
Tel: (202) 898-2578
Fax: (202) 898-2583
Website: www.nasua.org
E-Mail: info@nasua.org

National Clearinghouse on Elder
   Abuse (Literature)
University of Delaware
College of Human Resources,
   Education and Public Policy
Department of Consumer Studies
211 Allison Annex
Newark, DE 19716
Tel: (302) 831-3525
Fax: (302) 831-6081

National Committee for Prevention
   of Elder Abuse (Research)
Institute on Aging
UMASS Memorial Health Care
119 Belmont Street
Worcester, MA 01605
Tel: (508) 334-6166
Fax: (508) 334-6906
Website: www.preventelderabuse.org

National Senior Citizens Law
  Center
1101 14th Street, NW
Suite 400
Washington, DC 20005
Tel: (202) 289-6976
Fax: (202) 289-7224
Website: www.nsclc.org

RESOURCES ON SPECIFIC HEALTH PROBLEMS

Cancer

American Cancer Society, Inc.
National Headquarters
1599 Clifton Road, NE
Atlanta, GA 30329
Tel: (404) 320-3333
Fax: (404) 329-5787
Toll Free National Cancer
  Information Center: (800)
  227-2345
Website: www.cancer.org

National Cancer Institute
Public Inquiries Office
Building 31, Room 10A31
31 Center Drive, MSC 2580
Bethesda, MD 20892-2580
Tel: (301) 435-3848
Toll Free: (800) 4-CANCER
  (422-6237)
Website: www.nci.nih.gov

Diabetes Mellitus

American Diabetes Association
Attn: Customer Service
1701 North Beauregard Street
Alexandria, VA 22311
Tel: (703) 549-1500
Fax: (703) 549-6995
Toll Free: (800) DIABETES
  (232-3472)
Website: www.diabetes.org
E-Mail:
  customerservice@diabetes.org

National Diabetes Information
  Clearinghouse
1 Information Way
Bethesda, MD 20892-3560
Tel: (301) 654-3327
Fax: (301) 907-8906
Website: www.niddk.nih.gov
E-Mail: ndic@info.niddk.nih.gov

Digestive Problems

American Liver Foundation
75 Maiden Lane
Suite 603
New York, NY 10038
Toll Free: (800) GO LIVER
  (465-4837)
Website: www.liverfoundation.org
E-Mail:
  webmail@liverfoundation.org

National Digestive Disease
Information Clearinghouse
2 Information Way
Bethesda, MD 20892-2480
Tel: (301) 654-3810
Website: www.niddk.nih.gov
E-Mail: nddic@info.niddk.nih.gov

United Ostomy Association
19772 MacArthur Boulevard
Suite 200
Irvine, CA 92612-2405
Tel: (949) 660-8624
Fax: (949) 660-9262
Toll Free: (800) 826-0826
Website: www.uoa.org
E-Mail: info@uoa.org

Head and Neck Problems

American Academy of
  Otolaryngology—Head and Neck
  Surgery, Inc.
1 Prince Street
Alexandria, VA 22314-3357
Tel: (703) 836-4444
Fax: (703) 683-5100
TTY: (703) 519-1585
Website: www.entnet.org

American Council for Headache
  Education
19 Mantua Road
Mt. Royal, NJ 08061
Tel: (856) 423-0258
Toll Free: (800) 255-ACHE (2243)
Fax: (856) 423-0082
Website: www.achenet.org

American Dental Association
211 East Chicago Avenue
Chicago, IL 60611
Tel: (312) 440-2500
Fax: (312) 440-2800
Website: www.ada.org

American Society for Geriatric
  Dentistry
211 East Chicago Avenue
5th Floor
Chicago, IL 60611
Tel (312) 440-2660
Fax: (312) 440-2824
Website: www.foscod.org

National Headache Foundation
428 West St. James Place,
  2nd Floor
Chicago, IL 60614-2750
Tel: (773) 388-6399
Toll Free: (888) NHF-5552
Fax: (773) 525-7357
Website: www.headaches.org
E-Mail: info@headaches.org

National Institute of Dental &
  Craniofacial Research
National Institute of Health
Bethesda, MD 20892-2190
Tel: (301) 496-4261
Fax: (301) 496-9988
Website: www.nidcr.nih.gov
E-Mail: nidcrinfo@mail.nih.gov

Hearing Problems

American Tinnitus Association
PO Box 5
Portland, OR 97207-0005
Tel: (503) 248-9985
Fax: (503) 248-0024
Toll Free: (800) 634-8978
Website: www.ata.org
E-Mail: tinnitus@ata.org

Better Hearing Institute
515 King Street
Suite 420
Alexandria, VA 22314
Toll Free: (800) EARWELL
  (327-9355)
Fax: (703) 750-9302
Website: www.betterhearing.org
E-Mail: mail@betterhearing.org

International Hearing Society
16880 Middlebelt Road, Suite 4
Livonia, MI 48154
Tel: (734) 522-7200
Fax: (734) 522-0200
Toll Free Hearing Aid
Helpline:(800) 521-5247
Website: www.ihsinfo.org

National Institute on Deafness and
Other Communication Disorders
National Institute of Health
31 Center Drive, MSC 2320
Bethesda, MD 20892-2320
Tel: (301) 496-7243
Fax: (301) 402-0018
Toll Free NIDCD Information
Clearinghouse: (800) 241-1044
Website: www.nidcd.nih.gov
E-Mail:
webmaster@ms.nidcd.nih.gov

Self Help for Hard of Hearing
People
7910 Woodmont Avenue,
Suite 1200
Bethesda, MD 20814
Tel: (301) 657-2248
Fax: (301) 913-9413
TTY: (301) 657-2249
Website: www.shhh.org
E-Mail: national@shhh.org

Heart and Circulation Problems

American Association of
Cardiovascular and Pulmonary
Rehabilitation
7600 Terrace Avenue
Suite 203
Middleton, WI 53562
Tel: (608) 831-6989
Fax: (608) 831-5485
Website: www.aacvpr.org
E-Mail: accvpr@tmahq.com

American Heart Association
7272 Greenville Avenue
Dallas, TX 75231
Tel: (214) 373-6300
Toll Free Tel: (800) 242-8721
Website: www.americanheart.org
AHA's Stroke Connection: (800)
553-6321

Courage Stroke Network
3915 Golden Valley Road
Golden Valley, MN 55422
Tel: (763) 520-0520
Fax: (763) 520-0577

National Heart, Lung and Blood
Institute
Office of Prevention, Education and
Control
31 Center Drive
MSC 2480
Bethesda, MD 20892-2480
Tel: (301) 496-5437
Fax: (301) 402-2405
Website: www.nhlbi.nih.gov
E-Mail:
nhlbiinfo@rover.nhlbi.nih.gov

National Institute of Neurological
Disorders and Stroke
NIH Neurological Institute
PO Box 5801
Bethesda, MD 20824
Toll Free: (800) 352-9424
Website: www.ninds.nih.gov

National Stroke Association
9707 E. Easter Lane
Englewood, CO 80112
Tel: (303) 649-9299
Fax: (303) 649-1328
Toll Free: (800) STROKES
(787-6537)
Website: www.stroke.org

Joint, Muscle, and Bone Problems

American Academy of Orthopedic
Surgeons
6300 North River Road
Rosemont, IL 60018-4262
Tel: (847) 823-7186
Toll Free; (800) 346-AAOS (2267)
Fax: (847) 823-8125
Website: www.aaos.org
E-Mail: custserv@aaos.org

American Podiatric Medical
Association
9312 Old Georgetown Road
Bethesda, MD 20814
Tel: (301) 571-9200
Fax: (301) 530-2752
Toll Free for Patient Education
Literature only
(800) FOOT-CARE
Website: www.apma.org
E-Mail: askapma@apma.org

Arthritis Foundation
1330 West Peachtree Street
Atlanta, GA 30309
Tel: (404) 872-7100
Toll Free Information:
(800) 283-7800
Fax: (404) 872-0457
Website: www.arthritis.org
E-Mail: help@arthritis.org

Lupus Foundation of America
1300 Piccard Drive, Suite 200
Rockville, MD 20850-4303
Tel: (301) 670-9292
Toll Free Line for Information
Packet: English (800) 558-0121,
Spanish (800) 558-0231
Fax: (301) 670-9486
Website: www.lupus.org

National Arthritis and
Musculoskeletal and Skin
Diseases Information
Clearinghouse
National Institutes of Health
1AMS Circle
Bethesda, MD 20892-3675
Tel: (301) 495-4484
Toll Free: (877) 22-NIAMS
(64267)
Fax: (301) 718-6366
Website: www.nih.gov/niams
E-Mail: via website

National Osteoporosis Foundation
1232 22nd Street NW
Washington, DC 20037-1292
Tel: (202) 223-2226
Fax: (202) 223-2237
Toll Free Info: (800) 223-9994
Website: www.nof.org
E-Mail: customerservice@nof.org

Lung and Breathing Problems

American Association of
  Cardiovascular and Pulmonary
  Rehabilitation
7600 Terrace Avenue
Suite 203
Middleton, WI 53562
Tel: (608) 831-6989
Fax: (608) 831-5485
Website: www.aacvpr.org
E-Mail: accvpr@tmahq.com

American Lung Association
1740 Broadway
New York, NY 10019
Tel: (212) 315-8700
Fax: (212) 265-5642
Toll Free: (800) LUNG-USA
  (800-586-4872)
Website: www.lungusa.org
E-Mail: info@lungusa.org

National Heart, Lung and Blood
  Institute
Office of Prevention, Education and
  Control
31 Center Drive
MSC 2480
Bethesda, MD 20892-2480
Tel: (301) 496-5437
Fax: (301) 402-2405
Website: www.nhlbi.nih.gov
E-Mail:
  nhlbiinfo@rover.nhlbi.nih.gov

Memory and Thinking Problems

Alzheimer's Association
919 North Michigan Avenue
Suite 1100
Chicago, IL 60611-1676
Toll Free Information:
  (800) 272-3900
Tel: (312) 335-8700
TTY (312) 335-8882
Fax: (312) 335-1110
Website: http://www.alz.org/
E-Mail: info@alz.org
Safe Return Program
  (identification tags, medical alert
  bracelets) (888) 572-8566

Alzheimer's Disease Education and
  Referral Center
PO Box 8250
Silver Spring, MD 20907-8250
Tel: (301) 495-3311
Fax: (301) 495-3334
Toll Free Information Service: (800)
  438-4380
Website: www.alzheimers.org
E-Mail: adear@alzheimers.org

Neurologic Problems

American Academy of Neurology
1080 Montreal Avenue
St. Paul, MN 55116
Tel: (651) 695-1940
Fax: (651) 695-2791
Website: www.aan.com
E-Mail: web@aan.com

American Parkinson's Disease
  Association
1250 Hylan Boulevard
Suite 4B
Staten Island, NY 10305-1946
Tel: (718) 981-8001
Toll Free Information Hotline (800)
  223-2732
Fax: (718) 981-4399
Website: www.apdaparkinson.org
E-Mail: info@apdaparkinson.org

Epilepsy Foundation of America
4351 Garden City Drive
Landover, MD 20785
Tel: (301) 459-3700
Toll Free Information & Referral:
  (800) 332-1000
Fax: (301) 577-2684
Website: www.efa.org

Huntington's Disease Society of
  America
158 West 29th Street, 7th Floor
New York, NY 10001
Tel: (212) 242-1968
Fax: (212) 239-3430
Toll Free Hotline: (800) 345-4372
Website: www.hdsa.org
E-Mail: hdsainfo@hdsa.org

National Institute of Neurological
  Disorders and Stroke
NIH Neurological Institute
PO Box 5801
Bethesda, MD 20824
Toll Free: (800) 352-9424
Website: www.ninds.nih.gov
(for other stroke information,
  see Heart & Circulation)

Parkinson's Disease Foundation
William Black Medical Building
Columbia-Presbyterian Medical
  Center
710 West 168th Street
New York, NY 10032
Tel: (212) 923-4700
Toll Free: (800) 457-6676
Fax: (212) 923-4778
Website: www.pdf.org
E-Mail: info@pdf.org

Nutritional Concerns

Food and Nutrition Information
  Center
US Department of Agriculture
National Agriculture Library
  Building
10301 Baltimore Avenue
Room 304
Beltsville, MD 20705-2351
Tel: (301) 504-5719
Fax: (301) 504-6409
Website:
  http://www.nal.usda.gov/fnic
E-Mail: fnic@nal.usda.gov

Meals On Wheels Association of
  America
1414 Prince Street, Suite 202
Alexandria, VA 22314
Tel: (703) 548-5558
Fax: (703) 548-8024
Website: www.projectmeal.org
E-Mail: mowaa@tbq.dqsys.com

Pain

American Chronic Pain Association
PO Box 850
Rocklin, CA 95677
Tel: (916) 632-0922
Fax: (916) 632-3208
Website: www.theacpa.org
E-Mail: acpa@pacbell.net

American Geriatrics Society
The Empire State Building
350 Fifth Avenue, Suite 801
New York, NY 10118
Tel: (212) 308-1414
Fax: (212) 832-8646
Website: www.americangeriatrics.org
E-Mail:
    info.amger@americangeriatrics.org

American Pain Society
4700 West Lake Avenue
Glenview, IL 60025
Tel: (847) 375-4715
Fax: (847) 375-7777
Website: www.ampainsoc.org
E-Mail: info@ampainsoc.org

City of Hope Pain Resource Center
City of Hope National Medical
    Center
Dept. of Nursing Research &
    Education
1500 East Duarte Road
Duarte, CA 91010
Tel: (626) 359-8111 ext. 3829
Website: mayday.coh.org
E-Mail: bferrell@coh.org

National Chronic Pain Outreach
    Association
PO Box 274
Millboro, VA 24460-9606
Tel: (540) 862-9437
Fax: (540) 862-9485
Email: ncpoa@cfw.com

Psychological Problems

American Association for Geriatric
    Psychiatry
7910 Woodmont Avenue,
    Suite 1050
Bethesda, MD 20814-3004
Tel: (301) 654-7850
Fax: (301) 654-4137
Website: www.aagpgpa.org
E-Mail: main@aagpgpa.org

National Alliance for the Mentally
    Ill
Colonial Place Three
2107 Wilson Blvd.
Suite 300
Arlington, VA 22201-3042
Tel: (703) 524-7600
Fax: (703) 524-9094
Toll Free: (800) 950-6264
Website: www.nami.org

National Institute of Mental Health
Information Resources & Inquiries
6001 Executive Blvd.
Room 8184
MSC 9663
Bethesda, MD 20892-9663
Tel: (301) 443-4513
Fax for You: (301) 443-5158
Website: www.nimh.nih.gov
E-Mail: nimhinfo@nih.gov

National Mental Health Association
Information Center
1021 Prince Street
Alexandria, VA 22314-2971
Tel: (703) 684-7722
Fax: (703) 684-5968
Toll Free Information: (800)
    969-NMHA (6642)
Website: www.nmha.org

Sexuality and Sexual Concerns

American College of Obstetricians
    and Gynecologists
PO Box 96920
Washington, DC 20090-6920
Tel: (202) 863-2518
Fax: (202) 484-1595
Website: www.acog.com
E-Mail: resources@acog.org

American Urological Association
1120 North Charles Street
Baltimore, MD 21201
Tel: (410) 727-1100
Fax: (410) 223-4370
Website: www.auanet.org
E-Mail: aua@auanet.org

Hysterectomy Educational
    Resources and Services
    Foundation
422 Bryn Mawr Avenue
Bala Cynwyd, PA 19004
Tel: (610) 667-7757
Fax: (610) 667-8096
Website: http://ccon.com/hers/
E-Mail: HERSFdn@aol.com

Sexuality Information and
    Education Council of the
    United States
130 West 42nd Street, Suite 350
New York, NY 10036
Tel: (212) 819-9770
Fax: (212) 819-9776
Website: www.siecus.org
E-Mail: siecus@siecus.org

Sight Problems

American Academy of
    Ophthalmology
PO Box 7424
San Francisco, CA 94120
Tel: (415) 561-8500
Fax: (415) 561-8533
Toll Free: (800) 222-3937
Website: www.eyenet.org
E-Mail: comm@aao.org

American Foundation for the Blind
11 Penn Plaza, Suite 300
New York, NY 10001
Tel: (212) 502-7600
Toll Free: (800) AFB LINE
    (232-5463)
Fax: (212) 502-7777
Website: www.afb.org
E-Mail: afbinfo@afb.net

American Optometric Association
243 North Lindbergh Blvd.
St. Louis, MO 63141
Tel: (314) 991-4100
Fax: (314) 991-4101
Toll Free: (800) 365-2219
Website: http://www.aoanet.org

Better Vision Institute
1655 North Fort Meyer Drive,
   Suite 200
Arlington, VA 22209
Tel: (703) 243-1508
Toll Free: (800) 642-3253
Fax: (703) 243-1537
Website: www.visionsite.org
E-Mail: vca@visionsite.org

Foundation for Glaucoma Research
200 Pine Street
Suite 200
San Francisco, CA 94104
Tel: (415) 986-3162
Fax: (415) 986-3763
Website: www.glaucoma.org

National Eye Institute
Information Office
2020 Vision Place
Bethesda, MD 20892-3655
Tel: (301) 496-5248
Fax: (301) 402-1065
Website: www.nei.nih.gov
E-Mail: 2020@nei.nih.gov

Prevent Blindness America
500 East Remington Road
Schaumberg, IL 60173
Tel: (847) 843-2020
Fax: (847) 843-8458
Toll Free: (800) 331-2020
Website:
   http://www.preventblindness.org
E-Mail: info@preventblindness.org

Skin Problems

American Academy of Dermatology
930 North Meacham Road
Schaumberg, IL 60173
Tel: (847) 330-0230
Toll Free: (888) 462-DERM (3376)
Fax: (847) 330-0050
Website: www.aad.org

American Academy of Facial Plastic
   and Reconstructive Surgery
310 South Henry Street
Alexandria, VA 22314
Tel: (703) 299-9291
Fax: (703) 299-8898
Toll Free: (800) 332-FACE
Website: www.aafprs.org
E-Mail: info@aafprs.org

American Social Health Association
Herpes Resource Center
PO Box 13827
Research Triangle Park, NC 27709
Tel: (919) 361-8400
Fax: (919) 361-8425
Website: http://www.ashastd.org
E-Mail: phidra@ashastd.org

National Arthritis and
   Musculoskeletal and Skin Diseases
   Information Clearinghouse
National Institutes of Health
1 AMS Circle
Bethesda, MD 20892-3675
Tel: (301) 495-4484
Toll Free: (877) 22-NIAMS
   (64267)
Fax: (301) 718-6366
Website: www.nih.gov/niams
E-Mail: niamsinfo@mail.nih.gov

The Skin Cancer Foundation
PO Box 561
New York, NY 10156
Tel: (212) 725-5176
Toll Free: (800) SKIN-490
   (754-6490)
Fax: (212) 725-5751
Website: www.skincancer.org
E-Mail: info@skincancer.org

Urinary Problems

National Association for Continence
   (NAFC)
PO Box 8310
Spartanburg, SC 29305-8310
Tel: (864) 579-7900
Toll Free: (800) BLADDER
   (252-3337)
Fax: (864) 579-7902
Website: www.nafc.org

National Kidney and Urologic
   Diseases Information
   Clearinghouse
3 Information Way
Bethesda, MD 20892-3560
Tel: (301) 654-4415
Fax: (301) 907-8906
Website: www.niddk.nih.gov
E-Mail: ndic@info.niddk.nih.gov

National Kidney Foundation
30 East 33rd Street
Suite 1100
New York, NY 10016
Tel: (212) 889-2210
Toll Free: (800) 622-9010
Fax: (212) 689-9261
Website: www.kidney.org
E-Mail: info@kidney.org

The Simon Foundation for
   Continence
PO Box 835
Wilmette, IL 60091
Tel: (847) 864-3913
Toll Free: (800) 23-SIMON
   (237-4666)
Fax: (847) 864-9758
Website: www.simonfoundation.org
E-Mail:
   simoninfo@simonfoundation.org

Normal Laboratory Values*

For Blood, Plasma, and Serum Chemistries, Hematology, and Urine
Referenced in the Questions and Critiques

BLOOD, PLASMA, SERUM CHEMISTRIES

Aminotransferase, alanine (ALT, SGPT)   0–35 U/L

Aminotransferase, aspartate (AST, SGOT)   0–35 U/L

Bicarbonate (CO_2)   21–30 mEq/L

Blood gas studies:

  PO_2 83–108 mm Hg

  PCO_2 Female: 32–45 mm Hg; Male: 35–48 mm Hg

  pH   7.35–7.45

  Oxygen saturation   95%–98%

Calcium   8.8–10.3 mg/dL

Calcium, ionized   4.5–5.6 mEq/L

Carcinoembryonic antigen   < 2.5 ng/mL

Chloride   98–106 mEq/L

Cholesterol:

  Total   Recommended: < 200 mg/dL; Moderate risk:
  200–239 mg/dL; High risk: ≥ 240 mg/dL

  High-density lipoprotein (HDL)   Female: < 35 mg/dL;
  Male: < 29 mg/dL

  Low-density lipoprotein (LDL)   Recommended: < 130
  mg/dL; Moderate risk: 130–150 mg/dL; High risk:
  ≥ 160 mg/dL

Creatinine   0.7–1.5 mg/dL

Creatine kinase   Female: 26–140 U/L; Male: 38–174 U/L

Digoxin (therapeutic level)   0.8–2.0 ng/mL

Folate   2.2–17.3 ng/mL

Glucose   Fasting, 70–105 mg/dL; 2-h postprandial, < 140
mg/dL

Iron   50–150 µg/dL

Iron-binding capacity, total   250–450 µg/dL

Lactate dehydrogenase   60–100 U/L

Magnesium   1.8–3.0 mg/dL

Parathyroid hormone   10–65 pg/mL

Phosphatase, acid   0.5–5.5 U/L

Phosphatase, alkaline   20–135 U/L

Phosphorus (age 60 and over)   Female: 2.8–4.1 mg/dL;
Male: 2.3–3.7 mg/dL

Potassium   3.5–5 mEq/L

Prostate-specific antigen   < 4 ng/mL, normal; > 10
ng/mL, abnormal; 4–10 ng/mL, equivocal

Protein, total   6.4–8.3 g/dL

  Albumin   3.5–5.5 g/dL

  Globulin   2.0–3.5 g/dL

Rheumatoid factor, latest test   > 1:80 is abnormal

Sodium   136–145 mEq/L

Testosterone:

  Women   < 3.5 nmol/L

  Men   10–35 nmol/L

Thyrotropin (TSH)   0.5–5.0 µU/mL

Thyroxine (T_4)   Total, 5–12 µg/dL; free, 0.9–2.4 ng/dL

Triglycerides   Recommended: < 250 mg/dL

Urea nitrogen (BUN)   8–20 mg/dL

Uric acid   2.5–8.0 mg/dL

Vitamin B_{12} 190–900 pg/mL

HEMATOLOGY

Erythrocyte count   Female, 4.2–5.4 × 10^6/µL; Male,
4.7–6.1× 10^6/µL

Erythrocyte sedimentation rate (Westergren)   0–35 mm/h

Ferritin   Female 10–120 ng/mL; Male: 20–150 ng/mL

Hematocrit   Female, 33%–43%; Male, 39%–49%

Hemoglobin   Female, 11.5–15.5 g/dL; Male, 14.0–18.0
g/dL

Hemoglobin A_{1c} 5.3%–7.5%

Leukocyte count and differential   4800–10,800/µL;
54%–62% segmented neutrophils, 3%–5% band forms,
23%–33% lymphocytes, 3%–7% monocytes, 1%-3%
eosinophils, < 1% basophils

Mean corpuscular hemoglobin   28–32 pg

Mean corpuscular volume   86–98 fL (86–98 mm^3)

Platelet count   150,000–450,000/µL

URINE

Creatinine clearance   90–140 mL/min

Creatinine, urine   Female, 11–20 mg/kg per 24 h; Male,
14–26 mg/kg per 24 h

Urine, postvoid residual volume   < 50 mL, normal; > 200
mL, abnormal; 50–200 mL, equivocal

---

* Note: As normal ranges vary among laboratories, data in this table may not conform with all laboratories' data.

QUESTIONS

Directions: *Each of the questions or incomplete statements below is followed by four or five suggested answers or completions. Select the ONE answer or completion that is BEST in each case and place an "X" through the letter you have selected for each answer on the answer sheet. The table of Normal Laboratory Values on the facing page may be consulted for any of the questions in this book.*

1. A 74-year-old man has Parkinson's disease that is well controlled. However, his gait is unstable, with mild retropulsion and bradykinesia. The patient has had one minor fall and has reduced his activities because he fears falling again. He has no other neurologic or musculoskeletal problems. Which of the following adaptive mobility aides is most appropriate to facilitate safer ambulation for this patient?

   (A) Straight cane
   (B) Four-prong cane
   (C) Standard walker
   (D) Wheeled walker
   (E) Wheelchair

2. An 82-year-old female nursing-home resident has end-stage Alzheimer's dementia. She is mute, incontinent of urine and feces, and bedbound. Daily skin inspection reveals nonblanching erythema of the heels. Which of the following will best prevent a pressure ulcer in this patient?

   (A) Bladder catheterization
   (B) Massaging the sacral skin daily
   (C) Elevating the head of the bed to 45 degrees
   (D) Elevating the heels off the bed surface
   (E) Repositioning the patient every 4 hours

3. Which of the following figures, expressed as percentage of personal income, reflects average out-of-pocket spending on health care for Medicare beneficiaries aged 65 and older?

   (A) 64%
   (B) 45%
   (C) 19%
   (D) 8%
   (E) 3%

4. A 67-year-old woman asks you to prescribe sleeping pills for her. She reports initial insomnia and restless sleep with frequent awakenings. The patient is retired and leads a sedentary life style. She frequently reads or watches television in bed and often naps, despite caffeine intake throughout the day. Physical examination is unremarkable. Which of the following is most likely to ameliorate this patient's sleep disturbance?

   (A) Exposure to early morning daylight
   (B) Proper sleep habits
   (C) Sustained-release melatonin
   (D) Zolpidem
   (E) Referral for polysomnography

5. An 80-year-old woman comes to your office for an initial evaluation. She is accompanied by her daughter, who is concerned about the patient's memory. During the past year she has been repeating questions and statements; about 6 months ago she began to have infrequent problems "getting her words out." Symptoms "probably" have worsened. She is sometimes sad when talking about deceased relatives. The patient lives alone and does most of her own household chores. She completed the 10th grade. Her Mini–Mental State Examination (MMSE) score is 26/30, with two errors ("near-misses") in orientation and two in short-term recall. Physical examination is normal. Laboratory studies are normal. Which of the following is the most likely diagnosis?

   (A) Normal aging
   (B) Minimal cognitive impairment
   (C) Major depression
   (D) Delirium
   (E) Alzheimer's disease

6. An 81-year-old white man who recently was widowed is brought to your office by his daughter. She is concerned that he is losing weight and no longer attends the senior group he once enjoyed. The patient has many nonspecific somatic complaints. His appetite has decreased, and he has lost 2.5 kg (5.5 lb) in the past 6 months. He denies feeling depressed but admits to decreased interest and energy, and he has been waking early in the morning. Findings of physical examination are normal. Which of the following findings is characteristic of bereavement?

(A) Psychomotor retardation
(B) Suicidal thoughts
(C) Persistent dysphoria
(D) Pervasive guilt
(E) Functional disability

7. Which of the following is the primary source of funding for Medicare Part A (hospital insurance)?

(A) Monthly premiums paid by Medicare recipients
(B) Payroll taxes on all workers and employers
(C) General tax revenues
(D) Hospitals and health care facilities
(E) Social Security

8. An 80-year-old woman has fallen outside her home twice. She fractured a wrist 3 months ago and has arm and facial ecchymoses from a fall last week. She has a distant history of a myocardial infarction and is being treated with a diuretic for hypertension. She reports occasional difficulty with balance when walking. Which of the following is the most appropriate first step in evaluating the falls?

(A) Gather additional history and physical examination.
(B) Order laboratory studies, especially serum electrolytes.
(C) Perform electrocardiography.
(D) Order computed tomography of the head.
(E) Arrange for home-based assessment.

9. An 82-year-old woman with a history of hypertension, diabetes mellitus, and osteoporosis goes to the emergency department for evaluation of the acute onset of severe upper back pain. Evaluation demonstrates a new thoracic vertebral compression fracture. In addition to prescribing analgesia, you request a consultation to assist with discharge because the patient lives at home alone and has difficulty getting out of bed because of the pain. What factor is most likely to predict the admission of this patient to the hospital in the next month?

(A) Depressed mood
(B) Urinary incontinence
(C) Living alone
(D) Advanced age
(E) Functional impairment

10. An 83-year-old man who has Alzheimer's disease of moderate severity has lived in a skilled nursing facility for 2 years. He has had intermittent delusional thoughts and anxiety, but these have not been particularly distressing or persisted for prolonged periods. Medical history includes mild chronic renal failure and anemia; he also has had a fractured hip but now ambulates well. He takes no psychotropic medications and sleeps well. During the past 2 weeks, however, he has spent increasing amounts of time wandering the halls. Several times, he has entered another patient's room and rummaged through belongings. He also was found outside the building on one occasion. Which of the following is the most appropriate treatment strategy?

(A) Provide structured physical activity and accompanied outdoor walks.
(B) Use a vest restraint in a chair intermittently during the day.
(C) Use wrist restraints during episodes of particularly vigorous wandering.
(D) Prescribe risperidone, 1 mg orally twice daily.
(E) Transfer the patient to another skilled nursing facility.

11. A 95-year-old woman has advanced Alzheimer's disease and is admitted to a skilled nursing facility. After 5 months she no longer has the financial resources to pay for her care. She is a widow and has no assets; her primary source of income is Social Security benefits. Which of the following financing options will cover the costs of her ongoing skilled nursing care?

(A) Social Security
(B) Medicare
(C) Medicare Plus Choice
(D) Medicaid
(E) Medigap

12. A 79-year-old man, who has coronary artery disease and congestive heart failure, comes to the emergency department because of nausea, vomiting, headache, and abdominal pain. Symptoms began 3 days ago. Current medications are warfarin, furosemide, digoxin, captopril, vitamin E, and a multivitamin. The regimen had been stable for 10 years, until the furosemide dosage was increased last week to better control symptoms of heart failure. Which of the following toxicities is the most likely cause of this patient's problems?

(A) Digoxin
(B) Furosemide
(C) Warfarin
(D) Vitamin E
(E) Captopril

13. A 75-year-old man has hypertension, hyperlipidemia, type 2 diabetes mellitus, and osteoarthritis of the hips. He reports a fall 1 month ago, while in the bathroom in the middle of the night. Current medications are atenolol, 25 mg daily; atorvastatin, 10 mg daily; metformin, 500 mg twice daily; and acetaminophen, 650 mg three times daily. Pulse rate is 72 per minute, and rhythm is regular. Blood pressure is 130/74 mm Hg with no orthostatic changes. Visual acuity is 20/30. The patient uses his arms to rise from a chair. Stance is normal; gait is slow, symmetric, and steady. Which of the following is the best next step?

(A) Visiting nurse evaluation of vital signs
(B) In-home assessment of physical function
(C) Comprehensive geriatric assessment
(D) Prescription of an assistive device (cane or walker)

(E) Admission to a postacute-care facility for physical rehabilitation

14. An 84-year-old female nursing-home resident reports knee pain that developed overnight. She has osteoporosis and has sustained previous hip and pelvic fractures after falling out of bed, but no recent incidents have occurred. The patient is frail and thin. Temperature is 37.3C (99.1F). The right knee is warm and held in partial flexion. It is exquisitely painful on passive motion and palpation over the joint line and tibia. Musculoskeletal findings are otherwise normal except for osteoarthritis of the hands. Anteroposterior radiograph of the knee shows anterior joint-space narrowing. Arthrocentesis yields grossly bloody fluid. Hematocrit is 38%, leukocyte count 5600/μL, and platelet count 260,000/uL. Which of the following is most likely to identify the cause of this patient's knee pain?

(A) Microscopic examination of synovial fluid for crystals
(B) Culture of synovial fluid
(C) Magnetic resonance imaging (MRI) of the knee
(D) Bone scan

15. A 79-year-old man comes to you for a routine visit. He is accompanied by his daughter, who reports that the patient is having difficulty hearing. He denies this and explains that people around him do not speak clearly. The patient's ears are free of cerumen impaction. Which of the following is the most reliable and valid screening test for hearing loss?

(A) Tuning-fork test
(B) Finger-rub test
(C) Whisper test
(D) Rinné and Weber tests
(E) Audioscopy

16. An 85-year-old woman has not urinated in 12 hours. Medical history includes congestive heart failure and hypertension. Four days ago, she was seen in the emergency department because of a 1-week history of malaise, nausea, and vomiting. A diagnosis of "possible urinary tract infection" was made, and symptoms responded to the prescribed medication.

The patient reports some muscle aching today. She has lost 2.5 kg (5.5 lb) since her last visit 2 months ago. Pulse rate is 80 per minute sitting and 100 per minute standing; blood pressure is 120/84 mm Hg sitting and 110/84 mm Hg standing. The patient is "a little dizzy" when she stands. Mental status is at baseline.

Laboratory studies:

Blood urea nitrogen	76 mg/dL
Serum creatinine	3.0 mg/dL
Serum electrolytes:	
Sodium	140 mEq/L
Potassium	5.8 mEq/L
Chloride	90 mEq/L
Bicarbonate	28 mEq/L
Urinalysis	0–3 red blood cells, 0–3 white blood cells per high-power field; granular casts and needle-shaped crystals

Of the following medications taken by this patient, which is the most likely cause of acute renal failure?

(A) Digoxin
(B) Diphenhydramine
(C) Hydrochlorothiazide
(D) Lisinopril
(E) Trimethoprim–sulfamethizole

17. A 78-year-old woman comes to your office for an initial visit; she is accompanied by a niece, who lives in another city. The patient has not had medical care since her physician retired 5 years ago. She is well groomed, seems cheerful, and has no medical complaints. When examining the patient, you notice a slight odor of urine. Findings of physical examination are normal. Following the examination, the patient dresses without difficulty.

The niece phones your office the next day and asks your opinion about the patient's incontinence. As far as she can tell, the condition has been present for at least 3 years. She is surprised that her aunt did not mention the problem to you. Which of the following is the most appropriate next step?

(A) Assume that the patient is not bothered by the incontinence.
(B) Ask the patient to schedule another visit.
(C) Order urodynamic studies.
(D) Prescribe a course of antibiotics.
(E) Prescribe oral estrogen therapy.

18. A 75-year-old man has been hospitalized in the intensive care unit for 1 month because of an exacerbation of emphysema. A stage II pressure ulcer, 6.0 × 8.0 × 0.5 cm in depth, is noted over the sacrum. Examination reveals pink tissue and scant drainage, with no significant necrotic tissue or surrounding erythema. Which of the following is the most appropriate dressing for this pressure ulcer?

(A) Saline-moistened (wet-to-dry) gauze
(B) Calcium alginate
(C) Hydrocolloid
(D) Polyurethane foam

19. A 68-year-old man has severe vascular dementia and lives in a nursing home. A gastrostomy was placed 1 year ago because of severe dysphagia following a stroke. Recently, the patient has become increasingly agitated and pulled out the feeding tube several times. Efforts to conceal and anchor the tube have been unsuccessful. A change in environment and judicious use of medications also have been ineffective. Which of the following is the most appropriate action?

(A) Place mitts on the patient's hands.
(B) Place restraints on the patient's wrists.
(C) Increase medication dosage to sedate the patient.
(D) Replace the gastrostomy with a jejunostomy.
(E) Reevaluate the need for the gastrostomy.

20. A 75-year-old woman undergoes cystoscopy and transurethral resection of a bladder tumor. Postoperatively, she has delirium characterized by lethargy and inability to recognize family members. Psychoactive medications are discontinued, and the episode appears to be resolving. The patient is a retired professor who had mild forgetfulness but had been living independently.

On the fourth postoperative day, the patient is awake and able to follow simple commands. She requires assistance in rising from bed and is slightly unsteady on her feet. The Mini–Mental State Examination (MMSE) score is 17/30. Which of the following statements is correct regarding this patient's prognosis?

(A) It is excellent; she is recovering from a fully reversible event precipitated by major physiologic stress.

(B) It is good; delirium may take days or weeks to resolve, but the lack of agitation or psychotic features is an encouraging finding.

(C) It is guarded; functional and cognitive status should be monitored closely, and she will need restorative therapy.

(D) It is poor; she now has dementia.

21. A healthy, physically active, cognitively intact 79-year-old man is referred to you after serum prostate-specific antigen (PSA) is found to be 6.5 ng/mL. The patient has not seen a clinician in 15 years and underwent PSA testing at a health fair, after prompting by his wife. He reports nocturia once or twice per night, and physical examination reveals an enlarged, smooth prostate gland. The patient is aware of the controversies surrounding screening for and treatment of prostate cancer and suggests that he may ignore the test result and "just get on with life." Which of the following is the most appropriate approach to this patient?

(A) Recommend transrectal ultrasonography of the prostate gland.

(B) Tell him that doing nothing is reasonable but also explain more active options.

(C) Recommend repeat PSA testing in 6 months.

(D) Refer him to a urologist for biopsy.

22. A 65-year-old man who has been paraplegic since an automobile accident 5 years ago is admitted to a skilled nursing facility, following hospitalization for urosepsis. His other medical problems include type 2 diabetes mellitus, hypertension, and deconditioning. He mobilized independently in a wheelchair until this hospital admission. Which of the following is the best initial step in preventing ischial pressure ulcers?

(A) Instruct or assist the patient to shift his weight every hour.

(B) Instruct or assist the patient to shift his weight every 2 hours.

(C) Use an air-filled, doughnut-shaped seat cushion to protect the ischial tuberosities.

(D) Consult a physical therapist to develop a plan for wheelchair seating.

(E) Develop a written plan for skin care.

23. A 70-year-old man has a 2-month history of insomnia, weight loss, feelings of hopelessness, loss of interest, crying spells, and thoughts of suicide. The patient's wife describes a long, intermittent history of checking the door locks and windows 50 to 100 times a day. He also has a habit of counting his steps and multiplying the numbers he sees on license plates while he is driving. The wife reports that this counting and multiplying must end on an even number; otherwise, he will retrace his path repeatedly, whether driving or walking, until an even number occurs. The patient also saves newspapers, which now fill two rooms of their home. The patient recently began seeing a psychologist who initiated cognitive behavioral therapy and recommended adjunctive pharmacologic therapy. Which of the following medications is most appropriate?

(A) Bupropion
(B) Clomipramine
(C) Desipramine
(D) Lorazepam
(E) Sertraline

24. The daughter of a 74-year-old woman asks you to make a home visit because the patient is unwilling to leave the house. The daughter moved in with her mother 1 month ago, because the patient's ability to care for herself had declined in the previous 6 months. She is taking medications for blood pressure, a "heart condition," and to control "eye pressure." Since the daughter moved in, the patient feeds herself small amounts of food and drinks water, plus two or three cans of liquid supplement each day. The patient reports feeling weak and tired but claims to be eating enough. She does not feel sad or blue. Her daughter reports significant weight loss. The patient is normotensive and slightly tachycardic. She has poorly fitting dentures, a dense right cataract, squared shoulders, and wasting of the quadriceps. No focal findings are elicited on neurologic examination. Mental status examination reveals 3 of 3 in registration and 2 of 3 in recall; she correctly name the days of the week in reverse order. Which of the following should you do next?

(A) Obtain complete information on the medications prescribed for the patient.
(B) Obtain a thorough dietary history, including food preferences.
(C) Refer the patient to a psychiatrist to manage depression.
(D) Refer the patient to a dentist for better-fitting dentures.
(E) Contact Adult Protective Services (APS) to place the patient in a setting where she can receive adequate care.

25. Which of the following statements is correct concerning perpetrators of elder mistreatment?

(A) They are predominantly male.
(B) They often do not perceive their behavior as abnormal.
(C) Reproducible profiles are readily apparent.
(D) Few unifying characteristics exist because the most important risk factors tend to be victim-specific (eg, impairment in activities of daily living).
(E) Victims usually are dependent upon their abusers for housing or finances, or both.

26. A 69-year-old woman is 15% over ideal body weight and has mild hypertension. She smokes cigarettes and has a family history of premature heart disease. Which of the following screening maneuvers for this patient is best supported by medical evidence?

(A) Fasting plasma glucose
(B) Fasting serum lipid profile
(C) Hemoglobin A_{1C}
(D) Radiography of the chest
(E) Computed tomography of the chest

27. A 79-year-old woman has Alzheimer's disease of moderate severity, with impaired memory, visuospatial skills, and language. During the past week she has become increasingly anxious and preoccupied by thoughts that strangers are living in the basement. The patient lives with her daughter, who asks your advice in alleviating her mother's distress. Which of the following is the most effective behavioral management strategy?

(A) Allow the patient to rest alone in her room to minimize sensory input when she is most anxious.
(B) Eliminate stimuli that exacerbate the delusion, and reassure the patient.
(C) Remind the patient that her belief is not real.
(D) Consider moving to a new house where the patient may not have this delusion.
(E) Initiate nursing-home placement.

28. An 82-year-old man falls, sustains a right intertrochanteric fracture, and is admitted to the orthopedic service. The patient has dementia and systolic hypertension and resides in a long-term-care facility. He had an uncomplicated myocardial infarction 10 years ago but has had no clinical manifestations of coronary artery disease subsequently. Current medications are an angiotensin-converting enzyme inhibitor and aspirin. He ambulates without assistance, and his nutritional status is good. His advance directive requests active treatment of all medical conditions.

The patient is agitated and confused. Pulse rate is 84 per minute, and respirations are 16 per minute. Blood pressure is 150/90 mm Hg. Findings of physical examination are normal except for severe pain on rotation of the right lower extremity. Routine laboratory studies and chest radiograph also are normal. Electrocardiogram shows normal sinus rhythm and no ischemic changes; findings are unchanged from previous tracings. The orthopedic surgeon plans internal fixation and interoperative reduction of the fracture. Which of the following decisions regarding the timing of surgery is most appropriate?

(A) Medical management is indicated.
(B) Coronary angiography is indicated prior to surgery.
(C) Surgery should be deferred for 3 to 4 days to permit a more thorough evaluation.
(D) Surgery should be deferred to achieve better pain control.
(E) Surgery should be performed as soon as possible. ~

29. Health Care Financing Administration (in June 2001 renamed the Centers for Medicare & Medicaid Services) guidelines permit nursing homes to use psychotropic drugs without restrictions in which of the following situations?

(A) Uncooperative behavior
(B) Wandering
(C) Hiccups ~
(D) Disruptive vocalizations

30. After rising from bed in the morning, an elderly nursing-home resident with a history of recurrent falls is found to have a 30–mm Hg decline in systolic blood pressure. Which of the following statements is correct?

(A) The orthostatic change will persist throughout the day.
(B) Postprandial hypotension also is likely to be present.
(C) The patient probably does not have a history of hypertension.
(D) The patient's falls are probably related to orthostatic hypotension. ~
(E) The patient is at increased risk for rapid cognitive deterioration in the next 2 years.

31. A 75-year-old man has difficulty walking because of osteoarthritic pain in the right hip. You prescribe a cane, with the handle at the level of the wrist. Which of the following instructions is correct regarding use of the cane?

(A) Hold in the right hand and advance with the right leg.
(B) Hold in the right hand and advance with the left leg.
(C) Hold in the left hand and advance with the right leg. ~
(D) Hold in the left hand and advance with the left leg.

32. A previously sedentary 75-year-old obese woman with non-insulin-dependent diabetes mellitus has recently begun a program of brisk walking, plus flexibility and resistance exercises. She gradually increases her walking to 30 minutes per day. Which of the following statements about this patient after 3 months of this exercise program is most likely to be correct?

(A) Improvement in glucose tolerance precedes changes in abdominal adiposity. ~
(B) Improvement in glucose tolerance will occur only after a reduction in abdominal adiposity.
(C) Improvement in glucose tolerance is similar to that seen in a nondiabetic 75-year-old who follows the same program.
(D) Insulin sensitivity is unlikely to improve.

33. Functionally based exercises targeted at nursing-home patients with significant dementia and dependency in activities of daily living (ADLs) are likely to result in which of the following?

(A) Increased patient frustration and behavioral disturbances
(B) Slower decline in ADLs over time ~
(C) Decreased time to perform ADL tasks
(D) Decreased nursing time devoted to ADLs
(E) Decreased endurance in performance of ADLs over time

34. Which of the following changes in the external auditory canal contributes to an increased incidence of cerumen impaction with increasing age?

   (A) Atrophy of epithelial sebaceous glands
   (B) Shortening and thinning of hair follicles
   (C) Increased cerumen production
   (D) Reduced number and activity of cerumen glands
   (E) Increased tortuosity of the external auditory canal

35. Which of the following gastrointestinal functions is more likely caused by disease than by age-related changes?

   (A) Increase in diverticular disease
   (B) Oral motor dysfunction manifested by altered mastication
   (C) Decrease in small intestinal motility
   (D) Decrease in splanchnic blood flow
   (E) Decrease in upper and lower esophageal sphincter resting pressures

36. A patient who is recovering from a stroke is medically stable, follows one-step directions but errs with two-step directions, is able to sit for no more than 1 to 2 hours per day, and requires maximal assistance with most activities of daily living. Which of the following is the most appropriate site for postacute care?

   (A) Home care with home-health rehabilitation services
   (B) Outpatient rehabilitation program
   (C) Nursing home with no rehabilitation provided
   (D) Skilled nursing facility with rehabilitation services
   (E) Acute-level rehabilitation hospital

37. Which of the following is the best approach to the treatment of acute hip fracture in a frail 85-year-old woman who has stable coronary artery disease, ischemic cardiomyopathy (ejection fraction 35%), well-controlled hypertension, and mild dementia?

   (A) Perform surgery within 24 to 48 hours, postoperative physical therapy five or more times per week.
   (B) Perform surgery within 24 to 48 hours, postoperative physical therapy three to five times per week.
   (C) Perform surgery within 24 to 48 hours, postoperative physical therapy one to three times per week.
   (D) Delay surgery to assess the patient's cardiac condition, postoperative physical therapy five or more times per week.
   (E) Delay surgery to assess the patient's cardiac condition, postoperative physical therapy three to five times per week.

38. An 80-year-old woman who has moderately severe Alzheimer's dementia is found at home approximately 1 week after she confined herself to bed prior because of an upper respiratory tract infection. A stage III pressure ulcer, 10 × 12 × 2 cm in depth, is noted over the sacrum. The wound is covered with necrotic tissue and copious yellowish-green, foul-smelling exudate. The surrounding skin is erythematous and warm. Which of the following is the most appropriate initial management for this patient?

   (A) Swab cultures, chemical debridement, and topical antibiotics
   (B) Swab cultures, blood cultures, and oral antibiotics
   (C) Swab cultures, blood cultures, surgical debridement, and intravenous antibiotics
   (D) Blood cultures, chemical debridement, and intravenous antibiotics
   (E) Blood cultures, surgical debridement, and intravenous antibiotics

39. An 85-year-old woman is admitted to the hospital because of a left hemispheric stroke. Her only other medical problem is hypertension. The patient weighs 55 kg (121 lb). She is afebrile. Pulse rate is 88 per minute, and respirations are 18 per minute. Blood pressure is 160/84 mm Hg. Cardiopulmonary and abdominal examinations are normal. She has no evidence of a visual field defect or neglect. Muscle strength is 3/5 on the right side. Skin inspection reveals no areas of breakdown. Which of the following pressure-relieving surfaces is most appropriate for this patient?

    (A) 1.5-inch foam overlay
    (B) 4.0-inch foam overlay
    (C) Dynamic air-filled overlay
    (D) Low-air-loss mattress
    (E) Air-fluidized bed

40. A 78-year-old woman who has multiple serious medical conditions and is minimally responsive is admitted to the general medical service for palliative care. Her family is in agreement that her living will be honored, so no aggressive diagnostic or curative therapies will be pursued. The patient periodically becomes restless and moans when she is turned in bed but is unable to rate or describe her discomfort. Symptoms improve following administration of morphine sulfate, 2 to 4 mg intravenously as needed. Which of the following is the most appropriate management strategy during the next 24 to 48 hours?

    (A) Continuation of the current regimen
    (B) Fentanyl, 25 μg transdermally
    (C) Sustained-release morphine sulfate, 15 mg orally twice daily
    (D) Morphine sulfate elixir, 5 to 10 mg orally every 4 hours
    (E) Morphine sulfate, 1 mg hourly by continuous intravenous infusion

41. An 86-year-old woman with severe Alzheimer's disease is admitted from home to the hospital for treatment of a stroke. With the assistance of home-health aides, her daughter cares for her and wishes to continue to do so. The mother is dependent in all activities of daily living, incontinent of bowel and bladder, and alert intermittently. The patient is observed to cough with oral intake in the hospital. The patient's advance directives state that she does not want her life prolonged by the use of artificial food or hydration and does not wish to receive cardiopulmonary resuscitation.

    What is the most appropriate next step in the management of this patient?

    (A) Discharge to home with prior home-care services
    (B) Discharge to institutional long-term care
    (C) Discharge to a skilled nursing facility for rehabilitation
    (D) Discharge to a home hospice program
    (E) Discharge to an assisted-living facility

42. A 71-year-old woman who has been smoking approximately one and one-half packs of cigarettes daily for 40 years seeks your help to stop smoking. She has tried several times to quit "cold turkey" and experienced irritability, changes in sleep habits, and craving. She now has begun caring for a grandson in her home and has read that her smoking could harm his health. She has seen advertisements for nicotine patches and gum but is unsure which, if either, would be right for her. The patient also works outside the home part time, and she finds it difficult to remember to take medication when she is not at home. She has been in good health, except for a chronic cough that worsens with seasonal allergies and a history of "difficult-to-control" seizures. Her neurologist, who prescribed carbamazepine and gabapentin after phenytoin and phenobarbital were ineffective, advised her not to use bupropion.

    The patient is edentulous and has loose-fitting dentures. Pulse rate is 76 per minute, and blood pressure is 154/92 mm Hg. The nasal septum is deviated, and the mucosa is swollen and boggy. The lung fields are clear, with no adventitious sounds. Which of the following is the most appropriate form of nicotine replacement therapy for this patient?

(A) Nasal spray
(B) Oral inhaler
(C) Transdermal patch
(D) Gum
(E) Sublingual tablet

43. A 78-year-old man with a history of coronary artery disease, hypothyroidism, and osteoarthritis of the knees is admitted to the hospital from home for shortness of breath. He is treated successfully for an exacerbation of congestive heart failure, with changes in his medication regimen and a sodium-restricted diet. He lives alone, gets out of bed by himself, and ambulates independently with a cane. Folstein Mini–Mental State Examination score is 29. He wishes to return home when discharged from the hospital.

Which of the following interventions is most likely to reduce subsequent hospital utilization for this patient?

(A) Discharge to postacute care for rehabilitation
(B) Coordinated discharge planning with follow-up at home
(C) Prescription of home physical therapy
(D) Recommendation for a friendly visitor
(E) Recommendation to attend a senior center

44. The wife of a 79-year-old man phones you because her husband "has not been acting right" since breakfast. He is leaning forward, drooling, and producing large amounts of saliva. Food "comes right back up" when he eats, and he has been coughing but is not short of breath. The patient has severe dementia, and his speech has been garbled ever since he suffered a stroke several years ago. When the wife asks the patient what is wrong, he points to his sternum but cannot describe what he is feeling. The wife notes no change in speech and no new weakness. Which of the following is the most likely diagnosis?

(A) New stroke
(B) Esophageal foreign body
(C) Gastric ulcer with outlet obstruction
(D) Zenker's diverticulum
(E) Pneumonia

45. Which of the following describes the most likely effect of normal aging on basic personality?

(A) More rigid
(B) More irritable
(C) More mellow
(D) More childlike
(E) No change

46. An 82-year-old man comes to you for evaluation of unsteadiness when walking. This began gradually but has increased in severity during the past 3 years. His son, with whom he lives, has positioned furniture or handrails throughout the house to provide support. He takes hydrochlorothiazide for hypertension. The patient has not had lightheadedness, palpitations, syncope, or vertigo. On physical examination, Romberg sign is positive, and no dysdiadochokinesis is noted. Which of the following is the most likely cause of the disequilibrium?

(A) Cerebrovascular disease
(B) Postural hypotension
(C) Cardioinhibitory carotid sinus syndrome
(D) Vasodepressor carotid sinus syndrome
(E) Hydrochlorothiazide

47. Which of the following statements is correct regarding hypochondriacal symptoms?

(A) They are more common in elderly persons.
(B) They are a permanent condition in elderly persons.
(C) They commonly are associated with depression.
(D) They seldom have a psychologic meaning.

48. A 90-year-old woman falls at home and fractures her right hip. She is unable to rise from the floor and is not found for 24 hours. A stage II pressure ulcer, 3.0 × 2.0 × 0.5 cm in depth, is noted over the right greater trochanter. Assessment of the wound reveals pink tissue with scant necrotic areas at the periphery; a small amount of purulent-appearing, odorous drainage; and no erythema of the surrounding skin. Which of the following is the most appropriate cleansing agent for this pressure ulcer?

(A) Any skin cleanser
(B) Any wound cleanser
(C) Normal saline
(D) Hydrogen peroxide
(E) 1% silver sulfadiazine

49. A 75-year-old man comes to your office to establish a primary care relationship. When obtaining social history, you ask about his religious beliefs and practices. Which of the following statements is most correct regarding religious beliefs?

(A) They are associated with better physical health outcomes.
(B) They are associated with better emotional health outcomes.
(C) They are associated with better physical and emotional health outcomes.
(D) They have no demonstrable association with physical or emotional health outcomes.

50. Which of the following statements is correct regarding assisted-living settings?

(A) The median age of female residents is 74.
(B) Nearly 75% of residents are discharged to a nursing home.
(C) Continuous skilled nursing care is provided for residents who can pay privately.
(D) Medicaid programs do not subsidize assisted-living services through waiver programs.
(E) Regulations for assisted living are highly diverse from state to state.

51. A 65-year-old man has type 2 diabetes mellitus, systolic hypertension, and hypercholesterolemia but no evidence of target organ damage. He smokes cigarettes. Current medications are a statin, chlorthalidone, and metformin. The patient walks at a brisk pace for 30 minutes every day. Findings of physical examination are normal except for peripheral neuropathy. Electrocardiogram shows normal sinus rhythm without evidence of myocardial infarction. The patient tells you that his neighbor takes aspirin to prevent strokes, and he asks whether he should take it too. Which of the following should you advise?

(A) There is no evidence that aspirin will benefit him.
(B) The potential benefits of aspirin may outweigh the potential harms.
(C) The potential harms of aspirin may outweigh the potential benefits.
(D) The potential benefits of dipyridamole are greater than those of aspirin.

52. An 86-year-old man is brought to the emergency department because of shortness of breath. He is inattentive, combative, and unable to speak in full sentences. Pulse rate is 128 per minute, and respirations are 28 per minute; blood pressure is 180/100 mm Hg. Physical examination reveals audible wheezes, bilateral crackles, jugular venous distention, an S_3, and pitting 2+ pedal edema. The patient lives with his son, who tells you that his father has heart failure and was in the hospital last week for a similar episode. Current medications are digoxin, furosemide, and captopril. The son administers these, supervises his father, and runs a lucrative family business.

Electrocardiogram shows sinus tachycardia but no new ischemic changes. Chest radiograph shows pulmonary edema and several old rib fractures. Complete blood cell count and other routine laboratory studies are normal, but serum digoxin level is zero. A recent echocardiogram revealed an ejection fraction of 42%. The patient has been in the emergency department nine times in the past year with similar presentations. Which of the following statements is correct?

(A) You should confront the son immediately about abuse or neglect of his father.
(B) A toxicology screen would not be useful.
(C) A high socioeconomic level makes elder mistreatment unlikely.
(D) Frequent emergency department visits are rare in elder mistreatment.
(E) Evidence of physical abuse, such as rib fractures, may coexist with neglect.

53. You are asked to serve on the Patient Care Committee of a full-service community hospital with active medical and surgical services. In an effort to improve the quality of care and reduce operating expenses, the hospital has asked the committee to concentrate on reducing average length of stay. Data demonstrate that among Medicare patients (about 50% of all discharges), the most common contributor to excessive length of stay is the development of delirium. Approximately 60% of the delirious patients are on the surgical service. The committee is charged with developing a cost-effective strategy to prevent delirium and improve quality of care, while reducing of hospital costs. Which of the following would best meet these objectives?

(A) Institute a mandatory geriatric consultation for all Medicare patients.
(B) Establish an "early warning" surveillance system to identify patients with early signs of delirium and trigger targeted nursing intervention.
(C) Screen all Medicare patients for delirium on admission; implement targeted interventions for all patients, even those without evidence of delirium.
(D) Encourage greater family involvement with routine hospital care, including nighttime visitation.
(E) Require anesthesiologists to develop practice guidelines encouraging the use of local rather than general anesthesia.

54. An 83-year-old woman who resides in a long-term care facility complains of chronic insomnia. She is bedridden and is legally blind secondary to diabetes mellitus. Which of the following age-related changes most likely contributes to this patient's sleep disturbance?

(A) A reduction in total sleep time
(B) A reduction in melatonin secretion
(C) A reduction in the percentage of stage 3 and 4 sleep
(D) An increase in the percentage of rapid eye movement (REM) sleep
(E) A breakdown in the segregation of sleep and wakefulness

55. Which of the following statements is correct regarding the prevalence of mood disorders in persons aged 65 and over?

(A) It is higher than in younger adults.
(B) It is higher in community dwellers than in nursing-home residents.
(C) Manic episodes are as common as in younger adults.
(D) The burden of depressive symptoms within a birth cohort fluctuates throughout the life cycle.
(E) Lack of a sufficient social network is a risk factor for development of depression.

56. A 75-year-old white man has back pain after gardening and is found to have a T10 vertebral compression fracture. The patient has no other symptoms and has always been in good health except for mild hypertension that is treated with a diuretic. He is very active and does weight-bearing exercise for 1 to 2 hours each day. He does not smoke cigarettes and drinks alcohol only occasionally. Which of the following is the most likely cause of the fracture?

(A) Idiopathic osteoporosis
(B) Testosterone deficiency
(C) Longstanding corticosteroid use
(D) Chronic malabsorption
(E) Metastatic carcinoma

57. A 78-year-old man has longstanding urinary frequency and urgency that has worsened in the past month. He often cannot reach the toilet in time and must change clothes once or twice a day. The patient has a tremor of the left hand that has worsened during the past 2 months. His wife reports that he is "lazy and hardly moves around any more." Medical history also includes hypertension, coronary artery disease, and hypercholesterolemia.

The patient has masked facies, diminished arm swing with normal gait, and increased muscle tone on the left side. A resting tremor is present on the left. The abdomen and genitalia are normal. Rectal examination shows brown stool in the vault and no evidence of fecal impaction. The prostate gland seems slightly large, with partial obliteration of the median sulcus, but without nodules or masses. Urinalysis is normal. Plasma glucose and serum calcium levels are normal; serum creatinine is 1.2 mg/dL. Which of the following tests is the most appropriate next step?

(A) Urine cytology
(B) Serum prostate-specific antigen
(C) Postvoid residual volume (PVR)
(D) Cystometry
(E) Computed tomography of the head

58. Which of the following statements is correct regarding persons living beyond age 90?

(A) They have as many or more chronic conditions as persons in their 70s and 80s.
(B) They often have siblings and other first-degree relatives of a similar age.
(C) They typically have followed a healthier life style than persons who die at a younger age.
(D) They have higher health care costs in their terminal illnesses than persons who die at a younger age.

59. A 68-year-old woman has a 4-month history of progressive pain in the right shoulder. She is unable to wear pullover sweaters or comb the back of her hair and cannot reach items on high shelves. The patient has poorly controlled diabetes mellitus and a history of ulcer disease. Examination of the shoulder discloses no tenderness to palpation or crepitus. Passive abduction, forward flexion, and external rotation are limited and painful. There is no subacromial tenderness. Which of the following is the most likely diagnosis?

(A) Subacromial bursitis
(B) Rotator cuff tear
(C) Bicep tendonitis
(D) Adhesive capsulitis
(E) Osteoarthritis

60. A 76-year-woman, who recently relocated to your area to be near her daughter, comes to your office for an initial visit. She lives alone in an apartment and has no impairments of activities of daily living. Current medications are a thiazide diuretic, calcium and vitamin D supplements, and a multivitamin. Her pulse rate is 104 per minute. Generalized muscle weakness and 2+ ankle edema are noted. Her Mini–Mental State Examination score is 30/30. Serum thyroxine is 16.8 µg/dL, and thyrotropin is less than 0.01 µg/dL. Which of the following therapies is most appropriate for this patient?

(A) No treatment
(B) Propylthiouracil
(C) Tapazole
(D) Radioactive iodine
(E) Surgical ablation of the thyroid gland

61. A 70-year-old man has colon cancer with metastases to the liver and lungs. His advance directive states that he desires medical treatment only for conditions that could be easily reversed. His daughter, with whom he lives, has been designated with durable power of attorney for health care. Pain has been controlled with sustained-release morphine sulfate, 120 mg orally every 12 hours, and lorazepam, 1 mg orally at bedtime. The family asks you to make a home visit because the patient has become disoriented and is unable to follow commands. He has been agitated at night and had visual hallucinations. Oral intake has decreased during the past 12 hours, but he can still swallow liquids.

The patient is lethargic but rouses easily to voice. His attention wanders, and you must repeat commands several times. There is no grimacing or other obvious sign of pain. Temperature is 36.4C (97.5F). Respirations are 18 per minute. The mouth is dry but skin turgor appears normal. Cardiopulmonary and abdominal examinations are unremarkable. All four extremities show purposeful movement. The daughter desires a trial of simple measures to reverse this decline but wishes to avoid hospitalization. You substitute morphine elixir, every 4 hours, at a lower total dose of narcotic, and you instruct the daughter to rehydrate the patient orally. Which of the following is the most appropriate next step?

(A) Explain that this preterminal condition is unlikely to be reversed even with aggressive measures.
(B) Order computed tomography of the head before initiating further therapy.
(C) Administer naloxone to reverse the opiate effect and begin amoxicillin–clavulanate, orally, for possible early pneumonia.
(D) Discontinue lorazepam and begin haloperidol, 2 mg orally at bedtime.

62. A 70-year-old black American man notes gradually decreasing vision in the right eye. He has a 10-year history of non-insulin-dependent diabetes mellitus and a 3-year history of hypertension. Current medications are two oral hypoglycemic agents, a diuretic, and an angiotensin-converting enzyme inhibitor. He checks his blood glucose weekly and does not follow a strict diet. Cardiopulmonary, abdominal, and musculoskeletal findings are normal except for obesity. Neurologic examination shows decreased touch sensation in the fingertips. Urinalysis shows mild proteinuria. Fingerstick blood glucose level is greater than 200 mg/dL. Hgb A_{1c} is 10.2%. Which of the following is the least likely cause of the vision loss?

(A) Cataract
(B) Vitreous hemorrhage
(C) Macular edema
(D) Macular ischemia
(E) Age-related macular degeneration

63. An elderly man with multiple medical problems and dependencies in activities of daily living has been in an intensive care unit (ICU) for 1 week. He was admitted for treatment of pneumonia and received aggressive care, including ventilator support. The ICU team believes that the patient is very unlikely to survive this episode and probably will die within 1 week, even if life support is continued. The team has reached consensus that the medically appropriate approach is to discontinue life support and provide comfort care. The patient lacks decisional capacity and has not completed an advance directive. His wife has been involved in his care during hospitalization. An adult daughter is very close to her father but lives out of state and is unable to be present.

The ICU team discusses their decision with the patient's wife and asks her permission to discontinue life support and provide comfort care only. She listens carefully and asks that everything possible be done to keep her husband alive. She believes that he might recover. The team agrees to continue full life-support care.

Several days later, the patient's condition has deteriorated further. The ICU is full and more beds are needed. The team again discusses the situation with the wife. When asked to decide as if she were her husband, she thinks that he probably would want life support discontinued at this point but that she obviously is not him and cannot decide as if she were. She hesitantly tells the team that she feels pressured by the hospital to stop treatment for her husband, who may get better, and that this is wrong. Which of the following options is the best approach at this time?

(A) Continue life support without further discussion.
(B) Continue life support while pursuing discussions with the wife.
(C) Request psychiatric assistance to address the wife's use of denial as a defense mechanism.
(D) Seek permission from the patient's daughter to discontinue life support.
(E) Inform the wife that continued ICU care is medically futile and discontinue life support.

64. A 75-year-old woman comes to your office for a routine visit. She has mild hypertension for which she takes hydrochlorothiazide, 25 mg daily. She had a total abdominal hysterectomy and oophorectomy at age 48 because of leiomyomata associated with heavy irregular bleeding. She took perimenopausal hormone-replacement therapy briefly. Five years ago, bone mineral density was 1 standard deviation above the mean (Z score of +1) for age. The patient has no family history of cancer; her mother died of a myocardial infarction at age 80. Results of Papanicolaou testing prior to hysterectomy had been normal. She has no vaginal symptoms and has never noted any breast masses. In addition to annual clinical breast examination, which of the following screening tests should you recommend?

(A) Bimanual pelvic examination
(B) Bimanual pelvic examination and mammography
(C) Bimanual pelvic examination, Pap smear from the vaginal cuff, and mammography
(D) Mammography
(E) Pap smear from the vaginal cuff and mammography

65. A 67-year-old woman undergoes dual-energy x-ray absorptiometry (DEXA). Her bone mineral density in the lumbar spine and proximal femur are found to be in the osteopenic range, in comparison with young normal persons. The patient refuses pharmacologic treatment other than calcium and vitamin D. You recommend an increase in physical activity, which she is willing to do. Which of the following activities is most likely to help maintain bone density?

(A) Tai chi
(B) Swimming
(C) Resistance training
(D) Stationary bicycling

66. A 70-year-old Mexican American man comes to you for an initial visit. He recently moved to your area, following the death of his wife 14 months ago. The patient describes his overall health as "pretty good" but has fallen twice and had other "close calls" in the past 6 months. He has taken hydrochlorothiazide for many years, but his former primary clinician told him that a second medication might be required to control recurrent hypertension. The patient falls asleep without much difficulty but awakens several times nightly.

When you review the patient's health questionnaire, you note a positive response to the question on alcohol consumption. He claims to drink socially and denies any problem with drinking. He mentions that he drank heavily as a young man but "cut way back" when he married. You believe it would be worthwhile to know whether this patient now or has ever met the criteria for alcoholism or alcohol dependence, as well as how much and how often he currently drinks. Which of the following questionnaires is most appropriate to use in interviewing this patient?

(A) CAGE
(B) MAST
(C) PRIME-MD
(D) TWEAK
(E) AUDIT

67. A 72-year-old woman loses small amounts of urine when she coughs, sneezes, or laughs. She also loses a large volume when she gets out of bed in the morning. The patient is not always aware of the urine loss and usually changes incontinence pads about three times a day. The patient underwent a surgical procedure for urinary incontinence 6 years ago. Incontinence recurred about 1 year ago and has worsened in the past 3 months. Medical history also includes diabetes mellitus and hypertension. Her mother had breast cancer at age 82; the patient had a normal mammogram 2 months ago.

The patient is 160 cm (63 in) tall and weighs 88 kg (194 lb). Gait is normal. Orthostatic changes are noted in blood pressure, but she denies dizziness. Neuropathy is present in a stocking-and-glove pattern. Ankle jerks are absent bilaterally. Pelvic examination reveals first-degree uterine prolapse. Vaginal muscle squeeze is perceptible for less than 1 second and is barely felt around the fingers. When the patient coughs forcibly, a small amount of urine is lost. Postvoid residual volume is 375 mL. Which of the following treatment options should you recommend?

(A) Urodynamic studies
(B) Pelvic muscle (Kegel's) exercises
(C) Dicyclomine, 10 mg twice daily
(D) Oxybutynin, 2.5 mg twice daily
(E) Repeat surgical correction

68. A 76-year-old woman has a 6-month history of lower back pain that is present most of the day and has increased in the past 6 weeks. It worsens with exercise such as walking her dog, and she describes aching pain "like a toothache" in both thighs. She has little pain at night. Medical history includes a cholecystectomy many years ago and a L4–5 discectomy at age 60. Although she reports increasing difficulty with ambulation, she is able to walk "pretty well" at the supermarket when pushing a shopping cart. The patient stopped attending physical therapy because "it wasn't helping." Which of the following is the most likely diagnosis?

(A) Recurrent disc disease at L4–5
(B) Degenerative spinal stenosis at L4–5
(C) Ankylosing spondylitis
(D) Compression fracture
(E) Spasm of the paraspinous muscles

69. Which of the following is the most effective and least costly strategy to prevent exacerbation of chronic illness, hospitalization, and death due to influenza in elderly patients?

(A) Outbreak prophylaxis with oseltamivir or zanamivir for all residents and staff
(B) Outbreak prophylaxis with amantadine or rimantadine for all residents and staff
(C) Treatment with oseltamivir or zanamivir for all residents and staff
(D) Annual vaccination for all residents
(E) Annual vaccination for all residents and staff

70. According recommendations of the American Diabetes Association of 2001, which of the following criteria establishes a diagnosis of diabetes mellitus?

(A) Fasting plasma glucose of 110 to 126 mg/dL
(B) Fasting plasma glucose ≥ 110 mg/dL on two occasions
(C) Fasting plasma glucose ≥ 126 mg/dL on two occasions
(D) Classic symptoms of diabetes mellitus plus random plasma glucose ≥ 126 mg/dL
(E) Plasma glucose ≥ 120 mg/dL after 2 hours during a standard oral glucose tolerance test, on two occasions

71. The average length of stay in your hospital's medical unit has been increasing. Analysis of outliers among the most common diagnosis related groups (DRGs) reveals a number of patients who had prolonged hospitalizations secondary to acute confusional states. As a member of the quality improvement committee, you have been asked to suggest evidence-based measures to prevent this problem. Which of the following interventions should you recommend?

(A) Train nursing staff to perform serial Mini–Mental State Examination (MMSE).
(B) Establish a delirium consultation service to evaluate patients at the request of their attending physicians.
(C) Implement a clinical pathway to expedite neurologic imaging and other diagnostic tests in patients with delirium.
(D) Establish interdisciplinary protocols to address sensory impairment, immobility, dehydration, cognitive impairment, and sleep deprivation.
(E) Implement early discharge planning so that patients can be sent home before their predicted length of stay is exceeded.

72. Which of the following psychiatric disorders is most common in elderly persons?

(A) Anxiety disorders
(B) Personality disorders
(C) Mood disorders
(D) Somatoform disorders
(E) Substance abuse

73. A 71-year-old white woman who does not smoke cigarettes comes to the emergency department because of progressive dyspnea. She has had very mild shortness of breath on climbing stairs for 18 months but reports that this worsened after a "chest cold" 5 weeks ago. She now has a persistent nonproductive cough.

The patient is 172 cm (67 in) tall and weighs 82.0 kg (180.5 lb), for a body mass index of 28.3. Temperature is 36.7C (98.1F). Ear, nose, throat, and cardiovascular findings are normal. End-expiratory wheezing and cough with deep inspiration are noted. She has no cyanosis, clubbing, or edema. Chest radiograph and electrocardiogram are normal. Pulse oximetry indicates an Sao_2 of 97% with patient breathing room air. Which of the following should you do next?

(A) Order exercise electrocardiography.
(B) Prescribe a course of exercise to improve the deconditioning.
(C) Prescribe a 5-day course of oseltamivir.
(D) Perform pulmonary function tests.
(E) Admit the patient to the hospital for respiratory therapy and intravenous antibiotics.

74. A patient returns to the nursing home following hospitalization for pneumonia and superimposed delirium. A stage III sacral pressure ulcer developed during hospitalization because he was restrained to prevent him from removing an intravenous catheter. Weight in the hospital was 70 kg (154 lb), for a body mass index of 22.8; this is his "usual weight," but it is only 90% of ideal. Cognitive level is near baseline; Mini–Mental State Examination score is 16/30. He is able to follow a two-step command and to sit independently but requires assistance with transferring, dressing, grooming, and toileting. Muscular weakness is apparent in the deltoids, with some squaring of the shoulders. The quadriceps also are weak and wasted. The patient has no difficulty swallowing liquids or solids. The nursing-home dietitian recommends that the patient resume his previous diet, which provided 2100 kcal daily, with 70 g of protein. Which of the following should you advise?

(A) Institute oral liquid supplements with meals.
(B) Resume the previous diet.
(C) Increase protein intake to at least 105 g daily.
(D) Increase caloric intake to at least 2400 kcal daily.

75. A 72-year-old man has a "pimple" on his nose that occasionally bleeds and may have increased in size during the past year. The lesion is a 0.8-cm, dome-shaped, umbilicated papule with pearly translucence and telangiectasia. A small hemorrhagic crust covers the central portion. Which of the following is the most likely diagnonsis?

(A) Basal cell carcinoma
(B) Squamous cell carcinoma
(C) Sebaceous hyperplasia
(D) Molluscum contagiosum
(E) Keratoacanthoma

76. You are asked to evaluate an 85-year-old woman who has osteoarthritis of the right hip; she is scheduled to undergo elective total hip replacement. Her other medical problems are hypertension and anxiety disorder. Current medications are hydrochlorothiazide, 25 mg daily; atenolol, 50 mg daily; and alprazolam, 0.25 mg daily at bedtime. The patient is a pleasant, healthy-appearing woman who has a steady but antalgic gait. Pulse rate is 64 per minute, and blood pressure is 132/80 mm Hg. Cardiopulmonary and neurologic examinations are normal. Mini–Mental State Examination score is 29/30. Hematocrit, leukocyte count, blood urea nitrogen, plasma glucose, serum electrolytes, and urinalysis are within normal limits. Which of the following perioperative measures is most likely to reduce the risk for postoperative delirium?

(A) Immediate discontinuation of alprazolam
(B) Use of epidural rather than general anesthesia
(C) Avoidance of opiate analgesics postoperatively
(D) Insertion of a bladder catheter
(E) Maintenance of hematocrit at 30% or higher

77. Which of the following features predicts a good prognosis in late-life depression?

    (A) Presence of cerebral pathology
    (B) Slower recovery time
    (C) More severe initial symptoms
    (D) Duration of symptoms for more than 2 years
    (E) Younger age

78. An 84-year-old woman who lives in an intermediate-care facility has had several falls since she was discharged from a geropsychiatric unit. During that admission, medications were adjusted to manage depression with underlying psychotic features. Medical history also includes glaucoma, hypertension, and valvular heart disease.

    Which of the following medications is least likely to contribute to her falls?

    (A) Fluoxetine, 20 mg daily
    (B) Hydrochlorothiazide, 25 mg daily
    (C) Lorazepam, 0.5 mg three times daily
    (D) Risperidone, 2 mg at bedtime

79. An 83-year-old woman is brought to the emergency department because of dizziness on standing, followed by brief loss of consciousness. She has hypertension but is otherwise healthy. Current medications are metoprolol, 50 mg daily; captopril, 25 mg every morning; and nitroglycerin, 0.04 mg sublingually as needed.

    The patient now feels well. Blood pressure is 130/70 mm Hg sitting and 100/60 mm Hg standing. Physical examination is otherwise normal. Complete blood cell count, comprehensive metabolic panel, and blood urea nitrogen are normal, as is electrocardiogram. Which of the following is the most likely cause of the syncopal episode?

    (A) Sepsis
    (B) Drug-related event
    (C) Hypovolemic hypotensive episode
    (D) Cardiogenic shock
    (E) Unidentifiable cause

80. An 80-year-old woman has mild Alzheimer's disease. She lives with her husband, who assists with her care. She has most of her natural teeth and has no problems chewing. She has not had regular dental care, but a recent examination revealed caries at several root surfaces; restoration with fillings would be possible. Which of the following is the best management plan?

    (A) Dental radiographs to identify pulp cavities that should be treated
    (B) Treatment of symptomatic conditions only
    (C) Restorative dentistry and topical application of fluoride
    (D) Restorative dentistry and subsequent removal of teeth affected by periodontal disease secondary to poor oral hygiene
    (E) Prophylactic removal of remaining teeth and provision of well-fitting dentures

81. Which of the following statements regarding functional status is correct?

    (A) Approximately 10% of persons aged 65 and over have difficulty with one or more activities of daily living (ADLs) or instrumental activities of daily living (IADLs).
    (B) Approximately 75% of persons aged 85 and over have difficulty with one or more ADLs or IADLs.
    (C) In all age groups, men report a higher percentage of ADL limitations than women do.
    (D) White Americans have more ADL and IADL limitations than Hispanic Americans do.
    (E) Increased ADL limitation is associated with higher socioeconomic status.

82. Which of the following statements regarding ECT is correct?

    (A) It has limited usefulness in patients aged 75 and over.
    (B) It is as effective in elderly patients as in younger adults.
    (C) It is absolutely contraindicated in patients with a seizure disorder.
    (D) The presence of subcortical changes on magnetic resonance imaging of the head predicts a good response.
    (E) The risk of relapse after an adequate course of ECT is low.

83. A healthy 68-year-old man has no history of heart disease and currently walks about 20 minutes twice a day. He also works in his garden. The patient plans to begin an exercise program consisting of upper- and lower-extremity resistance exercises, stair climbing, and brisk walking 3 days per week. Which of the following statements describes the long-term effects of increased physical activity on this patient's risk for coronary artery disease (CAD) and mortality?

   (A) For someone already engaged in moderate daily exercise, further risk reduction is unlikely with more vigorous activity.
   (B) Risks are lower in older persons who engage in vigorous activity than in those who exercise moderately.
   (C) All-cause mortality is lower in older persons who exercise moderately, but risk for CAD is unaffected.
   (D) Risks for CAD and mortality increase in older persons who exercise vigorously.

84. A 73-year-old woman is brought to your office by her two nieces, who are her legal guardians, and with whom she has lived for more than 25 years. The patient has an intelligence quotient of 30 but is able to dress and bathe herself fairly independently. She has become increasingly irritable and seems physically uncomfortable in recent months, although her health always has been good. Her appetite has diminished and she had lost about 10 lb. She now sleeps only 4 or 5 hours per night. The patient has become less social with other family members and no longer spends time on her favorite activities. Her pleasant affect has been replaced by sadness or anger. On one occasion, she was found weeping in her room. The nieces have not been able to figure out what is bothering the patient; they are frustrated by her increased needs and problem behaviors and are not sure they can continue to provide a home for her.

   Findings of physical examination 6 months ago, including pelvic examination, were normal. The patient takes no medications routinely and has never used alcohol or tobacco. Which of the following is the most appropriate next step?

   (A) Recommend residential placement.
   (B) Refer the family to a psychiatrist experienced in developmental disabilities.
   (C) Arrange for home care services.
   (D) Begin a medical work-up for occult disease.
   (E) Prescribe an antidepressant.

85. An 81-year-old woman has fallen outside her home on two occasions. She experienced significant bruising from the second event. The patient is interested in exercises to reduce her fall risk. Which of the following is correct?

   (A) Exercises should be done with a group of people to be effective.
   (B) Ongoing physical therapy supervision is important.
   (C) Strength-training exercises are more important than balance-training exercises.
   (D) Regular exercise may reduce fall risk for a period of at least 2 years.
   (E) In patients age 80 and over, the effectiveness of exercise in reducing falls is unknown.

86. An 87-year-old woman is admitted to a nursing home because of increasing difficulties with self-care. She has been taking acetaminophen on an as-needed basis for joint pains in her knees, with incomplete effect. Her physical examination confirms degenerative joint disease in these joints. What is the most appropriate next step in management of her arthritis?

   (A) Obtain additional history regarding joint pain.
   (B) Order radiographs of all affected joints.
   (C) Prescribe propoxyphene, as needed, for pain.
   (D) Prescribe a course of corticosteroids.
   (E) Refer her to an orthopedic surgeon for consideration of a knee replacement.

87. You chair the infection-control committee at a 120-bed nursing home. In reviewing the facility's influenza immunization program, you find that almost all residents are immunized each September and that 20% of staff are immunized by their personal primary clinicians. The administration is skeptical but would consider providing a free immunization program for staff if research has shown evidence of benefit. Which of the following should you recommend?

(A) Continue to immunize residents in September; offer no special program for staff.
(B) Continue to immunize residents in September; establish an immunization program for all staff.
(C) Immunize residents in mid-October to mid-November; establish an immunization program for staff at high risk.
(D) Immunize residents in mid-October to mid-November; establish an immunization program for all staff.

88. A sedentary 73-year-old woman who has mild osteoarthritis of the hips and knees comes to you for a routine visit. She is accompanied by her daughter. The patient is 160 cm (63 in) tall and weighs 62 kg (150 lb), for a body mass index of 24.2. Her only medical complaint is morning joint stiffness that resolves in about 30 minutes. She takes acetaminophen, 1000 mg twice daily as needed for pain, and a daily multivitamin. Which of the following is the best recommendation for physical activity?

(A) Treadmill exercise electrocardiography before beginning an exercise program
(B) Walking, 30 minutes per day, 5 days per week
(C) Water aerobics, 3 days per week
(D) Determining what physical activities the patient likes to do and what prevents her from exercising
(E) Enlisting the daughter to help her mother engage in regular moderate physical activity

89. A 70-year-old white woman has a foreign body or gritty sensation in the left eye when she awakens, and the eyelashes occasionally are stuck together. Her eyes also are red but become clearer by the end of the day. Physical findings are otherwise normal except for broken capillaries on the cheeks and erythema of both eyelid margins. Which of the following treatments should you recommend?

(A) Antibiotic ointment
(B) Corticosteroid ointment
(C) Antibiotic plus corticosteroid ointment
(D) Oral antibiotics
(E) Oral corticosteroids

90. A 68-year-old woman has a history of Parkinson's disease, hypertension, and osteoarthritis. Current medications are carbidopa–levodopa (25 mg and 100 mg) three times daily; selegiline, 5 mg twice daily; losartan, 50 mg daily; celecoxib, 200 mg daily; and a multivitamin. In the past 3 weeks, she has been taking diphenhydramine at bedtime for insomnia. The patient now reports the onset of urinary incontinence. Which of the following is the most appropriate intervention?

(A) Discontinue celecoxib.
(B) Discontinue diphenhydramine.
(C) Discontinue losartan.
(D) Substitute fosinopril for losartan.
(E) Begin tolterodine.

91. Which of the following statements is correct regarding caregiver burden?

(A) Caregiver education has not been shown to reduce caregivers' subjective ratings of burden.
(B) Caregiver variables, such as perceived burden and physical health, are stronger predictors of institutionalization than are patient variables.
(C) Caregivers for patients who are more severely cognitively impaired tend to report greater burden.
(D) Men who are caregivers tend to report greater burden than do women who are caregivers.

92. An 84-year-old woman moved to a nursing home 6 months ago, following her husband's death. She has severe dementia and requires considerable assistance with eating. Since admission, she has lost 5 kg (11 lb), which is 20% below her ideal weight. No aspiration is noted on swallowing evaluation, but the patient eats very slowly. The staff confirm that a long period of time is required to feed the patient. Her dentures fit well, and a psychiatric evaluation reveals no evidence of depression. The patient never made any statements about artificial feeding and does not have the capacity to understand that option now. Which of the following is the most appropriate action?

(A) Order nutritional supplements.
(B) Develop interdisciplinary strategies to improve feeding.
(C) Arrange for temporary placement of a nasogastric feeding tube.
(D) Place a percutaneous endoscopic gastrostomy.
(E) Begin antidepressant therapy.

93. A 69-year-old man comes to your office for an initial visit. His medical problems include hypertension, benign prostatic hyperplasia, and obesity. He has been slightly depressed since his wife died 1 year ago. He asks you what he can do to make his "golden years really golden." Which of the following statements best describes this patient's chance of living a long and healthy life?

(A) It is genetically determined and resistant to change.
(B) It is related to his level of physical activity.
(C) It is independent of his depression.
(D) It is most strongly related to losing weight.

94. You are caring for an 86-year-old woman who lives in a long-term-care facility. The patient has osteoarthritis that has been treated intermittently with nonsteroidal anti-inflammatory agents. She also has residual left-sided weakness following a stroke 10 years ago and ambulates with a walker. Atrial fibrillation was detected at the time of the stroke, and warfarin was begun. INR was 2.0 several days ago. Her only other complaint is mild forgetfulness. The patient has received amantadine prophylaxis (200 mg once a day), as have other residents because of an influenza outbreak.

The patient is taken to the emergency department because of progressive confusion. She is only minimally responsive to voice commands but does recognize you. Temperature is 37.6C (99.7F). Pulse rate is 72 per minute, and rhythm is irregular. Respirations are 16 per minute. Blood pressure is 120/74 mm Hg. There is no nuchal rigidity. Lung findings are unremarkable; cardiac examination is normal except for the irregular rhythm. The abdomen is soft, and bowel sounds are normal. No pedal edema or venous cords are present. Except for the blunted sensorium, no new neurologic findings are noted. Cranial nerve examination is normal.

Laboratory studies:

Leukocyte count	10,000/cu mm; normal differential
Blood urea nitrogen	32 mg/dL
Serum creatinine	2.3 mg/dL
Serum electrolytes	Normal
Serum calcium	Normal
Serum phosphorus	Normal
Serum magnesium	Normal

Which of the following is the most likely explanation for the patient's condition?

(A) Embolic stroke secondary to atrial fibrillation
(B) Intracerebral bleeding
(C) Subarachnoid hemorrhage
(D) Adverse reaction to amantadine
(E) Influenza A encephalitis

95. You are asked to see a 78-year-old man who has a 6-week history of intermittent low-back pain that often occurs with bending but does not radiate into the legs. He obtains some relief when he takes acetaminophen or over-the-counter nonsteroidal anti-inflammatory agents. The patient has continued to take a daily walk of about one quarter mile, which is his only exercise. Another clinician ordered magnetic resonance imaging (MRI) of the lumbar spine, which showed "moderate spinal stenosis at L2–4 with bony foraminal encroachment on the nerve roots." The discs were described as deficient in water content, with some bulging and evidence of "degeneration." Which of the following should you recommend?

(A) A continuous regimen of high-dose nonsteroidal anti-inflammatory agents
(B) Referral to a chiropractor for a trial of spinal manipulation
(C) Referral to a physical therapist for a trial of flexibility exercises and sustained aerobic exercise
(D) Referral to an anesthesiologist for a course of facet-joint injections
(E) Referral to a surgeon for possible laminectomy

96. Which of the following is the most common pattern of hearing loss among older Americans?

(A) Symmetric high-frequency sensorineural
(B) Symmetric high-frequency conductive
(C) Asymmetric high-frequency conductive
(D) Symmetric low-frequency sensorineural
(E) Asymmetric high-frequency sensorineural

97. A 72-year-old woman has mitral valve prolapse with regurgitation. She has most of her natural teeth and has no problems chewing any foods. The patient has no drug allergies. Which of the following should you recommend prior to routine cleaning of the teeth?

(A) Amoxicillin, 2 g 1 hour before the procedure
(B) Clindamycin, 600 mg 1 hour before the procedure
(C) Erythromycin, 1 g 1 hour before the procedure
(D) Amoxicillin, 500 mg 1 hour before the procedure, then 4 and 8 hours after
(E) Cephalexin, 500 mg 1 hour before the procedure, then 4 and 8 hours after

98. A 75-year-old man comes to you for evaluation of dizziness. Symptoms began 8 weeks ago, when he had severe dizziness on rising from the bed. Since then, "everything is moving" when he turns his head quickly, rolls over in bed, or stands upright after bending forward. Episodes occur several times a day and last about 1 minute. He is fatigued and unsteady for up to 1 hour afterward. The patient has been less active recently because of this problem. Which of the following is most likely to be beneficial?

(A) Reduction of activity
(B) Epley maneuver
(C) Dix-Hallpike maneuver
(D) Diazepam
(E) Meclizine

99. An 82-year-old woman, who lives at home with her son, has diabetes mellitus and partial blindness. She has both Medicare and Medicaid coverage. She currently needs assistance with bathing, dressing, and medication management. The son provides this assistance but worries about her overall well-being and lack of socialization. Although he feels overwhelmed by the demands of caregiving, he would like his mother to remain at home as long as possible. Which of the following options is most appropriate?

(A) Assisted living
(B) Adult foster care
(C) "Swing bed"
(D) Program of All-Inclusive Care for the Elderly (PACE)
(E) Nursing home

100. A 69-year-old man who underwent radical prostatectomy 3 months ago consults you because he loses a small amount of urine when he coughs or lifts objects. Findings of physical examination are normal. He is able to rise from a chair and walk unassisted for 25 feet in less than 5 seconds. There is no evidence of obstruction or urethral stricture. Postvoid residual volume is 25 mL. Peak urine flow rate is 23 mL per second. Which of the following is the most appropriate initial approach?

(A) Reassurance and observation
(B) Comprehensive urodynamic evaluation
(C) Intermittent catheterization, three times daily
(D) Implantation of an artificial urethral sphincter
(E) Tamsulosin, 0.4 mg daily

101. A 68-year-old postmenopausal woman complains of vaginal dryness and urinary frequency and urgency. She has not had dysuria or urinary incontinence, and she takes no medications regularly. On pelvic examination, the vaginal epithelium is pale and thin, with a decrease in the height of the rugae. Urinalysis is normal. Topical treatment with which of the following agents is the most appropriate first step in management?

(A) Corticosteroids
(B) Estrogen
(C) Metronidazole
(D) Nystatin
(E) Testosterone

102. A 66-year-old woman has had recurrent urinary tract infections (UTI) for many years. The patient is otherwise healthy and is sexually active with one male partner on a regular basis, without pain or discomfort. Symptoms tend to occur a day or two following intercourse. She has not had pyelonephritis or required hospitalization. When urine cultures have been obtained, antibiotic-susceptible *Escherichia coli* and *Staphylococcus saprophyticus* have been isolated. Which of the following should you do first?

(A) Encourage the patient to drink cranberry juice.
(B) Perform pelvic examination and measure postvoid residual volume.
(C) Begin postcoital antibiotic prophylaxis.
(D) Begin daily, low-dose, suppressive antibiotic therapy.
(E) Begin estrogen supplementation.

103. An assessment of instrumental activities of daily living (IADLs) typically includes which of the following?

(A) Urinary continence
(B) Ability to take medications
(C) Recreational activities
(D) Use of assistive devices
(E) Social supports

104. A 68-year-old man has a 2-year history of progressive impairment of gait, posture, and balance. He walks with small, shuffling steps and has fallen repeatedly. Cognitive dysfunction developed in the past 6 months, although mentation sometimes is normal. The patient's wife describes episodes in which the patient seems to "go blank." Levodopa therapy was discontinued because of florid visual hallucinations. Which of the following is the most likely diagnosis?

(A) Normal-pressure hydrocephalus
(B) Parkinson's disease
(C) Alzheimer's disease
(D) Multi-infarct dementia
(E) Dementia with Lewy bodies (DLB)

105. Which of the following cancers is associated most strongly with heavy drinking?

(A) Skin
(B) Head and neck
(C) Renal
(D) Prostate
(E) Testicular cancer. It has been suggested that alcohol may increase the risk for stomach, pancreas, colon, lung, and breast cancer, although the evidence has been less clear.

106. An 84-year-old man is brought to the emergency department from a nursing home because of fever, cough, and a change in mental status. Temperature now is 38.1C (100.6F). Pulse rate is 110 per minute, and respirations are 28 per minute. Blood pressure is 110/60 mm Hg. The patient is unable to participate with mental status testing because of delirium. He has bilateral cataracts. Wasting is noted in the temporal areas and infrascapular fat pads; the deltoids are rounded. Crackles are heard at the right lung base with a focal area of tubular breath sounds. Skin findings are normal. Chest radiograph shows an infiltrate or atelectasis at the right lung base. Results of laboratory studies are within normal limits except for serum albumin of 2.0 g/dL.

The patient is admitted to the hospital. A dietitian reports: "Current weight not available, triceps skin fold indicates decreased fat stores, low albumin reflects significant visceral protein depletion; suggest tube feeding until swallowing evaluation is performed." The nurse manager tells you about a critical pathway for pneumonia that is being implemented. According to its guidelines, a serum albumin level below 2.5 g/dL is a risk factor for poorer outcomes. Which of the following should you recommend?

- (A) Weigh the patient and obtain baseline weight from the nursing home.
- (B) Encourage oral feeding.
- (C) Order liquid supplements with meals.
- (D) Begin peripheral parenteral nutrition.
- (E) Begin tube feedings.

107. An 87-year-old woman recently fell at home, after tripping over the telephone cord. She consults you because she is worried about another fall. The patient lives alone and is cognitively intact. She has cataracts and diminished visual acuity; osteoarthritic changes in the hands and knees; and absent Achilles' reflexes bilaterally with normal sensation to pinprick. She is unable to rise from a chair without using her arms. Romberg test is normal, but she is unable to do semi-tandem or tandem stances for more than 3 seconds and cannot stand on one leg. Gait is symmetric, with good foot clearance and steady turns. In addition to other measures, which of the following types of exercise is most likely to reduce her risk for falls?

- (A) A walking program, gradually increasing time and distance
- (B) A seated stretching program, 1 hour, 3 days per week
- (C) Stationary bicycling, gradually increasing time, to avoid impact on the knees
- (D) Balance and ankle-strengthening exercises, gradually increasing in difficulty

108. A 90-year-old man has chronic obstructive pulmonary disease, congestive heart failure, osteoarthritis, chronic urinary tract infections, and type 2 diabetes mellitus. Physical examination reveals a white coating over much of the intra-oral soft tissues. When the coating is wiped away with a gauze pad, the underlying site is reddish. Which of the following is the most likely diagnosis?

- (A) Candidiasis
- (B) Leukoplakia
- (C) Lichen planus
- (D) Squamous cell carcinoma

109. Research on group exercise programs in skilled nursing facilities supports which of the following statements?

  (A) Stretching, balance and strength exercises, and walking will improve strength and mobility.
  (B) Upper- and lower-extremity range-of-motion exercises performed while seated (for safety) will improve strength.
  (C) Resistance and flexibility exercises will reduce the incidence of falls.
  (D) Flexibility, balance, strength, and endurance exercises will result in fewer respiratory infections.

110. A 72-year-old woman has newly diagnosed stage 1 hypertension, with an average blood pressure of 152/96 mm Hg. She does not smoke cigarettes and does not have diabetes mellitus, dyslipidemia, clinically recognizable cardiovascular disease, or target organ damage. She is obese (body mass index 30) and does not exercise. Which of the following is the most appropriate initial treatment?

  (A) Regular exercise and weight loss
  (B) Fish oil supplementation
  (C) A thiazide diuretic
  (D) An angiotensin-converting enzyme (ACE) inhibitor
  (E) A calcium channel blocking agent

111. An 80-year-old woman must use her arms to rise from a chair. Her balance is good and gait is normal. Findings of the remainder of the physical examination are unremarkable. The patient has been less active in the past 2 months; she used to take daily walks but stopped because of inclement weather. Which is the best initial management for this patient?

  (A) Referral for physical therapy
  (B) Raised toilet seat
  (C) Single-point cane
  (D) Increased exercise

112. An occupational therapist makes a home visit to an 80-year-old man who has a history of falls. A number of hazards (eg, the seat of his favorite chair is low, the hallways are cluttered) are noted. Which of the following is the most likely outcome of a home assessment and subsequent suggestions for risk reduction?

  (A) It is likely to reduce falls at home but not those outside the home.
  (B) The presence of an environmental hazard is associated with increased fall risk.
  (C) The fall risk associated with an environmental hazard is related to the patient's interaction with the environment.
  (D) Environmental hazards are more likely to be found in the homes of disabled persons than in the homes of persons without disability.

113. A 73-year-old man comes to you for a routine visit. He has been seen twice before, for management of osteoarthritis of the knees, mild hypertension, and urinary hesitancy and nocturia. Prior to this visit, the patient's wife tells you privately that she is concerned about her husband's drinking. She thinks that it increased after his retirement 3 years ago.

Beginning with general open-ended questions, you initiate a discussion about the use of tobacco and alcohol, as well as other health habits. More detailed questioning leads the patient to report that he consumes about 21 to 25 drinks per week, including both beer and liquor. On some occasions he may have five drinks. He scores 0/4 on the CAGE questionnaire and consistently denies any symptoms suggestive of alcohol dependence. He also denies that alcohol has ever prevented him from fulfilling major obligations, drinking in situations when it might be dangerous, or legal problems related to drinking. However, when you mention the possibility of adverse health effects associated with drinking, he does express an interest in cutting down on his intake. He tells you that he was able to quit smoking 10 years ago. Which of the following is the most appropriate treatment option?

  (A) Brief intervention
  (B) Referral to Alcoholics Anonymous
  (C) Admission to an inpatient treatment center
  (D) Naltrexone

114. A 79-year-old woman who has Alzheimer's disease and resides in a skilled nursing facility has been angry, belligerent, and agitated for 3 days. She has had progressive dementia for 8 years and has resided in the facility for 2 years. Medical history also includes hypertension, congestive heart failure, and osteoporosis, all of which have been stable recently. She has no history of behavioral disturbances. The Mini–Mental State Examination score is 10/30. Which of the following is the most appropriate initial step in the care of this patient?

   (A) Ask the nursing staff to describe the specific behaviors that have occurred.
   (B) Perform a physical examination, including assessment of mental status.
   (C) Order complete blood cell count, serum electrolytes, and urinalysis.
   (D) Order chest radiograph.
   (E) Prescribe haloperidol, 0.5 mg orally twice daily, as needed for agitation.

115. Which of the following statements regarding the use of tube feeding in patients with severe dementia is correct?

   (A) It does not improve survival.
   (B) It protects against aspiration pneumonia.
   (C) It promotes the healing of pressure ulcers.
   (D) It improves patient comfort.
   (E) It improves functional status.

116. Which of the following demographic statements is correct?

   (A) The median income for persons aged 65 and over was $16,400 in 1998.
   (B) Approximately 45% of women aged 75 to 84 are widowed.
   (C) Approximately 55% of women aged 85 and over live alone.
   (D) The number of Americans aged 85 and over is expected to quadruple by 2025.
   (E) The percentage of older adults with college degrees is expected to increase from 15% to 35% by 2030.

QUESTIONS, ANSWERS, AND CRITIQUES

Directions: *Each of the questions or incomplete statements below is followed by four or five suggested answers or completions. Select the ONE answer or completion that is BEST in each case and fill in the circle containing the corresponding letter on the answer sheet. The table of Normal Laboratory Values on p 428 may be consulted for any of the questions in this book.*

1. A 74-year-old man has Parkinson's disease that is well controlled. However, his gait is unstable, with mild retropulsion and bradykinesia. The patient has had one minor fall and has reduced his activities because he fears falling again. He has no other neurologic or musculoskeletal problems. Which of the following adaptive mobility aides is most appropriate to facilitate safer ambulation for this patient?

   (A) Straight cane
   (B) Four-prong cane
   (C) Standard walker
   (D) Wheeled walker
   (E) Wheelchair

   ANSWER: D

   In a patient who curtails activity because of a fear of falling, it is important to respond quickly to avoid rapid deconditioning. This patient has mild retropulsion and would be able to advance a two-wheeled walker easily. If he began walking forward too quickly, applying weight on the walker would slow his speed. Patients with Parkinson's disease, particularly those with significant bradykinesia, often have difficulty initiating movement. Thus, the process of lifting and placing a cane or standard walker can be difficult. The continuous movement of advancing a wheeled walker obviates initiation of multiple movements. Some Parkinson's patients do even better with a four-wheeled walker than a two-wheeled walker because of this. A physical therapist can help determine whether a two- or four-wheeled walker would be better for a specific patient with parkinsonism. Canes offer less stability than walkers, which provide a wide base of stability, particularly when the patient turns—en bloc turning is a common finding in Parkinson's disease. A wheelchair would be appropriate if this patient were no longer able to walk at a speed consistent with effective ambulation and if ambulation were unsafe even with a walker.

2. An 82-year-old female nursing-home resident has end-stage Alzheimer's dementia. She is mute, incontinent of urine and feces, and bedbound. Daily skin inspection reveals nonblanching erythema of the heels. Which of the following will best prevent a pressure ulcer in this patient?

   (A) Bladder catheterization
   (B) Massaging the sacral skin daily
   (C) Elevating the head of the bed to 45 degrees
   (D) Elevating the heels off the bed surface
   (E) Repositioning the patient every 4 hours

   ANSWER: D

   The heels of a bedbound patient require extra protection, but it is difficult to redistribute pressure at the heels because of their small surface area. No pressure-relieving mattress surface adequately reduces pressure at the heels. The greater the weight and height of a patient, the greater the tissue-interface pressure at the heels and the greater the risk of skin breakdown. This patient's heels should be elevated off the bed surface. A readily available way to do this is to place plump pillows under the length of the lower legs.

   Urinary or fecal incontinence can cause skin maceration, which reduces the frictional coefficient of the skin and lowers the pressure–duration threshold for breakdown. However, bladder catheterization should be used only for urologic problems, such as urinary retention. A variety of absorbent pads and briefs will draw moisture away from the skin surface. Topical moisture-barrier creams also may be helpful. Massaging the skin over at-risk bony prominences previously was thought to stimulate blood and lymphatic flow and improve circulation. However, it is of no proven benefit and may damage dermal tissue. Elevation of the head of the patient's bed between 20 and 70 degrees puts additional pressure on the heels and ischial tuberosities and promotes shearing-force injury at the sacrum. Similar forces are produced when a patient is semi-recumbent in a chair. Shearing force is the presence of tangential pressure on the skin. It weakens the superficial fascial attachment of the skin to deeper tissues, causing tissue cleavage. Blood vessels are stretched and angulated in the area, leading to vessel thrombosis and reduced circulation. High shearing force deceases the amount of pressure required for vessel occlusion by one-half. All patients at risk for pressure ulcers require frequent turning. Optimal frequency depends on the patient's risk status and the pressure-relieving mattress surface used. Bedbound patients should be turned at least every 2 hours, and appropriate repositioning techniques should be used to avoid friction injuries.

3. Which of the following figures, expressed as percentage of personal income, reflects average out-of-pocket spending on health care for Medicare beneficiaries aged 65 and older?

    (A) 64%
    (B) 45%
    (C) 19%
    (D) 8%
    (E) 3%

ANSWER: C

Although Medicare is the primary health payer for older Americans, its coverage is not comprehensive. The current program requires cost sharing for many services, in addition to standard deductibles for Part A (hospital insurance) and Part B (outpatient or supplementary medical insurance) services. Further, services such as outpatient prescription drugs, vision care, dental care, and long-term nursing-home care are not covered. For an additional cost, the majority of Medicare beneficiaries purchase some type of private or public supplemental coverage (medigap) to pay for these services. Despite supplemental coverage,

substantial expenses still are incurred by many beneficiaries.

In 1999 Medicare beneficiaries aged 65 and over were projected to spend about $2430, or 19% of income, out of pocket for health care; one in four persons will have out-of-pocket costs exceeding $3000. Payments for health care goods and services—Medicare deductibles and co-insurance—and payments for goods and services not covered by Medicare, such as prescription drugs and dental care, account for 54% of this amount. The remaining 46% is spent on premium payments for Medicare Part B, private insurance, and Medicare Plus Choice plans. These estimates do not include the costs of home care or long-term nursing-home care.

The single largest component of out-of-pocket spending, after premium payments, is prescription drugs. On average, beneficiaries spend as much out of pocket for prescription drugs (17% of total out-of-pocket spending) as for physician care, vision services, and medical supplies combined. In contrast, inpatient and outpatient hospital care each account for about 3% of total out-of-pocket spending.

4. A 67-year-old woman asks you to prescribe sleeping pills for her. She reports initial insomnia and restless sleep with frequent awakenings. The patient is retired and leads a sedentary life style. She frequently reads or watches television in bed and often naps, despite caffeine intake throughout the day. Physical examination is unremarkable. Which of the following is most likely to ameliorate this patient's sleep disturbance?

    (A) Exposure to early morning daylight
    (B) Proper sleep habits
    (C) Sustained-release melatonin
    (D) Zolpidem
    (E) Referral for polysomnography

ANSWER: B

Poor sleep habits may be the most common cause of sleep problems in older adults. Irregular sleep–wake patterns, related to the life style in this patient, can undermine the ability of the circadian system to effectively provide sleepiness and wakefulness at appropriate times. Caffeine intake in the afternoon can have alerting effects for many hours, thus impairing night-time sleep. Excessive wake time in bed may cause increased arousal that is reinforced nightly. Other factors (eg, medical illness, medications, psychiatric disorders, and primary sleep disorders) also should be considered. However, proper sleep habits should be implemented. These include regularity of sleep and wake times; avoidance of excessive time in bed; relaxing bedtime routine; daily activity and exercise; avoidance of caffeine, alcohol, and nicotine in the afternoon and evening; and elimination of loud noise, excessive light, and uncomfortable room temperature. Even if poor sleep habits are not responsible for insomnia, their elimination minimizes any perpetuating influence.

Use of a short-acting hypnotic agent is not an appropriate first step in the management of simple insomnia. Hypnotics should be used only in limited circumstances, following evaluation of the patient's symptoms and in the context of proper sleep habits. Similarly, melatonin has not definitively been shown to benefit age-related sleep-maintenance insomnia. Exposure to early morning light can be useful for delayed or advanced sleep-phase syndrome or jet lag. Polysomnography can be useful for evaluating chronic insomnia or for suspicion of primary sleep disorders such as sleep apnea, periodic limb movement disorder, or rapid eye movement (REM)–behavior disorder, but referral to a sleep specialist is not warranted for this patient.

5. An 80-year-old woman comes to your office for an initial evaluation. She is accompanied by her daughter, who is concerned about the patient's memory. During the past year she has been repeating questions and statements; about 6 months ago she began to have infrequent problems "getting her words out." Symptoms "probably" have worsened. She is sometimes sad when talking about deceased relatives. The patient lives alone and does most of her own household chores. She completed the 10th grade. Her Mini–Mental State Examination (MMSE) score is 26/30, with two errors ("near-misses") in orientation and two in short-term recall. Physical examination is normal. Laboratory studies are normal. Which of the following is the most likely diagnosis?

(A) Normal aging
(B) Minimal cognitive impairment
(C) Major depression
(D) Delirium
(E) Alzheimer's disease

ANSWER: B

Minimal cognitive impairment is a syndrome of memory problems that worsen within 1 year, with limited functional impairment and no definite impairment in other cognitive domains. This patient has a 6- to 12-month history of worsening memory complaints, supported by screening assessment, with no evidence so far of other cognitive impairment. The MMSE score probably is normal for her age and education, but deficits may be more extensive on detailed evaluation. There is no evidence of any functional consequences. Treatment should include discontinuation of any medications known to cause cognitive changes; ensuring adequate nutrition; obtaining more information about her functional status, including driving abilities; and working with the family to enhance social stimulation. Her condition should be monitored closely for several months. It also might be reasonable to obtain neuropsychologic testing to help clarify the pattern of strengths and weaknesses.

The kinds of cognitive changes that can be expected in normal aging include some difficulty with recall of words and names, without extension to other domains and not obviously increasing in severity within the course of 1 year. The patient is not depressed or delirious. Alzheimer's disease may precede the clinical dementia syndrome by years, or even decades, and depressive features often are associated. Although this patient may have early dementia, most likely Alzheimer's disease, she does not meet the diagnostic criteria at this time. The research concept of "possible Alzheimer's disease" may be appropriate.

6. An 81-year-old white man who recently was widowed is brought to your office by his daughter. She is concerned that he is losing weight and no longer attends the senior group he once enjoyed. The patient has many nonspecific somatic complaints. His appetite has decreased, and he has lost 2.5 kg (5.5 lb) in the past 6 months. He denies feeling depressed but admits to decreased interest and energy, and he has been waking early in the morning. Findings of physical examination are normal. Which of the following findings is characteristic of bereavement?

(A) Psychomotor retardation
(B) Suicidal thoughts
(C) Persistent dysphoria
(D) Pervasive guilt
(E) Functional disability

ANSWER: C

Some grieving individuals, as part of their reaction to loss, have symptoms that are consistent with a major depressive episode, including depressed mood, insomnia, anorexia, and weight loss. The patient may view the depressed mood as a normal response but may seek relief for insomnia and loss of appetite. Although bereavement is not exclusively a problem of later life, it is more common and often means the end of a close relationship lasting many years. One stereotype holds that older people are better at handling loss because it is more expected and they have more experience dealing with it. However, the cumulative effects of multiple losses may make elderly persons more vulnerable to a depressive disorder. There are three phases of uncomplicated bereavement. The first is the stunned phase, lasting hours to weeks. This is followed by the mourning phase, which involves intense yearning and distress, feelings of futility, anorexia, insomnia, restlessness, irritability, preoccupation with the deceased, transient hallucinations, denial, and appropriate guilt. This phase may last for several months. It is followed by the acceptance and readjustment phase, which lasts several weeks to a year or more.

The duration of "normal" grief varies among cultures, but the diagnosis of major depressive disorder (MDD) generally is not made unless significant symptoms are present more than 2 months after the loss. Dysphoria is common in bereavement and often is persistent. Characteristic features of MDD which help distinguish it from bereavement are suicidal thoughts, pervasive guilt, morbid preoccupation with worthlessness, marked psychomotor retardation, prolonged disability, and functional impairment. Distinguishing between MDD and bereavement can be difficult, and recent bereavement is a risk factor for MDD. When in doubt, treatment is appropriate. Bereavement-associated MDD has been shown to respond to nortriptyline; the addition of psychotherapy further improves response rates.

7. Which of the following is the primary source of funding for Medicare Part A (hospital insurance)?

(A) Monthly premiums paid by Medicare recipients
(B) Payroll taxes on all workers and employers
(C) General tax revenues
(D) Hospitals and health care facilities
(E) Social Security

ANSWER: B

All financial operations for Medicare are handled through two trust funds in the U.S. Treasury, one for hospital insurance (HI or Part A) and one for supplementary medical insurance (SMI or Part B). These accounts are credited with all income received and charged with all expenditures for benefits and administration costs. Assets not needed for the payment of costs are invested in special Treasury securities. Financing is primarily through a mandatory payroll deduction (Federal Insurance Contributions Act or FICA). Almost all employees and self-employed workers in the United States pay taxes to support the cost of benefits for aged and disabled beneficiaries. Employers and employees each pay 1.45% of wage earnings; self-employed persons pay 2.90%. In 1994 the federal government removed income limits, so FICA now is paid on all covered wages and self-employment income. The money is used mainly to pay benefits for current beneficiaries. HI money can be used only for this program, and SMI funds cannot be transferred for HI use.

SMI is financed in two ways. The first source of financing is monthly premium payments ($50.00 per month in 2001) that usually are deducted from the Social Security benefits of enrollees. Premiums currently cover 25% of the average expenditures for aged beneficiaries. The second source is contributions from the general revenue of the U.S. Treasury.

Hospitals and health care facilities receive revenue from Part A services. Social Security provides pension payments to eligible retirees and disabled persons.

8. An 80-year-old woman has fallen outside her home twice. She fractured a wrist 3 months ago and has arm and facial ecchymoses from a fall last week. She has a distant history of a myocardial infarction and is being treated with a diuretic for hypertension. She reports occasional difficulty with balance when walking. Which of the following is the most appropriate first step in evaluating the falls?

(A) Gather additional history and physical examination.
(B) Order laboratory studies, especially serum electrolytes.
(C) Perform electrocardiography.
(D) Order computed tomography of the head.
(E) Arrange for home-based assessment.

ANSWER: A

The proper evaluation of a fall begins with the history and physical examination. For this patient, additional history is needed to assure that no syncope or dizziness (related to cardiac dysfunction or dehydration from the diuretic) occurred. Cardiac auscultation and orthostatic blood-pressure measurements are indicated. Since the patient has difficulty with balance while walking, history and physical examination should focus particularly on the neurologic and musculoskeletal system.

Some practitioners advocate obtaining laboratory tests for all patients who fall, because occult metabolic disturbances may be revealed. Few data justify an extensive laboratory and radiologic work-up; however, these may be warranted, depending on findings of the history and examination. For example, symptoms of weakness or confusion might suggest screening for the metabolic effects of the diuretic by

measuring serum electrolytes. A history of syncope may support the need for electrocardiography, and computed tomography would be appropriate for a patient with facial trauma and neurologic findings. Home-based assessment may be considered later, after a careful history and examination, if targeted interventions do not decrease the patient's falling.

9. An 82-year-old woman with a history of hypertension, diabetes mellitus, and osteoporosis goes to the emergency department for evaluation of the acute onset of severe upper back pain. Evaluation demonstrates a new thoracic vertebral compression fracture. In addition to prescribing analgesia, you request a consultation to assist with discharge because the patient lives at home alone and has difficulty getting out of bed because of the pain. What factor is most likely to predict the admission of this patient to the hospital in the next month?

(A) Depressed mood
(B) Urinary incontinence
(C) Living alone
(D) Advanced age
(E) Functional impairment

ANSWER: E

The promotion of functional independence is a primary goal of clinicians providing care to older persons. This goal may be achieved when older adults at high risk for functional decline are identified by the use of a screening instrument. Those found to be at high risk undergo a thorough assessment that identifies problems for which interventions can be prescribed to prevent functional impairment. One group of patients who may benefit from such screening is older adults discharged to home following an emergency department visit. One fifth of older patients discharged to home from the emergency department will return within the next 30 days, and a significant percentage of these will be admitted to the hospital.

The presence of impairments in activities of daily living (ADLs) or instrumental activities of daily living (IADLs) in this patient is most likely to predict hospitalization in the next 30 days. (See the Appendix, pp 384–385, for ADL and IADL screens.) Valid questions used in trials that were predictive of subsequent hospital admission included requiring the assistance of another person to care for oneself, an increase in the amount of help needed to care for oneself, requiring assistance in transportation, and requiring the assistance of a visiting nurse.

Cognitive factors associated with adverse outcomes in patients seen in the emergency department include memory impairment but not depressed mood. The presence of urinary incontinence, dependency in bladder function, fecal incontinence, or dependency in bowel functioning was not associated with hospital admission.

Advanced age without comorbidity in this patient population was not predictive of hospital admission following a visit to the emergency department. Community-dwelling older adults who live alone were not found to be at risk for hospital admission; either they are independent in their ADLs and IADLs, or they have identified the community resources needed to allow them to live alone successfully.

Additional variables that have been shown to be useful in identifying high-risk older patients in the emergency department include poor vision and the use of more than three medications.

10. An 83-year-old man who has Alzheimer's disease of moderate severity has lived in a skilled nursing facility for 2 years. He has had inter- mittent delusional thoughts and anxiety, but these have not been particularly distressing or persisted for prolonged periods. Medical history includes mild chronic renal failure and anemia; he also has had a fractured hip but now ambulates well. He takes no psychotropic medications and sleeps well. During the past 2 weeks, however, he has spent increasing amounts of time wandering the halls. Several times, he has entered another patient's room and rummaged through belongings. He also was found outside the building on one occasion. Which of the following is the most appropriate treatment strategy?

(A) Provide structured physical activity and accompanied outdoor walks.
(B) Use a vest restraint in a chair intermit- tently during the day.

(C) Use wrist restraints during episodes of particularly vigorous wandering.
(D) Prescribe risperidone, 1 mg orally twice daily.
(E) Transfer the patient to another skilled nursing facility.

ANSWER: A

Wandering and pacing behaviors are common in patients with Alzheimer's disease. It is important to recognize that wandering itself is not necessarily a problem, but the social and safety consequences warrant attention. Environ- mental interventions (eg, providing a safe place to wander, enhancing socialization opportu- nities, and moderately increasing sensory stimu- lation) can help reduce the behavior and promote safety. Providing structured physical activity and opportunities to take walks outdoors with family members or staff often is helpful.

Vest or wrist restraints usually are not effective. Research also indicates that use of physical restraints leads to increased falls and injury. Treatment with antipsychotic or other psychotropic medications may be warranted in cases of extreme motor activity, particularly when safety is compromised. Risperidone, 1 mg orally twice daily, is an excessive initial dosage. Transferring the patient to another facility may exacerbate wandering and other behavioral disturbances.

11. A 95-year-old woman has advanced Alzheimer's disease and is admitted to a skilled nursing facility. After 5 months she no longer has the financial resources to pay for her care. She is a widow and has no assets; her primary source of income is Social Security benefits. Which of the following financing options will cover the costs of her ongoing skilled nursing care?

(A) Social Security
(B) Medicare
(C) Medicare Plus Choice
(D) Medicaid
(E) Medigap

ANSWER: D

One of the most important benefits of the Medicaid program is its coverage of long-term care, especially in the nursing home. For older people with physical and cognitive limitations that impede their ability to live independently, Medicaid has become virtually the only insurer for institutional and community-based long-term-care services. In 1997 Medicaid financed 38% of the $115 billion in long-term-care expenditures and 47% of the $83 billion in nursing-home expenditures. Most of the long-term care paid for by Medicaid is delivered in nursing homes; Medicaid is the payer for about two thirds of the nearly 1.6 million nursing-home residents. Eligibility is determined by income and asset tests that are administered by state governments.

Social Security or Old Age Insurance (OAI) is an entitlement program funded through payroll taxes. It pays monthly benefits to retired workers who have qualified by having been employed for a minimum amount of time and by having made contributions to the program. Financial need is not a requirement. A person's OAI pension is applied to the cost of nursing-home care but usually covers only a small portion of the total expenses.

Medicare provides health insurance for 34 million older persons and 5 million disabled persons. Skilled nursing care is covered by Medicare when it follows within 30 days of hospitalization for 3 or more days and is certified as medically necessary. Coverage is similar to that for inpatient stays but also includes rehabilitation services and appliances. A maximum of 100 days can be covered per benefit period. Medicare does not pay for nursing-home care if the patient does not require skilled nursing or skilled rehabilitation services.

Medicare Plus Choice includes both the traditional managed-care plans as well as a broader range of plans similar to those now available through private insurance. It provides benefits covered under traditional Medicare without imposing out-of-pocket costs. Additional services such as prescription medications also may be covered. However, the long-term care benefits from most Medicare Plus Choice plans are no greater than from Medicare.

Medigap is private insurance that supplements or helps fill the "gaps" in Medicare coverage by paying health care expenses that fee-for-service Medicare covers only partially or not at all. The only long-term-care benefit provided by Medigap is the copayment for days 21 to 100 of skilled care in a nursing home.

12. A 79-year-old man, who has coronary artery disease and congestive heart failure, comes to the emergency department because of nausea, vomiting, headache, and abdominal pain. Symptoms began 3 days ago. Current medications are warfarin, furosemide, digoxin, captopril, vitamin E, and a multivitamin. The regimen had been stable for 10 years, until the furosemide dosage was increased last week to better control symptoms of heart failure. Which of the following toxicities is the most likely cause of this patient's problems?

(A) Digoxin
(B) Furosemide
(C) Warfarin
(D) Vitamin E
(E) Captopril

ANSWER: A

Gastrointestinal and neurologic effects are the most common symptoms of digoxin toxicity. Patients commonly experience anorexia, nausea, diarrhea, vomiting, abdominal pain, headache, fatigue, dizziness, delirium, malaise, and confusion. Cardiac and respiratory effects also are common. Geriatric patients are most susceptible to neuropsychiatric abnormalities. Patients with decreased renal function and electrolyte imbalances are at increased risk for toxicity. Concomitant use of furosemide and digoxin can cause digoxin toxicity secondary to hypokalemia and possibly hypomagnesemia. In a study of more than 2000 patients taking digoxin, just over 4% had at least one sign, symptom, or electrocardiographic change suggesting toxicity. To avoid misinterpretation of serum digoxin level, clinicians must know when the medication was taken and when the measurement was obtained.

Warfarin toxicity usually produces bleeding complications, although headache, chest and joint pain, dizziness, weakness, hypotension, and shortness of breath also may occur. Vitamin E can alter the effect of vitamin K on clotting factors, resulting in an increased hypoprothrombinemic response to warfarin. However, nausea does not occur in this

Questions/Answers/Critiques

situation. Although the presence of lasix and captopril may have increased the likelihood of fluid and electrolyte problems, these agents are not causing the digoxin toxic symptoms.

13. A 75-year-old man has hypertension, hyperlipidemia, type 2 diabetes mellitus, and osteoarthritis of the hips. He reports a fall 1 month ago, while in the bathroom in the middle of the night. Current medications are atenolol, 25 mg daily; atorvastatin, 10 mg daily; metformin, 500 mg twice daily; and acetaminophen, 650 mg three times daily. Pulse rate is 72 per minute, and rhythm is regular. Blood pressure is 130/74 mm Hg with no orthostatic changes. Visual acuity is 20/30. The patient uses his arms to rise from a chair. Stance is normal; gait is slow, symmetric, and steady. Which of the following is the best next step?

(A) Visiting nurse evaluation of vital signs
(B) In-home assessment of physical function
(C) Comprehensive geriatric assessment
(D) Prescription of an assistive device (cane or walker)
(E) Admission to a postacute-care facility for physical rehabilitation

ANSWER: B

A fall is a sentinel event in the life of an older adult. Without intervention, this patient is likely to have recurrent falls with the potential for serious injury (eg, fracture, head trauma) and loss of independence. The homes of older persons frequently contain environmental hazards that interfere with performance of activities of daily living, for example, objects that impact on the capacity to get out of bed or chair and walk safely. A randomized, controlled trial of comprehensive home assessment, with prescription of appropriate assistive devices and modification of environmental hazards, found that this approach slowed the rate of functional decline in cognitively intact, frail older adults without increasing health care costs.

Although an evaluation of vital signs by a visiting nurse may be helpful in assessing orthostasis and medication adherence, there is no evidence that this would reduce falls. Comprehensive geriatric assessment has been studied in multiple settings and has been shown to benefit targeted individuals. Given this

patient's lower-extremity weakness, which is revealed by use of arms to rise, a focused intervention would be a more appropriate first step. Assistive devices should be reserved for patients with impaired gait and balance. A cane improves balance by providing increased stability, especially for unilateral conditions; a walker provides more stability, for conditions affecting both lower extremities. Both devices are inappropriate for this patient. Furthermore, because he can transfer and walk without assistance, he does not require the intensity of inpatient rehabilitation; however, he would most likely benefit from an exercise regimen to increase his lower extremity strength.

14. An 84-year-old female nursing-home resident reports knee pain that developed overnight. She has osteoporosis and has sustained previous hip and pelvic fractures after falling out of bed, but no recent incidents have occurred. The patient is frail and thin. Temperature is 37.3C (99.1F). The right knee is warm and held in partial flexion. It is exquisitely painful on passive motion and palpation over the joint line and tibia. Musculoskeletal findings are otherwise normal except for osteoarthritis of the hands. Anteroposterior radiograph of the knee shows anterior joint-space narrowing. Arthrocentesis yields grossly bloody fluid. Hematocrit is 38%, leukocyte count 5600/µL, and platelet count 260,000/µL. Which of the following is most likely to identify the cause of this patient's knee pain?

(A) Microscopic examination of synovial fluid for crystals
(B) Culture of synovial fluid
(C) Magnetic resonance imaging (MRI) of the knee
(D) Bone scan

ANSWER: C

Arthrocentesis is appropriate to evaluate this patient's monoarthritis. Synovial fluid cell count would be helpful in determining whether the effusion is inflammatory (> 2000 white blood cells [WBCs]), noninflammatory (< 2000 WBCs), or hemorrhagic. Hemarthrosis develops as a result of trauma, internal derangement, anticoagulation or bleeding dyscrasia, gout or calcium pyrophosphate dihydrate deposition disease, tumor, or fracture of the patellar, femoral, or tibial plateau. The presence of tibial tenderness suggests that the subchondral bone as well as the joint are abnormal. Given this patient's history of fractures, a tibial plateau fracture is likely. MRI can characterize the fracture pattern and severity, while identifying associated intra- and peri-articular injuries, which are present in nearly 50% of cases. Fracture severity and the patient's comorbidities should be weighed in the decision to pursue surgical repair. However, degenerative changes and a poor functional outcome are common following tibial plateau fractures in patients aged 60 and over.

Crystalline-mediated arthritis can cause monoarthritis with or without a fever and can produce a bloody effusion that should be examined using polarized-light microscopy. Synovial fluid Gram's stain or culture should be obtained if an infectious arthritis is suspected, but this is not likely in an afebrile patient with a normal leukocyte count. Synovial fluid glucose level is of little clinical utility. Plain radiographs may not be sensitive enough to detect a tibial plateau fracture. Bone scan would permit diagnosis of a fracture but yields information that is neither sensitive nor specific.

15. A 79-year-old man comes to you for a routine visit. He is accompanied by his daughter, who reports that the patient is having difficulty hearing. He denies this and explains that people around him do not speak clearly. The patient's ears are free of cerumen impaction. Which of the following is the most reliable and valid screening test for hearing loss?

    (A) Tuning-fork test
    (B) Finger-rub test
    (C) Whisper test
    (D) Rinné and Weber tests
    (E) Audioscopy

ANSWER: E

Self-report is helpful in identifying hearing impairments that older adults perceive as handicapping or disabling. The most common cause of hearing impairment is presbycusis, which is a bilateral, symmetric, high-frequency sensorineural hearing loss. Persons with mild to moderate loss often complain that others mumble. This is because patients are unable to hear consonants, which are high-frequency sounds.

The hand-held audioscope permits reliable and valid screening for hearing loss. It is sensitive (87% to 90%) and specific (70% to 90%), when compared with the gold standard of audiometry performed by an audiologist. The audioscope, an otoscope with a built-in audiometer, is set at 40 dB to assess hearing in older persons. A test tone of 60 dB is delivered, then four tones (500, 100, 2000, and 4000 Hz) at 40 dB are delivered. Testing takes approximately 3 minutes. Patients fail the screen if they are unable to hear either the 1000- or 2000-Hz frequency in both ears, or both the 1000- and 2000-Hz frequency in one ear. The audioscope costs a little more than a standard otoscope and should be recalibrated annually.

The tuning-fork test is performed by striking the tines of the fork against the heel of the hand, then holding the vibrating fork 1 inch from the ear. The fork then is moved away from the ear at a rate of 1 foot per second. The patient indicates when the tone is no longer audible. Tuning forks assess hearing in the range of 512 to 1024 Hz. This is not sufficient to evaluate hearing loss in older persons, whose loss usually is in the range of 2000 Hz or higher. Testing also depends on the force with which the fork is struck, how quickly it is withdrawn, and assessment of the distance at which the tone is no longer heard. The finger-rub test is performed by rubbing the index finger and thumb together 1 inch from the ear, then slowly withdrawing until the sound no longer is heard by the patient. Its use has not been well studied in older patients. In the whisper test, the examiner whispers at the side of the patient. This is not reliable and correlates poorly with audiometry findings. Examiner variability is a concern when using the tuning-fork, finger-rub, or whisper tests.

The Rinné test compares conduction of sound in air and bone, to distinguish conductive from sensorineural loss. The Weber test is used to lateralize hearing loss, which is usually bilateral in older persons. Neither of these is a screen for hearing loss.

16. An 85-year-old woman has not urinated in 12 hours. Medical history includes congestive heart failure and hypertension. Four days ago, she was seen in the emergency department because of a 1-week history of malaise, nausea, and vomiting. A diagnosis of "possible urinary tract infection" was made, and symptoms responded to the prescribed medication.

The patient reports some muscle aching today. She has lost 2.5 kg (5.5 lb) since her last visit 2 months ago. Pulse rate is 80 per minute sitting and 100 per minute standing; blood pressure is 120/84 mm Hg sitting and 110/84 mm Hg standing. The patient is "a little dizzy" when she stands. Mental status is at baseline.

Laboratory studies:

Blood urea nitrogen	76 mg/dL
Serum creatinine	3.0 mg/dL
Serum electrolytes:	
Sodium	140 mEq/L
Potassium	5.8 mEq/L
Chloride	90 mEq/L
Bicarbonate	28 mEq/L
Urinalysis	0–3 red blood cells, 0–3 white blood cells per high-power field; granular casts and needle-shaped crystals

Of the following medications taken by this patient, which is the most likely cause of acute renal failure?

(A) Digoxin
(B) Diphenhydramine
(C) Hydrochlorothiazide
(D) Lisinopril
(E) Trimethoprim–sulfamethizole

ANSWER: E

This patient has crystal-induced acute renal failure (ARF) secondary to sulfonamide use. Several other medications, most notably methotrexate and triamterene, also produce crystals that are insoluble in urine. This patient is at increased risk for crystal deposition because of renal insufficiency and decreased intravascular volume. Renal failure often is reversible with discontinuation of the drug and volume expansion with high urinary rates; dialysis may be required, however.

This patient is at risk for digoxin toxicity because of decreased renal excretion, but this drug does not cause ARF. Standard doses of diphenhydramine are unlikely to cause ARF. Thiazides may impair the renal diluting systems to cause hyponatremia but not ARF. Angiotensin-converting enzyme inhibitors have become the standard of care in treatment of congestive heart failure and diabetic nephropathy. They cause pre-renal ARF in patients with renal artery stenosis, but the features are not consistent with this patient's presentation.

17. A 78-year-old woman comes to your office for an initial visit; she is accompanied by a niece, who lives in another city. The patient has not had medical care since her physician retired 5 years ago. She is well groomed, seems cheerful, and has no medical complaints. When examining the patient, you notice a slight odor of urine. Findings of physical examination are normal. Following the examination, the patient dresses without difficulty.

The niece phones your office the next day and asks your opinion about the patient's incontinence. As far as she can tell, the condition has been present for at least 3 years. She is surprised that her aunt did not mention the problem to you. Which of the following is the most appropriate next step?

(A) Assume that the patient is not bothered by the incontinence.
(B) Ask the patient to schedule another visit.
(C) Order urodynamic studies.
(D) Prescribe a course of antibiotics.
(E) Prescribe oral estrogen therapy.

ANSWER: B

Urinary incontinence (UI) is a common problem, affecting 24% of men and 49% of women. Among lower urinary tract symptoms (including urgency, frequency, nocturia), it is the problem for which patients are most likely to seek care. However, only 30% of men and 13% of women seek care for their symptoms. Therefore, clinicians should question patients routinely. Open-ended questions, such as "Tell me about any problems you are having with your bladder?" or "Tell me about any trouble you are having holding your urine (water)?" are useful. If the patient responds negatively, more specific questions, such as "How often do you lose urine when you don't want to?" or "How often do you wear a pad or other protective device to collect your urine?" may help to identify UI.

The vast majority of older patients with UI can be managed without urodynamic studies. Prescribing an antibiotic when there is no evidence of a urinary tract infection (UTI) is not appropriate. Decreased estrogen levels can produce atrophic vaginitis and urethritis, which can cause symptoms of dysuria and urgency. Although most investigators believe that estrogen deficiency predisposes older women to UTI and stress or urge incontinence, randomized, controlled trials of oral estrogen supplementation have not been shown to improve symptoms or decrease urine loss.

18. A 75-year-old man has been hospitalized in the intensive care unit for 1 month because of an exacerbation of emphysema. A stage II pressure ulcer, 6.0 × 8.0 × 0.5 cm in depth, is noted over the sacrum. Examination reveals pink tissue and scant drainage, with no significant necrotic tissue or surrounding erythema. Which of the following is the most appropriate dressing for this pressure ulcer?

(A) Saline-moistened (wet-to-dry) gauze
(B) Calcium alginate
(C) Hydrocolloid
(D) Polyurethane foam

ANSWER: C

Maintenance of a clean, moist wound surface promotes healing of pressure ulcers. Covering a wound promotes re-epithelization, provides a barrier to bacteria, and reduces pain. The ideal dressing should keep the wound bed moist while keeping the surrounding skin dry. Selection of an appropriate dressing is based on ulcer characteristics: location; dimensions; signs of infection; amount of granulation tissue and epithelialization; and presence of exudate or necrotic tissue, undermining, and sinus tracts. As an ulcer heals, dressing requirements may change. At this time, the most appropriate choice for this patient is a hydrocolloid dressing. These are mildly absorbent and not gas permeable. The surface of the dressing mixes with wound fluid to form a gel that allows migration of epithelial cells onto the ulcer surface. Hydrocolloids are available in sheets and in paste or granule forms for deeper wounds. They are contraindicated in the presence of infection. Depending upon the amount of exudate, hydrocolloid dressings should be changed every 3 to 7 days.

Newer dressing products have not been found to promote healing faster than saline-moistened gauze. However, the need to remoisten or change gauze dressings every 4 hours make them impractical in nonhospital settings and increase personnel costs in all settings. Thus, newer products usually are more cost-effective. Saline-moistened gauze also has a limited ability to control exudate and does not promote autolytic debridement (ie, release of self-degradative enzymes that aid in wound cleansing). Gauze dressings should be used only for mechanical debridement, which is not needed in this patient. Calcium alginate and polyurethane foam should be used on heavily draining wounds. Calcium alginate wicks moisture to keep the surrounding skin dry. In this patient, however, these types of dressings would desiccate the wound surface. Depending on the amount of drainage, these dressings should be changed as often as twice a day or as infrequently as every 1 to 2 days. Transparent thin-film dressings are semipermeable, nonabsorbent polyurethane sheets. They are suitable for superficial wounds with minimal drainage and are contraindicated in the presence of infection. These dressings are highly adherent, so removal may damage fragile skin. Depending on the amount of wound fluid, they should be changed every 1 to 3 days.

19. A 68-year-old man has severe vascular dementia and lives in a nursing home. A gastrostomy was placed 1 year ago because of severe dysphagia following a stroke. Recently, the patient has become increasingly agitated and pulled out the feeding tube several times. Efforts to conceal and anchor the tube have been unsuccessful. A change in environment and judicious use of medications also have been ineffective. Which of the following is the most appropriate action?

(A) Place mitts on the patient's hands.
(B) Place restraints on the patient's wrists.
(C) Increase medication dosage to sedate the patient.
(D) Replace the gastrostomy with a jejunostomy.
(E) Reevaluate the need for the gastrostomy.

ANSWER: E

The most appropriate action is to evaluate the need for a feeding tube. Although mortality rates are high in patients who have strokes complicated by dysphagia or aspiration, repeat examination in the weeks or months after the stroke can show improved swallowing and decreased aspiration. Tube feedings should be continued if dysphagia or aspiration persist and if consistent with the patient's wishes. However, it should be noted that at least two studies have failed to demonstrate any improvement with gastrostomy feedings in clinically important outcomes, including survival benefit. Thus, it is important to inform those involved in the substituted decision-making process of the lack of documented benefit. Every attempt should be made to conceal the feeding tube with clothing or nonintrusive wraps.

Mitts or gloves may be used sparingly for patients who are a significant danger to themselves or others; they are less restrictive than other types of restraints. Medications should be used to target specific behaviors or psychiatric disorders and not to sedate a patient. Changing to a jejunostomy will not prevent the patient from attempting to remove the tube.

20. A 75-year-old woman undergoes cystoscopy and transurethral resection of a bladder tumor. Postoperatively, she has delirium characterized by lethargy and inability to recognize family members. Psychoactive medications are discontinued, and the episode appears to be resolving. The patient is a retired professor who had mild forgetfulness but had been living independently.

On the fourth postoperative day, the patient is awake and able to follow simple commands. She requires assistance in rising from bed and is slightly unsteady on her feet. The Mini–Mental State Examination (MMSE) score is 17/30. Which of the following statements is correct regarding this patient's prognosis?

(A) It is excellent; she is recovering from a fully reversible event precipitated by major physiologic stress.
(B) It is good; delirium may take days or weeks to resolve, but the lack of agitation or psychotic features is an encouraging finding.
(C) It is guarded; functional and cognitive status should be monitored closely, and she will need restorative therapy.
(D) It is poor; she now has dementia.

ANSWER: C

Although potentially reversible, delirium in a hospitalized patient often leads to poor long-term outcomes, including increased mortality, prolonged hospitalization, loss of cognitive and functional abilities, and increased use of institutional long-term care. In various studies, this increased risk persists from 1 month to as long as 2 years following hospitalization. Delirium remains a predictor of poor outcomes even after controlling for potential confounding factors such as severity of illness or prior dementia. However, because of the difficulties in adjusting for all potential confounders, it is uncertain whether delirium itself causes the poor outcomes, or whether it is a marker for other disease processes. Thus, the prognosis in this patient is guarded. Patients should be monitored for cognitive and functional decline, with restorative therapy as needed. Poor outcomes may be related to complications of immobility, such as aspiration pneumonia, skin breakdown, loss of muscle strength, balance difficulties, and falls. Patients with agitation or disruptive behaviors may be at greater risk secondary to use of restraints and psychoactive medications. An emphasis on restorative care and maximization of cognitive and functional status may be particularly beneficial for this population.

There appears to be an interaction between underlying risk for delirium (determined by factors such as age, cognitive and functional status, and sensory abilities) and acute precipitating factors (such as psychoactive medications, dehydration, bladder catheterization, and major surgery). Delirium may develop in highly vulnerable patients following only minor physiologic stress, whereas patients with lower vulnerability would require a more noxious insult. In this patient, delirium followed a relatively mild physiologic stress. Thus, she likely had higher baseline vulnerability, which might make her long-term prognosis less positive.

Delirium most often presents as a quiet withdrawn state, as in this patient, or as a mixture of hypoactivity and hyperactivity. Hyperactive delirium, characterized by agitation and prominent psychotic features, is more common in younger patients. Case studies suggest that prognosis for full recovery may be better for patients with the hyperactive variant. This patient is still recovering from her episode of delirium, so the MMSE is not a valid indicator of the severity of any underlying dementia. Therefore, it is too early to determine that her prognosis is poor.

21. A healthy, physically active, cognitively intact 79-year-old man is referred to you after serum prostate-specific antigen (PSA) is found to be 6.5 ng/mL. The patient has not seen a clinician in 15 years and underwent PSA testing at a health fair, after prompting by his wife. He reports nocturia once or twice per night, and physical examination reveals an enlarged, smooth prostate gland. The patient is aware of the controversies surrounding screening for and treatment of prostate cancer and suggests that he may ignore the test result and "just get on with life." Which of the following is the most appropriate approach to this patient?

(A) Recommend transrectal ultrasonography of the prostate gland.
(B) Tell him that doing nothing is reasonable but also explain more active options.
(C) Recommend repeat PSA testing in 6 months.
(D) Refer him to a urologist for biopsy.

ANSWER: B

Controversy persists regarding screening for prostate cancer. For example, the American Cancer Society and the American Urological Association initially recommended screening but later modified their positions to be less dogmatic; the United States Preventive Services Task Force (USPSTF) recommends against it. This scenario also highlights uncertainty regarding age limits above which screening for

prostate (or other) cancer no longer is appropriate. Further, an upper age limit may exist for radical prostatectomy, if cancer is found.

The most appropriate action for this patient is to let him know that doing nothing is a reasonable option, given the lack of evidence to support any particular strategy. This lack of evidence, however, is not a reason to avoid discussing other options. Despite his past avoidance of the health care system, and although he may seem displeased with the medical interventions that may await him, the patient simply may be anxious about the situation. He might be familiar, for example, with a friend, relative, or public figure with prostate cancer, and he may follow your recommendations to pursue an evaluation if you justify the process.

Although age- and race-specific "normal ranges" for PSA have been published, these vary only the sensitivity and specificity of the test and do not provide evidence of effectiveness. Additional diagnostic tests have not been shown to improve clinical outcomes, and a urology referral would be premature at this time.

22. A 65-year-old man who has been paraplegic since an automobile accident 5 years ago is admitted to a skilled nursing facility, following hospitalization for urosepsis. His other medical problems include type 2 diabetes mellitus, hypertension, and deconditioning. He mobilized independently in a wheelchair until this hospital admission. Which of the following is the best initial step in preventing ischial pressure ulcers?

(A) Instruct or assist the patient to shift his weight every hour.
(B) Instruct or assist the patient to shift his weight every 2 hours.
(C) Use an air-filled, doughnut-shaped seat cushion to protect the ischial tuberosities.
(D) Consult a physical therapist to develop a plan for wheelchair seating.
(E) Develop a written plan for skin care.

ANSWER: E

This patient is at very high risk for pressure-ulcer development secondary to paraplegia, deconditioning, and diabetes. Most patients with a spinal cord injury will have a pressure ulcer at some time. The Agency for Health Care Policy and Research (AHCPR) convened a multidisciplinary panel to review the literature on pressure-ulcer prevention in the early 1990s. One of their strongest recommendations was for development of a written skin-care plan. This should include the results of a comprehensive risk assessment, ways to address each risk factor, the response to all interventions, and adjustments to the plan. Systematic skin inspection should be performed and documented at least once a day, with particular attention to the skin overlying bony prominences.

In a seated patient, the ischial tuberosities are of greatest concern. The pressure measured at the skin overlying this site is 150 to 500 mm Hg. Higher interstitial pressures develop at the bone–muscle interface. Much less pressure ($\geq$ 32 mm Hg) is required to compromise local microcirculation. Both the duration and degree of pressure are important in the development of tissue damage. If pressure is intermittently relieved, minimal tissue changes occur. Consequently, this high-risk patient should be instructed or assisted to shift his weight every 15 minutes and reposition himself every hour. Weight shifts can be accomplished by leaning forward or backward or performing a wheelchair push-up. Although a pressure-relieving seating surface is warranted, an air-filled doughnut-shaped cushion could cause venous congestion and edema and may decrease circulation to the central area. Overall, these cushions are more likely to cause pressure ulcers than prevent them. For a seated patient, a written plan for the use of positioning devices and a repositioning schedule is recommended. For an immobile seated patient, prevention of pressure ulcers involves an understanding of body positioning that will reduce pressure over bony prominences. Occupational therapists possess the expertise to develop a wheelchair seating plan that is based on assessment of the patient's individual anatomy, postural alignment, and weight distribution. As part of the seating plan, the occupational therapist determines the most appropriate pressure-relieving cushion to fit the patient's wheelchair, decrease tissue-interface pressure, promote sitting balance and stability, and improve the patient's comfort.

23. A 70-year-old man has a 2-month history of insomnia, weight loss, feelings of hopelessness, loss of interest, crying spells, and thoughts of suicide. The patient's wife describes a long, intermittent history of checking the door locks and windows 50 to 100 times a day. He also has a habit of counting his steps and multiplying the numbers he sees on license plates while he is driving. The wife reports that this counting and multiplying must end on an even number; otherwise, he will retrace his path repeatedly, whether driving or walking, until an even number occurs. The patient also saves newspapers, which now fill two rooms of their home. The patient recently began seeing a psychologist who initiated cognitive behavioral therapy and recommended adjunctive pharmacologic therapy. Which of the following medications is most appropriate?

(A) Bupropion
(B) Clomipramine
(C) Desipramine
(D) Lorazepam
(E) Sertraline

ANSWER: E

This patient has a typical presentation of obsessive-compulsive disorder (OCD) with coexisting depression. OCD usually begins early in life, waxes and wanes, but persists into old age. Patients may not seek treatment until a major depression develops. Optimal treatment of OCD requires both behavioral and pharmacologic therapy. Studies indicate that older patients benefit from the same agents that are effective in younger patients. Selective serotonin-reuptake inhibitors (SSRIs) generally are considered the first-line pharmacologic treatment of OCD in elderly adults. Sertraline is an excellent choice for this patient who has both OCD and major depression. Treatment response can be slow, so therapeutic trials should last at least 12 weeks.

Clomipramine is the treatment of choice for OCD, but elderly patients may be particularly vulnerable to its anticholinergic, hypotensive, and cardiac effects. There is no evidence that benzodiazepines such as lorazepam have any efficacy as primary treatment for OCD or major depression. Bupropion and desipramine are effective antidepressants but are not helpful for OCD.

24. The daughter of a 74-year-old woman asks you to make a home visit because the patient is unwilling to leave the house. The daughter moved in with her mother 1 month ago, because the patient's ability to care for herself had declined in the previous 6 months. She is taking medications for blood pressure, a "heart condition," and to control "eye pressure." Since the daughter moved in, the patient feeds herself small amounts of food and drinks water, plus two or three cans of liquid supplement each day. The patient reports feeling weak and tired but claims to be eating enough. She does not feel sad or blue. Her daughter reports significant weight loss. The patient is normotensive and slightly tachycardic. She has poorly fitting dentures, a dense right cataract, squared shoulders, and wasting of the quadriceps. No focal findings are elicited on neurologic examination. Mental status examination reveals 3 of 3 in registration and 2 of 3 in recall; she correctly name the days of the week in reverse order. Which of the following should you do next?

(A) Obtain complete information on the medications prescribed for the patient.
(B) Obtain a thorough dietary history, including food preferences.
(C) Refer the patient to a psychiatrist to manage depression.
(D) Refer the patient to a dentist for better-fitting dentures.
(E) Contact Adult Protective Services (APS) to place the patient in a setting where she can receive adequate care.

ANSWER: A

This patient has a number of risk factors for poor nutrition: ill-fitting dentures, decreased vision, impairments in activities of daily living, and multiple medications. Depression is a common underlying cause of both functional decline and malnutrition. Numerous medications can alter nutrient intake by affecting cognitive status or gastrointestinal function, producing anorexia or antagonizing nutrient absorption or function. The "eye pressure" drug could be an older carbonic anhydrase

inhibitor that can cause profound metabolic acidosis, resulting in anorexia, loss of function, and deconditioning. With proper encouragement, the patient should be able to maintain adequate food intake at home, while you complete the evaluation. Fluid needs generally are 20 to 30 mL/kg daily, or 1200 to 1800 mL, which she may be meeting. The daughter should learn to increase the caloric density of the patient's food, for example, by adding fat and protein to a milkshake. Food preferences are important to elicit, but a thorough dietary history at this point would add relatively little to the main goals of the assessment. The patient has a concerned caregiver living in the home and is taking in some nutrients, so action by APS would not be appropriate at this time.

25. Which of the following statements is correct concerning perpetrators of elder mistreatment?

(A) They are predominantly male.
(B) They often do not perceive their behavior as abnormal.
(C) Reproducible profiles are readily apparent.
(D) Few unifying characteristics exist because the most important risk factors tend to be victim-specific (eg, impairment in activities of daily living).
(E) Victims usually are dependent upon their abusers for housing or finances, or both.

ANSWER: B

Perpetrators of elder mistreatment commonly do not perceive their behavior as abusive or neglectful, especially in environments where they are isolated with the victim. Cultural variation also exits regarding what constitutes respectful behavior toward older adults. Clinicians can play an important educational role with neglectful caregivers (eg, emphasizing the importance of timely medication administration or the need for proper skin hygiene to prevent pressure ulcers).

There is no overwhelming gender predominance among elder abusers. Some studies have pointed to a higher prevalence among women, but this may reflect the fact that women more often are placed in a caregiving role. Reproducible risk factors for abusers have not emerged, probably because there are many different "typologies" of abusers. These include the adult child with poorly controlled schizo-phrenia, the lifelong abusive spouse who now has aged, and the patient with Alzheimer's disease whose dementia-related behavior includes assaultiveness. Functional disability and other victim-specific risk factors also have not consistently been identified. Such profiles also ignore features of the abuser, such as mental health problems, substance abuse, and dementia-related behaviors. Although younger victims of domestic violence (eg, battered spouses and children) commonly are financially dependent upon their abusers for shelter and housing, this is not typical of elder abuse. Substantial resources, such as home equity and retirement savings, often are available to older victims. These resources also may be the impetus for mistreatment in the case of abusing and exploitive adult children.

26. A 69-year-old woman is 15% over ideal body weight and has mild hypertension. She smokes cigarettes and has a family history of premature heart disease. Which of the following screening maneuvers for this patient is best supported by medical evidence?

    (A) Fasting plasma glucose
    (B) Fasting serum lipid profile
    (C) Hemoglobin A_{1C}
    (D) Radiography of the chest
    (E) Computed tomography of the chest

    ANSWER: B

    Little or no data from randomized trials are available to resolve much of the controversy regarding screening in older adults. Evidence supports obtaining a fasting lipid profile in patients aged 65 to 75 who have risk factors for coronary artery disease (CAD). Randomized trials have shown that treatment of hypercholesterolemia is beneficial for patients with CAD and for middle-aged men. Limited data concerning women and the young-old age group suggest potential benefits of lipid lowering for primary prevention. An analysis found dietary therapy to be cost-effective in older patients; treatment with 3-hydroxy-3-methylglutaryl–coenzyme A (HMG–CoA) reductase inhibitors (statins) were cost-effective in some higher-risk subgroups. The Air Force/Texas Coronary Atherosclerosis

Prevention (AFCAPS/TexCAPS) study found lovastatin to be effective in patients with normal serum low-density lipoprotein (LDL) cholesterol and decreased high-density lipoprotein (HDL) levels. Analyses did not show statistically significant results in older adults or women, but trends were favorable in these subgroups.

Treatment of type 2 diabetes mellitus has been shown to reduce complications, and the American Diabetes Association recommends measuring fasting blood glucose every 3 years in persons aged 45 and over. However, the potential benefits of treatment decrease with age because of shorter life expectancy. A 1998 cost-effectiveness analysis concluded that screening after age 65 would not result in any gain in life expectancy. No data support the screening of smokers with chest films, and very limited data support screening with computed tomography.

In this patient, screening for hypothyroidism may be indicated because the condition is common in elderly women and may be subtle. Mammography also is indicated in this age group.

27. A 79-year-old woman has Alzheimer's disease of moderate severity, with impaired memory, visuospatial skills, and language. During the past week she has become increasingly anxious and preoccupied by thoughts that strangers are living in the basement. The patient lives with her daughter, who asks your advice in alleviating her mother's distress. Which of the following is the most effective behavioral management strategy?

    (A) Allow the patient to rest alone in her room to minimize sensory input when she is most anxious.
    (B) Eliminate stimuli that exacerbate the delusion, and reassure the patient.
    (C) Remind the patient that her belief is not real.
    (D) Consider moving to a new house where the patient may not have this delusion.
    (E) Initiate nursing-home placement.

    ANSWER: B

    Delusions often occur in patients with moderate to advanced Alzheimer's disease, and the "phantom boarder syndrome" (ie, belief that strangers are living in the home) is common. Antipsychotic medications can be effective, but their adverse effects may be a problem. Behavioral interventions also can be effective, but a combined approach often is most beneficial. For this patient, the most effective strategy is to identify and eliminate stimuli that appear to contribute to the delusional thoughts and provide gentle reassurance. Distracting the patient by engaging her in another activity also can be helpful.

When patients are distressed by delusions, reassurance is important, and leaving the patient alone usually is not helpful. Distressed patients with Alzheimer's disease often seek out familiar caregivers and will not tolerate isolation. Reminding the patient that her belief is not real is unlikely to be effective, particularly if the delusion occurs frequently. Patients with Alzheimer's disease generally are aware of caregiver distress and irritability; patient anxiety often increases and behavior deteriorates in this situation. Language comprehension also may be impaired such that the patient does not entirely understand explanations. Moving to a new home or relocating the patient to a nursing home are not good strategies, because delusional thoughts often persist despite a change in environment. Moreover, moving may exacerbate distress and promote transient cognitive and functional decline.

28. An 82-year-old man falls, sustains a right intertrochanteric fracture, and is admitted to the orthopedic service. The patient has dementia and systolic hypertension and resides in a long-term-care facility. He had an uncomplicated myocardial infarction 10 years ago but has had no clinical manifestations of coronary artery disease subsequently. Current medications are an angiotensin-converting enzyme inhibitor and aspirin. He ambulates without assistance, and his nutritional status is good. His advance directive requests active treatment of all medical conditions.

The patient is agitated and confused. Pulse rate is 84 per minute, and respirations are 16 per minute. Blood pressure is 150/90 mm Hg. Findings of physical examination are normal except for severe pain on rotation of the right lower extremity. Routine laboratory studies and

chest radiograph also are normal. Electrocardiogram shows normal sinus rhythm and no ischemic changes; findings are unchanged from previous tracings. The orthopedic surgeon plans internal fixation and interoperative reduction of the fracture. Which of the following decisions regarding the timing of surgery is most appropriate?

(A) Medical management is indicated.
(B) Coronary angiography is indicated prior to surgery.
(C) Surgery should be deferred for 3 to 4 days to permit a more thorough evaluation.
(D) Surgery should be deferred to achieve better pain control.
(E) Surgery should be performed as soon as possible.

ANSWER: E

Hip fractures remain one of the most important causes of death and functional decline in older adults. For Medicare recipients 1-year mortality is 14%. Among survivors, only 54% walk unaided after 1 year. The timing of operative intervention can affect patient outcome in two ways: a delay may diminish functional recovery; however, failure to optimize and stabilize medical conditions may increase perioperative complications. Evidence from most cohort studies indicates that for stable patients who do not have active comorbid illnesses, surgical repair within the first 24 to 48 hours is associated with better return of function and reduced mortality. Considerable evidence supports careful medical evaluation to maximize outcome. The primary care clinician and orthopedist must form a partnership. Since most orthopedic services use practice guidelines, the more typical medical aspects of hip surgery (eg, prophylaxis for wound and urinary tract infections and for thromboembolism; nutritional management) often are routine. The primary clinician should provide critical expertise in recognition of functional status, the causes of delirium, and strategies for rehabilitation and early hospital discharge.

Medical management, which almost certainly would lead to permanent lack of independent ambulation, is not appropriate given this patient's previous ambulatory status and advance directive. Although an argument might be made for cardiac evaluation, the apparent clinical stability, lack of physical findings, and unchanged electrocardiogram suggest that his cardiovascular disease is well controlled. The agitated mental state is to be expected because of pain, fear, and the hospital environment. The underlying cause is the hip fracture, and surgical repair is the best "treatment" for this delirium. The demented patient is especially at risk because of communication difficulties and the failure to distinguish delirium from dementia. Studies also suggest that pain control following hip fracture is much less adequate for patients with dementia.

29. Health Care Financing Administration (in June 2001 renamed the Centers for Medicare & Medicaid Services) guidelines permit nursing homes to use psychotropic drugs without restrictions in which of the following situations?

    (A) Uncooperative behavior
    (B) Wandering
    (C) Hiccups
    (D) Disruptive vocalizations

    ANSWER: C

    The 1987 Omnibus Budget Reconciliation Act (OBRA) limited the use of psychotropic medications in treating nursing-home residents. Updates of OBRA guidelines have liberalized some dosing restrictions, but documentation of medical necessity and of periodic trials of withdrawal (attempts to reduce dosage at least twice per year) are mandated. Antipsychotics can be prescribed without restrictions to persons with psychosis or psychotic mood disorder, hiccups, nausea, vomiting, pruritus, Huntington's disease, or Tourette's syndrome. They also may be prescribed if the target behavior is documented, permanent, persistent, causing psychotic symptoms, or dangerous to the patient or others. Routine dosing is preferred to as-needed orders. Adverse effects such as tardive dyskinesia, cognitive or behavioral impairment, orthostatic hypotension, akathisia, and parkinsonism should be monitored carefully.

    Uncooperative behavior and wandering are not adequate indications for the use of psychotropic drugs. Behavior management techniques should be used first, including redirection, distraction, and environmental modification. A physical activity program has been used successfully for some wanderers. Agitated behavior secondary to dementia should be controlled with drugs only when the behavior is dangerous to the patient or others.

30. After rising from bed in the morning, an elderly nursing-home resident with a history of recurrent falls is found to have a 30–mm Hg decline in systolic blood pressure. Which of the following statements is correct?

    (A) The orthostatic change will persist throughout the day.
    (B) Postprandial hypotension also is likely to be present.
    (C) The patient probably does not have a history of hypertension.
    (D) The patient's falls are probably related to orthostatic hypotension.
    (E) The patient is at increased risk for rapid cognitive deterioration in the next 2 years.

    ANSWER: D

    Nearly 50% of elderly nursing-home residents experience orthostatic hypotension (OH) one or more times per day. At any given time, approximately 20% to 30% of residents experience OH. In the nursing home, it is associated with falls only in residents who have a history of falling in the past 6 months. The condition is highly variable, occurring most frequently before breakfast or after 1 minute of standing. It is more common in patients with hypertension. Although OH may occur after a meal and in patients with postprandial hypotension, these two abnormalities in blood-pressure regulation rarely occur together in the same patient. Longitudinal studies examining long-term outcomes have shown a relationship between OH and cardiovascular mortality in community-dwelling populations. Although transient hypotension might be expected to result in decreased cerebral perfusion and cause cognitive dysfunction, a Finnish study of community-dwelling and institutionalized elderly persons showed no association with cognitive deterioration during a 2-year follow-up period.

31. A 75-year-old man has difficulty walking because of osteoarthritic pain in the right hip. You prescribe a cane, with the handle at the level of the wrist. Which of the following instructions is correct regarding use of the cane?

(A) Hold in the right hand and advance with the right leg.
(B) Hold in the right hand and advance with the left leg.
(C) Hold in the left hand and advance with the right leg.
(D) Hold in the left hand and advance with the left leg.

ANSWER: C

Ideally, a cane or walker should fit the patient so that the center of gravity remains over the feet. This affords a biomechanical advantage when using the arms to help support the weight of the body. For a unilateral deficit, the cane should be held in the hand opposite the impaired leg, to bear some weight during the stance phase. The cane then is advanced with the impaired leg, taking advantage of the arm and leg opposition that occurs in normal gait. With the handle at the level of the wrist, the elbow will be flexed approximately 15 to 20 degrees during stance phase when the handle is grasped. This stretches the triceps slightly, allowing for maximal exertion of force by the muscle.

The choice of mobility aid should be guided by several principles, including versatility of the device, effectiveness, and cost. Most canes are cheaper than most walkers, which in turn are cheaper than most wheelchairs and scooters. Walkers, wheelchairs, and scooters are not helpful on stairs. In addition, both weight and width increase as one moves up the spectrum from canes to scooters. Most motorized scooters will not fit through most interior doors, and special lifts must be attached to a car to transport them. Specific subtypes of devices are designed to optimize the amount of support provided and to meet special needs. For example, a front-wheeled walker is easier to use than a four-prong walker because it can be pushed forward rather than lifted in time with the gait cycle. A front-wheeled walker is more stable than a four-wheeled walker because the rear posts act as brakes when patients increase weight on the walker (for example, if balance is lost). Front-wheeled walkers are most often prescribed, both for ease of use and safety reasons.

32. A previously sedentary 75-year-old obese woman with non-insulin-dependent diabetes mellitus has recently begun a program of brisk walking, plus flexibility and resistance exercises. She gradually increases her walking to 30 minutes per day. Which of the following statements about this patient after 3 months of this exercise program is most likely to be correct?

(A) Improvement in glucose tolerance precedes changes in abdominal adiposity.
(B) Improvement in glucose tolerance will occur only after a reduction in abdominal adiposity.
(C) Improvement in glucose tolerance is similar to that seen in a nondiabetic 75-year-old who follows the same program.
(D) Insulin sensitivity is unlikely to improve.

ANSWER: A

A number of studies have shown that glucose metabolism is enhanced by regular exercise. The relative risk of developing non-insulin-dependent diabetes mellitus is reduced incrementally with increased frequency of exercise. Increased insulin sensitivity and improved glucose tolerance occur within the first 4 months of increased activity, preceding changes in weight loss and body composition. This patient is most likely to have improvement in glucose tolerance before seeing a decrease in abdominal fat. Improvement in glucose metabolism is more likely to be seen in persons with impaired glucose metabolism.

33. Functionally based exercises targeted at nursing-home patients with significant dementia and dependency in activities of daily living (ADLs) are likely to result in which of the following?

(A) Increased patient frustration and behavioral disturbances
(B) Slower decline in ADLs over time
(C) Decreased time to perform ADL tasks
(D) Decreased nursing time devoted to ADLs
(E) Decreased endurance in performance of ADLs over time

ANSWER: B

Permitting functionally dependent, demented patients to help with ADL tasks rather than doing the task for them (eg, holding the pant leg open while the patient puts his or her leg into it instead of putting pants on the patient) takes more time. On the other hand, having patients assist with ADLs or perform additional practice ADL tasks (eg, doing two sit-to-stand maneuvers every time they transfer from chair to bed) decreases disruptive behavior and increases independence in ADLs. (See the Appendix, p 384, for an ADL Screen.) Educational programs for nurses and aides can change the way staff interact with patients during daily activities, and this in turn can slow functional decline.

In one randomized trial, patients undergoing "skills training" took, on average, twice as long to complete a given ADL task as did those in the control group. However, the incidence of disruptive behavior declined by more than 50%. Performance was well maintained during the "habit training" follow-up stage. Another randomized trial with demented nursing-home patients showed that an exercise program integrated into ADLs ("functional incidental training") resulted in improved endurance during ADLs. The intervention was a combination of prompted voiding four times per day with an additional one to two sit-to-stand maneuvers performed per prompted voiding event, plus walking or wheelchair propelling for 1 to 5 minutes. Estimates of added time for this training were not provided.

A quasi-experimental design compared nurses trained to elicit greater patient participation during daily care activities ("nursing rehabilitation") versus "exercise" (resistive exercise plus walking) versus "usual care." Six nursing homes were randomized to one of the three groups. Nurses and aides in facilities carrying out the nursing rehabilitation intervention underwent training in assessing ADL capacity and linked assessed capacity to specific rehabilitation protocols to be carried out by staff during daily care. Both the exercise and the nursing rehabilitation groups had significantly less decline in ADLs than did the usual-care group. However, the nursing rehabilitation group showed a trend ($P = 0.07$) for greater benefit in ADL activities than did the exercise group.

34. Which of the following changes in the external auditory canal contributes to an increased incidence of cerumen impaction with increasing age?

(A) Atrophy of epithelial sebaceous glands
(B) Shortening and thinning of hair follicles
(C) Increased cerumen production
(D) Reduced number and activity of cerumen glands
(E) Increased tortuosity of the external auditory canal

ANSWER: D

Cerumen is created by secretions from sebaceous and apocrine glands that mix with dust particles, desquamated epithelial cells, and dislodged hair follicles. It serves a protective function, lubricating the skin lining the ear canal and trapping unwanted materials and objects. The reduced activity and number of cerumen glands in older persons correlates with drier and less viscous cerumen. This may explain why cerumen impaction tends to be more common in older people.

Atrophy of the epithelial sebaceous glands causes a decrease in the epithelial oiliness and skin hydration. Dryness of the skin contributes to pruritus in the external auditory canal, which is a common complaint in older persons, but not to cerumen impaction. With age, thicker and longer hair follicles orient toward the tympanic membrane; this also may contribute to impaction. The anatomy of the external auditory canal does not change with age.

35. Which of the following gastrointestinal functions is more likely caused by disease than by age-related changes?

(A) Increase in diverticular disease
(B) Oral motor dysfunction manifested by altered mastication
(C) Decrease in small intestinal motility
(D) Decrease in splanchnic blood flow
(E) Decrease in upper and lower esophageal sphincter resting pressures

ANSWER: C

Many changes in gastrointestinal function have been shown to be associated with comorbid illness, rather than a natural consequence of aging. In healthy persons, motility of the small intestine does not decline with age. However, systemic diseases such as diabetes mellitus or the use of certain medications can adversely affect intestinal motility.

Diverticular disease increases with age and affects up to 60% of people age 80 and over. This may be related to changes in connective tissue elements or colonic pressure, or both. The colonic wall contains increased amounts of collagen and elastic fibers, both of which are present in tissues with reduced distensibility. This may account for the diminished ability of the colon to resist increases in intraluminal pressure. Studies of oral motor function have shown age-related alterations in mastication, swallowing, oral muscular posture, and tone. Altered mastication is reported most often, and even fully dentate older adults are less able than younger people to prepare food for swallowing. Splanchnic blood flow decreases with age—an important factor to consider when prescribing medications that are metabolized by the liver. Asymptomatic esophageal changes that occur with age include diminished upper and lower sphincter resting pressures, with delayed relaxation on swallowing. Up to 40% of asymptomatic 80-year-olds have abnormalities on swallowing studies.

36. A patient who is recovering from a stroke is medically stable, follows one-step directions but errs with two-step directions, is able to sit for no more than 1 to 2 hours per day, and requires maximal assistance with most activities of daily living. Which of the following is the most appropriate site for postacute care?

(A) Home care with home-health rehabilitation services
(B) Outpatient rehabilitation program
(C) Nursing home with no rehabilitation provided
(D) Skilled nursing facility with rehabilitation services
(E) Acute-level rehabilitation hospital

ANSWER: D

All stroke patients with residual disability should be considered for rehabilitation if they are medically stable and able to learn (ie, able to follow one-step directions or able to retain simple messages when repeated multiple times). Those who do not have functional disability do not need rehabilitation. Patients who are medically unstable should be stabilized before rehabilitation is considered. Patients who are unable to learn should receive care in a setting with adequate support services (eg, nursing home). As a patient's condition changes, the appropriateness of rehabilitation should be reassessed.

Among patients for whom rehabilitation is appropriate, the choice of site is based on the degree of disability, ability to tolerate being out of bed, and amount of home support that is available. Patients with minimal disability can be considered for home or outpatient rehabilitation if they are able to sit unsupported for 1 or more hours and have adequate support at home. The choice of home versus outpatient services is determined by whether the patient would be homebound. If a patient is able to transfer into a car and transportation is available, the outpatient setting would be preferred. If a patient has minimal disability but is unable to sit for 1 or more hours, the setting of choice would be a skilled nursing facility or home with home-health services, if adequate support is available. Patients with moderate to maximal disability should be considered for inpatient rehabilitation in either a skilled nursing facility, a rehabilitation hospital, or a nursing home with postacute care. Some nursing homes offer intensive rehabilitation resembling that of a rehabilitation hospital. An acute-level rehabilitation hospital is appropriate for patients who can tolerate 3 or more hours per day of therapy.

37. Which of the following is the best approach to the treatment of acute hip fracture in a frail 85-year-old woman who has stable coronary artery disease, ischemic cardiomyopathy (ejection fraction 35%), well-controlled hypertension, and mild dementia?

(A) Perform surgery within 24 to 48 hours, postoperative physical therapy five or more times per week.

(B) Perform surgery within 24 to 48 hours, postoperative physical therapy three to five times per week.

(C) Perform surgery within 24 to 48 hours, postoperative physical therapy one to three times per week.

(D) Delay surgery to assess the patient's cardiac condition, postoperative physical therapy five or more times per week.

(E) Delay surgery to assess the patient's cardiac condition, postoperative physical therapy three to five times per week.

ANSWER: A

More than 250,000 hip fractures occur annually in the United States, and that number is expected to increase. Mortality is substantial: 24% of patients die within 12 months. For patients who live 6 months or longer, only 60% regain their prefracture walking ability, and even fewer fully recover their ability to perform activities of daily living (ADLs) and instrumental activities of daily living (IADLs). (See the Appendix, p 384–385, for Screens.) Evidence from cohort studies indicates that for medically stable patients without active comorbid illness, surgical repair within 24 to 48 hours is associated with a decrease in 1-year mortality. In a cohort study that controlled for both comorbid conditions and quality of medical care, early surgery was associated with a shorter length of stay and earlier ambulation; patients whose surgery was delayed had more medical complications.

One randomized, controlled trial and several cohort studies found that more physical therapy sessions during the early postoperative period are associated with better functional outcomes. Both early surgery and frequent physical therapy promote early mobilization, which helps prevent deconditioning and other common postoperative complications (eg, aspiration pneumonia, pressure ulcers). Early mobilization is facilitated by activity orders that allow the patient to be out of bed and as active as possible. Many older patients have difficulty understanding and complying with orders such as "partial weight-bearing" or "touch-down weight-bearing," but they often can comply with a directive such as "weight-bearing as tolerated," which achieves the same effect.

The choice of surgical repair also should be directed by the patient's capacity to learn. Open reduction and internal fixation, which necessitates partial weight bearing, may be preferable for an intertrochanteric fracture in a patient who is cognitively intact. However, it probably is the wrong choice for an individual with significant cognitive impairments, because orders regarding weight bearing may not be understood by such a patient. Thus, a demented patient may be relegated to either no physical activity or activity that risks harming the orthopedic repair. Total hip replacement, which allows immediate weight bearing, usually is preferable for patients with significant cognitive impairments. The geriatric consultant must be sure that the orthopedic surgeon is aware of the patient's learning capacity. This does not require a lengthy evaluation and should not delay surgery.

38. An 80-year-old woman who has moderately severe Alzheimer's dementia is found at home approximately 1 week after she confined herself to bed prior because of an upper respiratory tract infection. A stage III pressure ulcer, $10 \times 12 \times 2$ cm in depth, is noted over the sacrum. The wound is covered with necrotic tissue and copious yellowish-green, foul-smelling exudate. The surrounding skin is erythematous and warm. Which of the following is the most appropriate initial management for this patient?

(A) Swab cultures, chemical debridement, and topical antibiotics
(B) Swab cultures, blood cultures, and oral antibiotics
(C) Swab cultures, blood cultures, surgical debridement, and intravenous antibiotics
(D) Blood cultures, chemical debridement, and intravenous antibiotics
(E) Blood cultures, surgical debridement, and intravenous antibiotics

ANSWER: E

This patient has at least local cellulitis related to the pressure ulcer and requires immediate debridement to remove bacteria-laden necrotic tissue. Use of a scalpel or scissors is the most rapid method and is appropriate in the presence of cellulitis or sepsis. A wound will not heal until inflammation resolves, and the presence of bacteria is a major cause of acute and chronic inflammation. Irrigation with normal saline also will reduce bacterial counts.

Cellulitis secondary to a pressure ulcer requires broad-spectrum intravenous antibiotics. Infection of stage III and IV ulcers often is polymicrobial. The presence of necrosis usually indicates a combination of aerobic and anaerobic organisms. A foul odor may indicate anaerobes or *Bacillus fragilis.* Blood cultures, both aerobic and anaerobic, are required to exclude bacteremia.

All open wounds are colonized with bacteria, so the presence of bacteria in a pressure ulcer does not necessarily indicate infection. Swab cultures usually reveal polymicrobial growth; further, they do not grow the same organisms as deep cultures, and they do not correlate with the presence of pathogenic bacteria. Three methods can be used to quantify bacterial levels in wound tissue: biopsy, needle aspiration, and quantitative swab culture. Quantitative swab cultures are obtained by cleansing the ulcer with saline, then twisting the end of a cotton-tipped swab over the ulcer with enough pressure to express fluid from the underlying tissue. The presence of more than 100,000 organisms indicates invasive infection that may impede healing.

39. An 85-year-old woman is admitted to the hospital because of a left hemispheric stroke. Her only other medical problem is hypertension. The patient weighs 55 kg (121 lb). She is afebrile. Pulse rate is 88 per minute, and respirations are 18 per minute. Blood pressure is 160/84 mm Hg. Cardiopulmonary and abdominal examinations are normal. She has no evidence of a visual field defect or neglect. Muscle strength is 3/5 on the right side. Skin inspection reveals no areas of breakdown. Which of the following pressure-relieving surfaces is most appropriate for this patient?

(A) 1.5-inch foam overlay
(B) 4.0-inch foam overlay
(C) Dynamic air-filled overlay
(D) Low-air-loss mattress
(E) Air-fluidized bed

ANSWER: B

A pressure-relieving mattress surface is indicated for all patients at risk for pressure-ulcer development. There is evidence that a support surface decreases the incidence and severity of pressure ulcers; however, it does not eliminate the need for repositioning. Pressure-relieving devices generally are classified as static (nonmoving) or dynamic. The choice for a particular patient is based on health status, care setting, ease of use, maintenance requirements, and cost. No support surface is clearly superior in all circumstances.

For this patient, a foam overlay is the most appropriate choice and is relatively inexpensive. Deep-cut, foam-cube mattress overlays, at least 4.0 inches thick, have been found to decrease healing time. A 1.5-inch overlay will not decrease pressure sufficiently. Bedsheets must be left somewhat loose over the foam, so that the pressure-distributing characteristics are maintained. The main problem with foam overlays is their potential for overcompression (*bottoming out*). When the surface is compressed to less than 1 inch, pressure-relieving properties are reduced. With prolonged use or with patients who weigh more than 114 kg (250 lb), bottoming out may occur. To assess for this, place an outstretched hand, palm up, under the overlay below the dependent body part. If less than 1 inch of foam is present, another type of surface is indicated.

A dynamic air-filled overlay provides alternating currents of air that redistribute or regulate pressure against the body. Dynamic overlays also reduce skin shear and retain moisture and heat. However, they are more expensive and have higher maintenance costs than static devices. They should be considered for patients who cannot assume a variety of positions or for those who have bottomed out on a static device. Low-air-loss and air-fluidized beds reduce skin-surface pressures below capillary filling pressures (< 32 mm Hg). They aid in skin-shear reduction and move air across the skin, which may help when skin moisture is a problem. However, insensible fluid loss may be promoted. Repositioning and transfers also may be difficult. These devices are expensive and should be reserved for use with patients who already have multiple pressure ulcers on more than one turning surface, who have bottomed out on a foam surface, or who have not responded to a dynamic overlay.

40. A 78-year-old woman who has multiple serious medical conditions and is minimally responsive is admitted to the general medical service for palliative care. Her family is in agreement that her living will be honored, so no aggressive diagnostic or curative therapies will be pursued. The patient periodically becomes restless and moans when she is turned in bed but is unable to rate or describe her discomfort. Symptoms improve following administration of morphine sulfate, 2 to 4 mg intravenously as needed. Which of the following is the most appropriate management strategy during the next 24 to 48 hours?

(A) Continuation of the current regimen
(B) Fentanyl, 25 μg transdermally
(C) Sustained-release morphine sulfate, 15 mg orally twice daily
(D) Morphine sulfate elixir, 5 to 10 mg orally every 4 hours
(E) Morphine sulfate, 1 mg hourly by continuous intravenous infusion

ANSWER: A

This patient's pain is well managed with as-needed dosing. It is appropriate to "start low and go slow" when beginning opioid use in elderly patients. For patients aged 70 and over, the usual adult dose should be reduced by 25% to 50%. Regular assessment of pain and reassessment after medication administration will help determine appropriate dosages, but this is difficult in minimally responsive patients who cannot participate in the assessment of their pain. Short-acting opioids can be titrated to provide pain relief without causing adverse side effects in patients with renal failure.

Transdermal administration of fentanyl provides steady-state drug levels and reduces the need for medication to control breakthrough pain. Transdermal therapy is very beneficial for patients with poor intravenous access or difficulty swallowing. Patients should have received the equivalent of 45 to 120 mg of oral morphine within a 24-hour period prior to application of a 25-μg patch. The proposed dose of sustained-release morphine is an appropriate conversion (3 oral:1 intravenous); however, this patient is not likely to be able to take oral medications for much longer. The as-needed dose of an immediate-release oral medication should be one fourth to one third of the sustained-release dose. Morphine elixir can be taken orally or given sublingually or buccally in unresponsive patients. Continuous infusion also provides steady-state drug levels; for patients who are at the end of life, however, decreasing liver and kidney function can cause an accumulation of metabolites and development of adverse effects. The *Education for Physicians on End-of-life Care (EPEC) Curriculum* recommends that, to minimize this risk, routine dosing or continuous infusions be stopped when urine output ceases; as-needed medications then can be used to manage expressions of pain. Subcutaneous infusions are excellent alternatives to the intravenous route when access is a problem. The dose remains the same; the concentration of the medication should be such that the volume does not exceed 2 to 5 mL per hour. The infusion site may be established with a butterfly needle or an intravenous catheter inserted into the subcutaneous tissue, and it should be changed weekly.

41. An 86-year-old woman with severe Alzheimer's disease is admitted from home to the hospital for treatment of a stroke. With the assistance of home-health aides, her daughter cares for her and wishes to continue to do so. The mother is dependent in all activities of daily living, incontinent of bowel and bladder, and alert intermittently. The patient is observed to cough with oral intake in the hospital. The patient's advance directives state that she does not want her life prolonged by the use of artificial food or hydration and does not wish to receive cardiopulmonary resuscitation.

What is the most appropriate next step in the management of this patient?

(A) Discharge to home with prior home-care services
(B) Discharge to institutional long-term care
(C) Discharge to a skilled nursing facility for rehabilitation
(D) Discharge to a home hospice program
(E) Discharge to an assisted-living facility

ANSWER: D

The most appropriate discharge plan for this patient is to a hospice program, either at home or in an institutional setting. Because the daughter wishes to continue to care for her mother, home is the most appropriate setting. The Medicare hospice benefit offers increased availability of palliative therapies, including bereavement services for the family.

The previous inability to predict survival of patients with end-stage dementia has served as a barrier to enrolling these patients in hospice care. Data from 1990 Medicare claims show that only 1.5% of patients enrolled in a hospice program had a primary diagnosis of dementia, with 35% of these patients surviving longer than 6 months. Recent research has identified criteria that may more accurately predict the survival of patients with severe dementia. Criteria have also been developed for other end-stage chronic diseases. This patient's dependency in activities of daily living, incontinence, decreased level of consciousness, and dysphagia make death very likely within the next 6 months.

In emphasizing end-of-life care rather than acute interventions, the focus of home hospice programs is more appropriate for this patient than that of usual home-care programs.

Discharge to institutional long-term care would be appropriate only if the current caregiver could no longer care for the patient at home because of increasing stress or inability to provide for the patient's activities of daily living. Many patients with end-stage dementia reside in nursing homes, which typically do not offer formal bereavement programs. The severity of this patient's dementia makes it highly unlikely that she would be able to benefit from a rehabilitation program. Residence in an assisted-living facility is appropriate for patients with dementia who require minimal supervision of activities of daily living or medication supervision, or both.

42. A 71-year-old woman who has been smoking approximately one and one-half packs of cigarettes daily for 40 years seeks your help to stop smoking. She has tried several times to quit "cold turkey" and experienced irritability, changes in sleep habits, and craving. She now has begun caring for a grandson in her home and has read that her smoking could harm his health. She has seen advertisements for nicotine patches and gum but is unsure which, if either, would be right for her. The patient also works outside the home part time, and she finds it difficult to remember to take medication when she is not at home. She has been in good health, except for a chronic cough that worsens with seasonal allergies and a history of "difficult-to-control" seizures. Her neurologist, who prescribed carbamazepine and gabapentin after phenytoin and phenobarbital were ineffective, advised her not to use bupropion.

The patient is edentulous and has loose-fitting dentures. Pulse rate is 76 per minute, and blood pressure is 154/92 mm Hg. The nasal septum is deviated, and the mucosa is swollen and boggy. The lung fields are clear, with no adventitious sounds. Which of the following is the most appropriate form of nicotine replacement therapy for this patient?

(A) Nasal spray
(B) Oral inhaler
(C) Transdermal patch
(D) Gum
(E) Sublingual tablet

ANSWER: C

A clinical trial comparing the different forms of nicotine replacement (ie, nasal spray, oral inhaler, transdermal patch, and gum) found no significant differences in abstinence rates after 12 weeks of therapy. All four products had success rates of just over 20%. However, differences were noted in adherence rates and adverse events. Experts recommend that the choice of product be based on patient preferences, comorbidities, and experiences with nicotine replacement therapy during past unsuccessful attempts, as well as information on adherence and adverse effects. The transdermal patch, in comparison with other products, had the highest rate of adherence and a relatively low rate of adverse events. This patient, who has trouble remembering to take medications, may find it easier to place a patch in the morning and not have to worry about additional doses during the rest of the day.

The nasal spray had a very low adherence rate and the highest rate of adverse events. For this patient, who has a deviated septum and seasonal allergic rhinitis, a nasal spray could be difficult to use. The oral inhaler had the lowest adherence rate and was rated as more embarrassing to use than the other forms. Nicotine polacrilex also had a low adherence rate, and gum is a suboptimal choice for this patient with ill-fitting dentures. Multiple doses of the spray, the inhaler, and the gum would be necessary during the day, raising the likelihood of nonadherence. Sublingual tablets have not yet been approved for use in the United States, although clinical trials are under way. Again, for this patient, they would be less appropriate because of the need for frequent use.

43. A 78-year-old man with a history of coronary artery disease, hypothyroidism, and osteoarthritis of the knees is admitted to the hospital from home for shortness of breath. He is treated successfully for an exacerbation of congestive heart failure, with changes in his medication regimen and a sodium-restricted diet. He lives alone, gets out of bed by himself, and ambulates independently with a cane. Folstein Mini–Mental State Examination score is 29. He wishes to return home when discharged from the hospital.

Which of the following interventions is most likely to reduce subsequent hospital utilization for this patient?

(A) Discharge to postacute care for rehabilitation
(B) Coordinated discharge planning with follow-up at home
(C) Prescription of home physical therapy
(D) Recommendation for a friendly visitor
(E) Recommendation to attend a senior center

ANSWER: B

Congestive heart failure is a common diagnosis for 30- and 90-day readmission to the hospital in Medicare patients. Patients who benefit from discharge planning services in the hospital are also those who are most at risk for rehospitalization. Characteristics common to these patients include advanced age, multiple comorbid conditions, cognitive impairment, depression, living alone, recent hospitalization, and impaired physical function.

Several clinical trials have demonstrated that coordinated discharge planning initiated in the hospital and carried through into the home setting can reduce subsequent hospitalization. Key components of these interventions are a multidisciplinary assessment of patients' needs and an ongoing review of medications, disease symptoms, and nutrition. The home visit provides an opportunity to assess a patient's adherence to the discharge plan and intervene in a timely fashion. In patients with congestive heart failure, medication assessment (an angiotensin-converting enzyme inhibitor, a β-blocker, and spironolactone, which have been demonstrated to improve important outcomes) and counseling are important features of the home visit.

There is some data to suggest that patients enrolled in interdisciplinary team–based programs of care, such as PACE, are hospitalized at a lower rate than usual Medicare beneficiaries.

This patient can transfer from bed to chair and walk independently at hospital discharge; therefore, transfer to a postacute care facility for rehabilitation is not required. Referral for physical therapy would be appropriate if further strengthening of the lower extremities is necessary or if the patient has a history of falls.

There is no evidence to suggest that physical rehabilitation by itself will reduce subsequent hospital utilization in patients at high risk for readmission.

Patients who live alone are at risk for social isolation. Interventions aimed at reducing this risk, such as a home visit from a volunteer or a visit to a senior center, lack the multidisciplinary assessment and coordinated follow-up by trained clinicians necessary to reduce hospital utilization.

44. The wife of a 79-year-old man phones you because her husband "has not been acting right" since breakfast. He is leaning forward, drooling, and producing large amounts of saliva. Food "comes right back up" when he eats, and he has been coughing but is not short of breath. The patient has severe dementia, and his speech has been garbled ever since he suffered a stroke several years ago. When the wife asks the patient what is wrong, he points to his sternum but cannot describe what he is feeling. The wife notes no change in speech and no new weakness. Which of the following is the most likely diagnosis?

(A) New stroke
(B) Esophageal foreign body
(C) Gastric ulcer with outlet obstruction
(D) Zenker's diverticulum
(E) Pneumonia

ANSWER: B

In older persons, food or pills can become lodged in the esophagus, resulting in difficulty handling secretions, drooling, and leaning forward. Patients often can localize the level of the obstruction by pointing to it. They also may report an inability to swallow and regurgitation of food into the mouth but no vomiting. Underlying causes include cancer, stricture, diverticulum, or ring formation.

A stroke can produce severe dysphagia, but this patient has no new neurologic deficits. Complications of gastric ulcer include hemorrhage, perforation, and obstruction. Obstruction usually does not present with hypersalivation, regurgitation, and retrosternal fullness; however, this diagnosis should be considered if evaluation reveals a normal esophagus. Zenker's diverticulum develops in a natural area of weakness in the posterior hypopharyngeal wall. It develops slowly, with gradually worsening symptoms of halitosis and regurgitation of food particles consumed several days previously. A large diverticulum can become filled with food and compress the esophagus, causing dysphagia or complete obstruction. Pneumonia is unlikely because of the acute onset and lack of preceding cough or other respiratory symptoms.

45. Which of the following describes the most likely effect of normal aging on basic personality?

(A) More rigid
(B) More irritable
(C) More mellow
(D) More childlike
(E) No change

ANSWER: E

Personality is an enduring pattern of inner experience and behavior. Although various stereotypes about personality and aging exist and empirical studies are limited, most authors agree that basic personality remains relatively unchanged throughout life, including the geriatric period. Personality may have somewhat different manifestations as the capabilities of the person change, but significant changes in personality most often herald an unrecognized psychiatric illness (eg, depression or dementia) or the onset of a medical illness. This is particularly evident in the new onset of carelessness, lack of discretion, or apathy that often accompanies the development of a frontal dementia syndrome.

The idea that aging persons become more mellow or more irritable reflects ageism and cultural stereotyping. Such observations frequently are the result of countertransference reactions of professionals or the lack of adequate longitudinal data or corroborating information from outside sources. The impression that older persons become more childlike most often reflects the reemergence of longstanding basic personality traits that were suppressed in midlife by social or other constraints. Studies have shown that birth cohorts may differ in degree of personal rigidity, but this trait also does not change within individuals over time. However, an obsessional personality may become more apparent as an individual becomes more dependent and involved with the health care system.

46. An 82-year-old man comes to you for evaluation of unsteadiness when walking. This began gradually but has increased in severity during the past 3 years. His son, with whom he lives, has positioned furniture or handrails throughout the house to provide support. He takes hydrochlorothiazide for hypertension. The patient has not had lightheadedness, palpitations, syncope, or vertigo. On physical examination, Romberg sign is positive, and no dysdiadochokinesis is noted. Which of the following is the most likely cause of the disequilibrium?

(A) Cerebrovascular disease
(B) Postural hypotension
(C) Cardioinhibitory carotid sinus syndrome
(D) Vasodepressor carotid sinus syndrome
(E) Hydrochlorothiazide

ANSWER: A

The first step in evaluating dizziness is determining whether the symptom involves a sensation of movement (vertigo), impending faint (presyncope), imbalance (disequilibrium), or vague lightheadedness. This patient has impaired balance and gait in the absence of any abnormal sensation in the head. In older persons, disequilibrium is very common; in isolation, it suggests neurologic disorders or multiple neurosensory impairments. Cerebrovascular disease probably is the most common cause of unsteadiness in older persons, particularly in the absence of acute labyrinthitis or other peripheral vestibular disease. In a study of 149 community-dwelling elderly persons with dizziness, "central vascular disease" was found to be a contributing factor in 105 (70%). The study's diagnostic criteria—"unsteadiness with or without lightheadedness in association with an abnormal gait (marche a petit pas) and increased reflexes and tone, with or without loss of power"—were nonspecific and, therefore, may have overestimated the prevalence. However, additional support for a cerebrovascular cause was provided by a 5-year longitudinal study in which 29 patients (aged 75 to 92) with disequilibrium were compared with age- and sex-matched controls. Affected persons were found to have a significantly greater frequency ($P < 0.001$) of subcortical white-matter lesions and frontal atrophy.

The absence of lightheadedness makes postural hypotension and hydrochlorothiazide use unlikely causes. Likewise, the absence of palpitations and syncope along with the gradual onset makes cardioinhibitory or vasodepressor carotid sinus syndrome unlikely.

47. Which of the following statements is correct regarding hypochondriacal symptoms?

(A) They are more common in elderly persons.
(B) They are a permanent condition in elderly persons.
(C) They commonly are associated with depression.
(D) They seldom have a psychologic meaning.

ANSWER: C

Hypochondriasis is defined by the fourth edition of the *Diagnostic and Statistical Manual of Mental Disorders* as "a preoccupation with fears of having or the idea that one has a serious disease based on the person's misinterpretation of bodily symptoms." It is one of seven somatoform disorders that share the phenomenon of identifying bodily concerns without a clear organic explanation. The preoccupation must persist for at least 6 months, despite medical reassurance to the contrary, and cause clinically significant distress or functional impairment. It also must not be of delusional intensity or be better explained by another psychiatric disorder. Hypochondriasis involves only one primary bodily concern, in contrast to somatization disorder, which must present with at least eight symptoms divided among four major systems.

Despite commonly held views, hypochondriasis is not part of the normal aging process and is not more common in older persons. Studies in primary care settings show the prevalence to be 2% to 3% of all patients; in patients who also have a major depressive disorder, however, it may be as high as 60%. Hypochondriasis can be transient and may respond to psychotherapeutic and psychopharmacologic treatment. Antidepressant medications commonly are used in the treatment of most somatoform disorders. Hypochondriasis may be related to psychosocial problems and may subside as situational stress resolves.

The hypochondriac's symptoms usually are considered a form of learned social behavior, related to early childhood trauma and learned sick-role behaviors. The behavior in adulthood may become a source of "secondary gain" and serve several functions, including facilitating interactions with others, creating a situation in which one is attended to and touched, communicating distress, and controlling the behavior of others.

48. A 90-year-old woman falls at home and fractures her right hip. She is unable to rise from the floor and is not found for 24 hours. A stage II pressure ulcer, 3.0 × 2.0 × 0.5 cm in depth, is noted over the right greater trochanter. Assessment of the wound reveals pink tissue with scant necrotic areas at the periphery; a small amount of purulent-appearing, odorous drainage; and no erythema of the surrounding skin. Which of the following is the most appropriate cleansing agent for this pressure ulcer?

(A) Any skin cleanser
(B) Any wound cleanser
(C) Normal saline
(D) Hydrogen peroxide
(E) 1% silver sulfadiazine

ANSWER: C

Appropriate cleansing of a pressure ulcer decreases the bacterial burden and promotes healing. Cleansing should remove loosely adherent necrotic tissue, exudate, and metabolic wastes. The most appropriate cleansing agent for a pressure ulcer is normal saline, which is not cytotoxic. To reduce local tissue damage, the saline should be delivered as an irrigating stream, delivered at 4 to 15 psi. Lower irrigation pressures may not cleanse the wound adequately, and higher pressures may cause tissue trauma and drive bacteria into the wound. The appropriate amount of irrigation pressure can be delivered using a 35-mL syringe with a 19-gauge angiocatheter, a dental irrigator (eg, Water Pik) at the lowest setting, or a 250-mL squeeze bottle.

Topical antiseptic agents are cytotoxic and may retard epithelialization; there is no evidence that their use significantly decreases bacterial counts in wound tissue. In fibroblast studies, 1% povidone iodine, 0.25% acetic acid, 3% hydrogen peroxide, and 0.5% sodium hypochlorite (Dakin's solution) were 100% cytotoxic. In animal models, nearly all of these agents delayed wound healing; only hydrogen peroxide was found to be minimally bactericidal. The role of topical antibiotics in pressure-ulcer care is unclear. Although they do not appear to be cytotoxic, their use may select for growth of resistant organisms and probably should be reserved for locally infected or nonhealing wounds that have not responded after 2 to 4 weeks of optimal care (including more aggressive cleansing and debridement). To decrease the potential for growth of antibiotic-resistant bacteria, use should be limited to a 2-week trial.

49. A 75-year-old man comes to your office to establish a primary care relationship. When obtaining social history, you ask about his religious beliefs and practices. Which of the following statements is most correct regarding religious beliefs?

(A) They are associated with better physical health outcomes.
(B) They are associated with better emotional health outcomes.
(C) They are associated with better physical and emotional health outcomes.
(D) They have no demonstrable association with physical or emotional health outcomes.

ANSWER: C

When obtaining patient history, it is appropriate to inquire, in a nonjudgmental way, about religious beliefs and practices. Understanding these beliefs may help in understanding how a patient approaches medical decision making. For example, it obviously is important to know if a patient is a Jehovah's Witness and precluded from blood transfusions or that a patient is a Christian Scientist and likely to resist taking medication. However, even in the absence of overt influences, religious beliefs have a significant effect on physical and emotional well-being.

Studies have indicated that as many as 96% of older persons believe in God or a universal spirit and 90% pray. In a study of hospitalized men aged 70 and over, 25% spontaneously stated that religion was the most important factor in helping them cope with health problems. Lower rates of depression are reported in those who have religious beliefs, and such beliefs are among five predictors of speed of recovery. It has been hypothesized that religious faith provides patients with a sense of control over uncontrollable problems such as illness. Also, the ability to reduce stress and worry by enlisting one's faith in the healing process is a probable factor in improved mood. Religious beliefs are also associated with reduced morbidity and prolonged survival. Religious involvement has been associated with increased life span by almost 7 years. Although this effect is not well understood from a physiologic perspective, persons who attend religious services have been found to have lower levels of interleukin-6, suggesting a stronger immune system. Similarly, in a study of 2812 older patients, those who attended religious services had better physical functioning than those who did not attend.

50. Which of the following statements is correct regarding assisted-living settings?

(A) The median age of female residents is 74.
(B) Nearly 75% of residents are discharged to a nursing home.
(C) Continuous skilled nursing care is provided for residents who can pay privately.
(D) Medicaid programs do not subsidize assisted-living services through waiver programs.
(E) Regulations for assisted living are highly diverse from state to state.

ANSWER: E

Assisted living comprises housing, personalized supportive services, and health care for persons needing assistance with activities of daily living (ADLs) and instrumental activities of daily living (IADLs). Services generally include 24-hour supervision, personal care, social services, medication management, meals, health-promotion activities, and other supports. Physical and psychosocial needs are assessed on admission and at regular intervals. A service agreement is developed to coordinate the delivery of services for each resident. Regulation of facilities varies substantially among the states. There is little standardization in the definition of what constitutes an assisted-living residence, although guidelines have been developed. All facilities must comply with local building and fire-safety codes, but only some states require training and certification of staff. Other regulations address environmental, service, staffing, or admission and retention standards.

Currently, more than 1 million people live in an estimated 20,000 assisted-living residences. Nearly 80% are women, with a median age of 84; the median age of men is 82. The median annual income is $25,000, with assets of $100,000. Although 26% of residents are completely independent in personal care activities, help is needed with an average of two ADLs. Approximately 80% need or accept assistance with medication management. Typically, facilities do not provide continuous skilled nursing care. Residents who experience extended periods of incapacity or require higher levels of medical care are relocated. Approximately 45% are discharged to a nursing home. The average length of stay in assisted living is about 3 years. Costs are highly variable, depending upon the residence, room size, and services provided. Approximately 25% of facilities have average monthly rent and fees of $1501 to $2000. About 90% of assisted-living services are paid for with private funds. Many states are experimenting with limited Medicaid reimbursements through waivers to pay for some service components. Depending on individual insurance, certain costs may be reimbursed.

51. A 65-year-old man has type 2 diabetes mellitus, systolic hypertension, and hypercholesterolemia but no evidence of target organ damage. He smokes cigarettes. Current medications are a statin, chlorthalidone, and metformin. The patient walks at a brisk pace for 30 minutes every day. Findings of physical examination are normal except for peripheral neuropathy. Electrocardiogram shows normal sinus rhythm without evidence of myocardial infarction. The patient tells you that his neighbor takes aspirin to prevent strokes, and he asks whether he should take it too. Which of the following should you advise?

(A) There is no evidence that aspirin will benefit him.
(B) The potential benefits of aspirin may outweigh the potential harms.
(C) The potential harms of aspirin may outweigh the potential benefits.
(D) The potential benefits of dipyridamole are greater than those of aspirin.

ANSWER: B

Four randomized trials in men without a history of myocardial infarction or stroke have shown that aspirin chemoprophylaxis prevents fatal and nonfatal cardiac events. The magnitude of potential benefit is related to underlying risk of coronary artery disease. This patient is at high ($> 5\%$) risk for a cardiovascular event in the next 5 years. Approximately 15 cardiovascular events could be prevented by treating 1000 such persons for 5 years. Persons who are at low ($< 1\%$) risk are less likely to benefit. Approximately three cardiovascular events could be prevented by treating 1000 such persons for 5 years.

Adverse effects of aspirin include hemorrhagic strokes and major gastrointestinal (GI) bleeding. These are not closely tied to the underlying risk of cardiovascular disease. It is estimated that daily low-dose (≤ 325 mg) aspirin would precipitate one to two hemorrhagic strokes and five to ten GI bleeds in 1000 persons taking aspirin for 5 years. Thus, in persons who are at low-risk of cardiovascular disease, aspirin is more likely to precipitate a stroke or major GI bleed than to prevent a cardiovascular event. However, the opposite is true for persons at higher risk, so aspirin therapy is indicated. There is no evidence from primary prevention trials that dipyridamole prevents cardiovascular events.

52. An 86-year-old man is brought to the emergency department because of shortness of breath. He is inattentive, combative, and unable to speak in full sentences. Pulse rate is 128 per minute, and respirations are 28 per minute; blood pressure is 180/100 mm Hg. Physical examination reveals audible wheezes, bilateral crackles, jugular venous distention, an S_3, and pitting 2+ pedal edema. The patient lives with his son, who tells you that his father has heart failure and was in the hospital last week for a similar episode. Current medications are digoxin, furosemide, and captopril. The son administers these, supervises his father, and runs a lucrative family business.

Electrocardiogram shows sinus tachycardia but no new ischemic changes. Chest radiograph shows pulmonary edema and several old rib fractures. Complete blood cell count and other routine laboratory studies are normal, but serum digoxin level is zero. A recent echocardiogram revealed an ejection fraction of 42%. The patient has been in the emergency department nine times in the past year with similar presentations. Which of the following statements is correct?

(A) You should confront the son immediately about abuse or neglect of his father.
(B) A toxicology screen would not be useful.
(C) A high socioeconomic level makes elder mistreatment unlikely.
(D) Frequent emergency department visits are rare in elder mistreatment.
(E) Evidence of physical abuse, such as rib fractures, may coexist with neglect.

ANSWER: E

Abuse and neglect affect 3% to 6% of patients aged 65 and over. A clinician may be the only person an abused elder sees, other than the perpetrator of mistreatment; thus, the role of clinicians in identifying and managing mistreatment is critical. Different forms of mistreatment (eg, physical abuse, verbal abuse, neglect, exploitation) often coexist. Several studies point to the frequent concurrence of abuse and neglect. This patient may have been physically abused, but other findings (ie, emergency department recidivism, nonadherence with medications, and an increase in caregiver burden) suggest that neglect also is occurring.

Confrontation with a suspected abuser in the information-gathering phase of an evaluation may result in sequestration of the victim. Loss of access to a vulnerable patient is worrisome. Abusers often are the primary caregivers for victims. Strategies to engage and support suspected perpetrators, rather than confront and punish them, may be appropriate. Digoxin has an extremely long half-life, so several doses must be missed for the level to be zero. The patient's altered mental status may reflect hypoxia from pulmonary edema but could reflect restraint with unprescribed sedatives. Toxicology screening is indicated. High socioeconomic level should not foster complacency in cases of suspected mistreatment. This problem crosses all ethnic groups, income levels, and geographic regions. A higher prevalence of nonwhite persons in Adult Protective Service databases probably reflects a reporting bias for disenfranchised minority patients. Abused elderly persons often have substantial contact with emergency departments before mistreatment is finally diagnosed, a pattern that represents missed opportunities for detection of mistreatment.

53. You are asked to serve on the Patient Care Committee of a full-service community hospital with active medical and surgical services. In an effort to improve the quality of care and reduce operating expenses, the hospital has asked the committee to concentrate on reducing average length of stay. Data demonstrate that among Medicare patients (about 50% of all discharges), the most common contributor to excessive length of stay is the development of delirium. Approximately 60% of the delirious patients are on the surgical service. The committee is charged with developing a cost-effective strategy to prevent delirium and improve quality of care, while reducing of hospital costs. Which of the following would best meet these objectives?

(A) Institute a mandatory geriatric consultation for all Medicare patients.
(B) Establish an "early warning" surveillance system to identify patients with early signs of delirium and trigger targeted nursing intervention.
(C) Screen all Medicare patients for delirium on admission; implement targeted interventions for all patients, even those without evidence of delirium.
(D) Encourage greater family involvement with routine hospital care, including nighttime visitation.
(E) Require anesthesiologists to develop practice guidelines encouraging the use of local rather than general anesthesia.

ANSWER: C

Delirium is a serious cause of morbidity and mortality among hospitalized older adults. The information from this hypothetical hospital is representative of national averages. Studies generally have focused on three approaches. First, a number of reliable predictors have been identified to assist in establishing the diagnosis of delirium. When these are used in combination, the operating characteristics of these tests are better than single-factor analysis. For example, the Confusion Assessment Method is one instrument to define delirium that assesses a combination of factors. (See Table 19.2 in "Delirium," p 128.) Its criteria are acute onset and a fluctuating course, inattention, and either disorganized thinking or an altered level of consciousness. When administered by trained personnel, it has a sensitivity of 94% to 100%, a specificity of 90% to 95%, and high interobserver reliability. The use of such screening tools should improve the ability of hospital personnel to identify delirium and distinguish it from dementia or depression.

A second research approach has been to devise treatment strategies, such as reduction in the use of multiple medications, especially the inappropriate use of restraints; correction of metabolic abnormalities; and better pain control. The third area of investigation centers on development of what might be called primary prevention strategies. Most interventional studies have focused on geriatric assessment, nursing approaches, and family intervention. Although there is some evidence that each of these can reduce delirium, they do not demonstrate statistical significance. Thus, a recommendation to provide geriatric consultation, targeted nursing, or family involvement has serious limitations. One major study describes a multicomponent intervention for patients aged 70 and over. All patients, both with and without clinical manifestations of delirium, received interventions aimed at six risk factors: cognitive impairment, sleep deprivation, immobility, visual impairment, hearing impairment, and dehydration. This resulted in significant reductions in the number and duration of episodes of delirium in hospitalized patients. The estimated cost per case of delirium prevented was $6341, which compares favorably with other accepted interventions in acute care medicine. This approach was not effective in reducing duration, severity, or recurrence in patients who already had signs of delirium, however, thus providing less rationale for an "early warning" approach. Many causes of delirium would not be influenced by changing the route of anesthetic administration.

54. An 83-year-old woman who resides in a long-term care facility complains of chronic insomnia. She is bedridden and is legally blind secondary to diabetes mellitus. Which of the following age-related changes most likely contributes to this patient's sleep disturbance?

(A) A reduction in total sleep time
(B) A reduction in melatonin secretion
(C) A reduction in the percentage of stage 3 and 4 sleep
(D) An increase in the percentage of rapid eye movement (REM) sleep
(E) A breakdown in the segregation of sleep and wakefulness

ANSWER: E

A fundamental change occurs in the circadian physiology of older adults. Decreased nocturnal sleep, the tendency to nap, and daytime sleepiness suggest that the segregation of sleep and wakefulness in the light–dark cycle breaks down with age. Moreover, older adults exhibit a "flattened" (ie, less prominent day–night demarcation) circadian rhythm with respect to basal body temperature and cortisol production. This patient, who is blind and bedridden, likely

has relatively few social and environmental cues to indicate day or night. Thus, she may sleep randomly during a 24-hour period and experience nighttime awakenings or insomnia.

Total sleep time decreases only moderately between the third and ninth decade, and older persons generally are able to maintain normal sleep patterns. Compared with a younger individual, an older person's sleep is less efficient, with substantial reduction in deep (stages 3 and 4) sleep, as well as a tendency to experience more awakenings because of environmental noise or temperature change. The relative percentage of REM sleep changes little with age, although the temporal distribution does "flatten" (ie, more uniform percentage of REM sleep in both halves of the night). Age-related changes in both REM and deep sleep may contribute to this patient's sleep disturbance, but these factors are not clinically significant. Although circulating levels of melatonin decrease with advancing age, the biologic and clinical implications of this change are not clear. In this patient, a relative deficiency of melatonin is not sufficient to explain the clinical presentation.

55. Which of the following statements is correct regarding the prevalence of mood disorders in persons aged 65 and over?

(A) It is higher than in younger adults.
(B) It is higher in community dwellers than in nursing-home residents.
(C) Manic episodes are as common as in younger adults.
(D) The burden of depressive symptoms within a birth cohort fluctuates throughout the life cycle.
(E) Lack of a sufficient social network is a risk factor for development of depression.

ANSWER: E

In prospective studies of elderly patients, one of the characteristics found to be correlated with the onset of depression is having an insufficient social network. Other risks are dementia and more than two depressive symptoms on initial evaluation. In a study of mood disorders in persons aged 65 to 100, the point prevalence of major depression was 4.4% in women and 2.7% in men. Other depressive syndromes were uncommon. These rates are significantly lower than the rate (8.29%) in persons aged 25 to 44. Depressive disorders are less common in community-dwelling elderly persons than in younger adults. Studies of depression in patients on medical floors of general hospitals and in nursing homes showed a higher than expected prevalence: 12% among inpatients and up to 16% in nursing-home residents. This points to the need for awareness of risk factors and the benefits of screening those at increased risk (eg, multiple recent stressors, previous history of depression). The burden of depressive symptoms seems to remain constant throughout the life cycle, and the cohort effect may be as important a predictor as age.

Although depressive disorders are fairly common in elderly patients, new-onset manic episodes are relatively uncommon. When an initial manic episode occurs in an older patient, it is important to rule out organic causes, such as medications (especially corticosteroids), illicit drug use, cerebrovascular disease (especially right-sided), alcoholism, head injury, systemic lupus erythematosus, or multiple sclerosis.

56. A 75-year-old white man has back pain after gardening and is found to have a T10 vertebral compression fracture. The patient has no other symptoms and has always been in good health except for mild hypertension that is treated with a diuretic. He is very active and does weight-bearing exercise for 1 to 2 hours each day. He does not smoke cigarettes and drinks alcohol only occasionally. Which of the following is the most likely cause of the fracture?

(A) Idiopathic osteoporosis
(B) Testosterone deficiency
(C) Longstanding corticosteroid use
(D) Chronic malabsorption
(E) Metastatic carcinoma

ANSWER: A

Approximately 20% of all osteoporotic fractures reported annually in the United States occur in men, and approximately one third of hip fractures in patients aged 75 and over occur in men. The majority (50% to 60%) of men with osteoporosis are found to have an underlying cause. Testosterone deficiency, longstanding

corticosteroid use, and malabsorption (such as celiac disease) are the most common secondary causes; primary or metastatic malignancy also should be considered. Chronic, excessive alcohol use can lead to low bone mass and fractures. The diagnosis of idiopathic osteoporosis is made after other causes have been excluded.

Treatment of idiopathic male osteoporosis includes adequate calcium and vitamin D (1500 mg of elemental calcium and 400 IU of vitamin D daily). Alendronate, 10 mg daily, currently is the most effective pharmacologic treatment. Other bisphosphonates (eg, risedronate) also may prove useful. Calcitonin has not been well studied in men and at present has no role in treatment. Studies of parathyroid hormone (PTH) found significant improvement in bone density of the lumbar spine after 18 months of treatment. Further studies are required to assess the effects on fracture reduction.

When male osteoporosis develops secondary to hypogonadism, therapy is aimed at treating the underlying pathophysiology. Studies have shown that older men with borderline to low testosterone levels have improved bone density after testosterone treatment. Patients also report improved muscular strength and sense of well-being. However, because of the potential to aggravate atherosclerotic disease or prostatic changes, testosterone should be used only after careful consideration of its potential risks and benefits.

This patient does not have a history of food idiosyncrasies and chronic diarrhea, so malabsorption is unlikely. He also has no history of corticosteroid use. The patient has no symptoms suggestive of metastatic carcinoma. Testosterone deficiency, while important to rule out, is not the most likely cause of a single compression fracture seen on plain film.

57. A 78-year-old man has longstanding urinary frequency and urgency that has worsened in the past month. He often cannot reach the toilet in time and must change clothes once or twice a day. The patient has a tremor of the left hand that has worsened during the past 2 months. His wife reports that he is "lazy and hardly moves around any more." Medical history also includes hypertension, coronary artery disease, and hypercholesterolemia.

The patient has masked facies, diminished arm swing with normal gait, and increased muscle tone on the left side. A resting tremor is present on the left. The abdomen and genitalia are normal. Rectal examination shows brown stool in the vault and no evidence of fecal impaction. The prostate gland seems slightly large, with partial obliteration of the median sulcus, but without nodules or masses. Urinalysis is normal. Plasma glucose and serum calcium levels are normal; serum creatinine is 1.2 mg/dL. Which of the following tests is the most appropriate next step?

(A) Urine cytology
(B) Serum prostate-specific antigen
(C) Postvoid residual volume (PVR)
(D) Cystometry
(E) Computed tomography of the head

ANSWER: C

Studies have shown that many older men experience urinary incontinence (UI). In a Veterans Administration primary-care setting, 32.3% reported UI within the past 12 months and 13.8% (43% of those who were incontinent) reported episodes at least weekly. Age did not correlate with frequency or amount of urine loss, while emotional health, social relationships, physical activity, and travel were related. Only about 30% of men discussed UI with their medical provider, but 75% desired evaluation and treatment.

The patient's resting tremor, bradykinesia, and rigidity are suggestive of Parkinson's disease. Their asymmetric nature is typical of early disease. Patients with neurologic conditions such as Parkinson's disease may present with UI. However, patients with UI are not more likely to have an underlying neurologic condition. In men, the differential diagnosis includes urge incontinence and overflow incontinence. In this patient with mobility impairment and poor fine-motor control of the upper extremities, functional incontinence is a likely contributory cause. Physical examination of the abdomen is a poorly sensitive test for detecting urinary retention (although it may be highly specific). PVR should be measured routinely in men with UI. This can be accomplished noninvasively by the use of ultrasonography of the bladder; if

catheterization is performed, a sample of the residual urine can be used for urinalysis and microscopic examination. PVR also should be part of the routine evaluation for UI in some women, especially those with diabetes mellitus.

Urine cytology is not recommended in the routine evaluation of UI but may be indicated if the patient has persistent hematuria (2 to 5 red blood cells per high-power field) in the absence of a urinary tract infection (UTI). Incontinence is not a risk factor for bladder cancer. Further, urine cytology is a poor screening test for bladder cancer, with sensitivities of 20% to 70%. Cystoscopy and cytology should be performed for patients with hematuria or the sudden onset of irritative voiding symptoms in the absence of UTI. Urine culture also is unnecessary. Dipstick testing can detect bacteriuria and pyuria with varying degrees of accuracy, depending on method and patient population. Cultures should be ordered when dipstick testing indicates infection or when symptoms suggest infection.

Prostatic enlargement or poor bladder contracting may be contributing to this patient's symptoms by causing bladder outlet obstruction, which would be confirmed by PVR. This patient's findings are suggestive of benign prostatic hyperplasia (BPH). Serum prostate-specific antigen may be elevated in BPH, yet PSA testing has no value in the evaluation of most lower urinary tract symptoms. This patient's age also places him outside the guideline for PSA screening for prostate cancer. Cystometry in this patient may demonstrate the presence of reduced bladder capacity or uninhibited bladder contractions with filling. Although these findings are suggestive of detrusor hyperactivity or urge incontinence, their specificity and sensitivity are poor. This patient's clinical features are consistent with Parkinson's disease, so computed tomography of the head would add little information.

58. Which of the following statements is correct regarding persons living beyond age 90?

(A) They have as many or more chronic conditions as persons in their 70s and 80s.
(B) They often have siblings and other first-degree relatives of a similar age.
(C) They typically have followed a healthier life style than persons who die at a younger age.
(D) They have higher health care costs in their terminal illnesses than persons who die at a younger age.

ANSWER: B

Perhaps the most important finding in studies of nonagenarians and centenarians, whose numbers are rapidly increasing, is the frequency of similarly aged persons in the same family. This strongly suggests a genetic predisposition to longevity. Family studies now are under way to identify the genes responsible and to understand their mechanisms of action. The APOE4 genotype, which is highly associated with Alzheimer's disease, is rare in centenarians. Another noteworthy finding, also probably related to genetic makeup, is the rarity of the usual chronic diseases of old age (eg, diabetes mellitus, cancer, arthritis, dementia, heart disease). Except for a decline in vision and hearing, very old persons typically are in reasonably good physical and mental health, despite having grown up when little attention was paid to what now is considered healthy nutrition. In contrast to the mortality rate in those younger than age 90, which rises exponentially with age, the mortality rate in the very old population declines. It also has been observed that the period of terminal illness among nonagenarians and centenarians is brief and not associated with the high costs seen in many persons dying at a younger age (60–80 years).

59. A 68-year-old woman has a 4-month history of progressive pain in the right shoulder. She is unable to wear pullover sweaters or comb the back of her hair and cannot reach items on high shelves. The patient has poorly controlled diabetes mellitus and a history of ulcer disease. Examination of the shoulder discloses no tenderness to palpation or crepitus. Passive abduction, forward flexion, and external rotation are limited and painful. There is no subacromial tenderness. Which of the following is the most likely diagnosis?

(A) Subacromial bursitis
(B) Rotator cuff tear
(C) Bicep tendonitis
(D) Adhesive capsulitis
(E) Osteoarthritis

ANSWER: D

The musculoskeletal complications of diabetes mellitus are numerous and associated with longstanding disease and poor or erratic control. This patient has evidence of adhesive capsulitis (AC) with limited passive range of motion in three directions. AC develops in approximately 30% of diabetic patients; it is associated with retinopathy but not neuropathy or macroproteinuria. The risk increases with age and duration of diabetes. Idiopathic AC usually responds to gentle physical therapy, including ultrasound. Some have suggested that intra-articular corticosteroid injection with capsular distention is more effective than injection alone. If the condition does not respond, closed manipulation with the patient under anesthesia is indicated. Some patients may be candidates for arthroscopic capsular release, which allows identification and treatment of associated pathology, such as impingement lesions and secondary subacromial space inflammation, calcific deposits, and acromioclavicular arthritis.

The absence of tenderness below the acromion excludes subacromial bursitis. Although range of motion is limited, this patient is able to abduct her arm actively. This suggests that the rotator cuff is competent. In biceps tendonitis, pain is reproduced with resisted forward flexion of the shoulder and forearm supination. Although osteoarthritis may limit range of motion, crepitus and tenderness at the joint line should be present.

60. A 76-year-woman, who recently relocated to your area to be near her daughter, comes to your office for an initial visit. She lives alone in an apartment and has no impairments of activities of daily living. Current medications are a thiazide diuretic, calcium and vitamin D supplements, and a multivitamin. Her pulse rate is 104 per minute. Generalized muscle weakness and 2+ ankle edema are noted. Her Mini–Mental State Examination score is 30/30. Serum thyroxine is 16.8 µg/dL, and thyrotropin is less than 0.01 µg/dL. Which of the following therapies is most appropriate for this patient?

(A) No treatment
(B) Propylthiouracil
(C) Tapazole
(D) Radioactive iodine
(E) Surgical ablation of the thyroid gland

ANSWER: D

Although many older adults with elevated levels of serum thyroid hormone are asymptomatic (*apathetic hyperthyroidism*), patients without cardiac conduction abnormalities will often have resting tachycardia. Treatment with radioactive iodine is indicated for this patient. Antithyroid drugs such as propylthiouracil and methimazole commonly are used in younger patients who may have spontaneous remission. In older adults, long-term complications of radiation (ie, malignancy) are less relevant, and the major goal is complete remission of hyperthyroidism. Surgery rarely is indicated in older patients, who are at high risk for complications; an exception might be the presence of a large toxic multinodular goiter.

61. A 70-year-old man has colon cancer with metastases to the liver and lungs. His advance directive states that he desires medical treatment only for conditions that could be easily reversed. His daughter, with whom he lives, has been designated with durable power of attorney for health care. Pain has been controlled with sustained-release morphine sulfate, 120 mg orally every 12 hours, and lorazepam, 1 mg orally at bedtime. The family asks you to make a home visit because the patient has become disoriented and is unable to follow commands. He has been agitated at night and had visual hallucinations. Oral intake has decreased during the past 12 hours, but he can still swallow liquids.

The patient is lethargic but rouses easily to voice. His attention wanders, and you must repeat commands several times. There is no grimacing or other obvious sign of pain. Temperature is 36.4C (97.5F). Respirations are 18 per minute. The mouth is dry but skin turgor appears normal. Cardiopulmonary and abdominal examinations are unremarkable. All four extremities show purposeful movement. The daughter desires a trial of simple measures to reverse this decline but wishes to avoid hospitalization. You substitute morphine elixir, every 4 hours, at a lower total dose of narcotic, and you instruct the daughter to rehydrate the patient orally. Which of the following is the most appropriate next step?

(A) Explain that this preterminal condition is unlikely to be reversed even with aggressive measures.
(B) Order computed tomography of the head before initiating further therapy.
(C) Administer naloxone to reverse the opiate effect and begin amoxicillin–clavulanate, orally, for possible early pneumonia.
(D) Discontinue lorazepam and begin haloperidol, 2 mg orally at bedtime.

ANSWER: D

Delirium is one of the most common neuropsychiatric complications of advanced cancer, affecting nearly 30% of patients with lung or colon cancer within the last 3 days of life and contributing to poor quality of life for patients and caregivers. Although delirium is a preterminal condition, it should not be ignored.

In a large case series of patients receiving hospice care, delirium was found to be treatable in nearly 50% of patients by the use of simple measures. The most successful treatments were reduction of opiate dosing, discontinuation of other psychoactive medications, and correction of dehydration with minimally invasive strategies (eg, oral hydration or hypodermoclysis). After morphine is reduced and this patient is rehydrated, lorazepam should be discontinued and haloperidol begun to control the psychotic manifestations. By calming the patient, haloperidol may work synergistically with analgesics to improve comfort at a lower total dose of morphine.

Most patients with preterminal delirium do not have brain metastases or other structural lesions in the central nervous system. Computed tomography would be indicated only if there were new focal neurologic findings or if simpler measures failed and it was deemed appropriate to pursue an aggressive evaluation. This patient is not experiencing hypopnea, so rapid reversal of opiate-induced sedation with naloxone is not indicated. Any potential benefit from reducing confusion will be far outweighed by the risk of precipitating opiate withdrawal and a marked increase in discomfort. Antibiotic therapy is inappropriate, since there are no obvious signs of pneumonia.

62. A 70-year-old black American man notes gradually decreasing vision in the right eye. He has a 10-year history of non-insulin-dependent diabetes mellitus and a 3-year history of hypertension. Current medications are two oral hypoglycemic agents, a diuretic, and an angiotensin-converting enzyme inhibitor. He checks his blood glucose weekly and does not follow a strict diet. Cardiopulmonary, abdominal, and musculoskeletal findings are normal except for obesity. Neurologic examination shows decreased touch sensation in the fingertips. Urinalysis shows mild proteinuria. Fingerstick blood glucose level is greater than 200 mg/dL. Hgb A_{1c} is 10.2%. Which of the following is the least likely cause of the vision loss?

(A) Cataract
(B) Vitreous hemorrhage
(C) Macular edema
(D) Macular ischemia
(E) Age-related macular degeneration

ANSWER: E

Age-related macular degeneration is the most common cause of vision loss in the elderly white population but is rare in black persons, who may be protected by their pigmentation. The most likely cause is longstanding, poorly controlled diabetes. Cataract is more prevalent among diabetic persons, in whom typical senile lenticular changes may develop earlier than in the nondiabetic persons. Caution must be exercised with cataract extraction in diabetic patients, who are more prone to develop visually debilitating macular edema. Vitreous hemorrhage may cause severe visual loss in diabetic patients with proliferative retinopathy. Panretinal photocoagulation or laser destruction of the peripheral retina will inhibit the stimulus for growth of new blood vessels (neovascularization). Vitrectomy may be indicated for a dense, noncleaning hemorrhage that has been present longer than 3 months. Macular edema is a common cause of moderate visual loss in diabetic patients. Argon laser therapy is beneficial in stabilizing or improving visual acuity. Macular ischemia may result from capillary nonperfusion and is not directly amenable to therapeutic intervention. Argon laser therapy also is indicated for ischemia associated with macular edema, although the prognosis for visual improvement is poor.

63. An elderly man with multiple medical problems and dependencies in activities of daily living has been in an intensive care unit (ICU) for 1 week. He was admitted for treatment of pneumonia and received aggressive care, including ventilator support. The ICU team believes that the patient is very unlikely to survive this episode and probably will die within 1 week, even if life support is continued. The team has reached consensus that the medically appropriate approach is to discontinue life support and provide comfort care. The patient lacks decisional capacity and has not completed an advance directive. His wife has been involved in his care during hospitalization. An adult daughter is very close to her father but lives out of state and is unable to be present.

The ICU team discusses their decision with the patient's wife and asks her permission to discontinue life support and provide comfort care only. She listens carefully and asks that everything possible be done to keep her husband alive. She believes that he might recover. The team agrees to continue full life-support care.

Several days later, the patient's condition has deteriorated further. The ICU is full and more beds are needed. The team again discusses the situation with the wife. When asked to decide as if she were her husband, she thinks that he probably would want life support discontinued at this point but that she obviously is not him and cannot decide as if she were. She hesitantly tells the team that she feels pressured by the hospital to stop treatment for her husband, who may get better, and that this is wrong. Which of the following options is the best approach at this time?

(A) Continue life support without further discussion.
(B) Continue life support while pursuing discussions with the wife.
(C) Request psychiatric assistance to address the wife's use of denial as a defense mechanism.
(D) Seek permission from the patient's daughter to discontinue life support.
(E) Inform the wife that continued ICU care is medically futile and discontinue life support.

ANSWER: B

Clinicians and patients bring different considerations and values to end-of-life discussions. In this case, the team is approaching the situation from a philosophical framework of Western medical ethics. In thinking about the benefits and harms to the patient, they consider the case from the ethical perspectives of *beneficence* (to maximize the good) and *nonmaleficence* (to not cause harm). They encourage the patient's wife to speak for her husband from the perspective of what he would have wanted in this situation (*substituted judgment*), an approach that emphasizes the preservation of the patient's *autonomy*. In considering the impact of this patient's continued ICU stay on the availability of ICU beds for other patients, they are considering issues of *justice* or overall fairness.

These are highly appropriate considerations. However, in this case, it appears that the wife's philosophical framework may be quite different, and the discussion may be proceeding at cross-purposes. The wife may be experiencing psychologic denial about the seriousness of her husband's condition, but it is equally possible that other factors account for her responses. The wife undoubtedly shares the team's desire to spare her husband discomfort, but she may not find this a compelling reason to discontinue life support. She may believe there is more to life than seeking pleasure and avoiding pain. She may believe that other considerations, such as role obligation, are much more important than autonomy. For example, she may believe that the greatest good occurs when people are true to their roles, and that the proper role of a wife is to ask that everything be done for her husband. Finally, although just allocation of scarce resources is an appropriate and important ethical concern for clinicians, who have responsibilities to society as well as to individual patients, this may not be a relevant concern for the wife, who naturally wonders why the team would think that someone else's life might be more important than her husband's.

It is helpful for clinicians to have some familiarity with philosophical traditions of various cultural groups. Role obligation is an important part of the ethical tradition in many Asian cultures. In the United States, black patients are likely to request more life-sustaining technological treatments at the end of life than are whites. Many black Americans would continue all measures until death rather than withdraw treatment because of a poor prognosis; longevity is valued as an intrinsic good. Attitudinal differences between black and white patients are not explained entirely by socioeconomic factors or by differences in familiarity with the treatments since the same pattern is observed among black and white clinicians. It is important to note that individual differences probably outweigh group attributes. The clinician should elicit a sense of a patient's framework of values and avoid stereotyping any patient on the basis of cultural group.

64. A 75-year-old woman comes to your office for a routine visit. She has mild hypertension for which she takes hydrochlorothiazide, 25 mg daily. She had a total abdominal hysterectomy and oophorectomy at age 48 because of leiomyomata associated with heavy irregular bleeding. She took perimenopausal hormone-replacement therapy briefly. Five years ago, bone mineral density was 1 standard deviation above the mean (Z score of +1) for age. The patient has no family history of cancer; her mother died of a myocardial infarction at age 80. Results of Papanicolaou testing prior to hysterectomy had been normal. She has no vaginal symptoms and has never noted any breast masses. In addition to annual clinical breast examination, which of the following screening tests should you recommend?

(A) Bimanual pelvic examination
(B) Bimanual pelvic examination and mammography
(C) Bimanual pelvic examination, Pap smear from the vaginal cuff, and mammography
(D) Mammography
(E) Pap smear from the vaginal cuff and mammography

ANSWER: D

Breast examination and mammography for women aged 50 to 70 are among the best established preventive interventions; however, data for women after age 70 are limited. Most authorities favor screening at least into the early 80s unless life expectancy is less than 5 years. The U.S. Preventive Services Task Force (USPSTF) rated the evidence as inadequate to recommend for or against screening. However,

continued screening may be appropriate for other reasons, including the ongoing burden of disease and the lack of evidence that mammography has different test characteristics in older women. Analysis suggests that most of the benefit of continued screening for women in their 70s would accrue to those whose bone mineral density was above the 25th percentile (upper three quartiles). Continued biennial screening of women in this age group is estimated to save 9.4 lives in a hypothetical cohort of 10,000 women. There is no specific information on continuing breast examinations in addition to mammograms; however, the examinations are simple and provide some complementary information in middle-aged women.

There is no good evidence for any benefit from pelvic examinations and vaginal cuff Pap smears in women who had a hysterectomy for a benign condition. The USPSTF recommends against such screening. Despite this, the American Cancer Society (ACS) continues to recommend regular pelvic examinations and Pap tests. Rates of vaginal cancer are very low (0.3 to 0.4 per 100,000 women). One study that enrolled a relatively high-risk population found no cancers and only a few cases of mild to moderate dysplasia in nearly 10,000 smears. Given this evidence, the best recommendation for women who had a hysterectomy for a benign condition is to limit pelvic examinations and Pap testing to patients with specific symptoms or to those who desire testing despite appropriate counseling. In women with ovaries, the ACS argues for continued bimanual examinations; again, the USPSTF found no good evidence to support this position.

65. A 67-year-old woman undergoes dual-energy x-ray absorptiometry (DEXA). Her bone mineral density in the lumbar spine and proximal femur are found to be in the osteopenic range, in comparison with young normal persons. The patient refuses pharmacologic treatment other than calcium and vitamin D. You recommend an increase in physical activity, which she is willing to do. Which of the following activities is most likely to help maintain bone density?

(A) Tai chi
(B) Swimming
(C) Resistance training
(D) Stationary bicycling

ANSWER: C

There is good evidence that higher peak bone mass is achieved partly by increased physical activity early in life. The role of activity in maintaining bone density in older women is less certain. Studies have shown that high-impact activities, such as resistance training with weights or weight-bearing aerobic exercise, are most likely to help maintain or improve bone density. Tai chi is not aerobic, and there have been no studies to support a beneficial effect on bone density. Swimming is not weight bearing and therefore has little impact on bone. Bicycling is low-impact aerobic exercise but is less likely to increase bone density than is resistance training.

66. A 70-year-old Mexican American man comes to you for an initial visit. He recently moved to your area, following the death of his wife 14 months ago. The patient describes his overall health as "pretty good" but has fallen twice and had other "close calls" in the past 6 months. He has taken hydrochlorothiazide for many years, but his former primary clinician told him that a second medication might be required to control recurrent hypertension. The patient falls asleep without much difficulty but awakens several times nightly.

When you review the patient's health questionnaire, you note a positive response to the question on alcohol consumption. He claims to drink socially and denies any problem with drinking. He mentions that he drank heavily as a young man but "cut way back" when he married. You believe it would be worthwhile to know whether this patient now or has ever met the criteria for alcoholism or alcohol dependence, as well as how much and how often he currently drinks. Which of the following questionnaires is most appropriate to use in interviewing this patient?

(A) CAGE
(B) MAST
(C) PRIME-MD
(D) TWEAK
(E) AUDIT

ANSWER: E

Different categories of alcohol use have been defined by various investigators and professional organizations. The American Psychiatric Association has published criteria for alcohol abuse and dependence, and the World Health Organization has sought to broaden the focus to include hazardous and harmful drinking, in addition to dependence. Hazardous drinking is defined as a quantity or pattern of alcohol consumption that exceeds a specific threshold and may increase risk for adverse health events. That threshold has been established at different levels by different organizations. The National Institute of Alcohol Abuse and Alcoholism set thresholds based on age and gender: more than 14 drinks per week or four per occasion for men aged 65 and under, and more than seven drinks per week or three per occasion for women aged 65 and under and all persons aged 65 and over. Harmful drinking has been defined as consumption that results in physical or psychological harm, or both.

The AUDIT (Alcohol Use Disorders Identification Test) is a ten-item questionnaire that measures average quantity and frequency of consumption, the presence of binge drinking, alcohol-dependence symptoms, and alcohol-related problems. It has been validated in a variety of settings and for many diverse populations and patient subgroups. It is the most appropriate questionnaire for this patient.

The MAST (Michigan Alcoholism Screening Test), the CAGE, and the TWEAK were developed primarily to detect alcohol dependence, rather than hazardous or harmful drinking. (See http://www.niaaa.nih.gov/publications/instable.htm for information about and access to copies of these and other alcohol screens.) They do not provide information about the quantity, frequency, or pattern of alcohol consumption. In addition, they do not discriminate between current and past drinking. The MAST also has been faulted for its excessive length. The newer MAST-G (geriatric version; see the Appendix, p 386), focuses on older adults but again fails to assess quantity or pattern of drinking. The CAGE is the most widely used screening test for alcohol use disorders, and its performance among older adults has been well studied. However, it has been shown to be less sensitive than the AUDIT for use with Mexican Americans. The TWEAK, derived from the CAGE, has shown strength in identifying alcohol dependence in women but has performed less well in men. The PRIME-MD (Primary Care Evaluation of Mental Disorders) was designed for screening, evaluating, and generating preliminary diagnoses for the mental disorders most commonly seen in primary care settings. It does contain questions on alcohol problems, but these were designed to identify alcohol dependence. The one question pertaining to the quantity and pattern of drinking addresses only binge drinking.

A useful approach in the primary care of older patients may be to combine quantity and frequency questions, such as those contained in the AUDIT, with a very brief instrument focused on alcohol dependence, such as the CAGE. This would provide current information on quantity and pattern of drinking, while taking advantage of the brevity and the validity of the CAGE.

67. A 72-year-old woman loses small amounts of urine when she coughs, sneezes, or laughs. She also loses a large volume when she gets out of bed in the morning. The patient is not always aware of the urine loss and usually changes incontinence pads about three times a day. The patient underwent a surgical procedure for urinary incontinence 6 years ago. Incontinence recurred about 1 year ago and has worsened in the past 3 months. Medical history also includes diabetes mellitus and hypertension. Her mother had breast cancer at age 82; the patient had a normal mammogram 2 months ago.

The patient is 160 cm (63 in) tall and weighs 88 kg (194 lb). Gait is normal. Orthostatic changes are noted in blood pressure, but she denies dizziness. Neuropathy is present in a stocking-and-glove pattern. Ankle jerks are absent bilaterally. Pelvic examination reveals first-degree uterine prolapse. Vaginal muscle squeeze is perceptible for less than 1 second and is barely felt around the fingers. When the patient coughs forcibly, a small amount of urine is lost. Postvoid residual volume is 375 mL. Which of the following treatment options should you recommend?

(A) Urodynamic studies
(B) Pelvic muscle (Kegel's) exercises
(C) Dicyclomine, 10 mg twice daily
(D) Oxybutynin, 2.5 mg twice daily
(E) Repeat surgical correction

ANSWER: A

The loss of small amounts of urine with position changes is consistent with stress incontinence. However, the postvoid residual volume (PVR) of 375 mL is well above the maximum normal of 100 mL. Thus, this patient has overflow incontinence and meets consensus criteria for urodynamic studies. She may have urinary retention secondary to bladder outlet obstruction from the previous surgery, a neurogenic bladder secondary to diabetes or another pathologic process, or detrusor hyperactivity with incomplete contractility. It is unlikely that the first-degree uterine prolapse is the precipitating cause. Urodynamic evaluation is essential to confirm the cause and to address the urinary retention, which increases her risk for urinary tract or systemic infection.

Pelvic muscle exercises would not be appropriate as first-line management for a patient with an elevated PVR. Dicyclomine and oxybutynin are effective for urge incontinence but can precipitate urinary retention. In this patient with an elevated PVR, they could worsen symptoms. Surgery for pelvic floor laxity is inappropriate because the patient has both overflow and stress incontinence.

68. A 76-year-old woman has a 6-month history of lower back pain that is present most of the day and has increased in the past 6 weeks. It worsens with exercise such as walking her dog, and she describes aching pain "like a toothache" in both thighs. She has little pain at night. Medical history includes a cholecystectomy many years ago and a L4–5 discectomy at age 60. Although she reports increasing difficulty with ambulation, she is able to walk "pretty well" at the supermarket when pushing a shopping cart. The patient stopped attending physical therapy because "it wasn't helping." Which of the following is the most likely diagnosis?

(A) Recurrent disc disease at L4–5
(B) Degenerative spinal stenosis at L4–5
(C) Ankylosing spondylitis
(D) Compression fracture
(E) Spasm of the paraspinous muscles

ANSWER: B

This patient has a classic presentation of degenerative spinal stenosis. This is an increasingly common diagnosis because of larger numbers of elderly patients, greater awareness of the condition, and the availability of sophisticated diagnostic technology such as computed tomography and magnetic resonance imaging. The cause of the pain is not completely clear, although some research indicates that pressure on the spinal nerve roots—caused by a combination of bony overgrowth, ligament hypertrophy, postoperative changes, and disc protrusion—leads to localized ischemia and pain. Physical factors that increase pressure on the nerve roots include walking and upright posture; thus, pain may be relieved by sitting or forward bending. If a patient can walk while bending forward, such as when pushing a shopping cart, pain decreases and the distance that can be walked increases. Radiation of pain to the thigh or buttocks is very common, although true sciatica (ie, pain radiating to the knee or below) is rare. Symptoms commonly are present for some time before the patient seeks medical attention.

This patient has had one disc herniation and is at risk for another. However, her symptoms are not typical for herniation. Ankylosing spondylitis (AS) is an inflammatory disease of the sacroiliac joints and axial skeleton that is much more common in men than in women. Onset in later life also is uncommon. AS is characterized by pain and stiffness on arising in the morning, which generally improves with exercise. Older women are at significant risk for compression fractures, but this patient has no history of trauma. Compression fractures can occur spontaneously, but this patient's pattern of pain on walking and relief with leaning forward is much more consistent with spinal stenosis. The identification of muscle spasm on clinical examination is difficult. Although muscular pain can cause back pain, it is difficult to determine with any specificity that pain is muscular in origin. However, the radiation pattern and the improvement with sitting described by this patient are not consistent with spasm, in which pain generally worsens with sitting.

69. Which of the following is the most effective and least costly strategy to prevent exacerbation of chronic illness, hospitalization, and death due to influenza in elderly patients?

(A) Outbreak prophylaxis with oseltamivir or zanamivir for all residents and staff
(B) Outbreak prophylaxis with amantadine or rimantadine for all residents and staff
(C) Treatment with oseltamivir or zanamivir for all residents and staff
(D) Annual vaccination for all residents
(E) Annual vaccination for all residents and staff

ANSWER: E

In frail older adults, influenza vaccine attenuates or prevents illness due to influenza A and B by 30% to 40%. More importantly, hospitalization for confirmed influenza, influenza-like illnesses, and cardiopulmonary complications are reduced by 60% during influenza season; mortality is reduced by 80% in older patients. Overall, vaccination is highly cost-effective. The efficacy is further enhanced if both patients and staff are vaccinated.

The neuraminidase inhibitors oseltamivir and zanamivir are active against both influenza A and B. Expectant treatment with these agents has not been assessed in frail older adults in the community or nursing home. In healthy young and older adults, treatment has reduced febrile illness, the duration of symptoms by several days, and the number of antibiotic prescriptions written. Currently, only amantadine and rimantadine are approved for prophylactic use in the United States. They are active only against influenza A, and resistance emerges in 30% of patients. These agents are considerably less expensive than the neuraminidase inhibitors. Amantadine requires careful dosing and monitoring of renal function.

70. According recommendations of the American Diabetes Association of 2001, which of the following criteria establishes a diagnosis of diabetes mellitus?

   (A) Fasting plasma glucose of 110 to 126 mg/dL
   (B) Fasting plasma glucose $\geq$ 110 mg/dL on two occasions
   (C) Fasting plasma glucose $\geq$ 126 mg/dL on two occasions
   (D) Classic symptoms of diabetes mellitus plus random plasma glucose $\geq$ 126 mg/dL
   (E) Plasma glucose $\geq$ 120 mg/dL after 2 hours during a standard oral glucose tolerance test, on two occasions

ANSWER: C

The current classification of diabetes mellitus is based upon cause rather than age of onset or type of treatment. Four major types are recognized: type 1, type 2, gestational, and hyperglycemia secondary to other causes. Measurement of fasting plasma glucose is the recommended diagnostic test; oral glucose tolerance testing no longer is recommended for diagnostic use except in testing for gestational diabetes. The criterion for diagnosis of diabetes mellitus is fasting plasma glucose $\geq$ 126 mg/dL on two occasions.

   Three unequivocal criteria for a diagnosis of diabetes mellitus have been defined: 1) Symptoms of hyperglycemia with a casual blood glucose of $\geq$ 200 mg/dL, 2) fasting blood glucose $\geq$ 126 mg/dL, and 3) a 2-hour blood glucose of $\geq$ 200 mg/dL after a 75-gram oral glucose tolerance test. These criteria should be confirmed by repeat testing on a different day.

   A separate category of "impaired glucose tolerance" is indicated by 1) fasting blood glucose of $\geq$ 110 mg/dL but $<$ 126 mg/dL, or 2) a 2-hour blood glucose of $\geq$ 140 mg/dL but $<$ 200 mg/dL with a 75-gram oral glucose challenge.

71. The average length of stay in your hospital's medical unit has been increasing. Analysis of outliers among the most common diagnosis related groups (DRGs) reveals a number of patients who had prolonged hospitalizations secondary to acute confusional states. As a member of the quality improvement committee, you have been asked to suggest evidence-based measures to prevent this problem. Which of the following interventions should you recommend?

   (A) Train nursing staff to perform serial Mini–Mental State Examination (MMSE).
   (B) Establish a delirium consultation service to evaluate patients at the request of their attending physicians.
   (C) Implement a clinical pathway to expedite neurologic imaging and other diagnostic tests in patients with delirium.
   (D) Establish interdisciplinary protocols to address sensory impairment, immobility, dehydration, cognitive impairment, and sleep deprivation.
   (E) Implement early discharge planning so that patients can be sent home before their predicted length of stay is exceeded.

ANSWER: D

Delirium in hospitalized patients is associated with increased morbidity, functional decline, greater hospital costs, increased length of stay, and greater rates of nursing-home placement. Thus, it is an appropriate target for quality-improvement efforts. Delirium is a multifactorial disorder occurring in frail older persons, and single-component interventions are not likely to be sufficient; therefore, multiple approaches must be implemented. In a controlled trial of a multicomponent intervention on a general medical service, the incidence of delirium was reduced by one third. The intervention involved the use of interdisciplinary protocols directed toward improving cognitive impairment, sleep hygiene, and mobility, and reducing visual impairment, hearing impairment, and dehydration.

Training nursing staff to recognize delirium in its earliest stages may allow therapies targeting its precipitants to be more successful. However, the MMSE does not distinguish delirium from dementia and takes significant time to administer. Better tools for identifying delirium are those directed toward global awareness and attention, such as the Confusion Assessment Method (see Table 19.2 in "Delirium," p 128). A delirium consultation service may be useful for managing complex presentations, but clinicians fail to detect confusion in one third to two thirds of cases. Most patients with delirium do not have structural changes in the central nervous system, so expedited neuroimaging is unlikely to be of benefit. Early discharge with home-care services may be appropriate for medically stable patients, but patients with delirium often have persistent symptoms of confusion and functional impairment and are inappropriate for early discharge.

72. Which of the following psychiatric disorders is most common in elderly persons?

    (A) Anxiety disorders
    (B) Personality disorders
    (C) Mood disorders
    (D) Somatoform disorders
    (E) Substance abuse

ANSWER: A

The anxiety disorders are the most common psychiatric disorders of late life. They include generalized anxiety disorders, phobias (agoraphobia, specific, social), panic disorder, obsessive-compulsive disorder, posttraumatic stress disorder, anxiety disorders secondary to general medical conditions, and substance-induced anxiety disorders. A series of epidemiologic studies have raised awareness of these conditions. For example, during one 6-month period a community-dwelling elderly population was found to have a 19.7% incidence of all anxiety disorders. Other studies have estimated that 17.1% of men and 21.5% of women experience symptoms warranting treatment. Previous studies often underreported the rates of anxiety disorders in elderly adults because of medical and psychiatric comorbidity. Some studies noted that at least one third of

elderly patients with depression have anxiety. Symptoms also may be caused by medications or bereavement.

Evaluation of older persons with symptoms of anxiety can be challenging. A thorough medical history and drug and alcohol inventory should be obtained. Physical examination and mental status evaluation are required. Symptom-focused laboratory studies (eg, complete blood cell count, plasma glucose, serum electrolytes and thyroid-stimulating hormone, and urinalysis) may be appropriate to assess for medical illness as the cause of anxiety. Other useful tests include a drug screen, pulse oximetry for hypoxia-driven anxiety, and electrocardiography for patients with cardiac symptoms associated with anxiety.

Mood and substance abuse disorders are common in elderly persons but not as common as anxiety disorders. Somatoform and personality disorders are much less common in older persons.

73. A 71-year-old white woman who does not smoke cigarettes comes to the emergency department because of progressive dyspnea. She has had very mild shortness of breath on climbing stairs for 18 months but reports that this worsened after a "chest cold" 5 weeks ago. She now has a persistent nonproductive cough.

The patient is 172 cm (67 in) tall and weighs 82.0 kg (180.5 lb), for a body mass index of 28.3. Temperature is 36.7C (98.1F). Ear, nose, throat, and cardiovascular findings are normal. End-expiratory wheezing and cough with deep inspiration are noted. She has no cyanosis, clubbing, or edema. Chest radiograph and electrocardiogram are normal. Pulse oximetry indicates an Sao_2 of 97% with patient breathing room air. Which of the following should you do next?

    (A) Order exercise electrocardiography.
    (B) Prescribe a course of exercise to improve the deconditioning.
    (C) Prescribe a 5-day course of oseltamivir.
    (D) Perform pulmonary function tests.
    (E) Admit the patient to the hospital for respiratory therapy and intravenous antibiotics.

ANSWER: D

Chronic obstructive pulmonary disease (COPD) is the fourth leading cause of death in patients aged 65 and over. The prevalence is increasing rapidly in older women but stabilizing in older men. Among the reasons for this trend are physiologic features in women, such as smaller lungs and airways, lower elastic recoil, more hyperactive airways (eg, response to methylcholine challenge). Also, cigarette smoking has increased among women, and COPD develops in women at a lower level of tobacco exposure. For reasons that are unclear, the first episode of COPD in older women is likely to occur after a bronchitic infection. Spirometry provides useful diagnostic and prognostic information. If the acute obstruction reverses, outpatient management may be appropriate for this patient.

The history, physical findings, and normal electrocardiogram argue strongly against intrinsic coronary artery disease. Dyspnea is not a normal part of aging. Mild decrements that accompany aging are not clinically relevant, although they do lower physiologic reserve. Admission for intensive respiratory therapy and antibiotics may be required if the patient's condition does not improve with outpatient treatment.

74. A patient returns to the nursing home following hospitalization for pneumonia and superimposed delirium. A stage III sacral pressure ulcer developed during hospitalization because he was restrained to prevent him from removing an intravenous catheter. Weight in the hospital was 70 kg (154 lb), for a body mass index of 22.8; this is his "usual weight," but it is only 90% of ideal. Cognitive level is near baseline; Mini–Mental State Examination score is 16/30. He is able to follow a two-step command and to sit independently but requires assistance with transferring, dressing, grooming, and toileting. Muscular weakness is apparent in the deltoids, with some squaring of the shoulders. The quadriceps also are weak and wasted. The patient has no difficulty swallowing liquids or solids. The nursing-home dietitian recommends that the patient resume his previous diet, which provided 2100 kcal daily, with 70 g of protein. Which of the following should you advise?

(A) Institute oral liquid supplements with meals.
(B) Resume the previous diet.
(C) Increase protein intake to at least 105 g daily.
(D) Increase caloric intake to at least 2400 kcal daily.

ANSWER: C

This patient's pressure ulcer, muscle breakdown, and functional decline are the results of the catabolic effects of illness during hospitalization, complicated by forced immobility. The previous diet provides inadequate protein, given the pressure ulcer; protein intake should be increased to promote wound healing. Current guidelines recommend at least 1.5 g/kg daily for stage III or IV wounds, although many would use 2 g/kg.

Supplements given with meals tend to substitute for food; they may be more effective if given between meals. The previous diet provides adequate calories, perhaps more than necessary. Caloric requirements for persons with a body mass index greater than 20 are 25 to 28 kcal/kg daily.

75. A 72-year-old man has a "pimple" on his nose that occasionally bleeds and may have increased in size during the past year. The lesion is a 0.8-cm, dome-shaped, umbilicated papule with pearly translucence and telangiectasia. A small hemorrhagic crust covers the central portion. Which of the following is the most likely diagnonsis?

(A) Basal cell carcinoma
(B) Squamous cell carcinoma
(C) Sebaceous hyperplasia
(D) Molluscum contagiosum
(E) Keratoacanthoma

ANSWER: A

Basal cell carcinoma arises in the basal cells of the epidermis. Although these cells rarely metastasize, their ability to invade local tissues accounts for their malignant nature. The nodular form is the most common. It has a pearly, translucent, papular appearance with a depressed crateriform central portion and multiple telangiectases. Many patients seek medical attention for a lesion that does not heal.

Sebaceous hyperplasia can be very difficult to differentiate from basal cell carcinoma. Lesions typically are 1- to 3-mm papules and have a yellowish hue, telangiectases, and a central pore. Squamous cell carcinoma usually appears on sun-exposed skin. It also can develop within the scar from an injury or burn. Lesions are firm, erythematous plaques with a hyperkeratotic, verrucal surface; ulceration or crusting also may be present. Molluscum contagiosum is caused by a DNA poxvirus. Lesions are smaller, dome-shaped papules with umbilicated centers, without telangiectasia or bleeding. Keratoacanthoma can resemble squamous cell carcinoma but develops rapidly, within 1 to 2 months. Lesions are round, flesh-colored papules with a central keratin-filled crater, but again without telangiectasia or bleeding.

76. You are asked to evaluate an 85-year-old woman who has osteoarthritis of the right hip; she is scheduled to undergo elective total hip replacement. Her other medical problems are hypertension and anxiety disorder. Current medications are hydrochlorothiazide, 25 mg daily; atenolol, 50 mg daily; and alprazolam, 0.25 mg daily at bedtime. The patient is a pleasant, healthy-appearing woman who has a steady but antalgic gait. Pulse rate is 64 per minute, and blood pressure is 132/80 mm Hg. Cardiopulmonary and neurologic examinations are normal. Mini–Mental State Examination score is 29/30. Hematocrit, leukocyte count, blood urea nitrogen, plasma glucose, serum electrolytes, and urinalysis are within normal limits. Which of the following perioperative measures is most likely to reduce the risk for postoperative delirium?

(A) Immediate discontinuation of alprazolam
(B) Use of epidural rather than general anesthesia
(C) Avoidance of opiate analgesics postoperatively
(D) Insertion of a bladder catheter
(E) Maintenance of hematocrit at 30% or higher

ANSWER: E

Delirium is a common complication of surgery in older persons and is associated with poor functional and cognitive recovery, increased length of hospital stay, and greater cost. Risk factors for postoperative delirium include increased age, cognitive and functional impairment, fluid and electrolyte abnormalities, and use of psychoactive medications. Translating these risk factors into strategies for preventing postoperative delirium remains a challenge, especially because there are few well-designed studies of the effect of interventions to prevent delirium. In the largest prospective study of risk factors for delirium in noncardiac surgery, the only potentially avoidable factor identified was a postoperative hematocrit below 30%. It is reasonable to assume that a low perioperative hematocrit can cause a central nervous system insult that predisposes to delirium. Careful monitoring in high-risk situations, avoidance of intraoperative blood loss, and transfusions as needed may reduce the risk of delirium.

Although benzodiazepines, particularly those with long half-lives, have been associated with delirium and falls, abrupt discontinuation of these medications can precipitate a potentially dangerous withdrawal syndrome that includes hyperactive delirium. Case reports suggest that delirium is particularly prevalent in alprazolam withdrawal; slow tapering, no more than 10% to 20% of total daily dosage, is recommended. Modern anesthetics are cleared from the central nervous system rapidly and do not directly cause significant cognitive impairment. Route of anesthesia has not been associated with risk for delirium, and recovery of postoperative function may be slower in patients receiving epidural anesthesia during hip surgery. Excessive narcotic use can cause postoperative delirium. The risk is particularly high with meperidine and fentanyl, which have anticholinergic metabolites that accumulate to toxic levels in patients with renal insufficiency. In contrast, patient-controlled morphine infusions generally can be titrated to control pain without inducing confusion. Undertreatment of pain has been associated with risk for delirium, so strict avoidance of opiates is inappropriate. Bladder catheterization is a recognized precipitant of delirium, most likely because of the increased likelihood of urinary tract infection. If the procedure is necessary, close monitoring is warranted.

77. Which of the following features predicts a good prognosis in late-life depression?

(A) Presence of cerebral pathology
(B) Slower recovery time
(C) More severe initial symptoms
(D) Duration of symptoms for more than 2 years
(E) Younger age

ANSWER: E

Depressive illness is prone to relapse, recurrence, and chronicity in patients of all ages. However, several studies have shown a higher frequency of relapse in elderly patients. In a study of first-episode patients who responded to nortriptyline, depression was found to recur in 61% when the drug was stopped after 2 years. These data add to the consensus that the outcome of late-life depression can be brittle and deserves careful monitoring.

Cerebral pathology, either coarse or subtle, or the occurrence of severe medical problems just prior to or during the episode of depression predicts a poorer long-term prognosis. Depressive symptoms that persist more than 2 years, a slower recovery time, more severe symptoms at the time of diagnosis, and a history of two or more episodes in the past 2 years also are associated with poor outcome. Early recognition of symptoms and aggressive treatment with medications as well as psychological and social interventions predicts a better long-term outcome. Relapse, which is most likely in the first 18 to 24 months, initially may be undetected unless follow-up is in place for at least 18 months. Antidepressant medication and psychological and social support should be included in the long-term management plan.

78. An 84-year-old woman who lives in an intermediate-care facility has had several falls since she was discharged from a geropsychiatric unit. During that admission, medications were adjusted to manage depression with underlying psychotic features. Medical history also includes glaucoma, hypertension, and valvular heart disease.

Which of the following medications is least likely to contribute to her falls?

(A) Fluoxetine, 20 mg daily
(B) Hydrochlorothiazide, 25 mg daily
(C) Lorazepam, 0.5 mg three times daily
(D) Risperidone, 2 mg at bedtime

ANSWER: B

Falls are a major cause of morbidity and mortality in elderly persons. Multiple studies have examined various medications as a cause of falls. Although uncontrolled confounding factors are a potential problem in most of these studies, diuretics have not been uniformly shown to cause falls. Psychotropic medications, however, appear to produce about a twofold increase in risk. In one study, both tricyclic antidepressants and selective serotonin-reuptake inhibitors were found to be associated with increased falls; adjusted risk ratios were 2.0 and 1.8, respectively. These two classes of antidepressant also confer an increased risk for hip fracture. Risperidone produces parkinsonian symptoms in 20% of nursing-home patients and is associated with an increased fall risk.

79. An 83-year-old woman is brought to the emergency department because of dizziness on standing, followed by brief loss of consciousness. She has hypertension but is otherwise healthy. Current medications are metoprolol, 50 mg daily; captopril, 25 mg every morning; and nitroglycerin, 0.04 mg sublingually as needed.

The patient now feels well. Blood pressure is 130/70 mm Hg sitting and 100/60 mm Hg standing. Physical examination is otherwise normal. Complete blood cell count, comprehensive metabolic panel, and blood urea nitrogen are normal, as is electrocardiogram. Which of the following is the most likely cause of the syncopal episode?

(A) Sepsis
(B) Drug-related event
(C) Hypovolemic hypotensive episode
(D) Cardiogenic shock
(E) Unidentifiable cause

ANSWER: B

Approximately 3% of emergency department visits are for syncope and associated falls, and 80% occur in patients aged 65 and over. Drug-related syncope is the most likely cause in this patient, who takes more than one drug that may cause or worsen orthostatic intolerance and lead to syncope. Decreased baroreceptor sensitivity, decreased renin and aldosterone levels, and increased atrial natriuretic hormone level leads to impaired sodium–water balance and hypotension. Captopril, an angiotensin-converting enzyme inhibitor, lowers peripheral vascular resistance. Metoprolol, a β-adrenergic blocking agent, has negative chronotropic and inotropic effects. Nitroglycerin, a vasodilator, also could be responsible. Other drugs that have been associated with orthostatic hypotension include α-adrenergic blocking agents, calcium channel blocking agents, diuretics, ganglionic blockers, opiates, bromocriptine, hydralazine, and ethanol.

One strategy to decrease the incidence of orthostatic hypotension is staggered dosing rather than administering all medications at the same time. Nonpharmacologic approaches include rising slowly from a sitting to standing position and dangling the feet over the side of the bed before rising from the supine to standing position. Sepsis, hypovolemia, and cardiogenic shock may cause dizziness, syncope, and orthostasis, but this patient has no evidence of systemic illness. A drug-related explanation is more likely.

80. An 80-year-old woman has mild Alzheimer's disease. She lives with her husband, who assists with her care. She has most of her natural teeth and has no problems chewing. She has not had regular dental care, but a recent examination revealed caries at several root surfaces; restoration with fillings would be possible. Which of the following is the best management plan?

(A) Dental radiographs to identify pulp cavities that should be treated
(B) Treatment of symptomatic conditions only
(C) Restorative dentistry and topical application of fluoride
(D) Restorative dentistry and subsequent removal of teeth affected by periodontal disease secondary to poor oral hygiene
(E) Prophylactic removal of remaining teeth and provision of well-fitting dentures

ANSWER: C

Maximum preventive efforts against caries and periodontal disease are indicated for this patient. Restorative dentistry (placement of fillings) should be done as soon as possible. This will minimize ongoing destruction of dental surfaces by active caries. Topical fluoride treatments, along with fluoride toothpaste, can help prevent new caries. With effective preventive care, she should be able to maintain her teeth for at least several years. Deterioration of mental status eventually will lead to the inability to cooperate with dental procedures.

Dental films are not indicated, because the majority of caries in older adults are at the root surface and generally are painless. Pulp cavities are rare and usually associated with pain. Treating only symptoms permits advancement of caries and periodontal disease and may produce unnecessary discomfort. Treatment at a later date also may be more difficult if behavior problems develop. Removal of teeth that can be restored leads to masticatory ineffectiveness and is strongly contraindicated, especially since patients with Alzheimer's disease often lose the capacity to use dentures.

81. Which of the following statements regarding functional status is correct?

(A) Approximately 10% of persons aged 65 and over have difficulty with one or more activities of daily living (ADLs) or instrumental activities of daily living (IADLs).

(B) Approximately 75% of persons aged 85 and over have difficulty with one or more ADLs or IADLs.

(C) In all age groups, men report a higher percentage of ADL limitations than women do.

(D) White Americans have more ADL and IADL limitations than Hispanic Americans do.

(E) Increased ADL limitation is associated with higher socioeconomic status.

ANSWER: B

Comprehensive assessment of function typically measures disabilities in the physical, mental, social, psychological, and economic domains. Physical functioning most often is determined by validated scales for ability to perform ADLs and IADLs. (See the Appendix pp 384–385, for screens.) ADL function includes tasks related to personal care: bathing, dressing, eating, toileting, transferring from bed to chair. IADL function addresses the ability to perform more complex tasks, such as handling finances, shopping, taking medications, and using the telephone. Measures include both the number of tasks for which assistance is required and the level of assistance. Research suggests that ADLs and IADLs are closely related, and integrated scales have been proposed.

ADL and IADL dependency is strongly associated with increased age. Only 28% of 65-year-olds have some ADL or IADL dependency, but this rises to 78% for those aged 85 and over. Rates of limitation differ by gender, race and ethnicity, and income. Women are more likely to report ADL needs at all ages over 65, and racial and ethnic minorities have greater needs at older ages. Higher proportions of persons who are poor or near-poor report difficulties than do those of middle or high income. Demographic trends in life expectancy suggest the potential for more years of functional incapacity, particularly in vulnerable groups. Consequently, interest is increasing in strategies to delay disability through health promotion and prevention. Functional status is strongly correlated with use of both formal and informal services, as well as key clinical outcomes. For example, it routinely predicts receipt of formal care in both community and institutional settings.

82. Which of the following statements regarding ECT is correct?

(A) It has limited usefulness in patients aged 75 and over.

(B) It is as effective in elderly patients as in younger adults.

(C) It is absolutely contraindicated in patients with a seizure disorder.

(D) The presence of subcortical changes on magnetic resonance imaging of the head predicts a good response.

(E) The risk of relapse after an adequate course of ECT is low.

ANSWER: B

ECT is an effective treatment for major depression, with response rates of up to 90%. It is especially effective for patients with psychotic features. There is no upper age limit for use of this treatment, and elderly patients respond as well as younger patients. ECT is particularly useful in elderly patients with profound disability, food and fluid refusal, suicidal behavior, and delusional depression. There are no absolute contraindications to ECT; greatest caution is required in the presence of increased intracranial pressure. Relative contraindications include cerebrovascular accident within 3 months, myocardial infarction within 6 weeks, uncontrolled hypertension, uncontrolled heart failure or arrhythmia, arterial aneurysm, and markedly impaired respiratory capacity. The presence of a pacemaker or anticoagulant therapy does not preclude its use. Patients with subcortical changes, who respond poorly to antidepressants, also may not respond well to ECT. In general, the presence of delusions, melancholia, and inappropriate guilt predict a good response. Elderly patients, unlike younger adults, seem to respond well when anxiety is the dominant feature. Even with an adequate course of treatment and good clinical response, the relapse rate is as high as 64% within 1 year; up to 30% of patients require rehospitalization.

83. A healthy 68-year-old man has no history of heart disease and currently walks about 20 minutes twice a day. He also works in his garden. The patient plans to begin an exercise program consisting of upper- and lower-extremity resistance exercises, stair climbing, and brisk walking 3 days per week. Which of the following statements describes the long-term effects of increased physical activity on this patient's risk for coronary artery disease (CAD) and mortality?

(A) For someone already engaged in moderate daily exercise, further risk reduction is unlikely with more vigorous activity.
(B) Risks are lower in older persons who engage in vigorous activity than in those who exercise moderately.
(C) All-cause mortality is lower in older persons who exercise moderately, but risk for CAD is unaffected.
(D) Risks for CAD and mortality increase in older persons who exercise vigorously.

ANSWER: B

Physical activity has important health benefits, particularly in reducing the risk of CAD and all-cause mortality. The greatest benefits are seen in sedentary persons who begin regular moderate physical activity, such as brisk walking (3 to 4 mph, at an intensity of 3 to 6 metabolic equivalents). This patient already is exercising at a moderate level, meeting the recommendation for 30 minutes of moderate physical activity at least 5 days per week. Persons who exceed the recommendation for moderate activity or those who engage in vigorous activity have lower risks. Supervised treadmill-exercise electrocardiography is recommended for previously sedentary persons aged 50 and over who want to begin a vigorous exercise program and who are unlikely to start with a low-intensity, short-duration program that gradually increases in duration and intensity.

84. A 73-year-old woman is brought to your office by her two nieces, who are her legal guardians, and with whom she has lived for more than 25 years. The patient has an intelligence quotient of 30 but is able to dress and bathe herself fairly independently. She has become increasingly irritable and seems physically uncomfortable in recent months, although her health always has been good. Her appetite has diminished and she had lost about 10 lb. She now sleeps only 4 or 5 hours per night. The patient has become less social with other family members and no longer spends time on her favorite activities. Her pleasant affect has been replaced by sadness or anger. On one occasion, she was found weeping in her room. The nieces have not been able to figure out what is bothering the patient; they are frustrated by her increased needs and problem behaviors and are not sure they can continue to provide a home for her.

Findings of physical examination 6 months ago, including pelvic examination, were normal. The patient takes no medications routinely and has never used alcohol or tobacco. Which of the following is the most appropriate next step?

(A) Recommend residential placement.
(B) Refer the family to a psychiatrist experienced in developmental disabilities.
(C) Arrange for home care services.
(D) Begin a medical work-up for occult disease.
(E) Prescribe an antidepressant.

ANSWER: E

Many of this patient's symptoms suggest a major depressive disorder, so the best initial action would be to begin an antidepressant medication such as a selective serotonin-reuptake inhibitor. If her health status were unknown, a delay in treatment to exclude physical causes would be prudent and could avoid the small risk of starting an unnecessary medication.

In general, experts believe it is important for adults with developmental disabilities to live in a community setting that can provide for their needs and continue to challenge them to develop new skills. This may be accomplished in the family home but may be compromised as the individual and family members age. A transition to residential care should be considered when persons are doing well, rather than when they are under significant physical or emotional distress. Under the latter circumstances, a decline in health or behavior may result. Residential care may be desirable for this patient but not at this time, if it can be avoided. There also are times when an older person with a developmental disability would benefit from in-home care to enhance quality of life; however, it is not likely to benefit someone who is primarily suffering from a depressive disorder. Referral to a psychiatrist who specializes in the care of geriatric patients and persons with mental retardation is not needed.

This patient has some physical symptoms that suggest that a disease process could be the cause of her behavioral changes. However, the recent physical examination makes this unlikely. Overall, the prevalence of morbidity and most causes of mortality for an aging population with developmental disabilities is comparable to that of persons without cognitive limitations. One longitudinal study compared autopsy findings to physical diagnoses of diseases made by a physician experienced in developmental disabilities and communication difficulties. The clinician diagnoses correlated well with autopsy results, and morbidity and mortality rates were comparable to a noncognitively impaired control group.

85. An 81-year-old woman has fallen outside her home on two occasions. She experienced significant bruising from the second event. The patient is interested in exercises to reduce her fall risk. Which of the following is correct?

(A) Exercises should be done with a group of people to be effective.
(B) Ongoing physical therapy supervision is important.
(C) Strength-training exercises are more important than balance-training exercises.
(D) Regular exercise may reduce fall risk for a period of at least 2 years.
(E) In patients age 80 and over, the effectiveness of exercise in reducing falls is unknown.

ANSWER: D

The reduction in fall risk with community-based exercise programs is becoming increasingly clear. The most successful programs are targeted at selected older adults at risk (such as those with mild strength or balance deficits), rather than unselected older adult populations. Controlled trials that are most successful in reducing falls use strength training, balance training, Tai Chi, or endurance training. Meta-analysis of a series of exercise trials indicates that balance training contributes more than strength training to the reduction of fall risk. Thus, choice C is incorrect. One caveat is that many exercise studies in the past have excluded severely impaired older adults, many of whom are at high risk for falls. On the other hand, therapy-induced reductions in balance, gait, and transferring problems were found to contribute significantly to the reduction in falls in a multifactorial (not limited to exercise) intervention.

After initial supervision, patients have performed these exercise programs safely at home, with reasonable adherence. Thus, choice A is incorrect. Studies indicate that exercises must be of sufficient intensity and must be performed regularly to have a significant, sustainable effect on fall reduction. Individualizing these exercises and providing a means to guide patients through them and to optimize adherence (eg, with pamphlets and instruction videos) have not been widely tested.

An individually tailored home-based program for women aged 80 and over demonstrated a reduction in falls for up to a 2-year period. Thus B is incorrect and D is correct. Other studies have included persons over 80 years old and have demonstrated similar effects on fall reduction.

86. An 87-year-old woman is admitted to a nursing home because of increasing difficulties with self-care. She has been taking acetaminophen on an as-needed basis for joint pains in her knees, with incomplete effect. Her physical examination confirms degenerative joint disease in these joints. What is the most appropriate next step in management of her arthritis?

(A)　Obtain additional history regarding joint pain.
(B)　Order radiographs of all affected joints.
(C)　Prescribe propoxyphene, as needed, for pain.
(D)　Prescribe a course of corticosteroids.
(E)　Refer her to an orthopedic surgeon for consideration of a knee replacement.

ANSWER: A

Additional history is needed to assess the intensity, severity, and impact of pain before determining the most appropriate course of treatment. Pain management should begin with a thorough assessment that includes medical history, physical examination, prior therapies and their effects, mental status evaluation, screening for depression, and assessment of activities of daily living. In addition, the location of pain, its intensity as measured on a pain scale, and factors that aggravate or improve it should be sought, documented, and reevaluated on a regular basis. Patients with decreased muscle strength or joint range of motion, or with weight-bearing pain, may benefit from exercises, gait aids, or physical therapy.

Studies indicate that propoxyphene has one half to one third the potency of codeine. At its recommended dose of 100 mg, propoxyphene is about equal to 60 mg of codeine—approximately equianalgesic to two 325 mg tablets of aspirin. Propoxyphene produces an active metabolite called norpropoxyphene, the half-life of which is 30 to 36 hours. With repeated propoxyphene dosing, norpropoxyphene accumulates. Norpropoxyphene can produce pulmonary edema and cardiotoxicity, apnea, cardiac arrest, and death.

For patients with ongoing chronic pain, analgesics are best prescribed on a regular schedule, with as-needed dosing used as an adjunct for breakthrough pain. COX-2 inhibitors may be preferred over nonsteroidal anti-inflammatory drugs (NSAIDs) because of their relative decrease in gastrointestinal toxicity. However, COX-2 inhibitors have been shown to impair renal function among the elderly patients much as traditional NSAIDs do, so caution and frequent monitoring are required in their use. Controlled-release oxycodone has also been shown to reduce osteoarthritis pain and improve sleep quality; however, typical

opioid-related adverse effects (eg, nausea and constipation) lead to discontinuation in many patients. In this patient, a trial of scheduled acetaminophen may be the next medication treatment, after a thorough evaluation of her pain.

Referral to an orthopedist for joint replacement is premature, given that the patient has not had a full assessment of pain and its effect on her physical status. An adequate trial of an analgesic also should be undertaken first, before surgery is considered.

Radiographs are useful in diagnosing specific conditions. Given this patient's classic findings of osteoarthritis, however, films are unlikely to change initial management.

Corticosteroids are inappropriate for treating this patient's osteoarthritis.

87. You chair the infection-control committee at a 120-bed nursing home. In reviewing the facility's influenza immunization program, you find that almost all residents are immunized each September and that 20% of staff are immunized by their personal primary clinicians. The administration is skeptical but would consider providing a free immunization program for staff if research has shown evidence of benefit. Which of the following should you recommend?

(A)　Continue to immunize residents in September; offer no special program for staff.
(B)　Continue to immunize residents in September; establish an immunization program for all staff.
(C)　Immunize residents in mid-October to mid-November; establish an immunization program for staff at high risk.
(D)　Immunize residents in mid-October to mid-November; establish an immunization program for all staff.

ANSWER: D

Influenza remains an important cause of morbidity and mortality in elderly persons; epidemics in long-term-care facilities are particularly troubling. Outbreaks usually occur from December through the spring, so the optimum time for immunization is October to mid-November. Earlier immunization risks the waning of immunity by the spring. Past studies of the benefit of immunization have reported mixed results. In community residents, both infection rates and complications decreased; in nursing homes, complications were reduced but not infection rates. However, two studies suggested that the most effective intervention to prevent influenza complications in nursing-home residents is to immunize staff. Scottish researchers found that mortality during an influenza season was reduced from 17% to 10% in facilities randomized to offer immunization of staff. Half of the facilities had routine policies favoring immunization of residents and half did not. In this study, resident immunization status did not correlate with outcomes. Another study found a significant mortality reduction in facilities that were randomized to offer immunizations to staff. Influenza virus was isolated less often at autopsy in residents who died in facilities with staff immunization programs, but there was no evidence of reduced infection overall. New vaccines undergoing testing ultimately may yield improved efficacy for immunizing residents. Meanwhile, immunization of both residents and staff is the most prudent policy.

88. A sedentary 73-year-old woman who has mild osteoarthritis of the hips and knees comes to you for a routine visit. She is accompanied by her daughter. The patient is 160 cm (63 in) tall and weighs 62 kg (150 lb), for a body mass index of 24.2. Her only medical complaint is morning joint stiffness that resolves in about 30 minutes. She takes acetaminophen, 1000 mg twice daily as needed for pain, and a daily multivitamin. Which of the following is the best recommendation for physical activity?

(A) Treadmill exercise electrocardiography before beginning an exercise program
(B) Walking, 30 minutes per day, 5 days per week
(C) Water aerobics, 3 days per week
(D) Determining what physical activities the patient likes to do and what prevents her from exercising
(E) Enlisting the daughter to help her mother engage in regular moderate physical activity

ANSWER: D

Many studies have shown the benefits of exercise in people of all ages, but many people engage in little or no physical activity. The percentage of sedentary persons increases with age. In the National Health and Nutrition Survey III, approximately 20% of men and 30% of women aged 45 to 64 reported no activity; the percentages increase to 35% of men and nearly 60% of women aged 75 and older. Clinicians, as sources of health information and advice, can play an important role in influencing health behavior, such as increasing physical activity. When discussing exercise, it is important to establish the patient's baseline activity level and willingness to change behavior. In this sedentary patient, the clinician should discuss exercise history to determine what activities has she participated in and enjoyed, what activities she currently does, and barriers to exercise (eg, time, arthritis pain, lack of support from friends or family). Finally, a plan to decrease barriers and gradually increase activity should be agreed on and monitored during subsequent visits.

The current recommendation is that older persons exercise moderately for 30 minutes per day, at least 5 days per week. While the walking program satisfies this recommendation, this patient probably is not ready to embark on a considerable life-style and activity change. Water aerobics provides moderate exercise that would be particularly beneficial, since she has osteoarthritis. However, her exercise preferences have not been explored; she may dislike swimming or group activities. A stress test is unnecessary for someone who has no cardiac risk factors and increases activity gradually. Finally, although the patient's daughter can provide support for life-style changes, the discussion must take place between clinician and patient.

89. A 70-year-old white woman has a foreign body or gritty sensation in the left eye when she awakens, and the eyelashes occasionally are stuck together. Her eyes also are red but become clearer by the end of the day. Physical findings are otherwise normal except for broken capillaries on the cheeks and erythema of both eyelid margins. Which of the following treatments should you recommend?

(A) Antibiotic ointment
(B) Corticosteroid ointment
(C) Antibiotic plus corticosteroid ointment
(D) Oral antibiotics
(E) Oral corticosteroids

ANSWER: D

There are two types of blepharitis: anterior (refers to the outer portion of the lid margin containing the cilia) and posterior (refers to the inner portion containing the meibomian glands). This patient has posterior blepharitis, which is a chronic intermittent inflammation of the inner eyelid margin. It commonly is seen in patients with rosacea, which explains the broken capillaries on the cheeks. The oil-producing meibomian glands that lie just posterior to the eyelashes are plugged with highly viscous secretions that build up during sleep and blur morning vision by changing the properties of the tear film. The condition improves but does not resolve with local treatment; a course of oral tetracycline or doxycycline will decrease the viscosity of the secretions and help resolve the condition.

Anterior blepharitis, which is a low-grade infection of the outer eyelid margin caused by *Staphylococcus aureus*, responds to washing the eyelids with soap. Intermittent use of topical antibiotics or topical antibiotics plus corticosteroids is useful for some cases. The combination ointment should be prescribed only by an ophthalmologist because corticosteroids can increase intraocular pressure or promote cataract formation. Topical corticosteroids may help with inflammation but will not resolve the infection. Oral corticosteroids are not helpful for either type of blepharitis.

90. A 68-year-old woman has a history of Parkinson's disease, hypertension, and osteoarthritis. Current medications are carbidopa–levodopa (25 mg and 100 mg) three times daily; selegiline, 5 mg twice daily; losartan, 50 mg daily; celecoxib, 200 mg daily; and a multivitamin. In the past 3 weeks, she has been taking diphenhydramine at bedtime for insomnia. The patient now reports the onset of urinary incontinence. Which of the following is the most appropriate intervention?

(A) Discontinue celecoxib.
(B) Discontinue diphenhydramine.
(C) Discontinue losartan.
(D) Substitute fosinopril for losartan.
(E) Begin tolterodine.

ANSWER: B

This patient most likely has overflow incontinence secondary to diphenhydramine. Urinary incontinence is a common problem in elderly patients. An estimated 15% to 30% of community-dwelling elderly patients have incontinence. Physicians rarely inquire about it, however, and patients rarely report the problem. Anticholinergics and older antihistamines can produce urinary retention by inhibiting bladder contraction. These agents are especially troublesome in elderly men with benign prostatic hyperplasia.

Celecoxib is unlikely to cause to incontinence. Losartan should have little effect on micturition, so discontinuing it or substituting fosinopril would do little to improve this patient's problem. Tolterodine is used to treat urinary frequency, urgency, or urge incontinence secondary to an overactive bladder. It would worsen urinary retention. Rather than adding another agent to the regimen, it would be more appropriate to treat the underlying cause.

91. Which of the following statements is correct regarding caregiver burden?

(A) Caregiver education has not been shown to reduce caregivers' subjective ratings of burden.
(B) Caregiver variables, such as perceived burden and physical health, are stronger predictors of institutionalization than are patient variables.
(C) Caregivers for patients who are more severely cognitively impaired tend to report greater burden.
(D) Men who are caregivers tend to report greater burden than do women who are caregivers.

ANSWER: B

Research does not support the prediction of caregiver burden by a simple positive linear relationship between degree of cognitive impairment and subjective sense of burden.

Among the important patient variables are behavioral problems, severity of cognitive impairment, and impairment in activities of daily living (especially incontinence). However, caregiver variables have been shown to be stronger than patient variables as predictors of institutionalization of the patient. The experience of burden appears to be mediated by several factors, including caregiver resources (eg, social support, finances), coping abilities, feelings of self-efficacy, and ethnicity. In most studies, the caregivers who are women report a higher level of burden than do men. The presence of a daughter is one of the most powerful predictors of continued community living.

92. An 84-year-old woman moved to a nursing home 6 months ago, following her husband's death. She has severe dementia and requires considerable assistance with eating. Since admission, she has lost 5 kg (11 lb), which is 20% below her ideal weight. No aspiration is noted on swallowing evaluation, but the patient eats very slowly. The staff confirm that a long period of time is required to feed the patient. Her dentures fit well, and a psychiatric evaluation reveals no evidence of depression. The patient never made any statements about artificial feeding and does not have the capacity to understand that option now. Which of the following is the most appropriate action?

(A) Order nutritional supplements.
(B) Develop interdisciplinary strategies to improve feeding.
(C) Arrange for temporary placement of a nasogastric feeding tube.
(D) Place a percutaneous endoscopic gastrostomy.
(E) Begin antidepressant therapy.

ANSWER: B

A multidisciplinary approach to this patient's care can be very effective in providing adequate nutrition. Valuable information about the patient's food preferences can be learned from the family. Changing the approach to feeding the patient, providing high-calorie foods, and removing any dietary restrictions can improve the chance of supplying adequate caloric intake. Every attempt should be made to understand

the effects of the environment on this patient and to alter it, if possible, to enhance feeding.

Nutritional supplements may be appropriate as part of an overall plan to ensure adequate assistance in feeding. A feeding tube should not be used to compensate for insufficient staffing in nursing homes; it also is inappropriate in this case, given this patient's ability to chew and swallow. Treatment for depression, which can present with failure to eat, is not appropriate at this time.

93. A 69-year-old man comes to your office for an initial visit. His medical problems include hypertension, benign prostatic hyperplasia, and obesity. He has been slightly depressed since his wife died 1 year ago. He asks you what he can do to make his "golden years really golden." Which of the following statements best describes this patient's chance of living a long and healthy life?

(A) It is genetically determined and resistant to change.
(B) It is related to his level of physical activity.
(C) It is independent of his depression.
(D) It is most strongly related to losing weight.

ANSWER: B

The concept of healthy aging includes three main components: low probability of disease and disability, high cognitive and physical functional capacity, and active engagement with life. Physical activity appears to have a protective effect in preventing or minimizing disability in late life. In a study of 1097 persons who died in late life, physical activity was found to be a key predictor of being nondisabled at the time of death. Healthy aging is not genetically driven and is amenable to change. A considerable body of literature demonstrates that, like younger adults, elderly persons are influenced by a multitude of factors, including social environment, attitudes toward aging, and activity level. In a study of over 5000 middle-aged and older adults, the presence of depressive symptoms was found to be a stronger predictor of functional problems, poor health perception, and lower well-being than was general medical condition. Although control of obesity is an important goal in maximizing function, physical activity probably is more highly related to improving function in older adults.

94. You are caring for an 86-year-old woman who lives in a long-term-care facility. The patient has osteoarthritis that has been treated intermittently with nonsteroidal anti-inflammatory agents. She also has residual left-sided weakness following a stroke 10 years ago and ambulates with a walker. Atrial fibrillation was detected at the time of the stroke, and warfarin was begun. INR was 2.0 several days ago. Her only other complaint is mild forgetfulness. The patient has received amantadine prophylaxis (200 mg once a day), as have other residents because of an influenza outbreak.

The patient is taken to the emergency department because of progressive confusion. She is only minimally responsive to voice commands but does recognize you. Temperature is 37.6C (99.7F). Pulse rate is 72 per minute, and rhythm is irregular. Respirations are 16 per minute. Blood pressure is 120/74 mm Hg. There is no nuchal rigidity. Lung findings are unremarkable; cardiac examination is normal except for the irregular rhythm. The abdomen is soft, and bowel sounds are normal. No pedal edema or venous cords are present. Except for the blunted sensorium, no new neurologic findings are noted. Cranial nerve examination is normal.

Laboratory studies:

Leukocyte count	10,000/cu mm; normal differential
Blood urea nitrogen	32 mg/dL
Serum creatinine	2.3 mg/dL
Serum electrolytes	Normal
Serum calcium	Normal
Serum phosphorus	Normal
Serum magnesium	Normal

Which of the following is the most likely explanation for the patient's condition?

(A) Embolic stroke secondary to atrial fibrillation
(B) Intracerebral bleeding
(C) Subarachnoid hemorrhage
(D) Adverse reaction to amantadine
(E) Influenza A encephalitis

ANSWER: D

This patient with a reduced creatinine clearance has had an adverse drug reaction (ADR) to amantadine. In one study, 18.6% of nursing-home residents experienced adverse effects with this drug, compared with 1% when rimantadine (a more costly agent) was used. ADRs currently are the fourth to sixth leading cause of death in the United States, higher than diabetes mellitus and pneumonia. Three fourths are dose dependent, but ADRs may occur at recommended doses, especially in older adults. Approximately half of all deaths attributed to ADRs occur in patients aged 60 and over. Although this age group represents 17% of the population, it accounts for 39% of hospitalizations; 10% to 17% of hospitalizations in older adults are believed to be directly related to ADRs. Because this agent is primarily renally excreted, reduced doses are indicated in the common setting of reduced renal clearance.

This patient has many risk factors for vascular disease, including atrial fibrillation and a history of stroke; however, anticoagulation has been adequate, and she has no focal neurologic findings. While she has an increased risk for bleeding secondary to warfarin therapy, INR is therapeutic, and she has no history of a fall. This patient's presentation does not suggest influenza, and cerebral involvement is an unusual complication of influenza A.

95. You are asked to see a 78-year-old man who has a 6-week history of intermittent low-back pain that often occurs with bending but does not radiate into the legs. He obtains some relief when he takes acetaminophen or over-the-counter nonsteroidal anti-inflammatory agents. The patient has continued to take a daily walk of about one quarter mile, which is his only exercise. Another clinician ordered magnetic resonance imaging (MRI) of the lumbar spine, which showed "moderate spinal stenosis at L2–4 with bony foraminal encroachment on the nerve roots." The discs were described as deficient in water content, with some bulging and evidence of "degeneration." Which of the following should you recommend?

(A) A continuous regimen of high-dose nonsteroidal anti-inflammatory agents
(B) Referral to a chiropractor for a trial of spinal manipulation
(C) Referral to a physical therapist for a trial of flexibility exercises and sustained aerobic exercise
(D) Referral to an anesthesiologist for a course of facet-joint injections
(E) Referral to a surgeon for possible laminectomy

ANSWER: C

Back pain is a common problem among persons of all ages, including those 65 and over. Serious causes (eg, metastatic disease and vertebral compression fracture) are more common in older patients, but in the majority of cases, back pain is of unclear and often nonspecific origin. Supportive care and maintenance of daily activities are adequate therapies for most patients, and about 90% of new-onset low-back pain will resolve within 1 to 2 months with conservative measures. The availability of new imaging technology, combined with a relative lack of appreciation for common anatomic changes associated with aging, can lead to over interpretation of common findings.

Results of a randomized trial confirm that bed rest is contraindicated in the treatment of most back pain. Patients with acute pain should be instructed to maintain their usual activities as much as possible. About 5% of patients progress to chronic pain and may need additional encouragement to maintain function. Several trials have demonstrated that active exercise is helpful in chronic, but probably not acute, pain. The type of exercise may be less important than the fact that exercise is occurring and function is being maintained. Referral to a physical therapist for an exercise program represents the best option for this patient.

Nonsteroidal anti-inflammatory agents may play a role in the care of patients with back pain; however, prolonged courses should be avoided in geriatric patients, especially those who do not have an inflammatory disease. Acetaminophen often gives a similar level of analgesia with less risk for gastric or renal toxicity.

Spinal manipulation has been studied in a number of randomized trials. Meta-analyses have demonstrated somewhat conflicting results regarding overall efficacy for acute low-back pain. One large prospective cohort study found it to be about as effective as conventional medical therapy but at a higher cost because of the numbers of visits (usually 10 to 15 visits). Little evidence is available regarding its effectiveness in chronic low-back pain. For this patient, who is relatively inactive, a conditioning program would be preferable.

Facet joint injections (corticosteroids and long-acting local anesthetic) and similar procedures (eg, epidural corticosteroid instillation), sometimes are used for sciatica caused by an acute herniated lumbar disc or in severe, chronic lower back pain. Limited randomized trials have demonstrated minimal, if any, response overall, but some subsets of patients may benefit.

Laminectomy also is inappropriate for this patient. Although the MRI findings are consistent with degenerative lumbar spinal stenosis, this patient's clinical presentation is not characteristic. The pain is relatively brief and does not worsen with ambulation or radiate to the legs (pseudoclaudication). Bony spinal stenosis commonly ($> 25\%$) is found in older persons who do not have any back pain, and the prevalence of this finding increases with age. The diagnosis of spinal stenosis must be made clinically, with imaging findings playing only a confirmatory role.

96. Which of the following is the most common pattern of hearing loss among older Americans?

(A) Symmetric high-frequency sensorineural
(B) Symmetric high-frequency conductive
(C) Asymmetric high-frequency conductive
(D) Symmetric low-frequency sensorineural
(E) Asymmetric high-frequency sensorineural

ANSWER: A

Hearing loss associated with aging affects nearly 40% of persons aged 65 and over. The prevalence is as high as 80% among nursing-home residents. Cross-sectional and longitudinal studies consistently reveal that hearing sensitivity declines with age, more prominently in high than in low frequencies. Presbycusis is the bilateral, symmetric, high-frequency sensorineural hearing loss that affects older adults. This tends to be gradual in onset and mild to moderate in severity. Risk factors include noise exposure and elevated systolic blood pressure. Overall, men have poorer hearing than women. Presbycusis is associated with difficulty understanding speech, especially in the presence of noise. Hence, the primary complaint of older adults is that they have difficulty understanding others, especially in a noisy room or when the speaker is standing at a distance. Older adults often blame hearing loss on an accumulation of cerumen, but this usually is not responsible. Asymmetric hearing loss raises concerns about less common conditions, such as acoustic neuroma.

97. A 72-year-old woman has mitral valve prolapse with regurgitation. She has most of her natural teeth and has no problems chewing any foods. The patient has no drug allergies. Which of the following should you recommend prior to routine cleaning of the teeth?

(A) Amoxicillin, 2 g 1 hour before the procedure
(B) Clindamycin, 600 mg 1 hour before the procedure
(C) Erythromycin, 1 g 1 hour before the procedure
(D) Amoxicillin, 500 mg 1 hour before the procedure, then 4 and 8 hours after
(E) Cephalexin, 500 mg 1 hour before the procedure, then 4 and 8 hours after

ANSWER: A

In patients with mitral regurgitation, antibiotic prophylaxis is recommended for procedures likely to induce bleeding. A thorough dental examination includes periodontal probing, which can produce bleeding; dental prophylaxis and scaling (teeth cleaning) nearly always produce some bleeding. Amoxicillin is recommended by the American Heart Association because of its rapid absorption and effectiveness against group A streptococci, which are the most likely cause of heart valve damage.

Clindamycin is recommended for persons allergic to penicillin derivatives; erythromycin is another alternative. Previous recommendations called for post-treatment doses, but these are not required if peak antibiotic levels are achieved at the time of the procedure. This

corresponds to the peak likelihood of bacteremia. A cephalosporin would be appropriate for prophylaxis when skin may be the source of infection (eg, hip surgery).

98. A 75-year-old man comes to you for evaluation of dizziness. Symptoms began 8 weeks ago, when he had severe dizziness on rising from the bed. Since then, "everything is moving" when he turns his head quickly, rolls over in bed, or stands upright after bending forward. Episodes occur several times a day and last about 1 minute. He is fatigued and unsteady for up to 1 hour afterward. The patient has been less active recently because of this problem. Which of the following is most likely to be beneficial?

(A) Reduction of activity
(B) Epley maneuver
(C) Dix-Hallpike maneuver
(D) Diazepam
(E) Meclizine

ANSWER: B

Dizziness can be classified by type: vertigo, presyncope, disequilibrium, or other. Vertigo is the illusion that the body or environment is moving, usually rotating. It often begins abruptly and is episodic; severe cases are associated with nausea, vomiting, and a staggering gait. True vertigo almost always arises from a disorder of the peripheral labyrinth or its central connections. The length of episodes provides a clue to the cause. The most common vestibular disorder producing vertigo in older persons is benign paroxysmal positional vertigo (BPPV), which is caused when otolith debris from the utricle gains access to the posterior semicircular canal. In BPPV, vertigo lasts less than 1 minute and occurs when a patient moves the head in the plane of the posterior semicircular canal (eg, rolling over in bed, standing after bending forward). Symptoms initially are severe but improve within a few days and typically resolve in days to weeks. Some cases persist 1 month or longer.

The Epley maneuver is a relatively new procedure that has replaced Brandt-Daroff exercises as the treatment of choice for severe cases of BPPV. The patient is placed in the head-hanging position, with the affected ear down. A series of head rotations are performed for approximately 10 minutes. These are designed to permit the displaced material to pass through the semicircular canal and return to the utricle. In a study, 18 of 28 patients (64%) using a modified Epley procedure had resolution within 1 week; Brandt-Daroff exercises were effective in 6 of 26 patients. (See Figures 23.1 and 23.2 in "Dizziness," p 154–155, for illustrated instructions for performing the Epley maneuver.)

Physical stimulation of the vestibular system appears to accelerate recovery; thus, inactivity leads to prolonged symptoms. The Dix-Hallpike maneuver is a diagnostic test for BPPV. It is performed by rapidly moving the patient from a sitting to a head-hanging supine position, while the head is turned 30 degrees to the right and then to the left, to assess each posterior semicircular canal. A classic positive response is induction of vertigo accompanied by rotatory nystagmus, with symptoms beginning a few seconds after the head-hanging position is achieved. The severity of the response decreases when the test is repeated immediately. Diazepam and meclizine rarely are helpful since symptoms usually are not severe. Both drugs also cause sedation.

99. An 82-year-old woman, who lives at home with her son, has diabetes mellitus and partial blindness. She has both Medicare and Medicaid coverage. She currently needs assistance with bathing, dressing, and medication management. The son provides this assistance but worries about her overall well-being and lack of socialization. Although he feels overwhelmed by the demands of caregiving, he would like his mother to remain at home as long as possible. Which of the following options is most appropriate?

(A) Assisted living
(B) Adult foster care
(C) "Swing bed"
(D) Program of All-Inclusive Care for the Elderly (PACE)
(E) Nursing home

ANSWER: D

PACE is a capitated benefit authorized by the Balanced Budget Act of 1997. It features a comprehensive service delivery system and integrated Medicare–Medicaid financing. PACE was developed to address the needs of long-term care clients, providers, and payers. The comprehensive service package permits most participants to continue living at home, rather than being institutionalized. Capitated financing allows providers to deliver all needed services, not just those reimbursable under the Medicare and Medicaid fee-for-service systems. Participants must be aged 55 or over, live in the PACE service area, and be certified by the appropriate state agency as eligible for nursing-home care. An interdisciplinary team of professionals and paraprofessionals assesses participant needs, develops care plans, and delivers all services (including acute care and nursing-home services), which are integrated for seamless provision of total care. PACE programs provide social and medical services primarily in an adult day health center, supplemented by in-home and referral services.

All of the other options would result in the patient leaving her home, which is not preferred by the family in this case. Assisted living offers a combination of housing, personal services, and health care designed to promote maximum independence for persons who need help with normal daily activities. Personal services, 24-hour supervision and assistance, activities, and health-related services are provided in a congregate residential setting. Costs, which can vary greatly, are not covered by Medicare or Medicaid and must be paid for out of pocket. Adult foster care is a licensed, adult-appropriate, sheltered-living arrangement provided in a family-like environment. Foster homes provide food, lodging, supervision, and household services. They also may provide personal care and medication assistance. Residents pay for their care by using Social Security, pensions, and income from savings or investments. "Swing beds" address the shortage of rural nursing-home beds for Medicare patients. Rural hospitals with fewer than 50 beds are reimbursed by Medicare for furnishing post-hospitalization extended-care services. Nursing-home placement is not indicated because the patient's son prefers that his mother remain at home.

100. A 69-year-old man who underwent radical prostatectomy 3 months ago consults you because he loses a small amount of urine when he coughs or lifts objects. Findings of physical examination are normal. He is able to rise from a chair and walk unassisted for 25 feet in less than 5 seconds. There is no evidence of obstruction or urethral stricture. Postvoid residual volume is 25 mL. Peak urine flow rate is 23 mL per second. Which of the following is the most appropriate initial approach?

(A) Reassurance and observation
(B) Comprehensive urodynamic evaluation
(C) Intermittent catheterization, three times daily
(D) Implantation of an artificial urethral sphincter
(E) Tamsulosin, 0.4 mg daily

ANSWER: A

Urinary incontinence in men usually is caused by urge incontinence or obstruction with overflow incontinence. Few men have stress incontinence, except following prostatic surgery, as in this patient. Total urinary control following surgery is rare, but incontinence in the initial postoperative period may resolve over time. In one study, total control was found to increase from 20.5% at 6 months to 31.9% at 24 months. Also at 24 months, 11.9% of patients had incontinence more than twice daily, and 3.3% three or more times daily. A measure of the level of associated bother improved over time, with 8.7% of patients reporting that incontinence was a moderate-to-big problem at 24 months.

Urodynamic studies may distinguish stress from urge incontinence, but results are unlikely to change the treatment plan, because symptoms often improve during the first postoperative year. This patient has no evidence of urinary obstruction, so intermittent catheterization is not indicated. Tamsulosin, a selective α_1-adrenergic blocking agent used to treat benign prostatic hypertrophy, also is not indicated.

101. A 68-year-old postmenopausal woman complains of vaginal dryness and urinary frequency and urgency. She has not had dysuria or urinary incontinence, and she takes no medications regularly. On pelvic examination, the vaginal epithelium is pale and thin, with a decrease in the height of the rugae. Urinalysis is normal. Topical treatment with which of the following agents is the most appropriate first step in management?

(A) Corticosteroids
(B) Estrogen
(C) Metronidazole
(D) Nystatin
(E) Testosterone

ANSWER: B

Common vulvovaginal disorders in postmenopausal women include atrophic vaginitis, vaginal candidiasis, squamous cell hyperplasia, and lichen sclerosus. Atrophic vaginitis is a consequence of estrogen deficiency and is common in women not taking hormone-replacement therapy. Symptoms include vulvar pruritus, dyspareunia, urinary urgency and frequency, and dysuria. The vagina has a pale, shiny, dry appearance with a decrease in height of the rugae. In more severe cases, the epithelium is erythematous, friable, and bleeds easily. The diagnosis is made on the basis of clinical findings. The treatment is estrogen given orally, topically, or both. Two commonly used forms are estradiol and conjugated equine estrogen. In patients with an intact uterus, a progestin should be given.

Symptoms of vaginal candidiasis include pruritus and burning of the vulva or vagina or both, as well as dysuria and dyspareunia. A thick, curd-like, white or yellow discharge is characteristic. The most common cause is *Candida albicans*. The diagnosis is made microscopically by visualizing candidal organisms in a specimen of the discharge that has been treated with 10% to 20% potassium hydroxide. Treatment consists of topical antifungal agents such as nystatin or clotrimazole. A single dose of fluconazole (150 mg orally) also can be used.

Squamous cell hyperplasia presents with pruritus and sometimes painful vulvar lesions, with epithelial thickening and hyperkeratosis. Thickened white or reddish patches involve the labia majora and outer aspects of the labia minora. Aggravating factors include inability to maintain good hygiene, candidiasis, or diabetes mellitus. The diagnosis is confirmed by punch biopsy. Treatment consists of a 4- to 6-week course of topical fluorinated corticosteroids. If symptoms persist after 6 weeks, 1% hydrocortisone should be used.

Lichen sclerosus is a pruritic condition characterized by white macules that frequently involve the entire vulva. The skin thins and takes on a "cigarette paper" appearance. The labia minora may fuse with the labia majora. Edema of the clitoral hood may be an early sign. A punch biopsy is needed to confirm the diagnosis. Treatment consists of topical 2% testosterone proprionate, twice daily for 1 to 2 weeks. A potent corticosteroid, 0.05% clobetasol, also has been used successfully.

Metronidazole is used for bacterial vaginosis, which is common in younger persons. This condition has varied presentations but does not mimic atrophy.

102. A 66-year-old woman has had recurrent urinary tract infections (UTI) for many years. The patient is otherwise healthy and is sexually active with one male partner on a regular basis, without pain or discomfort. Symptoms tend to occur a day or two following intercourse. She has not had pyelonephritis or required hospitalization. When urine cultures have been obtained, antibiotic-susceptible *Escherichia coli* and *Staphylococcus saprophyticus* have been isolated. Which of the following should you do first?

(A) Encourage the patient to drink cranberry juice.
(B) Perform pelvic examination and measure postvoid residual volume.
(C) Begin postcoital antibiotic prophylaxis.
(D) Begin daily, low-dose, suppressive antibiotic therapy.
(E) Begin estrogen supplementation.

ANSWER: B

In young women, risk factors for recurrent UTI are sexual intercourse, use of diaphragms or spermicides, and history of UTI. In frail older women, risk factors are poor functional status, requirement for skilled care, and catheterization.

Risk factors in healthy older women include prior history of UTI, genetic predisposition, cystocele, elevated postvoid residual volume, and incontinence. Lack of estrogen effect and sexual activity also may play a role, but these have not been fully evaluated in this age group. Initial examination of a patient should document the presence of incomplete voiding, incontinence, or gynecologic abnormalities. Treatment of incontinence, bladder obstruction, or urinary stasis may help to alleviate the condition.

The efficacy of cranberry juice in preventing adhesion of bacteria to urinary epithelial cells, bacteriuria, and UTI has not been proven convincingly. Postcoital antibiotic prophylaxis has been studied primarily in premenopausal women. Daily suppressive antibiotic therapy also has been assessed mostly in younger women; routine use should be avoided because of the potential to develop resistant organisms. Topical estrogens may be efficacious in restoring normal colonizing lactobacilli and reducing pathogenic gram-negative bacilli in the vaginal flora of older women. However, a pelvic examination and measurement of postvoid residual volume would be most likely to identify a treatable predisposing cause.

103. An assessment of instrumental activities of daily living (IADLs) typically includes which of the following?

(A) Urinary continence
(B) Ability to take medications
(C) Recreational activities
(D) Use of assistive devices
(E) Social supports

ANSWER: B

IADLs are tasks that are required for an older person to remain independent and to live alone in the community (see the Appendix, p 385, for a screen). They typically include using the telephone, managing transportation, shopping, preparing meals, doing housework, taking medicines, and managing money. Persons unable to perform these functions must rely on others, or they may need an assisted-living environment. Evaluating the ability to perform these functions and providing referrals to obtain needed assistance may allow a person to remain at home.

Basic activities of daily living (ADLs) include tasks essential to the performance of self-care or hygiene (see the Appendix, p 384, for a screen). They include being continent of urine and stool, bathing, dressing, being able to get on and off the toilet, transferring (for example, out of bed or from chair to bed without the use of assistive devices), and feeding. Persons dependent in basic ADLs usually cannot live alone in the community, even with supplemental services. Recreational activities are examples of advanced ADLs. These patient-specific activities, such as community service, occupational tasks, or avocational activities, are appropriate for functional assessment of many community-dwelling older persons. Social support is not an ADL or IADL but typically is evaluated as part of a comprehensive geriatric assessment.

104. A 68-year-old man has a 2-year history of progressive impairment of gait, posture, and balance. He walks with small, shuffling steps and has fallen repeatedly. Cognitive dysfunction developed in the past 6 months, although mentation sometimes is normal. The patient's wife describes episodes in which the patient seems to "go blank." Levodopa therapy was discontinued because of florid visual hallucinations. Which of the following is the most likely diagnosis?

(A) Normal-pressure hydrocephalus
(B) Parkinson's disease
(C) Alzheimer's disease
(D) Multi-infarct dementia
(E) Dementia with Lewy bodies (DLB)

ANSWER: E

Neuropathologic autopsy findings suggest that DLB may be the second largest cause of dementia, accounting for 15% to 25% of all cases. Three core features have been identified: fluctuation in cognitive function, visual hallucinations, and parkinsonism. Additional features include repeated falls, syncopal episodes, and neuroleptic sensitivity. Early in the illness, patients display periods of cognitive impairment that alternate with near-normal function. Detailed visual hallucinations help distinguish

DLB from Alzheimer's disease. The parkinsonism usually is characterized by rigidity and bradykinesia; tremor is less common. Cognitive impairment typically develops within 12 months of the appearance of parkinsonism.

Normal-pressure hydrocephalus is characterized by a triad of clinical features: progressive dementia, gait impairment, and urinary incontinence. Functional improvement may follow shunt implantation. Extrapyramidal dysfunction may develop as Alzheimer's disease progresses, but cognitive impairment remains the dominant feature. The dementia is of the "cortical" type, with memory loss and features such as apraxia, aphasia, and agnosia. Progressive cognitive impairment may develop in Parkinson's disease but usually not within the first 2 years. Multi-infarct dementia is characterized by step-wise deterioration in cognitive function and gait, presumably because of accumulating micro-infarcts. Neuroimaging studies reveal widespread lacunar infarcts.

105. Which of the following cancers is associated most strongly with heavy drinking?

(A) Skin
(B) Head and neck
(C) Renal
(D) Prostate
(E) Testicular

ANSWER: B

Heavy drinking has been associated with a number of adverse health effects, including cancer. A potential relationship with alcohol has been explored for many types of cancer; however, the strongest evidence exists for that affecting the head and neck. The risk for cancer of the mouth, pharynx, and larynx increases with alcohol consumption that exceeds two drinks per day, and the magnitude of risk continues to rise with increasing intake. Risk appears to be amplified in smokers. Alcohol consumption has not been linked with any of the major types of skin cancer or with either renal or testicular cancer. A possible relationship between heavy drinking and prostate cancer has been investigated, and alcohol does not appear to increase risk. Heavy drinking has been associated with hepatic cancer, almost always preceded by cirrhosis, and with esophageal cancer. It has been suggested that alcohol may increase the risk for stomach, pancreas, colon, lung, and breast cancer, although the evidence has been less clear.

106. An 84-year-old man is brought to the emergency department from a nursing home because of fever, cough, and a change in mental status. Temperature now is 38.1C (100.6F). Pulse rate is 110 per minute, and respirations are 28 per minute. Blood pressure is 110/60 mm Hg. The patient is unable to participate with mental status testing because of delirium. He has bilateral cataracts. Wasting is noted in the temporal areas and infrascapular fat pads; the deltoids are rounded. Crackles are heard at the right lung base with a focal area of tubular breath sounds. Skin findings are normal. Chest radiograph shows an infiltrate or atelectasis at the right lung base. Results of laboratory studies are within normal limits except for serum albumin of 2.0 g/dL.

The patient is admitted to the hospital. A dietitian reports: "Current weight not available, triceps skin fold indicates decreased fat stores, low albumin reflects significant visceral protein depletion; suggest tube feeding until swallowing evaluation is performed." The nurse manager tells you about a critical pathway for pneumonia that is being implemented. According to its guidelines, a serum albumin level below 2.5 g/dL is a risk factor for poorer outcomes. Which of the following should you recommend?

(A) Weigh the patient and obtain baseline weight from the nursing home.
(B) Encourage oral feeding.
(C) Order liquid supplements with meals.
(D) Begin peripheral parenteral nutrition.
(E) Begin tube feedings.

ANSWER: A

This patient does not show clear signs of malnutrition and reportedly had no previous difficulty eating. Although he has limited fat stores, the shoulders and quadriceps are not wasted. A pattern of weight loss would raise concern about diminished nutritional state, but the patient's current and baseline weights are unknown. The pattern and amount of weight loss are the two most important factors in predicting malnutrition-associated complications.

Although a low serum albumin level is associated with poor outcome in a large number of conditions, low serum protein levels may be a manifestation of an acute-phase response or of protein-energy undernutrition. In the absence of weight loss or muscle wasting, this patient's low protein level likely represents an acute-phase response. Supplements given with meals tend to substitute for food; they may be more effective if given between meals. Meeting caloric requirements with peripheral parenteral nutrition is more difficult than meeting protein needs, owing to the osmotic load. There is no evidence that tube feeding at this point would alter the clinical course. Because of mental status changes, this patient is unable to safely eat by himself.

107. An 87-year-old woman recently fell at home, after tripping over the telephone cord. She consults you because she is worried about another fall. The patient lives alone and is cognitively intact. She has cataracts and diminished visual acuity; osteoarthritic changes in the hands and knees; and absent Achilles' reflexes bilaterally with normal sensation to pinprick. She is unable to rise from a chair without using her arms. Romberg test is normal, but she is unable to do semi-tandem or tandem stances for more than 3 seconds and cannot stand on one leg. Gait is symmetric, with good foot clearance and steady turns. In addition to other measures, which of the following types of exercise is most likely to reduce her risk for falls?

(A) A walking program, gradually increasing time and distance
(B) A seated stretching program, 1 hour, 3 days per week
(C) Stationary bicycling, gradually increasing time, to avoid impact on the knees
(D) Balance and ankle-strengthening exercises, gradually increasing in difficulty

ANSWER: D

This patient has decreased mobility and impaired balance, and she is fearful of falling. An exercise program that includes balance and ankle-strengthening exercises is most likely to decrease her risk for future falls. In a meta-analysis of the Frailty and Injuries:

Cooperative Studies of Intervention Techniques (FICSIT) trials, interventions that included balance exercises were found to reduce the incidence of falls by 17% in community-dwelling older persons. Strength and endurance exercises were less effective. In a study of women aged 80 and over, a home-based program of strength and balance exercises resulted in a decreased incidence of falls at 1 and 2 years. A walking program would improve endurance and physical fitness and might indirectly affect balance. However, walking alone has not been shown to decrease the risk for falls. Exercises performed in a chair would not improve balance, strength, or endurance. Stationary bicycling would improve endurance but would not improve balance or decrease the risk for falls.

108. A 90-year-old man has chronic obstructive pulmonary disease, congestive heart failure, osteoarthritis, chronic urinary tract infections, and type 2 diabetes mellitus. Physical examination reveals a white coating over much of the intra-oral soft tissues. When the coating is wiped away with a gauze pad, the underlying site is reddish. Which of the following is the most likely diagnosis?

(A) Candidiasis
(B) Leukoplakia
(C) Lichen planus
(D) Squamous cell carcinoma

ANSWER: A

This patient has a number of chronic medical conditions and may be debilitated. Thus, he is more susceptible to overgrowth of *Candida albicans*. He also may be using inhaled corticosteroids, which is another risk factor for this condition. This organism is a normal oral inhabitant and usually becomes evident only if normal defenses are suppressed. The typical appearance is layers of white hyphae that are loosely attached to the mucosa. It is these hyphae that can be wiped away with gauze. The other listed conditions cannot be wiped away with gauze. Leukoplakia and squamous cell carcinoma usually are confined to one site. Lichen planus is most common on the buccal mucosae. Biopsy is indicated for any white lesion that is not clearly benign.

109. Research on group exercise programs in skilled nursing facilities supports which of the following statements?

(A) Stretching, balance and strength exercises, and walking will improve strength and mobility.
(B) Upper- and lower-extremity range-of-motion exercises performed while seated (for safety) will improve strength.
(C) Resistance and flexibility exercises will reduce the incidence of falls.
(D) Flexibility, balance, strength, and endurance exercises will result in fewer respiratory infections.

ANSWER: A

Effective group exercise in a skilled nursing facility requires close supervision with structured activities, frequent cuing, and commitment of involved staff. One study compared a program of strength, balance, flexibility, and mobility training to seated range-of-motion exercises. The more active group had improved mobility, lower-extremity strength, and balance. Seated range-of-motion exercises do not increase leg strength. Studies have shown increases in strength and improvements in gait with exercise interventions; however, a reduction in falls has not been shown. In one study of frail nursing-home residents, the incidence of falls was higher in the intervention group than in the control goup. The effect of exercise on respiratory infections has not been measured.

110. A 72-year-old woman has newly diagnosed stage 1 hypertension, with an average blood pressure of 152/96 mm Hg. She does not smoke cigarettes and does not have diabetes mellitus, dyslipidemia, clinically recognizable cardiovascular disease, or target organ damage. She is obese (body mass index 30) and does not exercise. Which of the following is the most appropriate initial treatment?

(A) Regular exercise and weight loss
(B) Fish oil supplementation
(C) A thiazide diuretic
(D) An angiotensin-converting enzyme (ACE) inhibitor
(E) A calcium channel blocking agent

ANSWER: A

In 18 randomized trials enrolling obese hypertensive patients, weight loss through calorie-restricted diet was found to decrease blood pressure. Caloric intakes ranged from 450 to 1500 kcal daily, with reductions of 3% to 9% of body weight; average blood-pressure decreases were approximately 3/3 mm Hg (systolic/diastolic). However, these trials included mostly middle-aged persons and may not be generalizable to the elderly population. A randomized trial of nonpharmacologic interventions in persons aged 60 to 80 showed reductions in blood pressure with reduced sodium intake or weight loss. The benefits of lower-extremity aerobic exercise were demonstrated in a meta-analysis of nine randomized trials that included subjects aged 29 to 72. The average exercise program was 45 minutes, 3 days per week, for 4 months; average intensity was 60% of VO_2max. Blood pressure in the exercisers decreased by approximately 7/5 mm Hg (systolic/diastolic).

Drug therapy is not recommended as initial therapy for stage 1 hypertension with no target-organ damage, cardiovascular disease, or diabetes. Fish oil supplementation (or daily consumption of 200 g of fish high in omega-2 polyunsaturated fatty acid) does lower blood pressure, but many people cannot maintain these doses for prolonged periods.

111. An 80-year-old woman must use her arms to rise from a chair. Her balance is good and gait is normal. Findings of the remainder of the physical examination are unremarkable. The patient has been less active in the past 2 months; she used to take daily walks but stopped because of inclement weather. Which is the best initial management for this patient?

(A) Referral for physical therapy
(B) Raised toilet seat
(C) Single-point cane
(D) Increased exercise

ANSWER: D

Deconditioning is the most likely cause for this patient's reduced quadriceps muscle strength. An exercise program such as walking often is the best initial recommendation. A written exercise prescription may be useful. She may be better able to adhere to the prescription if she

first is instructed to walk for 5 minutes, three times a week, then gradually increasing to 30 minutes daily. Another alternative may be use of an exercise video or audiotape in the home or group exercise at a local senior center or YMCA. If such an intervention is not followed, physical therapy for quadriceps-strengthening exercises should be recommended. Balance and gait are normal, so the patient does not need physical therapy or a cane. A raised toilet seat would be appropriate if she had quadriceps weakness that was unlikely to be corrected with exercise.

112. An occupational therapist makes a home visit to an 80-year-old man who has a history of falls. A number of hazards (eg, the seat of his favorite chair is low, the hallways are cluttered) are noted. Which of the following is the most likely outcome of a home assessment and subsequent suggestions for risk reduction?

(A) It is likely to reduce falls at home but not those outside the home.
(B) The presence of an environmental hazard is associated with increased fall risk.
(C) The fall risk associated with an environmental hazard is related to the patient's interaction with the environment.
(D) Environmental hazards are more likely to be found in the homes of disabled persons than in the homes of persons without disability.

ANSWER: C

Environmental hazards are equally prevalent in the homes of patients with and without impaired physical function. For example, a low chair is as commonly or even more commonly found in the homes of patients with difficulty rising from a chair as in homes of those without this difficulty. Results of a controlled prospective trial suggest that falls are reduced as a result of occupational therapy assessment and intervention; precisely how the environment (or its modification) contributes to this improvement is unclear. The intervention apparently reduces falls outside the home as well as inside, perhaps because strategies taught in the program carry over to increase a person's safety in general.

Case-controlled studies suggest that the presence of an environmental hazard itself is not associated with an increased fall risk. The risk associated with a hazard also depends upon the underlying impairment and how the patient interacts with the environment. For example, colliding with furniture in the dark may reflect a willingness to attempt to walk in the dark, lack of sufficient night vision to detect the furniture, or a problem with the furniture placement itself.

113. A 73-year-old man comes to you for a routine visit. He has been seen twice before, for management of osteoarthritis of the knees, mild hypertension, and urinary hesitancy and nocturia. Prior to this visit, the patient's wife tells you privately that she is concerned about her husband's drinking. She thinks that it increased after his retirement 3 years ago.

Beginning with general open-ended questions, you initiate a discussion about the use of tobacco and alcohol, as well as other health habits. More detailed questioning leads the patient to report that he consumes about 21 to 25 drinks per week, including both beer and liquor. On some occasions he may have five drinks. He scores 0/4 on the CAGE question-naire and consistently denies any symptoms suggestive of alcohol dependence. He also denies that alcohol has ever prevented him from fulfilling major obligations, drinking in situa-tions when it might be dangerous, or legal problems related to drinking. However, when you mention the possibility of adverse health effects associated with drinking, he does express an interest in cutting down on his intake. He tells you that he was able to quit smoking 10 years ago. Which of the following is the most appropriate treatment option?

(A) Brief intervention
(B) Referral to Alcoholics Anonymous
(C) Admission to an inpatient treatment center
(D) Naltrexone

ANSWER: A

The United States Department of Agriculture, in *Dietary Guidelines for Americans* (3rd edition), has set the threshold for safe or low-risk drinking in men at 14 drinks per week or four on any one occasion, regardless of age. The National Institute of Alcohol Abuse and Alcoholism, in *The Physician's Guide to Helping Patients with Alcohol Problems*, set a lower threshold for men aged 65 and over: seven drinks per week or three on any one occasion. Potential adverse health effects have been described when drinking exceeds these thresholds.

Randomized clinical trials have shown that brief intervention or counseling by primary care physicians and other providers can result in a significant reduction in alcohol consumption. Most studies have enrolled at-risk or hazardous drinkers (ie, those who exceed thresholds for safe or low-risk drinking but do not meet criteria for abuse or dependence). Key elements of such interventions include education about current and potential adverse effects of drinking and specific recommendations for safe limits on drinking. In a trial of brief physician advice for alcohol problems in older adults, significant reductions were found in 7-day alcohol use, episodes of binge drinking, and frequency of excessive drinking. The magnitude of reduction actually exceeded that seen in some trials with younger adults. For this patient, whose alcohol use can be categorized as at-risk or hazardous, brief intervention is the best approach.

Alcoholics Anonymous, inpatient alcohol treatment centers, and pharmacotherapy with naltrexone have proven value for treatment of alcohol use disorders, but their use has focused almost entirely on alcohol dependence. Directing a patient without evidence of abuse or dependence to one of these treatment options might not only be unnecessary but could lead to alienating the patient if he feels that the severity of his drinking problem has been overestimated. However, any or all of these options might be appropriate if the patient does not respond to brief intervention or if additional information suggests that the patient has alcohol dependence.

114. A 79-year-old woman who has Alzheimer's disease and resides in a skilled nursing facility has been angry, belligerent, and agitated for 3 days. She has had progressive dementia for 8 years and has resided in the facility for 2 years. Medical history also includes hypertension, congestive heart failure, and osteoporosis, all of which have been stable recently. She has no history of behavioral disturbances. The Mini–Mental State Examination score is 10/30. Which of the following is the most appropriate initial step in the care of this patient?

(A) Ask the nursing staff to describe the specific behaviors that have occurred.
(B) Perform a physical examination, including assessment of mental status.
(C) Order complete blood cell count, serum electrolytes, and urinalysis.
(D) Order chest radiograph.
(E) Prescribe haloperidol, 0.5 mg orally twice daily, as needed for agitation.

ANSWER: A

The term *agitation* is used by clinical staff and family caregivers to describe a variety of behaviors that occur in patients with moderate to advanced dementia. Agitation usually refers to inappropriate verbal or physical activities, including pacing, yelling, hitting, irritability, and oppositional behaviors. The most important initial step in the care of an agitated patient is to clarify what specific behaviors are occurring and under what circumstances. Changes in the environment, the presence of additional psychiatric symptoms (eg, insomnia, delusions, hallucinations, depression), the time course, precipitating factors, and changes in medical symptoms (eg, pain, shortness of breath, incontinence) should be noted.

   Laboratory studies and chest films may be appropriate in the evaluation of new-onset behavioral disturbance, particularly with preexisting medical problems, but the decision to pursue such testing should be directed by an initial understanding of the likely contributing factors. Further evaluation may be unnecessary if the behavior is driven by a specific change in the environment, for example. Similarly, a physical and mental status examination often is an essential part of the evaluation but also should be directed by a clear understanding of the behaviors. Pharmacologic intervention should occur only after the diagnostic evaluation is complete and behavioral interventions have been considered.

115. Which of the following statements regarding the use of tube feeding in patients with severe dementia is correct?

(A) It does not improve survival.
(B) It protects against aspiration pneumonia.
(C) It promotes the healing of pressure ulcers.
(D) It improves patient comfort.
(E) It improves functional status.

ANSWER: A

There is no evidence that tube feeding leads to a better or longer life in patients with severe dementia. Further, it does not prevent aspiration of oropharyngeal secretions; aspiration pneumonia is the most common complication of tube feeding. Other complications include occlusion, leakage, and local infection. Although no randomized, controlled studies have evaluated tube feeding, data are available from cohort studies, retrospective analyses, and case series. Initiation of tube feeding should be considered in the context of patient values, prognosis, and goals of therapy; continued use should be reevaluated periodically. Surrogate decision makers must be involved in these discussions.

116. Which of the following demographic statements is correct?

(A) The median income for persons aged 65 and over was $16,400 in 1998.
(B) Approximately 45% of women aged 75 to 84 are widowed.
(C) Approximately 55% of women aged 85 and over live alone.
(D) The number of Americans aged 85 and over is expected to quadruple by 2025.
(E) The percentage of older adults with college degrees is expected to increase from 15% to 35% by 2030.

ANSWER: C

About 33% of community-dwelling elderly persons lived alone in 1998. This percentage increases with age, and women are more likely than men to live alone. Almost 60% of women aged 85 and over live alone, compared with 28% of men in the same age group.

Since the early 1960s the overall financial status of elderly persons has improved because of economic growth, the creation of public-benefit programs such as Medicare and Medicaid, and private insurance. The biggest advance was a consequence of Social Security, which began paying benefits in 1940. Incomes are highest among younger, married white Americans and lowest among unmarried Hispanic American women. Although poverty rates have declined, some subgroups, particularly unmarried women aged 85 and over, remain vulnerable. In 1998 households headed by persons aged 65 and over reported a median income of $31,568. Considerable variability among racial and ethnic groups was reported: $32,398 for white Americans, $22,102 for black Americans, and $21,935 for Hispanic Americans. About 10% of elderly persons lived below the poverty level in 1998, although the proportion is much higher for black Americans (26%) and Hispanic Americans (21%). Another 6.8% were classified as near-poor (125% of poverty level).

About 75% of older men but 43% of older women are married. Women are four times more likely to be widowed than men, primarily because of age and sex differences in mortality.

Remarriage rates also differ by gender. The proportion of married persons declines significantly after age 85, to 51% for men and 14% for women. Eight percent of women aged 85 and older are widowed.

Expected alterations in the demographic profile of the United States in the coming decades have major implications for the provision of geriatric care. In 1998, 34.4 million persons aged 65 and over lived in the United States, representing 12.7% of the total population. Demographers project significant increases in both the absolute number of elderly persons and their proportion of the total population. The greatest growth will occur between 2010 and 2030, as the 76 million persons born between 1946 and 1964 (baby-boom generation) ages. The number of persons aged 85 and over (the oldest-old group) is expected to double by 2025 and increase fivefold by 2050.

The level of education of older persons has improved in the past several decades, and improvement is expected to continue. For example, the percentage of persons aged 60 to 70 who earned a high school diploma increased from 28% in 1970 to 67% in 1998. Improvements in educational level likely will have positive effects on health, use of health care, and changes in health habits.

INDEX

Page references followed by *t* and *f* indicate tables and figures, respectively. Those followed by "(q)" indicate pages with questions and critiques.

A

Abandonment, 53*t*
ABC-R (ATP-binding cassette protein of the retina), 170
Abdominal adiposity, 473 (q32)
Abdominal aortic aneurysm, 253
ABI. *See* Ankle-brachial index
Abnormal Involuntary Movement Scale (AIMS), 405–406
Abuse, elder, 53*t*, 485–486 (q52). *See also* Elder mistreatment
  agencies and organizations, 422–423
  psychologic, 54
  risk factors for, 52, 52*t*
Acarbose, 327–328, 328*t*
ACE. *See* Acute Care for Elders
ACE inhibitors. *See* Angiotensin-converting enzyme inhibitors
Acetaminophen (Tylenol)
  for mild pain, 106
  for osteoarthritis, 263
  perioperative, 80
  for persistent pain, 411
  for sleep problems, 207
Acetazolamide, 311*t*
α_1-Acid glycoprotein, 36
Acidosis, renal tubular, 365
Acquired immunodeficiency syndrome (AIDS), 300, 419, 420
Actinic cheilitis, 379
Actinic keratoses, 379, 379*f*
Actinobacillus, 298
Action tremors, 285, 289–290, 290*t*
Activities of daily living (ADLs), 47, 47*t*, 384–385, 459–460 (q9), 473–474 (q33), 504 (q81)
  difficulty of Medicare beneficiaries in, 10, 10*t*
  Instrumental Activities of Daily Living (IADLs), 47, 47*t*, 385, 504 (q81), 516–517 (q103)
  Physical Self-Maintenance Scale (ADLs), 384
Acute care. *See also* Hospital care
  interface with long-term care, 98–99
  multifactorial interventions for falls in, 391
Acute Care for Elders (ACE), 81
Acute confusional state, 127
Acute interstitial nephritis, 359, 363
Acute lumbar sacral strain, 274, 274*t*
Acute mental status change, 127
Acute myeloid leukemia, 355
Acute-phase response, 518 (q106)
Acute renal insufficiency or failure, 360–362
Acute tubular necrosis, 360, 361
Acute vertigo attacks, 158*t*

Acyclovir, 378
Adaptive behavioral difficulties, 241
Adaptive mobility aids, 455 (q1)
Adaptive rehabilitation techniques, 89, 90
Addiction, 108, 235. *See also* Substance abuse
  to opioids, 108
  pseudoaddiction, 108
Adenomas, colonic, 318–319
Adenosine stress echocardiography, 244–245
ADEs. *See* Adverse drug events
Adhesive capsulitis, 490–491 (q59)
Adiposity, abdominal, 473 (q32)
ADLs. *See* Activities of daily living
Adrenal androgens, 324
Adrenal cortex disorders, 324
β-Adrenergic receptor agonists, 303
α-Adrenergic receptor antagonists, 259, 366–367
β-Adrenergic receptor antagonists. *See* β-Blockers
Adrenocorticotropic hormone, 324
ADRs. *See* Adverse drug reactions
Adult day care, 94
Adult foster care, 96
Adult Protective Services (APS), 55–58, 93
Advance care plans, 20, 117, 190. *See also* Advance directives
Advance directives, 21, 23
Adverse drug events (ADEs), 38–39
  drug-disease interactions, 40
  risk factors for, 39, 40*t*
  upper gastrointestinal, 314, 315*t*
Adverse drug reactions (ADRs), 38–39, 511 (q94)
AEDs. *See* Antiepileptic drugs
Aerobic activities, 68
Affective disorders
  and continence, 134–135, 135*t*
  and mental retardation, 240
Age Page, 68
Age-related changes
  in auditory system, 163–164
  in body composition, 182
  in calcium homeostasis, 322, 322*t*
  cardiovascular, 243*t*
  cellular, 3
  in dental pulp, 307, 307*t*
  in drug metabolism, 36
  in energy requirements, 182
  in external auditory canal, 474 (q34)
  in feet, 275
  in female sexuality, 342–343
  in fluid needs, 183
  gastrointestinal, 475 (q35)
  in immune function, 293, 293*t*
  in lower urinary tract, 366
  in macronutrient needs, 182–183

  in male sexuality, 339
  in micturition, 134, 134*t*
  in nutrition, 182–183
  in oral tissues, 307, 307*t*
  in personality, 481–482 (q45)
  in pharmacodynamics, 37–38
  in pharmacokinetics, 35–37
  and pharmacologic treatment of dementia, 118
  in pulmonary physiology, 302
  in renal function, 357
  in salivary glands, 307, 307*t*
  in sleep, 201
  in teeth, 307, 307*t*
Age-related macular degeneration, 169–170, 492 (q62)
Age-related maculopathy, 169–170, 170*f*
Agency for Health Care Policy and Research (AHCPR). *See now* Agency for Healthcare Research and Quality (AHRQ)
  Pressure Ulcers in Adults: Prediction and Prevention, 195
  rehabilitation recommendations for stroke, 87, 87*t*
  Treatment of Pressure Ulcers, 196, 197
Agency for Healthcare Research and Quality (AHRQ), 418
Aggression, 126
Aging, 372, 510–511 (q93)
  agencies and organizations, 418–421
  biology of, 1–7
  cancer biology and, 349–350
  characteristics of, 1
  demographics, 7, 522–523 (q116)
  general principles of, 1–42
  increased prevalence of cancer with, 349–350
  photoaging, 372
  salivary function in, 309–310
  swallowing and, 191–192
  theories of, 1–3, 1*t*
Aging network, 93
Agitation, 117, 222, 522 (q114)
  treatment of, 126
AHRQ. *See* Agency for Healthcare Research and Quality
AIDS (acquired immunodeficiency syndrome), 300, 419, 420
AIMS. *See* Abnormal Involuntary Movement Scale
Air-flow limitation, 303
Albumin, 185, 328
Alcohol, 186*t*, 235–236
Alcohol abuse, 236
Alcohol dependency, 203, 235
Alcohol Use Disorders Identification Test (AUDIT), 237, 495–496 (q66)

Alcoholics Anonymous, 238

Alcoholics Victorious, 238

Alcoholism, 235
brief interventions for, 521 (q113)
and continence, 134–135, 135t
and delirium, 131, 132t
heavy drinking, 235, 517–518 (q105)
and mental health problems, 237
screening for, 60t, 61, 237, 237t, 386,
495–496 (q66)

Alendronate, 179, 179t

Alexithymia, 233

ALFs. *See* Assisted-living facilities

Alginate, 200t

Alkaline phosphatase, 315

Alkalosis, 365

Allopurinol, 264, 311t

Alpha-2U-globulin, 2t

Alpha-B-crystallin, 2t, 5

α-Blockers, 259, 366–367

Alprazolam, 132t

ALS. *See* Amyotrophic lateral sclerosis

Altered mental status, 127 *See also* Delirium

Alternative medicine, 42–45

Alzheimer's disease, 113, 241, 457 (q5), 460
(q10). *See also* Dementia
behavioral management in, 470–471 (q27)
brain imaging with, 116, 116t
deaths due to, 11, 11t
differential diagnosis of, 114–115
epidemiology of, 113–114
genetic factors, 114
genetic testing and, 23
initial stages of, 117
with mental retardation, 240
progression of, 115, 116t
resources, 425
risk factors and protective factors for, 114,
114t
treatment and prevention of, 331

Alzheimer's type dementia, 117
diagnostic criteria for, 115, 115t
mental retardation, 240

Amantadine, 132t, 288, 511 (q94)

Amaurosis fugax, 282

Ambulatory electrocardiographic monitoring,
161–162

American Academy of Family Practitioners,
186

American Academy of Orthopaedic Surgeons,
69t

American Association of Cardiovascular and
Pulmonary Rehabilitation Guidelines
Panel, 69t

American Cancer Society, 368

American College of Chest Physicians, 69t

American College of Physicians, 59, 63

American College of Rheumatology, 69t

American College of Sports Medicine, 66,
66t

American Diabetes Association, 69t, 327,
327t

American Dietetic Association, 186

American Geriatrics Society (AGS)
"Exercise: Feeling Fit for Life," 68
guidelines for research with cognitively
impaired persons as subjects, 22t
recommendations for physical activity, 69t
recommendations for prevention of falls,
391
Website resources, 417

American Heart Association, 251, 299

American Medical Association (AMA), 55

American Medical Directors Association, 99

American Urological Association (AUA),
368, 389

Ametropia, 169

Amiloride, 311t

Aminoglutethimide, 352t

Amitriptyline, 36, 132t, 311t

AML. *See* Acute myeloid leukemia

Amoxicillin, 36, 513 (q97). *See also*
Antibiotics

Amphetamines, 289–290, 290t, 311t

Amphotericin B, 311t

Ampicillin, 36, 311t

Amputation, 88–89
of lower extremity, 31t

Amyloidosis, 357, 359

Amyotrophic lateral sclerosis, 291

Analgesia. *See also* Pain management;
Palliative care
for back pain, 273–274
magnitude of use, 235
nonopioid, 274, 411
opioid, 107, 132t, 412
rescue, 107
three-step ladder, 106, 106f
for vertebral compression fracture, 274

Anastrozole, 352t

Androgen ablation, complete, 371

Androgen deficiency, 333

Androgens, 175–176, 324

Anemia, 345–347

Aneurysms, 253–254

Angina pectoris, 244
screening for, 63t
stable, 245
unstable, 245

Angiodysplasia, colonic, 318

Angioplasty, percutaneous transluminal
coronary, 245, 246, 254

Angiotensin-converting enzyme inhibitors
for acute MI, 246
for congestive heart failure, 248t, 249
drug interactions, 40t
for hypertension, 259
after myocardial infarction, 246
perioperative, 79–80

Angiotensin II type 1 receptor antagonists,
249

Angiotensin receptor antagonists, 259

Anhedonia, 212

Ankle-brachial index, 254

Ankle-strengthening exercises, 518–519
(q107)

Anorexia, 110

Antacids-drug interactions, 186t

Anterior ischemic optic neuropathy, 173

Anterior vaginal repair, 140t, 141

Anthropometrics, 183

Antiandrogens, 352t, 371

Antiarrhythmics, 40t

Antibiotics. *See also specific diseases; specific
drugs*
and delirium, 131, 132t
for endocarditis prophylaxis, 513 (q97)
for infections, 294–295
nutrient interactions, 186t
for posterior blepharitis, 508–509 (q89)
for pressure ulcers, 476–477 (q38)
for prostatitis, 371

Antibodies, monoclonal, 352

Anticholinergics
and delirium, 131, 132t
movement disorders associated with,
289–290, 290t

Anticoagulation, 387–388 *See also*
Coagulation
herbal preparation interactions, 44t
initiation and monitoring of, 388
oral anticoagulants, 387
reversal of, 388
when surgical procedure is planned, 388

Anticonvulsants
and delirium, 131, 132t
for mania, 218
for persistent pain, 411
and risk of osteoporosis, 176t

Antidepressants, 505–506 (q84)
for anxiety disorders, 222–223
and delirium, 131, 132t
for dementia, 119
for depression, 214–217
for depressive and other neuropsychiatric
disturbances in dementia, 124, 124t
drug interactions, 40t
for female sexual dysfunction, 344t
guidelines for selecting, 214–215, 215t
for sleep problems, 206, 206t
tricyclic, 124, 124t, 131, 132t, 215, 215t,
222t, 411

Antidiuretic hormone, 323
inappropriate secretion of, 364

Antiepileptic drugs, 283–284, 284t
movement disorders associated with,
289–290, 290t

Antiestrogens, 352t

Antifungals, imidazole, 36

Antiglomerular basement membrane disease,
361, 362

Antihistamines
for anxiety disorders, 223
and delirium, 131, 132t
for nausea and vomiting, 109–110, 109t

Antiparkinsonian drugs
and delirium, 131, 132t
movement disorders associated with,
289–290, 290t

Antiplatelets, 44t

Antipsychotic medications, 225–226, 226t
  for anxiety disorders, 223
  atypical, 223
  and delirium, 131, 132t
  for dementia, 124, 124t
  drug interactions, 40t
  movement disorders associated with, 289–290, 290t
Antisocial personality disorder
  features of, 228, 229t
  therapeutic strategies for, 230–231, 231t
Anxiety disorders, 220–223, 499 (q72)
  classes of, 220–221, 220t
  and continence, 134–135, 135t
  generalized anxiety disorder, 221, 222, 222t
  and medical disorders, 222
  and mental retardation, 240
  pharmacologic management of, 222–223, 222t
Anxious or fearful behaviors, 228, 229t
Aortic aneurysm, 253
Aortic regurgitation, 251
Aortic stenosis, valvular, 250–251
APACHE III, 19
Apathetic thyrotoxicosis, 321
Apnea, obstructive sleep, 304, 304t
APO-1, 2t
APOE gene, 114
Apoptosis, 6–7
APS. See Adult Protective Services
Arch pain, 278–279
Arginine vasopressin, 364
ARMD. See Age-related macular degeneration
Aromatase inhibitors, 352t
Arrhythmias, 252–253
Arteriovascular disease
  and continence, 134–135, 135t
  lower-extremity, 254
Arteriovenous malformation, 318
Arthritis
  activity recommendations for, 69t
  of foot, 280
  gait findings in, 149, 150t
  glucosamine and chondroitin for, 45, 263
  gout, 263–264, 280
  of knee, 69t, 462–463 (q14)
  osteoarthritis, 69t, 262–263, 280, 462–463 (q14), 506–507 (q86)
  physical activity and, 262
  prevalence of, 261–269
  resources, 424
  rheumatoid, 262, 263
Artificial feeding, 190
Artificial sphincters, 140t, 141
Ascites, 40
Asian Americans, burning mouth syndrome in, 310–311
Aspiration pneumonia, 192
Aspirin therapy, 60t, 63t, 64
  for acute MI, 246
  for angina pectoris and non-Q-wave MI, 245
  for atrial fibrillation, 253

for mild pain, 107
for peripheral vascular disease, 254
preventive, 80, 246, 282, 387, 485 (q51)
Assessment, 47–51. See also Screening
  cognitive, 48–49
  comprehensive geriatric assessment, 40
  in elder mistreatment, 53–54, 55, 56f
  financial, 54
  genetic testing, 23
  home, 462 (q13)
  home care, 91–92
  of hospitalized patients, 75–78, 75t
  nutrition, 183–186
  Outcome and Assessment Information Set (OASIS), 84, 91
  physical, 47–48, 53–54
  psychologic, 49, 54
  and rehabilitation planning, 86
  social, 49
  systematic, 75–78, 75t
Assisted-living facilities (ALFs), 9, 95, 484 (q50)
  multifactorial interventions for falls in, 391
Assistive devices, 89, 90, 473 (q31)
  for prevention of falls, 392
Assistive listening devices, 168
Asthma, 302–303
Asthmatic COPD, 303
Astigmatism, 169
At-risk drinking, 236–237
Atherosclerotic vascular disease, 254
ATP-binding cassette protein of the retina (ABC-R), 170
Atrial fibrillation, 247, 253
  in hospitalized patients, 75, 75t, 76
  oral anticoagulation for, 387
Atrophic vaginitis, 515–516 (q101)
Atrophy
  multisystem, 134–135, 135t
  urogenital, 335, 335f
  vulvovaginal, 335, 335f
Attending physicians, 99, 99t
Audiograms, 164, 165f
Audioscopy, 463 (q15)
AUDIT. See Alcohol Use Disorders Identification Test
Auditory system changes, 163–164
Autistic traits, 240
Autoimmune thrombocytopenia, 347
Autolytic debridement, 198, 199t
Autonomy, 22–23, 493–494 (q63)
Aventyl, 411. See also Nortriptyline
Average length of stay, 11, 486 (q53)
Avinza, 412. See also Morphine
Avoidant personality disorder
  features of, 228, 229t
  therapeutic strategies for, 230–231, 231t
Axillary lymphadenectomy, 354
Azathioprine, 311t
  for polymyositis and dermatomyositis, 269
  for rheumatoid arthritis, 266
  for systemic lupus erythematosus, 268
Azotemia, 365

B

B-Myb, 2t, 5
Back pain, 270–274, 511–512 (q95)
  causes of, 270–272, 270t, 271t
  management of, 273–274, 274t
Baclofen (Lioresal), 311t, 411
Bacteremia, 295
Bacteriuria, asymptomatic, 296–297
Balance exercises, 518–519 (q107)
Balance testing, 48, 407–408
Balance training, 68
Balanced Budget Act of 1997 (BBA 97), 33–34, 91
Balanced Budget Revision Act of 1999, 34, 91
Barbiturates, 131, 132t
BARD1, 2t, 5
Barium enema, 59–60, 60t
Basal cell carcinoma, 379–380, 380f, 500–501 (q75)
Basal energy expenditure, 182, 183t
Bathing, 208
bcl-2, 2t, 6
Bedsores. See Pressure ulcers
Behavior(s)
  anxious or fearful, 228, 229t
  dramatic, emotional, or erratic, 228, 229t
  healthy, 17
  maladaptive, 241
  odd or eccentric, 228, 229t
Behavioral disorders. See also Personality disorders
  in dementia, 121–126, 121t
  in mental retardation, 241
  REM sleep behavior disorder, 204
Behavioral management, 470–471 (q27)
Behavioral treatment
  for incontinence, 137, 139t, 141, 403–404
  for prevention of falls, 392
Bell's palsy, 300
Beneficence, 21, 493–494 (q63)
Benign paroxysmal positional dizziness, 513–514 (q98)
Benign positional vertigo, 153
  Epley's maneuver for, 154f, 155f
  management of, 158t
Benign prostatic hyperplasia, 366–367, 467 (q21), 488–489 (q57)
  International Prostate Symptom Score, 389
Benzodiazepines, 468–469 (q23), 501 (q76)
  for anxiety disorders, 222t, 223
  chronic use of, 206–207
  and delirium, 131, 132t
  for depression, 215
  drug interactions, 40t
  magnitude of use, 235
  for sleep problems, 205–206, 206t
Benztropine, 132t
Bereavement, 213, 458 (q6)
Best interest standard, 21
β-Blockers
  for acute MI, 246
  for atrial fibrillation, 253

for congestive heart failure, 248*t*, 249–250
for hypertension, 258–259
after myocardial infarction, 246
for stable angina pectoris, 245
for unstable angina pectoris and
non-Q-wave MI, 245
for ventricular arrhythmias, 252
β-Lactam, 295
β-Lactamase, 295
Betamethasone, 264
Bextra (valdecoxib), 411
Bicalutamide, 352*t*
Biguanides, 327–328, 328*t*
Biliary disease, 315
Bioavailability, 35
Biofeedback, 139*t*, 141
Biologic therapy, 352–353
Biology
of aging, 1–7
of cancer, 349–350
Biotin, 185*t*
Bipolar disorder, 212, 240
Bisoprolol, 249
Bisphosphonates, 179–180, 179*t*
Black Americans
causes of death, 11
congestive heart failure in, 247
intracerebral hemorrhage in, 282
life expectancy, 7–8, 8*t*
perceived health of, 10, 10*t*
poverty rates, 8
pressure ulcers in, 194
Bladder, overactive, 135–136
Bladder training, 137, 139*t*, 141, 403
Bladder urge control procedure, 404
Bleeding, 347–348
intracerebral hemorrhage, 282
occult gastrointestinal, 317–318
postmenopausal vaginal, 338–339
Bleomycin, 311*t*, 356
Blepharitis, 508–509 (q89)
Blepharochalasis, 173
Blepharoptosis, 173
Blindness, transient monocular, 282
Blood cultures of pressure ulcers, 476–477
(q38)
Blood glucose levels, 63*t*
Blood pressure. *See also* Hypertension;
Hypotension
classification of, 256, 256*t*
control in diabetes mellitus, 328
screening, 60*t*
transient decreases in, 159
Blood testing, fecal occult, 59, 60*t*
Blood urea nitrogen, 361
BMD. *See* Bone mineral density
BMI. *See* Body mass index
Body composition, 182
Body dysmorphic disorder, 232, 232*t*
Body mass index (BMI), 48, 183
Body size classification, 183, 185*t*
Body weight
and energy needs, 182, 183*t*
and protein needs, 182, 183*t*

Bone, Paget's disease of, 176*t*, 323
Bone formation, 176
Bone infections, 299
Bone loss, 174–175. *See also* Osteomalacia;
Osteoporosis
Bone mass measurement, 177
Bone mineral density, 174, 494–495 (q65)
Bone mineral density testing, 63*t*, 177
indications for, 177, 177*t*
Bone remodeling, 174
Bone turnover, 174, 177
Borderline personality disorder
features of, 228, 229*t*
therapeutic strategies for, 230–231, 231*t*
Bordetella pertussis infection, 302
Borrelia burgdorferi, 300
BPH. *See* Benign prostatic hyperplasia
BPV. *See* Benign positional vertigo
Brachytherapy, 370
Braden Scale for Predicting Pressure Sore
Risk, 195, 413–414
Bradykinesia, 286
Brain disease, structural, 213
Brain imaging techniques, 116, 116*t*
brca1, 2*t*
BRCA1-associated RING domain 1
(BARD1), 2*t*, 5
Breast cancer, 354
characteristics of, 350
and estrogen replacement therapy, 331
hormonal therapy for, 352, 352*t*
metastatic, 354
screening for, 59, 60*t*, 494 (q64)
Breast cancer 1 (*brca1*) gene, 2*t*
British Geriatrics Society, 69*t*
Bromocriptine, 288
Bronchodilator inhalers, 289–290, 290*t*
"Brown-bag" pharmacotherapy evaluation, 41
Bruce treadmill protocol, 244
Bulking injections, periurethral, 140*t*, 141
Bullous pemphigoid, 374–375, 374*f*
Bunions, 278
Bupropion
for dementia, 124, 124*t*
for depression, 215*t*, 216
Burning mouth syndrome, 310–311
Burns, 60*t*
Buspirone, 222*t*, 223
Butyrophenones, 109–110, 109*t*
Bypass graft surgery, coronary artery, 245,
289*t*

C

C-reactive protein, 265
Cachexia, 110, 187
CAGE Questionnaire, 237, 237*t*, 495–496
(q66)
Calcaneal spurs, 276*t*, 278–279
Calcitonin, 179*t*, 180
Calcium
disorders of metabolism of, 322–323
drug interactions, 186*t*

homeostasis, 322, 322*t*
intake, 60*t*
in osteoporosis prevention and treatment,
176*t*, 178
recommended daily allowances, 185*t*
Calcium channel blockers
for congestive heart failure, 248*t*, 250
drug interactions, 40*t*
for hypertension, 258
movement disorders associated with,
289–290, 290*t*
for stable angina pectoris, 245
Calcium deficiency, 175
Calcium pyrophosphate dihydrate (CPPD)
crystals, 264
Caloric requirements, 500 (q74)
CAM. *See* Complementary and alternative
therapies; Confusion Assessment Method
Canadian Task Force, 59, 62
Canadian Task Force on the Periodic Health
Examination, 368
Cancer
basal cell carcinoma, 379–380, 380*f*,
500–501 (q75)
biology of, 349–350
breast, 59, 60*t*, 331, 350, 352, 352*t*, 354,
494 (q64)
cervical, 60, 60*t*
characteristics of, 350
colon, 63*t*, 318–319, 355, 491–492 (q61)
colorectal cancer, 59–60, 60*t*
endometrial, 331–332, 352, 352*t*
esophageal, 314
general considerations for, 356*t*
heavy drinking and, 517–518 (q105)
lung, 354–355
management of, 350–354, 356, 356*t*
neuropsychiatric complications of, 491–492
(q61)
oral, 60*t*, 310
prostate, 63, 63*t*, 352, 352*t*, 367–371
quality-of-life issues, 353–354
recommended preventive services for, 60*t*
resources, 423
screening for, 351
skin, 63–64, 63*t*, 427, 500–501 (q75)
squamous cell carcinoma, 310, 379
thyroid, 322
of vulva, 336
Candidiasis, 378, 519 (q108)
oral, 310
between toes, 374, 374*f*
Canes, 89
Capitation structures, 24–25, 34
Capsulotomy, 169
Captopril, 311*t*
Carbamazepine (Tegretol), 311*t*
for epilepsy, 284*t*
for mania, 218
for mood disturbances in dementia, 125
for persistent pain, 411
Carbidopa. *See* Levodopa-carbidopa
Cardiac asthma, 302
Cardiac disorders. *See specific disorders*
Cardiobacterium, 298

Cardiomyopathy, 387
Cardiovascular diseases and disorders,
243–355. *See also* specific disorders
activity recommendations for, 69*t*
and continence, 134–135, 135*t*
prevention of, 330–331
resources, 424
Cardiovascular system changes, 243*t*
Caregivers, 509–510 (q91)
communication with, 117–118
resources, 421
risk factors, 52, 52*t*
support for, 92
Caregiving, 13, 52, 52*t*
Carotid endarterectomy, 282
Carotid stenosis, 282
Carvedilol, 250
Case management, 55, 57*f*, 93
Caspase-1, 2*t*
Caspase-2, 2*t*
Caspase-3, 2*t*
Cataracts, 169
Catechol-*O*-methyltransferase inhibitors, 288
Catheters, urinary, 141–142
Cationic drugs, 36
CCAs. *See* Calcium channel blockers
CCRCs. *See* Continuing care retirement
communities
CD28, 2*t*
CD95, 2*t*
CD152, 2*t*
CD154, 2*t*
CDC25B, 2*t*, 5
Cefotaxime, 295
Ceftriaxone, 36, 295
Celebrex, 411. *See also* Celecoxib
Celecoxib (Celebrex), 266, 411
Cell death, 6–7
Cellular changes, 3
Cellular defense mechanisms, 5–6
Cellulitis, 197*t*, 476–477 (q38)
Centenarians, 8, 490 (q58)
Centers for Disease Control and Prevention
(CDC), 66, 66*t*
Centers for Medicare & Medicaid Services
(CMS), 25, 27, 84, 472 (q29)
average adjusted per capita cost for FFS
Medicare beneficiaries, 34
capitation payments, 34
demonstration projects, 34
Web site, 28, 29, 34
Central nervous system medications, 235
Cephalosporin, 295
Cerebellar ataxia, 149–150, 150*t*
Cerebrovascular diseases, 281–283, 482
(q46)
deaths due to, 11, 11*t*
effects on continence, 134–135, 135*t*
gait findings in, 150–151, 150*t*
Cerumen impaction, 474 (q34)
Cervical cancer screening, 60, 60*t*
CGA. *See* Comprehensive geriatric assessment
Charles Bonnet syndrome, 227

Chemoprophylaxis, 64
potentially beneficial services lacking
evidence, 63*t*
recommended services, 60*t*, 62
Chemosensory perception, 311
Chemotherapy, 351–352, 351*t*
Chemstrip Micral, 358
Chinese Americans, intracerebral hemorrhage
in, 282
Chlamydia trachomatis, 371
Chloral hydrate, 132*t*, 206
Chlordiazepoxide, 132*t*
Chlorpheniramine maleate, 311*t*
Cholecalciferol (vitamin D₃), 175, 181
Cholesterol, 185. *See also* Hypercholesteremia
activity recommendations for, 69*t*
high-density lipoprotein (HDL), 243–244
low-density lipoprotein (LDL), 243, 328
Cholestyramine, 110
Choline, 185*t*
Choline magnesium trisalicylate (Tricosal,
Trilisate), 411
Cholinesterase inhibitors, 118–119
Chondrocalcinosis, 264
Chondroitin, glucosamine with, 45, 263
Chorea, 289–290, 289*t*, 290*t*
Choroidal neovascularization, 170, 170*f*
Chronic disease, anemia of, 346–347
Chronic lymphocytic leukemia, 355
Chronic obstructive pulmonary disease
(COPD), 303–304, 499–500 (q73)
activity recommendations for, 69*t*
deaths due to, 11, 11*t*
recommended preventive services for, 60*t*
Ciclopirox, 277
Ciprofloxacin
and delirium, 132*t*
for diverticulitis, 317
Circulation
age-related changes that affect, 243*t*
resources, 424
Citalopram
for depression, 215*t*, 216
for depressive and other neuropsychiatric
disturbances in dementia, 124, 124*t*
Claw toes, 278
Cleansing agents, 483 (q48)
CLL. *See* Chronic lymphocytic leukemia
Clonal senescence, 3
Clonazepam (Klonopin), 411
Clopidogrel
for acute MI, 246
for peripheral vascular disease, 254
for prevention of stroke, 282
for unstable angina pectoris and
non-Q-wave MI, 245
Clostridium difficile colitis, 301
Clotting factor deficiency, 348
Clozapine, 225–226, 226*t*
and delirium, 132*t*
for dementia, 124, 124*t*
for Parkinson's disease and hallucinations,
227
Clubbing, 304

Coagulation, 347–348. *See also*
Anticoagulation
Cochlear implants, 168
Cockroft and Gault equation, 37
Codeine, 107, 311*t*
Cognitive assessment, 48–49
Cognitive behavior therapy
for depression, 214
for pain management, 106
for sleep problems, 207–208, 208*t*
for somatoform disorders, 234
Cognitive enhancers, 117, 119
Cognitive impairment, 457 (q5). *See also*
Alzheimer's disease; Dementia
AGS guidelines for research with
cognitively impaired persons as
subjects, 22*t*
in hospitalized patients, 75*t*, 76–77
pain assessment in persons with, 108–109
resources, 425
treatment and prevention of, 331
Colchicine, 311*t*
for gout, 264
nutrient interactions, 186*t*
for pseudogout, 264
Colitis, 301
Collaborative practice agreements, 102
Colon cancer, 318–319, 355, 491–492 (q61)
prevention of, 63*t*
screening for, 59–60, 60*t*
Colon diseases and disorders, 315–319
Colonic angiodysplasia, 318
Colonic polyps, 318–319
Colonoscopy, 59, 60*t*, 319
"virtual," 60
Colorectal cancer. *See also* Colon cancer
screening for, 59–60, 60*t*
Colporrhaphy, 140*t*, 141
Communication
about dementia, 117–118
about physical activity, 70, 71*f*
of bad news, 103–104
clinician–patient, 50–51
with family and caregivers, 117–118
with hearing-impaired persons, 167, 167*t*
with nursing-home population, 97
strategies to enhance, 50–51, 51*t*, 167,
167*t*
Community-acquired pneumonia, 295, 296*f*
Community-based care, 91–96
Community-dwelling older persons, 391
Competence, 20
Complementary and alternative medicine
(CAM). *See* Complementary and
alternative therapies
Complementary and alternative therapies,
42–45
Complementary medicine, 42. *See also*
Complementary and alternative therapies
Comprehensive geriatric assessment, 40
Compression fractures, vertebral, 271*t*, 272
management of, 274, 274*t*
Conflicts of interest, 24

Confusion Assessment Method (CAM), 127–128, 128*t*

Confusional state, acute, 127

Confusional State Evaluation, 128

Congestive heart failure, 246–250, 480–481 (q43)
  and continence, 134–135, 135*t*
  drug treatment of, 248, 248*t*

Consent, informed, for research, 22

Conservative management, 370

Conservatorships, 21

Constipation, 109, 315–316

Continuing care retirement communities (CCRCs), 96

Conversion disorder, 232, 232*t*

Coombs' serum test, 346

COPD. *See* Chronic obstructive pulmonary disease

Coping strategies, 15

Copper-drug interaction, 186*t*

Corns, 278

Coronary angiography, 244

Coronary angioplasty, percutaneous transluminal, 245, 246, 254

Coronary artery bypass graft (CABG) surgery, 245, 289*t*

Coronary artery disease, 243–245
  exercise and, 505 (q83)
  recommended preventive services for, 60*t*
  rehabilitation care for, 85, 85*t*
  screening for, 60*t*

Coronary revascularization, 245

Corticosteroids
  for COPD, 303–304
  for giant cell arteritis, 266
  for idiopathic pulmonary fibrosis, 304
  for intertrigo, 374
  movement disorders associated with, 289–290, 290*t*
  for persistent pain, 411
  for polymyositis and dermatomyositis, 269
  for pseudogout, 264
  for psoriasis, 303, 304
  for rheumatoid arthritis, 266
  for systemic lupus erythematosus, 268
  for vulvar lesions, 336

Costs
  of complementary and alternative therapies, 43
  of health care, 26–35, 66
  of home-health care, 32
  of hospice care, 33
  of inpatient care, 30–31
  of nursing-home care, 32–33
  of outpatient care, 26–30
  of postacute rehabilitation, 31–32
  of skilled nursing care, 460–461 (q11)

Cough in terminal illness, 112

Counseling, 60*t*, 61
  about physical activity, 70, 71*f*

COX-2, 5

COX-2 inhibitors
  for gastrointestinal complications, 314
  for mild pain, 107

for osteoarthritis, 263
  renal diseases associated with, 363
  for rheumatoid arthritis, 266

CPP32, 2*t*, 6

CPPD (calcium pyrophosphate dihydrate) crystals, 264

Creatinine, 357, 361

Creatinine clearance (CrCl), 37, 357, 358

Credé's maneuver, 140, 141

Crescentic glomerulonephritis, 359, 361

Crutches, 89

Cruzan v. Director, Department of Health of Missouri, 18

Crystal-induced acute renal failure, 464 (q16)

CTLA-4. *See* CD152

Cushing's disease, 176*t*

Cutaneous horn, 379

Cyanocobalamin, 36

Cyclins, 2*t*, 4–5

Cyclophosphamide
  for non-Hodgkin's lymphoma, 355
  for rheumatoid arthritis, 266
  for systemic lupus erythematosus, 268

Cyclosporine
  for psoriasis, 376
  for rheumatoid arthritis, 267
  and risk of osteoporosis, 176*t*

Cystic erosion, 276*t*

Cystometry, 488–489 (q57)

Cytochrome P-450 2D6, 40

Cytochrome P-450 3A4, 39–40

D

D-dimer, 347

D-Penicillamine, 311*t*

Dacarbazine, 356

daf-2, 2*t*, 6

Dapsone, 268

Day care, adult, 94

Day hospitals, 94

DDIs. *See* Drug-drug interactions

Death
  ability to predict time of, 19
  causes of, 11, 11*t*
  interventions that may hasten, 18–19

Debridement, 198, 199*t*

Decision making
  about institutionalization, 93
  end-of-life, 18–19, 493–494 (q63)
  principles for patients who lack decisional capacity, 20–21
  role of incapacitated patient in, 21
  strategies for incapacitated patients, 20

Decisional capacity, lack of, 19–22

Deconditioning, 520 (q111)

Decubitus ulcers, 194. *See also* Pressure ulcers

Deep-vein thrombosis, 254, 387

Deep venous insufficiency, 254–255

Degenerative spinal stenosis, 497 (q68)

Deglutition examination, videofluoroscopic, 192

Dehydration, hypertonic, 364–365

Dehydroepiandrosterone, 324

Delirium, 127–133
  diagnosis of, 127–128, 128*t*
  drug-associated, 461–462 (q12)
  drugs to reduce or eliminate in, 131, 132*t*
  DSM-IV diagnostic criteria for, 127*t*
  effects on continence, 134–135, 135*t*
  geriatric syndrome management model of, 74
  in hospitalized patients, 77, 498–499 (q71)
  palliation of, 110
  postoperative, 130, 466–467 (q20), 471–472 (q28), 501 (q76)
  prevention of, 133, 498–499 (q71), 501 (q76)
  psychotic symptoms in, 226
  risk factors for, 129, 129*t*
  screening for, 486 (q53)

Delirium Rating Scale, 128

Delirium Severity Scale, 128

Deltasone, 411. *See also* Prednisone

Delusions, 470–471 (q27)
  in dementia, 125
  evaluation of, 224, 225*f*
  mood congruent, 226
  treatment of, 125

Dementia, 113–120, 471–472 (q28). *See also* Alzheimer's disease
  aggression in, 126
  agitation in, 117, 126, 222
  Alzheimer's type, 115, 115*t*, 117, 240
  anxiety in, 222
  assessment of, 116–117, 116*t*
  behavioral disturbances in, 121–126, 121*t*
  brain imaging with, 116, 116*t*
  changes in sleep with, 204
  delusions in, 125
  depression in, 124, 124*t*
  drug interactions, 40
  effects on continence, 134–135, 135*t*
  ethical issues in, 22–23
  hallucinations in, 125
  hypersexuality in, 125
  with Lewy bodies, 114, 117, 517 (q104)
  in mental retardation, 240, 241
  mood disturbances in, 124–125
  neuropsychiatric disturbances in, 121–126, 121*t*, 122*f*
  psychotic disturbances in, 125, 226
  reversible, 127
  screening for, 63*t*
  sleep disturbances in, 125
  sundowning in, 119, 120*t*
  symptoms of, 113, 113*t*
  tube feeding in, 522 (q115)

Demographics, 7–12, 522–523 (q116)

Dental anatomy, 308*f*

Dental care counseling, 60*t*, 61

Dental caries, 307–308

Dental pulp changes, 307, 307*t*

Dental resources, 423

Dentistry, restorative, 503 (q80)

Dentures, 309

Dependency
  alcohol, 203, 235
  drug, 203, 235. *See also* Substance abuse

opioid, 108
prevention of, 65
Dependent personality disorder
   features of, 228, 229*t*
   therapeutic strategies for, 230–231, 231*t*
Depression, 211–219
   brain imaging with, 116, 116*t*
   in dementia, 124, 124*t*
   diagnosis of, 211–212, 212*t*
   differential diagnosis of, 115, 212–213
   drugs for, 124, 124*t*
   DSM-IV diagnostic criteria for, 211*t*
   Geriatric Depression Scale (short form,
      GDS), 390
   in hospitalized patients, 75*t*, 77–78
   and hypochondriasis, 482–483 (q47)
   major, 505–506 (q84)
   major depressive disorder, 458 (q6)
   with mental retardation, 240
   mixed anxiety and, 222
   with obsessive-compulsive disorder,
      468–469 (q23)
   outcomes of, 213*t*
   palliation of, 110–111
   with parkinsonism, 287
   prevalence of, 211, 487–488 (q55)
   prognostic factors, 502 (q77)
   screening for, 49, 60*t*, 61, 63, 63*t*, 402
   vascular or executive dysfunction, 213
Depression questionnaire, 60*t*, 63*t*
Depressive personality disorder
   features of, 228, 229*t*
   therapeutic strategies for, 230–231, 231*t*
Depth shoe, 280
Dermatitis
   neurodermatitis, 373–374
   seborrheic, 372–373
Dermatologic diseases and disorders,
   372–381, 427
Dermatomyositis, 268–269
Desipramine (Norpramin)
   for depressive and other neuropsychiatric
      disturbances in dementia, 124, 124*t*
   distribution of, 36
   indications for, 215*t*
   for persistent pain, 411
Desmoplakin, 375
DETERMINE Your Nutritional Health
   Checklist, 186, 410
Detoxification, 238
Detrusor hyperactivity with impaired
   contractility, 136, 140
Detrusor overactivity, 135–136, 141
Developmental disabilities, 505–506 (q84)
Dexamethasone, 109–110, 109*t*, 311*t*
Dextroamphetamine, 107
DHEA. *See* Dehydroepiandrosterone
DHIC. *See* Detrusor hyperactivity with
   impaired contractility
Di Guglielmo's syndrome, 346
Diabetes mellitus, 326–328
   activity recommendations for, 69*t*
   complications of, 63, 63*t*, 490–491 (q59)
   and continence, 134–135, 135*t*
   deaths due to, 11, 11*t*

diagnosis of, 326–327, 498 (q70)
   and exercise, 473 (q32)
   foot problems in, 279–280
   glucose control in, 473 (q32)
   and macular degeneration, 491–492 (q61)
   management of, 327–328, 327*t*
   and pressure ulcers, 467–468 (q22)
   rehabilitation care for, 85, 85*t*
   resources, 423
   screening for, 63, 63*t*, 470 (q26)
   type 2, 327–328, 327*t*, 328*t*
   and urinary incontinence, 496 (q67)
Diabetic retinopathy, 170–171, 172*f*
*Diagnostic and Statistical Manual of Mental
   Disorders (DSM-IV)*
   diagnostic criteria for delirium, 127*t*
   diagnostic criteria for depression, 211*t*
   types of anxiety disorders, 220–221, 220*t*
Dialysis, renal, 363–364
Diarrhea
   infectious, 300–301
   palliation of, 110
Diazepam, 36, 132*t*
Diazoxide, 311*t*
Dietary counseling, 60*t*, 61
Dietary Guidelines for Americans, 183
Dietary interventions, 327, 500 (q74). *See
   also* Malnutrition
Diethylstilbestrol, 352*t*
Digestive problems. *See also* Gastrointestinal
   diseases and disorders
   resources, 423
Digital rectal examination, 63*t*, 368
Digitalis, 40*t*
Digiti flexus, 275, 276*t*
Digiti quinti varus, 276*t*
Digoxin
   for atrial fibrillation, 253
   for congestive heart failure, 248*t*, 250
   distribution of, 36
   herbal preparation interactions, 44*t*
   nutrient interactions, 186*t*
   toxicity, 461–462 (q12)
Dilaudid, 412. *See also* Hydromorphone
Diltiazem, 311*t*
Diphenhydramine, 132*t*, 509 (q90)
Dipyridamole, 311*t*
Disability
   excess, with substance use, 236–237
   in hospitalized patients, 75*t*, 78
   *International Classification of Impairments,
      Disabilities, and Handicaps*
      (ICIDH-2), 82–83, 82*f*
   screening for, 402
   trends in, 11
Disalcid, 411. *See also* Salsalate
Disc disease
   herniated nucleus pulposus, 271–272
   lumbar degenerative, 271*t*, 272
Discharge planning, 31, 31*t*, 480–481 (q43)
Discounted FFS, 29
Disequilibrium, 153, 156, 482 (q46)
   management of, 158*t*
Dissections, peripheral arterial, 253–254

Diuretics
   for congestive heart failure, 248–249, 248*t*
   drug interactions, 40*t*
   herbal preparation interactions, 44*t*
   for hypertension, 258
   nutrient interactions, 186*t*
Divalproex (valproic acid), 125, 218
Diverticular disease, 317
Diverticulitis, 317
Diverticulosis, 317
Dix-Hallpike test, 151, 157
Dizziness, 153–158. *See also* Syncope
   evaluation of, 156–157, 156*t*
   management of, 157–158, 158*t*
   psychogenic, 158*t*
DNA
   HSF1 binding, 6
   mitochondrial (mtDNA), 2, 4
   mutations or deletions, 3–4
DO. *See* Detrusor overactivity
"Dobutamine holiday," 19
Dobutamine stress echocardiography,
   244–245
Domperidone, 109–110, 109*t*
Donepezil, 118–119
Dopamine agonists
   and delirium, 132*t*
   movement disorders associated with,
      289–290, 290*t*
   for Parkinson's disease, 288
Dopamine replacement therapy, 289, 289*t*
Double effect, rule of, 18
Down syndrome, 240, 241, 242
Doxepin, 132*t*
Doxorubicin, 311*t*
   for Hodgkin's disease, 356
   for non-Hodgkin's lymphoma, 355
Dramatic, emotional, or erratic behaviors,
   228, 229*t*
Dressings, pressure ulcer, 198–199, 200*t*,
   465 (q18)
Drinking. *See also* Alcoholism
   at-risk, 236–237
   heavy, 235, 517–518 (q105)
Drinking Problems Index, 237
Driving, 25, 40
Drosophila, 6
Drug dependency, 235. *See also* Substance
   abuse
   opioid, 108
   prevention of, 65
   and sleep, 203
Drug-disease interactions, 40
Drug-drug interactions (DDIs), 39–40, 40*t*
Drug-induced movement disorders, 289–290
Drug-nutrient interactions, 185, 186*t*
Drug-related syncope, 502–503 (q79)
Drug use, 75*t*, 78, 235
Drugs. *See also* Pharmacotherapy; *specific
   drugs*
   absorption of, 35–36
   adverse drug events (ADEs), 38–39, 40*t*

adverse drug reactions (ADRs), 38, 511
    (q94)
  antiepileptic, 283–284, 284*t*
  antipsychotic, 225–226, 226*t*
  associated with chorea, 289*t*
  cationic, 36
  clearance of, 37
  delirium associated with, 461–462 (q12)
  distribution of, 36
  elimination of, 37
  and falls, 502 (q78)
  half-life of, 37
  herbal preparation interactions, 44*t*
  hydrophilic, 36
  lipophilic, 36
  metabolism of, 36
  movement disorders associated with,
      289–290, 290*t*
  psychotropic, 472 (q29)
  that increase risk of osteoporosis, 176*t*
  that interfere with gustation (taste), 311,
      311*t*
  that interfere with olfaction (smell), 311,
      311*t*
  trends in prescription drugs, 12
Dry eye syndrome, 173
Dry mouth, 309–310
*DSM-IV. See Diagnostic and Statistical
    Manual of Mental Disorders*
Duragesic (transdermal fentanyl), 412
Dynamic Gait Index, 148
Dysergastic reaction, 127
Dyslipidemia screening, 61
Dyspareunia, 343, 344
Dyspepsia, 314
Dysphagia, 191
  esophageal, 312
  oropharyngeal, 192, 312
Dysphoria, 458 (q6)
Dyspnea, 244, 302, 499–500 (q73)
  palliation of, 111–112
Dystonia, drug-induced, 289–290, 290*t*
Dystrophy
  onychodystrophy, 275
  Sorsby's fundus, 170
  vulvar, 336

E

Eating problems, 191–193
Eccentric behaviors, 228, 229*t*
Echocardiography, 244
  for aortic regurgitation, 251
  exercise, 244–245
  stress, 244–245
  for syncope, 162
  transthoracic, 299
Eczema craquelé, 373, 374*f*
Edentulism, 60*t*, 308–309
Education
  agencies and organizations, 422
  for prevention of falls, 392
Eikenella, 298
Elder mistreatment, 52–58, 469–470 (q25),
    485–486 (q52)
  agencies and organizations, 422–423

assessment for, 55, 56*f*
  case management in, 55, 57*f*
  in hospitalized patients, 75*t*, 78
  intervention in, 55, 57*f*
  risk factors for, 52, 52*t*
  signs that raise suspicion for, 53, 53*t*
Eldercare Locator, 93
Electrical stimulation, 139*t*, 141
Electrocardiography
  ambulatory monitoring, 161–162
  in Q-wave MI, 244
  in syncope, 161
Electroconvulsive therapy, 504–505 (q82)
  for depression, 215*t*, 217
  for mania, 218–219
Electrolyte balance, 323–324
Electrolyte disturbances, 364–365
Electronystagmography, 157
Electrophysiologic studies, 162
Elimination of drugs, 37
EM. *See* Elder mistreatment
E&M codes. *See* Evaluation and management
    codes
Embolism, systemic, 387
Emergencies and urgencies, hypertensive, 260
Emmetropia, 169
Emory Functional Ambulation Profile, 148
Emotional or erratic behaviors, 228, 229*t*
Emphysema, 303–304
Enalapril, 311*t*
Encephalopathy, toxic or metabolic, 127
End-of-life care, 478 (q40), 479 (q41). *See
    also* Hospice care, Palliative care
  agencies and organizations, 421–422
  decisions, 18–19, 493–494 (q63)
End-stage renal disease, 363–364
Endocarditis, infective, 298–299, 513 (q97)
Endocrine disorders, 319–329
Endometrial cancer
  and estrogen replacement therapy,
      331–332
  hormonal therapy for, 352, 352*t*
Endoscopic retrograde
      cholangiopancreatography, 315
Endoscopic ultrasonography, 315
Endoscopy, esophageal, 313, 314
Energy requirements
  age-related changes in, 182
  estimation of, 182, 183*t*
Enoxaparin, 80
Ensure HP, 193*t*
Ensure Plus HN, 193*t*
Enteral nutrition, 189
Entrapment syndrome, 275, 276*t*
Environmental assessment, 78
Environmental hazards, 520–521 (q112)
Environmental modifications
  for dementia, 118
  for prevention of falls, 392
  for rehabilitation, 89–90
Enzymatic debridement, 198, 199*t*

Epilepsy, 283–284
  antiepileptic therapy for, 283–284, 284*t*
  resources, 425
Epley's maneuver, 154*f*, 155*f*, 513–514
    (q98)
Erectile dysfunction, 339–340
  evaluation of, 340–341
  treatment of, 341–342, 343*t*
Erikson's theory of stages development, 16
Erratic behaviors, 228, 229*t*
Erythema, persistent, 194
Erythrocyte sedimentation rate, 262, 265
Erythromycin, 36
Erythroplakia, 310
Erythropoiesis, ineffective, 346
Escherichia coli, 300–301
Esophageal cancer, 314
Esophageal dysmotility, 191
Esophageal dysphagia, 191, 312
Esophageal foreign body, 481 (q44)
Esophageal injury, drug-induced, 313–314
Esophagus, 312–314
Essential tremor, 285–286
Estazolam, 205, 206*t*
Estradiol valerate, 329–330, 330*t*
Estrogen-androgen replacement, 344
Estrogen deficiency, 175, 515–516 (q101)
Estrogen-progesterone combinations,
    329–330, 330*t*, 331
Estrogen replacement therapy, 289*t*, 329
  adverse effects of, 332
  and breast cancer, 331
  for cancer, 352*t*
  for cardiovascular disease, 330–331
  for cognitive disorders, 331
  continuing, 332
  contraindications to, 332
  and endometrial cancer, 331–332
  for female sexual dysfunction, 343, 344,
      344*t*
  indications for, 332
  for lichen planus, 336
  movement disorders associated with,
      289–290, 290*t*
  for osteoporosis, 60*t*, 178, 329–330, 330*t*
  preparations and dosages, 330, 330*t*
  regimens, 332
  for urinary incontinence, 139*t*, 141
Etanercept, 267
Ethacrynic acid, 311*t*
Ethambutol hydrochloride, 311*t*
Ethanol, 36
Ethical issues, 18–25, 493–494 (q63)
  in home care, 93
  in malnutrition, 189–190
Etidronate, 179*t*, 180, 311*t*
Euthanasia, 18–19
Evaluation and management (E&M) codes,
    29, 30*t*
Executive dysfunction depression, 213
Exercise(s). *See also* Physical activity
  ankle-strengthening, 518–519 (q107)
  for back pain, 511–512 (q95)
  balance, 518–519 (q107)

benefits of, 473 (q32), 505 (q83)
definition of, 65
functionally based, 473–474 (q33)
for glucose control, 473 (q32)
group exercise programs, 519 (q109)
for hypertension with obesity, 519–520 (q110)
to improve sleep, 208
pelvic muscle (Kegel's), 137, 139t, 141, 336, 404
for polymyositis and dermatomyositis, 269
prescription for, 508 (q88)
for prevention of falls, 392, 506 (q85), 518–519 (q107)
quadriceps-strengthening, 520 (q111)
to reduce risk of osteoporosis, 176t
resistance training, 494–495 (q65)
role in osteoporosis prevention and treatment, 177–178
stretching, 70
Exercise: A Guide from the National Institute on Aging, 68
"Exercise: Feeling Fit for Life" (American Geriatrics Society and the National Institute on Aging), 68
Exercise echocardiography, 244–245
Exercise stress testing, 244–245
Expert Panel on Detection, Evaluation and Treatment of High Blood Cholesterol in Adults, 69t
External auditory canal changes, 474 (q34)
Extremity movements, abnormal, 405
Eyelid abnormalities, 173

F

Facial movements, abnormal, 405
Facial nerve palsy, 300
Failure to thrive, 187–188
Fainting. *See* Dizziness; Syncope
Falls, 143–148
activity recommendations for, 69t
assessment of, 144–146, 145f, 391
and drugs, 502 (q78)
due to orthostatic hypotension, 472 (q30)
environmental hazards, 520–521 (q112)
evaluation of, 459 (q8)
in hospitalized patients, 75t, 77
management of, 144–146, 145f
multifactorial interventions for, 391
physical activity and, 68
prevention of, 146–147, 392, 462 (q13), 506 (q85), 518–519 (q107)
recommendations for prevention of, 60t, 391
single interventions for, 392
Family, communication with, 117–118
Farsightedness, 169
Fas, 2t, 7
Fasting plasma glucose, 498 (q70)
Fasting serum lipid profile, 470 (q26)
FDA. *See* Food and Drug Administration
FDG-PET scan, 287
Fearful behaviors, 228, 229t
Fecal incontinence, 316–317

Fecal occult blood testing, 59, 60t
Federal financing of health care, 33–34
Fee for service (FFS)
discounted, 29
home-health care, 32
hospice care, 33
inpatient care, 30–31
Medicare, 24, 26, 27t, 28, 29–30, 29t, 30t, 31–32, 33, 34
nursing-home care, 33
outpatient care, 29–30
postacute rehabilitation coverage, 31–32
private plans, 33
structures, 24
Feeding, 192–193
artificial, 190
enteral, 189
percutaneous endoscopic gastrostomy, 192
tube, 188, 193t, 465–466 (q19), 522 (q115)
Feeding problems, 191–193, 510 (q92)
Female sexual dysfunction, 343–344, 344t
Female sexuality, 342–344
Femur procedures, 31t
Fentanyl
for breakthrough pain, 107
for dyspnea, 111
for persistent pain, 412
transdermal (Duragesic), 412
Fever
in frail, older residents in long-term care facilities, 294, 294t
of unknown origin, 301, 301t
FFS. *See* Fee for service (FFS)
Fibrosis, pulmonary, 304
Financial assessment, 54
Financial mistreatment, 54
Financing
federal, 33–34
health care, 24–25, 26–35, 26f
home-health care, 32
inpatient care, 30–31
nursing-home care, 32–33, 97–98
outpatient care, 26–30
postacute rehabilitation, 31–32
Fitness, low, 69–70
Flat feet (pes planus), 275, 276t, 278
Flexible sigmoidoscopy, 59, 60t
Fluid disturbances, 364–365
Fluid management, 79
Fluid needs, 183
Fluoride
for osteoporosis, 181
recommended daily allowances, 185t
topical, 503 (q80)
Fluoroquinolones, 295–296, 297
5-Fluorouracil, 355
Fluoxetine
for depression, 216
for depressive and other neuropsychiatric disturbances in dementia, 124, 124t
drug interactions, 216
indications for, 215t
Flurazepam, 36, 132t
Flutamide, 352t, 371

Fluvoxamine, 216
Foam islands, 200t
Foam overlays, 477 (q39)
FOBT. *See* Fecal occult blood testing
Folate, 186t, 348–349
Follicle-stimulating hormone, 325
Folstein Mini–Mental State Examination, 49, 116, 151
Food(s). *See also* Nutrition
modified Food Pyramid for 70+ adults, 184f
resources, 425
Food and Drug Administration (FDA), 43–44
Foot changes, 275
Foot diseases and disorders, 275–281, 276t, 424
Foot ulcers, 279
Foreign body, esophageal, 481 (q44)
Forgoing and discontinuing interventions, 18
Foster care, adult, 96
Fractures
of hip or pelvis, 31t
intertrochanteric, 471–472 (q28)
osteoporotic, 176, 272
physical activity and, 68
prediction of, 176–177
rib, 485–486 (q52)
tibial plateau, 462–463 (q14)
vertebral, 181, 271t, 272, 488 (q56)
Fresh frozen plasma, 388
FRGs. *See* Function Related Groups
Function Related Groups (FRGs), 84
Functional abilities, 504 (q81)
assessment of, 47–48
decline in hospitalized patients, 72
Functional Activities Questionnaire (FAQ), 116, 401
Functional Ambulation Classification, 148
Functional Obstacle Course, 148
"functional reach" test, 146
impairment of, 459–460 (q9)
prevention of limitations in, 65
trends in, 10–11
Functionally based exercises, 473–474 (q33)
FUO (fever of unknown origin), 301, 301t

G

G-regulatory protein, 2t, 6
Gabapentin (Neurontin)
for epilepsy, 284t
for mania, 218
for persistent pain, 411
Gait, cautious, 150–151, 150t
Gait assessment, 148–149, 408
Gait disturbances, 148–152, 482 (q46)
classification of, 149–151, 150t
frontal-related, 150–151, 150t
Gait speed, 48
Gallstones, 315
Gastaut-Geschwind syndrome, 241
Gastritis, *H. pylori*-induced, 314
Gastroesophageal reflux disease, 312–313

Gastrointestinal bleeding, occult, 317–318
Gastrointestinal diseases and disorders, 312–319, 475 (q35)
  effects on continence, 134–135, 135t
  infections, 300
  resources, 423
Gastrostomy, 465–466 (q19)
Gatifloxacin, 295
Gauze packing, 200t
Gaze-evoked nystagmus, 157
GDS. See Geriatric Depression Scale
Gender differences, 36
Gene expression, 4–5
Generalized anxiety disorder, 221, 222, 222t
Genetic predisposition to longevity, 490 (q58)
Genetic terminology, 2t
Genetic testing, 23
Genitourinary imaging, 359
GERD. See Gastroesophageal reflux disease
Geriatric assessment, comprehensive, 40
Geriatric Depression Scale (short form, GDS), 49, 390
Geriatric Institutional Assessment Profile (GIAP), 73–74
Geriatric nursing practitioners (GNPs), 101
Geriatric Resource Nurse (GRN) model, 74
Geriatric screening. See Screening
Geriatric Syndrome Management model, 74
Gerontological Nurse Specialists (GNSs), 74–75
Geschwind syndrome, 230
Get Up and Go test, 48, 148
Giant cell arteritis, 265–266
GIAP. See Geriatric Institutional Assessment Profile
Gingivitis, 308
Ginkgo biloba, 45, 119
Glaucoma, 171–172
  primary open-angle (POAG), 172–173
  resources, 427
GLC1A gene, 172
Gleason grading system, 368
Glimepiride, 327–328, 328t
Glipizide, 311t, 327–328, 328t
Glomerulonephritis, 361–362
Glucocorticoids, 176–177, 176t
Glucosamine and chondroitin, 45, 263
Glucose
  blood levels, 63t
  fasting plasma, 498 (q70)
Glucose control, 327, 327t, 473 (q32)
Glucose tolerance, 473 (q32)
α-Glucosidase inhibitors, 327–328, 328t
Glyburide, 327–328, 328t
GNPs. See Geriatric nursing practitioners
GNSs. See Gerontological Nurse Specialists
Goiter, 322
Gold, 311t
Goserelin, 352t, 370
Gottron's papules, 268

Gout, 263–264, 280
Gram-negative rods, 295, 296, 296f, 300
Granisetron, 109–110, 109t
Granulation, 197t
Grief, 13–14, 458 (q6)
Griseofulvin, 311t
GRN model. See Geriatric Resource Nurse model
Group exercise programs, 519 (q109)
Group homes, 96
Group therapy, 117
Growth hormone, 325–326
GTP-binding protein. See G-regulatory protein
Guardians, 21
Gustation (taste), 311, 311t
Gynecologic diseases and disorders, 334–339, 426

H

Habit training, 139t, 140, 141
HACEK organisms, 298
Haemophilis influenzae, 295, 296f, 298
Haglund's deformity, 275, 276t, 279
Hallucinations, 224
  in dementia, 125
  evaluation of, 224, 225f
  isolated, syndromes of, 227
  Parkinson's disease with, 227
  treatment of, 125
Hallucinosis, organic, 227
Hallux abducto valgus, 276t, 278, 278f
Hallux limitus, 275, 276t
Hallux rigidus, 275, 276t
Hallux valgus, 275, 276t
Haloperidol, 225–226, 226t, 491–492 (q61)
  for delirium, 107, 131
  for dementia, 124, 124t
  for nausea and vomiting, 109–110, 109t
Hammertoe, 278, 278f
Harris-Benedict equation, 182, 183t
HCFA (Health Care Financing Administration). See now Centers for Medicare & Medicaid Services (CMS)
HDL (high-density lipoprotein) cholesterol, 243–244. See also Cholesterol
Head and neck resources, 423
Headaches, 284–285, 423
Healing
  monitoring, 197–198
  Pressure Ulcer Healing Chart, 416
  Pressure Ulcer Scale for Healing (PUSH), 197, 415
Health care
  costs of, 26–35, 66
  financing of, 24–25, 26–35, 26f
  payment by Medicare HMOs, 29, 30t
  trends in, 10–11, 11–12
Health care agent or proxy, 21
Health Care Financing Administration (HCFA). See now Centers for Medicare & Medicaid Services (CMS)

Health insurance. See also Medicaid; Medicare
  advantages and disadvantages of, 29t
  coverage for older Americans, 26, 27t, 28
Health maintenance organizations (HMOs), 29
  home-health care coverage, 32
  hospice care, 33
  inpatient care coverage, 30
  Medicare, 29, 30, 30t, 31, 32–33
  nursing-home care coverage, 32–33
  outpatient care coverage, 29
  payments to providers of health care, 29, 30t
  postacute rehabilitation coverage, 31
Health Survey, SF-36™, 393–398
Healthcare Employers' Data Information System (HEDIS), 34
Healthy People 2010, 66, 66t, 70
Hearing, 163–164
Hearing aids, 165–167, 166t
Hearing assessment, 48, 60t, 463 (q15)
Hearing Handicap Inventory for the Elderly–Screening Version (HHIE-S), 165, 399
Hearing impairment, 163–168, 463 (q15)
  effects of, 165–166, 166t
  patterns of loss, 512–513 (q96)
  rehabilitation of, 165–166, 166t
  resources, 423–424
  screening for, 48, 60t, 61, 402
  sensorineural, 512–513 (q96)
  strategies to enhance communication with hearing-impaired persons, 167, 167t
Heart changes, 243t
Heart disease
  deaths due to, 11, 11t
  ischemic, 243–246
  resources, 424
  valvular, 250–252, 387
Heart failure, 246–250
  congestive, 134–135, 135t, 246–250, 248t, 480–481 (q43)
  and continence, 134–135, 135t
  drug treatment of, 248, 248t
Heart rate, maximal, 70
Heart valves
  mechanical, 387
  tissue prosthetic, 387
Heat-shock factor (HSF1), 5, 6
Heat shock protein 70 (HSP70), 2t, 6
"Heavy" drinking, 235
HEDIS. See Healthcare Employers' Data Information System
Heel pain, 278–279
Heel pressure ulcers, 196t, 455–456 (q2)
Height, 60t
Helicobacter pylori infection, 314
Heloma, subungual, 278
HELP. See Hospitalized Elderly Longitudinal Project
Hematocrit, 501 (q76)
Hematologic diseases and disorders, 345–349
Hematologic malignancies, 355–356
Hematoma, subdural, 292

Hematuria, 357–358
Hemiparesis, 149–150, 150t
Hemiplegia, 149–150, 150t
Hemolytic anemia, 346
Hemorrhage, intracerebral, 282
Henoch-Schönlein syndrome, 361
Heparin
   for acute MI, 246
   initiation of, 388
   low-molecular-weight, 80, 387, 388
   for prevention of systemic embolism, 387
   for prevention of venous
      thromboembolism, 80, 387
   for pulmonary thromboembolism, 305
   and risk of osteoporosis, 176t
   when surgical procedure is planned, 388
Herbal preparations, 44–45
   drug interactions, 44t
   regulation and research, 43–44
Herniated nucleus pulposus, 271–272
Herpes simplex virus, 300
Herpes zoster, 300, 377–378, 377f
   effects on continence, 134–135, 135t
   ophthalmicus, 173
HHIE-S. See Hearing Handicap Inventory
   for the Elderly–Screening Version
HHRGs. See Home Health Related Groups
HIAP (human inhibitor of apoptosis
   protein), 2t, 6
Hiccups, 472 (q29)
High-density lipoprotein (HDL) cholesterol,
   243–244. See also Cholesterol
Hip fracture, 31t, 88, 471–472 (q28), 476
   (q37)
Hip procedures, 31t
Hip replacement, 31t
Hispanic Americans
   causes of death, 11
   congestive heart failure in, 247
   perceived health of, 10, 10t
   poverty rates, 8
Histamine H₂-blocking agents, 132t, 313
History taking, 483–484 (q49)
Histrionic personality disorder
   features of, 228, 229t
   therapeutic strategies for, 230–231, 231t
HIV infection, 300
   effects on continence, 134–135, 135t
   resources, 419, 420
HMOs. See Health maintenance
   organizations
Hodgkin's disease, 350, 356
Home assessment, 462 (q13)
Home-health care, 12, 91–93, 480–481
   (q43)
   financing, coverage, and costs of, 32
   hospice programs, 479 (q41)
   Medicare benefits, 34
Home Health Related Groups (HHRGs), 91
Home hospitals, 95
Home Safety Checklist, 400
Homocysteine, 348–349

Hormonal therapy
   for breast cancer, 354
   for cancer, 352, 352t
Hormone replacement therapy, 60t, 62,
   329–333. See also Estrogen replacement
   therapy
   for cognitive disorders, 331
   for menopausal symptoms, 329
   for osteoporosis, 329–330, 330t
   for prevention of cardiovascular disease,
      330–331
   for urogenital symptoms, 329
Horner's syndrome, 282
Hospice care, 103, 479 (q41). See also
   End-of-life care; Palliative care
   financing, coverage, and costs of, 33
   resources, 422
Hospital-acquired pneumonia, 295, 296f
Hospital care, 72–81. See also Acute care;
   Discharge planning
   day hospitals, 94
   drug-drug adverse effects identified upon
      entry to, 39, 40t
   early discharges from, 31, 31t
   financing, coverage, and costs of, 30–31
   home hospitals, 95
   multifactorial interventions for falls in, 391
   trends in discharges, 11
Hospital insurance, 458–459 (q7)
Hospitalized Elderly Longitudinal Project
   (HELP), 112
Hospitalized patients
   assessment of, 75–78, 75t
   delirium in, 498–499 (q71)
   functional decline in, 72
   strategies for managing, 79–81
   systematic approaches to, 80–81
Hot flushes, 329
House calls, 92, 92t
Housing, sheltered, 96
HSF1 (heat shock factor 1), 5, 6
HSP70 (heat shock protein 70), 2t, 6
Human immunodeficiency virus infection,
   300
   effects on continence, 134–135, 135t
   resources, 419
Human inhibitor of apoptosis protein
   (HIAP), 2t, 6
Huntington's disease, 289t, 425
Hutchinson's sign, 173
Hyaluronan polymers, 263
Hyaluronic acid, 263
Hydralazine, isosorbide dinitrate plus, 248t,
   250
Hydrobromide, 109–110, 109t
Hydrocephalus, normal-pressure
   effects on continence, 134–135, 135t
   gait findings in, 150–151, 150t
Hydrochlorothiazide, 258, 502 (q78)
Hydrocodone (Lorcet, Lortab, Vicodin,
   Vicoprofen), 107, 412
Hydrocolloids, 198–199, 200t, 465 (q18)
Hydrocortisone, 311t, 374
Hydrogel, 200t

Hydromorphone (Dilaudid, Hydrostat), 107,
   412
Hydrophilic drugs, 36
Hydrostat, 412. See also Hydromorphone
3-Hydroxy-3-methylglutaryl coenzyme A
   reductase, 181
Hydroxychloroquine, 267, 268
Hyperadrenocorticoidism, 324
Hypercalcemia, 134–135, 135t, 322–323
Hypercholesteremia, 470 (q26). See also
   Lipids, serum
Hyperkalemia, 365
Hyperkeratosis, 275
Hyperkinesias, 285
Hyperlipidemia, 243
Hypernatremia, 364–365
Hyperopia, 169
Hyperparathyroidism, 323
   primary, 176, 176t
   secondary, 175
Hyperplasia
   benign prostatic, 366–367, 389, 467
      (q21), 488–489 (q57)
   squamous, 336
Hypersexuality, 125
Hypertension, 243, 256–261
   activity recommendations for, 69t
   classification of, 256, 256t
   in diabetes mellitus, 328
   follow-up visits, 259–260, 259t
   nonpharmacologic therapy for, 257–258,
      257t
   with obesity, 519–520 (q110)
   pharmacologic treatment of, 258–259, 258t
   screening for, 59, 60t
   stage 1, 256t, 257, 257t, 258, 258t
   treatment of, 257–260, 258t, 283
Hypertensive emergencies and urgencies, 260
Hyperthyroidism, 289t, 321–322
   apathetic, 491 (q60)
   screening for, 63, 63t
   screening for secondary osteoporosis in,
      176t
Hypertriglyceridemia, 243–244
Hyperuricemia, 264
Hypnotics, chronic use, 206–207
Hypoadrenocorticoidism, 324
Hypochondriasis, 232, 232t, 482–483 (q47)
Hypoglycemic agents, 44t
Hypogonadism, 176, 176t, 325
Hypokalemia, 365
Hypokinesias, 285
Hyponatremia, 364–365
Hypoproliferative anemia, 346
Hypotension, orthostatic, 158t, 472 (q30),
   502–503 (q79)
Hypothyroidism, 63, 63t, 320–321
Hysteria, 233

I

"I SNORED" screen, 304, 304t
IADLs. See Instrumental activities of daily
   living

ICE. *See* Interleukin-1 converting enzyme

ICH-1, 2*t*, 6

ICIDH-2. *See International Classification of Impairments, Disabilities, and Handicaps*

ICU care, 305, 493–494 (q63)

Idiopathic pulmonary fibrosis, 304

Idoxuridine, 311*t*

Imaging. *See also specific modalities*
- of back pain, 273
- brain imaging techniques, 116, 116*t*
- genitourinary, 359
- renal, 359

Imidazole antifungals, 36

Imipramine, 36, 132*t*

Immobility, 60*t*, 75*t*, 77

Immune function changes, 293, 293*t*

Immune senescence, 293, 293*t*

Immunizations, 60*t*, 62
- annual, 497–498 (q69)
- for influenza, 507–508 (q87)
- resources, 419

Immunoglobulin A nephropathy, 361, 362

Implants
- brachytherapy, 370
- cochlear, 168

Incompetence, decisional, 20, 21

Incontinence
- fecal, 316–317
- urinary. *See* Urinary incontinence

Indinavir, 36

Ineffective anemia, 346

Infections
- antibiotic management of, 294–295
- antibiotic prophylaxis for, 513 (q97)
- bone and joint, 299
- clinical presentation of, 294
- diagnosis and management of, 294–295
- gastrointestinal, 300
- HIV, 300
- periungual, 275
- predisposition to, 293–294
- in pressure ulcers, 198
- prosthetic device, 299
- urinary tract, 296–297
- vertebral, 270, 271*t*
- vulvovaginal, 335

Infectious diarrhea, 300–301

Infectious diseases, 293–301
- effects on continence, 134–135, 135*t*
- syndromes, 295–301

Infective endocarditis, 298–299

Infestations, louse, 378–379

Infliximab, 267

Influenza
- assessment of, 75*t*, 76
- deaths due to, 11, 11*t*
- vaccination against, 60*t*, 62, 75*t*, 76, 507–508 (q87)

Informed consent for research, 22

Injury
- deaths due to, 11, 11*t*
- drug-induced esophageal, 313–314
- recommended preventive services for, 60*t*, 61

Insomnia, 456–457 (q4), 487 (q54). *See also* Sleep problems

Inspection, skin, 63*t*

Institutionalization, 93, 509–510 (q91)

Instrumental Activities of Daily Living (IADLs), 47, 47*t*, 385, 504 (q81), 516–517 (q103)
- difficulty of Medicare beneficiaries in, 10, 10*t*

Insurance, hospital, 458–459 (q7). *See also* Health insurance; Medicaid; Medicare

Intensive care unit (ICU), 305, 493–494 (q63)

α-Interferon, 352

Interictal personality disorders, 230

Interleukin-1 converting enzyme, 2*t*, 6

Interleukin-2, 352

Internal carotid artery disease, 282

International Classification of Impairments, Disabilities, and Handicaps (ICIDH-2), 82–83, 82*f*

International Prostate Symptom Score (IPSS), 389

Interstitial nephritis, acute, 359, 363

Intertrigo, 374, 374*f*

Intertrochanteric fractures, 471–472 (q28)

Intervertebral disc herniation, 271–272

Intracerebral hemorrhage, 282

Intraocular lens, 169

Investigational agents, 180–181

Iodine, radioactive, 491 (q60)

Ipratropium bromide, 303

IPSS. *See* International Prostate Symptom Score

Iron-drug interactions, 186*t*, 347

Iron sorbitex, 311*t*

Iron supplements, 347

Ischemic heart disease, 243–246

Ischemic optic neuropathy, anterior, 173, 173*f*

Ischial pressure ulcers, 467–468 (q22)

Isoniazid, 186*t*, 298

Isosorbide dinitrate plus hydralazine, 248*t*, 250

Itching, 375

Ivermectin, 378

J

J-curve hypothesis, 259

Jevity Plus, 193*t*

Jewett-Whitmore staging system, 368–369, 369*t*

The John A. Hartford Foundation Institute for Geriatric Nursing
- Nurses Improving Care for Health System Elders (NICHE), 73–75
- *Try This: Best Practices in Care to Older Adults*, 47, 105
- Web site, 105

Joint National Committee on Prevention, Detection, Evaluation, and Treatment of High Blood Pressure, 69*t*

Joint problems
- infections, 299
- pain, 506–507 (q86)
- resources, 424

Judgment, substituted, 493–494 (q63)

K

Kadian, 107, 412. *See also* Morphine

Kava, 44–45

Kegel's exercises
- for incontinence, 137, 139*t*, 141, 404
- for prolapse, 336

Keratitis sicca, 173

Keratosis, subungual, 275

Kidney diseases, 359–364, 427

Kidney function changes, 357

Kidney stones, 357

Kingella, 298

Kip1, 2*t*

Klonopin (clonazepam), 411

Klüver-Bucy syndrome, 241

Knee osteoarthritis, 462–463 (q14). *See also* Osteoarthritis
- activity recommendations for, 69*t*

Koebner's phenomenon, 375

L

Laboratory testing
- in malnutrition, 185
- services not indicated in older adults, 64, 64*t*

Labyrinthitis, 153

Lacunar disease, 282

LaForte colpocleisis, 338

Lamotrigine, 218, 284*t*

Laxatives, 186*t*

LDL (low-density lipoprotein) cholesterol, 243, 328. *See also* Cholesterol

Leflunomide, 267

Left ventricular ejection fraction, 247

Leg mobility screening, 402

Leg movements during sleep, periodic, 203

Legs syndrome, restless, 203

Legal issues, 18–25
- agencies and organizations, 422–423
- in home care, 93
- in malnutrition, 189–190
- medical-legal interface, 55–58

Legionella, 296

Length of stay, 11

Lentigo maligna, 380

Letrozole, 352*t*

Leucovorin, 355

Leukemia, 350, 355

Leukoplakia, 310

Leuprolide, 125, 352*t*, 370

Levodopa, 186*t*, 311*t*

Levodopa-carbidopa, 132*t*, 287, 288

Levodopa replacement therapy, 289–290, 290*t*

Levofloxacin, 295

Lewy body dementia, 517 (q104). *See also* Alzheimer's disease; Dementia

Liability, 93

Lice, 378–379

Lichen planus, 336

Lichen sclerosus, 336

Lichen simplex chronicus, 373–374

Lidocaine, 36

Life expectancy, 7–8, 8*t*

Life-style modification, 257–258

Life support, continuation of, 493–494 (q63)

Light, to improve sleep, 208

Lightheadedness, 154

Lioresal, 411. *See also* Baclofen

Lipid-binding resins, 186*t*

Lipids, serum, 60*t*, 63*t*, 470 (q26)

Lipophilic drugs, 36

Liquid nitrogen, 379

Liquid Pred, 411. *See also* Prednisone

Listeria, 300

Lithium
  and delirium, 132*t*
  distribution of, 36
  for mania, 218
  movement disorders associated with, 289–290, 290*t*

Lithium carbonate, 311*t*

Liver disease, 347–348, 423

Living arrangements, 8–9, 9*t*

Living wills, 21, 478 (q40)

Long-term care
  and acute care, 98–99
  fever in frail, older residents in, 294, 294*t*
  hypertension in residents in, 260–261
  multifactorial interventions for falls in, 391
  pneumonia in, 295, 296*f*
  resources, 420

Longevity, 490 (q58)

Lorazepam, 491–492 (q61)
  distribution of, 36
  for sleep problems, 205, 206*t*

Lorcet, 412. *See also* Hydrocodone

Lortab, 412. *See also* Hydrocodone

Loss and grief, 13–14

Louse infestations, 378–379

Low-density lipoprotein (LDL) cholesterol, 243, 328. *See also* Cholesterol

Low-molecular-weight heparin, 80, 387, 388

Low T4 syndrome, 320

Low-vision aids, 174

Low-vision rehabilitation, 174

Lower-extremity amputation, 31*t*

Lower-extremity arterial disease, 254

Lower-extremity innervation, 271, 272*t*

Lower urinary tract, 366

Lubricants, 344, 344*t*

Lumbar degenerative disc disease, 272

Lumbar sacral strain, acute, 274, 274*t*

Lumbar spinal stenosis, 271, 271*t*, 274, 274*t*

Lumbar spine, unstable, 271*t*, 272, 274, 274*t*

Lumpectomy, 354. *See also* Breast cancer

Lung cancer, 354–355

Lung disease
  chronic, activity recommendations for, 69*t*
  chronic obstructive, 11, 11*t*, 303–304, 499–500 (q73)
  effects on continence, 134–135, 135*t*
  resources, 424, 425

Luteinizing hormone, 325

Luteinizing hormone-releasing hormone agonists, 370

Luteinizing hormone-releasing hormone analogs, 352*t*

Lyme disease, 300

Lymphadenectomy, axillary, 354

Lymphoma, non-Hodgkin's, 355

M

Macronutrient needs, 182–183

Macular degeneration, age-related, 169–170, 492 (q62)

Macular edema, 172, 172*f*

Maculopathy, age-related, 169–170, 170*f*

Magnesium, 185*t*
  -drug interactions, 186*t*

Magnetic resonance cholangiography, 315

Magnetic resonance imaging, 273

Major depressive disorder, 458 (q6). *See also* Depression

Maladaptive behaviors, 241

Malassezia furfur, 372

Male sexuality, 339–342

Malignancy. *See also* Cancer
  hematologic, 355–356
  neoplasms, 11, 11*t*

Mallet toes, 278

Malnutrition, 182–190, 469 (q24). *See also* Dietary interventions
  assessment of, 75*t*, 76
  and infection, 293–294
  resources, 425
  risk factors for, 185–186, 186*t*
  screening for, 60–61, 60*t*, 402

Mammography, 60*t*, 494 (q64)

Managed care
  home-health care coverage, 32
  inpatient care coverage, 30
  nursing-home care coverage, 32–33
  outpatient care coverage, 29
  postacute rehabilitation coverage, 31
  Quality Improvement System for Managed Care (QISMC), 34

Mania, 218

Marital status, 8–9, 9*t*

Marital therapy, 344, 344*t*

Marshall-Marchetti-Krantz abdominal procedure, 140*t*, 141

MAST-G (Michigan Alcoholism Screening Test–Geriatric Version), 237
  short (S-MAST-G), 237, 238*t*

Mattress surfaces, 477 (q39)

MDS. *See* Minimum Data Set

Mechanical debridement, 198, 199*t*

Mechanical heart valves, 387

Mechanical loading, 195–196

Mechanical ventilation, 305

Meclizine, 109–110, 109*t*

Mediators, stress, 14–16

Medicaid, 28, 460–461 (q11), 514 (q99)
  advantages and disadvantages of, 29*t*
  assisted living benefits, 95

Medical directors, 102

Medical disorders. *See also* specific disorders
  anxiety and, 222
  differentiation of depression from, 213
  with mental retardation, 242
  and sleep disturbances, 203

Medical-legal interface, 55–58

Medical savings accounts (MSAs), 33

Medicare, 27, 28
  capitation schedules, 34
  cochlear implant benefits, 168
  colorectal cancer screening benefits, 59
  difficulty in ADLs and IADLs of beneficiaries, 10, 10*t*
  FFS (fee-for-service), 24, 26, 27*t*, 28, 29–30, 29*t*, 30*t*, 31–32, 33, 34
  home-health care benefits, 32, 34, 84, 91, 92
  hospice benefits, 19, 33, 103
  inpatient care benefits, 30–31
  marital status and living arrangements of beneficiaries, 8–9, 9*t*
  nursing-home care benefits, 9–10, 33
  out-of-pocket expenses, 28, 456 (q3)
  outpatient care benefits, 29–30
  Part A, 27, 28, 458–459 (q7)
  Part B, 27–28
  perceived health of beneficiaries, 10, 10*t*
  postacute rehabilitation benefits, 31–32
  premiums for, 28
  rehabilitation care benefits, 83, 84
  skilled nursing benefits, 83, 98
  therapeutic shoe benefits, 281

Medicare Health Outcomes Survey, 34

Medicare HMOs, 28
  financing of, 33
  home-health care coverage, 32
  hospice care, 33
  inpatient care coverage, 30
  nursing-home care coverage, 32–33
  outpatient care coverage, 29
  payments to providers of health care, 29, 30*t*
  postacute rehabilitation coverage, 31

Medicare Plus Choice, 460–461 (q11)
  advantages and disadvantages of, 29*t*
  BBA provisions for, 34
  capitation structure, 25
  number of beneficiaries enrolled in, 33–34
  types of plans, 33

Medicare SELECT, 28

Medicated urethral system for erection (MUSE), 342, 342*t*

Medications. *See* Drugs; Pharmacotherapy; *specific medications*

Medigap, 26, 28, 29*t*, 460–461 (q11)

Medroxyprogesterone
  for cancer, 352t
  for osteoporosis, 329–330, 330t
Melanoma, 380–381, 380f
Melatonin, 207, 326
Membranous nephropathy, 359–360
Memorial Delirium Assessment Scale, 128
Memory problems, 402, 425, 457 (q5). *See also* Cognitive impairment
Men
  androgen deficiency in, 333
  androgens in, 175–176
  congestive heart failure in, 247
  difficulty in ADLs and IADLs, 10, 10t
  drug metabolism in, 36
  headaches in, 284
  life expectancy, 7–8, 8t
  marital status and living arrangements of, 8–9, 9t
  nursing-home population, 97
  obesity in, 60–61
  poverty rates, 8
  stroke in, 281
  suicide rates, 11
  systemic lupus erythematosus in, 267
  urinary tract infection in, 297
Mendelson's syndrome, 192
Ménière's disease, 158t
Menopausal symptoms, 329
Menopause, 329
Mental health
  impacts of robust social networks on, 15–16, 16t
  impacts of self-efficacy beliefs on, 14–15, 15t
  and mental retardation, 240–241
  and substance use, 237
Mental retardation, 240–242
Mental status, altered, 127
Mental status change, acute, 127
Mental status examination, 63t
Meperidine, 107, 132t
Merry Walker Ambulation Device, 89–90
Mesangioproliferative glomerulonephritis, 362
Messenger ribonucleic acid (mRNA), 4, 5
Metabolic disorders, 319–329
  effects on continence, 134–135, 135t
  encephalopathy, 127
Metabolism, 36
Metatarsal prolapse, 275, 276t
Metatarsalgia, 275, 276t, 279
Metformin
  nutrient interactions, 186t
  for type 2 diabetes mellitus, 327–328, 328t
Methimazole, 311t
Methotrexate, 311t
  for polymyositis and dermatomyositis, 269
  for psoriasis, 376
  for rheumatoid arthritis, 266, 267
  and risk of osteoporosis, 176t
  for SLE, 268
Methyldopa, 289–290, 290t

Methylmalonic acid, 348–349
Methylphenidate, 107, 215
Methylprednisolone
  for polymyalgia rheumatica, 265
  for polymyositis and dermatomyositis, 269
  for pseudogout, 264
Methyltestosterone, 344
Methylthiouracil, 311t
Methylxanthines, 289–290, 290t
Metoclopramide
  metabolism of, 36
  movement disorders associated with, 289–290, 290t
  for nausea and vomiting, 109–110, 109t
Metoprolol, 246, 249, 250
Metronidazole, 311t, 317
Metyrosine, 289
Mexiletine (Mexitil), 411
Mexitil (mexiletine), 411
Michigan Alcoholism Screening Test–Geriatric Version (MAST-G), 386, 495–496 (q66)
  short (S-MAST-G), 237, 238t
Miconazole powder, 374
Micronutrient requirements, 183
Micturition, 134, 134t
Migraines, 284–285
Mineral oil-drug interactions, 186t
Mini Nutritional Assessment, 186
Mini–Mental State Examination (MMSE), 20, 49, 77, 116
  in gait disturbances, 151
Minimum Data Set (MDS), 83, 183, 190, 197
Minocycline, 266–267
Mirtazapine
  for dementia, 124, 124t
  for depression, 215t, 217
Misoprostol, 107
Mistreatment, elder, 52–58, 469–470 (q25), 485–486 (q52)
  agencies and organizations, 422–423
  in hospitalized patients, 75t, 78
Mitochondrial DNA (mtDNA), 2, 4
Mitral regurgitation, 251–252
Mitral stenosis, 252
Mixed urge and stress incontinence, 139t
MMSE. *See* Mini–Mental State Examination
MND. *See* Motor neuron disease
Mobility aids, 89–90, 455 (q1), 473 (q31)
Mobility and movement, 405–408
  Abnormal Involuntary Movement Scale (AIMS), 405–406
  activities of daily living (IADLs), 10, 10t
  leg mobility screening, 402
  Performance Oriented Mobility Assessment (POMA), 148, 407–408
  periodic leg movements during sleep, 203
  restless legs syndrome, 203
Moderators, stress, 16–17
Modified Food Pyramid for 70+ adults, 184f
Modified Gait Abnormality Rating scale, 148
Mono-Gesic, 411. *See also* Salsalate

Monoamine oxidase inhibitors
  for anxiety disorders, 222t
  for depression, 217
  indications for, 215t
Monoclonal antibodies, 352
"Mood congruent" delusions, 226
Mood disorders, 211–219, 487–488 (q55). *See also* Depression
  psychotic symptoms in, 226
Mood disturbances, 124–125, 124t
Mood stabilizers, 218
Morphine (MSContin, Kadian, Avinza, MSIR, Roxanol), 478 (q40)
  for dyspnea, 111
  for moderate and severe pain, 107
  for persistent pain, 412
Morton's syndrome, 275, 276t
Motility agents, 109–110, 109t
Motor neuron disease, 290–291
Motor vehicle crashes, 60t
Movement disorders, 285–290
Moxifloxacin, 295
Moxisylyte, 342
MSAs. *See* Medical savings accounts
MSContin, 412. *See also* Morphine
MSIR, 412. *See also* Morphine
Multidisciplinary teams, 84–85
Multiple myeloma, 176t, 356
Multiple sclerosis, 134–135, 135t
Multisystem atrophy, 134–135, 135t
Multivitamin supplements, 347
Musculoskeletal diseases and disorders, 261–269
  effects on continence, 134–135, 135t
  rehabilitation care for, 85, 85t
  resources, 424
MUSE (medicated urethral system for erection), 342, 342t
Mycobacterium tuberculosis, 297, 298
Myelopathy, 290
Myelotoxicity, 351–352, 351t
Myocardial infarction
  acute, 244, 246, 387
  non-Q-wave, 245
  oral anticoagulation for, 387
  prevention of, 63t
  Q-wave, 244
  recommended preventive services for, 60t
  risk stratification after, 246, 247t
  screening for, 63t
  treatment after, 246
Myopathy, 149, 150t, 291–292
Myopia, 169

N

Nail problems, 277–278
Naloxone, 108
Narcissistic personality disorders
  features of, 228, 229t
  therapeutic strategies for, 230–231, 231t
Narcotics Anonymous, 238
National Center on Elder Abuse, 55

National Council on Aging, Inc., 186

National Family Caregiver Support Program (NFSCP), 93

National Heart, Lung and Blood Institute (NHLBI) Expert Panel on the Identification, Evaluation, and Treatment of Overweight and Obesity in Adults, 69*t*

National Institute on Aging, 68

National Institutes of Health (NIH)
Consensus Conference on Osteoporosis Prevention, Diagnosis and Therapy, 69*t*
Consensus Conference on Physical Activity and Cardiovascular Health, 69*t*
Consensus Statement on the Treatment of Sleep Disorders of Older People, 201
guidelines for body size classification, 183, 185*t*
recommendations for physical activity, 68, 69*t*

National Pressure Ulcer Advisory Panel (NPUAP), 197

Native Americans, 93, 310–311

Nausea and vomiting, 109–110, 109*t*

Nd:YAG laser, 314

Nearsightedness, 169

Necrosis, 197*t*, 360, 361*t*

Needle suspension, 140*t*, 141

Nefazodone
for depression, 215*t*, 217
for depressive and other neuropsychiatric disturbances in dementia, 124, 124*t*
drug interactions, 216
metabolism of, 36
for sleep problems, 125, 206, 206*t*

Neglect, 53*t*, 485–486 (q52). *See also* Elder mistreatment

Neisseria gonorrhea, 371

Neoplasia
malignant, 11, 11*t*
vulvar, 336

Neovascularization
choroidal, 170, 170*f*
with proliferative diabetic retinopathy, 172, 172*f*

Nephritis
acute interstitial, 359
deaths due to, 11, 11*t*

Nephropathy, 360, 362

Nephrosis, 11, 11*t*

Nephrotic syndrome, 357, 359
deaths due to, 11, 11*t*

Nepro, 193*t*

Neuralgia, post-herpetic, 173, 300, 377

Neurodermatitis, 373–374

Neurologic diseases and disorders, 281–292
effects on continence, 134–135, 135*t*

Neurologic signs, 281

Neurologic testing, 162

Neurontin, 411. *See also* Gabapentin

Neuropathy, 149, 150*t*

Neuropsychiatric disturbances in dementia, 121–126, 121*t*, 122*f*
drugs to treat, 123*t*, 124
nonbiologic interventions for, 123, 123*t*

Neurosyphilis, 134–135, 135*t*, 300

NF-kB, 2*t*, 5

NFSCP. *See* National Family Caregiver Support Program

NHLBI Expert Panel on the Identification, Evaluation, and Treatment of Overweight and Obesity in Adults, 69*t*

Niacin, 185*t*, 186*t*

Nicardipine, 258

NICHE Ready Sheet, 73, 409

Nicotine replacement therapy, 479–480 (q42)

Nifedipine, 35, 311*t*

Nitrates, 40*t*, 245, 246

Nitrazepam, 38

Nitrogen, liquid, 379

Nitroglycerin, 245, 311*t*

Nodular thyroid disease, 322

Non-Hodgkin's lymphoma, 355

Nonadherence, 41–42

Nonagenarians, 490 (q58)

Nonmaleficence, 493–494 (q63)

Nonsteroidal anti-inflammatory drugs (NSAIDs)
gastric complications, 314
for gout, 264
for mild pain, 106, 107
for osteoarthritis, 263
for polymyalgia rheumatica, 265
renal diseases associated with, 362–363
for rheumatoid arthritis, 266
risk factors for upper GI adverse events, 314, 315*t*

Norpramin, 411. *See also* Desipramine

Norton Scale, 195

Nortriptyline (Aventyl, Pamelor)
for depressive and other neuropsychiatric disturbances in dementia, 124, 124*t*
indications for, 215*t*
for persistent pain, 411

NSAIDs. *See* Nonsteroidal anti-inflammatory drugs

Nuclear factor kB (NF-kB), 2*t*, 5

Nurse, Geriatric Resource (GRN) model, 74

Nurse practitioners, 101–102

Nurse Specialists, Geronotological (GNSs), 74–75

Nurses Improving Care for Health System Elders (NICHE), 73–75, 409

Nursing care
costs of, 460–461 (q11)
trends in, 12

Nursing Home Bill of Rights, 55

Nursing-home care, 97–102
ethics in, 23–24
exercise programs, 519 (q109)
financing, coverage, and costs of, 32–33
HCFA restrictions on psychotropic drugs in, 472 (q29)

influenza immunization programs, 507–508 (q87)
prevention of pressure ulcers in, 455–456 (q2)
private practice model, 101
risk of admission to, 509–510 (q91)
sleep in, 204
treatment decisions in, 23–24
trends in use, 9–10
unacceptable weight loss in, 189

Nutriceuticals, 35, 263

Nutrient-drug interactions, 185, 186*t*

Nutrition, 186–188
age-related changes in, 182–183
assessment of, 48, 183–186
intake, 183–184
requirements, 182, 183*t*
resources, 425

Nutrition screening, 183–186, 402, 410

Nutritional interventions, 188–189, 469 (q24)
for chronic renal failure, 363
for infection, 294
for pressure ulcers, 199
to reduce risk of osteoporosis, 176*t*

Nutritional Program (OAA), 93

Nystagmus, 157

Nystatin cream, 374

O

OAA. *See* Older Americans Act

OASIS. *See* Outcome and Assessment Information Set

Obesity, 188, 519–520 (q110)
activity recommendations for, 69*t*
definition of, 60–61
drug interactions, 40
screening for, 60–61, 60*t*

OBRA. *See* Omnibus Budget Reconciliation Act

Obsessive-compulsive disorder, 221, 468–469 (q23)
features of, 228, 229*t*
pharmacologic management of, 222, 222*t*
therapeutic strategies for, 230–231, 231*t*

Obstructive nephropathy, 362

Obstructive sleep apnea, 304, 304*t*

Occlusive peripheral vascular disease, 254

Occult gastrointestinal bleeding, 317–318

Odd or eccentric behaviors, 228, 229*t*

Odynophagia, 312

Office-based house-call programs, 92

Olanzapine, 225–226, 226*t*
for dementia, 124, 124*t*
for Parkinson's disease and hallucinations, 227

Old Age Insurance, 460–461 (q11)

Older Americans Act (OAA), 93, 96, 188

Olfactory dysfunction, 311, 311*t*

Omeprazole, 107

Omnibus Budget Reconciliation Act (OBRA), 55, 99, 189

Oncology, 349–357

Ondansetron, 109–110, 109*t*

Onychauxis, 277, 277f
Onychia, 278
Onychodysplasia, 278f
Onychodystrophy, 275, 278f
Onychogryphosis, 277, 277t
Onycholysis, 278
Onychomycosis, 275, 277, 277f, 375–376, 375f
Onychopathy, 275
Onychophosis, 275
Onychorrhexis, 275
Open-angle glaucoma, primary, 172–173
Opioids, 478 (q40), 506–507 (q86)
    addiction to, 108
    analgesics, 107, 132t, 412
    and delirium, 131, 132t
    dependence on, 108
    for osteoarthritis, 263
    for pain, 107, 412
    pseudoaddiction to, 108
    side effects of, 107–108
    tolerance to, 108
Optic neuropathy, anterior ischemic, 173, 173f
Oral cancer, 60t, 310
Oral diseases and disorders, 307–311
Oral movements, abnormal, 405
Oral mucosal problems, 310–311
Oral supplements, 188
Oral tissue changes, 307, 307t
Orasone, 411. See also Prednisone
Orchiectomy, 370
Oregon Death with Dignity Act, 19
Organic brain syndrome, 127
Organic disturbances, 31t
Organic hallucinosis, 227
Oropharyngeal dysphagia, 192, 312
Oropharyngeal malignancy, 310
Orthostatic hypotension, 158t, 472 (q30), 502–503 (q79)
Orthotics, 90, 280–281
Osmolite, 193t
Osteoarthritis, 262–263, 506–507 (q86)
    of foot, 280
    of knee, 69t, 462–463 (q14)
Osteomalacia, 176t, 181
Osteopenia, 174, 494–495 (q65)
Osteoporosis, 174–182
    activity recommendations for, 69t
    hormone replacement therapy for, 329–330, 330t
    idiopathic, 488 (q56)
    pharmacologic options for, 178–181, 179t
    physical activity and, 68
    prevention of, 177–181, 329–330, 494–495 (q65)
    recommended preventive services for, 60t
    resources, 424
    risk factors for, 176, 176t
    sacral fractures of, 272
    screening for, 63, 63t
    secondary, 176–177, 176t

treatment of, 177–181, 329–330
vertebral compression fracture of, 271t, 272
Ostomy resources, 423
Outcome and Assessment Information Set (OASIS), 84, 91
Outpatient care, 26–30, 238
Over-the-counter sleeping agents, 207
Overactive bladder, 135–136
Overflow incontinence, 136, 141, 496 (q67), 509 (q90)
Oxazepam, 36
Oxidative stress theory of aging, 1–2
Oxybutynin, 132t, 139t, 140
Oxycodone (OxyIR, OxyContin), 107, 412
OxyContin, 412. See also Oxycodone
Oxygen therapy, 111, 245
OxyIR, 412. See also Oxycodone

P

P-glycoprotein, 40
p16, 2t
p27, 2t
PACE. See Program of All-inclusive Care of the Elderly
Pacing, 460 (q10)
Paget's disease, 176t, 323
Pain, 104–105
    assessment of, 108–109
    back, 270–274, 511–512 (q95)
    heel and arch, 278–279
    intensity scales, 104, 104f
    with intercourse, 344, 344t
    joint, 506–507 (q86)
    knee, 462–463 (q14)
    mild, 106–107
    moderate, 107
    resources, 425–426
    severe, 107
    shoulder, 490–491 (q59)
Pain disorder, 232, 232t
Pain management, 106–109, 411–412. See also Analgesia; Palliative care
    nonpharmacologic interventions, 106
    pharmacologic interventions, 106–108, 411–412, 478 (q40)
Painful diverticulosis, 317
Palliative care, 103–112, 478 (q40). See also Analgesia; Hospice care; Pain management
    endoscopic, of esophageal cancer, 314
    interventions that may hasten death, 18–19
Palsy
    facial nerve (Bell's), 300
    progressive supranuclear, 288–289
    vertical-gaze, 289
Pamelor, 411. See also Nortriptyline
Pamidronate, 180
Panic attack, 220
Panic disorder, 220, 222, 222t
Pantothenic acid, 185t
Pap smear, 60, 60t
Papaverine, 341

Paranoid personality disorder
    features of, 228, 229t
    therapeutic strategies for, 230–231, 231t
Paraparesis, 149–150, 150t
Paraplegia, 149–150, 150t
Parathyroid gland disorders, 322–323
Parathyroid hormone, 175, 322, 322t
    for osteoporosis prevention and treatment, 180–181
Parathyroid hormone-related peptide, 323
Parenteral nutrition, 189
Parkinsonism
    drug-induced, 289–290, 290t
    gait findings in, 149–150, 150t
Parkinson's disease, 117, 286–288, 488–489 (q57)
    adaptive mobility aids for, 455 (q1)
    brain imaging in, 116, 116t
    effects on continence, 134–135, 135t
    with hallucinations, 227
    resources, 425
Paronychia, 278
Paroxetine
    for depression, 215t, 216
    for depressive and other neuropsychiatric disturbances in dementia, 124, 124t
    drug interactions, 216
Paroxysmal atrial fibrillation, 253
Passive-aggressive personality disorder
    features of, 228, 229t
    therapeutic strategies for, 230–231, 231t
Patient history, 483–484 (q49)
Pauci-immune crescentic glomerulonephritis, 361
Pediculosis capitis, 378–379
Pediculosis corporis, 378–379
Pediculosis pubis, 378–379
PEG. See Percutaneous endoscopic gastrostomy
Pelvic examination, 334, 516 (q102)
Pelvic floor support disorders, 336–338
Pelvic fracture, 31t
Pelvic muscle exercises (Kegel's)
    for incontinence, 137, 139t, 141, 404
    for prolapse, 336
Pelvic organ prolapse, 336, 337t
Penicillin, 132t
Penile prosthesis, 342, 342t
Peptic ulcer disease, 314–315
Percutaneous endoscopic gastrostomy, 192
Percutaneous transluminal coronary angioplasty, 245, 246, 254
Performance Oriented Mobility Assessment (POMA), 148, 407–408
Pergolide, 288
Periodic leg movements during sleep, 203
Periodontal anatomy, 308f
Periodontal ligament, 308
Periodontitis, 308
Periodontium, diseases of, 308
Perioperative care, 79–80
Periostitis, 275, 276t
Peripheral arterial disease, 253–254

Peripheral neuropathy, 291
Peripheral vascular disease
    foot problems in, 280
    occlusive, 254
    rehabilitation care for, 85, 85t
Peripheral venous insufficiency, 134–135,
    135t
Periurethral bulking injections, 140t, 141
Permethrin, 378
Personality changes, 481–482 (q45)
Personality disorders, 228–232
    borderline, 228, 229t, 230–231, 231t
    features of, 228, 229t
    provisional, 228, 229t
    treatment of, 230–232, 231t
Pes cavus, 275, 276t, 278
Pes planus, 275, 276t, 278
Pes valgo planus, 275, 276t
Pessaries, 337–338, 337f, 338t
PEU. See Protein-energy undernutrition
Phacoemulsification, 169
Phantom boarder syndrome, 470–471 (q27)
Pharmacodynamic changes, 37–38
Pharmacokinetic changes, 35–37
Pharmacotherapy, 35–42. See also Drugs;
    specific agents
    age-related issues, 118
    "brown-bag" evaluation of, 41
    for congestive heart failure, 248, 248t
    and delirium, 131, 132t
    for dementia, 118–119
    for depressive disturbances in dementia,
        124, 124t
    for diabetes mellitus, 327–328, 328t
    for emphysema, 303
    and falls, 502 (q78)
    for hypertension, 258–259, 258t
    for mania, 218
    for neuropsychiatric disturbances in
        dementia, 124, 124t
    nonadherence to, 41–42
    optimizing prescribing, 38
    for osteoporosis, 178, 179t
    for osteoporosis prevention and treatment,
        178–181, 179t
    pain management, 106–108
    for persistent pain, 411–412
    polypharmacy, 469 (q24)
    prescribing cascade, 39, 39f
    for prevention of falls, 392
    principles of prescribing, 40–41, 41t
    for psychotic disturbances in dementia,
        124, 124t
    for schizophrenia and schizophrenia-like
        syndromes, 225–226
    for sleep problems, 205–206, 206t
    suboptimal, 78
    for substance abuse, 239
    and syncope, 502–503 (q79)
    trends in, 12
    for urinary incontinence, 139t
Phenelzine, 215t, 217
Phenobarbital, 284t
Phenothiazines, 109–110, 109t
Phentolamine, 341

Phenylbutazone, 311t
Phenytoin, 311t
    absorption of, 35
    and delirium, 132t
    distribution of, 36
    for epilepsy, 284t
    nutrient interactions, 186t
Phobia, social, 222, 222t
Phobic disorders, 220–221
Phosphorus, 185t
Photoaging, 372
Photodynamic therapy, 170
Physical abuse, 485–486 (q52). See also Elder
    mistreatment
Physical activity, 65–72. See also Exercise(s)
    benefits of, 510–511 (q93)
    counseling for, 60t, 61
    and diabetes mellitus, 327
    discussions with older patients about, 70,
        71f
    to improve sleep, 208–209
    long-term effects of, 505 (q83)
    to maintain bone density, 494–495 (q65)
    prescription for, 508 (q88)
    recommendations for, 66–67, 66t, 68, 69t
    and rheumatologic disorders, 262
Physical assessment, 47–48, 53–54
Physical disability
    excess, with substance use, 236–237
    in hospitalized patients, 75t
    International Classification of Impairments,
        Disabilities, and Handicaps
        (ICIDH-2), 82–83, 82f
    screening for, 402
    trends in, 11
Physical Self-Maintenance Scale (ADLs), 384
Physical therapy
    for back pain, 511–512 (q95)
    for hip fracture, 476 (q37)
Physician-assisted suicide, 18–19
Pilocarpine, 310
Pioglitazone, 327–328, 328t
Pityrosporum orbiculare, 372
Plantar fasciitis, 275, 276t, 278–279
Plasminogen, 283
PLMS. See Periodic leg movements during
    sleep
PM. See Polymyositis
Pneumococcal vaccination, 60t, 62
    in hospitalized patients, 75t, 76
Pneumonia, 295–296
    aspiration, 192
    causes of, 295, 296f
    deaths due to, 11, 11t
    in hospitalized patients, 75t
Polymyalgia rheumatica, 264–265
Polymyositis, 268–269
Polypharmacy, 39, 39f, 469 (q24)
Polyps, colonic, 318–319
Polysomnography, 202
POMA. See Performance Oriented Mobility
    Assessment
Positional dizziness, benign paroxysmal,
    513–514 (q98)

Positional vertigo, benign, 153
    Epley's maneuver for, 154f, 155f
    management of, 158t
Positron emission tomography, 287
Post-herpetic neuralgia, 173, 300, 377
Postacute care, 31–32, 31t
Posttraumatic stress disorder, 221, 222, 222t
Postvoid residual volume (PVR), 137,
    488–489 (q57)
Potassium, 40t, 186t
Potassium deficiency, 365
Potassium-titanyl-phosphate laser, 373
Poverty rates, 8
PPD skin tests, 296, 298
PPOs. See Preferred provider organizations
Prader-Willi syndrome, 241
Pramipexole, 288
Prealbumin, 185
Prednisone (Deltasone, Liquid Pred,
    Orasone)
    for giant cell arteritis, 266
    for multiple myeloma, 356
    for non-Hodgkin's lymphoma, 355
    for persistent pain, 411
    for polymyalgia rheumatica, 265
    for polymyositis and dermatomyositis, 269
    for rheumatoid arthritis, 266
Preferred provider organizations (PPOs), 33
Presbycusis, 164
Presbyesophagus, 191
Presbyopia, 169
Prescription drugs. See Drugs;
    Pharmacotherapy
Pressure-relieving surfaces, 477 (q39)
Pressure Sore Status Tool, 197
Pressure Ulcer Healing Chart, 416
Pressure Ulcer Scale for Healing (PUSH),
    197, 415
Pressure ulcers, 194–200, 413–416
    Braden Scale for Predicting Pressure Sore
        Risk, 195, 413–414
    cleansing agents for, 483 (q48)
    and diabetes, 467–468 (q22)
    dressings for, 198–199, 200t, 465 (q18)
    of heel, 455–456 (q2)
    ischial, 467–468 (q22)
    management of, 196–199, 197t
    prevention of, 195, 196t, 455–456 (q2),
        467–468 (q22), 477 (q39)
    sacral, 476–477 (q38)
    staging system for, 197, 198t
    status tool, 197
    support surfaces for persons at risk for,
        196, 196t
    surgical debridement of, 476–477 (q38)
Pressure Ulcers in Adults: Prediction and
    Prevention (AHCPR), 195
Prevention, 59–65. See also Screening
    potentially beneficial services lacking
        evidence, 62–63, 63t
    recommended services, 59–62, 60t
    services not indicated in older adults, 64,
        64t

Primary open-angle glaucoma (POAG), 172–173
PRIME-MD (Primary Care Evaluation of Mental Disorders), 495–496 (q66)
Probenecid, 264
Prochlorperazine, 109–110, 109*t*
Progesterone
 breast cancer and, 331
 endometrial cancer and, 331
 for hypersexuality, 125
 for osteoporosis, 329–330, 330*t*
Progestin, 332
Program of All-inclusive Care of the Elderly (PACE), 32, 94, 514 (q99)
Progressive supranuclear palsy, 288–289
Prokinetic agents, 109–110, 109*t*
Proliferative diabetic retinopathy, 172, 172*f*
Prompted voiding, 137, 139*t*, 141
Propranolol
 for congestive heart failure, 250
 distribution of, 36
 for ventricular arrhythmias, 252
Propyl uracil, 311*t*
Propylthiouracil, 311*t*
Prospective payment systems (PPSs), 91
Prostaglandin E^1, 341, 342*t*
Prostate, digital rectal examination of, 368
Prostate cancer, 367–371
 hormonal therapy for, 352, 352*t*
 screening for, 63, 63*t*, 368
 staging systems, 368–369, 369*t*
Prostate disease, 366–371, 389
Prostate-specific antigen
 screening, 63, 63*t*
 serum levels, 368, 369–370, 467 (q21)
Prostatectomy, radical, 370
Prostatic hyperplasia, benign, 366–367, 467 (q21), 488–489 (q57)
 International Prostate Symptom Score, 389
Prostatism, 366
Prostatitis, 371
Prostheses
 infections, 299
 penile, 342, 342*t*
 tissue heart valve, 387
Protectionism, 22–23
Protein-energy undernutrition, 187, 518 (q106)
Protein intake, 500 (q74)
Protein requirements, 182–183, 183*t*
Proteinuria, 358
Proton pump inhibitors, 313
Provider-sponsored organizations (PSOs), 33
Pruritus, 375
Pseudoaddiction, 108
Pseudoclaudication, 271
Pseudogout, 264
Pseudomonas, 300
Psoralen with UVA light (PUVA), 376
Psoriasis, 375–376, 376*f*
PSOs. *See* Provider-sponsored organizations

Psychiatric diseases and disorders, 211–242, 499 (q72). *See also specific disorders*
 with incontinence, 134–135, 135*t*
 with mental retardation, 240–241
 resources, 426
 and sleep problems, 202–203
Psychogenic dizziness, 158*t*
Psychologic assessment, 49, 54
"Psychologic autopsy" studies, 214
Psychosis, 134–135, 135*t*, 224
Psychosocial problems, 13–17, 202–203
Psychotherapy, 214, 223
Psychotic depression, 217
Psychotic disorders, 224–227
Psychotic disturbances in dementia, 124, 124*t*, 125
Psychotropic drug restrictions, 472 (q29)
PTCA. *See* Percutaneous transluminal coronary angioplasty
PTH. *See* Parathyroid hormone
Pulmocare, 193*t*
Pulmonary disease
 chronic, activity recommendations for, 69*t*
 chronic obstructive, 11, 11*t*, 303–304, 499–500 (q73)
 effects on continence, 134–135, 135*t*
 resources, 424
Pulmonary embolus, 387
Pulmonary evaluation, preoperative, 305–306
Pulmonary fibrosis, idiopathic, 304
Pulmonary function testing, 499–500 (q73)
Pulmonary physiology changes, 302
Pulmonary thromboembolism, 304–305
Purified protein derivative, 296, 298
PUSH. *See* Pressure Ulcer Scale for Healing
PUVA (psoralen with UVA light), 376
PVR. *See* Postvoid residual volume
Pyelonephritis, 297
Pyrazinamide, 298
Pyridoxine, 298

Q

QISMC. *See* Quality Improvement System for Managed Care
Quadriceps-strengthening exercise, 520 (q111)
Quality cost model of transitional care, 74–75
Quality Improvement System for Managed Care (QISMC), 34
Quality of care, 99
Quality of life, 49, 353–354
Quetiapine, 225–226, 226*t*, 227
Quinidine, 36

R

Radiation therapy
 for cancer, 353
 after lumpectomy, 354
 for prostate cancer, 370
Radiculopathy, 291
Radioactive iodine, 491 (q60)

Radionuclide ventriculography, 244
Raloxifene, 180
Rapid-eye-movement (REM) sleep, 201
ras1, 2*t*, 4
Rational Recovery, 238
Recombinant tissue-plasminogen, 283
Rectal examination, digital, 63*t*, 368
5α-Reductase, 367
Reflux, gastroesophageal, 312–313
Refractive errors, 169
Refusal of treatment, 18
Rehabilitation, 82–90
 care plans, 85, 85*t*
 low-vision, 174
 postacute, 31–32
 for stroke patients, 475–476 (q36)
Rehabilitation hospitals, acute-level, 475–476 (q36)
Relaxation techniques, 208, 208*t*, 209
Religious beliefs, 16–17, 483–484 (q49)
REM (rapid-eye-movement) sleep, 201
REM sleep behavior disorder, 204
Reminiscence therapy, 117
Renal artery stenosis, 357
Renal biopsy, 359
Renal dialysis, 363–364
Renal diseases and disorders, 357–365
Renal failure
 acute, 360–362
 acute, crystal-induced, 464 (q16)
 chronic, 363–364
Renal function changes, 357
Renal imaging techniques, 359
Renal insufficiency, 358, 360–362
Renal transplantation, 363–364
Renal tubular acidosis type IV, 365
Renal vascular disease, 362
Rescue analgesia, 107
Research
 with cognitively impaired persons as subjects, 22*t*
 on herbal preparations, 43–44
 informed consent for, 22
Reserpine, 289–290, 290*t*
Resident Assessment Protocols, 190
Resistance training, 67–68, 494–495 (q65)
Resources, 417–427
Respiratory diseases and disorders, 302–306
Respiratory symptoms and complaints, 302
Restless legs syndrome, 203
Restraints, 24
Resuscitation, 79
Retinopathy, diabetic, 170–171, 172*f*
Retropubic suspension, 140*t*, 141
Rheumatoid arthritis, 263, 266–267
 of foot problems, 280
 physical activity and, 262
Rheumatoid gout, 263
Rheumatologic disorders, 261–262
Rib fractures, 485–486 (q52)
Riboflavin, 185*t*
Ribonucleic acid, messenger (mRNA), 4

Ribosomal RNA (rRNA), 3–4
Rifampin, 298
Rinné test, 463 (q15)
Risedronate, 179–180, 179*t*
Risperidone, 225–226, 226*t*
  for opioid-induced delirium, 107
  for psychotic and other neuropsychiatric
    disturbances in dementia, 124, 124*t*
Rituximab, 352–353
Rivastigmine, 119
RNA
  messenger (mRNA), 4
  ribosomal (rRNA), 3–4
Rofecoxib (Vioxx), 266, 411
Role loss and acquisition, 14
Ropinirole, 288
Rosacea, 373, 373*f*
Rosiglitazone, 327–328, 328*t*
Roxanol, 412. *See also* Morphine

S

S-MAST-G (Short Michigan Alcoholism
    Screening Test–Geriatric Version), 237,
    238*t*
Sacral fractures, osteoporotic, 272
Sacral pressure ulcers, 476–477 (q38)
Safety
  and dementia, 118
  Home Safety Checklist, 400
Salflex (salsalate), 411
Salicylates, 186*t*
Salicylic acid, 36
Salivary function, 309–310
Salivary glands, 307, 307*t*
Salmonella, 300
Salsalate (Disalcid, Mono-Gesic, Salflex), 266,
    411
Sarcopenia, 67, 186–187
Saw palmetto, 45
Scabies, 378
Scheduled toileting, 137, 139*t*, 140, 141
Schizoid or schizotypal personality disorder
  features of, 228, 229*t*
  therapeutic strategies for, 230–231, 231*t*
Schizoid (socially isolated personality) traits,
    224
Schizophrenia, 224–226, 240
Schizophrenia-like psychosis, 224
Schizophrenia-like syndromes, 224–226
Schizotypal personality disorder
  features of, 228, 229*t*
  therapeutic strategies for, 230–231, 231*t*
Sciatica, 271, 271*t*
Scopolamine, 109–110, 109*t*
Screening
  for alcohol problems, 60*t*, 61, 237, 237*t*,
    386, 495–496 (q66)
  for breast cancer, 59, 60*t*, 494 (q64)
  for cancer, 351
  for delirium, 486 (q53)
  for depression, 49, 60*t*, 61, 63, 63*t*, 402
  for diabetes, 63, 63*t*, 470 (q26)
  geriatric, 402

Hearing Handicap Inventory for the
    Elderly–Screening Version (HHIE-S),
    165, 399
  for hearing loss, 48, 60*t*, 61, 402
  for hypercholesteremia, 470 (q26)
  leg mobility, 402
  nutrition, 183–186, 402, 410
  for obstructive sleep apnea, 304, 304*t*
  potentially beneficial services lacking
    evidence, 63–64, 63*t*
  in primary care, 402
  for prostate cancer, 63, 63*t*, 368
  recommended services, 59–61, 60*t*
  S-MAST-G (Short Michigan Alcoholism
    Screening Test–Geriatric Version),
    237, 238*t*
  for secondary osteoporosis, 176*t*
  services not indicated in older adults, 64,
    64*t*
  for visual impairment, 48, 402
Seborrheic dermatitis, 372–373
Sedentary behavior, 68–69
Seizures, 283
Selective estrogen receptor modulators, 179*t*,
    180
Selective serotonin-reuptake inhibitors
  for anxiety disorders, 222–223, 222*t*
  for depression, 215–216, 215*t*
  for depressive and other neuropsychiatric
    disturbances in dementia, 124, 124*t*
  drug interactions, 216
  nutrient interactions, 186*t*
Selegiline, 288
Selenium, 185*t*
Self-care, 10, 10*t*
Self-care testing, 48
Self-efficacy beliefs, 14–15, 15*t*
Self-management, 250
Self-neglect, 54
Senescence. *See also* Aging
  clonal, 3
  DNA mutations or deletions during, 3–4
  gene expression during, 4–5
  immune, 293, 293*t*
  telomeres during, 4
Senile chorea, 289, 289*t*
Sensorineural hearing loss, 512–513 (q96)
Sensory ataxia, 149, 150*t*
Sensory impairment. *See also* Hearing
    impairment; Visual impairment
  assessment of, 75*t*, 77
  rehabilitation care for, 85, 85*t*
  screening for, 60*t*
Sepsis, 295
Septicemia, 11, 11*t*
SERMs. *See* Selective estrogen receptor
    modulators
Serotonergic antagonists, 109–110, 109*t*
Serotonin antagonists, 109–110, 109*t*
Sertraline, 468–469 (q23)
  for depressive and other neuropsychiatric
    disturbances in dementia, 124, 124*t*
  drug interactions, 216
  indications for, 215*t*
Serum lipids, 60*t*, 63*t*, 470 (q26)

Sex hormone-binding globulin, 325
Sex therapy, 342*t*, 344, 344*t*
Sexual function disorders, 339–345, 426
Sexuality
  female, 342–344
  male, 339–342
  resources, 426
SF-36™ Health Survey, 49, 393–398
Sharp debridement, 198, 199*t*
Sheltered housing, 96
Shigella, 300–301
Shingles, 173, 300
SHMOs. *See* Social health maintenance
    organizations
Shoes, 280–281
Short Form-36 Health Survey (SF-36™),
    49, 393–398
Short Michigan Alcoholism Screening
    Test–Geriatric Version (S-MAST-G),
    237, 238*t*
Short Portable Mental Status Questionnaire
    (SPMSQ), 76–77
Shoulder pain, 490–491 (q59)
Shy-Drager syndrome, 288
Sight problems. *See* Visual impairment
Sigmoidoscopy, flexible, 59, 60*t*
Sildenafil, 341, 342*t*, 344
Sjögren's disease, 268
Sjögren's syndrome, 268, 309
Skilled nursing care costs, 460–461 (q11)
Skilled nursing facilities, 98, 519 (q109)
Skills training, 473–474 (q33)
Skin cancer, 500–501 (q75)
  resources, 427
  screening for, 63–64, 63*t*
Skin care, 195
Skin care plans, 467–468 (q22)
Skin dryness, 373, 374*f*
Skin grafts, 31*t*
Skin inspection, 63*t*
Skin problems. *See* Dermatologic diseases and
    disorders
SLE. *See* Systemic lupus erythematosus
Sleep, 456–457 (q4). *See also* Sleep problems
  age-related changes, 201
  changes with dementia, 204
  evaluation of, 201–202
  measures to improve, 204–205, 205*t*
  in nursing homes, 204
  periodic leg movements during, 203
  rapid-eye-movement (REM), 201
  REM sleep behavior disorder, 204
Sleep apnea, obstructive, 304, 304*t*
Sleep disorders, 202–204
Sleep problems, 201–209, 487 (q54)
  amelioration of, 456–457 (q4)
  management of, 125, 204–209
  National Institutes of Health Consensus
    Statement on the Treatment of Sleep
    Disorders of Older People, 201
  nonpharmacologic interventions for,
    207–209, 208*t*

Sleep restriction, 207–208, 208*t*

Sleep-wake cycle disturbances, 203–204, 487 (q54)

Sleeping agents, nonprescription, 207

Small intestinal motility changes, 475 (q35)

Smell dysfunction, 311, 311*t*

Smoking cessation, 479–480 (q42)
  counseling for, 60*t*, 61
  Four A's of, 303, 303*t*
  to reduce risk of osteoporosis, 176*t*

Snellen chart, 61

Social assessment, 49

Social health maintenance organizations (SHMOs), 94–95

Social networks, 15–16, 16*t*

Social phobia, 222, 222*t*

Social Security, 460–461 (q11)

Social status, 14, 242

Social support, 78

Socioeconomic status, 8

SOD (superoxide dismutase), 1, 2*t*

Sodium restriction, 257–258

Solar keratoses, 379, 379*f*

Somatoform disorders, 232–234
  clinical characteristics of, 232–233, 232*t*
  not otherwise specified, 232, 232*t*
  undifferentiated, 232, 232*t*

Sorsby's fundus dystrophy, 170

Sparfloxacin, 295

Spasticity, 149–150, 150*t*

Sphincter, artificial, 140*t*, 141

Spinal cord injury, 134–135, 135*t*

Spinal stenosis, 134–135, 135*t*, 497 (q68)

Spinal tumors, 270, 271*t*

Spiritual involvement, 16–17

Spironolactone, 248*t*, 249

SPMSQ. *See* Short Portable Mental Status Questionnaire

Spurs, 275
  calcaneal, 276*t*, 278–279

Squamous cell carcinoma, 310, 379

Squamous hyperplasia, 336

SSRIs. *See* Selective serotonin-reuptake inhibitors

St. John's wort, 44

Stabilization, 238

Staffing patterns, 98

Standards of care, 190

Staphylococcus aureus, 295, 296*f*, 299, 307

Statins, 181

Sticky or viscous personality, 230

Stimulus control, 207–208, 208*t*

Stomach disorders, 314–315. *See also* Gastrointestinal diseases and disorders

Streptococcus pneumoniae, 295, 296, 296*f*, 300

Streptomycin, 311*t*

Stress echocardiography, 244–245

Stress incontinence, 136, 496 (q67)
  behavioral and pharmacologic treatments for, 139*t*
  management of, 141

mixed urge and stress incontinence, 139*t*
  surgical treatments for, 140*t*, 141

Stress testing, 244

Stressors, 13–14

Stretching exercises, 70

Stroke, 86–88
  incidence of, 281
  management of, 86–88, 283
  postacute care, 475–476 (q36)
  prevention of, 63*t*, 485 (q51)
  recommended preventive services for, 60*t*
  resources, 424, 425
  risk factors for, 281
  transfers to postacute care facilities for, 31*t*

Stroke rehabilitation, 86–88, 87*t*

Subdural hematoma, 292

Substance abuse, 234–239. *See also* Addiction

Substance dependence, 234

Substance use, 236–237

Substance use disorders, 237

Substituted judgment, 493–494 (q63)

Subungual heloma, 278

Suicide, physician-assisted, 18–19

Suicide rates, 11

Sulfasalazine, 267, 311*t*

Sulfonylureas, 327–328, 328*t*

Sundowning, 119, 120*t*, 128

Superficial venous insufficiency, 255

Superoxide dismutase (SOD), 1, 2*t*

Supplements
  iron, 347
  multivitamin, 347
  oral, 188
  vitamin B$_{12}$, 348

Support surfaces, 196, 196*t*

Supranuclear palsy, progressive, 288–289

Surgery
  for benign prostatic hyperplasia, 367
  for cancer, 353
  coronary artery bypass graft (CABG), 245, 289*t*
  for hip fracture, 476 (q37)
  for osteoarthritis, 263
  postoperative delirium, 466–467 (q20), 501 (q76)
  postoperative incontinence, 515 (q100)
  preoperative pulmonary evaluation, 305–306
  for prostate cancer, 370
  repair of pressure ulcers, 199
  for stress incontinence, 140*t*, 141
  timing of, 471–472 (q28)
  for vaginal prolapse, 338

Surgical debridement, 198, 199*t*, 476–477 (q38)

Suspiciousness, 226–227, 470–471 (q27)

Swab cultures, 476–477 (q38)

Swallowing, 191–192

Syncope, 159–163. *See also* Dizziness
  causes of, 159, 159*t*
  characteristics of, 160, 161*t*
  drug-related, 502–503 (q79)

Syndrome of inappropriate antidiuretic hormone, 364

Syphilis, 300

Systemic lupus erythematosus, 267–268, 424

T

T-cell receptor (TCR), 2*t*

T$_3$. *See* Triiodothyronine

T$_4$. *See* Thyroxine

Tachykinesia, 286

Tailor's bunion, 275, 276*t*

Tamoxifen, 352*t*

Tardive dyskinesia, 289–290

Tardive dystonia, 289–290

Taste dysfunction, 311, 311*t*

TCR, 2*t*

Teaching nursing homes, 101

Technetium bone scan, 273

Teeth, 307, 307*t*

Tegretol, 411. *See also* Carbamazepine

Telomerase, 4

Telomeres, 4

Temazepam, 205, 206*t*

Temporal arteritis, 265

Tenosynovitis, 275, 276*t*

Terminal illness. *See* End-of-life care; Palliative care

Testamentary competence, 20

Testosterone, 324–325

Testosterone replacement therapy, 325, 333

Testosterone therapy
  for erectile dysfunction, 342
  for female sexual dysfunction, 343, 344, 344*t*
  for women, 333

Tetanus booster, 60*t*, 62

Tetracyclines, 311*t*

Thallium perfusion scintigraphy, 244

Theophylline
  for asthma, 303
  metabolism of, 36
  movement disorders associated with, 289–290, 290*t*
  nutrient interactions, 186*t*

Therapeutic shoes, 281

Thiamin, 185*t*

Thiazide diuretics, 258

Thiazolidinediones, 327–328, 328*t*

Thiopental, 36

Thiouracil, 311*t*

Thoracic aortic dissection, 253–254

Thoracic vertebral compression fracture, 459–460 (q9)

Thrombocytopenia, autoimmune, 347

Thromboembolism
  pulmonary, 304–305
  venous, 80, 387

Thrombolytic therapy, 246

Thyroid cancer, 322

Thyroid disorders, 63, 63*t*, 320–322

Thyroid hormone replacement, 176*t*, 320–321

Thyroid hormones, 289–290, 290*t*

Thyroid nodules, 322
Thyroid-stimulating hormone, 319–320
Thyrotoxicosis, 321
Thyrotropin, 63t
Thyroxine (T$_4$), 319–320
  high T$_4$ syndrome, 321
  for hypothyroidism, 320–321
  low T4 syndrome, 320
  for mood disturbances in dementia,
    124–125
Tiagabine, 284t
Tibial plateau fractures, 462–463 (q14)
Ticlopidine, 246
Tilt-table testing, 162
Timed Get Up and Go test, 48, 148
TIMP-3 (tissue inhibitor of metalloprotease),
    170
Tinea pedis, 277t
Tinea unguium, 275
Tinnitus resources, 423
Tissue inhibitor of metalloprotease
    (TIMP-3), 170
Tissue prosthetic heart valve, 387
TNM (tumor-node-metastasis) staging
    system, 368–369, 369t
α-Tocopherol, 185t . See also Vitamin E
Toenail problems, 275, 277–278
Toes, candidiasis between, 374, 374f
Toileting, scheduled, 137, 139t, 140, 141
Tolerance. See also Dependency
  to opioids, 108
Tolterodine, 139t, 140
Tooth dentin changes, 307, 307t
Toothlessness, 60t, 308–309
Topiramate, 284t
Toremifene, 352t
Toxic or metabolic encephalopathy, 127
Toxicity
  of chemotherapy, 351–352, 351t
  digoxin, 461–462 (q12)
  myelotoxicity, 351–352, 351t
Tracheostomy, 31t
Tramadol (Ultram), 412
Transdermal fentanyl (Duragesic), 412
Transfers to postacute care facilities, 31, 31t
Transient incontinence, 135, 136t
Transient ischemic attack, 60t
Transitional care, 74–75
Transparent film, 200t
Transplantation, renal, 363–364
Transthoracic echocardiography, 299
Tranylcypromine, 215t
Trastuzumab, 352–353
Trazodone
  distribution of, 36
  herbal preparation interactions, 44t
  for sleep problems, 125, 206, 206t
Treadmill testing, 244
Treatment of Pressure Ulcers (AHCPR), 196,
    197

Tremors
  action, 285, 289–290, 290t
  essential, 285–286
  "pill rolling," 117
Triamcinolone, 264, 336
Triazolam, 132t, 205
Tricosal (choline magnesium trisalicylate),
    411
Tricyclic antidepressants
  for anxiety disorders, 222t
  and delirium, 131, 132t
  for depression, 215, 215t
  for depressive and other neuropsychiatric
    disturbances in dementia, 124, 124t
  for persistent pain, 411
Trifluoperazine, 311t
Triiodothyronine (T$_3$), 320, 321
Triiodothyronine (T$_3$) thyrotoxicosis, 321
Trilisate (choline magnesium trisalicylate),
    411
Trimethoprim, 186t
Trimethoprim-sulfamethoxazole, 297, 464
    (q16)
"Triple As," 93
Trunk movements, abnormal, 406
Truth-telling, 22
Try This: Best Practices in Care to Older
    Adults (The John A. Hartford
    Foundation Institute for Geriatric
    Nursing), 47, 105
Tube feeding, 188, 465–466 (q19), 522
    (q115)
  refusal of, 18
  solutions, 193t
Tuberculosis, 297–298
  effects on continence, 134–135, 135t
  resources, 420
Tubular acidosis type IV, 365
Tubular necrosis, acute, 360, 361
Tumor-node-metastasis (TNM) staging
    system, 368–369, 369t
Tumors, spinal, 270, 271t
Tuning-fork test, 463 (q15)
TWEAK screen for alcohol dependence,
    495–496 (q56)
Two Cal HN, 193t
Tylenol, 411. See also Acetaminophen

U

UI. See Urinary incontinence
Ulcer care, 198
Ulcers
  decubitus, 194
  foot, 279
  peptic, 314–315
  pressure. See Pressure ulcers
Ultram (tramadol), 412
Ultraviolet A (UVA) radiation, 372, 376
Ultraviolet B (UVB) radiation, 372
Undernutrition. See also Malnutrition
  and infection, 293–294
  protein-energy, 187, 518 (q106)

Urge incontinence, 135–136, 488–489 (q57)
  behavioral treatment of, 137, 139t
  management of, 137–141
  mixed urge and stress incontinence, 139t
  pharmacologic treatment of, 139t
Urgencies, hypertensive, 260
Urinary incontinence, 134–142, 464–465
    (q17)
  assessment of, 137, 138t
  behavioral treatment of, 403–404
  medical conditions associated with,
    134–135, 135t
  mixed urge and stress incontinence, 139t
  overflow incontinence, 136, 141, 496
    (q67), 509 (q90)
  postoperative, 515 (q100)
  prevention and management of, 403–404
  resources, 427
  screening for, 402
  stress incontinence, 136, 139t, 140t, 141,
    496 (q67)
  transient incontinence, 135, 136t
  urge incontinence, 135–136, 137–141,
    488–489 (q57)
Urinary tract infection, 296–297, 516 (q102)
Urodynamic studies, 496 (q67)
Urogenital atrophy, 335, 335f
Urogenital symptoms, 329
U.S. Department of Agriculture (USDA),
    182, 184f
U.S. Preventive Services Task Force
    (USPSTF), 368
  preventive services to consider, 63–64
  recommended preventive services, 59, 61,
    62
U.S. Surgeon General, 66, 66t

V

Vaccinations, 60t, 62, 497–498 (q69)
Vacuum tumescence devices, 341, 342t
Vaginal bleeding, postmenopausal, 338–339,
    338t
Vaginal cones, 139t, 141
Vaginal pessaries, 337–338, 337f
Vaginal prolapse, 336–337, 338
Vaginal sling, 140t, 141
Vaginitis, atrophic, 515–516 (q101)
Valdecoxib (Bextra), 411
Valerian, 45
Valproate, 218. See also Valproic acid
Valproic acid (valproate, divalproex)
  distribution of, 36
  for epilepsy, 284t
  for mania, 218
  movement disorders associated with,
    289–290, 290t
Valsalva's maneuver, 140, 141
Valvular aortic stenosis, 250–251
Valvular heart disease, 250–252, 387
Varicella-zoster virus, 300, 377
Vascular chorea, 289t
Vascular depression, 213

Vascular disease
    peripheral, 85, 85*t*, 254, 280
    renal, 362
Vascular ectasia, 318
Vasoactive drugs, intracavernous injection of,
    341–342
Vasodilators, 40*t*
VDE. *See* Videofluoroscopic deglutition
    examination
Venlafaxine
    for depression, 215*t*, 216–217
    for depressive and other neuropsychiatric
        disturbances in dementia, 124, 124*t*
Venous disorders, 254–255
Venous insufficiency
    deep, 254–255
    superficial, 255
Venous thromboembolism, 80, 387
Ventilation, mechanical, 305
Ventricular arrhythmias, 252–253
Ventricular tachycardia, 252
Vertebral fractures
    compression, 271*t*, 272, 459–460 (q9),
        488 (q56)
    management of, 181, 274, 274*t*
Vertebral infections, 270, 271*t*
Vertebrobasilar arterial diseases, 282
Vertical-gaze palsy, 289
Vertigo, 153. *See also* Dizziness; Syncope
    acute attacks, 158*t*
    benign positional, 153, 154*f*, 155*f*, 158*t*
Vestibular ataxia, 149, 150*t*
Vestibular neuronitis, 153
Vestibulopathy, chronic, 158*t*
Vicodin, 412. *See also* Hydrocodone
Vicoprofen, 412. *See also* Hydrocodone
Videofluoroscopic deglutition examination,
    192
Vinblastine, 356
Vincristine, 311*t*, 355
Vioxx, 411. *See also* Rofecoxib
"Virtual" colonoscopy, 60
Viscous personality, 230
Vision loss. *See* Visual impairment
Vision testing, 48, 60*t*, 61
Visual aids, 174
Visual ataxia, 149, 150*t*
Visual impairment, 169–173, 492 (q62)
    resources, 426–427
    screening for, 48, 402
    transient monocular blindness, 282

Vitamin A, 186*t*
Vitamin B$_1$, 186*t*
Vitamin B$_2$, 186*t*
Vitamin B$_6$, 185*t*, 186*t*
Vitamin B$_{12}$, 186*t*, 348–349
Vitamin B$_{12}$ deficiency, 134–135, 135*t*
Vitamin B$_{12}$ replacement, 348
Vitamin B$_{12}$ supplements, 348
Vitamin D, 311*t*
    drug interactions, 186*t*
    for osteoporosis, 176*t*, 178
    recommended daily allowances, 185*t*
Vitamin D$_3$ (cholecalciferol), 175, 181
Vitamin E, 186*t*
Vitamin K, 186*t*, 388
Voiding, prompted, 139*t*, 140, 141
Vomiting, 109–110, 109*t*
Von Willebrand's factor, 347
Vulvar disorders, 335–336
Vulvar dystrophy, 336
Vulvar intraepithelial neoplasia, 336
Vulvar lesions, nonneoplastic, 336
Vulvar neoplasia, 336
Vulvovaginal atrophy, 335, 335*f*
Vulvovaginal infection and inflammation,
    335

W

Walkers, 89–90
Walking, 68. *See also* Exercise; Gait
    assessment; Gait disturbances
Walking canes, 473 (q31)
Wandering, 460 (q10)
Warfarin
    for atrial fibrillation, 253
    discontinuation of, 388
    distribution of, 36
    initiation of, 388
    metabolism of, 36
    for prevention of systemic embolism,
        387
    for prevention of venous
        thromboembolism, 80, 387
    for pulmonary thromboembolism, 305
    when surgical procedure is planned, 388
    withholding, 388
Wasting, 187
Water balance, 323–324
Weber test, 463 (q15)
Weight, 60*t*

Weight loss, 48
    for hypertension, 257–258, 519–520 (q110)
    screening for, 402
    unacceptable in nursing home, 189
Welch-Allyn pure-tone audioscope, 165
Wheelchairs, 90
White Americans
    causes of death, 11
    congestive heart failure in, 247
    life expectancy, 7–8, 8*t*
    perceived health, 10, 10*t*
    suicide rates, 11
Widower's syndrome, 340
Withholding treatment, 18
Women. *See also* Gynecologic diseases and
        disorders
    congestive heart failure in, 247
    difficulty in ADLs and IADLs of, 10, 10*t*
    drug metabolism in, 36
    estrogen deficiency in, 175
    headaches in, 284
    life expectancy, 7–8, 8*t*
    living alone, 522–523 (q116)
    marital status and living arrangements of,
        8–9, 9*t*
    nursing-home population, 97
    obesity in, 60–61
    poverty rates, 8
    stroke in, 281
    suicide rates, 11
    systemic lupus erythematosus in, 267
    testosterone therapy in, 333
    urinary tract infection in, 297
World Health Organization (WHO)
    *International Classification of Impairments,
        Disabilities, and Handicaps*
        (ICIDH-2), 82–83, 82*f*
    International Prostate Symptom Score
        (IPSS), 389
    three-step analgesic ladder, 106, 106*f*

X

Xerosis, 277, 373

Z

Zaleplon, 205–206, 206*t*
Zenker's diverticulum, 312
Zinc-drug interactions, 186*t*
Zoledronic acid, 180
Zolpidem, 125, 205–206, 206*t*

GRS5 CHAPTER AUTHORS

Sumaira Aasi, MD
Instructor, Department of Dermatology
Yale University School of Medicine
New Haven, CT

Marc E. Agronin, MD
Director of Mental Health Services
Miami Jewish Home and Hospital for the Aged
Voluntary Assistant Professor of Psychiatry
University of Miami School of Medicine
Miami, FL

Cathy A. Alessi, MD
Associate Professor
University of California, Los Angeles
Multicampus Program in Geriatric Medicine and
    Gerontology
Acting Clinical Associate Director, GRECC
Veterans Administration Greater Los Angeles Healthcare
    System
Sepulveda, CA

Neil B. Alexander, MD
Associate Professor
Division of Geriatric Medicine
Department of Internal Medicine
University of Michigan
Associate Director for Research, Research Scientist
VA Ann Arbor Health Care System GRECC
Ann Arbor, MI

Wilbert S. Aronow, MD
Professor of Medicine (Cardiology and Geriatrics)
New York Medical College
Valhalla, NY

Priscilla F. Bade, MD, MS
Associate Professor of Internal Medicine
University of South Dakota School of Medicine
Rapid City, SD

Harrison G. Bloom, MD
Vice Chairman for Clinical Affairs
Brookdale Department of Geriatrics
Mount Sinai School of Medicine
New York, NY

Chad Boult, MD, MPH, MBA
Director, Lipitz Center for Integrated Health Care
Bloomberg School of Public Health
Johns Hopkins University
Baltimore, MD

David M. Buchner, MD, MPH
Chief, Physical Activity and Health Branch
Division of Nutrition and Physical Activity
Centers for Disease Control and Prevention
Atlanta, GA

Lynda C. Burton, ScD
Associate Research Professor
The Johns Hopkins University
Bloomberg School of Public Health
Baltimore, MD

David Bush, MD
Director, Cardiac Catheterization Laboratory
Johns Hopkins Bayview Medical Center
Assistant Professor of Medicine
Division of Cardiology
Johns Hopkins University School of Medicine
Baltimore, MD

Erin L. Cassidy, PhD
Research Associate
Department of Psychiatry and Behavioral Sciences
Stanford University School of Medicine
Palo Alto, CA

Colleen Christmas, MD
Assistant Professor of Medicine
The Johns Hopkins University School of Medicine
Baltimore, MD

Brian Cook, MD, MBA
Chairman, Department of Dermatology
Northwestern Memorial Hospital
Northwestern University Medical School
Northwestern Medical Faculty Foundation

Leo M. Cooney, Jr, MD
Humana Foundation Professor of Geriatric Medicine
Professor and Chief, Section of General Internal Medicine
Yale University School of Medicine
New Haven, CT

G. Willy Davila, MD
Chairman, Department of Gynecology
Head, Section of Urogynecology and Reconstructive Pelvic
    Surgery
Cleveland Clinic Florida
Ft. Lauderdale, FL

Barbara J. de Lateur, MD, MS
Professor, Director and Lawrence Cardinal Shehan Chair
Department of Physical Medicine and Rehabilitation
The Johns Hopkins University School of Medicine
Good Samaritan Office Building

Margaret A. Drickamer, MD
Associate Professor of Medicine (Geriatrics)
Yale University School of Medicine
New Haven, CT

Catherine E. DuBeau, MD
Assistant Professor of Medicine
Harvard Medical School
Urban Medical Group
Boston, MA

Pamela W. Duncan, PhD
Professor of Health Policy and Management
Director of Research, Center on Aging
University of Kansas Medical Center
Kansas City, KS
Senior Health Research Scientist
Department of Veterans Affairs Medical Center
Kansas City, MO

Helen K. Edelberg, MD
Assistant Professor
Brookdale Department of Geriatrics and Adult Development
Mount Sinai School of Medicine
New York, NY

G. Paul Eleazer, MD
Director, Division of Geriatrics
University of South Carolina School of Medicine
Columbia, SC

E. Wesley Ely, MD, MPH
GRECC and Beeson Scholar
Assistant Professor
Divisions of Health Services Research and
Allergy, Pulmonary, and Critical Care Medicine
Vanderbilt University
Nashville, TN

William B. Ershler, MD
Director, Institute for Advanced Studies in Aging and
    Geriatric Medicine
Washington, DC

Terry T. Fulmer, PhD, RN
Professor of Nursing
Co-Director, Hartford Institute for Geriatric Nursing
New York University
New York, NY

Angela Gentili, MD
Director, Geriatrics Fellowship Training Program
Hunter Holmes McGuire VA Medical Center
Associate Professor of Medicine
Virginia Commonwealth University
Richmond, VA

Thomas M. Gill, MD
Associate Professor of Medicine
Yale University School of Medicine
New Haven, CT

Lisa J. Granville, MD
Associate Professor of Medicine
University of Miami School of Medicine
Clinical Investigator, VA Medical Center
Geriatric Research, Education, and Clinical Center
    (GRECC)
Miami, FL

David A. Gruenewald, MD
Associate Professor, Department of Medicine
University of Washington School of Medicine
Staff Physician, Geriatrics and Extended Care
VA Puget Sound Health Care System
Seattle, WA

Arthur E. Helfand, DPM, DABPPH
Professor of Community Health and Aging
Chair, Department of Community Health, Aging and
    Health Policy
Temple University School of Podiatric Medicine
Adjunct Professor of Medicine and Orthopedic Surgery
Jefferson Medical College
Thomas Jefferson University
Philadelphia, PA

Kenneth W. Hepburn, PhD
Associate Professor
Department of Family Practice and Community Health
University of Minnesota
Minneapolis, MN

Kevin P. High, MD, MSc
Associate Professor of Medicine
Sections of Infectious Diseases and Hematology/Oncology
Wake Forest University School of Medicine
Winston Salem, NC

Gordon L. Jensen, MD, PhD
Director, Vanderbilt Center for Human Nutrition
Associate Professor of Medicine
Vanderbilt University Medical Center
Nashville, TN

Don Jurivich, DO
Chief, Section of Geriatric Medicine
Vitoux Associate Professor of Medicine
University of Illinois at Chicago Medical School

Judith D. Kasper, PhD
Professor, Department of Health Policy and Management
The Johns Hopkins University
Bloomberg School of Public Health
Baltimore, MD

Jurgis Karuza, PhD
Visiting Professor of Rochester Medical Center
Rochester, NY
Professor and Chair, Psychology Department
State University College at Buffalo
Buffalo, NY

Paul R. Katz, MD
Professor of Medicine
University of Rochester School of Medicine
Medical Director, Monroe Community Hospital
Rochester, NY

Catherine Lee Kelleher, MD
Instructor in Medicine
Harvard Medical School
Beth Israel Deaconess Medical Center
Boston, MA

Anne Kenny, MD
Assistant Professor of Medicine
Traveler's Center on Aging
University of Connecticut Health Center
Farmington, CT

Douglas P. Kiel, MD, MPH
Associate Professor of Medicine
Harvard Medical School Division on Aging
Research Director, Beth Israel Deaconess Medical Center/
Hebrew Rehabilitation Center for Aged Joint Program on
    Aging
Boston, MA

Kurt Kroenke, MD
Senior Scientist, Regenstrief Institute for Health Care
Professor of Medicine
Indiana University School of Medicine
Indianapolis, IN

Helen Kuno, MD
Medical Director, Long-Term Care
Hunter Holmes McGuire VA Medical Center
Assistant Professor of Medicine
Virginia Commonwealth University
Richmond, VA

C. Seth Landefeld, MD
Professor of Medicine
Chief, Division of Geriatrics
Director, Mount Zion Center on Aging,
University of California, San Francisco
Associate Chief of Staff, Geriatrics and Extended Care
San Francisco VA Medical Center
San Francisco, CA

Robert Dean Lindeman, MD
Professor Emeritus of Medicine
University of New Mexico School of Medicine
Albuquerque, NM

David A. Lipschitz, MD, PhD
Professor of Geriatrics
Chair, Donald W. Reynolds Department of Geriatrics
Director, Donald W. Reynolds Center on Aging
University of Arkansas for Medical Sciences
Little Rock, AR

Dan L. Longo, MD
Scientific Director,
National Institute on Aging
Baltimore, MD

Elan D. Louis, MD, MS
Assistant Professor of Neurology
Gertrude H. Sergievsky Center
College of Physicians and Surgeons
Columbia University
New York, NY

Courtney H. Lyder, ND, GNP
Associate Professor and Director
Adult, Family, Gerontological & Women's Health Division
Yale University School of Nursing
Gerontological Nurse Consultant
Yale-New Haven Hospital
New Haven, CT

Constantine G. Lyketsos, MD, MHS
Professor of Psychiatry and Behavioral Sciences
Director, Neuropsychiatry Service
Johns Hopkins School of Medicine
Baltimore, MD

Edward R. Marcantonio, MD, SM
Director of Quality and Outcomes Research
Hebrew Rehabilitation Center for Aged
Assistant Professor of Medicine
Harvard Medical School
Boston, MA

Alvin M. Matsumoto, MD
Professor, Department of Medicine
University of Washington School of Medicine
Associate Director,
Geriatric Research, Education, and Clinical Center
VA Puget Sound Health Care System
Seattle, Washington

Barnett S. Meyers, MD
Professor of Psychiatry
Weill Medical College of Cornell University
Professor, Program in Clinical Epidemiology and Health
  Sciences
Weill Cornell University Graduate School of Medical
  Sciences
New York Presbyterian Hospital
White Plains, NY

R. Sean Morrison, MD
Associate Professor
Brookdale Department of Geriatrics and Adult Development
Director of Research,
Hertzberg Palliative Care Institute
Mount Sinai School of Medicine
New York, NY

Thomas Mulligan, MD
Service Line Chief, Geriatrics and Extended Care
Hunter Holmes McGuire VA Medical Center
Professor of Medicine
Virginia Commonwealth University
Richmond, VA

Michael J. Murphy, MD
Assistant Clinical Professor,
Department of Orthopaedics
Yale University School of Medicine
New Haven, CT

David W. Oslin, MD
Assistant Professor
University of Pennsylvania
Philadelphia VA Medical Center
Philadelphia, PA

Stacie T. Pinderhughes, MD
Assistant Professor
Brookdale Department of Geriatrics and Adult Development
The Mount Sinai School of Medicine
New York, NY

Peter Pompei, MD
Associate Professor of Medicine
Stanford University
Stanford, CA
Staff Physician
Palo Alto Veterans Affairs Health Care System
Palo Alto, CA

James S. Powers, MD
Clinical Associate Director,
Middle TN GRECC
Associate Professor of Medicine
Vanderbilt University Medical Center
Nashville, TN

Karen M. Prestwood, MD
Assistant Professor of Medicine (Geriatrics)
University of Connecticut Health Center
Farmington, CT

Peter V. Rabins, MD
Professor of Psychiatry and Behavioral Sciences
Johns Hopkins School of Medicine Baltimore, MD

John W. Rachow, MD, PhD
Assistant Clinical Professor
University of Iowa College of Medicine
Iowa City, IA

Paula A. Rochon, MD, MPH
Associate Professor
Department of Medicine and Public Health Sciences
University of Toronto
Scientist, Kunin-Lunenfeld Applied Research Unit
Scientist, Institute for Clinical Evaluative Sciences
Toronto, Ontario

David Sarraf, MD
Assistant Professor of Ophthalmology
Jules Stein Eye Institute, UCLA School of Medicine
Assistant Professor of Ophthalmology
Martin L. King Medical Center/Charles R. Drew University
   of Medicine
Los Angeles, CA

Todd P. Semla, PharmD, MS
Associate Director, Psychopharmacology Clinical and
   Research Center
Department of Psychiatry and Behavioral Health
Evanston Northwestern Healthcare
Evanston, IL
Assistant Clinical Professor
Section of Geriatric Medicine
University of Illinois at Chicago
Chicago, IL

Kenneth Shay, DDS, MS
Director, Geriatrics and Extended Care Service Line
Veterans Integrated Services Network #11
Section Chief, Dental Geriatrics
Ann Arbor VA Medical Center
Adjunct Associate Professor of Dentistry
University of Michigan School of Dentistry
Ann Arbor, MI

Javaid I. Sheikh, MD
Associate Professor
Department of Psychiatry and Behavioral Sciences
Stanford University School of Medicine
Stanford, CA
Chief of Staff, VA Palo Alto Health Care System
Palo Alto, CA

Gary W. Small, MD
Parlow-Solomon Professor of Psychiatry and Biobehavioral
   Sciences
Director, UCLA Center on Aging
Neuropsychiatric Institute and Hospital
Los Angeles, CA

Stephanie Studenski, MD, MPH
Professor and Director, Center on Aging
University of Kansas Medical Center
Kansas City, KS

Mark A. Supiano, MD
Director, Geriatric Research, Education and Clinical Center
VA Ann Arbor Healthcare System
Associate Professor of Internal Medicine
University of Michigan
Ann Arbor, MI

George Triadafilopoulos, MD
Professor of Medicine
Division of Gastroenterology and Hepatology
Stanford University School of Medicine
Stanford, CA
Chief, Gastroenterology Section
Palo Alto Veterans Affairs Health Care System
Palo Alto, CA

Bruce R. Troen, MD
Associate Professor of Geriatrics and Medicine
Mount Sinai School of Medicine
New York, NY

Andrew C. Warren, MB, BS, DPhil
Associate Professor
Department of Psychiatry
The Johns Hopkins University School of Medicine
Baltimore, MD

Melissa J. Webb, PharmD, CGP
Clinical Pharmacist
Orlando VA Outpatient Healthcare Center
Orlando, FL

Index

GRS5 QUESTION AND CRITIQUE AUTHORS

Neil B. Alexander, MD
Associate Professor
Division of Geriatric Medicine
Department of Internal Medicine
University of Michigan
Associate Director for Research, Research Scientist
VA Ann Arbor Health Care System GRECC
Ann Arbor, MI

Barbara L. Bayer, APRN
Advanced Practice Registered Nurse
University of Nebraska Medical Center
Omaha, NE

Lesley M. Blake, MD
Director, Division of Geriatric Psychiatry
Northwestern University Medical School
Chicago, IL

Suzanne F. Bradley, MD
Associate Professor of Internal Medicine
University of Michigan Medical School
Physician Scientist, GRECC
Veterans Affairs Ann Arbor Healthcare System
Ann Arbor, MI

Timothy S. Carey, MD, MPH
Professor of Medicine
University of North Carolina, Chapel Hill
Chapel Hill, NC

Charles Cefalu, MD, MS
Professor and Associate Chairman for Geriatric Program
   Development
Louisiana State University School of Medicine
Department of Family Medicine
New Orleans, LA

Elise M. Coletta, MD
Assistant Professor of Family Medicine
Brown University School of Medicine
Providence, RI

Anne L. Coleman, MD, PhD
Associate Professor of Ophthalmology
Jules Stein Eye Institute
UCLA School of Medicine
Los Angeles, CA

John Concato, MD
Associate Professor of Medicine
Yale University School of Medicine
New Haven, CT
Director, Clinical Epidemiology Unit
West Haven VA Medical Center
West Haven, CT

Leslie Curry, PhD, MPH
Director, Braceland Center for Mental Health & Aging
Associate Professor of Medicine,
University of Connecticut Health Center
Institute of Living, Hartford Hospital
Hartford, CT

Michelle S. Eslami, MD
Assistant Professor of Medicine,
Division of Geriatrics
UCLA School of Medicine
UCLA Fellowship Coordinator for
UCLA Multicampus Geriatric Fellowship Program
Los Angeles, CA

Mark H. Fleisher, MD
Associate Professor of Psychiatry
University of Nebraska College of Medicine
Omaha, NE

David G. Folks, MD
Professor and Chair, Department of Psychiatry
University of Nebraska Medical Center
Omaha, NE

Joseph Francis, Jr, MD, MPH
Vice President for Quality
St. Vincent's Hospital and Health System
Indianapolis, IN

Teri L. Gabel, PharmD
Vice President, Drug Therapy Consultants
Clinical Pharmacy Specialist—Psychiatry
VA Nebraska Western Iowa Health Care System
Omaha, NE

Mary K. Goldstein, MD, MS
Associate Director for Clinical Services,
Geriatrics Research, Education and Clinical Center
   (GRECC)
Palo Alto Veterans Affairs Health Care System
Palo Alto, CA
Associate Professor of Medicine
Stanford University
Stanford, CA

Cynthia A. Gruman, PhD
Interim Director,
Braceland Center for Mental Health and Aging
Hartford, CT
Assistant Professor of Medicine
University of Connecticut School of Medicine
Farmington, CT

Arthur E. Helfand, DPM, DABPPH
Professor of Community Health and Aging
Temple University School of Podiatry
Philadelphia, PA

Keela A. Herr, PhD, RN
Professor, College of Nursing
The University of Iowa
Adjunct Associate Professor
University of Iowa Hospitals and Clinics
Iowa City, IA

Helen M. Hoenig, MD, MPH
Assistant Professor, Division of Geriatrics
Duke University Medical Center
Chief, Physical Medicine and Rehabilitation Service
VA Medical Center
Durham, NC

Theodore M. Johnson, II, MD, MPH
Atlanta Site Director, Clinical and Educational Programs
Birmingham/Atlanta VA GRECC
Decatur, GA
Assistant Professor of Medicine
Division of Geriatrics, Emory University
Atlanta, GA

Thomas V. Jones, MD, MPH
Senior Assistant Editor,
The Merck Manuals
Merck & Company, Inc.
Blue Bell, PA

Fran E. Kaiser, MD
Senior Medical Director
Merck and Company, Inc.
Irving, TX
Clinical Professor of Medicine
UT Southwestern Medical Center
Dallas, TX

Anne Kenny, MD
Assistant Professor of Medicine
Traveler's Center on Aging
University of Connecticut Health Center
Farmington, CT

Mary B. King, MD
Assistant Professor, Medicine
University of Connecticut School of Medicine
Farmington, CT
Geriatrician
Hartford Hospital Geriatric Program
Hartford, CT

Bruce Kinosian, MD
Associate Professor of Medicine
Division of General Internal Medicine
University of Pennsylvania
Philadelphia, PA

Mark Lachs, MD, MPH
Associate Professor of Medicine
Weill Medical College of Cornell University
Director of Geriatrics
New York Presbyterian Health System
New York, NY

Shari M. Ling, MD
Staff Clinician
Gerontology Research Center
National Institute on Aging
Assistant Professor of Medicine
Division of Geriatric Medicine and Gerontology
Division of Rheumatology
The Johns Hopkins University School of Medicine
Baltimore, MD

Lewis A. Lipsitz, MD
Professor and Director
Harvard Division on Aging
Usen Co-Director of the Research and Training Institute
Hebrew Rehabilitation Center for Aged
Boston, MA

Robert Luchi, MD
Professor of Medicine
Baylor College of Medicine
Houston, TX

Kenneth W. Lyles, MD
GRECC, VA Medical Center
Professor of Medicine
Duke University Medical Center
Durham, NC

Robert M. McCann, MD
Associate Professor of Medicine
University of Rochester School of Medicine
Chief of Medicine
Highland Hospital
Rochester, NY

David W. Mai, MD
Affiliated Dermatologists, S.C.
Milwaukee, WI

Annette M. Medina-Walpole, MD
Assistant Professor of Medicine
University of Rochester
Rochester, NY

David R. Mehr, MD, MS
Associate Professor
Department of Family and Community Medicine
University of Missouri—Columbia
Columbia, MO

Daniel A. Mendelson, MD
Assistant Professor of Medicine,
Division of Geriatrics
University of Rochester
Medical Director, Acute Care for Elders Unit
Highland Hospital
Rochester, NY

Mark Monane, MD, MS
Vice President, Biotechnology
Needham and Company, Inc.
New York, NY
Clinical Adjunct Professor
Rutgers University College of Pharmacy
Piscataway, NJ

Alison A. Moore, MD, MPH
Assistant Professor of Medicine
UCLA Division of Geriatrics
Los Angeles, CA

Cynthia D. Mulrow, MD, MSc
Clinical Professor
Department of Medicine
The University of Texas Health Science Center at San Antonio
San Antonio, TX
Deputy Editor, *Annals of Internal Medicine*
Director, Robert Wood Johnson Foundation National Program
Office for Generalist Physician Scholars Program

Ronald F. Pfeiffer, MD
Professor and Vice Chair
Department of Neurology
University of Tennessee Health Science Center
Memphis, TN

Margaret O. Rathier, MD
Assistant Professor of Medicine, Geriatrics
University of Connecticut Health Center
Farmington, CT
Geriatrics and Extended Care
VA Connecticut Healthcare System
Newington, CT

George T. Reizner, MD
Professor of Medicine
Division of Dermatology
University of Wisconsin
Madison, WI

Christine S. Ritchie, MD, MSPH
Assistant Professor
University of Louisville
Division of General Internal Medicine and Geriatrics
Louisville, KY

Deepak M. Sahasrabudhe, MD
Associate Professor
University of Rochester
Rochester, NY

David Sarraf, MD
Assistant Professor of Ophthalmology
Jules Stein Eye Institute, UCLA School of Medicine
King/Drew Medical Center
Greater Los Angeles VA Healthcare Center
Los Angeles, CA

Ralph H. Saunders, DDS, MS
Associate Professor
University of Rochester School of Medicine and Dentistry
Rochester, NY

Susan K. Schultz, MD
Associate Professor of Psychiatry
University of Iowa College of Medicine
Iowa City, IA

Nancy Shafer-Clark, MD
Senior Instructor in Medicine and Geriatrics
University of Rochester School of Medicine
Rochester, NY

Philip D. Sloane, MD, MPH
Elizabeth and Oscar Goodwin Distinguished Professor of
    Family Medicine
University of North Carolina School of Medicine
Chapel Hill, NC

Jo-Anne Smith, MD
Assistant Professor of Medicine
Associate Director, Center for Osteoporosis
University of Connecticut School of Medicine
Farmington, CT

Monica Stallworth-Kolimas, MD
Assistant Professor of Family Medicine
Georgetown University School of Medicine
Washington, DC

David L. Sultzer, MD
Associate Professor
Department of Psychiatry and Biobehavioral Science
Director, Gero/Neuropsychiatry Division
VA Greater Los Angeles Healthcare System
Los Angeles, CA

Pierre N. Tariot, MD
Professor of Psychiatry, Medicine & Neurology
University of Rochester Medical Center
Director of Psychiatry
Monroe Community Hospital
Rochester, NY

Cheryl A. Vahl, RN, MSN, AOCN
Advanced Practice Nurse
Palliative Care Coordinator
University of Iowa Healthcare
University of Iowa
Iowa City, IA

Julia K. Warnock, MD, PhD
Professor of Psychiatry
University of Oklahoma Health Sciences Center
Tulsa, OK

James R. Webster, Jr, MD, MS
Professor of Medicine (Geriatrics)
Northwestern University Medical School
Emeritus Director, Buehler Center on Aging
Chicago, IL

Barbara E. Weinstein, PhD
Professor, Lehman College, CUNY
Bronx, NY
Professor, Graduate School and University Center
New York, NY

Steven P. Wengel, MD
Associate Professor of Psychiatry
University of Nebraska Medical Center
Omaha, NE

Robert J. Westlake, MD
Professor of Psychiatry and Human Behavior
Vice Chairman for Adult Psychiatry
Department of Psychiatry and Human Behavior
Brown University
Providence, RI

T. Franklin Williams, MD
Professor of Medicine Emeritus
University of Rochester
Rochester, NY